a **LANGE** clinical manual

Family Medicine
Ambulatory Care & Prevention

sixth edition

Edited by

Mindy A. Smith, MD, MS
Clinical Professor, Department of Family Medicine
Michigan State University, College of Human Medicine
East Lansing, Michigan

Leslie A. Shimp, PharmD, MS
Professor of Pharmacy
College of Pharmacy
Clinical Pharmacist, Ambulatory Care
University of Michigan
Ann Arbor, Michigan

Sarina Schrager, MD, MS
Professor, Department of Family Medicine
University of Wisconsin, School of Medicine and Public Health
Madison, Wisconsin

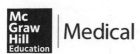 Medical

New York   Chicago   San Francisco   Athens   London   Madrid   Mexico City
New Delhi   Milan   San Juan   Singapore   Sydney   Toronto

Family Medicine: Ambulatory Care & Prevention, Sixth Edition

1 2 3 4 5 6 7 8 9 0 DOC/DOC 18 17 16 15 14

ISBN: 978-0-07-182073-8
MHID: 0-07-182073-6

ISSN # 1066-2715

This book was set in Futura Std by Aptara, Inc.
The editors were Sarah Henry and Christie Naglieri.
The production supervisor was Catherine Saggese.
Project Management was provided by Amit Kashyap, Aptara, Inc.
RR Donnellley was printer and binder.

This book is printed on acid-free paper.

International Edition ISBN 978-1-25-925250-1; MHID 1-25-925250-7. Copyright © 2014. Exclusive rights by McGraw-Hill Education, for manufacture and export. This book cannot be re-exported from the country to which it is consigned by McGraw-Hill Education. The International Edition is not available in North America.

Contents

Contributors ix
Preface xxi

Section I. Common Problems 1

1. Abdominal Pain 1
 Kalyanakrishnan Ramakrishnan, MD, MS, FRCS

2. The Abnormal Pap Smear 12
 Kathryn Reilly, MD, & Audra Fox, MD

3. Amenorrhea 17
 Amanda Kaufman, MD

4. Anemia 24
 Andrew D. Jones, MD, MBA, & Cary L. Clarke, MD

5. Ankle Injuries 31
 Philip R. Palmer, MD, FAAFP

6. Arm and Shoulder Complaints 37
 Brian R. Coleman, MD

7. Bites and Stings 44
 Brenda Powell, MD

8. Breast Lumps and Other Breast Conditions 54
 Diane J. Madlon-Kay, MD, MS

9. Cellulitis and Other Bacterial Skin Infections 58
 Donald B. Middleton, MD

10. Chest Pain 70
 George P.N. Samraj, MD, MRCOG

11. Confusion 78
 Robert C. Salinas, MD (CAQ-G, HPM), & Audra Fox, MD

12. Constipation 83
 Allen R. Last, MD, MPH, & Jonathan D. Ference, PharmD, BCPS

13. Cough 91
 Jennifer E. Lochner, MD, & David Holmes, MD

14. Dermatitis and Other Pruritic Dermatoses 103
 *A. Ildiko Martonffy, MD, Jie Wang, MD, Aleksandra Zgierska, MD, PhD,
 William G. Phillips, MD, & Marjorie Shaw Phillips, MS, RPh, FASHP*

15. Dermatologic Neoplasms 120
 Daniel L. Stulberg, MD, & Douglas G. Browning, MD, ATC-L

16. Diarrhea 131
Michael A. Noll, MD, Jeanne M. Ferrante, MD, MPH, &
Laura Hargro, MD, MBA

17. Dizziness.. 145
Suzanne L. Harrison, MD, & Lisa M. Johnson, MD

18. Dysmenorrhea... 149
Suzanne L. Harrison, MD, & Lisa M. Johnson, MD

19. Dyspepsia 154
Kalyanakrishnan Ramakrishnan, MD, MS, FRCS

20. Dyspnea... 161
James C. Chesnutt, MD, Mark R. Stephan, MD, Scott A. Fields, MD, &
William L. Toffler, MD

21. Dysuria in Women.. 166
L. Peter Schwiebert, MD

22. Earache 172
David Berkson, MD, FAAFP, Greeshma Naini, MD, & Carmelo DiSalvo, MD

23. Enuresis 183
Kalyanakrishnan Ramakrishnan, MD, MS, FRCS

24. Failure to Thrive 187
Jacqueline L. Gerhart, MD, & Cathy Kamens, MD

25. Fatigue... 193
Anthony F. Valdini, MD, MS

26. Fluid, Electrolyte, and Acid–Base Disturbances............................. 198
Mudit Gilotra, MD, Marc Altshuler, MD, & Lara Carson Weinstein, MD, MPH

27. Foot Conditions... 206
James R. Barrett, MD, CAQSM

28. Fractures 216
Ted C. Schaffer, MD, & Melanie C. Schaffer, MD

29. Gastrointestinal Bleeding.. 222
Erin C. Contratto, MD, & May S. Jennings, MD

30. Genital Lesions.. 228
Tomás P. Owens, Jr., MD

31. Hair and Nail Disorders.. 237
Amy D. Crawford-Faucher, MD, FAAFP

32. Hand and Wrist Complaints 251
Jessica T. Servey, MD, FAAFP, Col, USAF, Ted Boehm, MD, &
Nicole G. Stern, MD

33. Headaches.. 264
Dan F. Criswell, MD

34. Hearing Loss... 274
Robert C. Salinas, MD, & Audra Fox, MD

35. Hematuria 281
Cynthia M. Waickus, MD, PhD

36. Insomnia 287
Julianne Falleroni, DO, MPH

37. Jaundice.. 300
Kalyanakrishnan Ramakrishnan, MD, MS, FRCS, & L. Peter Schwiebert, MD

38. Joint Pain... 310
L. Peter Schwiebert, MD

39. Knee Complaints 317
Vimarie Rodriguez, MD, CAQSM, & Mitchell A. Kaminski, MD, MBA

40. Lacerations and Skin Biopsy 332
Jason Chao, MD, MS, & Rasai L. Ernst, MD

41. Leg and Hip Complaints.. 338
Geoffrey S. Kuhlman, MD, CAQSM, FAAFP

42. Liver Function Test Abnormalities 347
Angie Mathai, MD, & James P. McKenna, MD

43. Low Back Pain 352
Dan F. Criswell, MD

44. Lymphadenopathy 360
Jo Marie Reilly, MD, FAAFP, & Fred Kobylarz, MD, MPH

45. Myalgia 364
Tomás P. Owens, Jr., MD

46. Nausea and Vomiting 371
Nipa R. Shah, MD, & George R. Wilson, MD

47. Neck Pain 383
Michael P. Rowane, DO, MS, FAAFP, FAAO

48. Palpitations.. 387
Jose E. Rodríguez, MD, & Mike D. Hardin, Jr., MD

49. Pediatric Fever 395
Joanne Dempster, MD, & Urmi A. Desai, MD

50. Pelvic Pain... 400
*Guido Grasso-Knight, MD, MPH, Meredith A. Goodwin, MD, &
Niharika Khanna, MBBS, MD, DGO*

51. Perianal Complaints.. 410
Kalyanakrishnan Ramakrishnan, MD, MS, FRCS

52. Proteinuria... 418
Aamir Siddiqi, MD

53. The Red Eye... 423
Heidi S. Chumley, MD, Victor A. Diaz, Jr., MD, & Deborah K. Witt, MD

54. Rhinitis and Sinus Pain 432
*Jensena M. Carlson, MD, Melissa Stiles, MD, Robert G. Quattlebaum, MD,
Vanessa A. Diaz, MD, MS, & Arch G. Mainous III, PhD*

55. Scrotal Complaints 443
Michael N. Nduati, MD, MBA, MPH, & John A. Heydt, MD

56. Sore Throat.. 449
L. Peter Schwiebert, MD

57. Syncope.. 454
Brian H. Halstater, MD, John Ragsdale III, MD, LeRoy C. White, MD, JD, &
Felix Horng, MD, MBA

58. Tremors and Other Movement Disorders................................. 461
Aylin Yaman, MD, Hakan Yaman, MD, MS, & Goutham Rao, MD

59. Urinary Incontinence.. 471
Annette Sandretto, MSN, ANP-BC, RN, Karen D. Novielli, MD,
& Barry D. Weiss, MD

60. Urinary Symptoms in Men 479
Karl T. Rew, MD, & Linda L. Walker, MD, FAAFP

61. Urticaria.. 489
Robert Ellis, MD, Montiel Rosenthal, MD, & Laura Counsell, MD

62. Abnormal Vaginal Bleeding 500
Heather L. Paladine, MD, FAAFP & Pooja A. Shah, MD

63. Vaginal Discharge 506
L. Peter Schwiebert, MD

64. Venous Thromboembolism 512
Stefani A. Hudson, MD, &
Jeffrey M. Tingen, PharmD, MBA, BCPS, BCACP, CDE

65. Wheezing 518
Christopher Taggart, MD, & Judith Kerber Frazier, MD

Section II. Chronic Illness 525

66. Acne Vulgaris and Acne Rosacea.. 525
Paul C. Walker, PharmD, FASHP, Mindy A. Smith, MD, MS,
Brooke E. Farley, PharmD, BCPS, & Julie A. Murphy, PharmD, BCPS

67. Human Immunodeficiency Virus and Acquired
Immunodeficiency Syndrome.. 535
Parya Saberi, PharmD, MAS, Megan Mahoney, MD, &
Ronald H. Goldschmidt, MD

68. Asthma 548
Jonathan MacClements, MD, FAAFP

69. Cancers of the Breast, Lung, and Colon 562
Elizabeth R. Menzel, MD, & Kathryn Jacobe, MD

70. Chronic Obstructive Pulmonary Disease 576
H. Bruce Vogt, MD, FAAFP

71. Chronic (Persistent) Pain 596
Michael P. Temporal, MD

72. Cirrhosis 605
Mark C. Potter, MD, & Mari Egan, MD, MHPE

73. Congestive Heart Failure 614
Philip M. Diller, MD, PhD, & Christopher R. Bernheisel, MD

74. Dementia... 627
Radha Ramana Murthy Gokula, MD, CMD, & Leelasri Vanguru, MD

75. Diabetes Mellitus 643
Stuart D. Rockafellow, PharmD, BCACP, Caroline R. Richardson, MD, &
Mark B. Mengel, MD, MPH

76. Dyslipidemias 660
Trisha D. Wells, PharmD, Amanda M. Cox, MD, Mindy A. Smith, MD, MS, &
Michael A. Crouch, MD, MSPH

77. Hypertension 676
Ann E. Evensen, MD, FAAFP, & Charles B. Eaton, MD, MS

78. Inflammatory Bowel Disease 687
Russell Lemmon, DO, & David M. Lessens, MD, MPH

79. Ischemic Heart Disease and Acute Coronary Syndromes 697
Damon F. Lee, MD, Lovedhi Aggarwal, MD, & Allen L. Hixon, MD

80. Menopause 709
Linda M. Speer, MD, Tammy J. Lindsay, MD, & Mark Mengel, MD, MPH

81. Obesity 716
Radhika R. Hariharan, MD, MRCP (UK), Brian C. Reed, MD, &
Sarah R. Edmonson, MD, MS

82. Osteoarthritis 726
Charles Kodner, MD

83. Osteoporosis 737
William T. Manard, MD, FAAFP, &
Richard O. Schamp, MD, CMD, CHCQM

84. Peptic Ulcer Disease 747
Carol Stewart, MD, FAAFP, Nancy Tyre, MD, & Lesley D. Wilkinson, MD

85. Premenstrual Syndrome 755
Heather R. Pickett, DO, FAAFP, Abby L. Harris, MD, & Michael Michener, MD

86. Renal Failure 763
Terrence T. Truong, MD

87. Seizure Disorders 774
Mindy A. Smith, MD, MS, Shawn H. Blanchard, MD, &
William L. Toffler, MD

88. Stroke 786
Michael P. Temporal, MD

89. Thyroid Disease 797
Jeri R. Reid, MD, & Angela R. Wetherton, MD

Section III. Psychiatric Disorders 808

90. Alcohol and Drug Abuse 808
Robert Mallin, MD, & Kristen Hood Watson, MD

91. Anxiety 819
John C. Rogers, MD, MPH, MEd, & Alicia A. Kowalchuk, DO

92. Attention Deficit Hyperactivity Disorder 829
H. Russell Searight, PhD, MPH, Jennifer Gafford, PhD, &
Stephanie L. Evans, PharmD, BCPS

93. Family Violence: Child, Intimate Partner, and Elder Abuse 847
F. David Schneider, MD, MSPH, Nancy D. Kellogg, MD, &
Melissa A. Talamantes, MS

94. Depression 856
Rhonda A. Faulkner, PhD, & Luis T. Garcia, MD, A.B.F.M.

95. Eating Disorders 865
Brian C. Reed, MD

96. Somatization 873
Juliet Bradley, MD, & Tracy R. Juliao, PhD

Section IV. Reproductive Health 881

97. Contraception 881
Grant M. Greenberg, MD, MA, MHSA, Nell Kirst, MD, &
Margaret Dobson, MD

98. Infertility 892
Keith A. Frey, MD, MBA

99. Preconception and Prenatal Care 896
Kirsten Vitrikas, MD

100. Postpartum Care 909
Shami Goyal, MD, MS, & Jeannette E. South-Paul, MD

101. Sexual Dysfunction 915
Elizabeth H. Naumburg, MD, & Elizabeth J. Brown, MD, MPH

102. Sexually Transmitted Infections 932
Jessica Dalby, MD, & Jaime Marks, MD

Section V. Preventive Medicine and Health Promotion 943

103. Chemoprophylaxis 943
A. Ildiko Martonffy, MD, & Paul E. Lewis III, MD, MPH

104. Counseling for Behavioral Change 950
Mark R. Marnocha, PhD, David C. Pole, MPH, Ryan M. Niemiec, PsyD,
Laura Frankenstein, MD, & Shawn E. Boogaard, MSE

105. Immunizations 960
William E. Cayley, Jr., MD, MDiv

106. Screening Tests 967
Larry L. Dickey, MD, MPH

107. Travel Medicine 979
Mark K. Huntington, MD, PhD, FAAFP

108. Preoperative Evaluation 996
Jaime D. Marks, MD

Index 1007

Color insert appears between pages 586 and 587.

Contributors

Lovedhi Aggarwal, MD
Assistant Professor Department of Family Medicine and Community Health, University of Hawaii John A Burns School of Medicine, Honolulu, Hawaii

Marc Altshuler, MD
Associate Professor, Associate Residency Director, Department of Family and Community Medicine, Thomas Jefferson University, Philadelphia, Pennsylvania

James R. Barrett, MD, CAQSM
Professor of Family Medicine, University of Oklahoma Health Sciences Center, Oklahoma City, Oklahoma

David Berkson, MD, FAAFP
Associate Professor, Drexel University College of Medicine, Philadelphia, Pennsylvania

Christopher R. Bernheisel, MD
Assistant Professor of Family and Community Medicine, Director of UC/TCH Residency Program, The Christ Hospital Medical Office Building, Cincinnati, Ohio

Shawn H. Blanchard, MD
Assistant Professor, Department of Family Medicine, Associate Director, Predoctoral Education, Oregon Health & Science University, Portland, Oregon

Ted Boehm, MD
Volunteer Faculty, Primary Care Sports Medicine Fellowship, Department of Family Medicine, University of Oklahoma Health Sciences Center, Oklahoma City, Oklahoma; Primary Care Sports, Medicine Physician, Oklahoma Sports and Orthopedics Institute, Norman, Oklahoma

Shawn E. Boogaard, MSE
Health Educator/Counselor, University of Wisconsin Department of Family Medicine, Fox Valley Family Medicine Residency, Appleton, Wisconsin

Juliet Bradley, MD
Associate Professor of Clinical Medicine, Cook County-Loyola-Provident Family Medicine Residency Program, Chicago, Illinois

Douglas G. Browning, MD, ATC-L
Wake Forest Family Practice, Winston Salem, North Carolina

Elizabeth J. Brown, MD, MPH
Assistant Professor, Department of Family Medicine, University of Rochester, School of Medicine and Dentistry, Rochester, New York

Jensena M. Carlson, MD
Academic Fellow in Family Medicine, University of Wisconsin-Madison, Madison, Wisconsin

William E. Cayley, Jr., MD, MDiv
Professor, Department of Family Medicine, University of Wisconsin School of Medicine and Public Health, Eau Claire, Wisconsin

Jason Chao, MD, MS
Professor, Family Medicine and Community Health, Case Western Reserve University and University Hospitals Case Medical Center, Cleveland, Ohio

James C. Chesnutt, MD
Medical Director, Oregon Health and Science University Sports Medicine, Portland, Oregon

Heidi S. Chumley, MD
Executive Dean and Chief Academic Officer, American University of the Caribbean, Coral Gables, Florida

Cary L. Clarke, MD
Attending Faculty, Exempla Saint Joseph Hospital Family Medicine Residency, Denver, Colorado

Brian R. Coleman, MD
Associate Professor, University of Oklahoma, Department of Family Medicine, Oklahoma City, Oklahoma

Erin C. Contratto, MD
Assistant Professor of Internal Medicine, University of Alabama at Birmingham, Birmingham, Alabama

Laura Counsell, MD
Resident, St. Vincent Family Medicine Residency, Indianapolis, Indiana

Amanda M. Cox, MD
Instructor, Department of Internal Medicine, University of Michigan Medical School, Ann Arbor, Michigan

Amy D. Crawford-Faucher, MD, FAAFP
Assistant Clinical Professor, University of Pittsburgh Medical Center, Pittsburgh, Pennsylvania

Michael A. Crouch, MD, MSPH
Associate Professor, Family and Community Medicine, Baylor College of Medicine, Houston, Texas

Dan F. Criswell, MD
Staff Physician, Solutions Physicians/Duncan Regional Hospital, Duncan, Oklahoma

Jessica Dalby, MD
Assistant Professor, University of Wisconsin, Department of Family Medicine, Madison, Wisconsin

Joanne Dempster, MD
Chief of Service for Family Medicine at the Allen Hospital and Associate Residency Program Director for Family Medicine, New York Presbyterian Hospital/Columbia University Medical Center, New York, New York

Urmi A. Desai, MD
Assistant in Clinical Medicine and Research Fellow, Center for Family and Community Medicine, Columbia University Medical Center, New York, New York

Vanessa A. Diaz, MD, MS
Assistant Professor, Department of Family Medicine, Medical University of South Carolina, Charleston, South Carolina

Victor A. Diaz, Jr., MD
Assistant Professor, Family and Community Medicine, Jefferson Medical College, Assistant Medical Director, Jefferson Family Medicine Associates, Thomas Jefferson University Hospital, Philadelphia, Pennsylvania

Larry L. Dickey, MD, MPH
Associate Adjunct Professor, University of California, San Francisco, California, Medical Director, Office of Health Information Technology, California Department of Health Care Services, Sacramento, California

Philip M. Diller, MD, PhD
Fred Lazarus, Jr. Professor and Chair, Department of Family and Community Medicine, University of
Cincinnati College of Medicine, Cincinnati, Ohio

Carmelo DiSalvo, MD
Mid Atlantic Family Practice, Lewes, Delaware

Margaret Dobson, MD
Clinical Lecturer and Residency Program Director, University of Michigan Department of Family Medicine,
Ann Arbor, Michigan

Charles B. Eaton, MD, MS
Professor, Family Medicine, Department of Family Medicine, Director, Heart Disease Prevention Center,
Brown University School of Medicine, Pawtucket, Rhode Island

Sarah R. Edmonson, MD, MS
Instructor, Family and Community Medicine, Baylor College of Medicine, Houston, Texas

Mari Egan, MD, MHPE
Director of Medical Student Education, Associate Professor, Dept of Family Medicine, Pritzker School of
Medicine, University of Chicago, Chicago, Illinois

Robert Ellis, MD
Associate Professor, Department of Family and Community Medicine, University of Cincinnati College of
Medicine, Cincinnati, Ohio

Rasai L. Ernst, MD
Senior Instructor, Department of Family Medicine and Community Health, CaseWestern Reserve University
and University Hospitals Case Medical Center, Cleveland, Ohio

Stephanie L. Evans, PharmD, BCPS
Staff Pharmacist, Wal-Mart Pharmacy, Benton, Kentucky

Ann E. Evensen, MD , FAAFP
Associate Professor, Department of Family Medicine, University of Wisconsin School of Medicine and
Public Health, Madison, Wisconsin

Julianne Falleroni, DO, MPH
Assistant Professor of Family Medicine, UW Health Fox Valley Family Medicine Residency, Appleton,
Wisconsin

Rhonda A. Faulkner, PhD
Director of Behavioral Medicine, Department of Family Medicine, Saint Joseph Hospital, University of
Illinois College of Medicine, Chicago, Illinois

Jonathan D. Ference, PharmD, BCPS
Associate Professor, Department of Pharmacy Practice, Nesbitt College of Pharmacy and Nursing,
Wilkes-Barre, Pennsylvania; Director of Pharmacotherapy Education, The Wright Center for Graduate
Medical Education – Family Medicine Residency Program, Kingston, Pennsylvania

Jeanne M. Ferrante, MD, MPH
Associate Professor, Rutgers-Robert Wood Johnson Medical School, New Brunswick, New Jersey

Scott A. Fields, MD
Vice Chair, Family Medicine, Oregon Health Sciences University, Portland, Oregon

Audra Fox, MD
Assistant Professor, University of Oklahoma, Department of Family Medicine, Oklahoma City, Oklahoma

Brooke E. Farley, PharmD, BCPS
Clinical Pharmacist and Assistant Professor, Pharmacy Practice, Mercy Family Medicine, Saint John's
Mercy Family Medicine Residency Program and the Saint Louis College of Pharmacy, St. Louis, Missouri

Laura Frankenstein, MD
Clinical Assistant Professor, Department of Community and Family Medicine, Saint Louis University,
St. Louis, Missouri

Judith Kerber Frazier, MD
Family Medicine Physician, Mustang, Oklahoma

Keith A. Frey, MD, MBA
Professor of Family Medicine, Mayo Clinic, Scottsdale, Arizona

Jennifer Gafford, PhD
Assistant Professor, Saint Louis University Family Medicine Residency at SSM St. Mary's Health Center and
Director of Consultation Services, Family Care Health Centers, St. Louis, Missouri

Luis T. Garcia, MD, A.B.F.M.
Chairman and Program Director, Department of Family Medicine, Saint Joseph Hospital – University of
Illinois College of Medicine Master Affiliate, Chicago, Illinois

Jacqueline L. Gerhart, MD
Assistant Professor, UW School of Medicine and Public Health, University of Wisconsin-Madison,
Department of Family Medicine, Madison, Wisconsin

Mudit Gilotra, MD
Medical Director Lalmba Clinic, Chiri, Ethiopia (as of August 2013), (Participated in chapter as Chief
Resident, Jefferson Family Medicine, Philadelphia, Pennsylvania)

Radha Ramana Murthy Gokula, MD, CMD
Associate Professor/Program Director, Geriatrics Fellowship Program, University of Toledo, Toledo, Ohio

Ronald H. Goldschmidt, MD
Professor of Family and Community Medicine, Vice-Chair, University of California, San Francisco,
Department of Family and Community Medicine, San Francisco General Hospital, San Francisco,
California

Meredith A. Goodwin, MD
Assistant Professor, Family Medicine and Rural Health, Florida State University College of Medicine,
Resource Staff Physician, Tallahassee Memorial Hospital, Tallahassee, Florida

Shami Goyal, MD, MS
Assistant Professor, University of Pittsburgh, Department of Family Medicine, Pittsburgh, Pennsylvania

Guido Grasso-Knight, MD, MPH
Assistant Professor, Department of Family and Community, Medicine, University of Maryland School of
Medicine, Baltimore, Maryland

Grant M. Greenberg, MD, MA, MHSA
Assistant Professor and Associate Chair for Information Management and Quality, University of Michigan
Department of Family Medicine, Ann Arbor, Michigan

Brian H. Halstater, MD
Assistant Professor, Director of Duke Family Medicine Residency Program, Department of Community and
Family Medicine, Durham, North Carolina

Laura Hargro, MD, MBA
Assistant Professor, Dept. of Family Medicine, UMDNJ-New Jersey Medical School, Newark,
New Jersey

Mike D. Hardin, Jr., MD
Faculty Member, Department of Family Medicine, McLennan County Medical Education and Research Foundation, University of Texas Southwestern Medical School, Waco, Texas

John A. Heydt, MD
President and CEO, University Physicians & Surgeons, Senior Associate Dean of Clinical Affairs, University of California, Irvine

Radhika R. Hariharan MD, MRCP (UK)
Assistant Professor, Department of Internal Medicine, Baylor College of Medicine, Houston, Texas

Abby L. Harris, MD
Staff Family Physician, United States Air Force, Nellis AFB, Nevada

Suzanne L. Harrison, MD
Associate Professor, Director of Family Medicine Education, Department of Family Medicine and Rural Health, Florida State University College of Medicine, Tallahassee, Florida

Allen L. Hixon, MD
Associate Professor and Vice Chairman, Department of Family Medicine and Community Health, John A. Burns School of Medicine, University of Hawaii, Mililani, Hawaii

David Holmes, MD
Clinical Associate Professor, Family Medicine, University at Buffalo, State University of New York, Family Physician, Family Medicine, Kaleida Health, Buffalo, New York

Felix Horng, MD, MBA
Woodbury Medical Group, Irvine, California

Stefani A. Hudson, MD
Clinical Lecturer, Medical Director, Ypsilanti Health Center, Department of Family Medicine, University of Michigan Health System, Ypsilanti, Michigan

Mark K. Huntington, MD, PhD, FAAFP
Professor, Department of Family Medicine, University of South Dakota Sanford School of Medicine, Director, Sioux Falls Family Medicine Residency Program, Center for Family Medicine, Sioux Falls, South Dakota

Kathryn Jacobe, MD
Assistant Professor of Family Medicine, University of Wisconsin-Madison, Fox Valley Family Medicine Residency, Appleton, Wisconsin

May S. Jennings, MD
Associate Professor, University of Alabama at Birmingham, Birmingham, Alabama

Lisa M. Johnson, MD
Assistant Professor, Department of Family Medicine and Rural Health, Florida State University College of Medicine, Tallahassee, Florida

Andrew D. Jones, MD, MBA
Program Director, Exempla Saint Joseph Hospital Family Medicine, Denver, Colorado

Tracy R. Juliao, PhD
Counseling Psychology, Director, Psychology in Beaumont Weight Control Centers, Health Psychologist and Owner, Beaumont Health System, Total Health and Wellness Associates, PLLC, Royal Oak and Rochester Hills, MI Farmington Hills, Michigan

Amanda Kaufman, MD
Clinical Assistant Professor of Family Medicine, University of Michigan, Ann Arbor, Michigan

Cathy Kamens, MD
Lecturer, Department of Family and Community Medicine, University of Toronto, Family Physician, Women's College Hospital, Toronto, Ontario, Canada

Mitchell A. Kaminski, MD, MBA
Chairman, Department of Family Medicine, Clinical Associate Professor, Temple School of Medicine, Crozer-Chester Medical Center, Upland, Pennsylvania

Nancy D. Kellogg, MD
Professor, Division Chief of Child Abuse, University of Texas Health Science Center, Department of Pediatrics, San Antonio, Texas

Niharika Khanna, MBBS, MD, DGO
Associate Professor, Department of Family and Community Medicine, University of Maryland School of Medicine, Baltimore, Maryland

Nell Kirst, MD
Clinical Lecturer and Assistant Residency Program Director University of Michigan Department of Family Medicine, Ann Arbor, Michigan

Fred Kobylarz, MD, MPH
Associate Professor, Center for Healthy Aging, Department of Family Medicine, UMDNJ—Robert, Wood Johnson Medical School, Department of Family Medicine, Robert Wood Johnson University, Hospital, New Brunswick, New Jersey

Charles Kodner, MD
Associate Professor, University of Louisville School of Medicine, Department of Family and Geriatric Medicine, Louisville, Kentucky

Alicia A. Kowalchuk, DO
Assistant Professor of Family and Community Medicine, Baylor College of Medicine, Houston, Texas

Geoffrey S. Kuhlman, MD, CAQSM, FAAFP
Director of Sports Medicine, Hinsdale Family Medicine Residency, Private Practice, Bolingbrook, Illinois

Allen R. Last, MD, MPH
Residency Director, Fox Valley Family Medicine Residency, Appleton, Wisconsin

Damon F. Lee, MD
Assistant Director, Office of Student Affairs; Assistant Clinical Professor, Department of Family Medicine and Community Health, University of Hawaii, John A. Burns School of Medicine, Honolulu, Hawaii

Russell Lemmon, DO
Assistant Professor, University of Wisconsin, Department of Family Medicine, Madison, Wisconsin

David M. Lessens, MD, MPH
Integrative Family Physician, Southcentral Foundation, Anchorage, Alaska

Paul E. Lewis III, MD, MPH
Assistant Professor, SLU Family Medicine Residency Program, Saint Louis University, Belleville, Illinois

Tammy J. Lindsay, MD
Flight Commander; Interim Associate Program Director, SLU Family Medicine Residency Program, 375th MDOS and Saint Louis University, Belleville, Illinois

Jennifer E. Lochner, MD
Assistant Professor of Family Medicine, Department of Family Medicine, University of Wisconsin School of Medicine and Public Health, Madison, Wisconsin

Jonathan MacClements, MD, FAAFP
Professor, Director of Medical Education; Chairman Family Medicine Department, University of Texas Health Science Center at Tyler, Tyler, Texas

Diane J. Madlon-Kay, MD, MS
Professor, Department of Family Medicine and Community Health, University of Minnesota Medical School, Minneapolis, Minnesota

Megan Mahoney, MD
Associate Professor, University of California, San Francisco, San Francisco, California

Arch G. Mainous III, PhD
Professor, Department of Family Medicine, Medical University of South Carolina, Charleston, South Carolina

Robert Mallin, MD
Dean of Medical Education, College of Medicine, American University of Antigua, Antigua, West Indies

William T. Manard, MD, FAAFP
Assistant Professor and Director of Clinical Services, Department of Family and Community Medicine, Saint Louis University School of Medicine, St. Louis, Missouri

Jaime Marks, MD
Assistant Professor of Family Medicine, University of Wisconsin School of Medicine and Public Health, Madison, Wisconsin

Mark R. Marnocha, PhD
Professor and Clinical Psychologist, University of Wisconsin, Department of Family Medicine, Fox Valley Family Medicine, Appleton, Wisconsin

A. Ildiko Martonffy, MD
Assistant Professor of Family Medicine, Department of Family Medicine, University of Wisconsin School of Medicine and Public Health, Madison, Wisconsin

Angie Mathai, MD
Assistant Clinical Professor, East Carolina University, Greenville, North Carolina

James P. McKenna, MD
Residency Director, Family Medicine Residency, Hentage Valley Beaver, Beaver, Pennsylvania

Mark B. Mengel, MD, MPH
Vice Chancellor, Regional Programs, University of Arkansas for Medical Sciences, Professor, Family and Preventive Medicine, University of Arkansas for Medical Sciences, Little Rock, Arkansas

Elizabeth R. Menzel, MD
Assistant Professor of Family Medicine, University of Wisconsin-Madison, Fox Valley Family Medicine Residency, Appleton, Wisconsin

Michael Michener, MD
Associate Professor, SLU Family Medicine Residency Program, Saint Louis University, Belleville, Illinois

Donald B. Middleton, MD
Professor, Department of Family Medicine, Vice President for Residency Education, Pittsburgh, Pennsylvania

Julie A. Murphy, PharmD, BCPS
Clinical Pharmacist and Associate Professor of Pharmacy Practice, Mercy Family Medicine, Saint John's Mercy Family Medicine Residency Program and the Saint Louis College of Pharmacy, St. Louis, Missouri

Greeshma Naini, MD
Family Medicine Resident, Department of Family, Community, and Preventive Medicine, Drexel University College of Medicine, Philadelphia, Pennsylvania

Elizabeth H. Naumburg, MD
Associate Dean, Advising, Professor of Family Medicine, University of Rochester School of Medicine, Rochester, New York

Michael N. Nduati, MD, MBA, MPH
Associate Dean for Clinical Affairs, UC Riverside School of Medicine, Riverside, California

Ryan M. Niemiec, PsyD
Assistant Clinical Professor, Community and Family Medicine, Saint Louis University School of Medicine, Psychologist, Saint Louis Behavioral Medicine Institute, St. Louis, Missouri

Karen D. Novielli, MD
Senior Associate Dean for Faculty Affairs and Professional Development, Jefferson Medical College, Philadelphia, Pennsylvania

Michael A. Noll, MD
Instructor, Attending Hospitalist, Rutgers-Robert Wood Johnson Medical School, New Brunswick, New Jersey

Tomás P. Owens, Jr, MD
Chair of Family Medicine, INTEGRIS Baptist Medical Center, Clinical Professor, Departments of Internal Medicine, Geriatric Medicine, and Family and Preventive Medicine, University of Oklahoma Health Sciences Center, Oklahoma City, Oklahoma

Heather L. Paladine, MD, FAAFP
Assistant Professor of Medicine, Center for Family and Community Medicine, Columbia University Medical Center, New York, New York

Philip R. Palmer, MD, FAAFP
Faculty, Great Plains Family Medicine Residency, Oklahoma City, Oklahoma

Mark C. Potter, MD
Associate Professor and Residency Director, Department of Family Medicine, University of Illinois at Chicago, Chicago, Illinois

William G. Phillips, MD
Family Practice, Atlanta, Georgia

Marjorie Shaw Phillips, MS, RPh, FASHP
Clinical Research Pharmacist and Medication Safety Coordinator, Medical College of Georgia Health System and Clinical Professor, University of Georgia College of Pharmacy, Augusta, Georgia

Heather R. Pickett, DO FAAFP
Department of Physical Medicine and Rehabilitation, Veterans Administration, Southern Nevada Health System, Las Vegas, Nevada

David C. Pole, MPH
Deputy Director, Predoctoral and AHEC Programs, Community and Family Medicine, Saint Louis University, St. Louis, Missouri

Brenda Powell, MD
Assistant Medical Director University of Washington Neighborhood Clinics, Seattle, Washington

Robert G. Quattlebaum, MD
Trident Medical Center/Medical University of South Carolina, Family Medicine Residency Program, Charleston, South Carolina

Kalyanakrishnan Ramakrishnan, MD, MS, FRCS
Professor, Department of Family and Preventive Medicine, University of Oklahoma Health Sciences Center, Oklahoma City, Oklahoma

John Ragsdale III, MD
Assistant Professor, Director of Duke Family Medicine Residency Program, Department of Community and Family Medicine, Durham, North Carolina

Goutham Rao, MD
Clinical Director, Weight Management and Wellness Center, Associate Professor of Pediatrics and Family Medicine, University of Pittsburgh School of Medicine, Pittsburgh, Pennsylvania

Brian C. Reed, MD
Interim Chairman, Associate Professor, Department of Family and Community Medicine, Baylor College of Medicine, Waco, Texas

Jeri R. Reid, MD
Associate Professor, Department of Family and Geriatric Medicine, University of Louisville, Louisville, Kentucky

Kathryn Reilly, MD, MPH
Professor and Associate Residency Director, Department of Family and Community medicine, University of Oklahoma Health Science Center, Oklahoma City, Oklahoma

Jo Marie Reilly, MD, FAAFP
Associate Clinical Professor of Family Medicine, Keck School of Medicine at USC, Los Angeles, California

Karl T. Rew, MD
Assistant Professor, Departments of Family Medicine and Urology, University of Michigan Medical School, Ann Arbor, Michigan

Caroline R. Richardson, MD
Associate Professor, University of Michigan Department of Family Medicine, VA Center for Clinical Management Research, Ann Arbor, Michigan

Stuart D. Rockafellow, PharmD, BCACP
Clinical Assistant Professor, University of Michigan College of Pharmacy, Ann Arbor, Michigan

Jose E. Rodríguez, MD
Associate Professor, Department of Family Medicine and Rural Health, Florida State University, Tallahassee, Florida

Vimarie Rodriguez, MD, CAQSM
Assistant Professor, CCLP Family Medicine Residency Program, Loyola University Chicago, Stritch School of Medicine, Chicago, Illinois

John C. Rogers, MD, MPH, MEd
Professor of Family and Community Medicine, Baylor College of Medicine, Houston, Texas

Michael P. Rowane, DO, MS, FAAFP, FAAO
Associate Clinical Professor of Family Medicine and Psychiatry, Case Western Reserve University, Director of Medical Education, University Hospitals Regional Hospitals, Director of Osteopathic Medical Education, University Hospitals Case Medical Center, University Hospitals Regional Hospitals Department of Medical Education, Richmond Heights, Ohio

Parya Saberi, PharmD, MAS
Assistant Professor, University of California, San Francisco, San Francisco, California

Robert C. Salinas, MD
Associate Professor, OU Department of Family Medicine, Oklahoma City, Oklahoma

George P.N. Samraj, MD, MRCOG
Associate professor, University of Florida, College of Medicine, Gainesville, Florida

Annette Sandretto, MSN, ANP-BC, RN
Nurse Practitioner, University of Michigan Health System, Ann Arbor, Michigan

Ted C. Schaffer, MD
Program Director, UPMC St. Margaret Family Medicine Residency, Pittsburgh, Pennsylvania

Melanie C. Schaffer, MD
Senior Resident, UPMC St. Margaret Family Medicine Residency, Pittsburgh, Pennsylvania

Richard O. Schamp, MD, CMD, CHCQM
Chief Executive Officer, Capstone Performance Systems, St. Louis, Missouri

F. David Schneider, MD, MSPH
Professor and Chair, Department of Family and Community Medicine, Saint Louis University, St. Louis, Missouri

L. Peter Schwiebert, MD
Professor, University of Oklahoma Health Sciences Center, Department of Family and Preventive Medicine, Oklahoma City, Oklahoma

H. Russell Searight, PhD, MPH
Professor of Psychology, Lake Superior State University, Sault Sainte Marie, Michigan

Jessica T. Servey, MD, FAAFP, Col, USAF
Director, Family Medicine Clerkship, Vice Chair of Education, Dept of Family Medicine, Uniformed Services University of the Health Sciences, Bethesda, Maryland

Nipa R. Shah, MD
Associate Professor and Chair, Dept. of Community Health and Family Medicine, University of Florida, Jacksonville, Florida

Pooja A. Shah, MD
Assistant Professor of Medicine, Center for Family and Community Medicine, Columbia University Medical Center, New York, New York

Aamir Siddiqi, MD
Director of Clinical Services, Norris Health Center, University of Wisconsin-Milwaukee, Milwaukee, Wisconsin

Mindy A. Smith, MD, MS
Clinical Professor, Department of Family Medicine, Michigan State University, College of Human Medicine East Lansing, Michigan

Jeannette E. South-Paul, MD
Professor and Chair, University of Pittsburgh, Department of Family Medicine, Pittsburgh, Pennsylvania

Linda M. Speer, MD
Professor and Chair, Department of Family Medicine, University of Toledo, College of Medicine and Life Sciences, Toledo, Ohio

Nicole G. Stern, MD
Campus Health Service, Tucson, Arizona

Carol Stewart, MD, FAAFP
HS Clinical Associate Professor, David Geffen School of Medicine at UCLA, and Residency Program Director, Rio Bravo Family Medicine Residency, Santa Monica, California

Melissa Stiles, MD
Professor of Family Medicine, University of Wisconsin-Madison, Madison, Wisconsin

Daniel L. Stulberg, MD
Professor, Department of Family and Community Medicine, University of New Mexico, Albuquerque, New Mexico

Christopher Taggart, MD
Senior Instructor, University of Rochester, Rochester, New York

Melissa A. Talamantes, MS
Faculty, Department of Family Practice, University of Texas HSC, San Antonio, San Antonio, Texas

Michael P. Temporal, MD
Clinical Professor Family Medicine, Saint Louis University School of Medicine, Attending Physician Billings Clinic, Billings, Montana

Jeffrey M. Tingen, PharmD, MBA, BCPS, BCACP, CDE
Clinical Assistant Professor, University of Michigan College of Pharmacy, Ann Arbor, Michigan

William L. Toffler, MD
Professor, Department of Family Medicine, Director, Predoctoral Education, Oregon Health & Science University, Portland, Oregon

Terrence T. Truong, MD
Faculty, Great Plains Family Medicine Residency Program, Oklahoma, Oklahoma

Nancy Tyre, MD
Clinical Faculty Associate Physician Family Medicine, David Geffen School of Medicine at UCLA, Santa Monica, California

Anthony F. Valdini, MD, MS
Clinical Professor of Family Medicine and Community Health, Lawrence Family Medicine and University of Massachusetts, School of Medicine, City Lawrence, Massachusetts

Leelasri Vanguru, MD
Research Assistant, Department of Family Medicine, University of Toledo, Toledo, Ohio

Kirsten Vitrikas, MD
Associate Program Director, St Louis University Family Medicine Residency, Belleville, Illinois

H. Bruce Vogt, MD, FAAFP
Professor and Chair, Department of Family Medicine, Sanford School of Medicine, University of South Dakota, Program Director, South Dakota Area Health Education Center, Sioux Falls, South Dakota

Cynthia M. Waickus, MD, PhD
Associate Chair for Educational Programs, Director of Predoctoral Education, Department of Family Medicine, Rush Medical College, Chicago, Illinois

Linda L. Walker, MD, FAAFP
Associate Director, Family Medicine Program, The Medical Center, Columbus Georgia

Paul C. Walker, PharmD, FASHP
Clinical Professor, University of Michigan College of Pharmacy, Ann Arbor, Michigan

Jie Wang, MD
Clinical Assistant Professor, Department of Family Medicine, University of Wisconsin—Madison, Madison, Wisconsin

Kristen Hood Watson, MD
Chief Resident, Trident/Medical University of South Carolina, Department of Family Medicine, Charleston, South Carolina

Lara Carson Weinstein, MD, MPH
Assistant Professor, Department of Family and Community Medicine, Thomas Jefferson University, Philadelphia, Pennsylvania

Barry D. Weiss, MD
Professor of Family and Community Medicine, University of Arizona College of Medicine, Tucson, Arizona

Trisha D. Wells, PharmD
Clinical Assistant Professor, University of Michigan College of Pharmacy, Ann Arbor, Michigan

Angela R. Wetherton, MD
Assistant Professor, Department of Family and Geriatric Medicine, University of Louisville, Louisville, Kentucky

LeRoy C. White, MD, JD
Family Medicine—Enid, Oklahoma University Health Sciences Center, Oklahoma City, Oklahoma

Lesley D. Wilkinson, MD
Associate Clinical Professor, Family Medicine, David Geffen School of Medicine, at UCLA Los Angeles, California

George R. Wilson, MD,
Adjunct Professor, Senior Associate Dean for Clinical Affairs, University of Florida College of Medicine/ Jacksonville, Jacksonville, Florida

Deborah K. Witt, MD
Assistant Professor, Department of Family and Community Medicine, Jefferson Medical College, Thomas Jefferson University, Philadelphia, Pennsylvania

Aylin Yaman, MD
Specialist of Neurology, Deputy Chief Physician, MoH Antalya Education and Research Hospital, Antalya, Turkey

Hakan Yaman, MD, MS
Family Medicine, Professor, Akdeniz University Faculty of Medicine, Department of Family Medicine, Antalya, Turkey

Aleksandra Zgierska, MD, PhD
Clinical Instructor, Department of Family Medicine, University of Wisconsin School of Medicine and Public Health, Madison, Wisconsin

PURPOSE

This manual presents information on the most common complaints, problems, conditions, and diseases encountered by family medicine clinicians and other primary care providers who practice in the ambulatory settings. These common conditions, which have been selected from surveys taken from family medicine, internal medicine, and pediatrics, are arranged alphabetically in five sections. Evidence-based information and algorithms on diagnosis and treatment, including strength of recommendation ratings, is presented in such a way that busy clinicians can access information rapidly. Practical, specific treatment information, including medication dosing, side effects, and important drug interactions, is offered.

ORGANIZATION SCOPE

Although most medical books are organized by organ system, we have structured this manual according to typical patient presentations in primary care settings of common symptoms and signs (e.g., arm and shoulder complaints, chest pain, fatigue, or syncope), follow-up needs for chronic physical or mental illness, and reproductive health concerns. In addition, we provide information on screening and preventive healthcare recommendations.

New chapters in this edition are Deep Vein Thrombosis and Pulmonary Embolus (this replaces the Edema Chapter); Cancers of the Breast, Lung, and Colon; and Sexually Transmitted Infections.

Section I contains information on the most commonly encountered acute/undifferentiated problems in the primary care setting. Information is presented in such a way that a clinician can quickly form a list of diagnostic possibilities, perform a cost-effective evidence-based diagnostic workup, prescribe evidence-based treatment for the most common causes of these problems, and provide patients with patient education including preventive strategies.

Section II offers information on the treatment of patients with common chronic illnesses. Each chapter provides practical follow-up strategies for such patients, integrating cost-effective evidence-based clinical management with important psychosocial issues.

Section III is particularly important because many patients seen in the primary care settings have either a primary psychiatric disorder or a psychiatric disorder complicating the management of pre-existing medical conditions. Strategies that effectively identify and treat patients with psychiatric disorders are presented clearly and succinctly.

Section IV addresses common reproductive woman's health issues that present in the primary care setting including contraception, infertility, and prenatal and postnatal care.

Section V will assist primary care clinicians in the screening and prevention of important diseases in their patients. Authors of these chapters recommend interventions that can be easily applied in primary care practices including counseling, immunizations, screening tests, and chemoprophylaxis. Chapters on travel medicine and the preoperative evaluation complete this section.

In all chapters, authors have integrated principles of clinical decision-making, evidence-based medicine, and cost-effective clinical management and have considered psychosocial and contextual issues; where applicable, areas of controversy are identified. Where appropriate, complementary and alternative medical interventions are discussed.

Other useful features of this manual include the following:

- A convenient outline format and selective use of boldface type to afford quick, easy access to key aspects of diagnosis and treatment.
- Updated clinical content including recently released guidelines such as the 5th edition of the Diagnostic and Statistical Manual of Mental Disorders and the 2013 American College of Cardiology/American Heart Association Guideline on Treatment of Blood Cholesterol to Reduce Atherosclerotic Cardiovascular Risk in Adults.

- Over 30 additional color plates of photographs, provided by Dr. Richard Usatine and others from the Color Atlas of Family Medicine, that enhance diagnostic ability and prove once again that "a picture is worth a thousand words."
- Comprehensive drug tables that present dosing for adults, children, and the elderly where appropriate; common side effects; and important drug interactions.
- Algorithms facilitating the diagnostic workup and common management strategies for specific conditions.
- Links to important web resources including YouTube videos of common procedures, decision-support tools, and patient education materials. In addition to key references provided within each chapter, online references are provided for some chapters to support more detailed clinical material presented.
- Emphasis on cost-effective evidence-based strategies, with strength of recommendation ratings clearly visible.
- Each chapter is introduced by key point section that summarizes main issues.
- Sidebars in some chapters highlight specific unusual or particularly serious conditions.
- Streamline organizational framework makes it easy to find sections on screening and prevention, diagnosis, symptoms and signs, evaluation, and management strategies.

STRENGTH OF RECOMMENDATION TAXONOMIES

For this 6th edition, we have continued to ask all authors to use the strength of recommendation taxonomy used by major family medicine journals. Recommendations are graded as A, B, or C based on the quality and quantity of evidence as shown in the table below.

Strength of Recommendation	Basis for Recommendation
A	Consistent or good quality of patient-oriented evidence.
B	Inconsistent or limited quality of patient-oriented evidence.
C	Consensus, disease-oriented evidence, usual practice, expert opinion, or case series.

Patient-oriented evidence measures outcomes that matter to patients, such as morbidity, mortality, symptom improvement, cost reduction, and quality of life. Disease-oriented evidence measures intermediate physiologic or surrogate endpoints that may or may not reflect improvement in patient outcomes.

ACKNOWLEDGMENTS

First, we thank those of you who have used this manual. As the new editors for this 6th edition, we have carefully considered the feedback from medical students, residents, and practitioners in updating this manual to keep this edition of Family Medicine the quick, practical reference text that readers have come to expect. We have added links to excellent web resources and provided more standardized algorithms and drug tables for easy reference.

Second, we thank our authors of this 6th edition. Their excellent work and willingness to create new algorithms and provide original tables and figures is what makes this manual so valuable to our readers.

Third, we thank the outstanding University of Michigan pharmacy students (Andrew Chang, Rebecca Goldsmith, Shawna Ivancic, Ilene Izquierdo, Amanda Martell, Hsiao-Lan Ng, Rachel Rarus, and Katherine Veltman) who, under the guidance of Dr. Leslie Shimp, spent countless hours updating and checking the extensive material included in the drug tables.

Fourth, we thank the editors and their staff at McGraw Hill for their encouragement and support.

Lastly, but far from least, Mindy would like to acknowledge and thank her late husband, Gary Crakes, who always had time to listen, offer suggestions on phrasing, and teach her important life lessons about living in the present and creating happiness.

Mindy A. Smith, MD, MS
Leslie A. Shimp, PharmD, MS
Sarina Schrager, MD, MS
Editors, 2013

SECTION I. Common Problems

1   Abdominal Pain

Kalyanakrishnan Ramakrishnan, MD, MS, FRCS

KEY POINTS

- Most patients presenting with abdominal pain have minor, nonsurgical causes. Nonspecific abdominal pain (NSAP) is most common and accounts for 90% of pain in children. Chronic abdominal pain is most often gastrointestinal (GI) in origin. (SOR **C**)
- Proper history taking and a stepwise physical examination enable a diagnosis to be made in most patients. Laboratory tests help focus the differential diagnosis and confirm clinical suspicion of a disease process. (SOR **C**)
- Any woman of childbearing age presenting with abdominal pain should have a pregnancy test. Management in pregnancy should focus on both mother and fetus. (SOR **C**)
- Presentation of abdominal pain in the elderly is modified by comorbid illness and medications. Classical history and physical findings may be absent. (SOR **C**)
- Providing pain relief should not await a definitive diagnosis, because unrelieved acute pain produces adverse consequences and there is no evidence that immediate pain relief delays diagnosis or influences recovery. (SOR **A**)

I. **Definition.** Abdominal pain is defined as a subjective feeling of discomfort in the abdomen. When the pain duration is less than 6 hours, it is referred to as acute. Abdominal pain may be caused by luminal obstruction (renal or ureteric colic, bowel obstruction, diverticulitis), an inflamed organ (appendicitis, cholecystitis, pancreatitis, hepatitis), ischemia (mesenteric ischemia, ischemic colitis), hollow viscus perforation, or bowel motility disorders/multifactorial causes (irritable bowel syndrome [IBS], nonspecific abdominal pain [NSAP]).

II. **Common Diagnoses.** Abdominal pain accounts for 2.5 million office visits and 8 million emergency-department visits every year in the United States. It is the most frequent cause for gastroenterology consultation. Most patients have minor problems such as dyspepsia, although 20% to 25% are found to have a more serious condition requiring hospitalization. Table 1–1 lists the common causes of acute abdominal pain in adults and the elderly. In children, urinary tract disease, peptic ulcer, inflammatory bowel disease (IBD; see Chapter 78), and gastroesophageal reflux disease may present acutely; constipation, lactose intolerance, mid-cycle pain, and psychological (secondary gain, sexual abuse, school phobia) causes of abdominal pain are more chronic. Figure 1–1 presents an approach to the patient with acute abdominal pain beginning with determination of hemodynamic instability and triaging those patients with sudden severe pain, suggestive of perforated ulcer, to surgery. Localizing features assist in the differential diagnosis of the conditions listed below.

    A. **NSAP.** NSAP occurs in approximately one-third (35%) of patients presenting with acute abdominal pain. More than 90% of children who have abdominal pain have NSAP.

    B. **Appendicitis.** Appendicitis occurs in 7% of the US population (3% of women and 2% of men older than 50 years), with an incidence of 1.1/1000 people per year. It is the most frequent surgical cause of abdominal pain in children presenting to the emergency room or outpatient clinics and the most common nonobstetric cause of surgical emergency during pregnancy; more common in the second trimester. Perforation rates are higher in patients younger than 18 years and older than 50 years.

    C. **Gallstones.** Approximately 10% to 20% of adults aged 20 to 50 years have gallstones; older age groups, Native Americans, and younger women (where it is 2–6 times more frequent than in men) are at increased risk. Other risk factors include pregnancy, hormone replacement therapy (relative risk approximately doubled), obesity, rapid weight loss, diabetes mellitus, hepatic cirrhosis, Crohn disease, and sedentary lifestyle.

    D. **Pancreatitis.** The annual incidence of acute pancreatitis in the United States is approximately 10 new cases per 100,000. The most common causes include cholelithiasis (40%), alcohol abuse (40%), drugs (steroids, azathioprine, estrogens, diuretics), trauma, abdominal surgery or invasive procedures (endoscopic retrograde

TABLE 1–1. SITE-SPECIFIC CAUSES OF ACUTE ABDOMINAL PAIN

Right Upper Quadrant	Epigastrium	Left Upper Quadrant
Duodenal ulcer	Gastroduodenal ulcer	Peptic ulcer disease
Biliary tract disease (biliary colic, cholecystitis)[a]	Pancreatitis[b]	Splenic infarction, spontaneous splenic rupture
Hepatitis, congestive hepatomegaly[a]	Biliary tract disease[b]	Pancreatitis[a]
Subphrenic abscess	Esophagitis, esophageal perforation	Pneumonia, pneumothorax
Pneumonia[a], pneumothorax	Acute coronary syndrome[a]	Subphrenic abscess
Nephrolithiasis, pyelonephritis	Pericarditis	Nephrolithiasis, pyelonephritis
Colitis	Dissecting or leaking abdominal aortic aneurysm[a]	
Right-sided diverticulitis		
Herpes Zoster[a]		
Right Lumbar	**Periumbilical**	**Left Lumbar**
Urolithiasis, pyelonephritis	Appendicitis	Urolithiasis, pyelonephritis
Right-sided diverticulitis	Small-bowel obstruction	Left-sided diverticulitis
	Dissecting/leaking abdominal aortic aneurysm[a]	Ischemic colitis[a]
	Mesenteric ischemia[a]	
	Gastroenteritis[b]	
	Hernia	
Right Iliac Fossa	**Hypogastrium**	**Left Iliac Fossa**
Appendicitis[b]	Cystitis, prostatitis	Diverticulitis[a]
Crohn disease	Urolithiasis	Ischemic colitis
Twisted ovarian cyst[b]	Diverticulitis[a]	Urolithiasis
Ectopic gestation	Pelvic inflammatory disease	Twisted ovarian cyst[b]
Pelvic inflammatory disease		Ectopic gestation
Urolithiasis		Pelvic inflammatory disease
Right-sided diverticulitis		Sigmoid volvulus[a]
Cecal volvulus[a]		Inguinal/femoral hernia[a]
Inguinal/femoral hernia[a]		Testicular torsion[b]
Testicular torsion[b]		
Intussusception[b]		

Source: Information from Flasar MH, Goldberg E. Acute abdominal pain. *Med Clin North Am* 2006;90:481–503; Ragsdale L, Southerland L. Acute abdominal pain in the older adult. *Emerg Med Clin N Am* 2011;29:429–448; Marin JR, Alpern ER. Abdominal pain in children. *Emerg Med Clin N Am* 2011;29:401–428; Cartwright SL, Knudson MP. Evaluation of acute abdominal pain in adults. *Am Fam Physician.* 2008;77:971–978.
[a]More common in the elderly.
[b]More common in children.

cholangiopancreatogram [ERCP]), viral infections, and hypercalcemia or hypertriglyceridemia. Chronic pancreatitis usually follows prior recurrent acute attacks of pancreatitis and is more common following alcohol abuse.

E. **Diverticular disease.** The prevalence of diverticular disease is age dependent, increasing in the United States from <5% at age 40 years to 65% by age 85 years; men and women are equally affected. Most cases (70%) are discovered incidentally, in 15% to 25% diverticulitis develops, and 5% to 15% bleed. Risk factors, besides age, include low fiber intake; increased consumption of red meat, fat, alcohol and caffeine; sedentary lifestyle; and obesity.

F. **Mesenteric vascular occlusion.** Risk factors for mesenteric vascular occlusion include older age (>60 years) and atherosclerosis (embolic events in 50% and thrombotic or low-flow state with associated vasoconstriction). Hypercoagulable states, intra-abdominal sepsis, portal hypertension, and cancer increase risk for **mesenteric vein thrombosis,** although in 5% to 10% of patients, the cause remains unknown. In the elderly, arteriosclerosis, shock, congestive heart failure, and aortoiliac surgery can cause **ischemic colitis;** in younger patients, oral contraceptive use, vasculitis, and hypercoagulable states are risk factors.

G. **Bowel obstruction.** Obstruction of the large or small bowel is a major health problem in the elderly, accounting for approximately 12% of cases of abdominal pain. Risk factors for small-bowel obstruction are adhesions resulting from prior abdominal surgery, neoplasms, or hernia. For large-bowel obstruction, risk factors include colon cancer, diverticulitis, ischemic colitis, and sigmoid volvulus.

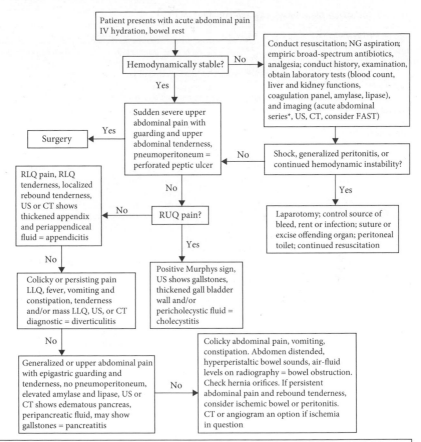

Abbreviations: IV = intravenous; NG = naso-gastric; RUQ = right upper quadrant; RLQ/LLQ = right/left lower quadrant; US = ultrasound; CT = computed axial tomography; FAST = focused abdominal sonographic technique
*Acute abdominal series=chest x-ray (erect), abdominal x-rays- erect and supine

Information from Millham FH. Acute abdominal pain. In: Feldman M, Friedman LS, Brandt LJ, eds. *Feldman, Sleisenger and Fordtran's Gastrointestinal and Liver Disease.* 9th ed. Philadelphia PA: Saunders; 2010:151–162.

FIGURE 1–1. Approach to the Patient with Acute Abdominal Pain.

    H. Hollow viscus perforation. Perforation may follow injury (trauma, surgery including endoscopy, contrast radiography), inflammation (colitis), bowel ischemia, bowel obstruction, cancer, sudden increases in intra-abdominal pressure (esophageal perforation) or after long-term administration of medications (potassium chloride, nonsteroidal anti-inflammatory drugs [NSAIDs]). Penetrating trauma accounts for most traumatic perforations.

    I. Other causes. Other common causes of abdominal pain not discussed here include dyspepsia (see Chapter 19), peptic ulcer disease (see Chapter 84), and pelvic inflammatory disease (see Chapter 50).

III. Symptoms. Proper history taking is the basis for making a correct diagnosis and should address a variety of features (Table 1–2). Prior history of peptic ulcer disease, biliary colic, or diverticulitis is helpful. Alcohol and drug use should be addressed. Alcohol abuse contributes to hepatitis, pancreatitis, hematemesis following esophageal varices or gastritis, esophageal rupture, and spontaneous bacterial peritonitis. Cocaine use may cause bowel ischemia. NSAIDs, prednisone, and immunosuppressants can cause bleeding and perforation; anticoagulants increase risk of bleeding. Medications, particularly in the elderly, can

TABLE 1–2. CORRELATION OF ABDOMINAL PAIN AND PATHOLOGY

Nature of Pain	Organ/Pathology
Acute or chronic (lasting weeks, months, years)	*Acute:* Biliary colic, renal colic, intestinal obstruction, perforated peptic ulcer, ruptured aneurysm, ruptured ectopic gestation *Chronic:* Peptic ulcer disease, chronic pancreatitis, diverticulosis
Onset of pain	*Sudden:* Sudden severe pain—perforated peptic ulcer, acute pancreatitis, ruptured aneurysm, ruptured ectopic gestation, renal/ureteric colic
Migration of pain	Appendicitis: Periumbilical, migrating to right iliac fossa Ureteric colic: From loin to groin
Referred pain	Biliary colic: Pain referred to the back and shoulder blades Pancreatitis: Referred to the back
Character of pain	*Burning pain:* Peptic ulcer *Colicky pain:* Biliary, renal, ureteric, intestinal colic (hollow organs) *Dull, continuous ache:* Solid organs (liver, spleen, kidneys)
Site of pain	*Epigastrium:* Stomach, liver, pancreas *Right hypochondrium:* Liver, biliary tree, hepatic flexure of colon *Left hypochondrium:* Spleen, tail of pancreas, splenic flexure of colon *Umbilicus:* Pancreas, transverse colon, small bowel *Right iliac fossa:* Appendix, cecum, ascending colon, terminal ileum, right fallopian tube and ovary, right ureter *Left iliac fossa:* Left fallopian tube and ovary, sigmoid colon, left ureter *Hypogastrium:* Urinary bladder, uterus *Back (renal angle):* Right/left kidney
Relieving factors	Antacids, food: Duodenal ulcer Sitting up, leaning forward: Pancreatitis Vomiting, antacids: Gastric ulcer
Associated symptoms	*Anorexia:* Gastric ulcer, appendicitis, peritonitis *Jaundice:* Biliary colic, cholecystitis, pancreatitis *Fever:* Appendicitis, cholecystitis *Vomiting:* Intestinal obstruction, pancreatitis, renal colic, ureteric colic, biliary colic, gastroenteritis *Hematemesis/melena:* Peptic ulcer disease *Diarrhea:* Gastroenteritis, colitis *Constipation:* Intestinal obstruction, appendicitis *Amenorrhea:* Pregnancy-related causes *Dysuria:* Urinary infection *Hematuria/smoky urine:* Renal/ureteric colic

induce nausea, vomiting, anorexia, and constipation and influence vital signs; in the elderly, atypical symptoms can also be misleading. Menstrual history is important in premenopausal women. Nausea, vomiting, constipation, urinary frequency, and pelvic or abdominal discomfort may all be experienced in normal pregnancy. Precise history taking in the elderly can be affected by cognitive impairment or decreased auditory and visual acuity.

A. NSAP and IBS. Pain may be colicky or persistent, and aggravated by meals. Most patients have a long history of recurrent abdominal pain relieved by defecation, a change in the frequency or consistency of the stool, abdominal bloating, and passage of excessive mucus (Manning criteria). Absence of abdominal pain can be used to rule out IBS. (SOR **G**) Weight loss, constitutional symptoms (fever, anorexia, nausea, arthralgia), or intestinal bleeding are uncommon.

B. Appendicitis. Anorexia and periumbilical pain followed by nausea, right lower quadrant (RLQ) pain, and vomiting occur in 50% of patients. Migration of pain has high sensitivity and specificity (approaching 80%). During pregnancy, the site of pain shifts progressively upward with increasing gestational age. Changes in bowel habits and hematuria/pyuria (pelvic appendicitis in 20%) can also be seen. Perforation results in generalized abdominal pain, fever, and tachycardia.

C. Cholelithiasis. More than 50% of patients with gallstones remain asymptomatic. Recurrent right upper quadrant or epigastric pain, radiating to the back or right shoulder blade, peaking over hours and resolving completely, suggests **biliary colic**. Upper abdominal pain in **cholecystitis** is severe, persistent, associated with constitutional symptoms and possibly jaundice. Perforation leading to **biliary peritonitis** causes spreading abdominal pain and worsening constitutional symptoms. **Stone in the common bile duct** may cause deepening jaundice, associated with fever, chills, and pain—**Charcot triad**. **Gallstone ileus** caused by migration of a gallstone into the small bowel following development of a cholecystenteric fistula presents with pain, distention, and vomiting—features of small-bowel obstruction.

D. **Pancreatitis.** Mid-epigastric or diffuse abdominal pain—relieved by bending forward; associated with gallstones, recent surgery, trauma, or invasive procedures; or occurring 1 to 3 days after a binge or cessation of drinking—suggests **pancreatitis**. Nausea, vomiting, restlessness, and agitation accompany the pain. Chronic pancreatitis causes pain, malabsorption, diarrhea (steatorrhea), weight loss, or diabetes mellitus.

E. **Diverticular disease.** Most diverticula are asymptomatic. **Diverticulitis** causes severe, abrupt, worsening left lower abdominal pain, fever, anorexia, nausea, vomiting, and constipation.

F. **Ischemic bowel disease** presents with severe localized or diffuse abdominal pain (out of proportion to physical findings), unexplained abdominal distention, or gastrointestinal (GI) bleeding (bloody diarrhea, hematemesis) indicating bowel infarction (SOR ●). Elderly individuals with chronic mesenteric ischemia **(intestinal angina)** experience recurrent upper abdominal cramps 10 to 15 minutes after meals gradually subsiding over 1 to 3 hours. Bloating, flatulence, episodic vomiting, constipation, or diarrhea and severe weight loss can occur. Steatorrhea develops in half of affected persons. A history of angina, claudication, or transient ischemic attacks may be present.

G. **Bowel obstruction.** Obstruction causes colicky pain, vomiting, abdominal distention, and constipation. In acute (small-bowel) obstruction, pain appears first followed by vomiting, distention, and constipation. In chronic (large-bowel) obstruction, constipation, followed by distention, pain, and vomiting, is seen (SOR ●).

H. **Hollow viscus perforation.** Abdominal pain worse on movement or increased intra-abdominal pressure, initially localized to the offending organ and then becoming generalized, is the hallmark of perforation (SOR ●). Nausea, vomiting, anorexia, fever, and abdominal distention can occur. Dysphagia is associated with esophageal injuries; jaundice with gallbladder perforations. Dizziness, weakness, and oliguria result from third spacing of large volumes of peritoneal fluid and resultant hypovolemia.

IV. **Signs** (Table 1–3). Clinical stability of the patient (pulse, respiration, blood pressure, oxygen saturation, level of consciousness) should be assessed initially (Figure 1–1). Shock, pallor, sweating, or syncope indicates serious intra-abdominal pathology. Rebound tenderness, guarding, and rigidity imply possible need for surgery. Operative scars suggest adhesions and bowel obstruction; umbilical, femoral, and inguinal sites should be checked for hernias. Rectal and vaginal examinations assess pelvic or rectal pathology. Guarding and rigidity may be absent during pregnancy, because of stretching of the abdominal wall, and the enlarging uterus preventing direct contact between the underlying inflamed organ and the parietal peritoneum. To distinguish uterine from extrauterine tenderness, pregnant women should be examined in the right or left lateral decubitus position.

A. In **NSAP,** bowel sounds may be increased; a fecal mass may palpated in either iliac fossa.

TABLE 1–3. PHYSICAL EXAMINATION IN ABDOMINAL PAIN

Inspection	Palpation	Percussion	Auscultation
Shape of the abdomen (scaphoid)	Guarding Rigidity	Tenderness Free fluid (ascites)	Bowel sounds
Whether all quadrants move equally with respiration	Of solid organs (liver, spleen, kidney, uterus, abdominal aorta, other palpable masses)	Organomegaly (liver, spleen, kidney, other masses)	Bruits (renal)
Engorged veins, visible abdominal pulsations, visible peristalsis	Testes, appendages (epididymis, spermatic cord)		
Hernial orifices (umbilical, inguinal, femoral)	Rectal/vaginal examination		
Scars of prior surgery			
Scrotum (testes, spermatic cord)			

B. Helpful findings in appendicitis include RLQ guarding or rigidity and tenderness, and rebound tenderness elicited on abdominal palpation or percussion. Nonspecific findings include a positive Rovsing sign (RLQ pain elicited by compression of the left iliac fossa—85%–95% specificity), Dunphy sign (RLQ pain elicited by coughing—95% sensitivity), positive iliopsoas sign (pain precipitated by extension of the ipsilateral hip), and a positive Cope obturator test (pain on internal rotation of the right hip). The triad of right lower abdominal pain, tenderness, and migration of pain from the umbilicus to the RLQ most likely suggests appendicitis. (SOR **Ⓐ**)

C. Cholecystitis is characterized by right upper quadrant tenderness worse on deep inspiration (Murphy sign – most reliable clinical indicator – 65% sensitivity), produced by the inflamed gallbladder coming in contact with the examiner's hand.

D. Patients with pancreatitis have epigastric or periumbilical guarding, abdominal distention, and ileus. Those with **hemorrhagic pancreatitis** can develop shock, and signs of retroperitoneal bleeding can be present as indicated by ecchymoses in the flanks (Grey Turner sign) or around the umbilicus (Cullen sign).

E. Localized peritonitis in diverticulitis can result in abdominal distention and ileus; rebound tenderness is sometimes elicited in the left iliac fossa.

F. Mesenteric ischemia produces few significant abdominal signs in the early stages. A systolic upper abdominal bruit is heard in half of patients with intestinal angina. Mild tenderness and guarding in the left flank or iliac fossa is usual in ischemic colitis.

G. Bowel obstruction produces abdominal distention with hyperperistaltic bowel sounds. Guarding and rigidity suggest strangulation, as do the features of sepsis or shock. Hernial orifices and scars can show a mass, suggesting an irreducible hernia. A tense and tender hernia with absent cough impulse indicates ischemic contents—bowel or omentum.

H. Hollow viscus perforation. Abdominal distention, guarding, rigidity, and rebound tenderness elicited on palpation and percussion are features of associated peritonitis. Bowel sounds are usually hypoactive or absent. Fever, tachycardia, tachypnea, and hypotension indicate sepsis and hypovolemia. The classic "Hippocratic Facies" of advanced peritonitis (drawn, pinched and pale face, sunken eyes, hollow cheeks and temples, and dry tongue) is rarely observed.

V. Laboratory Tests help focus the differential diagnosis and confirm clinical suspicion of a disease process. (SOR **Ⓖ**) The following approach relates to patients with **acute abdominal pain.** In **chronic abdominal pain,** testing must be individualized (Figure 1–2). In these patients, look for red flags (e.g., progressive pain awakening patient, fever, anorexia, dysphagia, vomiting, weight loss, dysuria or hematuria, anemia, abdominal mass, organomegaly, prior cancer) indicating a need to expedite a work-up.

ABDOMINAL WALL PAIN

Abdominal wall pain occurs in the young secondary to trauma, overexertion, or epigastric or incisional hernias. In the elderly, it may be secondary to herpes zoster and postherpetic neuralgia, or soft tissue tumors (neurofibroma). The pain often has an insidious onset, being sharp initially and becoming dull over time. Straining, as in sneezing, coughing, or lifting heavy objects, aggravates it; changing positions or applying heat may relieve it. A positive Carnett sign (tenderness reproduced by tensing the abdominal wall) may be present.

Useful measures include NSAIDs (e.g., oral ibuprofen 400–600 mg 3 times daily), muscle relaxants (e.g., cyclobenzaprine 10 mg 3 times daily, methocarbamol 1000 mg 4 times daily), antidepressants (e.g., amitriptyline), local application of ethyl chloride or capsaicin cream 0.025%, and trigger point injections of bupivacaine hydrochloride 0.35% plus triamcinolone 10 to 40 mg (most effective).

CHRONIC ABDOMINAL PAIN

Chronic pain implies persistent or intermittent pain for at least 6 months duration and impact on the patient's activities of daily living. Evaluation begins with ruling out GI causes. A blood count, sedimentation rate, chemistry panel, abdominal imaging (ultrasound, computed tomography) and upper and lower GI endoscopy rule out most serious causes. When the initial evaluation suggests the presence of a specific pathology, more specialized tests (e.g., endoscopic retrograde cholangiopancreatogram, angiography) can be considered.

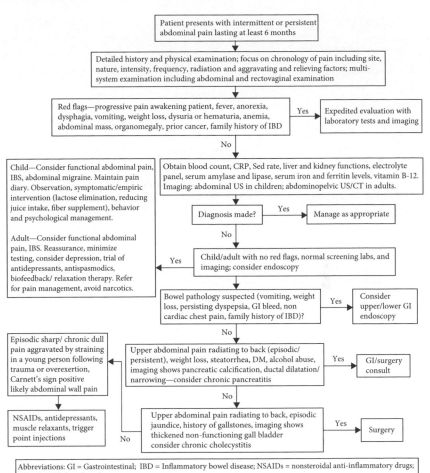

FIGURE 1-2. Approach to the Patient with Chronic Abdominal Pain.

In children, sonography of the abdomen and pelvis is usually performed first to exclude nonintestinal causes.

Optimal treatment incorporates acknowledging the reality of the pain, reassuring the patient that an underlying serious abnormality is unlikely to be missed, setting appropriate goals to minimize the impact of the pain on daily functioning, minimizing testing, and treating pain early using a multidisciplinary approach. Psychological evaluation and treatment, biofeedback and relaxation therapy, use of oral antidepressants (e.g., amitriptyline 25–50 mg at bedtime) as analgesic adjuncts, and referral to a pain management specialist may be indicated.

ABDOMINAL PAIN IN CHILDREN

Abdominal pain is one of the most common presenting symptoms in pediatric patients seeking emergency room care. History is obtained exclusively from the caregiver in preverbal children; older children contribute more. Adopting a soothing and calm approach helps elicit clinical findings from anxious and crying children. Menstrual and sexual histories are contributory in older children. Appendicitis followed by intussusceptions are the most common surgical emergencies. Nonsurgical causes (pneumonia, streptococcal tonsillitis [tonsil tummy], gastroenteritis, Henoch–Schönlein purpura, constipation) may also present acutely. **Recurrent abdominal pain syndrome** in children is vague, unrelated to meals, activity, or stool pattern, and does not awaken patients. An epigastric location is sometimes reported. Pallor, nausea, dizziness, headache, and fatigue can be present. Family history is often positive for functional bowel disorders. Indicators of serious disease in children include vomiting, localized pain away from midline, altered bowel habits, growth disturbance, nocturnal episodes, radiation of pain, incontinence, presence of systemic symptoms, and family history of peptic ulcer and IBD.

Response to empiric intervention (trial of lactose elimination, reduction of excessive juice intake, addition of a fiber supplement in constipation) and behavior and psychological management are helpful, as is educating the child and parents about diagnostic and treatment options. A symptom diary allows the child to play an active role in the diagnostic process. It is important for the child to maintain a normal routine, including school and extracurricular activities.

ABDOMINAL PAIN IN THE ELDERLY

Age-related pathophysiologic changes increase atypical presentations and prevalent dementia can make the elderly unreliable historians. Prior diabetes mellitus or abdominal surgery, NSAID, and anticoagulant or steroid use modify pain perception and immune response to infection and increase risk of bleeding, ulceration, and perforation. Many older patients present with spreading infection (peritonitis) and at a more advanced stage of inflammation, requiring more resuscitation and surgery. Pancreatitis is the most common nonsurgical cause. Increasing atherosclerosis and cardiac disease and medication use also increase risk of vascular catastrophes (ruptured aortic aneurysms, mesenteric arterial or venous occlusions, ischemic colitis, and rectus sheath hematomas). Cardiopulmonary (pneumonia, myocardial infarction), neuropathic (Herpes Zoster, nerve root irritation from osteoporotic spinal fractures or disc prolapse), metabolic derangements (diabetic ketoacidosis), and medications (antibiotics, oral hypoglycemic, NSAIDs, digoxin, colchicines, anti-depressants) can also cause abdominal pain in this age group. The anti-cholinergic action of many medications also predispose to functional large-bowel obstruction (Ogilvie syndrome). Malignancy (increasingly common) can also present with pain, bleeding, and perforation.

A. **Initial laboratory tests** in acute abdominal pain should include a complete blood count with differential, serum chemistries (electrolytes, serum glucose, liver and kidney function tests, amylase and lipase), urinalysis, coagulation panel in the elderly or if the drug history requires, and a pregnancy test in women of childbearing age. In children, investigations other than a complete blood count, urinalysis, urine culture, and stool Hemoccult are selected on the basis of clinical suspicion of specific pathology (sonography in pelvic pain or appendicitis, endoscopic evaluation with pain of GI origin suspected). Consider blood typing and cross-match before surgery or in patients with suspected bleeding. Blood cultures are considered in febrile patients. An electrocardiogram is often ordered in the elderly before surgery or if a cardiac source of pain is considered.

   1. **Blood count.** Anemia is a feature of bleeding peptic ulcers, ruptured aneurysm, IBD (along with raised sedimentation rate), and malignancies. Thrombocytopenia (platelets <50,000) may be seen in Henoch–Schönlein purpura in children. Leukocytosis (white cell count >12,000) is seen in appendicitis (sensitivity 91%, specificity 21%), cholecystitis (sensitivity 78%, specificity 11%), diverticulitis, and bowel ischemia. Leukocytosis is typical in the second and third trimesters of pregnancy and in early labor and hence less contributory in the diagnosis of abdominal pain during pregnancy; a normal white cell count does not rule out appendicitis (SOR **Ⓑ**).

   2. **Serum chemistry**

      a. Hypocalcemia and elevations in serum amylase (sensitivity 74%, specificity 50%) and lipase can be seen in pancreatitis. Amylase is elevated early (within 24 hours) in pancreatitis and lipase within a few days after symptom onset.

    b. Metabolic acidosis (in 50% of patients) and elevations of serum and peritoneal fluid amylase, alkaline phosphatase, and inorganic phosphate are seen in mesenteric ischemia.

    c. C-reactive protein can be elevated in appendicitis; normal levels in patients with symptoms lasting over 24 hours rules out appendicitis.

B. Radiologic tests

  1. X-rays in acute abdominal pain should include a flat plate and upright view of the abdomen, and an erect chest x-ray. X-rays have poor specificity (<15%), are of limited value, and in most instances do not change the clinical diagnosis. Cumulative radiation exposure adds to subsequent cancer risk and up to 2% of cancers may result from prior radiation exposure. Hence, imaging using ionizing radiation should be used only when necessary and techniques not entailing radiation should be used instead, when appropriate. Magnetic resonance imaging (MRI) has very little role in the initial evaluation of abdominal pain because of its expense, time commitment, and availability.

    a. Chest x-ray is useful in detecting pneumoperitoneum and cardiopulmonary pathology.

    b. Abdominal films also identify subdiaphragmatic or retroperitoneal gas associated with hollow viscus perforation, features of bowel obstruction (distended bowel, air-fluid levels), air in the biliary tree (gallstone ileus), calcium deposits (e.g., gallstones [10%–20% sensitivity], renal or ureteral stones, appendicolith, calcification in chronic pancreatitis, aortic aneurysm), foreign bodies, and pneumatosis (i.e., air in the bowel wall suggesting possible ischemia).

  2. Ultrasound (US) detects gallstones (sensitivity 85%–90%), sludge, gallbladder wall thickening (>5 mm is diagnostic in cholecystitis), pericholecystic fluid (in cholecystitis), and intrahepatic or extrahepatic bile duct dilatation associated with biliary obstruction (SOR Ⓒ). Focused abdominal sonography for trauma (FAST) can be performed at the bedside, in the emergency room, or in hospitalized patients and can detect free intraperitoneal fluid (evidence of bleeding or peritonitis), necessitating immediate laparotomy.

    a. US can also identify pancreatitis, pseudocysts and tumors, ascites, chronic liver disease (e.g., fatty liver or cirrhosis), gynecologic abnormalities, renal or adrenal pathologic findings, and acute appendicitis (sensitivity 85%–90%, specificity 92%–96%).

    b. Abdominal US is also useful in children with chronic abdominal pain and abdominal and pelvic US can be considered during the work-up of chronic abdominal pain in adults (Figure 1–2).

    c. Duplex ultrasonography is highly specific (92%–100%) for mesenteric arterial stenosis or occlusion.

  3. Computerized tomography (CT) is the most sensitive study in evaluating patients with acute abdominal pain, particularly obese patients. It has high sensitivities (pancreatitis, 65%–100%; appendicitis, 96%–98%; pancreatic tumors, 95%; high-grade bowel obstruction, 86%–100%; diverticulitis, 99%). (SOR Ⓑ) CT detects smaller volumes of free air as compared with plain x-rays, can detect loculated air, and is the diagnostic modality of choice in intraperitoneal and retroperitoneal abscess, diverticulitis, and in determining the presence and extent of diverticula-related complications, such as fistulas or sinus tracts.

C. Radionuclide scanning

  1. In acute cholecystitis, the cystic duct is obstructed; a technetium-labeled hepatic iminodiacetic acid (HIDA) scan showing nonvisualization of the gallbladder is 95% accurate in diagnosing acute cholecystitis. Poor fractional excretion on a HIDA scan (<15%) is characteristic of biliary dyskinesia (SOR Ⓒ).

  2. Preferential uptake of sodium Tc-pertechnetate by ectopic gastric tissue in a Meckel diverticulum (sensitivity 85% and specificity 95% in children) enables diagnosis of pathology related to diverticula (diverticulitis, bleeding).

D. Miscellaneous tests

  1. Magnetic resonance angiography, with and without gadolinium, detects severe narrowing or occlusion of the celiac axis and superior mesenteric artery. **Mesenteric angiography** can show the presence and site of emboli and thrombi and mesenteric vasoconstriction as well as adequacy of the splanchnic circulation. The angiographic catheter also provides a route for administration of intra-arterial vasodilators or thrombolytic agents.

2. **Barium enema or colonoscopy** is diagnostic in IBD and ischemic colitis; outlining ulcerations, thickened bowel, pseudopolyps, and strictures. **Water-soluble contrast medium** (meglumine diatrizoate [Gastrografin]) is preferred if contrast enema is to be performed in diverticulitis; it shows the diverticula and leakage and can outline a fistulous tract. Upper and lower GI endoscopy is considered in patients with chronic abdominal pain when bowel pathology is suspected (Figure 1–2).

3. **Endoscopic retrograde cholangiopancreatogram** is diagnostic in chronic pancreatitis, shows associated pseudocysts and glandular and ductal pathology (strictures, calculi), and helps rule out malignancy.

VI. **Treatment.** Once the patient's condition is stabilized, the physician can obtain a detailed history, perform a clinical examination and investigations, and formulate a treatment plan. **Providing pain relief** should not await a definitive diagnosis, because unrelieved acute pain produces adverse consequences and there is no evidence that immediate pain relief delays diagnosis or treatment. Multiple randomized controlled trials have demonstrated conclusively that administering analgesics to patients with abdominal pain results in early symptom relief without influencing subsequent appropriate management or resulting in worsening outcomes. (SOR **A**)

A. **NSAP.** Watchful waiting with close follow-up is recommended because most patients have a benign, self-limited illness. Providing reassurance, having patients avoid foods that precipitate the pain, and prescribing oral antispasmodics such as dicyclomine hydrochloride (e.g., Bentyl), 20 mg 4 times daily, or propantheline bromide (e.g., Pro-Banthine), 15 mg before meals and at bedtime, are useful. Narcotic analgesics should be avoided.

B. **IBS.** Treatment is directed at reducing anxiety and stress, increasing dietary fiber with bulk agents such as oral psyllium (e.g., Metamucil), avoiding foods that exacerbate or trigger IBS, and using antispasmodics such as dicyclomine hydrochloride. Psychotherapy may be useful. In patients with diarrhea, oral loperamide hydrochloride (e.g., Imodium) 2 to 4 mg, or diphenoxylate hydrochloride with atropine (e.g., Lomotil), 10 to 20 mg 4 times a day, is useful. Frequent follow-up is needed until symptoms stabilize. Alosetron (Lotronex) 1 mg once or twice daily and tegaserod (Zelnorm) 6 mg twice daily are useful in diarrhea-predominant and constipation-predominant IBS, respectively, in women. (SOR **B**) Linaclotide, 145 to 290 µg daily, is another option for patients over age 18 years with constipation-associated IBS.

C. **Appendicitis.** If the diagnosis of acute appendicitis is clear from the history and physical examination, no further testing is needed and immediate surgery is warranted. (SOR **C**) Diagnostic scoring systems (Table 1–4) used to predict the likelihood of appendicitis offer sensitivity and specificity >90% and reduce rates of perforation and negative laparotomy by half. Appendectomy is the treatment of choice with early diagnosis, if an abscess develops, or in recurrent appendicitis. A laparoscopic approach is less traumatic and has fewer complications (bleeding, wound infection, intra-abdominal sepsis) than open appendectomy. Other treatment measures include analgesics, intravenous (IV) fluids, and antibiotics. If an appendicular mass (inflamed appendix walled off by omentum) is noticed, nonoperative treatment (bowel rest, analgesics, IV fluids, and antibiotics) is continued until symptoms improve and the mass resolves, as in most patients. Interval appendectomy need not be offered to patients responding to conservative measures as the risk of recurrent appendicitis is low.

TABLE 1–4. THE ALVARADO SCORING SYSTEM FOR LIKELIHOOD OF ACUTE APPENDICITIS

Features	Score
Migratory right iliac fossa pain	1
Nausea/vomiting	1
Anorexia	1
Right iliac fossa tenderness	2
Fever >37.3°C	1
Rebound tenderness in right iliac fossa	1
Leukocytosis >10,000/mm^3	2
Neutrophilic shift to the left >75%	1
Total score	**10**

Score <4 indicates no appendicitis, 5 or 6 indicates compatible with acute appendicitis, 7 or 8 indicates probable acute appendicitis, 9 or 10 indicates very probable acute appendicitis.

D. Biliary disease
   1. Most patients with **biliary colic** respond to oral analgesics (hydrocodone/acetaminophen 5–7.5/500 mg, e.g., Lortab, every 4–6 hours) and clear liquids for 2 to 3 days.
   2. **Cholecystitis** responds to IV hydration, bowel rest, and broad-spectrum IV antibiotics (e.g., cefotaxime 2 g 3 times daily) for 2 to 3 days. Laparoscopic cholecystectomy during acute cholecystitis is safe and equally effective as delayed cholecystectomy, shortens hospital stay, and enables early return to regular activities. (SOR **Ⓐ**) Patients with chronic cholecystitis should also be referred for surgery (Figure 1–2).
   3. Chemical dissolution of gallstones using ursodiol 600 mg daily given in divided doses is reserved for patients declining surgery or in whom it is contraindicated, and is successful in 55% of patients older than 12 months. An oral cholecystogram is performed initially to confirm normal gallbladder function, a prerequisite for dissolution.

E. Pancreatitis
   1. Most patients improve with bowel rest, IV hydration, and pain relief for 2 to 3 days. Morphine sulfate 5 to 10 mg IV every 3 hours can be used in both biliary tract infections and pancreatitis; recent studies do not link morphine with causing or aggravating pancreatitis or cholecystitis.
   2. Once pancreatitis resolves, biliary stones should be removed and cholecystectomy performed. Alcohol intake should be avoided.
   3. Local complications include abscess formation, pseudocyst, bowel necrosis, pancreatic ascites, and splenic vein thrombosis. Shock or respiratory or renal failure is more likely in hemorrhagic pancreatitis. Initial leukocytosis ($>16,000/mm^3$), hyperglycemia (>200 mg/dL), elevated liver enzymes (lactate dehydrogenase >350 IU/L, aspartate aminotransferase >250 IU/L), and age >55 years are associated with a poorer prognosis **(Ranson criteria)**.
   4. Large pseudocysts can require consultation for percutaneous or internal drainage. Medication intake (e.g., steroids, antidiabetic agents, azathioprine) often needs modification and metabolic abnormalities (e.g., hypercalcemia) should be corrected to avoid recurrence and development of chronicity.
   5. Pain management in **chronic pancreatitis** is difficult and can require long-term narcotics (despite the strong predilection in alcoholics for addiction) or celiac plexus block with phenol or alcohol under CT guidance. A GI or surgery consult can be helpful for these patients (Figure 1–2). Steatorrhea should be treated with fat restriction (20 g/day) and Viokase (3 tablets with meals). Diabetes mellitus, if the condition occurs, is treated (see Chapter 75).

F. Diverticulitis
   1. Mild cases respond to a 7- to 10-day course of oral ciprofloxacin, 500 mg twice daily, plus metronidazole (e.g., Flagyl) 250 mg 3 times a day.
   2. Patients with vomiting, sepsis, or peritonitis require hospitalization for bowel rest, IV hydration, and antibiotics. Laparotomy and bowel resection is indicated in bowel perforation or obstruction, fistula, suspected cancer, massive hematochezia, or failed medical treatment. Percutaneous drainage of localized abdominal or pelvic abscesses by a radiologist under US or CT guidance is feasible.

G. Ischemic bowel disease requires hospitalization; patient stabilization; nasogastric aspiration; broad-spectrum antibiotics; interventional radiologist consultation for selective mesenteric arterial catheterization; possible vasodilator or thrombolytic infusion; and possible surgical consultation for embolectomy, bowel resection, or revascularization. Surgical resection is indicated in ischemic colitis if abdominal findings, fever, and leukocytosis suggest deterioration, or if the patient has diarrhea or bleeding for more than 2 weeks.

H. Patients with **obstruction of the large or small bowel** require hospitalization for IV hydration, correction of fluid and electrolyte imbalance, bowel rest, decompression through nasogastric aspiration, and administration of enemas to induce evacuation. Small-bowel obstruction caused by adhesions and incomplete large-bowel obstructions respond to this treatment. Endoscopic decompression relieves a sigmoid volvulus. Surgical consultation is indicated in patients not responding to conservative treatment, guarding and rigidity indicating bowel ischemia, or irreducible hernia.

I. Treatment of patients with **hollow viscus perforation** involves initial in-hospital resuscitation with large-volume crystalloids; correction of fluid, electrolyte, and acid–base imbalance; bowel rest; nasogastric suction; and IV broad-spectrum antibiotics effective against gram-negative rods, anaerobes, and oral flora. Definitive management is usually surgical and most often involves a laparotomy and suturing of the perforation or removal of the inflamed organ (cholecystectomy, appendectomy, segmental colectomy) and peritoneal toilet followed by continued bowel rest and antibiotics until return of bowel function and resolution of the infection.

SELECTED REFERENCES

Jackson PG, Raiji M. Evaluation and management of intestinal obstruction. *Am Fam Physician*. 2011; 83(2):159–165.

Marin JR, Alpern ER. Abdominal pain in children. *Emerg Med Clin North Am*. 2011;29(2):401–427.

McNamara R, Dean AJ. Approach to acute abdominal pain. *Emerg Med Clin North Am*. 2011; 29(2):159–173.

Millham FH. Acute abdominal pain. In: Feldman M, Friedman LS, Brandt LJ, eds. *Sleisenger and Fordtran's Gastrointestinal and Liver Disease*. 9th ed. Philadelphia, PA: Saunders Elsevier; 2010:151–162.

Panebianco NL, Jahnes K, Mills AM. Imaging and laboratory testing in acute abdominal pain. *Emerg Med Clin North Am*. 2011;29(2):175–193.

Ragsdale L, Southerland L. Acute abdominal pain in the older adult. *Emerg Med Clin N Am*. 2011; 29(2):429–448.

Wilkins T, Pepitone C, Alex B, Schade RR. Diagnosis and management of IBS in adults. *Am Fam Physician*. 2012;86(5):419–426.

---

2 The Abnormal Pap Smear

Kathryn Reilly, MD, & Audra Fox, MD

KEY POINTS

- Human papilloma virus (HPV) infection causes most abnormal Pap smears and virtually all cervical dysplasias. (SOR **C**)
- Many abnormal Pap smears resolve spontaneously as the underlying HPV infection clears. (SOR **B**)
- HPV testing is now widely available and can assist with decision making in many situations. (SOR **C**)

I. **Definition.** The Pap smear, a cytologic examination of exfoliated cervical and endocervical cells, was developed in the 1930s by Papanicolaou and is currently used as a screening tool for cervical neoplasia and carcinoma. Because of the increased use of Pap smear, deaths in the United States from cervical cancer fell 74% between 1955 and 1992; in 2010, approximately 12,200 new cases of cervical cancer were diagnosed and 4210 deaths from cervical cancer occurred.

Advances in our understanding of cervical disease, new reporting systems, and new diagnostic and treatment modalities make a systematic approach to the abnormal Pap smear very important. Recommendations for the frequency and method of the Pap smear can be found in Chapter 106.

    A. Several systems are used for reporting Pap smear results. The Bethesda system provides the most complete information and has been widely adopted; its classification scheme, updated in 2001, is used in this chapter. Equivalent classifications in the World Health Organization and cervical intraepithelial neoplasia (CIN) systems are provided. Because the systems are not interchangeable, it is essential that clinicians become familiar with the system used by their particular laboratory.

    B. Human papilloma virus (HPV) is a small DNA virus that replicates in the nuclei of epithelial cells. Some HPV types, which are termed "high risk," can cause malignant transformation by incorporation into the host DNA in chronic infections. Infection with HPV can be subclinical or can cause condylomata (by "low-risk" subtypes such as 6 and 11) or other lesions on the vulva, vagina, or cervix. HPV infection is generally contracted by sexual contact with an infected partner, who may be asymptomatic, although infection from nongenital lesions may also occur.

1. HPV infection is extremely common. At least 50% of sexually active men and women become infected by age 50 years. Most of them will clear the infection over time. Persistent infection with high-risk subtypes, especially 16 and 18, has been linked to development of cervical cancer (OR as high as 45). However, a large majority of those with persistent infection with high-risk subtypes do not develop high-grade dysplasia.

2. Because young women are known to resolve HPV infections at a high rate and are at a very low risk for developing cervical cancer, the management of abnormal Pap smears differs in many cases from that of women aged 25 years and older.

3. In the case of women aged 30 years and older, co-testing for high-risk HPV will alter the management of many types of abnormal Pap smear reports.

II. Screening and Prevention

A. Pap smear screening recommendations are provided in Chapter 106. See section V.B.4 for information on HPV testing.

B. As with other sexually transmitted infections, the risk of acquiring HPV infection increases with the number and risk status of sexual partners and may be reduced by the use of barrier contraception (e.g., condoms) (see Chapters 97 and 102).

C. Routine HPV vaccination is recommended for all adolescents at age 11 or 12 years. Detailed information on prevention of HPV is provided in Chapter 105.

III. Common Diagnoses.

Many types of cervical and vaginal abnormalities can be detected by the Pap smear, including the following:

A. Atypical squamous cells (ASCs). These cells are further classified as those "of uncertain significance" (ASC-US) or those that "cannot exclude HSIL" (ASC-H). (HSIL refers to high-grade squamous intraepithelial lesion.) ASC can be caused by infection, including HPV infection, or can occur in the absence of infection; in many cases, ASC is caused by atrophic changes in the vaginal epithelium. Under the Bethesda system, up to 5% of Pap smears can be read as ASC.

B. Low-grade squamous intraepithelial lesions (LSILs, mild dysplasia, or CIN 1). These are generally caused by transient **HPV** infection. In adolescents, 90% of LSILs regressed after 3 years. Even when teens were infected with high-risk HPV subtypes, their rate of regression to normal was 81%; only 6% progressed to high-grade lesions. The regression rate in adult women is 50% to 80%.

C. HSILs. These include moderate and severe dysplasias (CIN 2 and 3) and carcinoma in situ (CIN 3). They represent chronic HPV infection and are more likely to progress to more severe dysplasia or cancer. Twenty-two percent of CIN 2 and 14% of CIN 3 will progress to carcinoma in situ or invasive cancer; 43% of untreated CIN 2 will regress as will 32% of untreated CIN 3.

D. Atypical glandular cells (AGCs). These may be caused by inflammation or neoplasia in the endocervix, in the endometrium, or rarely in the fallopian tubes or ovary. They can be characterized as endocervical, endometrial, or not otherwise specified.

E. Frank cervical carcinomas. These include squamous cell carcinomas and adenocarcinomas, as well as noncervical carcinomas, including endocervical and vaginal carcinomas. Cervical carcinomas are discussed in Section VI E; the other carcinomas are beyond the scope of this chapter.

F. Organisms, including **bacteria** (e.g., *Chlamydia* or *Gardnerella*), **fungi** (e.g., *Candida*), and **protozoa** (e.g., *Trichomonas*), can colonize or infect the vaginal or cervical epithelium. This may occur without altering the mucosa or the infectious agent may elicit an inflammatory response and resultant cellular changes. Chlamydia and Trichomonas infections are sexually transmitted and multiple sexually transmitted infections can coexist. Candida infections are probably caused by alterations in the usual vaginal flora and may be triggered by antibiotics, altered host defenses, or other poorly understood causes. Frequent or severe candida infections occur in women with human immunodeficiency virus (HIV) infection or diabetes mellitus. Bacterial vaginosis is also caused by altered flora, but the cause of the alteration is not clear; it is generally believed not to be transmitted sexually.

IV. Symptoms

A. ASCs and **inflammation** are usually asymptomatic unless associated with an infection (see Section III.F); bleeding, especially after intercourse, may occur. Upon examination, the cervix can appear normal or may show redness, erosions, or friability, especially with some infections.

B. LSILs are usually asymptomatic. The cervix may appear normal or may show redness, erosions, friability, or gross lesions. Acetic acid application (see Section V.B.1) can identify lesions that are not grossly visible.

C. HSILs are usually asymptomatic, but may be associated with bleeding; large lesions may cause vaginal discharge. The cervix may appear normal or may show redness, erosions, friability, or gross lesions. Acetic acid application (see Section V.B.1) may identify lesions that are not grossly visible.

D. AGCs may be asymptomatic or may have symptoms related to the underlying disease (e.g., irregular bleeding with endometrial neoplasia).

E. Carcinomas may be asymptomatic or may cause bleeding, especially with intercourse, or vaginal discharge. Metastatic disease may be associated with abdominal fullness, weight loss, or other symptoms related to the sites and nature of the metastases.

F. Infections may be asymptomatic or may be associated with vaginal discharge, odor, or itching. Signs may include vaginal or cervical discharge or inflammation.

V. Laboratory Tests

A. The **Pap smear** report should include the following information:

1. Specimen adequacy. An unsatisfactory smear occurs in 1% or less of reports. Unsatisfactory indicates that insufficient squamous cells are present in the sample. A report of "negative with absent or inadequate cellularity" indicates that there is adequate cellularity for interpretation but there are no endocervical or metaplastic cells present in the specimen.

2. The report should specify any **epithelial cell abnormalities** using the terminology of the particular reporting system. Other findings may include organisms or other evidence of infection, reactive cellular changes (e.g., inflammation), or endometrial cells.

3. The report may include **educational notes and suggestions** regarding treatment, follow-up, or both. This information may be helpful, but the clinician should determine the plans for the patient, depending on the situation and his/her own clinical judgment.

B. Additional tests

1. Acetic acid application. Applying 5% acetic acid solution to the cervix for 1 minute will cause many condylomata or dysplastic areas to turn white (acetowhite lesions). These lesions should be evaluated by colposcopy and biopsy (see Section V.B.3).

2. Biopsy. Prior to the widespread use of colposcopy, cervical biopsies of suspicious areas, or random biopsies of visually normal areas, were used to evaluate abnormal smears. With the availability of colposcopy, biopsy should be done only in conjunction with colposcopy.

3. Colposcopy, cervical examination under stereoscopic magnification by an experienced examiner, along with endometrial sampling and biopsy of abnormal areas is the definitive procedure for assessing Pap smear abnormalities.

4. HPV testing can be done to determine whether one of the types likely to cause malignancy is present. This technology is now widely available and is a useful option in the management of ASC-US (see Section VI.C). Reflex testing can be performed if the Pap result is ASC-US when liquid-based Pap testing is done. Alternatively, many laboratories will hold the sample for a short period, which would allow HPV testing to be ordered if the Pap smear is abnormal. A third option is to have the patient return for HPV testing when the Pap result is ASC-US and the Pap was performed using conventional slide technology.

a. HPV testing is recommended for co-testing of women between 30 and 64 years of age as the preferred method of evaluation because it allows extending the Pap screening interval to 5 years if both are normal. Co-testing also assists with decisions on management of women in this age range who have abnormalities in their Pap smear.

b. A positive HPV test indicates infection with one of the high-risk subtypes of HPV. Many laboratories will automatically subtest a positive HPV for subtypes 16 and 18, which are responsible for a vast majority of cervical pathology.

VI. Evaluation of Abnormal Cytology. Evaluation and treatment of abnormal Pap smears has changed since the release of the 2012 Updated Consensus Guidelines for the Management of Abnormal Cervical Cancer Screening Tests and Cancer Precursors which were compiled by the American Society for Colposcopy and Cervical Pathology in 2013. The recommendations below are adapted from that document and summarized in Table 2–1.

TABLE 2–1. RECOMMENDED MANAGEMENT OF ABNORMAL PAP SMEARS[a]

Women Aged 21–24 Yrs	
ASCUS and HPV reflex positive or unknown	Repeat cytology at 12 and 24 mo If ASC-US or worse at 24 mo—colposcopy If ASC-H, HSIL, AGC at any time—colposcopy If negative twice—routine screening
ASC-US and HPV reflex negative	Routine screening
LSIL	Repeat cytology at 12 and 24 mo If ASC-H, HSIL, AGC at any time—colposcopy If ASC-US or worse at 24 mo—colposcopy If negative twice—routine screening
HSIL, ASC-H	Colposcopy
AGC	Colposcopy for all **PLUS** endometrial biopsy if abnormal bleeding or chronic anovulation
Women Aged 25 Yrs or More	
ASC-US	Reflex HPV testing (preferred) If positive HPV—colposcopy If negative HPV—repeat co-testing at 3 yrs **OR** Repeat cytology at 1 yr (acceptable) If negative—cytology at 3 yrs If ASC or worse—colposcopy
LSIL	Positive HPV test or no HPV test—colposcopy Negative HPV test—co-testing in 1 yr If both negative—repeat co-testing in 3 yrs If either abnormal—colposcopy Immediate colposcopy acceptable but not required
HSIL, ASC-H	Colposcopy
AGC	Colposcopy and endometrial biopsy

[a]For more details, see www.asccp.org.

A. Unsatisfactory cytology. Repeat cytology in 2 to 4 months. If co-testing with HPV is positive, either repeat cytology or colposcopy is acceptable. If repeat cytology is again unsatisfactory, colposcopy should be done. (SOR **B**)

B. Negative cytology with absent or insufficient cellularity. For women aged 21 to 29 years, the routine screening interval should be maintained. For women aged 30 to 64 years with unknown HPV status, repeat testing is preferred; however, repeat cytology in 3 years is acceptable. For women aged 30 to 64 years, who have known negative HPV testing, continue on the routine screening interval of every 5 years. For women aged 30 to 64 years who are HPV positive, either repeat cytology and HPV testing in 1 year or perform genotyping for HPV subtypes 16 and 18. (SOR **B**)

C. ASC-US. For women aged 21 to 24 years, repeat cytology at 12 months is recommended unless reflex testing (which does not need to be done in this age group) is negative. If the repeat cytology is negative, ASC-US or LSIL, cytology is again repeated in 1 year. If the repeat cytology is negative, the woman returns to routine screening. If the second repeat test is not normal or if either repeated test shows ASC-H, AGC, or HSIL, the woman should have a colposcopy. (SOR **B**)

　　1. For women aged 25 years and older, reflex HPV testing is preferred if co-testing has not been done. For women with HPV negative ASC-US, repeat co-testing in 3 years is recommended. (SOR **B**)

　　2. If the HPV test is positive, colposcopy should be done in women aged 25 to 64 years with endocervical sampling performed if no lesions are seen (SOR **B**) or the colposcopy is inadequate (SOR **A**).

D. ASC-H. Colposcopy should be performed on women with ASC-H results.

E. LSIL. For women aged 21 to 24 years who have LSIL, repeat cytology at 12-month intervals is recommended. If the 12-month repeat test shows ASC-H or HSIL, colposcopy should be done. For those whose 12-month test shows ASC-US or LSIL, colposcopy is recommended if the 24-month test is ASC-US or worse. (SOR **B**) For those with two consecutive negative results, return to the routine screening interval is recommended.

1. Colposcopy is recommended for women aged 25 years and older with LSIL who have no HPV test or who have a positive HPV test on co-testing. (SOR **Ⓐ**) If co-testing shows negative HPV, repeat co-testing after 1 year is recommended but colposcopy can be done if desired. If co-testing after 1 year shows both cytology and HPV test negative, co-testing at 3 years should be done and if still negative, return to regular screening interval. (SOR **Ⓑ**)

F. **HSIL.** Colposcopy should be performed for HSIL in women of all ages. (SOR **Ⓒ**)

G. **AGC and cytologic adenocarcinoma in situ.** Colposcopy and endocervical sampling should be performed for AGC and AIC in women of all ages. (SOR **Ⓐ**) Endometrial biopsy should be performed in women over 35 years of age and in those under 35 years of age who have unexplained vaginal bleeding or chronic anovulation. (SOR **Ⓑ**)

1. If CIN 2 or worse lesion is not identified, co-testing at 1 and 2 years is recommended. If both co-tests are negative, a repeat co-test after 3 years is recommended. If any of these tests are positive, colposcopy should be done. (SOR **Ⓑ**)

H. **Carcinomas.** The treatment for carcinomas is generally surgical; referral to a physician experienced in gynecologic oncology is indicated.

I. Specific **vaginal infections,** with confirmation as clinically appropriate, should be treated as described in Chapters 30 and 63. If the infection is sexually transmitted, the patient's partner(s) should be treated to prevent re-infection (Chapter 102). If reactive cellular changes, inflammation, or both are noted, re-examination of the patient may be appropriate to rule out infection. Empiric therapy with topical or systemic antimicrobial agents is not recommended.

J. **Endometrial cells** may be found on a Pap smear taken during or shortly after menstruation, but if they are found in the second half of the menstrual cycle or in a postmenopausal woman, endometrial biopsy or other endometrial sampling should be considered.

K. **HIV.** Although more intense evaluation was previously recommended for immunosuppressed women, data review in 2006 eliminated these guidelines. Women who have HIV or other conditions that suppress the immune system and who have abnormalities on Pap smear should be evaluated as outlined above.

L. **Pregnancy.** The management of pregnant women with ASC-US and LSIL are identical to those for nonpregnant women, except that endocervical curettage should not be done (SOR **Ⓐ**) and it is acceptable to postpone colposcopy until 6 weeks postpartum. (SOR **Ⓒ**)

M. **Adolescents.** Infection with HPV occurs in most adolescents within the first few years of sexual activity. The majority of these infections are transient, resolving on their own within 2 years. Pap screening is not recommended for women under the age of 21 years. (SOR **Ⓐ**) If adolescents have been inadvertently screened, they should have further evaluation, if needed, based on recommendations mentioned above for those aged 21 to 24 years.

N. **Postmenopausal women.** Postmenopausal women should be managed in the same manner as all women aged 30 to 64 years. Women who are being considered for exiting from screening at 65 years of age who have ASC-US or LSIL lesion should have repeat testing for the next 1 to 2 years, with no further screening after two consecutive negative tests.

VII. **Postcolposcopy Treatment.** Follow-up evaluation and treatment after colposcopy should be based on the colposcopist's evaluation, the guidelines of ASCCP, and the patient's wishes for future fertility and are beyond the scope of this chapter.

SELECTED REFERENCES

American Society for Colposcopy and Cervical Pathology. Consensus guidelines for managing abnormal cervical screening tests and cervical cancer precursors. www.asccp.org. Accessed June 15, 2013.

Apgar BS. Management of cervical cytologic abnormalities. *Am Fam Physician.* 2004;70(10): 1905–1916.

Apgar BS, Kaufman AJ, Bettcher C, Parker-Featherstone E. Gynecologic procedures: colposcopy, treatment of cervical intraepithelial neoplasia, and endometrial assessment. *Am Fam Physician.* 2013; 87(12):836–843.

Massad LS, Einstein MH, Huh WK, et al. 2012 Updated consensus guidelines for the management of abnormal cervical cancer screening tests and cancer precursors. *J Lower Gen Tract Dis.* 2013; 17(5):S1–S27.

Moyer VA for the US Preventive Services Task Force. Screening for cervical cancer: U.S. Preventive Services Task Force recommendation statement. *Ann Intern Med.* 2012;156:880–891.

3   Amenorrhea

Amanda Kaufman, MD

KEY POINTS

* Consider menses a female vital sign; investigate amenorrhea when a normal adult woman has absence of menses for 3 months, there is no menses by age 15 years in an adolescent with normal sexual development, or no menses by age 13 years in an adolescent without normal sexual development. (SOR **C**)
* Always consider pregnancy first in a woman with amenorrhea. (SOR **C**)
* The history and physical characteristics nearly always points to the etiology, although careful laboratory evaluation can distinguish between diagnoses. (SOR **C**)
* Target therapy to avoid long-term consequences of low estrogen states, polycystic ovarian syndrome, and neoplasms. (SOR **C**)

I. **Definition. Amenorrhea** is defined by when investigation should proceed: the absence of menses for 3 months in a normal adult woman, no menses by age 15 years in an adolescent with normal sexual development, or no menses by age 13 years in an adolescent without normal sexual development. **Primary amenorrhea** refers to women who have never menstruated, while **secondary amenorrhea** refers to cessation of menses in a previously menstruating woman. Oligomenorrhea of less than nine cycles a year should also be evaluated. (SOR **C**) The ages defining primary amenorrhea have changed as the average ages for thelarche and menarche have decreased; the ages of 13 years and 15 years are two standard deviations above the current average ages for thelarche and menarche in North America.

Normal menstruation depends on integrated hypothalamic, pituitary, ovarian follicular and endometrial function, and a patent outflow tract. Any hormonal disruption or anatomic blockage will prevent normal menstruation.

II. **Common Diagnoses.** Amenorrhea not caused by pregnancy, lactation, or menopause occurs in 3% to 5% of women.

   A. **Primary amenorrhea**

   1. **Hypogonadotropic/hypothalamic amenorrhea.** Among those with primary amenorrhea, the most common cause is constitutional delay of growth and puberty, a condition associated with low absolute height but normal height velocity prior to puberty. These children experience delayed pubertal development, including sexual maturation, and a delayed adolescent growth spurt. Most children with constitutional growth delay experience a late growth spurt and achieve a normal or near-normal height; a minority do not and may not reach their target height.

      a. **Obesity.** Obese girls progress more slowly through puberty despite earlier onset. Relative hypothalamic–pituitary suppression in obesity can cause hypogonadotropic hypogonadism. The causes are under investigation. These women will show signs of insulin resistance without elevated luteinizing hormone (LH) and are less likely to show hyperandrogenemia.

      b. Heterozygous mutations responsible for Kallmann syndrome (idiopathic hypogonadotropic hypogonadism) have been found in those with hypothalamic amenorrhea (HA) showing variable expression in these genes which can cause primary or secondary amenorrhea.

      c. Women with coexisting HA and polycystic ovarian syndrome (PCOS, see below) are more likely to have a higher body mass index and hyperandrogenemia and are at increased risk for loss of bone density.

   2. **Genetic defects.** Turner syndrome (XO karyotype) can present with primary amenorrhea because of failure of ovarian development. These patients typically have short stature, delayed puberty, and amenorrhea. In some cases, however, with chromosomal mosaicism, the phenotype may not be typical, and sexual maturity can occur spontaneously. Five percent of women with primary amenorrhea are found to have androgen insensitivity, also called testicular feminization (46XY karyotype).

3. **Anatomic defects.** The outflow tract may be blocked from **an imperforate hymen, a transverse vaginal septum, or a stenotic cervix**. Among those with primary amenorrhea, 10% are found to have Müllerian agenesis, with absence or partial development of the uterus or the vagina. This diagnosis is difficult prior to puberty as the uterus can be quite small and difficult to image.

B. **Secondary amenorrhea.** Secondary amenorrhea is commonly caused by **psychosocial and physical stress** including excessive strenuous **exercise or eating disorders associated with calorie-deficit states and weight loss**. Anorexia is present in 5% of females and 10% to 20% of female athletes.

FEMALE ATHLETE TRIAD

The **female athlete triad consists** of amenorrhea, eating disorder, and osteoporosis. The prevalence of eating disorders and amenorrhea in athletes is reported as high as 62%. Aesthetic sports (gymnastics, figure skating, and ballet) and endurance sports (distance running) share an increased risk of the female athlete triad. Other risk factors include self-esteem focused on athletic pursuits solely, presence of stress fractures, and social isolation caused by intensive involvement in sports. The negative caloric state of not ingesting enough calories for the exercise performed causes LH suppression or disorganization of its pulsatile release and results in amenorrhea. Resolution focuses on correcting this deficit.

1. **PCOS** is the most common cause of **normogonadotropic amenorrhea,** an endocrinopathy affecting 5% to 7% of premenopausal women and associated with obesity in 75% of North American patients. Women with PCOS are more likely to present with oligomenorrhea (76%) than with amenorrhea (24%).
   a. Features of PCOS are common in adolescence and transitory in nature, leading to stricter criteria for diagnosis in this population to avoid undue psychological stress and worry over future fertility. Consensus opinion suggests reserving the diagnosis of PCOS for adolescents meeting all criteria of hyperandrogenism defined as hirsutism and hyperandrogenemia, chronic anovulation more than 2 years post menarche, and polycystic ovaries defined as greater volume than 10 mL.
   b. Although some obese women with amenorrhea have PCOS, obese women in general report more amenorrhea and infertility than normal-weight women.
2. **Hyperprolactinemia. Pregnancy and lactation** elevate prolactin causing GnRH suppression and are the most common cause of amenorrhea in women of childbearing age. **Medications** (Table 3–1), renal failure, **hypothyroidism,** or prolactin-secreting tumors can elevate prolactin. In women with hyperprolactinemia, the prevalence of a pituitary tumor is 50% to 60%. The likelihood of a pituitary tumor

TABLE 3–1. MEDICATION CAUSES OF HYPERPROLACTINEMIA

Psychotropic drugs	**Drugs that work on the gastrointestinal tract**
Benzodiazepines	H₂ blockers
Selective serotonin reuptake inhibitors (SSRIs)	**Cardiovascular drugs**
Tricyclic antidepressants	Atenolol
Phenothiazines	Verapamil
Buspirone	Reserpine
Monoamine oxidase (MAO) inhibitors	Methyldopa
Neurologic drugs	**Herbal preparations**
Sumatriptan	Fenugreek seed
Valproic acid	Fennel
Dihydroergotamine	Anise
Hormonal medications	**Illicit drugs**
Danazol	Amphetamines
Estrogen	Cannabis (marijuana)
Depo-Provera	
Oral contraceptives	

is unrelated to the level of prolactin. The poor correlation between tumor presence and prolactin level indicates that magnetic resonance imaging (MRI) should be performed whenever prolactin levels are persistently elevated. (SOR ❸)

3. **Hypergonadotropic amenorrhea. Menopause occurs before 45 years of age in 5% of women, and before 40 years of age in 1% of women.** In women aged less than 40 years, genetic causes can be fragile X premutation and other X-chromosome mutations. Autoimmune thyroiditis, type-1 diabetes, myasthenia gravis, and other autoimmune conditions are associated. Iatrogenic causes include surgery, chemotherapy, or radiation.

4. **Asherman syndrome** is occasionally seen postpartum or after curettage of the uterus causing intrauterine synechiae blocking menstrual flow.

5. **Chronic debilitating diseases,** such as type-1 diabetes, end-stage kidney disease, malignancy, and AIDS are uncommon causes. These stressors disrupt the GnRH pulse generator, leading to a hypoestrogenic state. Recent research in GnRH receptor mutations reveals wide variations in susceptibility to these stressors.

III. **Symptoms/Signs.** A careful history and examination are essential for narrowing the differential diagnosis and should include the following:

A. A detailed **menstrual and puberty history,** including dates of last menstrual period, age at menarche, pubic hair growth, and breast development. **Oligomenorrhea progressing gradually to amenorrhea** characterizes PCOS, hypogonadotropic, or hyperprolactinemic amenorrhea. Chronic anovulation is common in the 5 years post menarche with only 23% to 35% of cycles being ovulatory in the first year progressing to 63% to 65% of cycles in the fifth year.

B. Gynecologic and obstetric history, especially infections and procedures.

C. **Medication history** (Table 3–1) for medication-induced hyperprolactinemia. After discontinuation of oral contraceptives (OCs), amenorrhea may occur for up to 12 months. Duration of post-pill amenorrhea of greater than 6 months occurs in less than 1% of women. The fertility rate also returns to normal by 1 year after discontinuation of OCs.

D. Family history including menstrual history of mother and sisters and genetic conditions.

E. Dietary history, excessive activity level (some studies suggest amenorrhea risk if more than 7 hours weekly), and fluctuations in weight to screen for an eating disorder.

F. **Psychosocial stressors.** Women exposed to violence such as war (including military personnel) or domestic violence can develop amenorrhea.

G. **Symptoms of pregnancy** including missed menses, nausea, fatigue, and breast tenderness (see Chapter 99).

H. **Galactorrhea** (milky discharge from the breasts) indicating hyperprolactinemia.

I. **Hyperandrogenism** (acne, hirsutism) and infertility increase the likelihood of PCOS.

J. Symptoms of **hypoestrogenic state** such as hot flashes, vaginal dryness, or decreased libido which may indicate premature ovarian failure or menopause.

K. Any history of **brain injury** (trauma, tumor, tuberculosis, syphilis, meningitis, and sarcoidosis), **pelvic radiation, or autoimmune disease can affect central or ovarian hormone production.** HIV has been associated with amenorrhea, though recent guidelines note common causes such as pregnancy being far more common, and evaluation should proceed the same as for other women.

L. **Genital examination.**
1. In women with primary amenorrhea, 15% will have an abnormal examination. Absent pubic hair and inguinal masses (testes) are signs of androgen insensitivity. Imperforate hymen can appear on examination as a distended bluish membrane at the introitus in young women with cyclic abdominal or pelvic pain and secondary sexual characteristics. If the patient or parent declines an examination, a transabdominal ultrasound is useful to confirm the presence or absence of a uterus and ovaries. (SOR ❸)
2. **Atrophic vaginal changes** and **vaginal dryness** suggest a hypoestrogenic state. **Clitoromegaly** is suggestive of androgen excess as is temporal balding and deepening voice.
3. If cervical stenosis is suspected, gentle penetration can be attempted with a uterine sound. (SOR ❸) Further investigation requires referral for hysteroscopy.

M. **Breast examination.** Normal breast development requires estrogen. **Galactorrhea** indicates a **hyperprolactinemic** state.

N. Thyroid examination for masses, enlargement, or tenderness.

O. Obesity, **hirsutism,** acne, or acanthosis nigricans may be present in PCOS.

P. Signs of emotional distress (depression, agitation) or any severe chronic illness.

Q. Visual field defect or headaches suspicious of intracranial cause suggest pituitary adenoma.

R. Short stature, widely spaced nipples, and neck webbing characterize Turner syndrome.

S. Striae, buffalo hump, significant central obesity, easy bruising, hypertension, and proximal muscle weakness as signs of Cushing disease.

IV. Diagnostic Tests. The workup can be done in a stepwise fashion (Figure 3–1) to avoid unnecessary testing.

A. A **pregnancy test** is always indicated. (SOR **C**)

B. Thyroid-stimulating hormone (TSH) level. Only 4.2% of amenorrheic adult women in a recent study had an abnormal TSH level; however, given the ease of treatment and the impact of thyroid dysfunction on prolactin levels, testing is recommended. (SOR **B**) Morning samples are preferred as afternoon levels may be artificially low.

C. Serum prolactin level should be tested, because 7.5% of cases of amenorrhea are associated with hyperprolactinemia. (SOR **B**) In a Korean population with secondary amenorrhea, an elevated prolactin level was found in 5.5% of those aged 11 to 20 years and 13.8% of those aged 21 to 30 years. Macroprolactin, an inactive prolactin bound to IgG, can falsely elevate the prolactin level and should be tested in asymptomatic women.

D. Brain MRI should be performed for persistent hyperprolactinemia to evaluate for pituitary adenoma. (SOR **B**) If amenorrhea because of hypothalamic causes

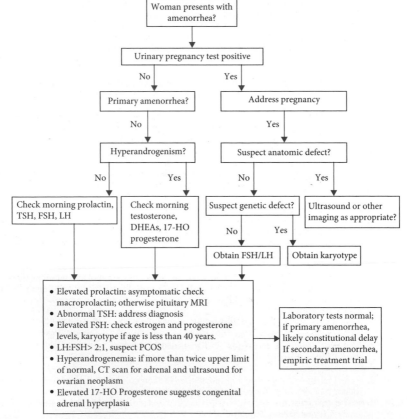

FIGURE 3–1. Suggested evaluation of women with amenorrhea. FSH, follicle-stimulating hormone; LH, luteinizing hormone; MRI, magnetic resonance imaging; PCOS, polycystic ovarian syndrome; TSH, thyroid-stimulating hormone.

persists despite long-term correction of stressors or calorie deficits, MRI should be considered to evaluate for possible hypothalamic or pituitary disease.

E. Gonadotropin levels. A follicle-stimulating hormone (FSH) level persistently greater than 40 mIU/mL suggests menopause. Because of the gravity of the diagnosis, experts recommend checking FSH level on initial evaluation. (SOR ❻) An LH level may be useful if PCOS is suspected, as the LH:FSH ratio can be >2:1. Anti-Müllerian hormone can be elevated in PCOS and will be low in premature ovarian failure.

F. Androgen testing (testosterone, androstenedione, dehydroepiandrosterone sulfate [DHEA-S], 17-hydroxyprogesterone) should be done in amenorrheic women with signs of androgen excess (virilization, hirsutism, acne). (SOR ❻) Samples should be drawn early morning as the levels will be higher at this time due to adrenocorticotropic hormone stimulation. If testing due to oligomenorrhea, testing in the early follicular phase is recommended. Testosterone levels >200 ng/dL and DHEA-S levels >700 ng/dL necessitate CT scan of the adrenals and ultrasound testing of the ovaries to rule out neoplasm. (SOR ❹) Elevated 17-hydroxyprogesterone can help diagnose adult-onset congenital adrenal hyperplasia. A testosterone level can differentiate between genital abnormalities caused by Müllerian agenesis (normal female range) or androgen insensitivity (normal male range or elevated).

G. Consider screening for diabetes mellitus in women suspected of having PCOS, even those with normal weight. (SOR ❸)

H. Karyotyping should be performed in women with menopause before 40 years of age or with stigmata of Turner syndrome. (SOR ❻)

I. Pelvic ultrasound should be performed for suspected structural abnormalities and considered in the diagnosis of PCOS in adolescents; however, 30% of asymptomatic women will have PCOS-like features on ultrasound and, due to decreased transmission via transabdominal scan, experts recommend use of a total ovarian volume of more than 10 cm^3 as a cut off for the diagnosis of PCOS in adolescents. (SOR ❻) PCOS-like findings in the setting of HA is not PCOS.

J. Referral for **hysteroscopy** may be needed to evaluate intrauterine defects.

K. Bone densitometry is indicated in any women with amenorrhea of >6 to 12 months duration. (SOR ❻)

L. The **progestin challenge** test is performed by giving medroxyprogesterone acetate (Provera), 10 mg daily for 7 to 10 days. Any bleeding during the week following the final dose is a positive test. Consensus opinion is that the test correlates poorly with estrogen status and imposes a 1-month delay in the diagnostic process. Up to 20% of women with oligomenorrhea or amenorrhea in whom estrogen is present have no withdrawal bleeding, and withdrawal bleeding occurs in up to 40% of women with amenorrhea caused by stress, weight loss, exercise, or hyperprolactinemia (where estrogen production is usually reduced) and in up to 50% of women with ovarian failure. This can be used when estrogen use is contraindicated, though otherwise the estrogen–progestin challenge test is preferred.

M. The **estrogen–progestin challenge test** is performed by giving estrogen (Estradiol 1 mg) for 21 to 25 days and a progestational agent (Provera 10 mg) for the final 5 to 7 days of estrogen therapy to stimulate withdrawal bleeding. If no bleeding occurs, an anatomic abnormality exists.

V. Treatment should be based on a firm diagnosis and attempt to resolve **underlying problems** while restoring menses, treating symptoms associated with estrogen deficiency, and addressing fertility when applicable.

A. Primary amenorrhea

    1. Hypogonadotropic/hypothalamic amenorrhea. In constitutional delay of growth and puberty, no treatment is necessary although careful measurements of growth every 6 months can be helpful to determine linear height velocity and to estimate final adult height.

        a. The psychological distress of appearing different than peers may warrant counseling or consideration of use of sex hormones to hasten the development of sex characteristics. Use of combined OCs is standard.

        b. It is not clear whether bone density monitoring is needed or not. Low-dose OCs have been shown to reduce serum bone turnover biomarkers but it is not clear whether this is clinically important or not. Low bone density is of a concern in patients with anorexia, but osteopenia normalizes with return to normal body weight. Consider measures to assist in achieving full bone density such as

weight-bearing activity, adequate dietary or supplemental calcium intake (600–1400 mg daily), and supplemental vitamin D as needed.
   c. If delayed puberty due to obesity is considered, diet and exercise counseling may be helpful.
2. **Genetic defects.** Referral to genetic counseling is essential for patients and their families to understand the scope of any genetic diagnosis. Many will need to undergo surgery to remove residual gonadal tissue as this tissue often carries a risk of malignancy. Typically, women with Turner syndrome and androgen insensitivity will need lifelong hormone therapy starting after the removal of gonadal tissue.
3. **Anatomic defects.** Suspected outflow tract obstructions will require a definitive procedure. In suspected Müllerian agenesis, exploratory laparotomy may be considered; if abnormal gonadal tissue is present, it should be removed. In these cases, hormone therapy will usually begin after surgery.

B. **Secondary amenorrhea**
   1. **Normogonadotropic amenorrhea** manifested as PCOS may require multifaceted therapy including the following:
      a. **Reduction of insulin resistance.** Insulin-sensitizing agents such as metformin have been shown to reduce hyperinsulinemia and restore ovulation. Oral metformin (up to 2550 mg daily) has been shown to enhance ovulation. (SOR **A**) Weight loss is recommended for obesity. (SOR **A**)
      b. Women with PCOS should be screened for diabetes mellitus with a fasting glucose. (SOR **B**)
      c. If pregnancy is desired, patients with PCOS are candidates for **induction of ovulation** with medications such as clomiphene citrate (Clomid).
      d. If pregnancy is not desired, therapy should be directed at **interruption of unopposed** estrogen and its effects. Use of OCs suppresses ovarian androgens and thus minimizes hirsutism, as well as providing a progestational agent to oppose estrogen and provide withdrawal bleeding.
      e. Spironolactone, an aldosterone antagonist, is an androgen blocker used for the **treatment of hirsutism**. Oral doses of 100 mg daily or twice daily are usually effective. (SOR **B**) Spironolactone works through a different mechanism than that of OCs, and, therefore, using these agents concomitantly improves their effectiveness. An OC containing progestin drospirenone is also an effective agent for the management of hirsutism.
   2. **Hyperprolactinemic amenorrhea**
      a. If medications, thyroid abnormality, or other etiology (e.g., exercise induced, tumor, chronic renal failure) is suspected, the underlying cause should be corrected and prolactin level repeated in 2 to 3 months.
      b. **Pituitary macroadenoma.** If a pituitary adenoma is identified, the goals of treatment are to suppress prolactin, decrease tumor size, prevent recurrence, and induce ovulation. In the absence of another organic condition, dopamine agonists are the preferred treatment of hyperprolactinemia with or without a pituitary tumor.
         (1) **Bromocriptine** is the drug most often used for the first-line therapy for hyperprolactinemia because it inhibits the secretion of prolactin, shrinks prolactinomas, eliminates galactorrhea, and reestablishes menses and fertility. (SOR **A**) Menses usually return 6 to 12 weeks after prolactin levels are normalized.
         (2) **Medroxyprogesterone acetate** (Provera), 10 mg per day taken for 10 days each month, is useful to induce menses if a woman does not desire fertility, does not have galactorrhea, or cannot tolerate bromocriptine. Provera does not affect prolactinoma size or prolactin levels.
         (3) In the past, treatment of pituitary adenoma was commonly **transsphenoidal resection.** However, recurrence of these tumors is common and therefore bromocriptine is the usual first-line therapy for both microadenomas and macroadenomas. (SOR **A**) Microadenomas grow slowly; prolactin levels should be monitored yearly and neuroimaging should be done every 2 to 3 years. (SOR **C**)
   3. **Hypogonadotropic/HA** is resolved when the stress causing the decreased GnRH secretion is lessened. Understanding the role of GnRH receptor mutations can be useful if an apparently less significant stressor causes amenorrhea.

      a. Dietary modification to reverse a calorie deficit and maintain at least 90% of ideal body weight is critical. (SOR **❸**) Eighty-six percent of women who maintain their ideal body weight will see resumption of menses within 6 months.

      b. To protect the patient from bone loss, **estrogen supplementation** with OCs should be provided until normal menstruation is established. (SOR **❹**) Several studies have found that OCs prevent further bone loss and improve spine bone density measurements but do not improve hip bone density measurements. Use of 20 μg ethinylestradiol pills is as effective as 35 μg pills. (SOR **❹**)

      c. Smoking should be discouraged and **adequate calcium intake** (1 g/day) and vitamin D (600 IU/day) encouraged to **prevent bone loss**. (SOR **❸**)

      d. Antiresorptive therapy (e.g., alendronate 70 mg orally weekly) should be initiated if osteoporosis is identified. (SOR **❹**) Bisphosphonates are all pregnancy category C drugs.

  C. Hypergonadotropic amenorrhea occurring prematurely has significant health implications with most current data showing increased cardiovascular risks. Estrogen has been recommended to prevent bone loss at least until the average age of menopause. (SOR **❹**) Vitamin D supplementation should be initiated for prevention of **osteoporosis**. (SOR **❸**) If a genetic abnormality is found, referral for genetic counseling should be considered. (SOR **❸**)

VI. Patient Education

  A. What is amenorrhea? Amenorrhea is the term used when a woman or an adolescent girl is not having menstrual periods. There are two types of amenorrhea. Primary amenorrhea: when a girl has not started having periods by age 15 (or without any signs of puberty by age 13). Secondary amenorrhea: when a girl or woman has been having periods but then stops having them for at least 3 months.

  B. Why does amenorrhea occur? Menstrual periods occur after puberty when various parts of the body release hormones in the correct way. A part of the brain releases a hormone that tells the pituitary gland to produce hormones called FSH and LH. The pituitary also secretes prolactin, which stimulates breast milk production after childbirth, and TSH, which regulates thyroid hormone production. Anything that blocks these hormones (such as pregnancy, breastfeeding, menopause, too much exercise, too little food) will cause amenorrhea. Hormonal birth control can also cause amenorrhea.

  C. What other symptoms are associated? There are many causes of amenorrhea, each with different other symptoms. Tell your health care provider if you have hot flashes, vaginal symptoms, milky discharge from your nipples, headaches, vision changes, acne, or abnormal hair growth. Nausea, feeling tired, and breast tenderness could be signs of pregnancy.

  D. What tests might I need? After talking to your health care provider and an examination, you will likely be tested for pregnancy. Other blood tests can measure different hormone levels to understand what part might not be functioning correctly. If early menopause is suspected, genetic causes might be considered and tested. If you have very high prolactin levels without other causes, a brain MRI will be useful.

  E. What treatments are available? The cause of the amenorrhea will determine which treatments are right for you. If you are underweight or overweight, keeping a healthy weight may correct amenorrhea. Medicines may need to be changed or may be useful to correct hormone levels. Vitamin D and calcium might be important to protect your bones.

  F. When should you consult your health care provider? If a girl has not had her period by age 15 years or shows no signs of puberty by age 13 years, she should consult a health care provider about primary amenorrhea. If you haven't had your period for more than 3 months, investigation into the causes of and then treatment of secondary amenorrhea is important.

SELECTED REFERENCES

Carmina E, Oberfield SE, Lobo RA. The diagnosis of polycystic ovary syndrome in adolescents. *Am J Obstet Gynecol.* 2010;203(3):201.e1–e5.

Caronia LM, Martin C, Welt CK, et al. A genetic basis for functional hypothalamic **amenorrhea**. *N Engl J Med.* 2011;364(3):215–225.

Committee opinion no. 502: primary ovarian insufficiency in the adolescent. *Obstet Gynecol.* 2011; 118(3):741–745.

Golden NH, Iglesias EA, Jacobson MS, et al. Alendronate for the treatment of osteopenia in anorexia nervosa: a randomized, double-blind, placebo-controlled trial. *J Clin Endocrinol Metab.* 2005;90(6): 3179–3185.

Lee DY, Oh YK, Yoon BK, Choi D. Prevalence of hyperprolactinemia in adolescents and young women with menstruation-related problems. *Am J Obstet Gynecol.* 2012;206(3):213.e1–e5.

New York State Department of Health. *Menstrual Disorders in HIV Infected Women.* New York, NY: New York State Department of Health; 2010, 5p.

Pehlivanov B, Mitkov M. Efficacy of an oral contraceptive containing drospirenone in the treatment of women with polycystic ovary syndrome. *Eur J Contracept Reprod Health Care.* 2007;12(1):30–35.

Poyrazoglu S, Gunoz H, Darendeliler F. Constitutional delay of growth and puberty: from presentation to final height. *J Pediatr Endocrinol Metab.* 2005;18:171–179.

Robin G, Gallo C, Catteau-Jonard S, et al. Polycystic Ovary-Like Abnormalities (PCO-L) in women with functional hypothalamic amenorrhea. *J Clin Endocrinol Metab.* 2012;97(11):4236–4243.

Santoro N. Update in hyper- and hypogonadotropic amenorrhea. *J Clin Endocrinol Metab.* 2011; 96(11):3281–3288.

Vescovi JD, VanHeest JL, De Souza MJ. Short-term response of bone turnover to low-dose oral contraceptives in exercising women with hypothalamic amenorrhea. *Contraception.* 2008;77(2):97–104.

---

4   Anemia

Andrew D. Jones, MD, MBA, & Cary L. Clarke, MD

KEY POINTS

- Anemia is not a normal state and a cause should always be sought; iron deficiency is the most common cause. (SOR **C**)
- Screening for anemia is recommended only in pregnant women. (SOR **A**)
- Ferritin is the best test to diagnose iron-deficiency anemia. (SOR **C**)
- For stable patients with acute blood loss anemia, a transfusion cut-off of 7 to 8 g/dL best balances benefits and harms. (SOR **A**)

I. **Definition.** Anemia is an abnormally low hemoglobin (Hb) or hematocrit (Hct) value compared with age-matched norms. In general, anemia is defined in adult men as Hb <13 g/dL and in adult women as Hb <12 g/dL. Anemia in pregnancy occurs at Hb <10 g/dL. Anemia in childhood occurs at Hb <10.5 g/dL. Hb is considered a better measure of anemia than Hct.

II. **Screening and Prevention**

   A. **Adults.** Screening for anemia is not recommended in non-pregnant adults. Screening for Hb products in the stool is a recommended strategy for detecting colorectal cancer (see Chapter 69). (SOR **A**)

   B. **Pregnant women.** The United States Preventive Services Task Force (USPSTF) recommends screening pregnant women for iron-deficiency anemia and prescribing iron therapy to those who are anemic. (SOR **B**)

   C. **Children**

      1. **Screening.** USPSTF does not recommend screening asymptomatic children aged 6 to 12 months for iron-deficiency anemia, but does recommend that children aged 6 to 12 months at an increased risk for iron deficiency be provided iron supplementation. Although there is no validated tool to evaluate infants for high risk of iron deficiency, risk factors include low socioeconomic status, Mexican American descent, history of prematurity or low birth weight (LBW), exposure to lead, and weaning to noniron-containing foods.

      2. **Prevention.** Iron-deficiency anemia in children is often caused by early initiation of cow's milk feedings. To prevent this, the American Academy of Pediatrics recommends: (1) supplementing exclusively or partially breast-feeding infants with iron after 4 months of age for 6 to 12 months, (2) using only iron-fortified formulas,

(3) avoiding cow's milk during the first year of life, and (4) eating iron-enriched cereals with the initiation of solid foods. High-risk infants (poor, black, Native American, Alaskan Native, immigrant from a developing country, preterm or LBW, or if the primary dietary intake is unfortified cow's milk) aged 6 to 12 months should be given routine iron supplementation. (SOR **B**)

III. **Common Diagnoses.** The prevalence of anemia is estimated to approach 25% of the world's population. The highest actual number of people diagnosed is the demographic segment of nonpregnant women. Preschool-aged children have the highest prevalence, and men are least commonly diagnosed.

Anemia can be thought of as a problem of red blood cell (RBC) production, destruction, or loss. Decreased red cell production occurs in conditions with deficiencies in substrate availability, as in malnutrition or malabsorption, or problems affecting bone marrow such as viral or chemical bone marrow suppression and malignancy of or infiltration into the marrow. Anemia from red cell destruction occurs either because of a defect within one or more components of the red cell structure itself, as is the case of both classes of thalassemia and glucose-6-phosphate dehydrogenase (G6PD) deficiency, or because of factors outside of the RBC such as overzealous cell segregation in the enlarged spleen, autoimmune destruction, and the traumatic encounter with a mechanical prosthetic heart valve. Red cell loss can be obvious, as in the patient who is bleeding from trauma or disordered clotting, or occult from a gastritis or gut malignancy.

A. **Disorders of red blood cell production**

1. **Iron deficiency** secondary to reduced iron intake is the most common cause of nutritional anemia worldwide. However, iron-deficiency anemia from nutritional deficiencies is uncommon in adults in developed countries because such deficiencies must occur for at least 5 years to produce iron-deficiency anemia in the presence of normal iron physiology. Newborn infants who are breast-fed or who are taking noniron-enriched formulas are an exception and can become iron deficient in the first year of life. Children aged 12 to 24 months can also become iron deficient as they transition from iron-fortified formula to cow's milk and solid foods. Malabsorption resulting from disease, resection of the small bowel, or partial gastric resection accounts for a small percentage of iron-deficiency anemia.

2. **Vitamin B$_{12}$ deficiency** causes anemia in 5% to 10% of elderly patients. Vitamin B$_{12}$ deficiency is often caused by malabsorption related to atrophic gastritis. Pernicious anemia (PA), or failure to absorb vitamin B$_{12}$ because of reduced production or secretion of intrinsic factor, occurs commonly; chronic use of histamine blockers or proton pump inhibitors and *Helicobacter pylori* gastritis can also play a role in development of PA. Other less common causes of vitamin B$_{12}$ malabsorption include small-bowel overgrowth, ileal malfunction, acidification of the small intestine, pancreatic disease, and certain drugs (e.g., metformin, p-aminosalicylic acid, neomycin, and potassium chloride). Vitamin B$_{12}$ deficiency increases the likelihood of subsequent development of gastric cancer or polyps, which is thought to be related to the gastritis associated with vitamin B$_{12}$ malabsorption. The only source of cobalamin is animal products; thus, strict vegetarians and vegans who eat no meat, eggs, or cheese for a number of years may develop a nutritional-deficiency state. Chronic alcoholics can also develop a nutritional deficiency of vitamin B$_{12}$.

3. **Folate deficiency** occurs because average dietary folic acid intake does not greatly exceed nutritional requirements, and body folate reserves are relatively small, depleting in 4 months. Deficiency thus occurs in patients who either do not consume or absorb enough folic acid or who have some condition that depletes their body reserves. Folate deficiency can be caused by decreased folate intake which can occur when the diet is deficient in fresh green vegetables, nuts, yeast, and liver. Decreased intake may occur in the elderly, in alcoholics, and because of loss of food folate through excessive cooking. Folate deficiency can also be caused by gastrointestinal (GI) conditions such as jejunal atrophy from celiac disease and drugs such as phenytoin or sulfasalazine. Folate antagonists include certain chemotherapeutic agents, antiviral drugs (e.g., azidothymidine [AZT] and zidovudine), folate antagonists (e.g., methotrexate), trimethoprim, nitrous oxide, primidone, and phenobarbital. Individuals on methotrexate should be supplemented with 1 mg of folic acid daily. Finally, increased demand for folate is caused by the increased nutritional demands of pregnancy and the increased requirements of chronic hemolytic anemia, and exfoliative psoriasis may deplete folic acid reserves.

4. Anemia of chronic disease (ACD) is present in up to 6% of adults hospitalized by family physicians and is caused by reduced ability to incorporate stored iron into Hb, despite adequate iron stores. It is most commonly associated with chronic kidney disease, cancer, chronic infections, and autoimmune disorders. ACD may also be exacerbated by features of the underlying disease including blood loss, hemolysis, malabsorption, malnutrition, or bone marrow replacement or suppression by infection or drugs.

5. Aplastic anemia occurs because of a marrow disturbance resulting in defective RBC synthesis. This may be caused by marrow infiltration by tumor or fibrosis; dose-related, idiosyncratic, or hypersensitivity effects of drugs (e.g., antithyroid medications, gold, chemotherapeutic agents, AZT, phenytoin); radiation; autoimmune suppression (e.g., with systemic lupus erythematosus); and infections such as tuberculosis, atypical mycobacterial infections, brucellosis, hepatitis A and B, and, rarely, mumps, rubella, infectious mononucleosis, influenza, human immunodeficiency virus, parvovirus, and fungal and parasitic infections.

6. Myelodysplastic syndromes (MDSs) are diagnosed in 1 to 10 per 100,000 people every year and are more common in elderly males. MDSs are stem-cell disorders resulting in abnormal hematopoietic precursors causing disturbances of RBCs, white blood cells, and platelets. Previous treatment with radiation or mutagenic chemicals may result in MDSs.

B. Disorders of red blood cell destruction

1. Sickle cell disease is inherited as an autosomal trait; it occurs in the heterozygous state as sickle trait in 8% to 10% of blacks in the United States. Sickle trait rarely occurs in Eastern Mediterranean people or people of Indian or Saudi Arabian ancestry. Sickle cell disease develops in persons who are homozygous for the sickle gene (*HbSS*) and affects approximately 2% of blacks in the United States. Other sickle syndromes, such as sickle β-thalassemia and sickle C disease, are uncommon in the United States.

2. Thalassemia is most common in Mediterranean and Asian populations. Sporadic cases of thalassemia are found among Africans and American blacks.

3. Hereditary elliptocytosis and spherocytosis are autosomal dominant disorders affecting approximately 200 to 300 million people worldwide, although these conditions are uncommon in the United States. These membrane defects cause intravascular hemolysis of RBCs.

4. G6PD deficiency is one of the most common disorders causing hemolysis worldwide, affecting 10% of black males in the United States. The gene for G6PD is carried on the X chromosome, and female carriers are rarely affected.

5. Pyruvate kinase deficiency is another common RBC enzyme deficiency. The intravascular hemolysis caused by these conditions is particularly worsened by illness, stress, and G6PD; large doses of salicylates should be avoided.

6. Autoimmune hemolytic anemia is rare and can occur idiopathically or secondary to other disorders such as systemic lupus erythematosus, chronic lymphocytic leukemia, non-Hodgkin lymphoma, Hodgkin disease, and cancer. Drugs such as methyldopa, penicillin, rifampin, sulfonamides, and quinidine can induce an immune hemolysis, clinically indistinguishable from immune hemolytic anemia. Autoimmune hemolytic anemia can have a dramatic clinical presentation. At times, anemia occurs rapidly and can be life threatening; patients can present with angina or congestive heart failure associated with jaundice developing over a 1- to 3-day period. Patients with thrombotic thrombocytopenic purpura, a type of autoimmune hemolytic anemia, can present with petechiae, fever, altered mental status, or focal neurologic findings.

C. Disorders of red blood cell loss

1. Acute blood loss. Acute hemorrhage is a potentially life-threatening cause of anemia and is essentially a problem of low circulating blood volume. Acute blood loss can present with minimal to no reduction in Hb/Hct, yet still be clinically significant. Acute hemorrhage can be asymptomatic or present with severe shock including fatigue, lightheadedness, or alteration in level of consciousness. Acute hemorrhage can also present as menorrhagia, melena, hematochezia, hematemesis, or hemoptysis. Acute hemorrhage is associated with orthostasis (positive tilt test) and is treated with hospitalization for fluid resuscitation, transfusion, and identification and management of underlying causes.

TABLE 4–1. FINDINGS IN COMMON ANEMIAS

Diagnosis	Abnormal Findings
Iron deficiency	Pica, esophageal webs (Plummer–Vinson syndrome), pallor of mucosa and nail beds, atrophic glossitis, angular stomatitis, cheilosis
Vitamin B$_{12}$ deficiency	Tongue burning/soreness, numbness/paresthesias, yellow skin, vitiligo, glossitis, hepatomegaly, splenomegaly, mental status changes
Hemolytic anemia	Fever, pain, jaundice, hepatomegaly, cardiomegaly, murmur
Folate deficiency	Malnourishment, diarrhea, glossitis, cheilosis; no neurologic abnormalities but mild mental status changes
Thalassemia	Bony deformities, growth failure, hepatosplenomegaly

    2. Chronic blood loss often causes iron-deficiency anemia. In young women, most cases are caused by menstrual blood loss and increased iron requirements of pregnancy. GI bleeding is another common source of blood loss; this is often due to the erosive effects of nonsteroidal anti-inflammatory drugs. In elderly patients, colonic carcinomas, diverticular disease, and vascular malformations are other major causes of GI bleeding. Rare causes of blood loss include chronic hemolysis, hemoptysis, and bleeding disorders.

IV. Symptoms and Signs. Clinical presentation can be as vague as fatigue, weakness, dyspnea on exertion, or syncope and palpitations. Acute blood loss is usually more dramatic in presentation with signs such as lethargy, tachycardia, coma, and end organ failure including myocardial infarction. Physical examination can reveal pallor, particularly evident in the mucous membranes, jaundice in the case of hemolytic anemia, or enlarged spleen. Some symptoms are more common in particular age groups and some syndromes have characteristic symptoms and signs (Table 4–1).

V. Diagnostic Tests. One approach to the diagnosis of anemia using Hb, mean corpuscular volume (MCV), RBC indices, and other tests is presented in Figures 4–1 and 4–2.

    A. Laboratory tests

        1. Complete blood count. This is the most useful initial test in the diagnosis and management of anemia. It quantifies the magnitude of anemia via Hb measurement, provides the MCV that is crucial in most diagnostic approaches to anemia, and allows for monitoring treatment. The MCV helps characterize anemia as microcytic (MCV <80 fL), normocytic (MCV 80–100 fL), or macrocytic (MCV >100 fL), which is the first step in narrowing the list of possible diagnoses. Most RBC indices are not particularly helpful but a normal RBC distribution width (RDW) effectively eliminates iron deficiency as a cause of microcytic anemia (Figure 4–1). Normocytic anemia is most often anemia of chronic disease or of iron deficiency. Vitamin B$_{12}$ and folate deficiencies cause macrocytic anemia.

        2. Ferritin. Low serum ferritin is an essential diagnostic criterion for iron-deficiency anemia; <30 ng/mL reflects deficient iron stores, low serum iron, and high iron-binding capacity. Microcytic and hypochromic peripheral RBCs occur later due to absent marrow iron stores. Values >100 ng/mL indicate adequate iron stores and a low likelihood of an iron-deficient state.

        3. Iron studies. Total iron-binding capacity (TIBC), serum iron level, and transferrin saturation can help confirm the diagnosis of iron-deficiency anemia when the ferritin level is equivocal (31–99 ng/mL). Typical findings in iron deficiency are increased TIBC, low serum iron, and low transferrin saturation. Conflicting findings on the iron panel are common in patients with ACD.

        4. Soluble transferrin receptor test and erythrocyte protoporphyrin test can be helpful when iron deficiency is suspected and both the ferritin and iron studies are equivocal. Both these tests will be elevated in cases of iron-deficiency anemia (Figure 4–2).

        5. Reticulocyte count assesses the response of the bone marrow to an anemic state. If the marrow is working properly, the reticulocyte count will be high as the marrow mounts a prompt response. The cardinal diagnostic feature of hemolytic anemia is significant reticulocytosis. It is also useful in monitoring therapy for anemia as the reticulocyte count should show response to effective treatment in as little as 2 weeks.

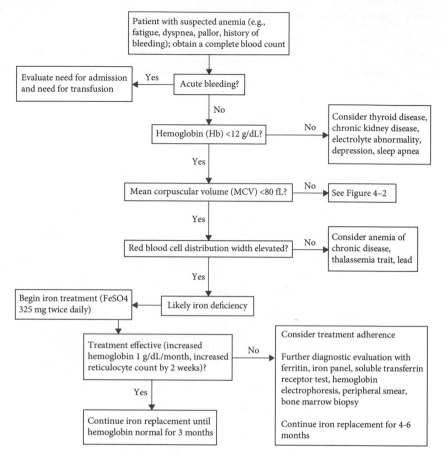

FIGURE 4–1. Approach to the patient with suspected anemia.

6. **Immunologic tests.** Immunohemolysis is diagnosed based on Coombs testing; a positive direct Coombs test indicates surface RBC antibodies and a positive indirect Coombs test indicates circulating RBC antibodies. Cold agglutinins will be found in patients with immune hemolysis caused by cold-reactive antibodies.

7. **Hemoglobin (Hb) electrophoresis** is used to diagnose sickle cell anemia (SCA) and sickle cell trait. In SCA, Hb electrophoresis shows RBCs containing 85% to 95% Hb S and, in homozygous S disease, no Hb A. Elevated levels of Hb A_2 on Hb electrophoresis and a positive family history of thalassemia are characteristic of sickle β-thalassemia.

8. **Peripheral blood smear** provides interesting but often nondiagnostic information. The peripheral smear in thalassemia shows hypochromia and microcytosis with basophilic stippling, potentially confusing these conditions with iron-deficiency anemia. Peripheral smears can be useful in cases of diagnostic uncertainty where hematology evaluation or bone marrow biopsy is under consideration.

9. **Vitamin B_{12}, folate, methylmalonic acid, and homocysteine.** These tests are critical in the evaluation of macrocytic anemia. If vitamin B_{12} and folate levels are not diagnostic, elevated methylmalonic acid can indicate a vitamin B_{12} deficiency and elevated homocysteine a folate deficiency.

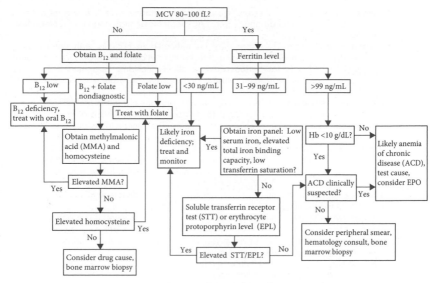

FIGURE 4–2. **Patients with anemia and MCV ≥80 fL.**

B. Invasive testing

1. **Bone marrow biopsy** is sometimes necessary to rule out MDSs and malignancy if levels of vitamin B_{12}, folate, and metabolites are normal, because these disorders can present with peripheral megaloblastosis. It can also diagnose iron deficiency when no other means are effective. Bone marrow biopsy is invasive but a crucial test and the gold standard in cases of diagnostic uncertainty.

2. **GI endoscopy.** Men and women older than 65 years with iron deficiency require GI endoscopy to screen for malignancy, as do men and nonmenstruating women younger than 65 years with unexplained iron deficiency. (SOR **☉**)

VI. Treatment. The treatment of anemia generally involves addressing the underlying etiology.

A. **Iron-deficiency anemia.** A trial of iron is a reasonable approach in children, adolescents, and women of reproductive age if the history, review of systems, and physical examination are negative.

1. **Iron preparations** such as ferrous sulfate, ferrous gluconate, ferrous fumarate, and polysaccharide–iron complexes (ferric polymaltose) can replenish iron deficiency. The usual dose is 120 mg of elemental iron daily (e.g., ferrous sulfate, 325 mg, twice daily). Reticulocytosis follows within a few days. An increase in the Hb of 1 g/dL should be expected every month with iron therapy. Once the Hb has corrected, therapy with iron should continue for 3 months to replenish iron stores. If a rise of 1 to 2 g of Hb is not seen within 4 weeks, the possibilities include iron malabsorption, bleeding, or an unknown lesion. Therapy should continue for 4 to 6 months to replenish iron stores.

2. **Prenatal vitamins with iron** are recommended during pregnancy. Supplemental iron therapy is recommended at Hb <11 g/dL in the first trimester and 10.5 g/dL in the third trimester.

3. **Iron deficiency in children.** In children, iron is replaced with once-daily dosing of 3 mg/kg per day of elemental iron for 3 months.

4. **GI side effects.** Cramping, nausea, constipation, and diarrhea can be side effects of iron therapy. Rinsing the mouth is suggested to prevent tooth staining from liquid preparations. To minimize GI side effects, iron therapy should begin with one tablet a day with meals, and the dose should be gradually increased. Ferrous gluconate, ferrous fumarate, and ferric polymaltose, while touted as less likely to cause GI side effects, have similar side effects when equal doses of elemental iron are used and are more expensive than ferrous sulfate.

5. **Nonresponse** to iron therapy is usually from nonadherence to treatment but may be caused by incorrect diagnosis (e.g., ACD or thalassemia), ongoing GI blood loss, or, rarely, poor absorption.

6. **Intravenous iron therapy** may be indicated in patients with inflammatory bowel disease, chronic bleeding, malabsorption, intolerance to oral iron, or renal-failure–induced anemia. Serious adverse effects including anaphylaxis and mild side effects such as headache, nausea, and diarrhea have been associated with IV iron therapy.

7. **RBC transfusion** is the most direct way to treat anemia but is problematic due to cost, inconvenience, and significant safety risks. There are limited data showing the superiority of transfusion over other treatments. The American Association of Blood Banks evidence-based guideline suggests a transfusion threshold of 7 to 8 g/dL.

B. **Vitamin B$_{12}$ deficiency.** Confirmed vitamin B$_{12}$ deficiency can be treated with oral, intramuscular, or intranasal forms of vitamin B$_{12}$. Oral administration with 2000 µg on day 1 and 1000 µg daily after that may be as effective as other treatment options. There is no conclusive evidence that replacement improves cognitive symptoms of vitamin B$_{12}$ deficiency. However, among women with low baseline dietary intake of B vitamins, replacement may significantly slow cognitive decline.

For patients with low vitamin B$_{12}$ intake, fortified breakfast cereals are one of the few plant-based sources for this vitamin. Exclusively breast-fed infants of women who are strict vegetarians/vegans can develop vitamin B$_{12}$ deficiency within months of birth that places them at risk for severe and permanent neurologic damage.

C. **Folate deficiency** is treated with oral folic acid, 1 mg per day. Folate-rich foods such as beef, spinach, asparagus, beans, and broccoli may be of use. Some cereals, rice, and breads are supplemented with folate.

D. **ACD/chronic kidney disease/chemotherapy.** There is no specific treatment except treating the underlying illness. Recombinant erythropoietin can be considered for all patients with anemia due to renal failure or for patients undergoing chemotherapy. IV iron and erythrocyte receptor activating agents can also play a role in managing patients with chronic kidney disease.

E. **Hemolytic processes**
1. **Sickle cell disease.** Patients with sickle cell disease should be immunized against *Streptococcus pneumoniae*, *Haemophilus influenzae*, and influenza according to Centers for Disease Control and Prevention. Infections should be treated early and aggressively. Antibiotic prophylaxis with penicillin should be given to children between the ages of 2 months and 5 years because of the high risk of pneumococcal infection. A typical regimen is oral penicillin, 125 mg twice daily until age 2 to 3 years, then 250 mg twice daily. Regular ophthalmologic examination is recommended.

The most common hemolytic condition requiring treatment is sickle cell crisis. Treatment of sickle cell crises consists of rest, hydration, and analgesia. Transfusions should be reserved for aplastic or hemolytic crisis and for patients in the third trimester of pregnancy. No treatment is required for patients with sickle trait. (SOR **C**)

F. **Acute blood loss** necessitates treatment with intravenous crystalloids to replete intravascular volume as well as transfusion of packed RBCs. In a stable nonbleeding patient, a transfusion cut-off of an Hb measurement of 7 to 8 g/dL or Hct of 21 mg/dL best balances benefits and harms of transfusion. (SOR **A**)

SELECTED REFERENCES

American Congress of Obstetricians and Gynecologists. ACOG Practice Bulletin No. 95; anemia in pregnancy. *Obstet Gynecol.* 2008;112(1):201–207.

Baker RD, Greer FR; The Committee on Nutrition. Diagnosis and prevention of iron deficiency and iron-deficiency anemia in infants and young children (0–3 years of age). *Pediatrics.* 2010;126: 1040.

Carson JL, Grossman BJ, Kleinman S, et al. Red blood cell transfusion: a clinical practice guideline from the AABB. *Ann Intern Med.* 2012;157(1):49–58.

Malouf R, Areosa Sastre A. Vitamin B12 for cognition. *Cochrane Database Syst Rev.* 2003;(3): CD004326.

National Institute of Health, National Heart Lung and Blood Institute, Division of Blood Diseases and Resources. The management of sickle cell disease. http://www.nhlbi.nih.gov/health/prof/blood/sickle/sc_mngt.pdf. Accessed January 29, 2013.

Office of Dietary Supplements. http://ods.od.nih.gov/factsheets/vitaminb12-HealthProfessional. Accessed February 28, 2013.

Short MW, Domagalski JE. Iron deficiency anemia: evaluation and management. *Am Fam Physician.* 2013;87(2):98–104.

United States Preventive Task Force. Screening for iron deficiency anemia in children and pregnant women and iron supplementation for children and pregnant women. www.ahrq.gov/clinic/pocket gd2012/gcp12s3.htm#anemia. Accessed January 28, 2013.

5   Ankle Injuries

Philip R. Palmer, MD, FAAFP

KEY POINTS

- Ankle sprains are among the most common injuries in sports and recreational activities. (SOR **C**)
- Progressive exercise programs and use of an ankle brace will help reduce the risk of an ankle sprain. (SOR **B**)
- The Ottawa Ankle Rules should be used to rule out fractures and make decisions about the need for x-rays. (SOR **A**)
- Other problems such as Achilles tendon rupture, fractures of the proximal fifth metatarsal, and navicular fractures can present as suspected ankle sprains. Careful history and examination with selected imaging can help differentiate them. (SOR **C**)

I. **Definition and Anatomy.** Ankle injuries are very common among active individuals, though evaluating pain about the ankle can be a challenging undertaking. To develop a proper differential diagnosis, it is important to have an understanding of the major bones, ligaments, and tendons comprising and surrounding the ankle joint (Figures 5–1 and 5–2).

   A. **Basic anatomy.** Range of motion occurs primarily in one plane—plantar flexion and dorsiflexion. Dorsiflexion is somewhat restricted as a result of the anterior widening of the talar dome. There is minimal inversion and eversion at the true ankle joint with most of this motion occurring at the subtalar joint. The subtalar joint of the foot allows for the full range of inversion, eversion, supination, and pronation. The medial malleolus (distal tibia) and the longer lateral malleolus (distal fibula) provide a significant amount of bony stability to the ankle joint through their downward extension along the talar dome.

   Ligaments provide medial and lateral stability (resisting eversion and inversion). The tibiofibular ligament and syndesmosis, which run between the tibia and fibula, maintain mortise stability; a variety of tendons traversing the joint serve as secondary stabilizers.

   B. **Ankle injuries** involve trauma to the bony or soft tissue structures of the ankle. Sprains involve tears to the ligaments whereas **strains** involve tears of the muscle–tendon unit. **Contusions** are bruises; **tenosynovitis** is the inflammation of the tendon and its sheath. **Fractures** are disruptions of the bony anatomy.

II. **Prevention of Sprains**

   a. Functional drills, proprioceptive training, and strengthening of the ankle all play a role in reducing the occurrence or reoccurrence of an ankle sprain. Attention to the peroneal muscles (evertors) is one of the keys to preventing a lateral ankle sprain. Progressive exercise programs, especially when proprioceptive training is incorporated, will help reduce the risk of an ankle sprain. (SOR **B**)

   b. The use of a semirigid ankle brace during high-risk sports will reduce the risk of a recurrent sprain in a previously injured ankle. (SOR **A**) There is also some evidence that the use of braces will reduce the risk of a sprain in uninjured ankles as well. (SOR **B**)

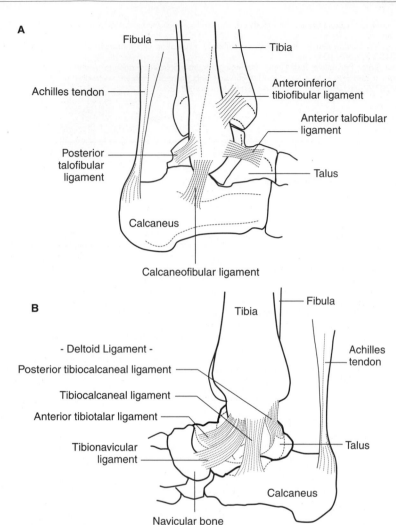

FIGURE 5-1. **Ankle ligaments: A. lateral views; B. medial views.**

III. Common Diagnoses. Ankle injuries represent approximately 20% of all sports injuries.
  A. Sprains (85% of all ankle injuries) are particularly common in individuals who participate in basketball, volleyball, ice-skating, or soccer. Most ankle sprains involve the ligaments of the lateral compartment. Less than 10% of ankle sprains involve the medial compartment, and this is usually a more serious injury than a lateral sprain.
  B. Strains (5% of all ankle injuries) are common in persons who engage in ballistic activities, such as track and field events. These injuries can also result from overuse of the muscle–tendon unit, particularly in endurance running, dancing, or gymnastics.
  C. Tenosynovitis (5% of all ankle injuries) most often occurs in individuals who are running, jumping, or dancing. This condition results from either a direct blow to the tendon or overuse with repetitive overloads and faulty technique.

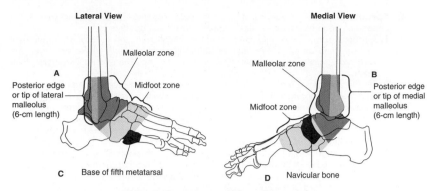

FIGURE 5–2. The Ottawa Ankle and Foot Rules.

D. Fractures (<5% of all ankle injuries) are more common than sprains in prepubertal children because the ligamentous structures are typically stronger than the bones, especially at the growth plates. Fractures occur most frequently in persons who engage in high-velocity, high-impact sports (e.g., football, soccer, skiing, hockey, and skateboarding).

　　1. Stress fractures occur most frequently in running, gymnastics, or dancing.

　　2. Salter–Harris type I and II fractures of the distal fibula are the most common ankle injuries in children. (For discussion of the Salter–Harris classification, see Chapter 28.)

E. Contusions (<5% of all ankle injuries) involving the ankle are significantly underreported and often occur in persons who participate in contact sports. Such injuries may also result from faulty footwear and poor field conditions. Contusions are primarily a diagnosis of exclusion and will not be discussed further.

IV. Symptoms and Signs. An approach to the patient with ankle pain is shown in Figure 5–3. With acute symptom onset, consider fracture and apply the Ottawa Ankle and Foot Rules (see V.A.) to determine the need for x-rays.

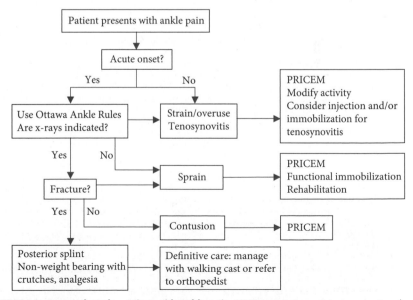

FIGURE 5–3. Approach to the patient with ankle pain. PRICEM: protection, rest, ice, compression, elevation, medications.

A. Sprains present with varying degrees of pain, swelling, disability, and joint laxity depending upon how severely the ligaments have been damaged.

   1. Grade 1 sprains are mild injuries with minimal pain and usually no impairment of weight bearing. These injuries manifest with minimal tenderness over the involved ligament and present with minimal swelling. There is no associated joint laxity.

   2. Grade 2 sprains are a more significant injury. Individuals experience moderate pain, and weight bearing will be impaired causing them to walk with a limp. There is moderate tenderness and swelling, and swelling may extend beyond the area of the injured ligaments. Ecchymosis may be present and joint laxity will be demonstrated with anterior drawer testing, which involves drawing the calcaneus and talus anteriorly while stabilizing the tibia (http://www.youtube.com/watch?v=zjauu5gXF2A). Movement of 3 to 14 mm indicates grade 2 sprain. Talar tilt testing (stressing the lateral ankle by stabilizing the subtalar joint and inverting the foot) will show 5 to 10 degrees greater motion in the injured versus the unaffected ankle (http://www.youtube.com/watch?v=2qF_DOe2jPE).

   3. Grade 3 sprains are the most significant injury. Affected athletes will often be unable to bear weight because of extreme pain. There will be marked diffuse swelling and significant tenderness. Ecchymosis will typically be present. Laxity will be present with anterior drawer testing (>14 mm) and talar tilt testing (>10 degree difference between ankles), although many individuals will not tolerate such stress tests initially because of extreme pain and swelling.

   4. Syndesmotic ankle sprains (also known as a high ankle sprain) involve the syndesmotic ligaments that connect the tibia and fibula in the lower leg. They typically present as a grade 2 or 3 lateral ankle sprain. Pain and swelling may be pronounced and weight bearing is very limited, if not impossible. A squeeze test (compressing the distal thirds of the tibia and fibula together) will produce pain at the ankle.

B. Strains also present with pain and swelling, although the pain is typically noticed only with activity and swelling is usually minimal. The location of the pain provides a clue to the diagnosis of strains.

   1. Posterior pain on ambulation indicates a strain of the Achilles tendon.

   2. Pain posterior and inferior to the medial malleolus suggests a strain of the tibialis posterior tendon.

   3. A painful anterior tibia and ankle and medial foot indicate a strain of the tibialis anterior tendon.

   4. Pain posterior and inferior to the lateral malleolus suggests a strain of the peroneal tendons.

   5. Chronic inflammation of a tendon can result in rupture. Classic findings are an inability to actively move in the plane controlled by that muscle–tendon unit. For example, individuals with a ruptured Achilles tendon cannot plantar flex their foot against resistance. These patients would also demonstrate a positive Thompson test where compression of the calf musculature (with the patient either prone or kneeling) does not produce plantar flexion of the foot.

C. Tenosynovitis. Pain and swelling over an affected tendon suggests tenosynovitis. Additional signs include tenderness with palpation, a thickening of the tendon, and weakness of involved muscle groups. Crepitus (described as a "packed snow" sensation) over the involved tendon is a classic finding, though it is often not present.

D. Fractures are frequently associated with immediate disability and a patient report of an audible pop or crack (see Chapter 28). Abrupt moderate-to-severe pain and swelling, localized bony tenderness, and possible crepitus and ecchymosis are signs of an **acute** fracture. An avulsion fracture of the base of the fifth metatarsal typically presents with symptoms and a mechanism of injury identical to an ankle sprain. **Occult** fractures typically present with a history of a "sprained" ankle that resists all treatment, dull ache with slight swelling after excessive walking, increased pain with activity, and complete relief with rest.

V. Imaging. Routine studies need not be performed. Imaging may be warranted in the following circumstances:

A. Plain films. The Ottawa Ankle and Foot Rules are used to determine the need for radiography in ankle or foot injury (see Chapter 28, Figure 28–1). Studies indicate that if a patient does not meet these criteria, radiographs are unnecessary. (SOR **A**)

1. **X-rays** are indicated if there is an **inability to bear weight** both immediately after an injury and in the emergency department (four steps) **OR** for the following findings:
   a. **Ankle.** Pain is present near the malleoli **PLUS bone tenderness** in the posterior half of the lower 6 cm of the tibia or fibula or at the tip of either malleolus.
   b. **Foot.** Pain is present in the midfoot **PLUS bone tenderness** at the navicular or the base of the fifth metatarsal.
2. **Appropriate** x-rays to evaluate the bony anatomy of the ankle include an anteroposterior, a lateral, and a mortise view. A mortise view is obtained by adducting the foot 15 degrees from its position for the anteroposterior view.
3. Comparing anteroposterior, lateral, and mortise views between affected and uninjured ankles helps demonstrate fracture fragments and is useful in identifying Salter–Harris fractures in children. **Oblique views** are useful for detecting **osteochondral fragments**. Routine films will not show stress fractures for the first 2 to 3 weeks following injury.
B. **Computerized tomography and magnetic resonance imaging (MRI)** are >80% sensitive and specific in detecting soft-tissue damage. These tests are recommended for locating fragments and determining the percentage of joint surface involved in osteochondral fractures. They are not routinely indicated for acute ankle injuries.
C. **Bone scans** can be helpful in detecting **stress fractures** in individuals with suggestive symptoms and normal plain films. MRI is often utilized for suspected stress fractures as well.

VI. **Treatment.** Treatment is based on presumptive diagnosis as displayed in Figure 5–3.
A. **Sprains**
   1. **Acute management**
      a. **Protection, rest, ice, compression, elevation, and medications (PRICEM)** are the keys for treating any ankle injury. Ice reduces edema and works better than heat to speed recovery to activity in moderate-to-severe sprains. (SOR **Ⓑ**) Functional compression with a semirigid brace (Aircast) or a soft lace-up brace helps manage swelling. These braces protect against inversion and eversion while allowing dorsiflexion and plantar flexion. This type of functional treatment for acute sprains is recommended over immobilization. (SOR **Ⓐ**)
      b. Ultrasound has been mentioned as a therapeutic modality to treat ankle sprains. A recent review, however, does not support the use of ultrasound. Any benefits are small and of limited clinical significance. (SOR **Ⓐ**)
      c. Nonsteroidal anti-inflammatory drugs (NSAIDs) (e.g., nonprescription naproxen 440 mg initially then 220 mg 8–12 hours later and for subsequent doses, with food) and analgesics (e.g., acetaminophen, 500–650 mg every 4–6 hours) should be given until edema and pain subside. NSAIDs not only reduce swelling and pain but may also decrease the time it takes to return to usual activities. (SOR **Ⓑ**)
   2. **Rehabilitation**
      a. **Range of motion** (ROM) exercises should begin within 48 hours of injury and weight bearing should progress as tolerated while wearing a functional brace. ROM includes controlled stretching of the Achilles tendon to help regain full dorsiflexion.
      b. **Strengthening.** Isometric exercises are started when pain and swelling have subsided and ROM is progressing. All four planes of motion (dorsiflexion, plantar flexion, inversion, and eversion) are worked against an immovable object. Progressive resistive exercises (PREs) in the same planes of motion follow and are readily accomplished by the use of elastic tubing. Toe raises and heel and toe walking are also introduced.
      c. **Proprioceptive exercises** (balance/wobble board) are started when the patient can walk pain-free. Walking on a variety of surfaces (flat floor to level ground to uneven terrain) in a progressive fashion and single leg balancing can also be used to help develop proprioception.
      d. **Functional training.** The next phase involves exercises that are more dynamic. The exercises are a mix of walking and jogging in both a straight line (forward and backward) and in patterns such as a figure of eight. Athletic individuals would then progress onto these exercises with a mix of jogging and running, and

finally incorporate sport-specific drills to further strengthen the ankle prior to a return to competition.

B. Strains should be managed as described earlier for sprains (see Section VI.A).

C. Tenosynovitis
1. **Initial treatment** includes **PRICEM, NSAIDs, and analgesics** as needed. **Corticosteroid injection** (e.g., methylprednisolone acetate, 4 mg, with an equal volume of 1% to 2% lidocaine [Xylocaine]) along the tendon may be helpful. This treatment is **contraindicated in Achilles tendinitis,** in the presence of infection, or if the patient has received a similar injection within the past 4 weeks or has a history of more than three such injections.
2. **Longer-term management** for persistent symptoms includes application of a **short leg, nonweight-bearing cast for 1 to 3 weeks**. ROM and PRE should be used for 1 to 3 weeks after cast removal (see Section VI.A.2).
3. **Surgical consultation** is indicated in cases of refractory pain and disability that are unresponsive to conservative therapy. Tenolysis and debridement may prove helpful in such cases.

D. Fractures
1. **Initial management** of all fractures includes **PRICEM using NSAIDs or analgesics** (hydrocodone/APAP 5/325 three to four times daily as needed) for pain management (Figure 5–3). See Chapter 28 for management. Consultation is advised for unstable, epiphyseal, and osteochondral fractures.
2. **Rehabilitation after immobilization** includes 2 to 4 weeks of ROM, PRE, and proprioceptive and functional exercises, as already described for ankle sprains (see Section VI.A.2).
3. Avulsion fractures of the base of the fifth metatarsal and small avulsion fractures of the distal fibula heal very well and can often be managed similar to an ankle sprain with the understanding that the recovery will be somewhat slower.

VII. Patient Education. Most ankle sprains heal within a few weeks. It is vital for patients to understand the importance of rest, ice, compression, and elevation. These measures are crucial for managing swelling which will result in significant pain relief. Minor sprains may not warrant formal rehabilitation, but moderate to severe sprains necessitate educating the patient about the benefits of rehabilitation and the need for a gradual return to activity as the ankle recovers.

SELECTED REFERENCES

Gravlee JR, Van Durme DJ. Braces and splints for musculoskeletal conditions. *Am Fam Physician.* 2007;75(3):342–348.

Nugent PJ. Ottawa Ankle Rules accurately assess injuries and reduce reliance on radiographs. *J Fam Practice.* 2004;53(10):785–788.

Ottawa Health and Research Institute. Ottawa Ankle Rules. http://www.ohri.ca/emerg/cdr/docs/cdr_ankle_poster.pdf. Accessed May 2013.

Safran MR, Zachazewski JE, Benedetti RS, et al. Lateral ankle sprains: a comprehensive review. *Med Sci Sports Exerc.* 1999;31(7 Suppl):S429–S437.

Stiell IG, McKnight RD, Greenberg GH, et al. Implementation of the Ottawa Ankle Rules. *JAMA.* 1994;271(11):827–832.

Thompson C, Kelsberg G, St Anna L, et al. Heat or ice for acute ankle sprain? *J Fam Practice.* 2003; 52(8):642–643.

Tiemstra JD. Update on acute ankle sprains. *Am Fam Physician.* 2012;85(12):1170–1176.

Van den Berkerom MP, van der Windt DA, Ter Riet G, et al. Therapeutic ultrasound for acute ankle sprains. *Cochrane Database Syst Reviews.* 2011;(6):CD001250.

Veenema KR. Ankle sprain: primary care evaluation and rehabilitation. *J Musculoskel Med.* 2000;17: 563–576.

Wolfe MW, Uhl TL, Mattacola CG, McCluskey LC. Management of ankle sprains. *Am Fam Physician.* 2001;63(1):93–104.

6   Arm and Shoulder Complaints

Brian R. Coleman, MD

KEY POINTS

- History and physical examination are very important in accurate diagnosis. (SOR Ⓒ)
- Specific testing can lead to more accurate diagnosis. (SOR Ⓒ)
- Shoulder-specific exercises can be preventive or reparative of many injuries. (SOR Ⓒ)

I. **Arm and shoulder complaints** comprise generalized or localized discomfort in the upper extremity. These can result from **direct trauma** (e.g., acromioclavicular injuries, shoulder dislocation/subluxation, olecranon bursitis, fractures) or from **overuse** (e.g., rotator cuff impingement/subacromial bursitis, olecranon bursitis, medial/lateral epicondylitis). Overuse of the musculotendinous unit evolves through several stages beginning with inflammation (pain, swelling, erythema, warmth) and followed by reparation (proliferative and maturation stages). Often, with continued overuse, fibrosis occurs which features histologically disorganized restructuring of the musculotendinous unit predisposing to degeneration, stenosing tenosynovitis, and even rupture. Aging also predisposes patients to these degenerative musculotendinous changes.

   A. **Anatomy and function.** The shoulder consists of four joints (glenohumeral, acromioclavicular, sternoclavicular, and scapulothoracic), which allow for movement in multiple planes. Unlike the hip, which is a stable joint having a deep acetabular socket, the shoulder is a mobile joint with a shallow glenoid fossa. The humerus has only minimal osseous support and is suspended from the glenoid by soft tissue, muscles, ligaments, and a joint capsule.

   Glenohumeral stability is owing to a combination of ligamentous and capsular constraints, musculature, and the glenoid labrum. **Static shoulder stability** is owing to the joint surfaces and the capsulolabral complex. **Dynamic shoulder stability** results from rotator cuff muscles and the scapular rotators (trapezius, serratus anterior, rhomboids, and levator scapulae).

   The **rotator cuff** is composed of four muscles, which assist in motion and depress the humeral head in the glenoid. The subscapularis assists internal rotation, the supraspinatus facilitates abduction, and the infraspinatus and teres minor assist in external rotation.

II. **Common Diagnoses** (Table 6–1). Arm and shoulder complaints are very common in family medicine. Causes of these complaints are based on patient age and activity level.

   A. **Rotator cuff impingement** and **subacromial bursitis** form a continuum, beginning with impingement with arm elevation, resulting in soft tissue edema/inflammation. **Before the age of 25 years,** ligamentous laxity predisposes to impingement; **beyond 25 years of age,** impingement is usually related to overuse and frequently results in partial- or full-thickness rotator cuff tears after the age of 40 years. Rotator cuff problems are the most common source of shoulder pain and may be the cause of two-third of the cases of shoulder complaints.

   B. **Dislocations and subluxations** of the shoulder are common and account for 45% of all joint dislocations. Anterior dislocations account for approximately 90% of glenohumeral dislocations. Active patients younger than 25 years of age with a history of previous dislocation have an 85% risk of recurrence.

   C. **Glenohumeral instability** is an increase in translation of the glenohumeral joint that can occur in one or multiple directions. Generalized ligamentous laxity can also contribute to instability, especially in young athletic women and individuals with Marfan syndrome.

   D. **Acromioclavicular (AC) injuries** are rare in skeletally immature individuals; they are most often caused by direct trauma.

TABLE 6–1. DIFFERENTIAL DIAGNOSIS OF COMMON ARM/SHOULDER COMPLAINTS

Condition	Risk Factors	Symptoms	Signs	Testing
AC injuries	Male:female, 5:1; 16–30 years Direct blow to tip of shoulder (e.g., football, lacrosse, wrestling)	Pain with shoulder forward flexion/adduction	AC joint tenderness without gross deformity and with abnormal cross-arm test (Table 6–2) in grade I or II dislocation; clavicular displacement (mildly and superiorly with grade III and markedly superiorly or inferiorly or posteriorly accompanied by neurovascular or muscle compromise with grades IV–VI)	Plain AP/lateral shoulder radiographs; stress radiographs are not recommended because they do not affect treatment
Glenohumeral instability	History of previous dislocation; adolescent girl athletes; repetitive overhead activity (e.g., gymnasts, swimmers, tennis, baseball pitching)	Vague pain referred to deltoid; feeling of impending dislocation or worse pain with overhead/abducted/extended rotated shoulder; "dead arm" after repetitive motion (e.g., pitching)	Abnormal apprehension/sulcus tests (Table 6–2)	Results from AP/lateral shoulder radiographs are usually negative, but may show anteroinferior glenoid rim fracture (Bankart lesion)
Dislocation/ subluxation	Contact sports (e.g., football, lacrosse, rugby); fall on outstretched arm (e.g., skaters, skiers, motorcyclists)	Pain, inability to abduct arm, possible arm paresthesias	Asymmetry compared to unaffected shoulder (prominent humeral head, sulcus between acromion and humerus)	AP/transscapular lateral Y and axillary lateral views should be obtained; postreduction x-rays indicated to detect Bankart lesion
Impingement/bursitis continuum	Repetitive overhead motion (e.g., throwing, racquet sports, swimming); overuse (e.g., carpenters, painters, plumbers); age >40 years	Pain with overhead activities, worse at night; anterolateral shoulder pain, possibly radiating to elbow	Abnormal Apley scratch, Neer, Hawkin, "empty can," or drop-arm tests (Table 6–2)	AP and transscapular lateral plain radiographs for degenerative changes; outlet or Alexander view visualizes subacromial space to grade acromial impingement; MRI 95% sensitive/specific detecting partial/complete tears, cuff degeneration, and chronic tendinitis

Condition	Epidemiology	Symptoms	Physical Examination	Imaging/Testing
Adhesive capsulitis	Highest incidence in 40- to 50-year-olds, shoulder immobilization, involves nondominant arm more often and in women more often than men	Painful loss of motion progressing to relatively pain-free restricted motion	Deltoid atrophy; decreased ROM, especially external rotation	AP/lateral radiographs useful to detect alternate diagnoses (fracture or calcification); arthrography may be helpful in diagnosis but is still controversial because of associated risks; currently, MRI is a diagnostic test of choice
Olecranon bursitis	Direct contusion (e.g., skaters, skateboarders, football players)	Swollen/fluctuant elbow extensor surface with or without pain	Fluctuant/tender or nontender mass over olecranon	Plain lateral radiograph may demonstrate bone spur or fracture with a history of trauma or in recurrent, poorly responsive cases
Medial epicondylitis ("golfer's elbow")	Golfers; Little League pitchers	Pain medial elbow/forearm; decreased pitch control	Tender medial epicondyle	No testing unless atypical presentation; plain radiographs can show fracture, OA, intra-articular loose bodies; EMG can document radiculopathy/neuropathy; MRI helpful in documenting soft tissue fraying or tear if surgical referral is considered
Lateral epicondylitis ("tennis elbow")	Age 40–60 years; 7 times as common as medial epicondylitis, 75% involve dominant arm; found in carpenters/painters/tennis players, or persons using poor equipment (wrong grip sizes, weight of racquet)	Pain lateral elbow/forearm (e.g., holding a telephone, opening a door, or picking up a coffee cup); decreased grip	Tender lateral epicondyle, worse with resisted extension of middle digit	

AC, acromioclavicular; AP, anteroposterior; EMG, electromyography; MRI, magnetic resonance imaging; OA, osteoarthritis; ROM, range of motion.

  E. Adhesive capsulitis is thickening and contraction of the capsule around the glenohumeral joint leading to significantly reduced range of motion (ROM) in the glenohumeral joint.

  F. Olecranon bursitis is inflammation of the superficial olecranon bursa caused by acute or chronic elbow trauma.

  G. Medial epicondylitis (also called golfer's elbow) is inflammation of tendons and ligaments attaching to the medial side of the elbow.

  H. Lateral epicondylitis (also called tennis elbow) is pain over the lateral elbow precipitated by repetitive forearm dorsiflexion, supination, and radial deviation.

BURNERS/STINGERS

Burners/stingers are stretching/compression brachial plexus injuries caused by a blow to the patient's extended or flexed neck while in rotation. These injuries are most common in contact sports (e.g., football, hockey, and lacrosse), are more common in males, and can also result from bicycling or motorcycle accidents.

Patients typically complain of burning/paresthesias of the arm and may experience some arm weakness hours to days after the injury, but should not have neck pain. Patients should have a thorough but brief neurologic examination of the affected extremity, as well as a cervical spine examination. Patients complaining of neck pain should be managed as if they have potential cervical spine injuries, with immobilization and emergency department evaluation. For uncomplicated stingers, radiographs are typically not required, and electromyography is required only if symptoms persist for 2 to 3 weeks (which occurs in <5%–10% of patients). Stingers usually resolve spontaneously; in athletic play situations, the patient may return to play once burning resolves, provided there is no neck pain, weakness, or concussion.

THORACIC OUTLET SYNDROME

Thoracic outlet syndrome results from the compression of the neurovascular supply to the upper limb in the supraclavicular area and shoulder girdle. It tends to occur in young adults, particularly women, and has been associated with cervical ribs, diabetes, thyroid disease, alcoholism, and obesity.

Patients may complain of pain in the neck or shoulder with numbness involving the entire upper extremity or forearm and hand; symptoms may be exacerbated by overhead activity. Nocturnal pain and paresthesias are common and should be distinguished from carpal tunnel syndrome. Thoracic outlet symptoms can often be reproduced and the condition is diagnosed using the following maneuvers: Adson maneuver (with the arm at the side and the neck hyperextended and turned to the affected side) and Wright maneuver (with the arm abducted and externally rotated). Rib films will rule out cervical ribs or long transverse processes; if clinical evaluation is suggestive, cervical magnetic resonance imaging (MRI) may help rule out discogenic disease, and chest radiographs can be used to evaluate for apical lung masses. Treatment for thoracic outlet syndrome involves management of underlying causes (e.g., thoracic surgery consultation for cervical rib).

ACUTE BRACHIAL PLEXUS NEURITIS

Acute brachial plexus neuritis is an uncommon disorder, which can be confused with more common causes of shoulder pain. Brachial plexus neuritis most often affects those between ages 20 and 60 years, with a male-to-female ratio ranging from 2:1 to 11.5:1. A viral or other infectious cause has been suggested.

Patients present with severe acute burning shoulder/upper arm pain without a known precipitant; the pain usually diminishes over days to weeks, replaced by upper arm weakness. Neck or arm movements typically do not affect pain. Brachial plexus neuritis must also be differentiated from cervical radiculopathy (see Chapter 47), which radiates from the neck down the arm, may be related to trauma or exertion, and is exacerbated by neck movements. In brachial plexus neuritis, electromyography and nerve conduction studies 3 to 4 weeks after symptom onset reveal abnormalities in more than one nerve (i.e., the brachial plexus); in contrast, cervical radiculopathy may feature osteophytes and interspace narrowing on cervical spine radiography and neuroforaminal disk impingement on MRI scan. Treatment for acute brachial plexus neuritis is supportive, with physical therapy to maintain shoulder strength/ mobility, analgesics as needed for pain, and reassurance that the condition generally will improve, albeit slowly.

III. **Symptoms** (Table 6–1). Important elements include a careful history of the mechanism of acute injury, the patient's occupational/recreational activities, as well as location, precipitants, and any symptoms associated with the patient's shoulder/arm complaint.
   A. **Location**
      1. Anterolateral shoulder pain possibly radiating to the elbow is consistent with **rotator cuff impingement/subacromial bursitis**.
      2. Vague pain radiating to the deltoid insertion occurs in patients with **glenohumeral instability**.
      3. Pain at the top of the shoulder near the distal clavicle may represent **AC joint** pathology.
      4. Lateral elbow pain characterizes **lateral epicondylitis;** medial elbow pain characterizes **medial epicondylitis**.
   B. **Precipitants/causes**
      1. Shoulder pain with overhead activities and worsening at night is a clue to **rotator cuff impingement/subacromial bursitis**.
      2. Pain with the shoulder overhead, abducted, and externally rotated occurs with **glenohumeral instability**. Pain worsens with repetitive activity such as pitching, tumbling.
      3. Pain with shoulder forward flexion/adduction characterizes AC **joint injury**. Injury can occur with a direct fall onto the shoulder.
      4. Pain following a direct blow to the elbow may indicate **olecranon bursitis**.
      5. Pain following repetitive forearm motion such as golf, tennis, and hammering may **indicate lateral or medial epicondylitis**.
   C. **Associated symptoms**
      1. A feeling of impending dislocation with the shoulder overhead, abducted, and externally rotated points toward **glenohumeral instability,** as does "dead arm" after repetitive shoulder motion.
      2. Painful decreased ROM, developing over time into relatively pain-free restricted ROM, is consistent with **adhesive capsulitis**.
      3. Extensor elbow swelling indicates **olecranon bursitis**.
      4. Patients with **lateral epicondylitis** complain of decreased/weakened grip.
IV. **Signs** (Table 6–1). Examination of the patient with arm/shoulder complaints should always include inspection (for asymmetry in AC or shoulder dislocations), palpation (for localized tenderness), and ROM/special maneuvers (Table 6–2).
V. **Laboratory Tests** (Table 6–1). In most patients with arm and shoulder complaints, a careful history and physical examination should clarify the diagnosis. Further testing, including imaging, should be undertaken on a case-by-case basis (Table 6–1).

USE OF ULTRASOUND IN THE DIAGNOSIS OF SHOULDER PAIN

Ultrasonography has many potential advantages in the diagnosis of causes of shoulder pain. Ultrasound has a lower operating cost and has the potential to have portable equipment to perform the examinations. It is a noninvasive technique with no ionizing radiation and no risk to pace makers or metal implants. It can also be useful in evaluation of the shoulder as it is able to visualize during dynamic phases, where plain film, computed tomography, and MRI are all static scans.

Sonography is effective in evaluation of Hill–Sachs lesions, AC joint arthritis and dislocation, biceps tendon pathology and is most effective in the evaluation of suspected rotator cuff pathology. It allows early detection of small changes in tendons and enables the location, measurement, and visualization of rotator cuff tears.

Ultrasonography is also frequently used to guide injection placement for glenohumeral injections or subacromial injections. As with all diagnostic modalities, it is important to know the equipment, technologists, and who is reading the studies. At some institutions, it may be recommended for specific studies based on availability.

TABLE 6–2. MANEUVERS USED IN EVALUATING COMMON ARM AND SHOULDER COMPLAINTS

Test Name	Description of Maneuver	Testing For	Positive Test
Apley scratch test	Patient reaches (a) above/behind the head, then (b) behind the back, attempting to touch contralateral scapula	Rotator cuff (a) Abduction/external rotation (b) Adduction/internal rotation	Diminished motion, pain
Neer sign	Forced shoulder flexion with forearm extended/pronated (scapula stabilized)	Subacromial impingement	Pain
Hawkin test	Forced shoulder internal rotation with arm forward elevated to 90 degrees	Subacromial impingement/rotator cuff tendinitis	Pain
"Empty can" test	With elbows extended, thumbs pointing downward and arms abducted to 90 degrees in forward flexion, patient attempts to elevate arms against examiner's resistance	Rotator cuff (supraspinatus)	Weakness, pain
Drop-arm test	After passive arm abduction, patient attempts to slowly lower arm to side	Rotator cuff tear/supraspinatus dysfunction (arm drops after 90 degrees)	Weakness
Cross-arm test	Patient raises arm to 90 degrees, then actively abducts, attempting to touch opposite shoulder	AC joint dysfunction	Pain, crepitus
Sulcus test	With arm extended and resting at patient's side, examiner exerts downward traction on humerus, watching for sulcus or depression lateral/inferior to acromion	Glenohumeral instability	Noted depression, subluxing of humeral head
Anterior/posterior apprehension test	With patient's arm abducted to 90 degrees and elbow bent, examiner externally rotates arm and exerts (a) anterior or (b) posterior pressure on humeral head	(a) Anterior and (b) posterior glenohumeral instability	Feeling of impending dislocation
Yergason test	With patient's arm at side, elbow flexed to 90 degrees and thumb pointing up, examiner resists patient's attempts to supinate forearm and flex elbow	Biceps tendinitis (may be concomitant or confused with rotator cuff tendinitis)	Pain and weakness
Spurling test	Patient extends neck; examiner axially compresses head and rotates it toward side of shoulder/arm complaint	Cervical nerve root compression	Shooting pain in arm, reproduction of symptoms

VI. Treatment of arm and shoulder complaints is directed at the underlying condition, which can be established through a careful focused history, examination, and selective testing.

    A. Rotator cuff injuries can be very difficult to treat. Initial therapy consists of rest, ice, and nonsteroidal anti-inflammatory drugs (NSAIDs). Early physical therapy consultation is recommended for ROM and strengthening exercises. A sling may provide some comfort, but could lead to decreased ROM.

        1. If a complete tear is noted, surgical intervention is needed; surgery is considered in partial tears only after physical therapy has failed. (SOR **C**) There appear to be no important differences between open or arthroscopic subacromial decompression and active nonoperative treatment for impingement. Results are also similar between arthroscopic and open subacromial decompression, although there appears to be earlier recovery with arthroscopic decompression. (SOR **B**)

    B. Dislocations are initially treated with relocation and sling immobilization followed by physical therapy with active and passive range of motion exercise (at about 3 weeks). Nonsteroidal anti-inflammatory medications (NSAIDs) (e.g., oral ibuprofen 600 mg 3 times daily with meals, or naproxen 550 mg twice daily with meals) are used to decrease pain and inflammation. A history of recurrent dislocation warrants orthopedic consultation for consideration of surgical reconstruction. (SOR **B**) **Subluxations** are managed with local application of ice, several days of rest and specific exercise to strengthen the shoulder muscles. Surgery is considered with repeated subluxation.

C. **Glenohumeral instability** is treated primarily with physical therapy consultation for rotator cuff strengthening exercises. NSAIDs as noted above can be used for pain, but are not often necessary.

D. Grade I–II **AC joint injuries** are often treated with several days' rest and a shoulder sling for comfort. Ice and analgesics for pain and early ROM exercises are important. Grade III–VI (severe) AC sprains or dislocations warrant orthopedic consultation for surgical consideration. (SOR **A**)

E. **Subacromial bursitis** is treated with relative rest, ice, ROM exercises, and possible injection in the bursa (http://www.youtube.com/watch?v=wr_FBVjHJY8 or http://www.youtube.com/watch?v=6DvdBNAozxs).

F. **Adhesive capsulitis** often resolves spontaneously, and treatment should focus on symptom relief. Gentle ROM exercises, stretching, and graded resistance training have been shown effective. (SOR **B**) **Manipulation under anesthesia** requires orthopedic referral and is a very controversial treatment of capsulitis; it should be reserved for cases refractory to the foregoing measures. Corticosteroid injections (subacromial and intra-articular) may reduce pain, but have not been shown to affect recovery. (SOR **B**)

G. **Olecranon bursitis** is treated with ice, NSAIDs, and close monitoring. Aspiration is performed only when swelling causes significant pain and loss of motion. Aspirated fluid should be analyzed for cell count, crystals, and Gram stain (see Chapter 38). Steroid injections have been used with mixed results and should only be performed if no infection is present.

H. **Medial epicondylitis** is most easily treated conservatively with rest, ice, NSAIDs, and gradual increase in stretching-and-strengthening exercises. (SOR **B**) Local steroid injections should be considered if there is a poor response to 2 to 3 weeks of conservative therapy.

I. For **lateral epicondylitis,** conservative initial management involves NSAIDs, ice after activities or three times daily, emphasis on proper technique for work or sports activities, forearm or counterforce bracing, and physical therapy referral for stretching-and-strengthening exercises with a goal of pain-free ROM. (SOR **C**) Steroid injection (1 mL of betamethasone mixed with 3–5 mL of bupivacaine into point of maximum tenerness in a spoke-and-wheel fashion) should be considered if there is poor response to 2 to 3 weeks of conservative management. Poor response to 6 to 12 months' treatment warrants consideration of orthopedic referral for possible debridement and tenotomy.

SELECTED REFERENCES

Anderson BC, Anderson RJ. Evaluation of the patient with shoulder complaints. Up To Date, 2012. www.uptodate.com. Accessed March 2013.

Blankstein A. Ultrasound in the diagnosis of clinical orthopedics: the orthopedic stethoscope. *World J Orthop.* 2011:2(2):13–24.

Coghlan JA, Buchbinder R, Green S, Johnston RV, Bell SN. Surgery for rotator cuff disease. *Cochrane Database of Syst Rev.* 2008;(1):CD005619.

Chumbly EM, O'Connor FG, Nirschl RP. Evaluation of overuse elbow injuries. *Am Fam Physician.* 2000; 61(3):691–700.

Ejnisman B, Andreoli CV, Soares BGO, et al. Interventions for tears of the rotator cuff in adults. *Cochrane Database Syst Rev.* 2004;(1):CD002758.

Green S, Buchbinder R, Hetrick SA. Some physiotherapy interventions are effective for shoulder pain in some cases. *Cochrane Database Syst Rev.* 2003;(2):CD004258.

Miller JD, Pruitt S, McDonald TJ. Acute brachial plexus neuritis: an uncommon cause of shoulder pain. *Am Fam Physician.* 2000;62(9):2067–2072.

Spencer EE Jr. Treatment of grade III acromioclavicular joint injuries: a systematic review. *Clin Orthop Relat Res.* 2007;455:38–44.

Tallia AF, Cardone DA. Diagnostic and therapeutic injection of the shoulder region. *Am Fam Physician.* 2003;67(6):1271–1276.

Woodward TW, Best TM. The painful shoulder: part I. Clinical evaluation. *Am Fam Physician.* 2000; 61(10):3079–3088.

Woodward TW, Best TM. The painful shoulder: part II. Acute and chronic disorders. *Am Fam Physician.* 2000;61(11):3291–3300.

7   Bites and Stings

Brenda Powell, MD

KEY POINTS

- Mammalian bites cause morbidity from tissue destruction and introduction of pathogens. (SOR **C**)
- Insect and arachnid bites cause morbidity from hypersensitivity reactions, toxins, and introduction of pathogens. (SOR **C**)
- Treatment is based on the reaction type and the introduced infectious agent. (SOR **C**)

I. **Definition.** A **mammalian bite** is a skin wound caused by the teeth of a human or other mammal. Mammalian bites cause morbidity from both mechanical disruption and introduction of pathogens, which include oral aerobic and anaerobic flora and viruses such as hepatitis B and rabies, a fatal viral encephalitis.

Insect and arachnid bites and stings involve penetration of the victim's skin by some part of the animal, with host reaction depending on the type of bite. Hypersensitivity to the organism itself occurs with lice, mosquito saliva, scabies, and hymenoptera stings. Spider bites cause neurotoxicity and local necrosis with hemorrhage and thrombosis. Bites can transmit other diseases (e.g., malaria and encephalitis from mosquitoes, Lyme disease and Rocky Mountain spotted fever from ticks, plague, and typhus from fleas).

II. **Prevention**

A. **Hepatitis B.** Persons at occupational risk for human bites, including health and dental workers and employees of institutions for the mentally retarded, should receive hepatitis B vaccine.

B. **Rabies.** Veterinary workers occupationally exposed to animal bites and people traveling to areas where rabid dogs are common should be immunized with 1 mL of human diploid cell rabies vaccine intramuscularly on days 0, 7, 21, or 28.

C. **Outdoor insect bites. Outdoor insect bites** can be prevented by avoiding their habitats, covering the skin with clothing, and using effective insect repellents that contain diethyltoluamide (DEET 30%). **Permethrin** (permenone tick repellent) sprayed on clothing protects against mosquitoes and ticks.

D. **Bedbugs. Bedbugs** first should be prevented from entering the home. Do not bring discarded furniture into the home. To search for bedbugs, use white bedding and search for them at their most active time of night, about 4 AM. Encasing the mattress in a plastic enclosed cover can prevent the bug from reaching the sleeper. Sleeping in 40% DEET or permethrin cream may prevent bedbug bites during the night.

III. **Common Diagnoses.** Approximately 1 million animal bites require medical attention each year in the United States. Lice and scabies are increasing in prevalence and are becoming more resistant to available treatments. Tick-borne diseases are the most common vector-borne illness in the United States. Hymenoptera is the largest order of insects including sawflies, wasps, bees, and ants. Hymenoptera stings cause more deaths than any other venomous animal (6 deaths per 100,000 people per year).

The following inflict the majority of bites and sting injuries to humans in the United States:

A. **Mammals,** including humans and other mammals, both domestic and wild. Approximately 90% of these bites are from dogs.

1. **Bite injuries from humans** are common in fights; these injuries involve primarily teenagers and alcohol-intoxicated adults. Abused children, children who live in shelters for the homeless, and residents and staff of institutions for the cognitively impaired are especially at a high risk for human bites.

2. Seventy-five percent of **animal bites** are considered "unprovoked." Sixty percent of dog bites involve neighborhood pets; 40% of these bites are superficial. Half of dog bite victims are children younger than 15 years. In the United States, rabies is found in unvaccinated domestic animals and wild animals such as skunks, raccoons, and bats.

B. Insects encompass diptera (mosquitoes, flies, and gnats); fleas and bedbugs; hymenoptera (bees, wasps, hornets, yellow jackets, and ants); and pubic, head, and body lice. **Mosquitoes** breed in stagnant water during the warm season. **Fleas** can be found in grass, rugs, upholstery, floor cracks, and pet bedding, especially during warm, humid months; the majority of flea bites usually result from contact with dogs or cats. **Bedbugs'** primary host is humans, but they feed on other mammals and birds. Bites are on exposed areas of the person during sleep. Multiple bedbugs may feed at night on the sleeping host and are often linear in arrangement, creating the classic three-bite line of "breakfast, lunch, and dinner." Bedbugs can survive in clothing, furniture, and bedding for 6 to 8 weeks without a blood meal. **Bee and wasp stings** are common in suburbs and rural areas. The bites of **fire ants** are a significant problem in the southeastern United States. **Pubic lice** are usually transmitted by close body contact and are rarely spread by fomites. **Head lice,** which are commonly transmitted by the exchange of hats, combs, and brushes, may also be spread by close personal contact. Epidemics occur in schools. Body lice, associated with poor hygiene, are rare.

C. Arachnids include mites that cause scabies, chiggers, hard and soft ticks, brown recluse, and black widow spiders.

    1. Scabies (adult mites or eggs) are readily transmitted by personal contact, especially within families or in crowded living situations. These parasitic mites burrow into the epidermis and lay eggs. It takes about 30 minutes from the time of contact for the mite to form a burrow. **Chiggers (harvest mites)** are prevalent in the southern and Midwestern United States and most often bite gardeners, hikers, and campers.

    2. Ticks can be acquired by contact with pets, vegetation, or the burrows of host animals such as mice. Several human diseases are transmitted by ticks. Rocky Mountain spotted fever and tick-borne relapsing fever are endemic to the western mountain states. Tularemia from tick bites occurs mainly in western states. Lyme disease, which is endemic to semiwooded areas in New England, New York, and Wisconsin, occurs sporadically in the Midwest and the West. There has been an increase in the tick population over the past decade likely due to a combination of factors such as warmer winters, increasing white-tail deer and wild turkey populations, migratory birds carrying ticks to new areas, and less use of insecticides.

    3. Spiders. The bites of **brown recluse, *Loxosceles,*** and **black widow spiders, *Latrodectus,*** cause serious morbidity and result in approximately 5% of all deaths from venomous animals. **Brown recluse spiders** are endemic to the south central United States. These spiders, which are active nocturnally, hide both indoors and outdoors. They bite humans only when they are disturbed. **Black widow spiders** are found throughout the United States and Canada. They nest outdoors in crevices near the ground, especially where flies are present (e.g., outhouses).

D. Less common bites and stings not discussed in this chapter include **marine envenomations** and **snakebites**.

IV. Symptoms and Signs

    A. Mammalian bite wounds. These bites may be superficial abrasions; puncture wounds that are sometimes arcuate (curvilinear); lacerations, often with crushed and macerated edges, or wounds that may involve avulsion of tissue. The wound should be examined for visible evidence of damage to underlying structures; diminished circulation or excessive bleeding; and decreased sensation, weakness, limited movement, or pain with movement. Signs of infection may become evident within hours of a bite. Rabies begins with pain and numbness in the area of the bite, followed by fever, dysphagia, pharyngeal spasms (hydrophobia), paralysis, convulsions, and death.

    B. Insect-bite wounds. Itching is a symptom of **mosquito, flea, bedbug, lice, mite,** and **tick bites**.

        1. The bites of **mosquitoes** are **pruritic, red papules,** or **vesicles**.

        2. The bites of **fleas and bedbugs** are also **pruritic, red papules, or vesicles**. They often occur in clusters or in a linear pattern on exposed areas, especially the wrists, ankles, and legs (fleas), and the hands, face, and neck (bedbugs). Bedbug bites can become wheals or bullae. They can be initially misdiagnosed as scabies, drug reactions, or chicken pox.

        3. The normal local reaction to **hymenoptera venom** is heat, redness, and tenderness. A **local allergic reaction** consists of a red papule surrounded by a pale zone of edema with varying amounts of local swelling. More severe **immediate**

hypersensitivity reactions manifest the signs of generalized urticaria (see Chapter 62), redness, swelling, and anaphylaxis. A **delayed hypersensitivity reaction (serum sickness)** with fever, arthralgias, and malaise may occur 10 to 14 days after the sting. **Fire ants** cause multiple papules, which become necrotic pustules within several hours.

4. The bites of **lice** are **pruritic, red papules, or vesicles**. The itching from lice begins approximately 21 days after infestation. Pubic lice live in pubic and axillary hair and skin, but move all over the body and may be found in eyelashes, eyebrows, and the hairline, especially in children. **Head lice** live on the scalp. The seams of clothing and folds of bedding should be searched for **body lice**. Nits of pubic and head lice attach to hairs at the skin level; since hairs grow 1 mm every 3 days, one can determine how recently nits were deposited by their distance from the skin on the hair shaft. This information is particularly helpful in deciding whether nits represent a new infestation following a course of treatment.

C. **Arachnid-bite wounds**
   1. **Mites**
      a. The female mite's burrow in **scabies** typically takes the form of a short, serpiginous lesion on wrists, elbows, finger webs, or intertriginous areas. Myriad other skin lesions, including erythematous papules, nodules, scaly patches, excoriations, and secondary impetigo, can occur. Except in infants, scabies does not infest the scalp or the face. Scabies mites can live for 4 days off of the host.
      b. The bites of **chiggers** are **pruritic, red papules, or vesicles**. They often occur in clusters or in a linear pattern on the exposed areas, especially the wrists, ankles, and legs. The bites of chiggers and flies have central puncta or vesicles, which may become hemorrhagic.
   2. After a **hard tick** has been attached for several days, its neurotoxin can cause an ascending, progressive paralysis, similar to Guillain–Barré syndrome, with hyporeflexia.
      a. **Lyme disease, caused by the spirochete *Borrelia burgdorferi,*** is the most common vector-borne illness in the United States. Illness usually begins with a slowly spreading, annular skin lesion—erythema chronicum migrans (Figure 7–1)—accompanied by regional lymphadenopathy and minor constitutional symptoms, fatigue, myalgias, arthralgias headache, and fever. Early

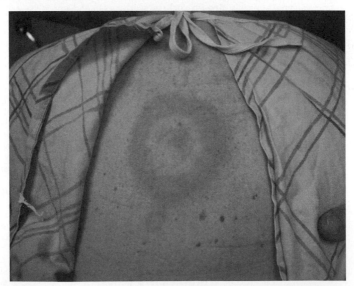

FIGURE 7–1. A 32-year-old woman presents having 5 days of low-grade fevers and the typical eruption of erythema migrans on her upper back. Note the expanding annular lesion with a target-like morphology (see color insert). (Used with permission from Gil Shlamovitz, MD.) (www.VisualDxSeries.com)

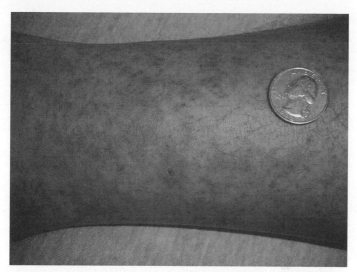

FIGURE 7–2. Rocky Mountain spotted fever with many petechiae visible around the original tick bite. This rickettsial disease looks similar to vasculitis (see color insert). (Used with permission of Tom Moore, MD.)

disseminated disease consists of multiple system involvement, lymphadenopathy, musculoskeletal pain, attacks of arthritis, cranial nerve palsies, meningitis, cardiac conduction defects or pericarditis, and myocarditis. Late Lyme disease is most often seen as a chronic arthritis involving a large joint. The neurologic system may be involved.

b. Rocky Mountain spotted fever is caused by _Rickettsia rickettsii._ Patients present with fever, headache, malaise, and myalgias. A rash, typically of red macules begins on the extremities and becomes purpuric, spreading to the trunk, palms, and soles (Figure 7–2).

c. Tularemia, _Francisella tularensis,_ is characterized by pain and ulceration at the bite site, with acutely inflamed, sometimes draining lymph nodes, or occasionally by severe pharyngeal inflammation with exudate, conjunctivitis, hepatosplenomegaly, or pneumonia.

3. Spiders

a. A **brown recluse spider bite is** often unnoticed until local pain and itching begin; it becomes a hemorrhagic bulla surrounded by induration and erythema after 6 to 12 hours. The area of skin and subcutaneous necrosis may progress over a few days, forming an ulcer, which heals slowly over 2 to 4 months. Systemic symptoms include headache, fever, chills, malaise, weakness, nausea, vomiting, and joint pains. Signs of systemic intoxication, including morbilliform rash, tachycardia, hypotension, intravascular coagulopathy (petechiae, purpura, and bleeding diathesis), and hemolysis, may appear 1 to 3 days after the bite and is termed loxoscelism. Brown recluse spiders have a 3- to 5-cm leg span and a 1- to 2-cm brown, fuzzy body, with a violin-shaped dark band on the dorsum.

b. The **black widow spider bite** is a mild prick, followed in 1 to 3 hours by severe, cramping pain at the bite site, spreading to adjacent parts of the body. Pain, abdominal wall rigidity, muscle cramps, anxiety, weakness, sweating, salivation, lacrimation, bronchorrhea, nausea, vomiting, and fever may occur in hours. Latrodectism is severe muscle cramping, nausea, and vomiting. The skin lesion develops a pale center with a reddish-blue border. Muscle rigidity, with tremor and fibrillations, develops in body parts near the bite. Signs of **cholinergic excess** (fever, lacrimation, rhinorrhea, and bradycardia) and **sympathetic activation** (hypertension and tachyarrhythmias) intensify over the next several hours, but may recur for up to 3 days. Black widow spiders have 1- to 2-cm shiny, black bodies, with a red hourglass mark on the underside.

V. Laboratory Tests
  A. Mammalian bites
   1. Culture with sensitivity studies. More than one-third of deeper human bite wounds and a smaller proportion of animal bites become infected; abrasions seldom reach that stage. Even apparently insignificant bites on the hand are prone to infection. Therefore, **culture with sensitivity studies** is recommended for the following types of mammalian bite wounds: deep puncture wounds, all bite wounds that are sutured, wounds that are clinically infected or require hospital treatment, and full-thickness bites on the hand.
   2. Radiograph. A plain radiograph should be obtained when osteomyelitis is suspected. Forceful injuries, such as a hand bite from a blow to a tooth, require an x-ray to look for fractures and embedded tooth fragments.
   3. Fluorescent antibody staining. An **animal suspected of being rabid** should be killed and its head sent to a health department laboratory, where the brain will be examined for rabies antigens by fluorescent antibody staining.
  B. Tests for possible scabies infestation. Scabies mites, eggs, or feces may be found by scraping open a pruritic lesion (especially the end of a burrow) with a no. 15 scalpel blade dipped in mineral oil, and then examining this material microscopically under a coverslip.
  C. Tests for suspected tick-borne diseases
   1. In the presence of **erythema chronicum migrans,** routine serologic testing for antibodies is not necessary and the patient should receive treatment with antibiotics. Otherwise, acute and convalescent titers of IgM and IgG to *B. burgdorferi* can be drawn.
   2. Spirochetes can be seen in the blood smear in 70% of cases of **tick-borne relapsing fever**.
   3. Rocky Mountain spotted fever and **tularemia** are diagnosed by antibody titers to *R. rickettsii* and *F. tularensis*, respectively. Serology will be positive at 2 weeks. Treatment is started based on signs and symptoms. In **Rocky Mountain spotted fever,** the initial laboratory tests often demonstrate normal or slightly depressed WBC, thrombocytopenia, elevated transaminases, and hyponatremia. In **tularemia,** the WBC and erythrocyte sedimentation rate may be normal or slightly elevated. The organism can be cultured, but this is not often done because of the risk of transmission to laboratory workers.
  D. Tests for brown recluse spider bite with systemic involvement. If this kind of bite is suspected, order blood type and screen, coagulation studies, complete blood cell count, electrolytes, blood urea nitrogen, creatinine, and urinalysis.
VI. Treatment
  A. Mammalian bites
   1. Wound care is similar for human and other mammalian bites.
    a. Thorough cleansing is necessary. At home, this means repeatedly flushing the wound with soap and water, 3% hydrogen peroxide, or iodine solution. In the office, this involves pressure irrigation or scrubbing with gauze sponges (under local anesthesia, if necessary) and 1% benzalkonium or povidone–iodine solution. The edges of a full-thickness wound should be debrided (see Chapter 40). Pressure irrigation should follow.
    b. Closure
     (1) Primary closure with sutures or wound tapes (Steri-Strips) may be considered for dog bites and for human and other animal bites on the face if the patient is treated within 3 to 6 hours after injury and if the wound appears to be uninfected. Subcutaneous sutures should be avoided. A pressure dressing should be applied for 24 hours, and the wound should be inspected for signs of infection after 48 hours. A single layer of skin sutures may be replaced with Steri-Strips after 5 to 7 days.
     (2) Bite wounds on the hands should never be closed primarily. A bitten hand should be immobilized, by splinting from the fingertips to the mid forearm, and elevated. Because of the risk of infection, the wound should be reexamined within 24 hours. After approximately 5 days, movement should be encouraged to minimize swelling and stiffness.
     (3) Other bite wounds should be packed with gauze impregnated with an antibacterial agent and seen on day 2 and 4 to 7 days later. Revision and delayed primary closure can be considered at that time.

     c. The reporting of animal bites (and of human bites in some locales) to the local health department is mandatory.

2. Antibiotic therapy

  a. Indications

    (1) Infected bite wounds require antibiotic therapy. Patients with such bites on the hand should be hospitalized to receive intravenous antibiotics.

    (2) Prophylactic antibiotics should be considered for cat and human bites (SOR **©**) and for dog bites that are >8 hours old.

    (3) It is reasonable to treat with antibiotics bite wounds that have been sutured or followed up for possible delayed closure, all bites on the hand, all human bites, bites causing deep puncture wounds, and all bites in patients with diabetes or immunosuppression. (SOR **©**)

  b. Agents of choice and treatment regimens (Table 7–1). Animal bites (especially cat bites) may become infected with *Pasteurella multocida*. Human bites are more likely to become infected than animal bites and be polymicrobial in nature. *Staphylococcus aureus, Streptococci, Eikenella corrodens* and *Bacteroides* spp., *Staphylococci,* and other penicillinase-producing organisms are present in up to 41% of bite wound infections. First-generation cephalosporins are not effective as monotherapy because *E. corrodens* and anaerobes are often resistant.

    (1) Amoxicillin with clavulanic acid (Augmentin) is the oral drug of choice for treatment (10-day course) or prevention (5-day course) of bite wound infection.

    (2) Penicillin V may be adequate initial therapy for animal bites but not for human bites. Infection developing within the first 24 hours suggests *Pasteurella* infection and constitutes an indication for penicillin.

    (3) Patients allergic to penicillin may receive the following antibiotics:

      (a) For adults and children aged 8 years or older: **erythromycin** (e.g., **erythromycin ethylsuccinate)** *and* **tetracycline hydrochloride** *or* **doxycycline.** Another regimen can be clindamycin plus either fluoroquinolone or trimethoprim-sulfamethoxazole.

      (b) For children younger than 8 years, for whom tetracycline is contraindicated: **erythromycin** *alone,* 30 to 50 mg/kg per day in three divided doses.

3. Hospitalization is indicated in the following situations:

  a. Bites to the hand if infected or more than superficial.

  b. Bites involving tendon, joint capsule, bone, or facial cartilage.

  c. Signs of infection despite antibiotics or when treatment has been delayed.

  d. Severe disfigurement or tissue loss that may require plastic surgery or grafting.

  e. Potential poor compliance with outpatient therapy.

4. Rabies postexposure prophylaxis

  a. Indications (Table 7–2). Contact the local health department or the Rabies Investigation Unit, Centers for Disease Control and Prevention, Atlanta, Georgia, at (404) 639 to 3534 or (800) 311 to 3435 for additional information.

  b. Regimen. Human rabies immune globulin, 20 immunizing units per kilogram is given, half intramuscularly and half infiltrated around the wound, up to 8 days after exposure. Active immunization with human diploid cell rabies vaccine, 1 mL intramuscularly, is given on days 0, 3, 7, 14, and 28. Pregnancy is not a contraindication. Immunosuppressive drugs such as corticosteroids should be avoided, if possible.

5. Tetanus prophylaxis. Tetanus prophylaxis should be administered according to the indications outlined in Chapter 40 (Table 40–2).

B. Insect bites. Symptomatic relief is all that is needed for most bug bites, including those of mosquitoes, flies, fleas, and bedbugs. Topical lotions or creams such as **calamine** or **0.5% hydrocortisone** or applications of ice may relieve itching. Occasionally, an oral antihistamine, such as **diphenhydramine** (Benadryl), 25 mg three times a day for adults, ameliorates the urticarial reaction. Other, more specific treatments are discussed below.

1. For flea and mite infestations, thorough **housecleaning,** including vacuuming, along with washing clothes and bedclothes, is indicated. All bedding, towels, and clothing must be put in the dryer for more than 10 minutes at 60°C. (SOR **Ⓐ**)

TABLE 7–1. TREATMENT OPTIONS FOR PATIENTS WITH ANIMAL BITES

Drug[a]	Dose	Common and Major Side Effects	Contraindications	Drug Interactions
Amoxicillin with clavulanic acid	Adult: 875 mg twice daily Pediatric: 20–40 mg/kg per d divided three times daily (based on severity)	Rash/diaper rash, diarrhea, Stevens-Johnson S, cholestasis, hepatotoxicity	Cholestatic jaundice, hepatic dysfunction, hemodialysis, CrCl <30 mL/min	Methotrexate (methotrexate toxicity), venlafaxine (serotonin S), warfarin (bleeding)
Erythromycin **plus** (doxycycline **or** tetracycline)	Adult: 400 mg three times daily **plus** (100 mg twice daily **or** 250 mg orally every 6 h)	See Erythromycin (below) Photosensitivity, teeth staining (children <8 yr), eosinophilia, hepatotoxicity		Multiple interactions See Erythromycin (below)
Erythromycin	Adult: 250–500 mg four times daily Pediatric: 30–50 mg/kg/d divided three times daily	Diarrhea, loss of appetite, nausea QT prolongation, ototoxicity, cholestatic hepatitis, Stevens-Johnson S		**Multiple drug interactions** Statins (myopathy); Astemizole, cisapride, Class 1A antiarrhythmics, antipsychotics, quinolones, macrolide antibiotics, mifepristone (QT prolongation); digoxin (digoxin toxicity); warfarin (bleeding)
Penicillin V	Adult: 250 mg orally every 6 h Pediatric: 25–50 mg/kg/d orally in 3–4 divided doses to a maximum of 3 g/d			

[a]Available as generic.
CrCl, creatinine clearance; S, syndrome.

TABLE 7–2. RABIES POSTEXPOSURE PROPHYLAXIS FOR NONIMMUNIZED PATIENTS

Animal	Animal Condition	Appropriate Treatment
Wild carnivores (e.g., skunks, bats, or raccoons)	Available Unknown	Obtain fluorescent rabies antibody (FRA) test on animal. Begin HRIG[a] and HDCV or PCECV.[b] Discontinue HDCV, if FRA test is negative. Assume rabid. Begin HRIG[a] and HDCV or PCECV.[b]
Domestic dog or cat	Healthy/available Rabid/suspected rabid or Unknown	Observe animal for 10 d. If animal stays healthy, no treatment is necessary. Obtain FRA test on animal. Begin HRIG[a] and HDCV or PCEV.[b] Discontinue HDCV, if FRA test is negative. Low risk of rabies in most areas. Consult local health department.
Rodents	Generally unknown	Prophylaxis rarely indicated. Consult local health department.

Source: Information from the Centers for Disease Control and Prevention. http://www.cdc.gov/rabies/medical_care/index.html. Accessed August 2013.
[a]Human rabies immune globulin, 20 IU/kg, thoroughly infiltrated in the area around and into the wounds with the remainder injected intramuscularly at a site distant from vaccine administration on day 0. Before HRIG is given, serum should be drawn for measurement of rabies antibody titer. HRIG can be administered up to 7 days after administration of the first dose of vaccine.
[b]Human diploid cell vaccine or purified chick embryo cell vaccine, 1 mL intramuscularly (deltoid area) on days 0, 3, 7, and 14.

2. **Eradication of fleas and bedbugs** is best performed by a professional exterminator. After **fumigation,** pets, children, and pregnant women should stay away for at least 4 hours. Keeping a room vacant is not practical for bedbug eradication since they can live up to 135 days at room temperature. (SOR **Ⓐ**)
3. **Pets with fleas should be treated with insecticide** (e.g., pyrethrum or malathion) after consultation with a veterinarian.
4. **Hymenoptera**
   a. The **stinger** (if present) **should be removed** by scraping sideways so as not to squeeze the attached venom sac.
   b. **Local pain and swelling** may be controlled by applying ice and a protease (e.g., a paste of meat tenderizer and water) to the site.
      Local allergic reactions should be treated with elevation to reduce swelling. **Antihistamines,** such as **diphenhydramine,** 25 to 50 mg (not recommended in infants; up to age 6 years, 6.25–12.5 mg and aged 6–12 years, 12.5–25 mg) orally every 4 to 6 hours. **Prednisone,** 1 mg/kg per day for 3 days, may also be effective.
   c. If **cellulitis** is present, an antibiotic, such as erythromycin, should be added to the above regimen (see Chapter 9).
   d. **Immediate hypersensitivity reactions** must be treated promptly with **epinephrine,** 1:1000, 0.01 mL/kg, up to 0.5 mL, injected subcutaneously, and repeated, if necessary, in 5 to 10 minutes. A large-bore intravenous line should be started and the patient should be observed for at least 6 to 8 hours, since the vast majority of rebound or biphasic anaphylactic reactions will occur during this period. Additional measures for treatment of anaphylaxis should be available, if necessary. Intravenous diphenhydramine, 50 mg, is given to block H_1 receptor sites. Aerosolized bronchodilators, such as albuterol, 2.5 mg (0.5 mL of 5 mg/mL solution) in 3 mL of normal saline, should be used for bronchospasm. Simultaneous use of H_2 blockers (e.g., ranitidine, 50 mg intravenously every 8 hours, or cimetidine, 300 mg intravenously every 6 hours) provides an additional benefit.
   e. For **serum sickness** that occurs 10 to 14 days after hymenoptera stings, **prednisone,** 1 to 2 mg/kg per day orally in divided doses, should be used and tapered over 2 weeks.
   f. **Prophylaxis.** Any individual who has had *any* systemic allergic symptoms or progressively severe local reactions from hymenoptera stings should carry a kit with injectable epinephrine (e.g., **Epi-Pen**), wear a medical identification bracelet, and avoid walking barefoot or wearing bright-colored clothing, flowers, or

TABLE 7-3. TREATMENT OPTIONS FOR PATIENTS WITH LICE OR SCABIES

Drug[a]	Dose	Common and Major Side Effects	Contraindications	Drug Interactions
Lice				
Permethrin 1% to the hair	Saturate hair and scalp	Skin discomfort, itching, edema		None
Lindane 1%	One ounce (do not use more than two ounces)	Dizziness, insomnia, anxiety, rash, skin irritation, seizure, myelosuppression	Premature infants, seizure disorders, skin conditions that may increase systemic absorption; do not use during lactation	None
Malathion 0.5%	Thoroughly wet hair and scalp	Skin irritation, chemical burn	Avoid use in infants and neonates due to potential for increased absorption	None
Scabies				
Permethrin 5%	1 ounce per person neck to toes. Leave on 8–14 h then wash off with soap and water	See above	See above	N/A
Lindane lotion 1%	One ounce neck to toes (do not use more than two ounces). Leave on 8–14 h then wash off with soap and water	See above	See above	
Ivermectin oral	Adults: 200 µg/kg × 1 dose, repeat in 2 weeks	Pruritus, dizziness, seizure, Mazzotti reaction[a]	Safety has not been established in children less than 15 kg and 6 mo	None

[a]Reaction characterized by fever, urticaria, lymphadenopathy, tachycardia, hypotension, arthralgias, edema, and abdominal pain that occurs within 7 days of treatment.

scent outdoors. Patients with allergic reactions can be evaluated by an allergist for desensitization treatment with venom extracts.

5. **Lice**
   a. **Pediculosis capitis** should be treated with a topical scabicide applied to dry hair and left on for 10 minutes before rinsing. Permethrin 1% is preferred (Table 7–3). (SOR **Ⓐ**) Pyrethrum insecticides are pregnancy category B; lindane 1% is an option, but not for children younger than 2 years or for pregnant women.
      (1) After treatment, nits may be loosened by wrapping the hair for 30 to 60 minutes with a towel soaked in vinegar or using a 50% water and vinegar rinse. Nits can be combed out with a fine-tooth comb. Parents should check for treatment failure (new nits visible close to the skin) at 12 hours and every 2 days for 2 weeks; if failure occurs, a second line medication should be used such as 0.5% malathion lotion. (SOR **Ⓐ**)
      (2) **Insecticides should be kept away from the eyes;** on eyelashes, a thick coating of petroleum jelly should be applied twice a day for 8 days.
      (3) Furniture should be vacuumed and all clothing laundered and then dried at >60°C for 10 minutes. Any items that cannot be laundered should be put in sealed plastic bags and set aside for more than 3 days, (SOR **Ⓐ**) or 13 days if nits are present. All combs should be boiled.
   b. **Pediculosis corporis** responds to a hot shower and laundering clothing/bed linens in hot water (60°C) and heated drying. (SOR **Ⓐ**)
   c. **Pediculosis pubis** responds to the same measures as pediculosis capitis (i.e., permethrin 1% as preferred agent; permethrin 5%, a second option; and lindane 1%, a third option). (SOR **Ⓐ**) It is important to treat all contacts. Bedding and

clothing should be washed and dried in a hot dryer, or dry cleaned or bagged in plastic for 72 hours. (SOR **C**)

6. **Scabies.** All household members should be treated simultaneously; bed linens and clothing used in the previous 4 days should be washed in hot water. Items that cannot be washed should be dry cleaned or sealed in a plastic bag for 5 days. (SOR **C**) Mites can live for 24 to 36 hours at room temperature without a meal. (SOR **A**)

   a. **Permethrin 5%** (Elimite cream) (Table 7–3). (SOR **A**) Treatment should be repeated 4 days later. (SOR **C**)

   b. A less expensive and equally effective treatment is **1% gamma-benzene hexachloride** (lindane [Kwell or Scabene]) **lotion** (Table 7–3). Because systemic absorption and neurotoxicity can occur, it should not be used on children younger than 2 years, pregnant or lactating women, patients with seizures or other neurologic disease, or those with extensively inflamed skin.

   c. Malathion 0.5% lotion is an alternative treatment. This is applied in the same manner as above. (SOR **A**)

   d. Despite elimination of live mites, pruritus and existing skin lesions may persist for several weeks. Itching can be treated with **hydrocortisone** or **0.1% triamcinolone cream, with or without oral antihistamines**.

   e. **Oral ivermectin** (Stromectol) is effective in eradicating scabies (Table 7–3), but is not approved by the US Food and Drug Administration for routine use. It should probably be reserved for scabies crustosa (Norwegian scabies), (SOR **B**) or in cases of treatment failure.

7. **Ticks**

   a. **Hard ticks should be removed.** The tick should be grasped very close to the skin with blunt forceps, and pulled upward with slow constant traction (see http://www.cdc.gov/ticks/removing_a_tick.html). If the tick is not completely removed, it should be excised (e.g., using a skin biopsy punch). Sometimes a diligent search is required to locate an attached tick.

   b. **Skin infections** should be treated with antibiotics (see Chapter 9).

   c. For **Lyme disease,** the length of treatment is dependent on the stage of the disease.

      (1) **Early localized Lyme disease** may be treated for 14 to 21 days with **doxycycline,** 100 mg twice a day, or **amoxicillin,** 500 mg three times a day 50 mg/kg per day for children).

      (2) **Early disseminated disease** is treated with intravenous therapy for 2 to 3 weeks. Options are ceftriaxone 2 g daily for 14 days or cefotaxime 2 g three times daily for 14 days. The risk of transmission of the disease is low, less than 5%, even in areas where the disease is hyperendemic; it is therefore probably not cost-effective to treat prophylactically with antibiotics after a tick bite.

   d. For **Rocky Mountain spotted fever,** treatment should be started promptly with oral tetracycline (if the patient is older than 8 years), 25 to 30 mg/kg per day in four divided doses, or with 1 dose of **chloramphenicol,** 50 mg/kg, followed by 50 mg/kg per day in four divided doses. When the patient becomes afebrile, the dose should be halved, and then discontinued after 2 to 3 days. If untreated, death may occur in 8 to 15 days. Untreated Rocky Mountain spotted fever has a fatality rate of 25% and 5% in treated cases.

   e. Adults with **tularemia** can be treated with **streptomycin,** 0.5 g intramuscularly twice a day for 1 week. (SOR **C**)

   f. **Tick-borne relapsing fever** in adults is treated with **tetracycline,** 500 mg orally four times daily for 10 days.

8. **Spider bites**

   a. **Hospitalization** is indicated for patients with black widow spider bites who are symptomatic, elderly, or very young. Hospital treatment may also be necessary for patients with brown recluse spider bites if they have systemic symptoms or if laboratory evidence of intravascular coagulation and hemolysis is present.

   b. For **local lesions caused by brown recluse spider bites,** good wound care is important. (SOR **C**) A bitten extremity should be splinted and elevated. Soaks and sterile dressings, and possibly topical antibacterial agents, such as silver sulfadiazine, are applied to the necrotic ulcer. Systemic antibiotics such as **erythromycin ethylsuccinate,** 400 mg orally four times a day, have been used but are not routinely indicated. **Excision** of the bite wound is ineffective

and **contraindicated.** Local and systemic corticosteroids are of no benefit. The following treatments are **experimental:** antivenom, hyperbaric oxygen, and dapsone, (SOR **B**) a polymorphonuclear cell inhibitor (dosage 50–200 mg per day). The latter agent has potentially serious side effects.
  c. Tetanus prophylaxis should be given (see Chapter 40). (SOR **C**)
  d. Initial therapy for **black widow spider bites** consists of application of ice and extremity elevation. Calcium gluconate in a 10% solution (10 mL given by intravenous push over 5 minutes) may provide relief from muscle spasm. (SOR **A**) Narcotics and diazepam in standard doses can be initiated to relieve pain and muscle spasm.
  e. Antivenom is recommended for significant symptoms of widow bites. (SOR **B**) Before administering **black widow spider antivenom,** testing for sensitivity to horse serum should be done. The test packaged with the antivenom can be used. One 2.5-mL ampule of black widow spider antivenom intramuscularly or intravenously with 10 to 15 mL of normal saline over 10 to 15 minutes can then be administered.

SELECTED REFERENCES

Depietropaola D, Powers JH, Gill JM, Foy AJ. Diagnosis of Lyme disease. *Am Fam Physician.* 2005; 72(2):297–304.
Doggett SL, Dwyer D, Peñas PF, Russell RC. Bed bugs: clinical relevance and control options. *Clin Microbiol Rev.* 2012;25(1):164–192.
Flinders D. Pediculosis and scabies. *Am Fam Physician.* 2004;69(2):341–348.
Graham J, Stockley K, Goldman R. Tick-borne illnesses: a CME update. *Pediatr Emerg Care.* 2011; 27(2):141–147.
Medeiros I, Saconato H. Antibiotic prophylaxis for mammalian bites. *Cochrane Database Syst Rev.* 2001; (2):C001738.
Shmidt E, Levitt J. Dermatologic infestations. *Int J Dermatol.* 2012;51:131–141.

---

8   Breast Lumps and Other Breast Conditions

Diane J. Madlon-Kay, MD, MS

KEY POINTS

- Benign breast disease affects almost all women. (SOR **C**)
- Mammograms are not recommended for women younger than 30 years. (SOR **B**)
- Family physicians can do needle aspirations of breast masses to determine whether they are cystic or not. (SOR **C**)

  I. Definition. Breast lumps are any areas of the breast that feel different from surrounding breast tissue. The normal breast is lumpy because of its cyst-like architecture.
  II. Screening and Prevention
  A. Screening. There is consensus among many organizations that routine screening mammography should be offered to women aged 50 to 69 years. There is controversy about routine screening mammography among women aged 40 to 49 years or women over 70 years of age. Consensus is also lacking regarding screening with clinical breast examination or breast self-examination or how frequently to screen with any of these modalities.
  B. Prevention
  1. Lifestyle changes. Women can make lifestyle choices that can decrease their risk of breast cancer, such as breastfeeding for at least 6 months, avoiding adult weight gain, limiting alcohol intake, avoiding smoking, getting regular exercise, childbearing at a young age, and avoiding prolonged use (i.e., >5 years) of postmenopausal hormones.

2. Chemoprevention. Women at very high risk of breast cancer can consider preventive therapy with raloxifene or tamoxifen.

III. Common Diagnoses
   A. Fibrocystic changes are the most common benign condition of the breast. The incidence of this disorder increases with age; approximately 25% of premenopausal women and up to 50% of postmenopausal women have this condition. Cysts range in size from 1 mm to large macrocysts >1 cm.
   B. Breast cancer will eventually develop in one of every nine women. Risk factors include age, genetic factors, and hormonal factors (see Chapter 69).
   C. Fibroadenomas are most prevalent in women younger than 25 years and in black women.
   D. Mastitis is almost always associated with lactation. This condition results from the entrance of *Staphylococcus aureus* or streptococci into the breast tissue through abraded skin or a cracked nipple. Streptococcal infection usually leads to cellulitis, whereas staphylococcal infection may lead to abscess formation.
   E. Gynecomastia is a benign enlargement of the male breast. It may be asymptomatic or painful, unilateral or bilateral. It commonly occurs during puberty. It also occurs in adults, with the highest prevalence among 50- to 80-year-old patients. Most patients seeing a physician for gynecomastia will have idiopathic gynecomastia (25%) or gynecomastia because of puberty (25%), drugs (10%–20%), cirrhosis or malnutrition (8%), or primary hypogonadism (8%).
   F. Mastalgia (breast pain) is the most common breast symptom causing women to consult physicians. Although fibrocystic disease is often present in the biopsy specimens of women with breast pain, fibrocystic changes are also present in the breasts of 50% to 90% of asymptomatic women.
IV. Symptoms and Signs
   A. Breast lump. In approximately 70% to 80% of women in whom breast cancer develops, the first and only symptom is the incidental discovery of a mass by the patient. Ideally, breast examination should take place 7 to 9 days after the onset of menstrual flow. In general, fibrocystic areas are slightly irregular, easily movable, bilateral, and in the upper outer quadrants. Compression often causes tenderness, especially premenstrually.
      1. On palpation, a cancerous lesion is usually solitary, irregular or stellate, hard, nontender, fixed, and not clearly delineated from surrounding tissues.
      2. Fibroadenomas are usually rubbery, smooth, well-circumscribed, nontender, and freely mobile.
   B. Breast pain is most commonly associated with the menstrual cycle (cyclic), but it can be unrelated to the menstrual cycle or can occur postmenopausally. Cyclic breast pain is usually bilateral and poorly localized. It is often described as a heaviness that radiates to the axilla and the arm and is relieved with the onset of menses. Cyclic mastalgia occurs more often in younger women. Noncyclic mastalgia is most common in women aged 40 to 50 years. It is often unilateral and is described as a sharp, burning pain that appears to be localized in the breast. Breast pain has a spontaneous remission rate of 60% to 80%.
   C. Nipple discharge of a yellow or greenish-brown color occurs in up to one-third of patients with mastitis. The second most frequent symptom of breast cancer, nipple discharge in women older than 50 years is of more concern than it is in younger women. If the discharge is associated with a mass, the mass is the primary concern. Spontaneous, recurrent, or persistent discharge requires surgical exploration. The character of the discharge cannot be used to distinguish benign from malignant causes. However, bloody, serous, serosanguineous, or watery discharges should be regarded with suspicion.
   D. Breast inflammation. Mastitis is characterized by inflamed, edematous, erythematous, indurated tender areas of the breast.
   E. Surface of the breast
      1. Retraction. Breast cancer frequently causes fibrosis. Contraction of this fibrotic tissue may produce dimpling of the skin, alteration of the breast contours, and flattening or deviation of the nipple.
      2. Edema of the skin. Lymphatic blockage produces thickened skin with enlarged pores characteristic of the so-called pigskin or orange peel (*peau d'orange*) appearance in breast cancer.
      3. Venous pattern. This may be prominent unilaterally in breast cancer.

V. Laboratory Tests and Imaging. Diagnostic testing is unnecessary in women with multiple, bilateral, diffuse, symmetric breast lumps without dominant masses.

A. Mammography

1. **Indication.** A woman older than 30 to 35 years with a solitary or dominant mass, or an area of asymmetric thickening in the breast, should undergo mammography. A breast lump is described as a dominant mass when the breasts are diffusely nodular, but one mass is clearly larger, firmer, or asymmetric in location. The mammogram can help characterize the mass and identify any other abnormalities.

2. **Contraindication.** Since breast tissue is very dense in young women, mammograms are *not* recommended in women younger than 30 years. In older women, some fatty displacement of breast tissue has occurred, and mammograms may be more worthwhile.

3. **Efficacy.** Although 85% of all breast cancers are documented by mammography, as many as 15% of women with breast cancers have a normal mammogram. Therefore, a palpable mass is of concern even if a mammographic report shows no evidence of malignancy. Use of postmenopausal hormone therapy can increase breast density impairing the ability of mammograms to detect cancers. **A biopsy is the only test that definitively excludes cancer.**

4. **Interpretation.** Mammogram results are reported using the Breast Imaging Reporting and Data System (BI-RADS):

   1. **Incomplete assessment.** Additional imaging is required.
   2. **Negative.** Routine follow-up.
   3. **Benign findings.** Routine follow-up.
   4. **Probably benign finding.** Short interval follow-up suggested.
   5. **Suspicious abnormality.** Biopsy should be considered.
   6. **Highly suggestive of malignancy.** Biopsy or surgical referral.
   7. **Biopsy proven malignancy.** Surgical and Oncology referral.

B. Other imaging techniques. Although ultrasonography is not useful as a screening tool for breast cancer, it is useful for discriminating solid from cystic lesions. Magnetic resonance imaging is not currently recommended for the evaluation of breast masses. Other imaging techniques considered experimental or of no proven benefit for evaluation of breast conditions include thermography, diaphanography, and computerized tomography.

C. Aspiration of a suspected breast cyst. Needle aspiration can be used to define the cystic nature of any breast mass.

A 20- or 22-gauge needle attached to a 10- or 20-mL syringe should be used. After the skin is cleaned with alcohol, the cyst is fixed between the fingers of one hand while the needle is directed into the cyst with the other. The aspirated fluid is usually amber to green in color. If the fluid is bloody or if the mass is still palpable or reappears within 1 month of observation, a biopsy is necessary. (SOR ❸) The fluid is usually discarded.

D. Breast biopsy. The cytologic or histologic characteristics of a clearly dominant breast mass should be confirmed by biopsy, regardless of other clinical or mammographic findings.

1. **Fine-needle aspiration biopsy** is used to determine the cytology of suspected breast cancer. Accurate interpretation requires proper smearing and fixation of the slides, as well as an experienced pathologist. In expert hands, the false-negative rate is 1.4% and the false-positive rate is near 0%.

2. **Excisional biopsy**
   a. Excisional biopsy is indicated if the results of the physical examination or mammogram suggest cancer even when the cytologic findings of aspiration are benign, or if a breast mass may be cancerous and fine-needle aspiration biopsy and cytologic evaluation are not available.
   b. The biopsy is usually performed as an outpatient procedure using local anesthesia. Removal of the entire mass is the objective.

3. **Incisional biopsy** may be performed in the following circumstances:
   1. To confirm the diagnosis of advanced cancer. If the mass is strongly suspected of being malignant, a cutting-edge core needle can be used.
   2. To evaluate a breast mass that is too large to be excised easily and completely.

E. Genetic testing for breast cancer. Women at risk for genetic mutations should be identified by taking a thorough personal and family history for breast or ovarian cancer, or both. Women at low risk for a genetic mutation should not undergo genetic testing because of the risk of indeterminate or false-positive results and the psychologic and social risks associated with testing. A helpful tool to calculate breast cancer risk is the Breast Cancer Risk Assessment Tool developed by the National Cancer Institute, available at http://www.cancer.gov/bcrisktool/. For women in whom genetic testing is warranted, testing should be done only in the context of genetic counseling.

F. **Gynecomastia** appearing during mid-to-late puberty requires only a history and physical examination, including careful palpation of the testicles and, if the results are normal, reassurance and periodic follow-up. In most boys, the condition resolves spontaneously within a year and no further evaluation is necessary. Since gynecomastia is so common in men, the presence of nontender, palpable breast tissue on a routine examination should not lead to a major laboratory evaluation.

   1. In most instances, taking a careful history is sufficient to uncover most of the conditions associated with gynecomastia. If no abnormalities are found on physical examination or after the assessment of hepatic, renal, and thyroid function by serum chemistry profiles, further specific evaluation is unlikely to be useful.
   2. The patient should be reexamined in 6 months. If a patient reports the recent onset of progressive breast enlargement and no underlying cause is apparent, measurements of serum beta-human chorionic gonadotropin, testosterone, estradiol, luteinizing hormone, follicle-stimulating hormone, and prolactin can help elucidate the cause.

VI. Treatment
A. Fibrocystic changes that are painful
   1. **Nonpharmacologic therapy**
      a. **Supportive measures** that may be helpful include the use of loose, light clothing, and a comfortable, supportive, well-padded bra.
      b. **Caffeine intake.** Although studies of dietary restriction of **caffeine** and other methylxanthines are conflicting, some reports suggest that eliminating consumption of such substances may be efficacious.
      c. **Evening primrose oil** is often used because of its low incidence of side effects, and nonhormonal composition. However, study results are conflicting regarding its effectiveness. The average dose is 3000 mg per day in divided doses for a minimum of 3 to 4 months. Evening primrose oil can be obtained without a prescription and costs less than $1 a day. (SOR Ⓑ)
   2. **Pharmacologic therapy.** Before beginning treatment, the woman's symptoms should be carefully evaluated. Minimal symptoms for only a few days of the month do not require daily drug therapy. It may take 3 to 4 months for evidence of improvement with any treatment regimen.
      a. **Analgesics** such as acetaminophen and nonsteroidal anti-inflammatory medications can be helpful. Topical diclofenac has been found to be effective in treating mastalgia in a randomized controlled trial. (SOR Ⓐ)
      b. **Danazol** is the only pharmacologic agent approved by the US Food and Drug Administration for use in the treatment of fibrocystic changes. Since danazol therapy is associated with significant side effects, this agent should be administered only by a physician familiar with its use. (SOR Ⓑ)
      c. **Tamoxifen** has been found to be effective in decreasing pain in randomized controlled trials. (SOR Ⓐ) It has significant side effects including an increased risk of endometrial cancer and deep venous thrombosis.
   3. **Surgery.** A subcutaneous mastectomy with implants or bilateral reduction mastectomies could be considered for the following patients:
      1. In women with an extremely high risk of breast cancer (e.g., a history of breast cancer in a mother and a sister).
      2. In women with ductal or lobular, atypical hyperplasia on biopsy. The risk of breast cancer is increased by a factor of approximately 5 in these women.
      3. In women with breast pain that is resistant to nonsurgical treatment.

B. Breast cancer.
The objective of treatment is to provide the greatest chance for cure or long-term survival. Whether this objective can be met while preserving the major portion of the breast is controversial. Radical mastectomy is now performed rarely, since modified radical mastectomy results in comparable survival. Lumpectomy is an option for some women (see Chapter 69).

C. Fibroadenoma. Surgical excision,
preserving as much normal breast tissue as possible, is the preferred treatment. After excision, the patient should be reassured that she is at no increased risk for cancer.

D. Mastitis. Lactating women should be encouraged to continue nursing.
  1. Ten days of an antibiotic effective against *S. aureus* and streptococci should be sufficient.
     a. A penicillinase-resistant synthetic penicillin, such as dicloxacillin, 500 mg orally every 6 hours, should be used.
     b. For patients who are allergic to penicillin, erythromycin, 500 mg orally every 6 hours, is a reasonable alternative.
  2. Local heat (e.g., heated gel pack) is also of benefit.
  3. Failure of symptoms to respond to treatment in 48 hours or the development of a mass may indicate a breast abscess that requires incision and drainage. Inflammatory breast cancer must be considered in any mastitis that does not respond to treatment after 5 days or in nonnursing women with mastitis. A biopsy will establish the diagnosis.
E. Gynecomastia. Most patients require no therapy other than the removal of any identified inciting cause. Specific treatment is indicated if the gynecomastia causes sufficient pain or embarrassment. Several medical regimens have been tried, including dihydrotestosterone, danazol, clomiphene citrate, tamoxifen, and testolactone. Surgical removal is also an option.

VII. Patient Education
  A. Changes in the breasts may be caused either by benign conditions or cancer. The most common symptoms are likely to be caused by benign conditions. Still, it is important to let your doctor know about any changes you notice. The younger a woman is, the more likely it is that a breast lump will be benign. Although most lumps are not breast cancer, there is always a chance that a lump may be breast cancer, even in a younger woman. **Regardless of a woman's age, lumps and other changes must be checked to be sure they are not breast cancer.**
  B. There is no sure way to prevent breast cancer. But there are things women can do that might reduce their risk: get regular, intentional physical activity; reduce your lifetime weight gain; and avoid or limit your alcohol intake. Women who breastfeed for at least several months may also get an added benefit of reducing their breast cancer risk. Not using long-term hormone therapy after menopause can help you avoid increasing your risk.

SELECTED REFERENCES

Dickson G. Gynecomastia. *Am Fam Physician.* 2012;85:716–722.
Institute for Clinical Systems Improvement Health Care Guideline: Diagnosis of breast disease. https://www.icsi.org/_asset/v9l91q/DxBrDis-Interactive0112.pdf. Accessed January 23, 2013.
Salzman B, Fleegle S, Tully AS. Common breast problems. *Am Fam Physician.* 2012;86:343–349.

---

9   Cellulitis and Other Bacterial Skin Infections

Donald B. Middleton, MD

KEY POINTS

- Skin infections, including cellulitis and impetigo, are most commonly caused by *Staphylococcus aureus* (which is often methicillin resistant) or *Streptococcus pyogenes* (which remains sensitive to all first-line cephalosporins and penicillins). (SOR **⊕**)
- Abscesses should be managed with incision and drainage. (SOR **⊕**)
- Hospitalization is indicated for those who fail to respond to appropriate outpatient treatment, show signs of major systemic illness, or have high-risk medical conditions. (SOR **⊕**)

I. Definition and Pathogenesis. Bacterial infection of the superficial or deep layers or specialized structures of the dermis is common. Infection may be a primary process resulting from an often trivial breach of the skin's surface allowing bacteria to penetrate or may reflect lymphatic or hematogenous spread from infection elsewhere.

A. Factors contributing to infection include **primary skin diseases** (e.g., eczema or psoriasis), **trauma** (e.g., abrasions, burns, and bites), **immunologic defects** (e.g., AIDS, alcoholism, multiple myeloma, and diabetes mellitus), **contaminated wounds** (e.g., from dirty water, soil, and feces), concurrent or preexisting **viral or fungal infections** (e.g., herpes simplex cold sore and athlete's foot), **bacterial infection** in structures contiguous to the skin (e.g., osteomyelitis, tooth abscess, and sinusitis), **circulatory dysfunction** (e.g., edema and lymphedema), **bacteremia** (e.g., sexually transmitted infection or subacute bacterial endocarditis); **pruritus** (uremia), **neuropathy** (failure to feel trauma), and **psychologic distress** (neuro-dermatitis).

B. Bacterial exotoxins enhance invasion and promote excretion of cytokines and lympho-kines that cause inflammatory warmth and erythema. Out of the more than 100 different bacterial pathogens reported to produce skin infection, the most common by far are *Staphylococcus aureus* or *Streptococcus pyogenes*. The likelihood of other organisms depends on host factors (e.g., age or immune status), source of inoculum (e.g., human or animal bite), and lesion morphology (e.g., erythema migrans in Lyme disease).

II. Common Diagnoses. In the primary care setting, bacterial skin infections account for at least 3% of ambulatory visits and are the 28th most common diagnosis in hospitalized persons, accounting for more than 300,000 admissions per year. Common bacterial skin infections are as follows.

A. Superficial infection (above or into the upper dermal papillae).

   1. Impetigo (Figure 9–1) is endemic in children, especially preschoolers. At least 20% of children have one or more bouts of this infection. The incidence peaks in late summer and early fall, when minor trauma from insect bites or abrasions promotes infection. Close person-to-person contact or scratching from winter dryness, hives, chickenpox, scabies, pediculosis, or tinea can initiate the infection and enhance spread. Epidemics of impetigo occur occasionally, for example, infecting a whole wrestling team. Underlying chronic disorders such as eczema or vascular stasis ulcers promote secondary infection. Impetigo can complicate surgical wounds.

   2. Erythrasma (Figure 9–2) is a *Corynebacterium* infection affecting mainly young men. In tropical climates, up to 20% of men often develop this chronic infection.

B. Deep infection (epidermis and full dermal layer down into the subcutaneous fat).

   1. Cellulitis (Figure 9–3) follows trauma to the skin or occurs seemingly spontaneously in the young, elderly, diabetic, alcoholic, edematous, or immunocompromised patients. Recurrent cellulitis is common in those with an underlying chronic, dermatologic process such as chronic leg edema, lymphedema (e.g., after axillary

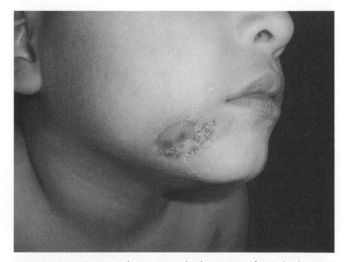

FIGURE 9–1. Impetigo (see color insert). (Used with permission of Dr. Richard Usatine.)

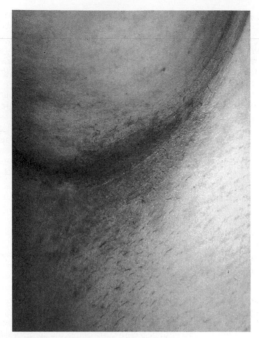

FIGURE 9–2. Erythrasma (see color insert). (Used with permission of Dr. Richard Usatine.)

dissection), and eczema. Cases occur year round. Among the many recognized subtypes, **necrotizing fasciitis** occurs most commonly in elderly patients, especially those with diabetes mellitus or myxedema. Persons with malignancy, anal fissure, hemorrhoids, peripheral vascular disease, or penetrating trauma and intravenous drug abusers are also at higher risk. Most cases are caused by *Streptococcus*

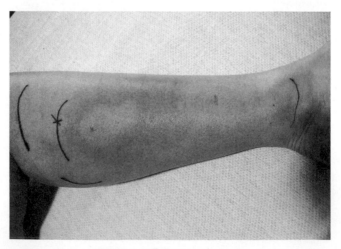

FIGURE 9–3. Cellulitis (see color insert).

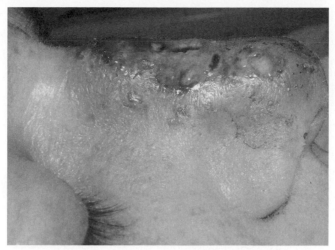

FIGURE 9–4. **Carbuncle of the nose** (see color insert).

pyogenes or *Staphylococcus aureus* or are polymicrobial. *Streptococcus pyogenes* fasciitis often follows other skin infections such as chickenpox.

2. A **furuncle (boil)** often arises in an area prone to perspiration and friction and is most common in adults. Obesity, immunocompromise, and self-trauma, including squeezing a pimple, are important etiologic factors.

3. A **carbuncle** (Figure 9–4) usually develops in persons with immunodeficiency owing to alcoholism or diabetes mellitus or in those who self-traumatize a furuncle.

4. Ecthyma is an ulcerated pyoderma that occurs in children or neglected elderly patients, often after insect bites or skin excoriation.

5. Erysipelas (Figure 9–5; a superficial cellulitis with prominent lymphatic involvement) is common in alcoholics, patients with diabetes, or immunocompromised hosts, but occasionally arises spontaneously in preschool children or older adults. Roughly 30% of patients have recurrences.

C. Specialized skin structure infection (initially localized to a hair follicle, sebaceous cyst, or sweat gland).

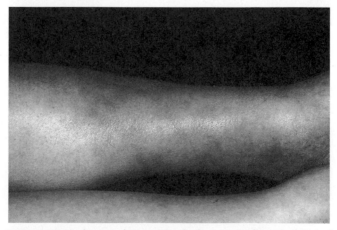

FIGURE 9–5. **Erysipelas** (see color insert). (Used with permission of Dr. Richard Usatine.)

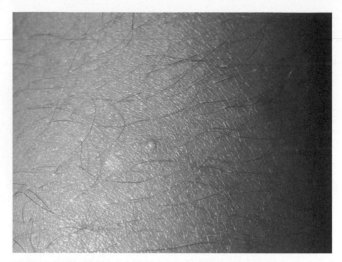

FIGURE 9–6. **Folliculitis** (see color insert). (Used with permission of Dr. Richard Usatine.)

1. **Folliculitis** (Figure 9–6) develops in moist areas with traumatized hair follicles. It often follows shaving, rubbing from tight clothing, or immersion in a hot tub and is usually caused by *Pseudomonas*.
2. **Sebaceous gland abscess** occurs in those with repetitive sebaceous cyst trauma from squeezing or rubbing.
3. **Hidradenitis suppurativa** (Figure 9–7), a sweat gland infection, does not occur prepubertally and usually follows axillary or groin shaving, particularly in obese persons. Men are more likely to have perianal infection and women are more likely to have axillary disease.

   Some less common but important infections are listed in Table 9–1.
III. **Symptoms and Signs** (Table 9–2). The hallmarks of infection are pain and tenderness, swelling, redness, and warmth. Most bacterial skin infections have a pathognomonic

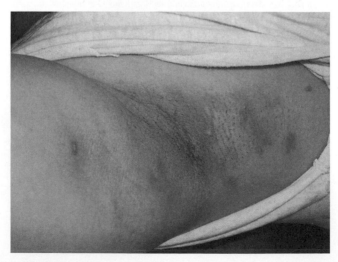

FIGURE 9–7. **Hidradenitis suppurativa** (see color insert). (Used with permission of Dr. Richard Usatine.)

TABLE 9-1. DIAGNOSING AND TREATING LESS COMMON BACTERIAL SKIN INFECTIONS

Condition	Findings	Treatment
Anthrax (*Bacillus anthracis*)	Painless papule progressing to vesicle to ulcer over 3–5 days Best diagnosed with punch biopsy of indurated plaque	Penicillin, ciprofloxacin, or doxycycline ≥10 days
Gangrene (*Clostridium perfringens* or mixed)	Gas in wound	Debride, oxygen; penicillin or clindamycin; a carbapenem; metronidazole
Erysipeloid (*Erysipelothrix rhusiopathiae*)	Contaminated animals or fish	Erythromycin or penicillin
Bacillary angiomatosis (*Rochalimaea henselae* or *R. quintana*)	Typically AIDS/HIV patient with cherry angiomatous or pyogenic granuloma-like lesions	Erythromycin or doxycycline for 2 weeks
Chancriform lesions (venereal [syphilis or chancroid or mycobacterial])	Ulcerative lesions (syphilitic are painless; chancroid are painful)	Based on cause
Lyme disease (*Borrelia burgdorferi*)	Red ≥5 cm circinate macule or target lesion at site of tick bite; similar distant lesions occur with hematogenous spread	Doxycycline or amoxicillin for 14–21 days
Paronychia or felon (*Staphylococcus aureus, Streptococcus pyogenes*)	Red, swollen digit tip or nail bed	Warm soaks; incision and drainage for felon; clindamycin or amoxicillin-clavulanate

AIDS/HIV, acquired immunodeficiency syndrome/human immunodeficiency virus.

appearance, but some must be distinguished from stasis dermatitis, allergic conditions (e.g., eczema), contact dermatitis (e.g., poison ivy), insect stings (e.g., fire ant), bites (e.g., brown recluse spider), trauma, and viral or fungal infections. A standing guideline to manage patients with suspected cellulitis can reduce diagnostic error and length of antibiotic treatment. An approach to the patient with cellulitis is shown in Figure 9–8.

A. General issues
 1. **Pain/tenderness** at the site of infection occurs with most infections, except perhaps impetigo, Lyme disease, and erythrasma.
 2. **Pruritus** is common in impetigo, cellulitis, folliculitis, and erythrasma. Scratching often causes further trauma and promotes spread of infection.
 3. **Feverishness/fever, chills,** and **malaise** can develop acutely. These symptoms often reflect invasion of deeper tissues or the bloodstream, especially with cellulitis, erysipelas, or a carbuncle. Severely ill patients can become septic or die. Erysipelas is especially prone to causing high fever.
 4. A red streak emanating from the rash suggests lymphangitic spread.
 5. Scattered purple or red skin papules or macules may reflect underlying bacteremia with agents such as *Pseudomonas* or gonorrhea.

B. Superficial infection
 1. Streptococcal **impetigo** presents as small vesicles with a red halo that gradually enlarge to ≥1 cm and develop central honey crusts. "Kissing" lesions occur where two skin surfaces touch. Autoinoculation and multiple lesions are common, particularly on the face. Classically, *Staphylococcus* causes bullous lesions with little surrounding erythema, but it is often grown from nonbullous lesions. A varnish-like finish often coats ruptured bullae (Figure 9–1). Underlying viral or fungal infections can be distinguished from impetigo by the appearance of the primary lesions (the smaller vesicles of chickenpox or the circinate raised edge and central clearing of tinea corporis).
 2. **Erythrasma** is usually located in intertriginous areas, especially the groin or sometimes the feet, is colored reddish-brown, and is finely scaled. Secondary to *Corynebacterium minutissimum* invasion, it is often mistaken for *Candida*.

C. Deep infection
 1. **Cellulitis** is acutely tender, red, and hot. The leading edge is not raised but margins are often well defined. Propagation from a central traumatic lesion is centripetal and rapid,

TABLE 9-2. DIAGNOSIS AND TREATMENT FOR COMMON SKIN INFECTIONS

Class	Condition	Findings	Treatment (Table 9-3)
Superficial infections	Impetigo	Small vesicles, enlarging to 1–2 cm with red halo and central "honey" crust (strep) versus bullous lesions with minimal surrounding erythema (staph)	Penicillinase-resistant penicillin, macrolide, or first-generation cephalosporin; doxycycline, TMP/SMX, clindamycin for MRSA; topical agents (mupirocin, retapamulin) for small areas or nasal carriage; good hygiene (avoid scrubbing)
	Erythrasma	Finely scaled red-brown lesions, especially in genital folds	Erythromycin for 14–21 days; single 1 g dose clarithromycin; topical econazole
Deep infections	Cellulitis	Typically, poorly demarcated; warmth/erythema/tenderness	Cephalosporin, fluoroquinolone, amoxicillin-clavulanate, azithromycin, clarithromycin, clindamycin for 5 days; supportive care (limb elevation, warm/cool soaks, and analgesics); hospitalization if severely ill, immunocompromised, or gram-negative or mixed aerobic/anaerobic cellulitis
	Erysipelas	Ill patient with well-demarcated erythema (70% involve lower extremity) with central peau d'orange appearance	Penicillin or erythromycin
	Preseptal orbital cellulitis	Red, swollen, tender eyelids	Amoxicillin-clavulanate, cefuroxime; hospitalization if ill-appearing
	Postseptal orbital cellulitis	Red, swollen, tender eyelids with proptosis, dysconiugate gaze, painful eye movement	Hospitalization for parenteral antibiotics
	Necrotizing fasciitis	Abrupt, painful onset; ill patient with initially only mildly abnormal skin or following trauma or chickenpox	Multiple drug regimen; hospitalize for surgical debridement
	Furuncle	Hot/tender deep purulent boil; typically neck, axilla, buttock, thigh	Moist heat, avoid squeezing; if fluctuant, office incision and drainage (I&D); antibiotic (cephalosporin) if toxic
	Ecthyma	Deep ulcerating lesions, especially in children or neglected elderly patients	Penicillin, cephalosporin; antipseudomonal, if testing warrants
	Carbuncle	Conglomeration of boils, with multiple purulent sites	Hospitalization for parenteral antistaphylococcal antibiotics and possible I&D
Special skin structure	Folliculitis	Red dome-shaped pustule(s) involving hair follicle(s)	Antistaphylococcal antibiotics (antipseudomonal with warm compresses and avoidance of cosmetics, if hot-tub folliculitis)
	Sebaceous cyst abscess	Painful, warm nodule with central black punctum	Office I&D, packing, 24-h follow-up; possibly antistaphylococcal antibiotics for 3–7 days
	Hidradenitis suppurativa	Carbuncle in axilla or groin, varying from acute/tender to chronically draining lesions	Acute: antistreptococcal or antistaphylococcal antibiotics, warm compress, topical isotretinoin, avoid shaving or deodorants, surgical referral Chronic: may respond to ≥3 months of tetracycline

TMP/SMX, trimethoprim/sulfamethoxazole; MRSA, methicillin-resistant Staphylococcus aureus.

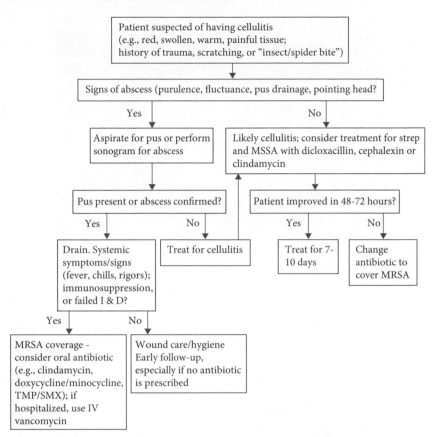

Information modified from Centers for Disease Control and Prevention. Outpatient management of skin and soft tissue infections in the era of community-associated MRSA. 2007. Available at http://www.cdc.gov/mrsa/treatment/outpatient-management.html. Accessed March 2013.

FIGURE 9–8. Approach to the patient with cellulitis. MSSA, methicillin-sensitive *Staphylococcus aureus*; MRSA, methicillin-resistant *Staphylococcus aureus*; TMP/SMX, trimethoprim/sulfamethoxazole; IV, intravenous.

often resulting in lymphangitis or lymphadenopathy. An allergic reaction is seldom as warm, tender, or well demarcated. Infection is occasionally indolent or can spread to regional lymph nodes, blood, fascia, or muscle, creating a life-threatening situation.

a. Cellulitis of the head. **Preseptal orbital cellulitis** (Figure 9–9) involves only the eyelids and **postseptal orbital cellulitis** includes orbital structures. Both make the eyelids red and swollen. Postseptal cellulitis presents with dysconjugate gaze, proptosis, and painful eye movements. Cheeks that are marked by a bluish discoloration and woody consistency indicate facial or buccal cellulitis, often secondary to *Haemophilus influenzae* type b (Hib) or pneumococcus.

b. **Hand cellulitis** often follows puncture wounds such as animal bites or foreign body insertion. Cat or dog bites often produce infection with *Pasteurella multocida*. **Cellulitis of the foot or the leg** often coexists with osteomyelitis in the immunocompromised host.

c. **Cellulitis** with a tense firm portion may indicate subcutaneous abscess formation.

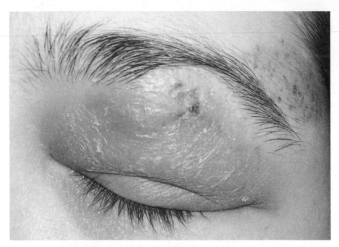

FIGURE 9–9. Periorbital cellulitis (see color insert).

    d. Necrotizing fasciitis has an abrupt, exquisitely painful onset that evolves over 1 to 3 days from cyanosis and edema into necrosis, sometimes accompanied by subcutaneous crepitance indicating gas-forming agents.

    e. Gas gangrene due to *Clostridia perfringens* develops rapidly and is diagnosed by crepitance of the infected skin.

  2. A **furuncle (boil)** is a localized, deep-seated, hot, tender pus-containing abscess commonly found on the neck, axillae, buttock, or thigh.

  3. A **carbuncle** is a conglomeration of boils with suppuration and many pus-draining ports.

  4. Erysipelas (Figure 9–5) is a fulminating cellulitis with a raised, demarcated edge, and fever. Seventy percent of cases are on the lower extremity, but erysipelas can occur on the forehead, face, and abdomen. A central *peau d'orange* (orange peel) appearance is typical.

D. Special skin structure infection

  1. Folliculitis produces small, red, domed-shaped pustules over the hair follicles that can be acute or chronic.

  2. Sebaceous cyst abscess is a raised, painful, hot boil in a sebaceous cyst. A black dot in the center of the lesion is a pore indicative of sebaceous gland involvement.

  3. Hidradenitis suppurativa is a carbuncle of the axilla or groin involving the apocrine sweat glands. It has a highly variable clinical course from an acute, red, tender infection with multiple drainage sites to a chronic scarified slowly draining lesion.

IV. Diagnostic Tests. Most skin infections, such as impetigo or cellulitis, can be treated empirically based on morphology and likely causative agents. Cultures of the leading edge (10%–15% positive), central abrasions (15%–50% positive), blood (a small percentage positive), or skin biopsies are minimally beneficial.

  A. Cultures are warranted in certain situations.

    1. Blood cultures are positive in 80% of patients with Hib and in approximately 20% of cases of pneumococcal cellulitis of the eye or face. Blood cultures should be obtained from patients who are toxic or immunocompromised; who have preseptal or postseptal orbital cellulitis, necrotizing fasciitis, diabetes, facial cellulitis, or fever with scattered papules/macules; or who fail to respond to treatment.

    2. Needle aspiration of unruptured bullae or pus from incised abscesses provides a reliable culture specimen, especially with **paronychia** (infection next to a nail) or a **boil.** However, cultures are unnecessary in most cases. **Gram stain** and **culture** are most often helpful in severely ill patients.

    3. Conjunctival cultures can be useful in preseptal or postseptal cellulitis.

    4. Skin biopsy can help with atypical lesions. For example, anthrax is best diagnosed with a **punch biopsy** of the indurated plaque.

TABLE 9–3. ANTIBIOTICS FOR SKIN INFECTIONS (USUAL COURSE 5–14 DAYS)

Drug (Trade Name)	Route of Administration[a]	Pediatric Dose (mg/kg/d)[b,c]	Adult Dose (g/d)[b]	Interval (Dose/day)
Penicillins				
Amoxicillin	po	20–40	0.75–1.5	3
Ampicillin	po, IV, IM	25–200	1–12	4
Ampicillin-clavulanate	po	20–40	0.75–1.5	3
Ampicillin-sulbactam	IV	100–400	6–12	4
Dicloxacillin	po	12.5–25	1–2	4
Nafcillin	po, IV, IM	50–200	1–12	4–6
Oxacillin	po, IV, IM	50–200	1–12	4
Penicillin G	IV	250,000–400,000 units	8–24 million units	4
Penicillin V	po	25–50	1–2	4
Piperacillin-tazobactam	IV	300 over age 9 mo	13.5	3–4
Cephalosporins				
For use against gram-positive cocci and some gram-negative agents				
Cefadroxil (Duricef)	po	30	1–2	1–2
Cefazolin (Ancef)	IV	30	1.5–6	3–4
Cephalexin (Keflex)	po	25–100	1–4	4
For use against above plus Haemophilus influenzae				
Cefaclor (Ceclor)	po	20–40	0.750–4	2–3
Cefprozil (Cefzil)	po	15–30	0.5–2	1–2
Ceftibuten (Cedax)	po	9	0.09–0.4	1
Cefuroxime axetil (Ceftin)	po	20–30 or 125 or 250 mg/dose	0.5–1	2
Loracarbef (Lorabid)	po	15–30	0.4–0.8	2
For use against primarily gram-negative agents and most gram-positive cocci				
Cefixime (Lupin)	po	8	0.4	1
Cefpodoxime (Vantin)	po	10	0.2–0.8	1–2
Ceftriaxone (Rocephin)	IV, IM	50–100	1–4	1–2
Fluoroquinolones (Over Age 18 Years Only)				
Ciprofloxacin (Cipro)	po, IV	Not used	0.5–1.5	2
Levofloxacin (Levaquin)	po, IV	Not used	0.25–0.75	1
Moxifloxacin (Avelox)	po, IV	Not used	0.4	1
Ofloxacin (Floxin)	po, IV	Not used	0.4–0.8	2
Other Antibiotics				
Azithromycin	po	5–10	0.5 initial, then 0.25	1
Clarithromycin (Biaxin)	po	15	0.5–1	2
Clindamycin (Cleocin)	po, IV	10–40	0.6–2.7	3–4
Doxycycline (many)	Po, IV	Over age 8 yr	200 mg	2
Minocycline (many)	po, IV	Over age 8 yr	200 mg	2
Tetracycline (many)	po	Over age 8 yr 25–50	1–2	4
Erythromycin (many)	po, IV	30–50	1–2	3–4
Linezolid (Zyvox)	po, IV	30	800–1200 mg	2–3
Daptomycin (Cubicin)	IV	Not used	4–6 mg/kg/d	1
Metronidazole (Flagyl)	po, IV	15–30	0.75–2	3
Tigecycline (Tygacil)	IV	Not used	100 mg initial then 50 mg	2
Trimethoprim/sulfamethox-azole (Bactrim)	po, IV	5 mL syrup/10 kg/dose (maximum 20 mL)	320/1600 mg	2
Vancomycin (Vancocin)	IV	10–15	0.5–2	1–4
Topical Agents				
Bacitracin (many)	Topical			3–5
Mupirocin (Bactroban)	Topical			2–5
Retapamulin (Altabax)	Topical			2

[a]po, oral; IV, intravenous; IM, intramuscular.
[b]Dosage may require adjustment in renal failure.
[c]Not to exceed the adult dose.

5. **Bone biopsy** with culture is the definitive test to diagnose coexistent osteomyelitis. Orthopedic consultation is required for bone biopsy, although some neuropathic patients with open wounds may have protruding fractured bone fragments that can be removed for culture.

B. **Special procedures** are sometimes helpful.

   1. **Plain radiographs** can detect tissue gas or foreign bodies, as well as bone, tooth socket, or sinus infection.
   2. **Sonograms** have proven value to detect underlying abscess or pus collection.
   3. **Magnetic resonance imaging (MRI) or computerized tomography scans** can distinguish preseptal from postseptal cellulitis. MRI is useful to detect underlying osteomyelitis, abscess formation, or free air, especially in patients with diabetes or in immunocompromised hosts.
   4. **Bone scans** in selected cases (e.g., patients with diabetes and foot infection, cases of extremity cellulitis that fail to improve, or trauma victims with crush injury) can detect concomitant osteomyelitis.
   5. **Wood lamp** illumination is useful in erythrasma; the infected skin fluoresces coral red.

V. **Treatment** (Tables 9–1 to 9–3). A 7- to 10-day course of antibiotics is required for nearly all bacterial skin infections, (SOR **Ⓐ**) most of which can be managed as outpatient therapy. Ordinarily, complete resolution is achievable, but recurrences are common. Therapeutic decisions include whether to hospitalize or seek consultation. Toxic patients or those with rapidly spreading infections, neutropenia, asplenia, cirrhosis, mixed aerobic and anaerobic infections, postseptal cellulitis, necrotizing fasciitis, or gram-negative cellulitis, especially that caused by *Pseudomonas*, or inadequate social supports are best hospitalized. Unfamiliar lesions are best handled through consultation. Patients with preseptal cellulitis, cellulitis of the hand, or immunocompromised status have been successfully treated as outpatients.

A. **Superficial infection**

   1. **Impetigo** is best treated with a penicillinase-resistant penicillin, macrolide, or first-generation cephalosporin. (SOR **Ⓐ**) Recent studies suggest that *Staphylococcus aureus*, usually phage group II, is a major culprit. **Cephalexin** seems ideal, but alternatives include any agent that eradicates Streptococci and Staphylococci, such as **clindamycin, azithromycin, clarithromycin,** or **amoxicillin-clavulanate**. Streptococcus has been reported to be resistant to erythromycin. Unfortunately, methicillin-resistant *Staphylococcus aureus* (MRSA) is becoming much more common causing up to 50% of cellulitis and skin abscesses in some series. Persons who fail to respond to oral cephalosporins in 48 to 72 hours should be considered to have MRSA and treated appropriately (see below).

      a. Topical agents, especially **mupirocin** ointment (Bactroban) (SOR **Ⓐ**) applied thrice daily and **retapamulin** (Altabax) applied twice daily are effective for small areas. Other topical antibiotics and agents such as hexachlorophene are not highly efficacious.

      b. With treatment, impetigo responds rapidly in more than 90% of cases; the spontaneous resolution rate is 60% in 10 days. Glomerulonephritis or, rarely, toxic shock, can complicate streptococcal impetigo. Scalded skin syndrome or, rarely, toxic shock may follow staphylococcal disease. Parents and patients should be warned to look for hematuria and peeling skin in the week following treatment. Although good hygiene with regular soap and water is helpful, scrubbing tends to spread infection.

      c. Eradication of nasal carriage of Staphylococci or Streptococci with topical **mupirocin** or oral **rifampin** may interrupt repetitive infections.

   2. Topical **isotretinoin (Retin A)** applied to areas of recurrent infection once a day and doxycycline orally have proven prophylactic value for **hidradenitis suppurativa**.

   3. **Erythrasma** is treated with macrolide antibiotics (14–21 days of erythromycin or a single 1 g dose of clarithromycin) and topical azole antifungals (econazole cream applied twice daily) but can relapse into asymptomatic infection lasting for years.

B. **Deep infection.** Although the major pathogens in **cellulitis** are group A (rarely group C or G) *Streptococcus pyogenes* and *Staphylococcus aureus*, numerous other bacteria are capable of producing cellulitis including Hib (buccal cellulitis in young infants), *Streptococcus pneumoniae* (preseptal or postseptal orbital cellulitis), mouth anaerobes such as *Peptostreptococcus* (human bites), soil bacteria such as *Clostridia* (necrotizing fasciitis), *P. multocida* (cat bites), and coliform organisms (decubitus ulcers).

   1. In selecting an antibiotic for cellulitis, likely etiologic agents, cost, and side-effect profile should be considered. Cellulitis responds well to **cephalosporins,**

fluoroquinolones, amoxicillin-clavulanate, azithromycin, clarithromycin, and **clindamycin. Cephalexin, cefadroxil, cefaclor, cefuroxime,** and **cefixime** are the most often utilized cephalosporins, but cefixime is not effective for *Staphylococcus.*

a. MRSA usually responds to **clindamycin, doxycycline,** or **sulfamethoxazole/trimethoprim** (which does not cover strep). Scattered reports of community-acquired MRSA resistant to **clindamycin, fluoroquinolones, minocycline,** and **doxycycline** exist. Intravenous **vancomycin, linezolid,** or **daptomycin** is warranted for systemically-ill patients with MRSA. (SOR **Ⓐ**)

b. In streptococcal disease, penicillin or cephalexin are the drugs of choice, whereas synthetic penicillins such as **dicloxacillin** or **nafcillin** are highly effective for both *Staphylococcus* and *Streptococcus.*

c. Severely ill or immunocompromised patients should be broadly treated initially, preferably with vancomycin until culture results direct narrowing the antibiotic regimen. Oral follow-up therapy with **cefadroxil** or **cephradine** for non-MRSA cases or linezolid or clindamycin for MRSA cases offers a satisfactory alternative to prolonged hospitalization. Twice daily nasal treatment with mupirocin (5 to 7 days) and washes with chlorhexidine may reduce risk of recurrent MRSA infection.

d. Necrotizing (flesh-eating) fasciitis usually reflects group A streptococcus infection alone or mixed with other, usually anaerobic, bacteria. If the infection is gas producing, **Clostridia** should be suspected. **Necrotizing fasciitis** requires hospitalization for surgical debridement and treatment with parental clindamycin and penicillin. (SOR **Ⓐ**)

e. Cellulitis of the diabetic foot is often multifactorial so warrants treatment with **ampicillin-sulbactam, meropenem,** or **imipenem-cilastatin** and often co-coverage with vancomycin as well if MRSA is suspected.

2. Supportive care includes limb elevation, moist warm or cool soaks, and analgesics (e.g., acetaminophen, aspirin, or ibuprofen in appropriate doses). However, some nonsteroidal anti-inflammatory drugs (NSAIDs) may actually delay recovery. Patients with underlying congestive heart failure, stasis ulceration, or diabetes mellitus frequently develop recurrent cellulitis of the legs. Support stockings or Unna boot therapy can help. Hyperbaric oxygen is of limited value for routine cellulitis but may benefit patients with clostridial infections.

3. Carbuncles should be treated with systemic antibiotics directed against *Staphylococci* (e.g., **nafcillin, cefazolin, clindamycin,** and **vancomycin**), incision and drainage, and hospitalization.

4. Erysipelas is treated with penicillins or cephalosporins and usually defervesces within 24 to 48 hours of initiation of appropriate treatment but recurs in up to 30% of cases.

5. Ecthyma is treated with penicillin, a cephalosporin or, in appropriate instances, an antipseudomonal antibiotic.

C. Specialized skin structure infection

1. Recurrent **folliculitis** can be treated prophylactically with chronic topical antibiotics. Normal saline compresses and avoidance of hot tubs or cosmetics help in some cases. **Sycosis barbae,** a deep folliculitis of the beard, is treated with saline compresses, topical mupirocin or bacitracin and, if recalcitrant, with oral cephalosporins for 7 to 10 days.

2. Incision, drainage, and packing alone may be adequate for **sebaceous cyst abscess** or boils. Some advise antistaphylococcal antibiotics (e.g., cephalexin) for 3 to 7 days to reduce the chance of spread.

3. Hidradenitis suppurativa is treated with doxycycline or minocycline, warm compresses, referral for surgical excision, avoidance of shaving and deodorants, topical daily isotretinoin, and occasionally prednisone, 40 to 60 mg orally daily for 5 to 10 days, to diminish scarring. Chronic infection may respond to tetracycline (e.g., doxycycline) orally for ≥3 months.

VI. Patient Education

A. Prevention. Use moisturizers to prevent the skin from cracking. Should a break in the skin occur, wash daily with soap and water and cover the break with an appropriate dressing. A topical antibiotic like bacitracin can be helpful for open wounds. Make certain that shoes fit properly and take care to trim nails without injuring the fingers or toes.

B. Infection. An infection of the skin called cellulitis causes redness, warmth, and pain. Cellulitis can develop on any area of the body and on occasion can spread rapidly. Persons with diabetes mellitus, cancer, or chronic swelling of the arms or legs are particularly at risk. Report the symptoms of cellulitis to your physician promptly, especially if you develop a fever. Many special forms of cellulitis exist. Hand washing helps to prevent spread.

Should you develop cellulitis, you can treat it by elevating the infected arm or leg above the level of your heart, applying compresses, taking an antibiotic, and taking acetaminophen or ibuprofen to reduce pain. If you become severely ill, you may need to be admitted to the hospital for intravenous antibiotics.

Even if you are being treated, you should call your doctor immediately if you develop a fever over 100.5°F especially with chills, if you become severely ill, if the cellulitis seems to be spreading rapidly, or if a boil develops.

With appropriate treatment cellulitis is totally curable.

SELECTED REFERENCES

CDC. Outpatient management of MRSA skin and soft tissues infections. http://www.cdc.gov/mrsa/pdf/Flowchart-k.pdf. Accessed March 2013.

Daly JM, Levy BT, Ely JW, et al. Management of skin and soft tissue infections in community practice before and after implementing a "best practice" approach: an Iowa Research Network (Irene) Intervention Study. *J Am Board Fam Med.* 2011;24(5):524–533.

Kilburn SA, Featherstone P, Higgins B, Brindle R. Interventions for cellulitis and erysipelas. *Cochrane Database Syst Rev.* 2010;(6):CD004299.

Liu C, Bayer A, Cosgrove SE, et al. Clinical practice guidelines by the Infectious Diseases Society of America for the treatment of methicillin-resistant *Staphylococcus aureus* infections in adults and children. *Clin Infect Dis.* 2011;52:1–38.

Jenkins TC, Knepper BC, Sabel AL, et al. Decreased antibiotic utilization after implementation of a guideline for impatient cellulitis and cutaneous abscess. *Arch Intern Med.* 2011;171(12):1072–1079.

---

10   Chest Pain

George P.N. Samraj, MD, MRCOG

KEY POINTS

- In most cases, the chest pain (CP) encountered in ambulatory primary care is not life-threatening and is related to the chest wall or gastrointestinal system. (SOR **C**)
- Most causes of CP can be managed in the primary care ambulatory setting. (SOR **C**)
- A careful and comprehensive history and physical examination with risk factor assessment and focused testing (laboratory studies, imaging studies) can uncover potentially serious conditions, including ischemia and pulmonary embolism (PE). (SOR **C**)
- Missed diagnosis of coronary artery disease (about 15% of CP cases) is common and further testing should be pursued when the etiology remains unclear after focused history and examination or in patients with severe CP. (SOR **C**)

I. **Definition.** Chest pain (CP) is discomfort or pain that is experienced anywhere along the front of the body between neck and the upper abdomen. CP can be acute (<72 hours), subacute (3 days to a month), chronic (more than a month), or chronic with an acute exacerbation and can be produced by a plethora of conditions including cardiac, pulmonary, musculoskeletal, upper gastrointestinal (GI), and psychologic.

II. **Common Diagnoses.** CP is one of the most common symptoms (approximately 1% of all outpatient visits and 10% of emergency department [ED] visits) for which patients seek medical attention. CP is a common presentation of nonlife-threatening conditions as well as life-threatening ones, including myocardial infarction (MI), aortic dissection, pneumothorax, pulmonary embolism (PE), and esophageal rupture. CP is one of the few symptoms where patients may appear well despite having an underlying life-threatening condition.

Approximately 50% to 60% of patients with CP visiting an ED are diagnosed with non-cardiac CP. The most common causes of noncardiac CP are gastroesophageal disorders followed by chest wall syndromes and psychosomatic disorders. Despite advancements in diagnostic technology, history and risk assessment is critically important in the initial evaluation of CP.

A. About 36% to 38% of cases are due to **chest wall pain** (neuromusculoskeletal disorders); 20% is owing to muscle pain; 13% to costochondritis; 2% to broken ribs; and <1% each to fibrocystic breast disease, sickle cell crisis, herpes zoster, and chest wall bruising or trauma. Protracted cough or vomiting may contribute to chest wall syndromes. Chest wall pain is most common in active, young men and women, especially with a history of chest trauma or work/recreational activities involving repetitive upper extremity motion, lifting, or range of motion extremes.

B. GI sources account for 20% to 30% of cases of CP, including gastroesophageal reflux disease (GERD) and esophagitis (13%), achalasia and esophageal spasm (4%), dyspepsia (1%–2%), peptic ulcer disease and gallbladder disease (1% each), and hiatal hernia, and other esophageal motility disorders (<1% each). Factors increasing the likelihood of a GI source of CP include past history of ulcers or dyspepsia, cigarette use, use of nonsteroidal anti-inflammatory drugs (NSAIDs), or use of other gastric irritants (e.g., ethanol, aspirin, erythromycin, tetracycline, or alendronate). Clinicians should specifically inquire about nonprescription NSAID and aspirin products, which patients often fail to report but which carry similar GI risk as prescription products.

C. Cardiovascular (CV) conditions account for approximately 20% of all CPs. The most common CV causes include angina (10%), MI (2%–3%), unstable angina (1.5%), cardiac arrhythmia (1%), and mitral valve prolapse (MVP) (2%); CP caused by aortic dissection or aortic aneurysm, pericarditis, and pericardial tamponade are substantially less frequent (each <1%). Heart disease is the leading cause of death for both women and men in the United States and accounts for 29% of all deaths. Each year over one million people in the United States suffer from MI. The likelihood of CV causes of CP increases in older patients, those with previous history of coronary artery disease (CAD), and persons with a burden of CV risk factors such as hypertension, dyslipidemia, smoking, and diabetes. Illicit substance use, particularly cocaine, is increasingly recognized as a contributor to acute CP, including MI, especially in younger persons, even in the absence of traditional CV risk factors. Within 1 hour of cocaine use, the risk of MI is increased 24-fold compared with risk in nonusers.

THORACIC AORTIC DISSECTION/ANEURYSM

Aortic dissection often presents with an abrupt onset of unremitting excruciating, ripping or tearing, and knifelike CP, radiating through to the back. Less commonly, dissection presents as less severe nagging midchest discomfort and occasionally painlessly. Aortic arch dissection can present with neck pain. Risk factors are hypertension, tobacco abuse, congenital aortic valvular or ascending aortic disease, atherosclerotic inflammatory/collagen aortic disease, pregnancy, and cocaine use. Physical examination may reveal an anxious, dyspneic patient with hypo- or hypertension, differences between right and left arm blood pressures, absent arm or other pulses, a harsh/holosystolic heart murmur associated with aortic insufficiency, pulsus paradoxus, and less often, paralysis.

When dissection is suspected by clinical history, the patient should be hospitalized with emergent cardiothoracic surgery consult and imaging studies (e.g., chest computed tomography [CT] scan, echocardiography) to confirm the diagnosis.

PERICARDITIS

Pericarditis is inflammation of the pericardium caused by various factors including infection (e.g., tuberculosis, HIV, or viral), inflammatory conditions (e.g., connective tissue disease), malignancy (e.g., leukemia, other cancers), endocrinologic disorders (e.g., hypothyroidism), renal disorders (e.g., kidney failure), postmyocardial infarction, and medications (e.g., procainamide, hydralazine, isoniazid). Pericarditis usually presents with substernal CP that is relieved by sitting up and leaning forward. The pain is typically pleuritic with a sharp and stabbing character, which can radiate to the neck, shoulder, back, or abdomen. Pericarditis pain often increases with deep breathing or lying flat, and can also increase with coughing and swallowing. Patients may experience dyspnea, including orthopnea, fever, fatigue, anxiety, and cough may be seen, and heart failure secondary to tamponade may lead to lower extremity edema.

Cardiac examination may reveal a pericardial rub. Heart sounds may be heard as muffled or distant. Lung examination may reveal signs of pleural effusion. Appropriate evaluations include chest x-ray (which may reveal cardiomegaly or a bottle-shaped heart in myocarditis, but is sometimes completely normal), electrocardiogram (ECG; manifesting abnormalities in voltage and ST-segment elevation in up to 90% of patients), complete blood count (CBC), cardiac enzymes, C-reactive protein, erythrocyte sedimentation rate, and blood cultures. Echocardiogram is of great help in identifying pericardial effusion. Sometimes CT, magnetic resonance imaging (MRI), or radionuclide scanning assists in clarifying the etiology and therapy. Pericardiocentesis can be both diagnostic and therapeutic. Treatment is supportive with serial monitoring, use of oral NSAIDs, and treatment of underlying disease processes.

D. Psychosocial sources account for **10% to 20%** of all CPs; these include stress-related sources (8%) and panic disorder and somatization disorder (<1% each). As many as 75% of patients with panic disorder present to the ED with CP. Emotional stress can also exacerbate GERD, cardiac CP, and asthma.

E. About 5% to 10% of CP is **pulmonary,** including bronchitis (2%); pleurisy (1%–2%); pneumonia (1%); and pneumonitis, sarcoidosis, obstructive lung mass, PE, pulmonary abscess, ruptured bullae, pneumothorax, asthma, or viral upper respiratory infection (<1% each). Risk factors for **bronchitis/pneumonia** include chronic lung disease, altered consciousness/impaired gag reflex, immunodeficiency, neuromuscular disease, and thoracic cage deformity. **Pneumonitis** tends to occur with occupational or chemical irritant exposure (e.g., farming, factory/foundry work, cleaning). Teens who recreationally sniff chemicals are at high risk for pneumonitis. Risk factors for **deep venous thrombosis and PE** include prolonged immobilization, pregnancy or recent delivery, pelvic or lower extremity trauma, hypercoagulability, estrogen use, and malignancy (see Chapters 41 and 64).

PULMONARY EMBOLISM

PE often presents with shortness of breath (either active or at rest) and/or CP that is worse with deep breathing and unrelieved by rest. CP can be sharp, stabbing, or dull aching. It may be associated with tachycardia, dyspnea, tachypnea, occasional hemoptysis, sweating, or lightheadedness.

Physical findings range from normal to tachypnea, isolated rales, and occasionally a pulmonary rub (end-inspiratory rubbing sound). Pulmonary hypertension associated with PE can produce left heart failure (fine bibasilar lung rales) or may be restricted to echocardiographic or angiographic abnormalities. Clinical scoring systems can be helpful in determining the risk for PE and the need for further testing, which should be done in the hospital setting (see Chapter 64).

F. Although rare in the office setting, **major trauma** (e.g., cardiac tamponade, tension pneumothorax) can also produce CP.

III. Symptoms. A careful history can narrow the differential diagnosis of CP and should address location and quality of pain, risk factors, exacerbating/alleviating factors, and associated symptoms.

A. Location/quality of pain

1. Patients with **ischemic heart disease (IHD)** can present with substernal tightness, pressure, or both, which can radiate to either the arm or to the jaw, the back, or both. The CP may be associated with shortness of breath, nausea, vomiting, dizziness, syncope, and diaphoresis. **Mitral valve prolapse (MVP)** produces an often sudden onset of chest discomfort/pain with palpitations.

2. **Acute thoracic aortic dissection** pain can present as sharp, stabbing, tearing, or ripping quality pain of the chest or back, especially in between the scapula. The pain can radiate to the neck, jaw, arm, abdomen, or hips. Change in position or movement of the arms or legs may worsen the pain.
3. **Pleuritic pain** is often sharp, stabbing, and localized within the left or right hemithorax and aggravated by breathing and coughing.
4. **Chest wall/muscle pain** can range from a sharp to dull ache and may be localized anywhere on the chest wall.
5. **GI pain** can be substernal and burning (dyspepsia/GERD) or squeezing, substernal pressure (achalasia/esophageal spasm). Achalasia presents with pain behind the sternum or midchest. Peptic ulcer and pancreatitis may present with pain in the epigastrium and sometimes in the back.
6. **Some psychiatric conditions** present with precordial CP. **Hyperventilation presents with** precordial pain associated with dyspnea, tingling and numbness of the limbs, and dizziness, whereas depression may present with constant or intermittent heaviness unrelated to activity or meals.

B. Risk factors (see Sections II.A–E)

C. Exacerbating/alleviating factors
1. **Pain from IHD** is worsened with activity or stress and alleviated by rest or by oxygen, nitrates, or both.
2. **Chest wall/muscle strain pain** is worsened with arm movements or deep inspiration. **Pleuritic CP** can also be produced or exacerbated by deep inspiration or cough.
3. **GI pain** is exacerbated by meals (particularly large meals) and supine positioning; antacids, protein pump inhibitors, or histamine-2 (H_2) blockers typically alleviate this pain. **Gallbladder pain** is classically brought on by high-fat meals.

D. Associated symptoms
1. Nausea, dyspnea, diaphoresis, or sudden severe overwhelming fatigue (particularly in women) can accompany **IHD**.
2. **MVP** may be associated with **palpitations** (especially when supine), lightheadedness, dyspnea, anxiety, or headaches.
3. **Cough** frequently accompanies **pulmonary CP** or **heart failure;** fever with productive or nonproductive cough occurs in **pneumonia;** insidious-onset cough with dyspnea and occasionally fever characterizes **pneumonitis**.
4. **Syncope and hypotension** may be seen with myocardial ischemia, aortic dissection, or PE.
5. **Fatigue with CP** is a presentation of ischemia.
6. **Associated arrhythmia.** Palpitations (e.g., owing to ventricular ectopy, atrial fibrillation) may be associated with CAD. In a patient with new onset of atrial fibrillation and CP, **PE** should be considered as a diagnosis (see Chapter 64).
7. **GI CP** is often associated with nocturnal/morning cough, flatus, belching, hoarseness, halitosis, dysphagia, or odynophagia.
8. A sensation of dyspnea, an inability to breathe deeply, or frank hyperventilation often accompanies **psychogenic CP**. Such pain is frequently associated with other somatic pain (chronic headaches, abdominal or pelvic pain). Panic disorder may feature the foregoing, along with paresthesias, dizziness, trembling, diaphoresis, and a sense of "impending doom."

E. Patient characteristics such as age, gender, ethnicity, culture, and comorbid medical conditions are pertinent in the evaluation of CP. For example, younger patients are less likely to have underlying CAD, while women and older individuals (>70 years) are more likely to have "atypical" presentations.

F. Location and nature of pain
1. **Ischemic pain** tends to be nonlocalized, involves a larger area, and can be difficult to describe (diffused discomfort, ill-defined area), whereas **musculoskeletal and pleuritic pain** are easy to describe and localized (can point to the pain with one finger).
2. **Referred pain** may follow a nerve distribution and is sometimes difficult to localize.
3. **Radiation to both arms** (left or right, but left more than the right), neck, throat, lower jaw, teeth, upper extremity, and shoulders is strong predictor of myocardial ischemic pain.

G. Time of onset and duration of pain

1. **Abrupt CP of great intensity** is more common with PE, aortic dissection, or pneumothorax. Myocardial ischemic pain (and esophageal disease) is usually more gradual, with crescendo intensity over time.

2. **Persistent pain of longer duration (days)** without progression is associated with functional disease.

3. **Fleeting pain** lasting only a few seconds is unlikely to be ischemic. Similarly, **enduring pain (weeks)** is probably not ischemic in origin. Ischemic pain, although it may occur at any time, is disproportionately frequent in the **early morning hours.**

4. **Cold weather, emotional stress, or sexual activities** are commonly recognized triggers for myocardial ischemia.

IV. Signs. Important aspects of the focused physical examination in all patients with CP include general appearance and vital signs, palpation (chest wall and epigastrium), and cardiopulmonary auscultation.

A. General appearance/vital signs. Those with **acute cardiac ischemia** (crescendo angina or MI) and those with **panic/anxiety** may appear anxious and dyspneic; **IHD** can also cause hyper- or hypotension and diaphoresis. **Panic/anxiety** can cause tremor.

B. Palpation

1. In **chest wall pain,** opposed movement or palpation of affected muscles or ligaments reproduces pain, while palpation of the costochondral junction (especially of the third and fourth ribs) reproduces **costochondral chest wall pain**. Chest wall tenderness may be present in patients suffering from myocardial ischemia. **Herpes zoster** is associated with rash and hyperalgesia. Pain can precede the rash of zoster; uncommonly, zoster pain can occur without rash.

2. **GI pain** can be associated with midepigastric tenderness.

C. Auscultation

1. **Cardiac auscultation** in **IHD** may be normal or reveal a new murmur or an S_3 or S_4 gallop. In individuals with **MVP,** auscultation classically reveals a mid-to-late systolic click and a late systolic murmur. Pericardial friction rub can be present in pericarditis.

2. **Pulmonary auscultation**

   a. **Pleuritic pain** may feature a friction rub—an end-inspiratory sound consistent with the rubbing of one's hand against rubber.

   b. Findings in **pneumonia** include localized rales, egophony ("e" to "a" changes), and expiratory sounds such as wheezes or more course rhonchi, which may decrease or be brought out by coughing.

   c. **Pneumonitis** can be accompanied by fine bibasilar rales.

V. Laboratory Testing (Figure 10–1). When a common cause of CP is highly probable based on focused history and examination (e.g., chest wall pain or costochondritis), further testing is unnecessary and treatment can be initiated. Further testing is necessary when the etiology remains unclear after focused history and examination or in patients with severe CP, as is often the case with IHD and pulmonary diseases.

A. Hematologic tests

1. **Complete blood count** can show leukocytosis and left shift with bacterial pneumonia and lymphocytosis with viral pneumonia or reduced hemoglobin suggestive of anemia.

2. A **metabolic panel** is obtained to assess kidney function (before imaging with contrast).

3. **Cardiac biomarkers** such as troponin, creatinine kinase (CK), and CK-MB (isoenzymes of muscle type [M] and brain type [B]) (serial testing) are essential in the management of acute coronary syndromes (ACS) (see Chapter 79).

4. **Thyroid-stimulating hormone levels** may be low or undetectable in hyperthyroidism, which can contribute to anxiety states (see Chapter 89).

5. *Helicobacter pylori* **stool antigen or urea breath test** can be used to evaluate for this potential cause of refractory dyspepsia (see Chapter 84).

B. ECG is often normal in IHD; in a setting compatible with acute IHD, ST-segment elevation or depression can assist the decision to hospitalize.

C. Chest radiography is helpful in both suspected cardiac and pulmonary causes of CP.

1. **Cardiomegaly** may be seen in dilated cardiomyopathy because of chronic IHD.

2. **Infiltrates** may be apparent in pneumonia or pneumonitis.

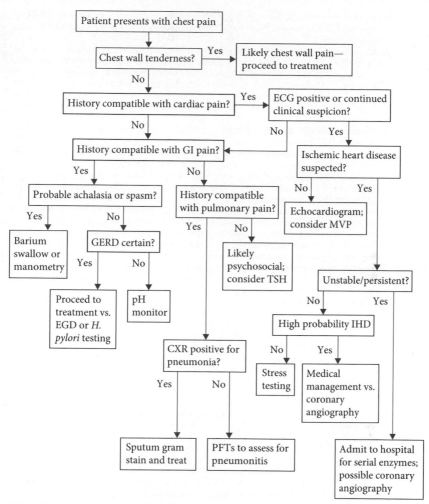

FIGURE 10–1. Approach to the patient with chest pain. ECG, electrocardiogram; EGD, esophagogastroduodenoscopy; CXR, chest x-ray; GERD, gastroesophageal reflux; GI, gastrointestinal; IHD, ischemic heart disease; MVP, mitral valve prolapse; PFTs, pulmonary function tests; TSH, thyroid-stimulating hormone.

      a. Lobar consolidation (bacterial pneumonia) or diffuse infiltrates (atypical or early pneumonia) can occur, but they generally lag behind clinical symptoms by hours-to-days and may be better visualized after rehydration.

      b. Diffuse infiltrates can be seen in pneumonitis.

      c. In **tension pneumothorax,** the CXR can show increased thoracic volume, ipsilateral heart border flattening, contralateral mediastinal deviation, and depression of hemidiaphragm.

      d. In **congestive heart failure,** there may be signs of fluid collection in the lungs (see Chapter 73).

      e. Rib fractures may be evident following trauma.

D. Stress testing

    1. Exercise stress electrocardiography detects ECG changes occurring during exercise that are absent on resting ECG. Dramatic ST-segment changes (>2 mm), particularly at low workloads (i.e., <6 minutes on Bruce protocol or at <70% of age-predicted maximum heart rate), indicate severe IHD and the need for coronary angiography.

2. **Exercise stress echocardiography** allows for similar evaluation as exercise stress ECG; however, echocardiography is preferred in certain patients, including women and those with obesity, pendulous breasts, left ventricular hypertrophy, or previous ECG changes (such as a bundle branch block, pacemaker, or previous MI) precluding evaluation for ischemia using ECG alone. In addition to ECG changes, stress echocardiography can evaluate wall motion abnormalities and ventricular ejection fraction.

3. **Pharmacologic stress testing** is preferred in individuals unable to achieve adequate heart rate through exercise; this inability may be because of severe arthritis, neurologic or vascular disease, obesity, pulmonary disease, or simply severe deconditioning. Pharmacologic stress tests employ either coronary vasodilators (e.g., dipyridamole, adenosine) or agents that increase heart rate (e.g., dobutamine). Either stressor will accentuate inadequacies in coronary flow. Because vasodilators preferentially dilate the nonstenotic coronary circulation, adenosine/dipyridamole will magnify the circulatory deficit seen under exercise by preferentially shunting flow to the nonstenotic areas. By increasing heart rate, a pharmacologic agent simulates exercise without the patient exercising. Intravenous administration of a radioisotope (e.g., thallium, technetium-sestamibi) at the time of stress testing provides additional information about myocardial perfusion.

E. **Coronary angiography,** which delineates coronary artery anatomy, is the gold standard for confirming abnormal stress testing and guiding therapy (i.e., medical versus surgical management, including stenting and coronary artery bypass grafting).

F. **Additional cardiac imaging,** including screening and diagnostic tests, is performed in some institutions as part of a comprehensive evaluation for ACS. The tests include computed tomographic coronary angiography, echocardiography, cardiac MRI, and myocardial perfusion studies. Wall motion abnormalities and perfusion abnormalities can be early signs of MI before the detection of cardiac biomarkers.

G. **Pulmonary function tests (PFTs)** can be helpful in patients with pulmonary CP in clarifying obstructive versus restrictive disease and its severity.

H. **GI studies**
1. **Esophageal pH probe** can help confirm GERD in cases where symptoms are atypical or cardiac evaluation is normal.
2. In patients with known GERD, **esophagogastroduodenoscopy** can be used to assess complications or severity of disease (e.g., Barrett esophagus, erosive esophagitis) and allow gastric biopsy to diagnose infection with *H. pylori*.
3. **Upper GI barium study** allows detection of fixed anatomic esophageal lesions (e.g., Schatzki ring, tumors) and can also help detect motility disorders and hiatal hernia; manometry increases sensitivity in detecting motility disorders.

VI. **Treatment.** Treatment of various CV and pulmonary conditions should include **specific management, discussion about lifestyle changes** (smoking cessation, stress reduction, diet, sleep hygiene, lipid-lowering agents, and planned exercise based on the disease), **and follow-up.**

A. **Chest wall pain/muscle strains**
1. Treatment includes rest initially, avoidance if possible of precipitating activities, warm moist compresses, and local ice packs after activity.
2. **Oral NSAIDs** (e.g., ibuprofen, 400–600 mg with meals) can provide relief.
3. Pain that is localized (e.g., trigger point or costochondral), disabling, and/or resistant to the foregoing measures may be alleviated with an injection (e.g., administration of a local anesthetic, such as 0.5–1 cm^3 of bupivacaine or 1% to 2% lidocaine, into a trigger point, or a mixture of 0.5–1 cm^3 local anesthetic and 0.5 cm^3 of Aristocort to 40 into a costochondral joint). Particularly with intercostal trigger point injection, care must be taken to avoid pleural penetration.

B. **GI.** See Chapters 19 and 84.

C. **Cardiovascular**
1. **Acute angina or escalating unstable or crescendo angina** or **suspected MI** is a medical emergency demanding immediate hospitalization for close monitoring, serial cardiac enzymes, oxygen, nitrates, pain management, aspirin, or other

anticoagulation. Mortality is reduced through risk factor identification/modification (e.g., lipid panel assessment and statin administration) and early use of beta-blockers, if not contraindicated. (SOR **Ⓐ**) For myocardial ischemia management, refer to the American Heart Association 2012 guidelines and Chapter 79.

2. Chronic stable angina (see Chapter 79)

3. Miral valve prolapse

   a. Explanation of the diagnosis and **reassurance** may be sufficient in those with minimal symptoms.

   b. Those bothered with palpitations, anxiety, or CP may be helped by counseling to minimize caffeine/ethanol intake and use of a beta-blocker (e.g., atenolol, 25–50 mg orally daily, with a gradual upward titration of dose based on symptoms and heart rate).

   c. Endocarditis prophylaxis is not indicated in MVP. (SOR **Ⓐ**)

D. Treatment of CP from **psychiatric disease** involves addressing underlying disorders (see Chapters 91, 94, and 96).

E. Pulmonary

1. Pneumonia (see Chapter 13).

2. Pleurisy may respond to NSAIDs (see Section VI.A.2). Incentive spirometry or deep breathing 10 to 20 times every few hours helps prevent atelectasis or secondary pneumonia from the splinting occurring with pleuritic pain.

3. Pneumonitis

   a. With normal PFTs, pneumonitis requires avoidance of precipitants and periodic monitoring of symptoms/PFTs.

   b. Symptomatic pneumonitis with abnormal PFTs generally should be evaluated and initially managed by a pulmonologist, who may initiate oral steroids (e.g., prednisone, 40–100 mg daily).

SELECTED REFERENCES

Chagnon I, Bounameaux H, Aujesky D, et al. Comparison of two clinical prediction rules and implicit assessment among patients with suspected pulmonary embolism. *Am J Med.* 2002;113(4): 269–275.

Jneid H, Anderson JL, Wright RS, et al. 2012 ACCF/AHA focused update of the guideline for the management of patients with unstable angina/non-ST-elevation myocardial infarction (updating the 2007 guideline and replacing the 2011 focused update): a report of the American College of Cardiology Foundation/American Heart Association Task Force on Practice Guidelines. *J Am Coll Cardiol.* 2012; 60(7):645–681.

Kontos CM, Diercks DB, Kirk JD. Emergency department and office-based evaluation of patients with chest pain. *Mayo Clin Proc.* 2010;85(3):284–299.

Lee TH, Goldman L. Evaluation of the patient with acute chest pain. *New Engl J Med.* 2000;342(16): 1187–1195.

Lenfant C. Chest pain of cardiac and noncardiac origin. *Metabolism.* 2010;59(suppl 1):S41–S46.

Mark DB. Risk stratification in patients with chest pain. *Prim Care.* 2001;28(1):99–118.

Nilsson S, Scheike M, Engblom D, et al. Chest pain and ischemic heart disease in primary care. *Br J Gen Pract.* 2003;53:378–382.

Schmermund A, Möhlenkamp S, Stang A, et al. Assessment of clinically silent atherosclerotic disease and established and novel risk factors for predicting myocardial infarction and cardiac death in healthy middle-aged subjects: rationale and design of the Heinz Nixdorf RECALL Study. Risk factors, evaluation of coronary calcium and lifestyle. *Am Heart J.* 2002;144(2):212–218.

Swap CJ, Nagurney JT. Value and limitations of chest pain history in the evaluation of patients with suspected acute coronary syndromes. *JAMA.* 2005;294(20):2623–2629.

11   Confusion

Robert C. Salinas, MD (CAQ-G, HPM), & Audra Fox, MD

KEY POINTS

- Delirium or acute confusional state is a syndrome for which an underlying cause must be found; it represents a true medical emergency. (SOR **C**)
- Delirium may be caused by a medical condition, drug abuse, prescription medication, toxin, or a combination of these. (SOR **C**)
- The elderly and those with underlying dementia are most susceptible to developing delirium. (SOR **C**)
- Evaluation of patients with delirium includes assessment of mental status; attention to vital signs for evidence of hypoxia, metabolic derangement or infection; funduscopic examination; laboratory testing including toxicology screen and urinalysis; and consideration of specialized testing such as imaging or lumbar puncture. (SOR **C**)
- Management usually includes hospitalization for identification and treatment of specific reversible underlying causes. (SOR **C**)

I. **Definition.** This chapter focuses on the assessment and management of a patient who is experiencing **delirium (acute confusional state)**. Delirium is a medical term used to describe a constellation of clinical symptoms that include the following:
  - Disturbance of consciousness with reduced ability to focus, sustain, or shift attention;
  - Change in cognition (e.g., memory deficit) or the development of a perceptual disturbance that is not better accounted for by a preexisting, established, or evolving dementia;
  - Acute onset (usually hours to days) with a tendency to fluctuate over the course of the day;
  - Evidence from clinical or laboratory findings that the disturbance is likely caused by the direct physiologic consequences of one or more specific medical conditions, substance intoxication, substance withdrawal, or from other reasons such as sensory deprivation.

  Delirium is often precipitated by one or more underlying medically-related causes and should be seen as a true emergency. Dementia and other chronic confusional states are discussed in Chapter 74, but remain strong risk factors for the development of acute delirium.

II. **Common Diagnoses.** The prevalence of delirium in the outpatient setting is unknown; it is thought that between 10% and 52% of elderly patients aged 65 years and older who are admitted to the hospital meet the criteria for delirium. Prevalence rates are even higher among older hospitalized adults with dementia. Delirium increases the length of hospital stay, morbidity and mortality, and the likelihood of being discharged to a long-term care institution for post-acute care. (SOR **B**)

  Delirium can be of the hyperactive type, hypoactive type, or of the mixed type (both hypo- and hyperactive), which makes the diagnosis more challenging.

  A. **Specific conditions predisposing to delirium.** There is a complex interplay between different patient predisposing vulnerabilities and environmental insults (iatrogenic) causing delirium, particularly in the acute and post-acute hospital setting.
    1. **General medical conditions** (Table 11–1). There are many illnesses that predispose a patient to develop acute delirium in any setting. Often, there are multiple factors that place a patient at higher risk.
    2. **Drug intoxication,** most often from cannabis, cocaine, or hallucinogens, is the most common cause of acute confusional state in older adolescents and young adults in the ambulatory care setting.
       a. **Substance-withdrawal delirium** is most often caused by previous use of high-dose ethanol, sedative hypnotics, or anxiolytic agents and an abrupt cessation.
       b. **Substance-induced delirium** is caused by exposure to medications or toxins (e.g., carbon monoxide, insecticides, and industrial solvents).
       c. **Prescription medications** (Table 11–2). Delirium from medication use should always be considered in the elderly, who account for approximately 30% of all prescribed medications and 40% of all nonprescription medications, some of which have centrally-acting anticholinergic properties.

TABLE 11-1. GENERAL MEDICAL CONDITIONS OFTEN CAUSING DELIRIUM

Metabolic disturbances	Hyponatremia, hypo-/hyperkalemia, hypo-/hyperthyroidism, anemia, hypercarbia, hypo-/hyperglycemia, dehydration, malnutrition, hypothermia, heat stroke
Neurologic	Head trauma, CVA, normal pressure hydrocephalus, subdural hematoma, meningitis, encephalitis, brain abscess, neurosyphilis, seizure disorders (ictal and postictal states)
Neoplastic	Primary intracranial neoplasm, metastatic disease to the brain
Cardiovascular	MI, CHF, arrhythmia, severe aortic stenosis, hypertensive encephalopathy
Pulmonary	Pneumonia, COPD exacerbation, respiratory failure
Gastrointestinal	Fecal impaction, intra-abdominal infection, liver failure
Urinary	Urinary tract infection, urinary retention

CVA, cerebrovascular accident; MI, myocardial infarction; CHF, congestive heart failure; COPD, chronic obstructive pulmonary disease.

3. **Change in environmental setting** (e.g., transfer to hospital or a new place of residence following acute hospitalization).
4. **Structural brain disease** (Alzheimer disease, vascular dementia, Lewy body dementia, Parkinson disease).
5. **Depression** coexists in more than one-third of outpatients diagnosed with dementia and even more so in nursing home residents with dementia, which can place a person at a higher risk for developing delirium during a hospital stay.
    B. Conditions that often mimic delirium include dementia (see Chapter 74), depression (see Chapter 94), other psychiatric disturbances, age-associated memory disorder (minimal cognitive impairment), malingering, and factitious disorder.

III. Symptoms. During an episode of delirium, obtaining a careful history from a caregiver familiar with the patient's underlying medical problems; medication use including those that were recently prescribed, herbal or natural products, and purchased nonprescription drugs; and functional independence baseline may shed light on likely reversible causes. History details should include the following:
    A. Onset and course of the confusional state (Table 11-3) clarify whether delirium is present, along with its severity, and help differentiate delirium from dementia.
    B. Risk factors. Table 11-4 highlights risk factors for development of delirium; vulnerable populations particularly at risk include (1) the **elderly** because of sensory/cognitive impairment, underlying chronic illness, polypharmacy, and possible changes in the synthesis of neurotransmitters (e.g., a decrease in acetylcholine and an increase in dopamine) felt vital to attention, learning, and memory; (2) **abusers of ethanol and other illicit drugs** (e.g., cocaine and hallucinogens) because of drug-induced imbalances in neurotransmitters such as acetylcholine, serotonin, and gamma-aminobutyric acid; (3) those with **chronic underlying structural brain disease** (dementia, Parkinson disease); and (4) the **terminally ill** because of medications (e.g., opiates) and anxiety/depression/sleep disturbance associated with the severity of disease progression, particularly during the last 48 hours of life. In addition, postoperative hospitalized patients are at risk for developing delirium as well as patients admitted to the surgical and medical intensive care units.

TABLE 11-2. DRUGS WITH ANTICHOLINERGIC PROPERTIES THAT CAN CAUSE DELIRIUM

Classical anticholinergics (e.g., atropine, scopolamine)
Antidepressants (e.g., tricyclic)
Antiemetics (e.g., dimenhydrinate, meclizine, prochlorperazine)
Antihistamines (e.g., diphenhydramine, hydroxyzine)
Antihypertensives
Antiparkinsonian (e.g., benztropine)
Antipsychotics
Antispasmodics
    Gastrointestinal (e.g., dicyclomine, hyoscyamine)
    Urinary tract (e.g., oxybutynin, tolterodine, solifenacin)
H2-blockers (e.g., cimetidine, ranitidine)
Muscle relaxants (e.g., cyclobenzaprine)
Opioids
Prednisone

TABLE 11–3. FEATURES OF DELIRIUM AND DEMENTIA

Feature	Delirium	Dementia
Onset	Abrupt	Insidious
Duration	Acute illness, generally days to weeks	Chronic illness, characteristically progressing over years
Reversibility	Usually reversible	Usually irreversible, often chronically progressive
Orientation	Disorientation early	Disorientation later in the illness, often after months or years
Stability	Variability from moment to moment, hour to hour, throughout the day	Much more stable day to day (unless superimposed delirium develops)
Physiologic changes	Prominent physiologic changes	Less prominent physiologic changes
Consciousness	Clouded, altered, and changing level of consciousness	Consciousness not clouded until terminal
Attention span	Strikingly short attention span	Attention span not characteristically reduced
Sleep–wake cycle	Disturbed sleep–wake cycle with hour-to-hour variation	Disturbed sleep–wake cycle with day–night reversal, but not hour-to-hour variation
Psychomotor changes	Marked psychomotor changes (hyperactive or hypoactive)	Psychomotor changes characteristically late (unless superimposed depression)

    C. Chronic illnesses (Table 11–1).
    D. Drug use (Table 11–2). Thorough assessment of a patient with delirium requires a careful review of all current prescription and nonprescription medications including those that were recently stopped or started. Special attention is given to medications with central-acting anticholinergic properties or those that potentially lead to electrolyte disturbance.
IV. Signs. A systematic review of precipitating factors and physical examination might yield clues to underlying causes of delirium and in addition should include the following:
    A. Evaluation of Mental Status
        1. The **Mini-Mental State Examination (MMSE)** (Table 11–5) has high sensitivity and specificity in evaluating memory loss and cognitive impairment; using a cut-off score of 23 or less, the MMSE has a sensitivity of 87% and a specificity of 82%.

TABLE 11–4. RISK FACTORS FOR DELIRIUM

Age	• Reduced capacity for homeostasis • Impairments in vision/hearing • Age-related changes in pharmacokinetics and pharmacodynamics • Chronic diseases • Psychosocial precipitants such as sleep loss, sensory deprivation, sensory overload, bereavement, or relocation • Structural brain disease
Preexisting dementia	• Imbalance of noradrenergic/cholinergic neurotransmission • Inflammatory mechanisms • HPA axis abnormalities • Disrupted circadian rhythm
Hospitalization	• Relocation • Euthyroid sick syndrome • Severe illness • Disrupted sleep–wake cycle • Physical restraints • Bladder catheterization • Addition of new medications
Polypharmacy	• Drug interactions • Additive effects
Surgical factors	• Significant intraoperative blood loss • Hemodynamic instability • Emergent versus elective surgery • History of noncardiac thoracic surgery or AAA repair
History of drug abuse	• Especially alcohol, cannabis, cocaine, hallucinogens

TABLE 11-5. MINI-MENTAL STATE EXAMINATION (MMSE) SAMPLE ITEMS

Orientation to Time
"What is the date?"
Registration
"Listen carefully. I am going to say three words. You say them back after I stop.
Ready? Here they are . . .
APPLE (pause), PENNY (pause), TABLE (pause). Now repeat those words back to me." [Repeat up to 5 times, but score only the first trial.]
Naming
"What is this?" [Point to a pencil or pen.]
Reading
"Please read this and do what it says." [Show examinee the words on the stimulus form.]
CLOSE YOUR EYES

Source: Reproduced by special permission of the publisher, Psychological Assessment Resources, Inc., 16204 North Florida Avenue, Lutz, Florida 33549, from the Mini Mental State Examination, by Marshal Folstein and Susan Folstein, Copyright 1975, 1998, 2001 by Mini Mental LLC, Inc. Published 2001 by Psychological Assessment Resources, Inc. Further reproduction is prohibited without permission of PAR, Inc. The MMSE can be purchased from PAR, Inc. by calling (813) 968-3003.

The MMSE cannot be used itself to diagnose dementia or delirium and results should be considered in the context of hearing, vision problems, physical disabilities, age, educational level, and cultural influences.

2. The **Confusion Assessment Method (CAM)** instrument (http://www.medscape.com/viewarticle/481726) has been used to evaluate hospitalized patients with suspected delirium and has a sensitivity of 94% to 100% and a specificity of 90% to 95%. The tool takes approximately 5 minutes to administer and a positive diagnosis requires that both acute onset, fluctuating course and inattention be present, along with either disorganized thinking or altered level of consciousness. (SOR ◉)

3. An **agitated confusional state without focal signs** can occur following head trauma. Hyperalert confusion can result from alcohol withdrawal. A person who is excited, hyperalert, and hallucinating may be experiencing toxicity from amphetamine, lysergic acid diethylamide (LSD), cocaine, or phencyclidine (PCP).

B. **Vital signs**

1. If **diastolic blood pressure is >120 mmHg,** hypertensive encephalopathy should be considered.

2. If **systolic blood pressure is <90 mmHg,** confusion may be from impaired cerebral perfusion secondary to shock. Drug overdose, adrenal insufficiency, and hyponatremia should also be considered.

3. **Tachycardia** suggests sepsis, dehydration, delirium tremens from alcohol withdrawal, hyperthyroidism, hypoglycemia, or an agitated, anxious patient.

4. **Fever** can indicate infection, delirium tremens, cerebral vasculitis, or fat embolism syndrome. **Hypothermia** is defined as a core temperature (rectal or esophageal) below 35°C (95°F) and can cause confusion.

5. **Tachypnea** suggests hypoxia. A patient with chronic obstructive lung disease receiving fractional inspiratory oxygen >0.28 can be confused from hypercarbia.

C. **Eye examination**

1. **Papilledema** suggests hypertensive encephalopathy or an intracranial mass.

2. **Dilated pupils** suggest sympathetic outflow, which is common with delirium tremens. **Pinpoint pupils** suggest narcotic excess or constricting eye drops.

D. **Other findings**

1. **Bibasilar crackles** on lung auscultation indicate pulmonary edema with potential accompanying hypoxia due to acute heart or lung disease.

2. **Acute confusion, ataxia, bilateral sixth-nerve palsy, and diarrhea** suggest Wernicke–Korsakoff encephalitis.

V. **Laboratory Tests.** Unless the cause of the acute confusional state is obvious from the history and physical examination, further diagnostic testing is important.

A. **Initial workup** may include complete blood cell count with differential; erythrocyte sedimentation rate; serum chemistry profile, magnesium, and calcium; toxicologic screen of urine, blood, or both; urine analysis; chest x-ray; electrocardiogram; and serum drug levels of prescribed medication as indicated.

B. A **lumbar puncture** should be considered in any delirious patient for whom the possibility of bacterial or viral meningitis is entertained. Relative contraindications include rapid improvement in the patient's clinical status and concerns about increased intracranial pressure from a mass lesion.

C. An **electroencephalogram** can identify partial complex seizures disorder, metabolic encephalopathy, or sedative use and should be considered in patients suspected of these disorders.

D. Imaging. Computerized tomography (CT) of the head is the test of choice for the initial evaluation of confused obtunded patients to rule out subdural hematoma, epidural hematoma, stroke, cerebral abscess, or neoplasm. Repeat CT after 24 to 48 hours should be done if acute infarct is suspected. **Magnetic resonance imaging** with magnetic resonance arteriography may be useful to rule out chronic subdural hematoma, regional blood flow abnormalities, or aneurysm.

E. Additional tests to consider are arterial blood gas analysis, blood cultures, serum ammonia levels, liver function studies, thyroid function tests, cortisone levels, antinuclear antibodies, serum protein electrophoresis, serum vitamin B_{12} and folate levels, syphilis test (venereal disease research laboratory), serum and urine osmolality, HIV titer, and urine tests for heavy metals and metanephrines.

VI. Treatment

A. General principles. Patients with acute delirium should usually be hospitalized for identification and management of any reversible underlying causes. Terminally ill hospice patients with delirium can often be managed at home or in an inpatient hospice setting, depending on patient and family desires. Principles of management include the following:

1. Supportive care while workup progresses includes a quiet private room with familiar objects, presence of a family member, maintenance of a normal sleep–wake pattern, review of medications, pain assessment, regular bowel and bladder program, avoidance of physical restraints, and if possible an interdisciplinary approach to care.

2. Drug therapy. Agitation and behavioral problems posing harm to the patient or others may require the use of neuroleptic agents for sedation. When considering such medication, the goal should be control of dangerous behavior or harm to self and others, while avoiding excessive sedation.

    a. Haloperidol. A recent Cochrane review suggests that low-dose haloperidol (0.25–2 mg) given intramuscularly can be helpful in the urgent setting. Occasionally, maintenance doses of haloperidol (0.25–0.5 mg orally two or three times daily) are used to control agitation while the underlying cause of delirium is determined and treated. (SOR **A**)

    b. Some of the newer atypical neuroleptic agents may be reasonable options and can also be used for maintenance or add-on purposes, in the critically ill. In such cases, Quetiapine (25 mg orally every 12 hours) can be used for acute delirium that has not responded to haloperidol.

    c. Paradoxical physiologic reactions can occur with any of these medications through anticholinergic properties and can worsen extrapyramidal symptoms.

    d. Benzodiazepines can be useful in delirium from ethanol withdrawal. If a benzodiazepine is used, **lorazepam** is usually the drug of choice because of its relatively short half-life. However, this too can paradoxically worsen agitation in patients with preexisting dementia.

    e. In hospice patients, the above medications can be of benefit in treating confusion; treatment of pain, anxiety, and depression is also indicated. Forgoing a search for a reversible underlying cause of the delirium may be appropriate in the terminally ill.

3. Open communication with family members about suspected causes and prognosis of the delirium is essential as caregivers may experience great distress in observing a patient's behavioral changes associated with acute cognitive impairment.

B. Treatment of specific conditions (see Chapters 74 and 94).

C. Prevention and education. Understanding that intrinsic and extrinsic factors predispose patients in certain age groups to delirium will help develop preventive strategies. The incidence of delirium can be decreased by limiting polypharmacy, closely monitoring drug usage by the elderly, and recognizing prodromal symptoms of insomnia, nightmares, fleeting hallucinations, and anxiety. (SOR **B**) In addition, identifying patients predisposed to developing delirium (Table 11–4) and instituting careful monitoring of exposure to potential precipitants can be key to preventing delirium in hospitalized patients.

SELECTED REFERENCES

Han JH, Wilber ST. Altered mental status in older patients in the emergency department. *Clin Geriatr Med.* 2013;29(1):101–136.

Han JH, Zimmerman EE, Cutler N, et al. Delirium in older emergency department patients: recognition, risk factors, and psychomotor types. *Acad Emerg Med.* 2009;16(3):193–200.

Huang LW, Inouye S, Jones R, et al. Identifying indicators of important diagnostic features of delirium. *J Am Geriatr Soc.* 2012;60(6):1044–1050.

Powney MJ, Adams CE, Jones H. Haloperidol for psychosis-induced aggression or agitation (rapid tranquillisation). *Cochrane Database Syst Rev.* 2012;(11):CD009377.

12 Constipation

Allen R. Last, MD, MPH, & Jonathan D. Ference, PharmD, BCPS

KEY POINTS

- Constipation is a common problem with more than 33% of people aged 60 years and older reporting these symptoms at any given time. (SOR **C**)
- Constipation can be categorized as normal- or slow-transit constipation, pelvic floor dysfunction or defecatory disorder constipation, and constipation due to secondary causes. These categories can be helpful in tailoring treatment. (SOR **C**)
- When constipation does not respond to initial therapy, a thorough history and abdominal and rectal examination is needed to rule out secondary causes (Tables 12–1 and 12–2) and define the underlying process. (SOR **C**)
- Laboratory testing is only indicated if alarm symptoms (Table 12–3) are present. (SOR **C**) Other diagnostic tests to consider to further define the cause are anorectal manometry, balloon expulsion test, barium or magnetic resonance defecography, and/or colonic transit testing. (SOR **C**)
- When no alarm symptoms are present, empiric treatment should be tried initially including increasing fiber in diet, exercise for fitness, and fluids. (SOR **C**)
- If constipation continues, options include fiber supplements, osmotic agents or polyethylene glycol 3350, stimulant laxatives, intestinal secretoagogues, or enemas. (SOR **C**)

I. **Definition.** Constipation is either the actual or a perceived difficulty with defecation. This can be from infrequent stools or difficult passage of stool or both. Classically, constipation has been defined as having fewer than three bowel movements per week. Often patients report being constipated in spite of having more than three weekly bowel movements; these patients usually have some problem with the passage of stool. The American Gastroenterological Association defines constipation as "difficult or infrequent passage of stool, hardness of stool or a feeling of incomplete evacuation." Chronic constipation should include some combination of these symptoms for at least 3 of the previous 12 months.

II. **Common Diagnosis.** Constipation is a common problem in Western cultures, with 15% of the general population and more than 33% of people aged 60 years and older reporting these symptoms at any given time. It is reported more commonly among women, elderly persons, those of non-Caucasian ethnicity, institutionalized patients, individuals from lower socioeconomic groups, and those living in northern states and rural areas. Constipation results in 8 million office visits to physicians and 92,000 hospital admissions annually in the United States. Nearly 5% of all pediatric office visits are for constipation.

Constipation can be categorized as normal-transit constipation (NTC), slow-transit constipation (STC), pelvic floor dysfunction or defecatory disorder constipation, and as due to secondary causes.

A. **NTC, the most common form of constipation,** was formerly referred to as "functional constipation." Patients with NTC have normal stooling frequency but perceive constipation because of symptoms of bloating, abdominal pain, and hard

TABLE 12–1. SECONDARY CAUSES OF CONSTIPATION

Drug Effects	See Table 12–2
Mechanical obstruction	Colon cancer
	External compression from malignancy
	Strictures
	Rectocele
	Postsurgical changes
	Megacolon
	Anal fissure or hemorrhoid
	Inflammatory bowel disease
Metabolic conditions	Diabetes mellitus
	Hypothyroidism
	Hypercalcemia
	Hypokalemia
	Hypomagnesemia
	Uremia
	Cystic fibrosis
	Heavy metal poisoning
Myopathies	Amyloidosis
	Myotonic dystrophy
	Scleroderma
Neuropathies	Parkinson disease
	Spinal cord injury or tumor
	Cerebrovascular accident
	Autonomic neuropathy
	Hirschsprung disease
	Multiple sclerosis
Other conditions	Anxiety
	Depression
	Somatization
	Cognitive impairment
	Immobility
	Pregnancy

stools. Causes include poor fiber intake, dehydration, physical inactivity, motility disorders such as irritable bowel syndrome, and suppressing the defecation reflex, as sometimes seen in children who have had previous painful experiences with bowel movements.

B. **STC** is typically seen in young women, often beginning with the onset of puberty. These patients often have fewer high-amplitude peristaltic waves than patients without constipation, resulting in colonic contents not being advanced effectively. The cause is unknown, but it is theorized that STC is a disorder of the autonomic or enteric nervous system and/or a dysfunctional neuroendocrine system.

C. **Pelvic floor dysfunction or defecatory disorder constipation** results from abnormal anal sphincter tone or pelvic floor muscle tension and contraction. Stool accumulates in the distal colon normally, but patients are unable to relax the perineum and anal sphincter or produce strong enough rectal propulsive force to allow stool to pass normally. Risk factors include multiparity, perineal surgeries, and a prolonged history of straining to stool.

D. **Secondary causes** should be considered in the diagnosis of constipation (Table 12–1). Included among the secondary causes are medications (Table 12–2), mechanical or anatomical obstruction (rectoceles, cancers, and postsurgical scarring), metabolic derangements (hypothyroidism, diabetes mellitus, and hypercalcemia), myopathies (amyloidosis and scleroderma), neuropathies (Parkinson disease, multiple sclerosis, cerebrovascular events), and other conditions.

TABLE 12–2. MEDICATIONS ASSOCIATED WITH CONSTIPATION

Examples

Nonprescription medications

Sympathomimetics	Ephedrine
Nonsteroidal anti-inflammatory drugs	Ibuprofen, naproxen
Antacids	Aluminum hydroxide, calcium carbonate
Calcium supplements	Calcium carbonate/citrate
Iron supplements	Ferrous sulfate/gluconate
Antidiarrheals	Loperamide, bismuth salicylate

Prescription medications

Anticholinergics	Benztropine, trihexylphenidate
Antihistamines	Diphenhydramine
Antidepressants	Tricyclics, amitriptyline
Antiparkinson agents	Levodopa, benztropine
Calcium-channel blockers	Verapamil, nifedipine
Antispasmodics	Dicyclomine
Antipsychotics	Chlorpromazine, haloperidol, risperidone
Diuretics	Furosemide
Opiates	Codeine, morphine, oxycodone, hydrocodone

1. **Hirschsprung disease** should be considered in any neonate who does not have a bowel movement within 48 hours of birth. It is typically diagnosed in newborns, but if not identified until infancy often presents with abdominal bloating, pencil-thin stools, failure to thrive, and bilious vomiting. The rectum will be empty on examination. A delay in diagnosis can lead to enterocolitis (fever, bloody diarrhea, and abdominal distension) in the second or third month of life.

   E. **Fecal impaction** is the presence of stool that cannot be evacuated by the patient. Prolonged and chronic constipation can lead to impaction. Fecal impaction typically occurs in the rectum and should be removed by manual disimpaction (scooping or scissoring motion of the fingers in the rectum). Higher impactions should be loosened with enemas. Avoid oral laxative agents until after an impaction has been resolved. Endoscopy is sometimes needed to remove higher impactions.

III. Symptoms and Signs

   A. **History.** A thorough history is needed to rule out secondary causes and define the underlying process when constipation does not respond to initial therapy. Symptoms suggesting constipation include abdominal bloating and/or pain, infrequent bowel movements, straining to defecate, hard stools, infrequent defecation, inability to defecate at will, and sometimes nausea.

      1. The clinician should elicit details about the problem such as the frequency and consistency of bowel movements, whether straining or external manipulation is necessary to induce a bowel movement, what attempts at treatment have been made, and the effectiveness of these attempts. A review of systems to rule out the presence of secondary causes should be performed.

      2. The presence of any **alarm symptoms** (Table 12–3) should prompt a thorough evaluation.

TABLE 12–3. ALARM SYMPTOMS/SIGNS REQUIRING DIAGNOSTIC EVALUATION

- Hematochezia
- Family history of colon cancer
- Family history of inflammatory bowel disease
- Anemia
- Positive fecal occult blood test
- Weight loss ≥10 pounds
- Severe, persistent constipation that is not responsive to treatment
- New onset constipation in people over 50 years of age without prior colon cancer screening

    B. Abdominal examination. Normal or hypoactive bowel sounds may be auscultated. Palpation may reveal an abdominal mass, typically in the left lower quadrant, which represents a stool bolus or more rarely a tumor or intussusception. Serial examinations should be performed to rule out a fixed mass.

    C. Rectal examination. A careful rectal examination is often the most helpful portion of the clinical evaluation. The perianal skin should be assessed for scars, fissures, hemorrhoids, and fistulas. The perineum should be observed at rest and during straining to evaluate the degree of perineal descent (2–4 cm is normal). A digital rectal examination should be performed to determine sphincter tone and rule out impaction, anal strictures, and masses. Women should be evaluated for a rectocele as a potential cause of constipation. Rectal examination in newborns should only be performed by those with expertise to interpret anatomical abnormalities.

IV. Laboratory Tests

    A. Laboratory testing is **only indicated if alarm symptoms are present,** including lack of response to initial therapy or if specific medical disorders are identified from the history and physical examination. A complete blood count is recommended. Thyroid-stimulating hormone, serum electrolytes, calcium, glucose, and urinalysis may be useful in patients with constipation. (SOR **⊙**)

    B. Fecal occult blood testing is a quick, inexpensive screening test for colon cancer, but suffers from a relatively high rate of false positives and negatives.

    C. Colonic imaging. Plain film radiographs will reliably diagnose fecal impactions, but are less useful for routine constipation. Colonoscopy or barium enema should be pursued in patients older than 50 years of age or with alarm symptoms (Table 12–3). (SOR **⊙**)

    D. Specialized testing. Anorectal manometry can be used to measure the pressures generated in the rectum to diagnose pelvic floor dysfunction and defecatory disorders and Hirschsprung disease. Balloon expulsion testing (a balloon filled with 50 cm^3 of air or water) can reveal a defecatory disorder. Defecography (an expulsion of a barium enema under fluoroscopy, magnetic resonance imaging, or scintigraphy), which evaluates the emptying mechanism of the rectum, is most useful when anorectal testing is inconsistent with the clinical impression. Colonic-transit testing can be measured when the etiology is still unclear even after laboratory evaluation, colonic imaging, and anorectal evaluation. Normal transit time is less than 72 hours. (SOR **⊙**)

V. Treatment. Treatment of constipation should be directed by history, physical examination, and diagnostic testing. The principal goals of therapy are to identify and treat secondary causes, relieve symptoms, and restore normal bowel function. Treatment of underlying disorders or discontinuation of offending agents may improve constipation. **When no alarm symptoms are present, empiric treatment should be tried initially.** The basis of therapy includes nonpharmacologic therapy, such as lifestyle modification, and pharmacologic therapy if needed. Figure 12–1 describes an initial approach to the patient with constipation.

    A. Lifestyle modifications of increasing fiber, fitness, and fluids (The 3 Fs) are simple measures to improve bowel function. These may be employed alone or in addition to pharmacologic therapy. Patient education and appropriate lifestyle modifications are the basis of maintenance of normal bowel function.

        1. Bowel training may be a simple first-line approach. Patients should be instructed to attempt to move their bowels at the same time each day. Optimal times to have a bowel movement are typically after waking, eating, or physical activity. Colonic activity is the greatest during these times. A stool diary may be helpful to record frequency, consistency, size, and degree of straining. (SOR **⊙**)

        2. Increasing **dietary fiber bulk** is considered a mainstay of nonpharmacologic therapy. Increased dietary fiber increases fecal bulk by promoting movement of water into the feces and bacterial proliferation. Foods high in fiber include beans, whole grains, bran cereals, fresh fruits, and certain vegetables (asparagus, Brussels sprouts, cabbage, and carrots) (http://www.nlm.nih.gov/medlineplus/dietaryfiber.html). Adding dietary or supplemental fiber is easy and inexpensive. The daily recommended fiber intake is 20 to 35 g, but most Americans consume 5 to 10 g. Patients should increase fiber slowly by 5 g per day each week until reaching the daily recommended intake to avoid gas, cramping, malabsorption, diarrhea, or constipation. Advise patients with constipation to avoid processed low-fiber foods (e.g., luncheon meats, hot dogs, certain cheeses, ice cream). (SOR **⊙**)

        3. Patients should be encouraged to be as **physically active** as possible because a low activity level is associated with a twofold increased risk of constipation. Walking

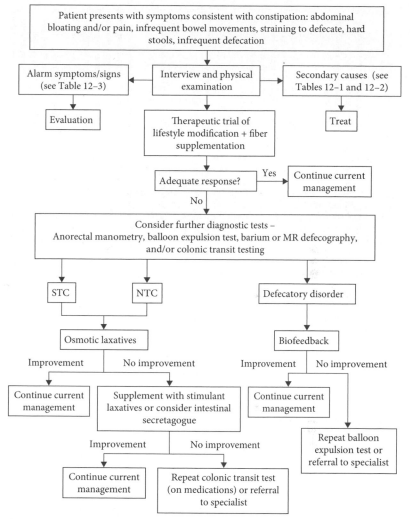

FIGURE 12–1. Approach to the patient with constipation. STC, slow-transit constipation; NTC, normal-transit constipation. (*Source:* Data from Bharucha AE, Dorn SD, Lembo A, Pressman A. American Gastroenterological Association medical position statement on constipation. *Gastroenterology.* 2013;144(1):211–217.)

and other aerobic exercises help to tone the muscles of the lower abdominal area, promoting propulsion in the bowel. (SOR **C**)

4. Adequate **fluid** intake is considered important to maintain normal bowel motility. A general recommendation of 32 oz of water daily may help maintain normal stool frequency. (SOR **C**)

5. **Biofeedback** therapy is considered by some to be the cornerstone for managing pelvic floor dysfunction. However, while therapy may improve symptoms in some patients with defecatory disorder, no high-quality research studies currently support its use. (SOR **C**)

B. **Pharmacologic therapy** (Table 12–4) may be employed when nonpharmacologic measures fail. Guidelines suggest the treatment for NTC and STC begin with a gradual increase of fiber intake (as both foods included in the diet and as supplements). If there is

TABLE 12–4. PHARMACOLOGIC THERAPY OPTIONS FOR CONSTIPATION

Drug[a]	Dose	Major Side Effects	Contraindications	Drug Interactions
Bulk-forming Agents				
Psyllium[a]	Adult: 2.5–30 g per day in divided doses Pediatric: 1.25–15 g per day in divided doses	Impaction above strictures, fluid overload, gas, and bloating	Fecal impaction, gastrointestinal obstruction	There are no known significant interactions
Methylcellulose[a]	Adult: Two caplets up to six times per day or 1 tablespoon up to three times per day Pediatric: One caplet up to six times per day or 2.5 teaspoons up to three times per day			There are no known significant interactions
Polycarbophil[a]	Adult: 1250 mg one to four times per day Pediatric (6–12 years): 625 mg one to four times per day			Bisphosphonates (↓ concentration), quinolone antibiotics (↓ absorption), thyroid products (diminished therapeutic effect)
Wheat dextrin powder	Adult: Stir well two teaspoons into 4–8 oz of any beverage or soft food (hot or cold), three times daily. Pediatric (6–11 years): One teaspoon three times per day			There are no known significant interactions
Osmotic Laxatives				
Polyethylene glycol[a]	Adult: 17 g of powder (~1 heaping tablespoon) dissolved in 4–8 oz of beverage, once daily Pediatric: 0.5–1.5 g/kg daily (initial dose: 0.5–1 g/kg; titrate to effect); not to exceed 17 g per day	Nausea, bloating, cramping	Use with caution in patients with electrolyte disturbances or bowel obstruction	There are no known significant interactions
Lactulose[a]	Adult: 10–20 g (15–30 mL) daily; may increase to 40 g (60 mL) daily if necessary Pediatric: No dosing recommendations	Abdominal bloating, flatulence	Patients requiring a low galactose diet	There are no known significant interactions
Sorbitol[a]	Adult: 30–150 mL (as 70% solution) Pediatric: 2 mL/kg (as 70% solution)	Abdominal bloating, flatulence	Anuria; use with caution in patients with electrolyte disturbances, cardiopulmonary disease, or renal impairment	There are no known significant interactions
Glycerin (glycerol)[a]	Adult: One adult suppository once daily as needed Elderly: Refer to adult dosing Pediatric: One pediatric suppository once daily as needed	Rectal irritation	None	Calcium polystyrene sulfonate (enhanced adverse/toxic effect), sodium polystyrene sulfonate (enhanced adverse/toxic effect)
Magnesium sulfate[a]	Adult: Two to six teaspoons of granules dissolved in water once daily Pediatric: One to two teaspoons of granules dissolved in water once daily	Watery stools and urgency	Heart block, myocardial damage; use with caution in renal impairment (magnesium toxicity)	Bisphosphonates (↓ concentration), calcitriol (↑ concentration of magnesium salts), calcium polystyrene sulfonate (enhanced adverse/toxic effect)
Magnesium citrate[a]	Adult: 195–300 mL given once or in divided doses Pediatric: 60–90 mL given once or in divided doses (2–6 years), 90–210 mL given once or in divided doses (6–12 years)		Low sodium diet; use with caution in patients with neuromuscular disease and renal impairment	

Drug	Dose	Side effects	Contraindications	Drug interactions
Stimulant Laxatives				
Bisacodyl[a] (oral medication or rectal suppositories)	Adult: Oral: 5–15 mg as single dose, Rectal: 10 mg as single dose. Pediatric: Oral: Children >6 yrs: 5–10 mg (0.3 mg/kg) at bedtime or before breakfast; Rectal: 5 mg as a single dose (<2 yrs), 10 mg (>2 yrs)	Gastric irritation (oral), rectal irritation (suppository)	Abdominal pain or obstruction, nausea, or vomiting	Antacids (diminished therapeutic effect)
Senna[a]	Adult: Sennosides 15 mg once daily (maximum: 70–100 mg per day, divided twice daily). Pediatric: Sennosides: Initial: 3.75 mg once daily (maximum: 15 mg/day, divided twice daily) (2–6 yrs), Sennosides: Initial: 8.6 mg once daily (maximum: 50 mg per day, divided twice daily) (6–12 yrs)	Melanosis coli	Intestinal obstruction, acute intestinal inflammation (e.g., Crohn disease), colitis ulcerosa, appendicitis, abdominal pain of unknown origin	There are no known significant interactions
Intestinal Secretagogues				
Lubiprostone[a] (Amitiza)	Adult: 24 μg twice daily. Pediatric: No dosing recommendations	Nausea, diarrhea	Known or suspected mechanical bowel obstruction	Methadone: (diminished therapeutic effect of lubiprostone)
Linaclotide (Linzess)	Adult: 145 μg once daily. Elderly: Refer to adult dosing (not adequately studied). Pediatric: No dosing recommendation	Diarrhea, bloating	Known or suspected mechanical gastrointestinal obstruction	There are no known significant interactions
Surfactants (Softeners)				
Docusate sodium[a] Docusate calcium[a]	Adult: 50–500 mg per day in one to four divided doses. Pediatric: 10–40 mg per day in one to four divided doses (infants and children aged <3 yrs), 20–60 mg per day in one to four divided doses (3–6 yrs), 40–150 mg per day in one to four divided doses (6–12 years)	Well tolerated; use lower dose if administered with another laxative; contact dermatitis reported	Concomitant use of mineral oil; intestinal obstruction, acute abdominal pain, nausea, or vomiting	There are no known significant interactions
Other				
Methylnaltrexone (Relistor)	Adult: Subcutaneous: Dosing is according to body weight: Administer one dose every other day as needed; maximum: one dose per 24 h, <38 kg: 0.15 mg/kg (round dose up to nearest 0.1 mL of volume), 38 to <62 kg: 8 mg, 62–114 kg: 12 mg, >114 kg: 0.15 mg/kg (round dose up to nearest 0.1 mL of volume). Elderly: Refer to adult dosing. Pediatric: No dosing recommendations	Abdominal pain, flatulence, nausea	Known or suspected mechanical bowel obstruction	Peginterferon Alfa-2b (may decrease the serum concentration of methylnaltrexone)

[a]Available as generic.

no improvement in symptoms, inexpensive osmotic agents or polyethylene glycol 3350 (PEG 3350) may be initiated. Depending on response and stool consistency, supplementation with a stimulant laxative may be considered. Newer agents, lubiprostone and linaclotide, should be considered when symptoms do not respond to laxative therapy. NTC and STC can be safely managed with long-term use of laxatives. However, aggressive laxative use may obscure underlying pathology; if constipation is refractory to medical treatment further evaluation is warranted, including possible referral. Patients with defecatory disorder may be initially treated with biofeedback. If there is no symptom improvement, repeat balloon expulsion testing and a referral for further evaluation is warranted.

1. **Bulk-forming agents** (fiber supplements) including psyllium (natural), calcium polycarbophil, methylcellulose (synthetic), and wheat fiber (natural) increase stool mass and soften stool consistency by absorbing water from the intestinal lumen. Generally these agents are well tolerated, but synthetic agents may cause less bloating and flatulence because they are indigestible. However, psyllium may be more effective in increasing stool frequency than synthetic agents. Patients should be instructed to increase daily fluid intake (up to 2–3 quarts of water) to maintain adequate hydration. While generally less effective than other agents (e.g. PEG 3350, lubiprostone), due to their low cost and favorable side-effect profile, fiber supplements are reasonable first-line options. (SOR **B**)

2. **Surfactants** (stool softeners) lower surface tension and allow more water to be incorporated into stool. Although these agents are well tolerated, they may not be as effective as psyllium in increasing stool frequency and are ineffective as monotherapy in the treatment of opioid-induced constipation. Mineral oil is not routinely recommended because of the potential risk of aspiration or depletion of fat-soluble vitamins A, D, E, K. (SOR **B**)

3. **Osmotic laxatives** cause secretion of water into the intestinal lumen by osmotic activity. These agents may be **saline laxatives** (magnesium hydroxide [milk of magnesia] or magnesium citrate and sodium phosphate) or **hyperosmolar** agents (lactulose, sorbitol, PEG 3350).

   a. **Saline laxatives** work within the lumen and are not systemically absorbed, but may cause electrolyte disturbances within the lumen resulting in hypokalemia and salt overload. Hypermagnesemia can result from chronic use of magnesium products, especially in patients with renal insufficiency. There are insufficient data to make a recommendation about the effectiveness of milk of magnesia for chronic constipation. (SOR **B**)

   b. **Hyperosmolar agents.** Lactulose is available as prescription and sorbitol and PEG 3350 as nonprescription products. Poor systemic absorption of these agents often causes flatulence and abdominal pain. Large doses of hyperosmolar agents are frequently used to evacuate the bowel for colonoscopy or surgery. Glycerin suppositories are locally active when inserted in the rectum. PEG 3350, and to a lesser extent lactulose, are effective in improving stool frequency and consistency in patients with chronic constipation. (SOR **A**)

4. **Stimulant laxatives** are the most common products used for acute symptomatic relief. Senna and bisacodyl exhibit their effects within hours by stimulating the colonic myenteric plexus, increasing motility. Bedtime administration may be beneficial in producing a morning bowel movement. Stimulant laxatives should not be used in patients with suspected intestinal obstruction, and research is not available to support their routine use for the treatment of chronic constipation. (SOR **B**)

5. **Intestinal secretagogues** stimulate net efflux of ions and water into the intestinal lumen, accelerate transit, and facilitate ease of defecation. These newer agents may be beneficial in the treatment of adults with chronic constipation refractory to other treatments.

   a. **Lubiprostone (Amitiza)** and **linaclotide (Linzess)** are FDA approved for the treatment of adults with chronic idiopathic constipation lasting at least 12 weeks. They activate chloride channels of the small intestine resulting in increased intestinal secretion. These agents increase the frequency of spontaneous bowel movements and may lower the risk of treatment failure in adults with chronic idiopathic constipation, but expense limits their routine use. (SOR **B**)

6. **Enemas** are useful for evacuating the distal colon and the rectum. Various agents are used, but plain warm water suffices in most cases. Enemas are usually the

treatment of choice for fecal impactions, but there is insufficient evidence to support their routine use for chronic constipation. (SOR **C**)

7. **Methylnaltrexone** (Relistor), a selective antagonist of peripheral mu-opioid receptors, is labeled for the treatment of opioid-induced constipation in patients with advanced illness who have not responded to laxative therapies. In clinical trials, discontinuation rates of methylnaltrexone have been lower than placebo with the most common adverse effects reported to be flatulence and nausea. In patients with at least a 2-week history of opioid-induced constipation who have failed laxative therapy, a significantly greater percentage of patients experienced a bowel movement within 4 hours of administration compared with placebo (NNT = 2). (SOR **B**)

SELECTED REFERENCES

Auth MKH, Vora R, Farrelly P, Baillie C. Childhood constipation. *BMJ.* 2012;345:e7309.
Bharucha AE, Dorn SD, Lembo A, Pressman A. American Gastroenterological Association medical position statement on constipation. *Gastroenterology.* 2013;144(1):211–217.
Bharucha AE, Pemberton JH, Locke GR 3rd. American Gastroenterological Association technical review on constipation. *Gastroenterology.* 2013;144(1):218–238.
Fratini JC, Nogueras JJ. Slow transit constipation: as review of a colonic functional disorder. *Clin Colon Rectal Surg.* 2008;21(2):146–152.

---

13 Cough

Jennifer E. Lochner, MD, & David Holmes, MD

KEY POINTS

- The most common cause of acute cough is viral upper respiratory illness. (SOR **C**)
- The most common causes of chronic cough are postnasal drainage in nonsmokers and tobacco irritants/chronic bronchitis in smokers. Other common causes are asthma and gastroesophageal reflux disease (GERD). (SOR **C**)
- Treatment of cough is directed at the underlying disease. (SOR **C**) Antibiotics are not indicated for viral infections. (SOR **A**)

I. Definition. A cough is a sudden explosive forcing of air through the glottis, occurring immediately on opening the previously closed glottis. It is initiated by airway inflammation, mechanical/chemical irritation of airways, or pressure from adjacent structures.

    A. The following classification of cough is used: **acute cough** lasts <3 weeks, **subacute cough** lasts 3 to 8 weeks, and **chronic cough** lasts >8 weeks.

II. Common Diagnoses. Cough is the most common presenting symptom in primary care, accounting for approximately 30 million office visits each year in the United States.

    A. Acute cough. The most common cause of acute cough in adults and children is viral infection, including upper respiratory infection (URI), sinusitis, bronchitis, and bronchiolitis. At times, cough may represent a more serious condition such as pneumonia, pulmonary embolism (PE), or heart failure. Exacerbations of asthma or chronic obstructive pulmonary disease (COPD) are other considerations. Environmental or occupational exposures including tobacco smoke, allergens, pollutants, and medications can contribute to acute (or chronic) cough. Inhalation of a foreign body must always be considered with sudden onset of cough in children.

        1. Viral URIs. Viral URIs are the most frequent illnesses in humans, with a prevalence as high as 35% worldwide. Thirty to fifty percent of all common colds are caused by rhinovirus; well over 200 other viruses may cause URI; the most common include echovirus, coxsackievirus, influenza virus, respiratory syncytial virus, parainfluenza virus, coronavirus, and adenovirus. Risk factors for development of URIs include exposure to URI, cigarette smoke, and other irritants.

2. **Acute bronchitis.** Acute bronchitis is one of the most common diagnoses in primary care. Up to 95% is viral, most commonly influenza (types A and B), respiratory syncytial virus, parainfluenza, coronavirus, and adenovirus; less common causes include *Mycobacterium pneumoniae*, *Bordetella pertussis*, and *Chlamydia pneumoniae*. Risk factors for acute bronchitis include exposure to viral URI, cigarette smoke and other irritants, and history of COPD.

3. **Sinusitis.** Sinusitis is very common in the United States, resulting in 25 million office visits annually. Acute sinusitis lasting less than 3 weeks is most often viral; other identified causative organisms include *Streptococcus pneumoniae* (most common bacterial etiology), *Haemophilis influenzae*, *Moraxella catarrhalis*, Group A *Streptococci*, *Staphylococcus aureus*, and anaerobes. Risk factors for sinusitis include history of URI, allergic rhinitis, nasotracheal or nasogastric intubation, dental infections, barotrauma (deep-sea diving, air travel), cystic fibrosis, irritants, nasal polyps, and tumors.

4. **Asthma exacerbation.** Approximately 26 million adults and children in the United States have asthma and 3000 to 4000 die each year because of it. Risk factors for asthma exacerbation include allergen exposure (e.g., mold, pollen, dust, animal dander, cosmetics), respiratory infection, exposure to irritants (e.g., smoke), exercise, and gastroesophageal reflux disease (GERD).

5. **COPD exacerbation.** COPD is common in the United States and worldwide; it is the third leading cause of deaths in the United States. It is estimated that up to 60% to 85% of people with COPD (mostly mild/moderate severity) are undiagnosed. Besides tobacco smoking, biomass exposure (wood-burning stoves), secondhand smoke, air pollution, and work exposures to fumes and dusts cause COPD in susceptible people. Infections (both viral and bacterial) cause the majority (~80%) of COPD exacerbations (see Chapter 71).

6. **Irritants.** Cigarette smoke is the most common offending irritant; the 40–50 million Americans who smoke and those breathing their smoke are at risk for this cause of coughing. Other irritants include pollutants and allergens.

7. **Allergic rhinitis.** Allergies to dust mites, molds, animals, and pollen occur in 8% of US residents, predominantly children and adolescents. Risk factors for allergic rhinitis include asthma, eczema, urticaria, and a family history of related symptoms.

8. **Angiotensin-converting enzyme inhibitor (ACE-I).** Up to one-third of patients taking an ACE-I develop a persistent dry cough. Onset of cough is usually within 2 weeks of starting the medication but may be delayed up to 6 months.

9. **Pneumonia.** Each year there are over 5 million cases of pneumonia in the United States, 1.1 million hospitalizations, and 50,000 deaths, making pneumonia the ninth most common cause of deaths in the United States. Persons at highest risk for pneumonia include smokers; those with chronic lung disease; the elderly; the immunocompromised; those with renal or hepatic failure, diabetes, or malignancy; and those in nursing homes or hospitals. A patient's age helps determine likely causative organisms:

   a. **Less than 6 months.** Group B *Streptococcus*, *Listeria monocytogenes*, *C. trachomatis*, and respiratory syncytial virus

   b. **Six months to 5 years.** *S. pneumoniae* and *H. influenza*

   c. **Young adults.** *S. pneumoniae*, *Mycoplasma pneumoniae*, and *C. pneumonia*

   d. **Elderly:** *S. pneumoniae*, *H. influenzae*, *Moraxella catarrhalis*, and *Legionella pneumophila*

10. **PE.** Cough is reported in about 20% of patients with PE. Dyspnea is the more common presenting symptom. Predisposing factors include recent orthopedic injury or surgery, malignancy, and estrogen use (see Chapter 64).

11. **Congestive heart failure (CHF).** Cough may be triggered by volume overload and pulmonary edema in a patient with CHF (see Chapter 73). CHF is most commonly associated with hypertension, diabetes, ischemic heart disease, and valvular heart disease.

12. **Aspiration.** Virtually everyone aspirates oral secretions or what they are eating or drinking at some point in their lives, but subsequent cough reflex protects the airway. Risk factors for more serious aspiration include being very old or very young (younger than 3 years) or having impaired gag or swallowing reflex. Foreign body aspiration is most common in young children and can be life-threatening if obstruction of large airways occurs.

B. **Subacute and chronic cough** (see Table 13–1).

   1. **Postinfectious cough** due to airway hyperresponsiveness, persisting inflammation, and excess mucus production following URI is a common cause of **subacute**

TABLE 13–1. DIFFERENTIAL DIAGNOSIS OF SUBACUTE AND CHRONIC COUGH

Differential Diagnosis	Etiology/Mechanism of Action	Risk Factors/History	Signs on Physical Examination	Testing
Postinfectious cough	URI → extensive inflammation → airway epithelial damage → hypersensitivity of the airway receptors to inhaled irritants	Recent URI; cough usually resolves in 3 weeks but may persist up to 7 weeks	Usually absent; possible wheezing	None
Pertussis	Inflammation of the larynx, trachea, and bronchi caused by *Bordetella pertussis*; attacks and damages cilia	Occurs in 5.5% of patients ≥16 years with persistent cough; initially: URI symptoms; 10–14 days after paroxysmal cough often, but not necessarily, followed by an inspiratory "whooping" sound, post-tussive vomiting lasting 2–12 weeks	Afebrile or mild fever, weight loss, lung consolidation (in 20%–25% of cases), post-tussive cyanosis	PCR testing of a nasopharyngeal specimen and serologic assays; WBC count (usually 15–20,000 and lymphocytosis >70%)
Postnasal drainage (PND or "upper airway cough syndrome")	Rhinitis (allergic and nonallergic) and sinusitis cause PND, which is aspirated Bacterial causes of chronic sinusitis include *H. influenzae, S. pneumoniae,* and oral anaerobes	Most common cause of chronic cough in nonsmokers; persistent URI symptoms, history of seasonal allergies, feeling something dripping/tickling in back of throat, frequent throat clearing, hoarseness, facial pain, tooth pain **Allergic:** red, itchy eyes, tearing, itching roof of mouth, otherwise unexplained cough, symptoms made worse by rhinitis or sinusitis, lying down, allergens, temperature changes, and pregnancy	Erythematous, swollen nasal mucosa and turbinates, nasal polyps, deviated nasal septum, purulent nasal discharge, sinus tenderness; pharyngeal cobblestoning/postnasal drainage **Allergic:** boggy nasal mucosa, conjunctivitis, tearing	Sinus CT
Smoking and other environmental irritants	Irritation of airways	Smoker or exposure to secondhand smoke or other irritants, cough worse in specific environments such as work or home	Often absent; possible wheezing	In a smoker with chronic cough, consider evaluation for COPD, infection, or cancer with spirometry, CXR, sputum assessment
Gastroesophageal reflux disease (GERD)	Transient loss of LES tone → increase in acid reflux and aspiration of gastric contents → irritation and airway inflammation	Chronic cough is the sole symptom in up to 75% of patients; heartburn, sour taste in back of throat, sore throat, regurgitation, laryngitis, dysphonia; symptoms worse with lying down, exercise, caffeine, alcohol, acidic foods; GERD causes chronic cough in up to 41% of adults	Usually absent, possible epigastric tenderness	24-h pH monitoring (consider if symptoms do not resolve after 3–6 months of therapy); upper GI series and upper endoscopy in those chronically symptomatic to assess complications of GERD

(continued)

TABLE 13–1. DIFFERENTIAL DIAGNOSIS OF SUBACUTE AND CHRONIC COUGH (Continued)

Differential Diagnosis	Etiology/Mechanism of Action	Risk Factors/History	Signs on Physical Examination	Testing
Asthma	Inflammation (mast cells infiltrate the smooth muscle cells in the airways) and hyperresponsiveness of airways result in airflow obstruction	Nonproductive cough is sole symptom in 50%; history of allergies and atopy; family history, wheezing, dyspnea, chest tightness, disturbed sleep; symptoms exacerbated by exercise, cold air, night-time, allergens, and respiratory infection	Bilateral expiratory wheezing and prolonged expiratory phase; respiratory distress, dyspnea, tachypnea, use of accessory respiratory muscles	PFTs (pre- and post-bronchodilator therapy); consider methacholine challenge test, pulse oximetry, sputum for eosinophils (should be high); sinus CT for concomitant sinusitis
COPD	Bronchial inflammation, excessive mucous production, and decreased ability of mucociliary system to clear secretions	Most common cause of chronic cough in smokers; history of smoking, ↑ sputum production, worse in morning, shortness of breath, dyspnea on exertion, wheezing; chronic bronchitis is diagnosed with a productive cough for at least 3 mo/yr for two consecutive yrs	Scattered rhonchi, wheezes (especially forced expiration), crackles, prolonged expiration or distant breath sounds, though lungs may be clear, no evidence of pulmonary consolidation	CXR, pulse oximetry, PFTs (pre- and post-bronchodilator therapy), ABG
Eosinophilic bronchitis (nonasthmatic)	Eosinophilic airway inflammation, similar to asthma, but with no airflow obstruction or airway hyperreactivity; mast cells localize within airway epithelium, unlike in asthma where the mast cells infiltrate smooth muscle cells	Cough, but no wheeze; exposure to allergens and occupational chemicals	Often absent; lung sounds are clear	Induced sputum for eosinophils (should be high), CXR (should be negative), PFTs (should be normal)
ACE inhibitors (ACE-Is) and other medications	ACE-I: unclear mechanism, Beta-blockers → bronchospasm, Nitrofurantoin → pulmonary fibrosis	Five to 30% of those taking ACE-I develop cough; if onset of cough is within 2 weeks of starting medication, suspect medication; reaction may be delayed up to 6 months	Usually absent	None
Cancer (primary pulmonary, Hodgkin lymphoma, metastatic disease)	Mechanical compression of airways	Rarely presents solely with cough; other symptoms include weight loss, dyspnea, hemoptysis, often a history of smoking	Weight loss, cachexia, fever, dyspnea	CXR, CT scan, MRI, bronchoscopy with biopsy, sputum cytology
Tuberculosis (TB)	Mycobacterium tuberculosis infection transmitted by inhaling airborne bacilli from a person with active TB	History of TB exposure, HIV, immigration from countries with high prevalence, homelessness, substance abuse, in prison or nursing home; fatigue, fever, night sweats, weight loss, anorexia, dyspnea, hemoptysis, pleuritic chest pain	Fever, crackles near lung apices, extrapulmonary TB may involve almost any organ and produce signs related to the specific site (such as recurrent UTIs, adenopathy, and meningitis)	Testing for extrapulmonary TB as directed by history and examination

ABG, arterial blood gases; BNP, B-type natriuretic peptide; CHF, congestive heart failure; COPD, chronic obstructive pulmonary disease; CT, computerized tomography; CXR, chest x-ray; HIV, human immunodeficiency virus; LES, lower esophageal sphincter; MRI, magnetic resonance imaging; PCR, polymerase chain reaction; PFTs, pulmonary function tests; PPD, purified protein derivative; URI, upper respiratory infection; UTI, urinary tract infection.

cough, usually resolving by 7 weeks after the URI. **Pertussis** must be considered with prolonged URI with prominent cough.

2. The prevalence of **chronic cough** in the United States is 14% to 23% in nonsmoking adults and children; it is three times higher in smokers. Chronic cough is also more common in the elderly, school-aged children, and people exposed to air pollution in urban areas.

   a. In more than 90% of persons, chronic cough is caused by **postnasal drip** (**PND**—referred to as upper airway cough syndrome or UACS in some literature), **asthma, smoking,** or **GERD**. Often, chronic cough is caused by a combination of diagnoses and some diagnoses commonly overlap as in GERD contributing to PND and upper airway inflammation.

   b. Other considerations for chronic cough are nonasthmatic eosinophilic bronchitis, ACE-I-induced cough, cancer (lung, lymphoma, metastatic disease), tuberculosis, and psychogenic or "habit cough."

3. **Less common causes of subacute and chronic cough** include pulmonary conditions such as pulmonary abscess, fungal infection, sarcoidosis, and bronchiectasis (irreversible dilation of bronchi/bronchioles because of inflammation or obstruction). Upper airway causes include compression from a goiter, Zenker (hypopharyngeal) diverticulum, or cancer. In children, laryngotracheomalacia is a consideration. Psychogenic causes include habit cough and Tourette syndrome (with a cough tic). External auditory canal irritation is another possibility (i.e., Arnold reflex—cerumen or hair on the tympanic membrane stimulating cough receptors).

4. **In infants with chronic cough** consider congenital vascular anomalies; **asthma is most common in older children**. Also common are GERD, respiratory infections, and psychogenic causes. Less common are cystic fibrosis, immunologic and fungal disorders, Tourette syndrome, and primary ciliary dyskinesia.

III. **Symptoms and Signs.** Diagnosis can be made by history alone in 70% to 80% of individuals with cough. Characteristics of cough, such as paroxysmal, barking, honking, brassy, self-propagating; productiveness; and timing during the day have not proved reliable in determining the cause. Associated symptoms of PND, heartburn, or wheezing can be important clues to a diagnosis.

The physical examination in patients with acute or chronic cough should focus on **vital signs** (higher temperature tends to indicate bacterial infection; tachypnea and tachycardia can indicate a more serious cause of cough as can hypoxemia as evaluated by pulse oximetry); **ear canals** (for hairs/cerumen on tympanic membrane [Arnold reflex]); **nares** (for edema, drainage, polyps, erythema); **sinuses** (for tenderness, indicative of URI or sinusitis); **oropharynx** (for cobblestoning, indicative of PND); **neck** (for masses/lymphadenopathy, indicative of infection or cancer); **lungs** (for localized inspiratory wheeze [foreign body or masses], diffused expiratory wheeze [bronchospasm], basilar fine crackles [pulmonary edema], percussion dullness, egophony, decreased breath sounds [pneumonia], or rhonchi [nonspecific], though absence of these findings does not exclude lung disease); **heart** (for S3 [CHF], or murmur [valvular disease]).

A. **Acute cough**

1. **Viral URI.** Viral URI features coryza, malaise, chills, rhinorrhea, fever, sore throat, sneezing, and nasal congestion. Examination findings often include clear rhinorrhea, pharyngeal erythema, cervical adenopathy, low-grade fever, and clear lungs (see Chapter 54).

2. **Acute bronchitis.** Following URI symptoms, a nonproductive cough may become productive. This occurs in 90% of patients with acute bronchitis. Cough persists ≤3 weeks in 50% of patients, but more than a month in 25%. Other symptoms include wheezing, fatigue, hemoptysis, and mild dyspnea. The lung examination may reveal crackles, rhonchi, or wheezing (especially with forced expiration), but often lungs are clear. Fever, injected pharynx, or cervical lymphadenopathy may also occur. Acute bronchitis should not be diagnosed until viral URI, asthma, and an acute exacerbation of chronic bronchitis have been ruled out.

3. **Sinusitis.** Sinusitis is suggested by URI symptoms lasting >10 days, nasal congestion, PND, maxillary or frontal headaches, and purulent rhinorrhea (see Chapter 54). Fever is uncommon.

4. **Asthma exacerbation.** In asthma, wheezing and shortness of breath usually accompany cough, though sometimes cough is the only symptom (see Chapter 68). Wheezes are often heard on lung examination.

5. **COPD exacerbation.** In a patient with known COPD, an exacerbation is typically signaled by increasing cough, dyspnea, and sputum production (see Chapter 71). If the exacerbation is triggered by infection, there also may be URI symptoms. Rhonchi and/or wheezes are heard on examination.

6. With **irritants,** there may be few symptoms other than cough. Chemical gas irritant exposure may in addition cause headache, lightheadedness, or confusion.

7. **Allergic rhinitis** presents with clear rhinorrhea, sneezing, watery eyes, and itching, often in the spring or fall when allergens are most common. On examination, pale boggy nasal mucosa is often noted along with red watery eyes and postnasal drainage.

8. **ACE-I cough** typically presents as a dry hacking cough that begins within 2 weeks of starting an ACE-I. It may however present much later after starting the medication.

9. **Pneumonia.** Symptoms include fever, chills, pleuritic chest pain, dyspnea, and myalgia; the elderly may also or predominantly present with confusion or delirium. Signs include fever, tachypnea, hypoxia, cyanosis, and evidence of pulmonary consolidation, or localized crackles or rhonchi. Atypical pneumonia may have minimal or no lung findings.

10. **PE.** Dyspnea and pleuritic chest pain are the most common symptoms in PE. Common signs include tachypnea, tachycardia, and sometimes a painful swollen leg, indicating lower extremity deep vein thrombosis (DVT) as a source (see Chapter 64).

11. **CHF.** A patient with decompensated heart failure typically presents with symptoms and signs of volume overload: cough and dyspnea, lower extremity edema, and fatigue (see Chapter 73).

12. In **aspiration,** there is sudden intractable cough, which may be accompanied by choking, vomiting, wheezing, shortness of breath, dysphagia, and acute anxiety. Examination findings with aspiration range from minimal localized wheezing to severe tachypnea and respiratory distress with hypoxemia.

B. **Subacute/chronic cough** (see Table 13–1).

1. **Postinfectious cough** follows URI and tends to have few other signs or symptoms. It may persist up to 7 weeks.

2. **Pertussis** should be considered in a patient with URI symptoms who also has episodes of paroxysmal coughing, sometimes followed by an inspiratory "whooping" sound or posttussive emesis. Signs may include low-grade fever with either normal lung examination or rhonchi or signs of consolidation.

3. **PND** is the most common cause of chronic cough in nonsmoking adults. It is usually associated with sinusitis or allergic rhinitis but GERD may also contribute to airway inflammation and mucus production. Patients usually report a sense of drainage down the back of the throat with frequent throat clearing and hoarseness, but up to 20% of PND may be clinically "silent." Examination findings typically include swollen nasal mucosa and either clear or purulent nasal discharge.

4. **Exposure to smoke and other irritants** as a cause of chronic cough is assessed via history. The examination is usually normal.

5. **GERD** may present as isolated cough in up to 75% of patients. Others report the classic heartburn and sour taste in the back of the throat. The examination is usually normal.

6. **Asthma** may also present as isolated cough in up to 50% of patients (see Chapter 68). Often there is a personal or family history of atopy or allergic disease. Dyspnea and chest tightness may also be reported. Wheezing is the classic physical examination finding.

7. **COPD** is usually found in tobacco smokers but other environmental exposures such as smoke from wood burning stoves are risk factors as well (see Chapter 71). Dyspnea, especially with exertion, tends to be a prominent symptom to accompany cough. Signs include rhonchi, wheezes, and prolonged expiratory phase. In more severe disease, there may be decreased breath sounds as airway obstruction worsens.

8. **Non-asthmatic eosinophilic bronchitis** is a condition of airway inflammation similar to asthma but with no airway obstruction or hyperreactivity. Patients typically cough but do not wheeze. Lungs are typically clear to examination.

9. **ACE-I-induced cough** is diagnosed based on history; there are no examination findings to support this diagnosis.

10. Cough due to **cancer** (primary lung or metastatic disease) is often associated with systemic symptoms such as fever or weight loss and also other pulmonary symptoms including dyspnea and hemoptysis. Tobacco exposure is a risk factor for many cancers.

Examination may be normal or may reveal cachexia or signs of consolidation on lung examination.

11. Risk factors for **TB** include immigration from a country with a high incidence of TB, homelessness, and incarceration. Classic presenting symptoms are fevers, night sweats, dyspnea, anorexia, and hemoptysis. On examination, lungs may sound clear or may reveal apical rales or rhonchi.

12. Psychogenic cough should be considered in patients with a history of depression or anxiety and no other localizing signs or symptoms.

IV. Laboratory Tests. Tests are directed by history and examination findings (see Table 13–1). In patients with acute cough, where a cause is clear, treatment can generally be initiated without further testing. Further testing in acute cough is generally reserved for the very ill, atypical presentations, or poor response to standard treatment (see below).

A. Hematologic tests

1. **White blood cell (WBC) count** may assist in assessing febrile patients to support or refute a diagnosis of bacterial infection (increased neutrophils) or viral infection (increased lymphocytes).

2. **Antibody titers** may be helpful in suspected fungal infection (aspergillosis, histoplasmosis, or coccidioidomycosis).

3. **Arterial blood gases** can assist assessment of hypoxemia in patients with severe asthma, pneumonia, COPD, or other pulmonary disease.

4. **Serologic testing (e.g., enzyme-linked immunosorbent assay [ELISA])** helps confirm suspected human immunodeficiency virus (HIV) infection.

5. **B-type natriuretic peptide (BNP),** a cardiac neurohormone produced by the ventricles in response to ventricular volume expansion and pressure overload, may assist in differentiating a cardiac from a pulmonary origin of cough. Levels >100 pg/mL indicate CHF and those >480 pg/mL correlate with a nearly 30-fold increase in cardiac events over the next 6 months.

B. Spirometry can differentiate obstructive from restrictive disease (asthma or COPD from sarcoidosis, pulmonary fibrosis, or interstitial lung disease, respectively).

1. **Pre- and postbronchodilator testing** evaluates for fixed as compared with reversible airway obstruction (e.g., asthma vs. COPD).

2. **Bronchoprovocative testing** with methacholine inhalation uncovers subtle reversible airway obstruction in suspected patients with asthma and normal or near-normal spirometry. Methacholine challenge is not widely available; its sensitivity approaches 100% in ruling out asthma, but its specificity is 60% to 80%, so positive testing does not conclusively rule in asthma.

3. **Spirometry** is difficult to perform in children younger than 5 years, so diagnosis in these patients is based on history, examination, and response to treatment.

4. **Peak expiratory flow rate (PEFR)** testing is an office procedure helpful in quantifying severity of airflow obstruction and response to treatment in acute asthma exacerbations.

C. Radiography/special imaging

1. **Chest x-ray (CXR)** is helpful in evaluating for pneumonia or complicated aspiration (localized infiltrates), bronchiectasis, COPD (hyperinflation/flat diaphragms), TB (fibro-nodular upper lobe infiltrates, cavitary lesions, hilar adenopathy, pleural effusion), sarcoidosis (hilar adenopathy), and pulmonary edema/CHF (vascular congestion, Kerley B-lines, perihilar infiltrates, pleural effusion, cardiomegaly). This testing should be ordered early in the evaluation of unexplained cough.

2. **Barium swallow** may be helpful in adults or young children with chronic cough to assess for GERD or vascular anomalies.

3. **Upper GI series** assists in evaluating those with chronic cough and poorly responsive GERD (for hiatal hernia or complications, such as ulceration and stricture).

4. **Computerized tomographic (CT) or magnetic resonance imaging (MRI)** of the chest assists in evaluating for bronchiectasis, interstitial lung disease, mass lesions of sarcoidosis, or neoplasms in patients whose clinical evaluation raises suspicion for these problems. CXR should precede CT or MRI. **Sinus CT** is the gold standard for diagnosing chronic sinusitis and should be considered with chronic PND, recurrent episodes of sinusitis, or pediatric asthma. Approximately 50% of children with asthma have radiographic evidence of sinusitis, and studies have shown that treatment of sinusitis decreases bronchial hyperresponsiveness. Therefore, all children with asthma should be evaluated for concurrent sinusitis.

5. Echocardiogram assesses left ventricular function and ejection fraction in suspected CHF.

D. Endoscopy

1. Referral for **bronchoscopy** is indicated in patients with (1) recurrent hemoptysis, (2) CT/MRI suggesting malignancy, or (3) chronic cough without diagnosis after evaluation for common causes.

2. **Nasopharyngoscopy** can be helpful in visualizing the turbinates/sinus ostia, pharynx, and larynx in individuals suspected of having cough originating in these structures (e.g., those with chronic sinusitis).

3. **Esophagogastroduodenoscopy (EGD)** is used to evaluate for GERD complications (such as esophagitis, ulceration and stricture, Barrett esophagus, and adenocarcinoma).

E. Other tests

1. **Sputum cytology** may be helpful if history or CT/MRI suggest malignancy.

2. **Sputum gram stain, culture, and smears** may also be used. The presence of many eosinophils suggests nonasthmatic eosinophilic bronchitis. Gram stain and culture of induced sputum may be useful in identifying a causative organism in pneumonia.

3. **A 24-hour esophageal pH monitoring** is 92% sensitive for GERD but is invasive. It should therefore be performed only after failure of empiric GERD treatment and a negative evaluation for asthma and sinusitis.

4. **Pulse oximetry** allows easy, noninvasive assessment of arterial oxygen saturation and is helpful in assessing the severity of acute disease or response to therapy in patients with asthma, pneumonia, or COPD.

5. **Purified protein derivative (PPD)** skin testing is a useful screen for pulmonary TB and should be considered in all patients with chronic cough, especially those at high risk. A PPD must be read within 48 to 72 hours of placement. A test is considered positive if the diameter of the reaction measures ≥5 mm for HIV-infected and other immunocompromised individuals, ≥10 mm for those at high risk, and ≥15 mm for all others. If a PPD test is positive, a CXR should be ordered. Symptomatic patients should be placed in respiratory isolation, pending results of a sputum smear with acid-fast stain and *Mycobacterium* culture. The Centers for Disease Control and Prevention no longer recommends routine anergy testing in conjunction with PPD skin testing among HIV-infected individuals.

6. **Nasal smear** may be helpful in differentiating allergic from nonallergic rhinitis (showing eosinophils and white blood cells, respectively).

7. **Skin testing** for allergies may be helpful in clarifying the role of allergens in cough and in evaluating severe, poorly controlled perennial allergic symptoms for possible benefit from desensitization.

8. **Polymerase chain reaction** testing of a nasopharyngeal specimen is helpful in diagnosing pertussis in individuals with suggestive clinical findings.

9. **Sweat chloride testing** is necessary in evaluating children with cough and other features suggestive of cystic fibrosis (failure to thrive, gastrointestinal abnormalities, and recurrent infections).

V. Treatment directed at the underlying disease is reported to be successful 80% to 95% of the times. For most conditions, management should include hydration, humidification, and rest. (SOR **C**) If the diagnosis is initially unclear, empiric treatment for the most likely cause may be preferable to extensive investigation, because such treatment may provide relief as well as diagnosis (Figure 13–1). Adequate treatment is important. In one study, many patients were correctly diagnosed by their primary care physician before pulmonology referral, but treatment was not aggressive enough to stop the cough.

A. Cough suppressants

1. **Prescription medications.** There is no evidence for the use of beta-2 agonists (e.g., albuterol), leukotriene inhibitors, or inhaled steroids in treating nonspecific cough in children or adults who do not have airflow obstruction. (SOR **A**) There are no randomized, controlled studies assessing the efficacy of prescription benzonatate (Tessalon Perles) compared with placebo.

2. **Most nonprescription medications** for cough of presumed viral origin are no better than placebo. (SOR **A**) However, there is some evidence that the older, sedating antihistamine–decongestant combination medications are useful in treating cough in adults, but not in children. (SOR **B**) Treatment should take effect within 1 week. The newer, nonsedating antihistamines have not been shown to be efficacious in adults or children.

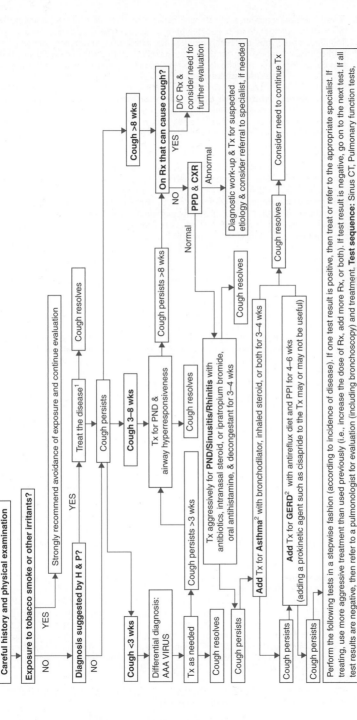

FIGURE 13–1. Cough management algorithm. [1]Or discontinue medication, such as ACE-I, if that is thought to be the cause of cough. [2]Treatment for asthma and GERD are added, not substituted, based on the fairly high prevalence of patients having two (23% to 42%) or even three (3% to 15%) causes of chronic cough. ACE-I, angiotensin-converting enzyme inhibitor; CT, computerized tomography; CXR, chest x-ray; GERD, gastroesophageal reflux disease; PND, postnasal drainage; PPI, proton pump inhibitor; PPD, purified protein derivative; Rx, prescription; Tx, therapy.

    a. Several nonprescription products are associated with side effects, particularly in children younger than 6 years where some adverse effects of nonprescription medications may be life-threatening. Reported adverse reactions of common medications include hypertension, tachycardia, central nervous system (CNS) stimulation (agitation, psychosis, seizures, insomnia), dysrhythmias, and myocardial infarction **(pseudoephedrine)**; CNS depression and anticholinergic symptoms, tachycardia, blurred vision, agitation, hyperactivity, seizures, torsades de pointes **(chlorpheniramine and brompheniramine)**; and lethargy, stupor, hyperexcitability, abnormal limb movements, and coma **(dextromethorphan)**.

    b. If patients want to try a nonprescription cough suppressant or expectorant (and are older than 6 years), they may experience a beneficial effect, including a placebo effect. Sucking on hard candies may have a similar effect.

B. Acute cough

  1. Viral URI (see Chapter 54). Central cough suppressants, such as codeine and dextromethorphan, are not recommended for cough caused by URI (SOR ®) and neither is zinc. (SOR ®) As noted above, older sedating antihistamine–decongestant combination medications and naproxen can be useful in treating cough in adults, but not in children. (SOR ®) Antibiotics are not indicated. Patients often underestimate the expected duration of cough with URI which can last 17.8 days (mean duration).

  2. Acute bronchitis. Supportive treatment for acute bronchitis includes rest, fluids (3 to 4 L/day, especially with fever). Beta-2 agonists (i.e., albuterol) are not effective if there is no bronchospasm. (SOR ®) Patients should expect to have a cough for 10 to 14 days. Patient satisfaction with the office visit does not depend on receiving an antibiotic, but instead on effective physician–patient communication. Patients should be advised that antibiotics are probably not going to be beneficial and that antibiotic treatment is associated with significant risks and side effects. To help patients understand the viral nature of their illness, it is helpful to refer to acute bronchitis as a "chest cold." Initial antibiotic prescription may be considered in patients with significant COPD, immunocompromised patients, patients with CHF, the elderly, and those appearing very ill or with high fever. (SOR ®) The American College of Chest Physicians recommends considering an antibiotic if there is not at least some improvement of the cough by day 7. [SOR ®]

  3. Sinusitis/postnasal drainage (see Chapter 54).

  4. Asthma exacerbation (see Chapter 68).

  5. COPD exacerbation (see Chapter 71).

  6. Irritant-related cough. Avoidance of the offending agent and smoking cessation should be encouraged. Approximately 75% of people stop coughing within a month of eliminating offensive exposures. (See Chapter 104 for suggestions on effective smoking cessation techniques.)

  7. Allergic rhinitis (see Chapter 54).

  8. ACE-I cough. ACE-Is and other medicines causing cough should be eliminated or changed (e.g., substituting an angiotensin receptor blocker for an ACE-I). Cough should resolve within 4 weeks after these changes.

  9. Pneumonia

    a. Antibiotics for outpatient treatment of community-acquired pneumonia include a macrolide (e.g., erythromycin, azithromycin, or clarithromycin) for suspected *M. pneumoniae* or trimethoprim-sulfamethoxazole or amoxicillin clavulanate for other causes. (SOR ®) Treatment should generally continue for 10 to 14 days, and symptomatic improvement should occur within 2 to 3 days.

    b. Supportive treatment includes antipyretics/analgesia and hydration.

    c. Hospitalization may be necessary, depending on comorbidities, support at home, and severity of illness. Indicators of severe illness include age older than 65 years, multiple medical problems, altered mental status, hypoxia (O_2 saturation <90% or PaO_2 <60 mmHg on room air), hypercapnia ($PaCO_2$ >45 mmHg), acidosis (arterial pH <7.35), hypotension, tachypnea, tachycardia, multi-organ dysfunction, anemia (Hb <9 g/dL), significant leukopenia or leukocytosis (<4000 WBC/mm^3 or >30,000 WBC/mm^3, respectively), or multi-lobe densities or large pleural effusion on CXR.

  10. PE (see Chapter 64).

  11. CHF. Medical management of CHF involves ACE-Is or ARBs, diuretics, beta-blockers, and aldosterone antagonists (see Chapter 73).

12. **Aspiration.** Inhaled foreign bodies may be dislodged with back slaps, chest thrusts, or the Heimlich maneuver. If concern remains for an inhaled foreign body, bronchoscopy is recommended for diagnosis and treatment.

C. **Subacute/chronic cough**

1. **Postinfectious cough.** Hyperresponsiveness of airways persists for up to 8 weeks after URI and resolves without treatment. Significant cough warrants a trial of a bronchodilator and an antihistamine, with addition of an inhaled steroid. (SOR ❸) If cough persists, oral steroids (SOR ❸) and/or inhaled ipratropium bromide (SOR ❸) can be used.

2. **Pertussis**

a. **Antibiotics.** Antibiotics do not alter the course of the illness, unless initiated early in its course; however, antibiotics do prevent transmission and decrease the need for respiratory isolation from 4 weeks to 1 week.

b. **Suggested regimens.**

(1) **Macrolide antibiotics** are the treatment of choice. (SOR ❹) One option is 14 days of **oral erythromycin,** 500 mg four times a day for adults and 40–50 mg/kg per day divided into four doses for pediatric patients, with a maximum of 2 g per day. Side effects include nausea, vomiting, diarrhea, and, in infants, pyloric stenosis.

(2) **Azithromycin** 500 mg on day 1 and 250 g on days 2 to 5 for adults and 10 mg/kg per day for 5 days in pediatric patients is also effective. Azithromycin is the safest therapy for infants younger than 1 month. (SOR ❸)

(3) **Clarithromycin** 500 mg twice daily for 7 days or 15 mg/kg divided bid in pediatric patients can also be used effectively.

c. **Alternative regimen. Oral trimethoprim-sulfamethoxazole-DS** twice daily in adults and 8 mg trimethoprim plus 40 mg sulfamethoxazole/kg day divided into twice-daily doses in pediatric patients for 14 days is also effective. (SOR ❹) It should be used only in patients who are allergic or have an intolerance to macrolides. It is **contraindicated** in women who have a term pregnancy or are breastfeeding, and in infants <2 months old.

d. **Hospitalization** is recommended for seriously ill patients, especially infants. (SOR ❸)

e. **Close household contacts should** be treated with antibiotics to prevent transmission of the disease. (SOR ❸)

f. **Vaccine.** Adolescents should receive Tdap instead of the Td booster. (SOR ❸) Adults should receive a Tdap booster one time instead of Td. (SOR ❸)

3. **Smoking and other environmental irritants.** Smoking cessation (see Chapters 71 and 104) and removal of irritants if possible or protective equipment if occupational exposure.

4. **Gastroesophageal reflux disease (GERD)** (see Chapter 19). Four to six weeks of treatment with a proton pump inhibitor successfully diagnoses and treats the vast majority of patients with GERD-related cough. (SOR ❹) Lifestyle interventions including avoidance of dietary triggers may also be helpful.

5. **Asthma** (see Chapter 68).

6. **COPD** (see Chapter 71). According to a Cochrane review of patients with COPD exacerbations, antibiotic therapy significantly reduced short-term mortality by 77%, treatment failure by 53%, and sputum purulence by 44%, regardless of the specific antibiotic used. Antibiotics did not affect arterial blood gases and peak flows. Antibiotics are recommended to treat moderately or severely ill patients with COPD exacerbations and a cough with purulent sputum. (SOR ❹) Salmeterol has been shown to decrease symptoms of cough, sputum, and shortness of breath in patients with COPD. (SOR ❸) Codeine and dextromethorphan are recommended for short-term symptomatic relief of cough. (SOR ❸)

7. **Postnasal drainage (PND)** (see Chapter 54). Treat underlying conditions such as allergic rhinitis, sinusitis, and irritant exposure. Postinfectious cough in adults can be treated with an antihistamine and decongestant combination. This is successful in >50% of nonsmokers with PND and chronic cough. (SOR ❸) Persisting cough thought to be due to PND can also be treated with nasal steroids or nasal ipratropium.

8. **Eosinophilic bronchitis (nonasthmatic).** If an allergen or specific occupational exposure is identified as the cause, it should be avoided. (SOR ❸) Inhaled corticosteroids have been shown to be effective. (SOR ❸) If they are not effective, oral steroids should be given. (SOR ❸)

9. **ACE-I and other medicines potentially causing cough.** Eliminating or changing medications (e.g., substituting an angiotensin receptor blocker for an ACE-I) should be attempted. Cough should resolve within 4 weeks after these changes.
10. **Cancer.** Referral to an oncologist is indicated.
11. **Tuberculosis**
    a. **Latent TB** (positive PPD and normal CXR) is treated with oral isoniazid (INH), 5 mg/kg up to 300 mg daily for 9 months, with addition of oral pyridoxine (Vitamin B_6), 25 mg daily, to prevent neuropathy in those older than 35 years. (SOR **A**) Six months of INH therapy can be considered for adults who are not HIV infected and have no fibrotic lesions on CXR. (SOR **B**)
    b. **Active TB** (positive PPD test and abnormal CXR or positive acid-fast bacilli culture/smear) requires reporting to the local health department, respiratory isolation, and multidrug therapy (e.g., oral isoniazid combined with rifampin, pyrazinamide, streptomycin, or ethambutol). (SOR **A**) Because of variable resistance, consultation with an infectious-disease specialist for assistance in drug selection and monitoring is prudent. During therapy, liver function tests should be monitored in those older than 35 years or with a history of drug/alcohol abuse or liver disease.
    c. To ensure compliance and effective treatment and to minimize the emergence of resistant strains, **directly observed therapy** should be implemented throughout treatment.
12. **Psychogenic** (habit cough). Providing reassurance of normal test results can alleviate patient anxiety, increase patient acceptance of diagnosis, and decrease cough symptoms. Persistent psychogenic cough warrants psychological therapy such as counseling, behavior modification, and biofeedback. (SOR **C**)
13. **Idiopathic (or "unexplained").** If no etiology can be determined, options for adults are limited to nonspecific therapies such as dextromethorphan, inhaled ipratropium, and codeine. (SOR **B**) It is important to periodically reevaluate the patient for new signs and symptoms, which may suggest an underlying illness.
14. **In children with chronic cough,** underlying disease should be treated. If the cough is thought to be psychogenic, a referral of the child and family for counseling should be considered. Children with vascular anomalies should be referred to a vascular surgeon.
    a. In general, medications to treat nonspecific cough in children (<15 years old) have not been shown to be effective and are therefore not recommended. (SOR **B**) However, a little improvement has been demonstrated in children with chronic nocturnal cough who were treated with high-dose inhaled steroids. (SOR **B**) Also, a Cochrane review of two studies supported a trial of antibiotics in children <7 years old with chronic cough. (SOR **B**)
    b. It is important to discuss with parents their expectations and fears regarding their child's condition. Education and reassurance may be valuable in the management of cough. (SOR **C**)

SELECTED REFERENCES

Benich JJ, Carek PJ. Evaluation of the patient with chronic cough. *Am Fam Physician.* 2011;84(8): 887–892.
Bolser D. Cough suppressant and pharmacologic protussive therapy, ACCP evidence-based clinical practice guidelines. *Chest.* 2006;129:238S–249S.
Ebell MH, Lundgren J, Youngpairoj S. How long does a cough last? Comparing patients' expectations with data from a systematic review of the literature. *Ann Fam Med.* 2013;11:5–13.
Irwin RS, Baumann MH, Bosler DC, et al. Diagnosis and management of cough executive summary— ACCP evidence-based clinical practice guidelines. *Chest.* 2006;129(1 Suppl):1S–23S.
Smith SM, Schroeder K, Fahey T. Over-the-counter (OTC) medications for acute cough in children and adults in ambulatory settings. *Cochrane Database Syst Rev.* 2012;(8):CD001831.

14   Dermatitis and Other Pruritic Dermatoses

A. Ildiko Martonffy, MD, Jie Wang, MD, Aleksandra Zgierska, MD, PhD, William G. Phillips, MD, & Marjorie Shaw Phillips, MS, RPh, FASHP

KEY POINTS

- Generalized pruritus requires as specific a diagnosis and treatment plan as possible. (SOR ⊙)
- Many serious systemic diseases produce generalized pruritus without skin manifestations. (SOR ⊙)
- Chronic pruritus has a variety of psychological explanations and consequences. (SOR ⊙)

I. **Definition. Pruritus** is an irritating sensation in the skin that causes one to itch and arouses the desire to scratch. **Dermatitis** is inflammation of the skin, whereas **dermatosis** is defined as any disease of the skin in which inflammation is not necessarily a feature.

For the purposes of this chapter, dermatitis and pruritic dermatoses will be considered in terms of the following: (1) primary dermatoses, (2) symptoms of significant internal medical or surgical illness, and (3) primary psychological disturbances.

II. **Common Diagnoses.** Approximately 15% of all patients presenting to primary care providers do so for care of a skin disease or lesion, and pruritic dermatoses are a significant proportion of these. Severe and chronic pruritus may significantly affect quality of life, including causing insomnia/daytime drowsiness, anxiety, distraction from one's daily social functioning, and personal embarrassment.

A. **Pruritic dermatoses**

1. **Atopic eczema** (Figure 14–1), a chronic inflammatory pruritic skin disease, is found in approximately 7 to 24 individuals per 1000 in the United States. It affects children and adults; however, it is more common in infancy and childhood. In 50% of affected children, the condition persists into adulthood. According to the PRAC-TALL Consensus Report, risk factors for developing and predicting the severity of the atopic dermatitis are parental atopy, exposure to aeroallergens (pets, mites, and pollens), sensitization to food allergens, and severity of disease in infancy.

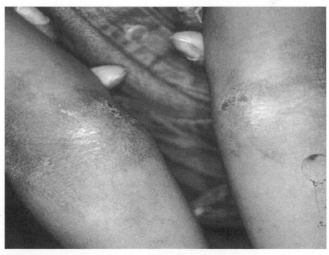

FIGURE 14–1. Atopic dermatitis (see color insert). (This photograph has been taken by and is the property of Dick Anstett, MD, MPH. Faculty, Family Medicine Residency of Idaho, Boise, Idaho.)

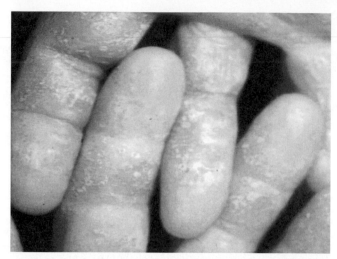

FIGURE 14–2. Contact dermatitis from dishwasher water (see color insert). (This photograph has been taken by and is the property of Dick Anstett, MD, MPH. Faculty, Family Medicine Residency of Idaho, Boise, Idaho.)

2. Contact dermatitis (Figure 14–2) affects 1 in 1000 workers annually and accounts for 50% of occupational illness. Those particularly at risk include workers in manufacturing, food production, construction, machine tool operation, printing, metal plating, and leather processing. The majority of occupational contact dermatitis is irritant-related; however, approximately 40% of cases are believed to be **allergic**. Allergic contact dermatitis is uncommon in young children and less common in deeply pigmented individuals.

3. Scabies (Figure 14–3), caused by the mite *Sarcoptes scabiei,* is an extremely common pruritic infestation with an estimated global prevalence of 300 million. It occurs in both genders and across all ages and is transmitted by close skin-to-skin

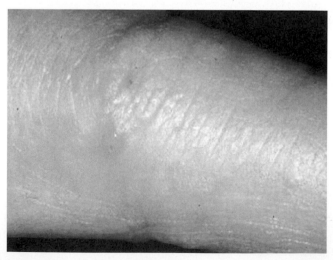

FIGURE 14–3. Scabies (see color insert). (This photograph has been taken by and is the property of Dick Anstett, MD, MPH. Faculty, Family Medicine Residency of Idaho, Boise, Idaho.)

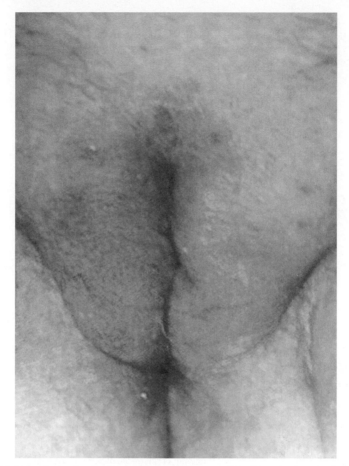

FIGURE 14–4. Lichen simplex chronicus (see color insert). (This photograph has been taken by and is the property of Dick Anstett, MD, MPH. Faculty, Family Medicine Residency of Idaho, Boise, Idaho.)

contact. Scabies should always be considered when multiple family members develop an intense pruritic rash contemporaneously.

4. **Head lice (pediculosis capitis)** affect 6 to 12 million people in the United States annually, occur most frequently in school or daycare settings, and can be spread via direct contact to the head or hair of an infested individual or through the sharing of personal items such as hats or brushes. It is also possible to spread head lice through use of a pillow or head rest that was previously used by an infested individual. Head lice infest all levels of societal and ethnic groups but infestation is less common in African-American children as compared with other races. **Pediculosis pubis** is usually transmitted sexually; it is often seen in the context of venereal disease clinics and student health services. **Body lice (pediculosis humanus)** are much less common than pediculosis pubis or capitis and are usually seen in a setting of poor hygiene, homelessness, and crowded conditions.

5. **Lichen simplex chronicus** (Figure 14–4) is more common in adults than in children; it preferentially affects middle-aged women, atopic individuals, and those experiencing substantial stress.

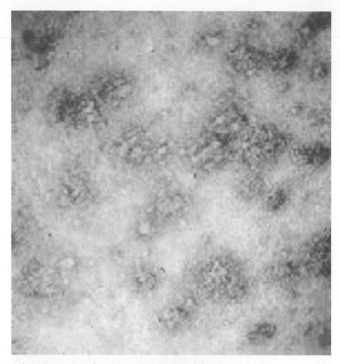

FIGURE 14–5. Lichen planus (see color insert). (This photograph has been taken by and is the property of Dick Anstett, MD, MPH. Faculty, Family Medicine Residency of Idaho, Boise, Idaho.)

6. **Lichen planus** (Figure 14–5) typically begins in the fourth decade. It is associated with a positive family history in approximately 10% of cases. It has also been linked to liver disease (e.g., hepatitis C) and use of certain medications, especially thiazides, captopril, and antimalarials. It is rare in children younger than 5 years.

7. **Xerosis (dry skin)** is common in northern climates, particularly during the winter months with indoor heating and low relative humidity. It is a common problem in the elderly, but can also affect younger individuals and children. It is seen particularly in atopic individuals, those who bathe frequently (especially using strong soaps), those with chemical or solvent exposure, as well as those with hypothyroidism, antiandrogen or diuretic therapy.

8. **Dyshidrosis** (Figure 14–6) accounts for 5% to 20% of all hand dermatitis, is more common during spring and summer in warmer climates, and may be associated with stress.

9. **Pityriasis rosea** (Figure 14–7) is seen more frequently in women than in men, and mostly in persons 10 to 35 years old. The incidence of the disease is higher during the colder months, and some patients have a recent history of viral upper respiratory infection associated with fatigue, headache, sore throat, and fever.

10. **Psoriasis** (Figure 14–8) affects 2% of people of European ancestry. It has a presumed autoimmune etiology and 40% of patients have a positive family history. Summer season, sunlight, and relaxation can improve psoriatic lesions, while upper respiratory and streptococcal infections, trauma to the skin, stress, and certain medications (e.g., lithium, beta-blockers, angiotensin-converting enzyme inhibitors, and indomethacin) can exacerbate psoriasis. Approximately 15% of affected patients develop a seronegative inflammatory arthritis that clinically resembles rheumatoid arthritis. **Guttate psoriasis** occurs in 2% of patients with psoriasis, typically begins before 30 years of age, and affects individuals of all races.

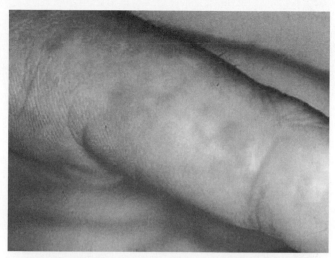

FIGURE 14–6. Dyshidrotic eczema (see color insert). (This photograph has been taken by and is the property of Dick Anstett, MD, MPH. Faculty, Family Medicine Residency of Idaho, Boise, Idaho.)

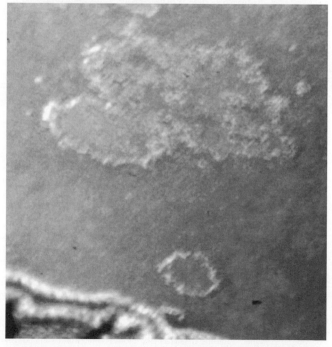

FIGURE 14–7. Herald patch, pityriasis rosea (see color insert). (This photograph has been taken by and is the property of Dick Anstett, MD, MPH. Faculty, Family Medicine Residency of Idaho, Boise, Idaho.)

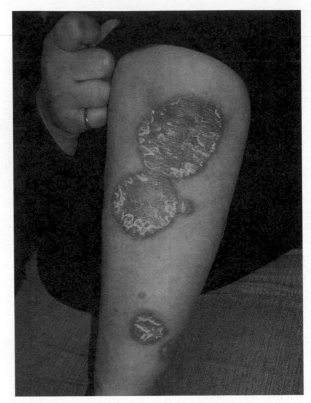

FIGURE 14–8. Typical plaque psoriasis on the elbow and arm (see color insert). (Used with permission from Richard P. Usatine, MD.) (*Source*: From Usatine R, Smith MA, Mayeaux EJ Jr, Chumley H, Tysinger J. The Color Atlas of Family Medicine.1st ed. New York, NY: McGraw-Hill Professional Publishing. Figure 145–1. p. 620.)

11. **Dermatophyte infection** is common, with 10% to 20% estimated lifetime risk of acquisition. **Tinea capitis** (Figure 14–9) is most common in 3- to 8-year-old boys and may occur in epidemics. **Tinea corporis** (Figure 14–10) is frequently seen in farmers and people who have pets. **Tinea cruris** is four times more common in young adults and men than in other groups. Obesity, heat, humidity, perspiration, and chafing predispose individuals to this condition. **Tinea pedis** (Figure 14–11) affects mostly adults (children are rarely infected) and more men than women. Acquisition of the disease appears to depend on a susceptibility factor.

12. **Seborrhea, a chronic inflammatory skin disease** (Figure 14–12), is often familial and most commonly occurs in adult men. It can be associated with hyper-androgenicity (e.g., polycystic ovarian syndrome, hirsutism), diabetes mellitus, Celiac disease, Parkinson disease, and epilepsy; severe seborrhea can be a symptom of human immunodeficiency virus (HIV) infection before other more specific symptoms of this illness occur.

13. **Nummular eczema** (Figure 14–13) typically occurs in young adults and, less commonly, in children. Its etiology is unknown, although the history is often positive for asthma or seasonal allergies, and, in the elderly, a low-protein diet.

B. **Pruritus in systemic disease**

1. **Pruritus can be a presenting symptom of systemic disease** in 10% to 50% of elderly patients. Systemic diseases associated with pruritus include hyperthyroidism, hypothyroidism, polycythemia vera, iron deficiency, obstructive biliary disease, multiple myeloma, HIV, lymphoma, Hodgkin disease (up to 30% of Hodgkin disease

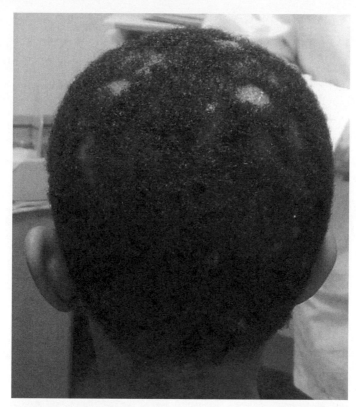

FIGURE 14–9. Tinea capitis in a young black boy (see color insert). (Used with permission from Richard P. Usatine, MD.) (*Source*: From Usatine R, Smith MA, Mayeaux EJ, Chumley H, Tysinger J. The Color Atlas of Family Medicine. 1st ed. New York, NY: McGraw-Hill Professional Publishing. Figure 131–1. p. 549.)

patients present with generalized pruritus), and end-stage renal failure (severe pruritus affects up to 25% of patients with chronic renal failure).

2. **Pruritic urticarial papules and plaques of pregnancy** (PUPP) (Figure 14–14) is the most common skin condition of pregnancy, usually appearing in the late third trimester.

C. **Pruritus with a prominent psychogenic component**

1. **Delusions of parasitosis** (Figure 14–15) are an example of a primary psychiatric disorder with dermatologic manifestations. Those affected by this disorder experience delusions of being infested by bugs, mites, worms, or other creatures, and experience a severe itching as a result of "infestation." Delusions of parasitosis can be symptoms of a primary mental health disorder (e.g., schizophrenia, psychotic depression, hypochondriasis, or some of the addictive disorders, such as alcohol withdrawal, amphetamine, and cocaine effects); they can also be associated with medical conditions (e.g., vitamin B_{12} deficiency, cerebrovascular disease, neurosyphilis, multiple sclerosis), or caused by medication side effects (e.g., glucocorticoids) or medication-related allergic reactions.

2. **Localized psychogenic pruritus** or localized itchiness with subsequent scratching, without identifiable organic pathology, occurs in 9% of patients with pruritus. It typically begins between ages 30 and 45 years and is more prevalent in women (52%–92% of patients). Depression, anxiety, and other mental health disorders can play a significant role in the etiology of the behavior.

III. **Symptoms and Signs** (Table 14–1). The intensity of pruritus in the pruritic dermatoses may vary from mild and annoying to intense. All patients presenting with pruritus, especially

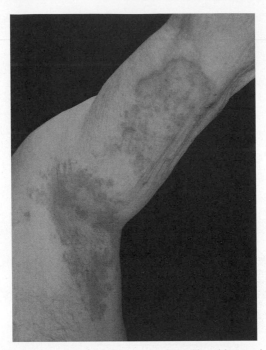

FIGURE 14–10. Extensive tinea corporis in the axilla and arm of this older adult (see color insert). (Used with permission from Richard P. Usatine, MD.) (*Source*: From Usatine R, Smith MA Jr, Mayeaux EJ, Chumley H, Tysinger J. The Color Atlas of Family Medicine. 1st ed. New York, NY: McGraw-Hill Professional Publishing. Figure 132–3. p. 554.)

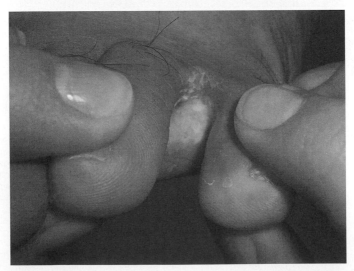

FIGURE 14–11. Tinea pedis seen in the interdigital space between the fourth and fifth digits. This is the most common area to see tinea pedis (see color insert). (Used with permission from Richard P. Usatine, MD.) (*Source*: From Usatine R, Smith MA, Mayeaux EJ, Chumley H, Tysinger J. The Color Atlas of Family Medicine. 1st ed. New York, NY: McGraw-Hill Professional Publishing. Figure 134–3. p. 561)

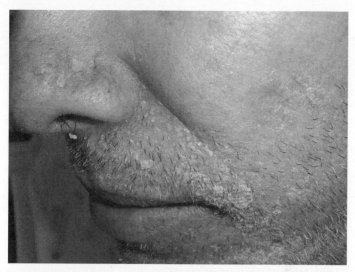

FIGURE 14–12. Severe seborrheic dermatitis on the face of a hospitalized man. The stress of his illness has worsened the otherwise mild seborrhea (see color insert). (Used with permission from Richard P. Usatine, MD.) (*Source:* From Usatine R, Smith MA, Mayeaux EJ, Chumley H, Tysinger J. The Color Atlas of Family Medicine.1st ed. New York, NY: McGraw-Hill Professional Publishing. Figure 144–4. p. 617.)

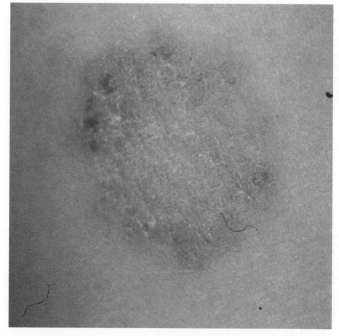

FIGURE 14–13. Nummular eczema (see color insert). (This photograph has been taken by and is the property of Dick Anstett, MD, MPH. Faculty, Family Medicine Residency of Idaho, Boise, Idaho.)

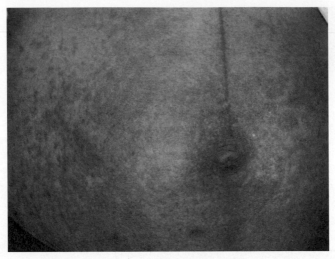

FIGURE 14–14. PUPP (see color insert). (This photograph has been taken by and is the property of Dick Anstett, MD, MPH. Faculty, Family Medicine Residency of Idaho, Boise, Idaho.)

when it is chronic and without characteristic features of common dermatoses (Table 14–1), should be assessed for systemic disease or psychiatric disorders (e.g., anxiety/depression, obsessive–compulsive disorder, or somatoform disorder).

A. Pruritic dermatoses. As with many dermatologic conditions, the diagnosis of most pruritic dermatoses is made on the basis of pattern recognition of skin lesions. **Pattern recognition** is the ability to identify a skin condition by its basic morphology, shape, size, color, distribution, and presence or absence of secondary features, such as pruritus. At times, a particular feature of a lesion or the history of the lesion can be extremely helpful in forming a diagnosis. Examples include (1) the presence of a "herald patch" in pityriasis rosea, (2) the classic distribution of lichen simplex chronicus on the back of the neck, (3) the presence of lice or nits in pediculosis, (4) the presence of mite eggs or feces in scabies, and (5) the linear vesicles or symmetric lesions of contact dermatitis.

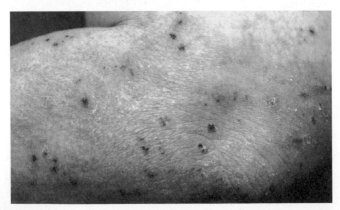

FIGURE 14–15. Delusion of parasitosis (see color insert). (This photograph has been taken by and is the property of Dick Anstett, MD, MPH. Faculty, Family Medicine Residency of Idaho, Boise, Idaho.)

TABLE 14–1. DIFFERENTIAL DIAGNOSES OF COMMON PRURITIC DERMATOSES

Diagnosis	Locations(s) Affected	Usual Morphology
Atopic eczema	Symmetric—cheeks/scalp/chest/ extensor (infants); lichenified flexural/eyelids/perioral (children); flexural hands/forearms/wrists/feet (teen/adult)	Thickened dry plaques
Contact dermatitis	At sites of irritant exposure; shape of irritant (e.g., watchband)	Vesicles (acute) Crusty, lichenification (chronic)
Scabies	Web spaces of fingers, hands, wrists, axillae, buttocks, groin; facial/scalp (infants)	Linear vesicles, erythematous papules Lichenified, excoriated
Lice	Scalp, pelvic, pubic	Nits on hairs ¼ inch from skin (capitis/pubis) Excoriation (body lice)
Lichen simplex chronicus	Back of neck, shoulders, forearms, lower legs, cheeks, perianal	Liner excoriations, scabs, scars
Lichen planus	Flexural wrists, scalp, trunk, ankles, genital, buccal mucosa	Violaceous flat-topped polygonal plaques White streaks on buccal mucosa (Wickham striae)
Xerosis	Especially lower legs	Exaggerated skin lines, plaques with superficial fissures
Dyshidrosis	Palms/web spaces (80% of patients) Feet (10%) Feet and hands (10%)	Burning or itching, followed by deep (tapioca-like) vesicles
Pityriasis rosea	Chest and trunk	Initially papulosquamous oval scaly 2- to 10-cm diameter pink "herald patch" followed by "Christmas tree" pink, scaly oval, salmon-colored macules on back
Psoriasis	Symmetric—elbows/knees/ears/ scalp/umbilicus/gluteal cleft/ genitalia/nails	Sharply demarcated erythematous plaque covered with grayish-white or silver-white scale; pitting/thickened nails 1- to 10-mm pink/red papules with fine scale (guttate)
Tinea corporis	Extremities, face, trunk	Flat scaly papules spreading radially into circinate lesion with raised scaly edge and central clearing
Tinea pedis	Interdigital; plantar	Interdigital scale/fissures Scaling plantar surface (moccasin) Vesiculobullous
Tinea cruris	Groin folds	Radially expanding raised edge with central clearing, slight scale
Seborrhea	Scalp, nasolabial folds, upper chest, postauricular creases, brows, eyelashes	Occasional dry flakes to thick greasy scale Diffuse erythema to oozing cracks
Nummular eczema	Extremities	Coin-red plaques 1–5 cm in diameter with minimal scaling
Primary psychological disorders	Face/scalp/trunk/arms/legs	Excoriations because of scratching or self-inflicted damage from cigarettes, chemicals, or sharp instruments without evidence of underlying skin disorder
Localized psychogenic pruritus	Localized lesions (neck, trunk, extremities)	Linear excoriations, scab, scar

1. **Dyshidrosis** presents with many deep-seated, small, intense pruritic vesicles, most commonly occurring on the hands and the feet. These acute lesions usually last for 3 to 4 weeks and spontaneously resolve, often with associated scaling. Dyshidrosis can recur or progress into chronic lesions that include lichenification and fissuring.
2. **Pityriasis rosea** generally starts as a single large patch (herald patch) followed several days later by more lesions that often follow cleavage lines or appear in a "Christmas tree" pattern on the back and the trunk. These oval lesions, usually with some scaling

at the edges, can take 6 to 12 weeks to spontaneously resolve. Instead of characteristic truncal lesions, African-American individuals can have facial or extremity lesions.

   3. **PUPP** presents with intensely pruritic papules that usually develop on the gravid abdomen near the umbilical area and spreads to the thighs and extremities, sparing the face, palms, and soles. The lesions usually resolve spontaneously within 1 week of parturition.

   B. In patients whose lesions lack the morphology of primary dermatoses (Table 14–1), especially in the elderly, signs of underlying systemic disease (e.g., cholestasis, chronic renal failure, lymphoma, HIV, multiple myeloma) should be carefully sought.

   C. **Primary psychiatric disorders.** Patients with **delusions of parasitosis** often have a positive "matchbox" sign: The patient brings in a matchbox or other container with bits of excoriated skin, debris, or "insect parts" as a "proof" of infestation.

IV. **Diagnostic Tests**

   A. The history and the physical examination are generally all that is necessary to correctly diagnose common primary dermatoses. The tests listed below can be useful to confirm a particular diagnosis.

   1. **Microscopic examination**
      a. With **mineral oil.** In suspected scabies, scrapings of suspected mite burrows should be microscopically examined (with mineral oil); findings of mites and their eggs or feces confirm the diagnosis.
      b. With **potassium hydroxide (KOH).** In tinea, microscopic examination with KOH is a diagnostic test. Skin scrapings are placed on a glass slide, one or two drops of 10% to 20% KOH are added, and the slide is heated gently to dissolve cellular material. Hyphae or spores are characteristic of tinea.

   2. **Wood light examination** is useful in the differential diagnosis of tinea capitis from other conditions. Some forms of tinea capitis fluoresce bright yellow–green under the Wood lamp light. Erythrasma, a skin condition resembling tinea and caused by *Corynebacterium minutissimum*, will fluoresce red.

   3. **Patch testing** is done for allergic contact dermatitis. A patch containing the suspected allergen is applied to the skin for 48 hours and then removed. The skin is observed 20 minutes later for skin reaction in the "patched" area.

   4. **Biopsy**
      a. If an eczema-like lesion involves the nipple and does not subside with simple treatment, biopsy should be performed to evaluate for Paget disease. More than 95% of people with Paget disease of the nipple also have breast cancer.
      b. When the diagnosis is in doubt, a biopsy should be considered.

   5. **Serologic testing** should be considered in cases of pityriasis rosea to rule out syphilis in high risk patients, as the rash of secondary syphilis can mimic pityriasis rosea.

   B. When the diagnosis of a common primary pruritic dermatosis is questionable and the above tests fail to confirm a diagnosis, additional tests should be considered. Further testing is especially indicated in the absence of reassuring factors that help clarify the diagnosis (e.g., localized lesions, cases with recent travel, contacts with a person displaying similar lesions, occupational exposure) in elderly patients or in those with suspected underlying systemic disease. Additional tests include thyroid-stimulating hormone, bilirubin, alkaline phosphatase, blood urea nitrogen, creatinine, complete blood count, HIV testing, and chest radiographs.

V. **Treatment.** Treatment goals include (1) appropriate management of diseases causing pruritus, (2) symptomatic relief, and (3) cosmetic improvement, if indicated.

   A. **General measures**
      1. **Non-medication measures** (SOR **☉**) include some or all of the following:
         a. **Bathing** no more frequently than daily, for 5 to 10 minutes, using warm (not hot) water.
         b. **Using mild soap** (e.g., Alpha-Keri, Cetaphil, Dove, Nivea Cream, Oilatum, Purpose, Basis) or soap-free cleansers (e.g., Cetaphil lotion, Aquanil lotion, SFC lotion, Lowila, Aveeno cleansing), and limiting soap use to specific body areas only (e.g., axillae, genitals, feet, etc.) to avoid drying out the skin excessively.
         c. **Patting** (not rubbing) the skin during drying.
         d. **Applying emollients** within a few minutes of bathing. Emollients range from lotions (least occlusive) to creams (most cosmetically acceptable) to ointments (most occlusive, but also greasy). Additives such as urea (e.g., Carmol, Aqua Care, and

Ureacin) or lactic acid (e.g., Lac-Hydrin, Penecare) can decrease dryness and promote skin hydration.

  e. Using a humidifier during cold months.

  f. Soaking dry, pruritic areas in cool solution of colloidal oatmeal (Aveeno) or baking soda.

  g. Cutting fingernails and wearing cotton gloves during sleep (for individuals who have difficulty controlling scratching).

  h. Avoiding known irritants, for example, alcohol, caffeine, rubber shoes, dyed socks, cosmetics, hairspray, or jewelry.

2. Medications. In individuals with more severe symptoms or lesions that have been refractory to non-medication measures (Section V.A.1), one or a combination of the following medications can be beneficial.

  a. Topical medications

  (1) Corticosteroids (SOR Ⓖ) (Table 14–2)

  (a) The efficacy and side effects of topical corticosteroids depend on several factors, including steroid **potency** (ranging from group 1 to 7, where 1 indicates most potent), **vehicle** potency (ointment > cream > lotions), **anatomic area** (for a given agent, the greatest penetration occurs on the face and groin, the lowest on palms and soles), and lesion **thickness** (thickened plaques are more resistant to treatment than thinner lesions).

  (b) As a general rule, the least potent, effective medication and vehicle should be chosen first to treat the lesion; this preparation should be used for as short a time as necessary. For example, in pediatric patients or those with intertriginous lesions, a group 6 or 7 (the least potent) topical corticosteroid should be prescribed; group 1 or 2 (the most potent) agents are appropriate for thickened lesions on the palm or sole.

  (c) Side effects associated with use of topical corticosteroids are mainly localized to the area of application and are listed in Table 14–2. The risk of systemic side effects (e.g., cataracts, Cushing syndrome, hypothalamic–pituitary–adrenal suppression) increases with the percentage of treated body surface, duration of treatment, and steroid potency.

  (2) Topical antihistamines (e.g., diphenhydramine) or **topical doxepin** (a tricyclic antidepressant), applied to affected areas three to four times daily (doxepin for maximum of 8 days), can be used to relieve pruritus. However, these drugs can cause allergic contact dermatitis.

  b. Oral medications

  (1) Antihistamines. The value of antihistamines in the treatment of pruritus is mainly from their sedative properties. (SOR Ⓖ) They can be useful as a short-term, adjuvant therapy added to topical treatment. The newer second-generation antihistamines are not only less sedating, but also less effective in controlling pruritus when compared with older sedating agents.

  (a) First-generation antihistamines can be sedating and are associated with decreased alertness and worsening of psychomotor performance. Examples include **hydroxyzine** (prescription drug; adults: 25–100 mg orally every 6–8 hours; children older than 12 years: adult dosing, but start with lower doses; children 6–12 years old: 12.5–25 mg orally every 6–8 hours; children younger than 6 years: 2 mg/kg/d orally in three to four divided doses) and **diphenhydramine** (nonprescription agent; administer as needed, adults: 25–50 mg orally every 4–6 hours, maximum 400 mg/day; children older than 12 years: adult dosing, but start with lower doses, maximum 300 mg/day; children 6–12 years old: 12.5–25 mg orally every 4–6 hours, maximum 150 mg/day; children 2–6 years old: 6.25–12.5 mg orally every 4–6 hours, maximum 37.5 mg/d; not recommended in infants or neonates).

  (b) Second-generation antihistamines (all nonprescription) are less sedating but generally less effective in controlling pruritus than older agents. Examples include **loratadine** (adults and children older than 6 years: 10 mg orally once daily; children 2–6 years old: 5 mg orally once daily), **fexofenadine** (adults and children older than 12 years: 180 mg orally once daily or 60 mg orally twice a day; children 6–11 years old: 30 mg orally twice a day; children 6 months to 5 years old:

TABLE 14–2. STEROIDS FOR DERMATOSES

Generic Name of Product	Dosing[a]	Side Effects	Contra-Indications	Drug Interactions
Lowest potency				
Hydrocortisone (cream, ointment, lotion) 0.5%–2.5%	Daily to four times daily	Skin atrophy, hypopigmentation, striae, telangiectasia, steroid rosacea (face), allergy, glaucoma (with prolonged use around the eyes)	Caution: if infection present; application on children risks systemic toxicity	No significant interactions
0.5%–1% available nonprescription				
Low potency				
Betamethasone valerate (cream) 0.01%	Daily to three or four times daily	High potency steroids used over large body surface risks hyperglycemia, Cushing syndrome	Avoid use of high potency on face	
Fluocinolone acetonide (cream, ointment) 0.01%				
Flurandrenolide (cream, [b]ointment, [b]lotion) 0.025%				
Triamcinolone acetonide (cream, ointment, lotion, aerosol) 0.025%				
High potency (for acute, self-limited dermatosis)				
Fluocinolone acetonide (cream) 0.01%–0.025%	Daily to three or four times daily			
Fluocinonide (cream, gel, ointment, solution) 0.05%				
Triamcinolone acetonide (cream, ointment) 0.5%				
Halcinonide (cream, ointment, solution) 0.1%				
Systemic steroids (for recalcitrant cases or cases involving >20% of skin surface)	0.5–1 mg/kg daily for 5–7 d followed by taper over the next 1–2 wks	Cataracts, glaucoma, hypertension, weight gain, CHF, osteoporosis, PUD, nausea, vomiting, immune suppression, child growth suppression, emotional instability (euphoria, insomnia, depression)	Systemic fungal infection, active infection (TB, recent varicella, measles history of ocular HSV); pregnancy class D	Bupropion (seizure risk), fluoroquinolones (risk of tendon rupture), montelukast (severe peripheral edema), aspirin (additive risk of GI toxicity), phenobarbital, phenytoin, rifampin, fluconazole (decreased effect of prednisone)
Prednisone				
Adult and pediatric dose 5–60 mg daily				

CHF, congestive heart failure; PUD, peptic ulcer disease; GI, gastrointestinal.
[a]Usual adult doses. Patients should be instructed to apply sparingly to skin in a light film and rub in gently.
[b]Available as a 58 g spray.

15–30 mg orally twice a day), **cetirizine** (adults and children older than 6 years: 5–10 mg orally once daily; children 2–6 years old: 2.5–5 mg orally daily; children 12–24 months old: 2.5 mg orally once–twice daily, maximum 5 mg/d; children 6–12 months old: 2.5 mg orally once daily).

    (c) Tricyclic antidepressants have antihistaminic and sedative effects and can be beneficial in reducing pruritus, as well as promoting sleep (e.g., **doxepin,** adults: 10 mg orally once daily at bedtime, may gradually increase to 25 mg at bedtime; it is not approved for use in pediatric patients). Tricyclic antidepressants should be used with caution in persons receiving other sedative medications, in the elderly, and in patients with cardiac conduction defects or prostatic hypertrophy.

  (2) Oral corticosteroids (SOR ⊙) can be beneficial for acute flare-ups or pruritic lesions that are refractory to other therapies. Prednisone can be prescribed as a short "burst" (4–5 days, 40–60 mg per day on average—this dosing can be stopped without tapering) or longer therapy, if needed (e.g., starting with 60 mg per day for 1–3 days, followed by tapering). "Burst" therapy minimizes side effects complicating long-term oral steroid therapy (Table 14–2). Systemic corticosteroid therapy should be used particularly cautiously in children.

B. Therapies for specific dermatoses

  1. Atopic dermatitis (atopic eczema)

    a. The foundation of treatment is regular use of emollients and conscientious **skin hydration** (see Section V.A.1), as well as avoidance of irritants and specific triggers. (SOR ⊙)

    b. For mild breakthrough symptoms despite the foregoing treatment, a **low-to-moderate-potency steroid** can be added; (SOR ⊙) for persistent or more severe breakthrough symptoms, a higher-potency topical steroid can also be used (see Table 14–2).

    c. Oral antihistamines, especially the first-generation sedating agents, can be beneficial as a short-term, adjuvant therapy in relieving pruritus, in conjunction with topical therapy.

    d. Topical immunosuppressants, tacrolimus and **pimecrolimus,** are approximately as effective as medium-potency topical corticosteroids. They can be used when glucocorticoids are ineffective or contraindicated, and are considered a second-line therapy for moderate-to-severe atopic dermatitis. (SOR ⊙) Common side effects associated with use of these medications include skin burning, erythema, and pruritus that are usually minor and self-limited, resolving after a few days of therapy. Tacrolimus and pimecrolimus do not cause skin atrophy, but have received a "black box warning" due to their association with rare cases of malignancies (e.g., skin cancer and lymphoma). Therefore, current recommendations (SOR ⊙) include avoiding continuous long-term use of topical tacrolimus and pimecrolimus, and their use should be limited to areas affected by atopic dermatitis. **Dosage of tacrolimus:** adults can apply thin layer of 0.03% or 0.1% ointment topically to affected areas twice daily; children older than 2 years can apply a thin layer of 0.03% ointment twice a day; **dosage of pimecrolimus:** adults can apply 1% cream topically to affected areas twice daily; children 2 years and older can use 1% cream twice daily. Tacrolimus and pimecrolimus are not approved for topical use in children younger than 2 years.

    e. Dilute bleach baths have been shown to reduce bacterial superinfection of eczematous lesions and eczema severity for patients with atopic dermatitis and frequent superinfection caused by *Staphylococcus aureus.* Two to four ounces (four to eight tablespoons) of regular household bleach is mixed into a full bathtub creating a solution of diluted bleach (about 0.005%), which is just slightly stronger than chlorinated swimming pool water. The patient should soak in the water for 10 minutes and then rinse off with fresh, lukewarm water before exiting the bath. This can be done several times per week.

    f. Patients who are compliant with prescribed treatment, but respond poorly, should generally be evaluated by a dermatologist for consideration of ultraviolet phototherapy or oral immunosuppressant therapy (e.g., cyclosporine).

  2. Contact dermatitis is best treated by identifying and removing the offending agent. Existing evidence supports use of barrier creams containing dimethicone, short-term use of high-lipid content moisturizers, and use of cotton liners if occlusive gloves are worn for prevention and treatment of irritant contact dermatitis. (SOR **Ⓑ**) Barrier creams with aluminum chlorohydrate seem to be ineffective. (SOR **Ⓑ**) **Acute** contact dermatitis (weepy, edematous, vesicular lesions) can be soothed by cotton dressings soaked in Burrow solution (aluminum acetate diluted 1:40 with cool water), applied four to six times daily. **Chronic** contact dermatitis (dry, scaly, thickened lesions) can be treated with emollients (Section V.A.1) and topical corticosteroids (Section V.A.2.a.(1) and Table 14–2).

3. **Scabies** and **lice**—for treatment details, see Chapter 7.

4. **Lichen simplex chronicus.** Treatment involves managing underlying mood disorders if present (see Chapters 90, 91, and 94), and educating patients about the itch–scratch cycle and ways to control it (see Section V.A). In addition, topical and systemic antipruritic medications and general measures can be used to alleviate symptoms.

5. **Lichen planus** should be treated with general measures (Section V.A) and topical corticosteroids (Section V.A.2.a.(1) and Table 14–2). Steroid gels (e.g., 0.05% fluocinonide applied twice daily) can be effective for intraoral lesions.

6. **Dry skin (xerosis).** Elimination of aggravating factors (e.g., certain medications) is an essential aspect of treatment. Good skin hydration and lubrication (as outlined in Section V.A.1) can alleviate symptoms.

7. **Dyshidrosis.** Nonpharmacologic management includes use of mild cleansers, wearing protective gloves, and avoiding known hand irritants. Burrow solution (Section V.B.2) can help improve bullous lesions. Medium- and high-potency topical corticosteroids can be used for flare-ups (Section V.A.2.a.(1) and Table 14–2. Oral steroids (Section V.A.2.b.(2)) can benefit more severe or acute symptoms. Those with persistent or refractory dyshidrosis should be referred to a dermatologist for psoralen plus ultraviolet A or low-dose methotrexate therapy.

8. **Pityriasis rosea** does not have a specific treatment. Oral antihistamines as well as Aveeno baths can reduce pruritus. Patients should be reassured that the condition is benign and self-limited, but can last for up to 6 to 12 weeks.

9. **Psoriasis.** Treatment of psoriatic lesions aims at the reduction of epidermal cell turnover and consists of topical, systemic, and phototherapy.

   a. Topical therapy

     (1) Emollients (e.g., Desitin ointment or A and D ointment, applied three times a day) should be applied chronically to affected areas.

     (2) Keratolytic agents, such as salicylic acid (e.g., salicylic acid soap), applied daily can not only bring limited improvement, but also irritate inflamed skin.
       Topical steroid ointments, mild to moderate potency (see Table 14–2), are one of the mainstays of treatment, (SOR **Ⓒ**) but can cause localized skin atrophy with prolonged use.

     (3) Tar preparations (e.g., Estar applied at bedtime to affected areas, allowing the gel to remain for 5 minutes and then removing any excess by patting with tissues) can also be used. (SOR **Ⓒ**)

     (4) Calcipotriene (Dovonex), a topical treatment for psoriasis of mild to moderate severity, (SOR **Ⓒ**) is a vitamin D derivative that inhibits epidermal cell proliferation in vitro. Calcipotriene should be applied twice daily to psoriatic plaques on the trunk or the extremities. Application with occlusion should be avoided as should application to the face or groin where it can cause irritation. Topical calcipotriene is approximately as effective as moderate-to-high-potency topical steroids, but can require 6 to 8 weeks of use before lesion improvement is noted. Absorption of calcipotriene is a problem only if large quantities (>100 g per week) are applied. Calcipotriene should not be used by patients with hypercalcemia or evidence of vitamin D toxicity.

   b. Patients with generalized psoriasis and psoriatic arthritis and who are acutely ill or requiring specialized treatments should be referred to a dermatologist. Dermatology consultation should also be considered for localized psoriasis requiring specialized treatment or uncontrolled with topical corticosteroids, calcipotriene, or coal tar products. Those with psoriatic arthritis can benefit from seeing a rheumatologist as well.

10. **Dermatophyte infection**

   a. Tinea capitis and barbae—for treatment, see Chapter 31.

   b. Tinea corporis. Superficial and localized lesions respond well to topical antifungal agents (SOR **Ⓒ**) applied once or twice daily for 1 to 2 weeks beyond when clinical response is first noted. These agents include topical clotrimazole, econazole, ketoconazole, miconazole, and terbinafine. More extensive lesions or lesions unresponsive to a topical therapy should be treated for 2 to 4 weeks with an oral agent (e.g., griseofulvin ultramicrosize, adults: 375 mg daily; children 2 years old and older: 5–10 mg/kg/day divided into one or two doses). (SOR ❸)

    c. Tinea pedis can be treated with topical antifungal preparations, although sometimes 4 to 8 weeks of concomitant oral antifungal treatment is required (e.g., griseofulvin ultramicrosize, adults: 250 mg three times daily; children 2 years and older: 5–10 mg/kg per day divided into one or two doses). (SOR ❸)

11. Seborrhea

    a. In adults, conventional therapy for **seborrheic dermatitis** of the scalp is a shampoo containing one of the following compounds: **salicylic acid** (e.g., X-Seb T or Sebulex), **selenium sulfide** (e.g., Selsun or Excel), **coal tar** (e.g., DHS Tar, Neutrogena T-Gel, or Polytar), or **pyrithione zinc** (e.g., DHS Zinc, Danex, or Sebulon). (SOR ❸) Each of these shampoos can be used two or three times a week. After application, shampoos should be left on the hair and scalp for at least 5 minutes to ensure that the medication reaches the skin. In more severe cases, adults may massage topical steroid lotions such as **2.5% hydrocortisone** lotion into the scalp once or twice daily.

    b. Flares or more resistant cases can respond to antifungal preparations (e.g., 2% ketoconazole shampoo used daily on affected scalp or beard for at least a month; 2% ketoconazole cream used topically to affected area twice a day for 4 weeks or until clinical clearing; 2% ketoconazole gel used topically to affected area once daily for 2 weeks). Scalp scaling can be treated with 2% salicylic acid shampoo. A peanut oil/mineral oil/corticosteroid preparation (Derma Smoothe/FS) is helpful in individuals with dry scalp who are unable to tolerate daily shampooing with other products.

    c. Facial seborrheic dermatitis often responds well to 1% metronidazole gel. (SOR ❸) One percent pimecrolimus cream can also be effective in treating moderate to severe facial seborrhea and is usually well tolerated (see Section V.B.1.d for description of FDA "black-box warning").

    d. Infantile seborrheic dermatitis. The usual treatment approach is conservative, with the use of a mild, nonmedicated shampoo first (e.g., baby shampoo twice a week), followed by the use of a shampoo with coal tar in resistant cases. Topical steroids should be avoided in infants if possible, because of significant percutaneous absorption.

  12. Nummular eczema usually responds to the same measures as **atopic dermatitis**.

VI. Patient Education

  A. Atopic dermatitis. The general measures listed above (in Section V.A) should be recommended to all patients with atopic dermatitis and can help those with xerosis and generalized pruritus as well. Prevention of triggers is paramount as is the importance of emphasizing to the patient that atopic dermatitis is a chronic condition that requires proper skin care even when lesions are not present. Patients should be educated on the proper use of corticosteroids with clear guidelines given for which agent to use on each affected part of the body.

  B. Contact dermatitis. Patients with contact dermatitis should be taught to avoid known triggers. As this can be difficult if they come into contact with their triggers for work or other unavoidable activities, advise them to modify activities (wear gloves or use other barriers) to avoid exacerbating their symptoms (e.g., for patients with contact dermatitis triggered by certain metals, nail polish painted over the metal such as the insides of the snaps on pants can prevent contact). Depending on the triggering agent, educate patients that products labeled "all natural" can still trigger a reaction.

  C. Scabies and lice. Prevention is best, but once a patient has scabies or lice he/she should be taught how to avoid spreading it. For scabies, affected individuals should be instructed to wash all clothes worn within the past 4 to 5 days in hot water and to dry them in a dryer on high heat. Any bedclothes and towels recently used should also be washed. Stuffed animals and other fabric toys an affected child has recently played with should be washed, too. If washing is not possible, contaminated items should be placed in a sealed plastic bag for at least 3 days as scabies mites will die without contact with human skin after a few days. Children can return to school after one day of treatment with permethrin. For lice, washing instructions are the same as those for scabies. If the plastic bag method is used, items should be kept sealed for 2 weeks. Those who live with the affected individual should be examined and treated if needed. Any bed partners of the affected individual should be treated even if no lice are seen.

SELECTED REFERENCES

Akdis CA, Akdis M, Bieber T, et al. Diagnosis and treatment of atopic dermatitis in children and adults: European Academy of Allergology and Clinical Immunology/American Academy of Allergy, Asthma and Immunology/PRACTALL consensus report. *Allergy.* 2006;61(8):969–987.

Fleischer AB, Jr. Black box warning for topical calcineurin inhibitors and the death of common sense. *Dermatol Online J.* 2006;12(6):2.

Saary J, Qureshi R, Palda V, et al. A systematic review of contact dermatitis treatment and prevention. *J Am Acad Dermatol.* 2005;53(5):845.

Usatine RP, Riojas M. Diagnosis and management of contact dermatitis. *Am Fam Physician.* 2010;82(3): 249–255.

Wollina U, Hansel G, Koch A, Abdel-Naser MB. Topical pimecrolimus for skin disease other than atopic dermatitis. *Expert Opin Pharmacother.* 2006;7(15):1967–1975.

---

15   Dermatologic Neoplasms

Daniel L. Stulberg, MD, & Douglas G. Browning, MD, ATC-L

KEY POINTS

- For any lesion appearing suspicious or if uncertain about the diagnosis, perform a biopsy to rule out malignancy. (SOR **C**)
- The primary preventable cause of skin malignancies is chronic sun exposure. (SOR **C**)
- A person with a history of a skin malignancy should have regular skin examinations to evaluate any suspicious lesions. (SOR **C**)
- Actinic keratoses are squamous cell carcinoma in situ and are seen in association with basal and squamous cell cancers elsewhere. (SOR **C**)
- Malignant melanoma can readily metastasize and is the skin malignancy with the poorest prognosis. (SOR **A**)

I. **Definition. Neoplasm** means new growth. A **dermatologic neoplasm** occurs when skin or subcutaneous cells begin to abnormally proliferate. Such new growths are extremely common and may be benign, premalignant, or malignant. They may arise in the **epidermis** (e.g., acrochordon, keratoacanthoma, seborrheic keratoses, basal and squamous cell carcinomas, malignant melanoma, nevi, actinic keratoses), the **dermis** (e.g., sebaceous hyperplasia, dermatofibromas, pyogenic granulomas, cherry angiomas, epidermoid cyst), or **subcutaneous tissue** (e.g., lipomas).

II. **Screening and Prevention**

A. **Screening in patients without prior skin cancer.** The Cochrane database authors and the United States Preventive Services Task Force (USPSTF) have not found conclusive evidence for recommending annual screening examinations for melanoma. The American Cancer Society recommends that patients who have any concerns about moles that are symptomatic, changing, or display any of the characteristics in their ABCDE rules (Table 15–1) should have a clinician evaluate those lesions.

B. **Screening in patients with prior skin cancer.** Patients with a **history of non-melanoma skin cancer** are at much higher risk for having already developed other skin cancers as well as at higher risk for developing future skin cancers. They should be examined closely at the time of diagnosis for additional lesions and every 6 to 12 months. Patients with a **history of melanoma** should have skin examinations annually to look for any new melanomas or local recurrence.

C. **Prevention.** Ultraviolet B (UVB) light is the primary inducer of skin cancers. The USPSTF recommends that fair-skinned individuals, ages 10 through 24 years, should reduce their sun exposure to lower their future risk of skin cancers. This can be done by covering

TABLE 15–1. AMERICAN CANCER SOCIETY ABCDE GUIDELINES FOR SUSPICIOUS LESION CHARACTERISTICS PROMPTING FURTHER EVALUATION

A—Asymmetry	Lesions with one portion looking different than the rest
B—Border	Borders that are ill defined or spreading in appearance
C—Color	The colors of the US flag (red, white, and blue) plus black
D—Diameter	Greater than 6 mm (approximately the size of a pencil's eraser)
E—Enlarging or evolution	Lesion growing in size or changing over time

exposed areas, use of sunscreens with a sun protection factor (SPF) of 30 or more, avoidance of sun exposure between 10 AM and 4 PM, and avoidance of tanning salons.

1. The SPF of a sunscreen denotes the product's ability to block UVB. A sunscreen with an SPF of 15 blocks 93% of UVB and an SPF of 30 blocks 96.7% of UVB.
2. There are two types of sunscreens, physical and chemical. Physical sunscreens (zinc oxide, titanium dioxide) reflect UV radiation and chemical sunscreens absorb and block UV radiation from reaching the skin.
3. To provide adequate protection against UVB skin damage, a sunscreen needs to be applied in sufficient quantity (a heaping tablespoonful for an average adult in a bathing suit) and frequency (15 minutes prior to sun exposure and every 2 hours for nonwater-resistant sunscreen or every 40 to 80 minutes [per product label] for water-resistant products during swimming).

III. **Common Diagnoses.** Of patients who consult primary care physicians for skin problems, approximately 20% are diagnosed as having skin neoplasm or tumor.

    A. **Macular lesions.** Please note nevi may be macular (flat) or may develop a vertical component.

        1. **Nevi** (moles) are aberrant collections of melanocytes in the epidermis, dermis, or dermoepidermal junction. Approximately 1% of infants have one or more nevi at birth. They can be flat (macular) or raised (papular) and be benign, atypical, dysplastic, or develop into malignant melanoma. The number of nevi increases during adolescence to an average of 20 to 40 lesions by the third decade. These lesions are more prevalent in whites, and sun exposure increases their number.

        2. **Ephelides (freckles) and lentigines** are hyperpigmented macular lesions that increase with sun exposure. Ephelides are found most commonly in children or young adults with light complexions. In elderly individuals, lentigines become more prevalent in sun-exposed areas, where they are called age or "liver spots."

        3. **Congenital nevi** occur in approximately 1% of the population.

        4. **Familial atypical mole and melanoma syndrome (FAMMS),** previously known as dysplastic nevus syndrome and part of atypical mole syndrome (AMS), is a familial autosomal dominant syndrome in which individuals have multiple nevi (macular or papular) increasing in size and number with age (Figure 15–1). The risk for the development of cutaneous melanoma is 15% if there is one first-degree relative and is nearly 100% if there are two first-degree relatives with melanomas.

        5. **Malignant melanomas** account for <5% of all skin cancers, but cause most of the skin cancer mortalities. The American Cancer Society estimates that there will be 76,690 new cases in the United States in 2013. Melanoma rates are highest in developed countries and in areas closer to the equator. Greater UV light exposure through depletion of the ozone layer may contribute to the increasing incidence of melanoma; however, correlation with sun exposure is weaker for melanoma than for basal and squamous cell cancers. Rather than duration, *intensity* of sun exposure is more relevant (i.e., a history of blistering sunburn before 20 years of age doubles the risk of melanoma). Other risk factors include congenital nevi, AMS, and personal history of previous melanoma. The relative incidence of the four histologic subtypes of melanoma is as follows:

- **Superficial spreading** (70% of melanomas)
- **Lentigo maligna** (12% of melanomas)
- **Nodular** (10% of melanomas)
- **Acral lentiginous** (8% of melanomas)

    B. **Papular lesions**

        1. **Nevi** can be macular or papular, see above.

        2. **Cherry angiomas,** dilated capillaries and postcapillary venules, occur in up to 50% of adults, beginning in adulthood and increasing with age (Figure 15–2).

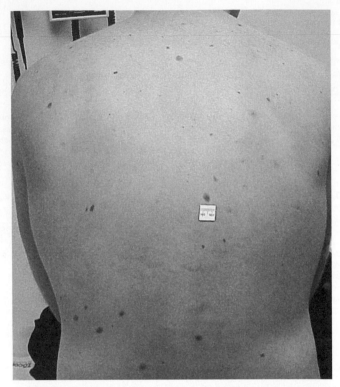

FIGURE 15–1. AMS; note multiple macular to papular lesions with variable coloring and size (see color insert).

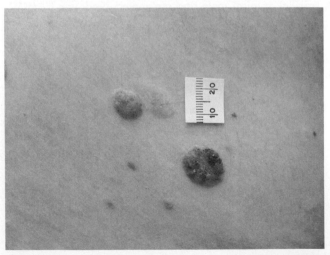

FIGURE 15–2. Multiple macular cherry angiomas. More advanced lesions may be raised or even polypoid. Note several verrucous irregularly pigmented seborrheic keratoses which are also age related (see color insert).

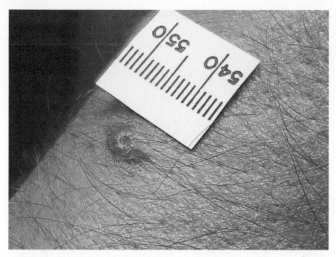

FIGURE 15–3. Keratoacanthoma with raised borders and central keratin plug (see color insert).

3. **Seborrheic keratoses** (less commonly called seborrheic or senile warts—although not a viral process) are common in middle-aged and older individuals, occurring equally in men and women (Figure 15–2).
4. **Verrucae (warts)** can occur at any age, but are more common in children and young adults. Their incidence, severity, and prevalence are greater in immunocompromised patients.
5. **Keratoacanthoma,** considered by some to be a form of low grade although commonly large squamous cell cancer, tend to occur in older individuals and can be related to sun exposure (Figure 15–3).
6. **Pyogenic granulomas** are associated with skin irritation, damage, or pregnancy. They are a proliferation of fragile vascular and epithelial tissues that are commonly seen at the newborn umbilicus and on the gums of pregnant women (Figure 15–4).

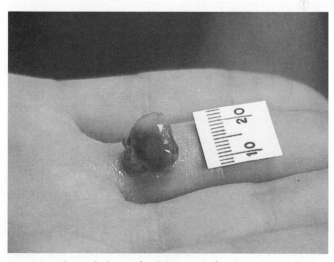

FIGURE 15–4. Pyogenic granuloma with glistening fragile overgrowth of capillaries and epithelium (see color insert).

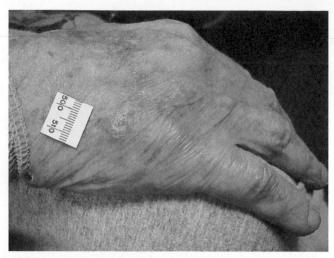

FIGURE 15–5. Actinic keratosis which has reached the raised actinic horn stage and also note the diffuse raised erythematous base of progression to squamous cell cancer (see color insert).

7. **Actinic keratoses** were formerly considered premalignant skin lesions. They are now considered squamous carcinoma in situ. They are mostly found on sun-exposed areas in middle-aged and older persons with light complexions and a history of chronic sun exposure. The lifetime risk of a cutaneous squamous cell carcinoma developing in an individual with actinic keratoses (Figure 15–5) is approximately 20%.

8. **Basal cell carcinoma** (Figure 15–6) is the most common skin cancer occurring mostly but not exclusively on sun-exposed skin. The American Cancer Society estimates that there were 3.5 million cases of basal and squamous cell cancers diagnosed in the United States in 2006.

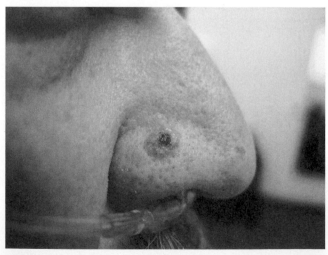

FIGURE 15–6. Basal cell cancer. Note similar appearance to keratoacanthoma with raised borders, but has telangiectasias and central ulceration (see color insert).

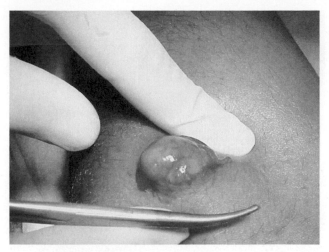

FIGURE 15–7. Lipoma with capsule being expressed after blunt dissection from a relatively small incision (see color insert).

9. **Squamous cell carcinoma** usually develops in sun-exposed areas of the body. The incidence of squamous cell cancer (Figure 15–5) is higher in individuals with fair skin, immune disorders, outdoor occupations, and exposure to hydrocarbons such as soot, coal tar, and lubricating oils.

10. **Acrochordon, or skin tags,** can occur as single or multiple lesions. They are found in 25% of individuals; increase with age and obesity; and frequently occur on the neck, axillae, and under the breasts.

C. Nodular lesions

1. **Lipomas,** subcutaneous encapsulated tumors of adipose cells, occur in 1 of 1000 individuals. They are solitary in 80% of cases, but may be multiple, especially in young men (Figure 15–7).

2. **Dermatofibromas,** subcutaneous scar tissue, can occur in reaction to trauma, insect sting, or folliculitis; multiple lesions can be associated with autoimmune disease (Figure 15–8).

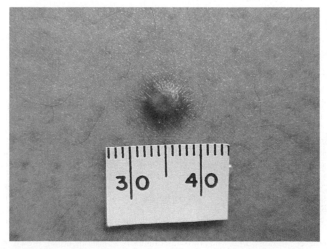

FIGURE 15–8. Dermatofibroma typically pigmented and sometimes raised (see color insert).

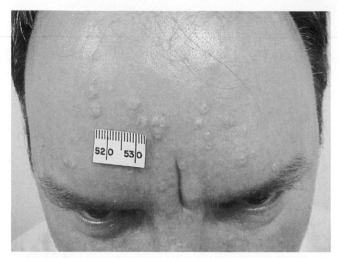

FIGURE 15–9. Sebaceous hyperplasia, common on the forehead and face looks similar to early BCCs, but is often seen as multiple lesions (see color insert).

     3. Epidermal cysts are smooth, pearl-colored cysts akin to very large comedones. Multiple epidermal cysts are associated with Gardner syndrome, a subtype of familial adenomatous polyposis.

     4. Sebaceous hyperplasia, enlarged sebaceous glands, is most common in middle-aged and older individuals (Figure 15–9).

IV. Symptoms. Dermatologic neoplasms are often asymptomatic. When symptoms occur, they can include the following:

    A. Cosmetic change or disfigurement.

    B. Local irritation with friction from clothing (collars, bras, belts), jewelry, skin folds, or trauma with shaving.

    C. Anxiety over changes in size or number of lesions, local discomfort, bleeding, discharge, or ulceration.

V. Signs

    A. Common types of **verrucae (warts),** which can occur as single or grouped lesions:

      1. Flat warts (verruca plana), 1- to 3-mm lesions with smooth, flesh-colored surfaces, generally found on the face, neck, hands, and lower legs in a linear distribution.

      2. Periungual warts, rough-surfaced lesions, found adjacent to and sometimes extending beneath the nails.

      3. Plantar warts, thick, sometimes coalescing lesions (Mosaic warts), typically on the heels or balls of the feet revealing pinpoint-sized bleeding capillaries when pared.

      4. Genital warts (condylomata acuminata or venereal warts), velvety, moist, slightly raised, cauliflower-like lesions occurring singularly or in clusters genitally or perianally.

    B. Melanomas can arise from moles that have been present or appear as a new lesion. The American Cancer Society ABCDE guidelines (see Table 15–1) for suspicious characteristics are useful for the general public and as a starting point for practitioners' evaluations. (SOR **❸**) AMS occurs spontaneously and also runs in families. Affected individuals have multiple atypical nevi with a high risk of melanoma. This encompasses the previously named FAMMS and dysplastic nevus syndrome. These nevi differ from common nevi in size (5–10 mm or more compared with <6 mm for common nevi), shape and contour (irregular borders with poor margination compared with symmetric, uniform borders for common nevi), and color (intra- and inter-lesional variations of brown, black, or red compared with more homogeneous variations of tan, brown, or black for common nevi).

TABLE 15–2. CONGENITAL NEVI

	Size	Malignant Potential	Treatment
Small	<1.5 cm	Low and rare before puberty	Follow clinically. If desired, prophylactic excision before puberty.
Medium	1.5–19.9 cm	Varies by depth of lesion epidermal versus deeper	Can biopsy: If epidermal, follow clinically or excise. If dermal, then excise as lesion cannot be accurately followed clinically.
Large	>20 cm or >5% of body surface area	Up to 7%	Excise prophylactically as early as possible. Half of melanomas develop by age 3–5 years and cannot be accurately followed clinically. If on the head or neck, check magnetic resonance imaging (MRI) for neural involvement.

    Congenital nevi are classified according to size into small, medium, and large with varying degrees of malignant potential (see Table 15–2).
    C. Epidermoid cysts may become fluctuant and tender if inflamed (Figure 15–10).
VI. Laboratory Tests. In most cases, when physical examination clarifies the nature of a lesion, no further testing is necessary. Dermoscopy by an experienced clinician using a handheld magnifier can increase the accuracy delineating between benign and malignant nevi. (SOR Ⓒ) Biopsies of suspicious lesions should be done. Suspicious lesions include the following:
    A. Any lesion that the clinician is suspicious about based on clinical appearance or history.
    B. Lesions with unexplained tenderness, itching, bleeding, or ulceration.
    C. Lesions with recent growth, ulceration, or characteristics suggestive of basal cell carcinoma, squamous cell carcinoma, or melanoma.
VII. Treatment
    A. Benign neoplasms
        1. Benign appearing nevi usually require no treatment except for cosmetic or diagnostic purposes. Most are easily removed by shave, punch, or excisional biopsy.
            a. Superficial shave excision is useful for elevated lesions and those in which depth of excision is unimportant.

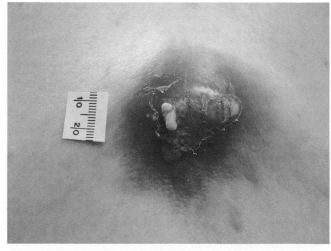

FIGURE 15–10. Epidermal cyst which has become infected, inflamed, and painful which requires incision and drainage (see color insert).

    b. Deep shave excision can be used to completely remove thin basal cell cancers (BCCs) and squamous cell carcinomas (SCCs) and is now considered appropriate for pigmented lesions suspicious for melanoma, with the provider attempting to get completely under the suspicious/pigmented tissue.

    c. Punch biopsy is an easy way to obtain a full-thickness diagnostic specimen; although irregular, large, or cystic lesions may be more appropriately excised.

    d. Excisional biopsy by scalpel, electrosurgery, or punch larger than the lesion allows for a complete, full-thickness excision of a worrisome skin lesion.

2. Removal of **seborrheic keratoses** can be achieved by cryosurgery without anesthetic or by shave excision or curettage after anesthetizing the skin with a local anesthetic.

3. Warts

    a. Common warts can be treated by many different methods. Starting with nonprescription salicylic acid liquids or "wart stick" applicators (daily) or tapes (every 2–3 days) is prudent and approximately 60% effective. It may take weeks to months, but is one of the most benign and inexpensive therapies available other than watchful waiting. (SOR Ⓐ) Soaking the wart for 10 to 15 minutes before application, debriding any dead or peeling skin from the lesion, and occluding the application of acid can all increase treatment success. Weekly occlusion of the lesion with **duct tape,** with removal of the devitalized skin between applications was initially reported to be 85% effective in a small trial but subsequent studies show much lower efficacy.

        Office-based cryotherapy with liquid nitrogen, compressed nitrous oxide, or liquid refrigerants have similar efficacy. Home-based nonprescription cryotherapy is up to 50% effective. Candida antigen mixed 10% in lidocaine and injected into the base of the wart can induce an immune response and resolution of the wart(s.) Weekly applications of bi- or tri-chloroacetic acid in the office can be used as well as sensitization with dinitrochlorobenzene via consultation with a specialist.

        More aggressive destruction can be achieved with electrodesiccation and curettage or laser, but there is no guarantee of an increased rate of resolution of the wart and there are associated surgical side effects.

    b. Flat warts tend to be numerous and are often present on the face or forehead making treatment with **cryosurgery, bichloracetic acid,** or over-the-counter **salicylic acid** more difficult because of the amount of inflammation and potential for noticeable pigmentation changes. Imiquimod 5% cream (Aldara) applied daily or every other day for several weeks can be useful. Alternatively, **tretinoin (retinoic acid)** cream or lotion (0.025%, 0.05%, or 0.1%) can be applied once or twice daily to produce mild inflammation and subsequent regression (often requires several weeks). **Fluorouracil** (Efudex) cream, 5%, applied once or twice a day for 3 to 5 weeks, is also effective.

    c. Periungual warts should be treated cautiously because of the proximity of the nail bed. **Cryosurgery** can be done, taking care to avoid injury to the nail matrix and superficial nerves. Alternatively, **topical keratolytics** (listed above for common warts) can be applied until the wart regresses. Occasionally, eradication can only be achieved by blunt dissection.

    d. Plantar warts can cause foot pain. Topical keratolytic agents (listed above for common warts) are used, but treatment usually requires several weeks to months. Paring down the lesion can reduce the painful sensation of "walking on a rock in my shoe." See the recommendations above for treatment of common warts as they are treated similarly but, **cryosurgery** or **excision** of these warts tends to temporarily cause pain with walking due to their location.

    e. Treatment of **anogenital warts (condylomata acuminata** or venereal warts) is discussed in Chapter 30.

4. Lentigines pose no health threat. Removal by topical or surgical techniques is unnecessary, and lesions tend to recur. Routine use of sunscreens can reduce the rate of additional lesions. Creams containing hydroquinone to bleach the skin may make these lesions less noticeable, and gentle cryotherapy can selectively damage melanocytes in relation to keratinocytes, decreasing pigmentation, without much destruction to other tissue.

5. Cherry angiomas can be electrocauterized or removed by shave excision after local anesthesia, if necessary, but are usually left untreated.

6. **Sebaceous hyperplasia** does not require treatment except for cosmetic purposes. Individual lesions can be removed by curetting or light cauterization, but at the risk of leaving a pit or indentation. When they are severe, extensive, or disfiguring, oral isotretinoin (or in females, antiandrogens) can help improve their appearance, at least temporarily.

7. **Acrochordon** (skin tags) can be removed by cryosurgery with liquid nitrogen, or special tweezers dipped in liquid nitrogen, electrosurgery, or by snip excision with sharp iris scissors.

8. **Dermatofibromas** require no treatment unless the diagnosis is uncertain, the lesion is symptomatic from repeated trauma, or is in an undesirable location from a cosmetic standpoint. Pigmentation and the raised portion can be reduced with cryotherapy. If excision is desired, dermatofibromas require a full-thickness approach because of the depth of the lesion.

9. Although **keratoacanthoma** usually eventually resolve spontaneously, excision or destruction is recommended to prevent the long duration of disease and the usual scarring. Electrodesiccation and curettage can be used for small lesions. Larger lesions can be surgically excised or the patient referred for topical 5-fluorouracil, or imiquimod, or intralesional 5-fluorouracil, methotrexate, interferon alfa-2a, or isotretinoin.

10. **For pyogenic granuloma,** shave or snip excision is used for diagnosis or to rule out amelanotic melanoma. The base is treated with electrodesiccation and thorough curettage or topical application of silver nitrate.

11. **Epidermoid (also known as sebaceous) cysts** can recur if there are adjacent cysts or if they are not completely excised. Traditionally, if desired, these lesions are excised via an incision down to the capsule and blunt dissection around the capsule to remove the cyst intact. A newer technique uses a smaller incision into the cyst, expressing the contents and then inverting and removing the cyst wall. If the lesion is friable and intact removal is not possible, the cyst wall can be curetted out or removed with forceps. If the cyst becomes infected, it should be sharply incised, drained, and packed using a gauze strip with appropriate follow-up care.

12. **Lipomas** generally require no treatment except for cosmesis, unless they interfere with the movement of adjacent muscles; in this case, they may be removed by simple surgical excision or liposuction. If there is pain, rapid growth, or attachment to adjacent tissues, they should be evaluated for liposarcoma.

B. **Premalignant lesions** are usually treated to prevent malignant degeneration. Patients with these lesions should be educated regarding **sun protection** (i.e., covering exposed areas), **use of sunscreens** with an SPF of 30 or more, **avoidance of sun exposure** between 10 am and 4 pm, performance of regular **skin self-examination,** and avoidance of tanning salons.

1. **Actinic keratoses.** Untreated actinic keratoses can progress from the in situ phase to squamous cell carcinomas. **Cryotherapy, or electrodesiccation with curettage,** is practical if there are a limited number of lesions. For areas with extensive lesions, **5% topical 5-fluorouracil** (Efudex) is used twice daily until marked inflammation occurs. Treatment for the face and lips is approximately 2 weeks. Treatment for thicker skin can require 4 or more weeks. More recently, diclofenac gel 3% (Solaraze) applied twice daily for 60 to 90 days or imiquimod 5% cream (Aldara) applied topically for 8 hours twice weekly for 16 weeks (SOR **Ⓐ**) are also effective for the majority of lesions, and the remaining lesions can be treated as above. Topical steroids or petrolatum (Vaseline) can be used to decrease post-treatment inflammation as needed.

   Tretinoin (0.05% or 0.1%) **cream,** applied daily, can be used in patients with mild actinic damage. **Dermabrasion** and **chemical peel** are also effective, but should be performed only by physicians trained and experienced in these techniques.

2. **AMS.** This syndrome requires frequent examinations, a low threshold for biopsy of suspicious lesions, and consideration for body mapping (serial photographs).

C. **Malignant lesions**

1. **BCCs.** Untreated BCC grows slowly, but if left untreated can invade contiguous soft tissue, bone, and cartilage. The method of removal depends on lesion size, location, and physician and patient preference. Treatment technique for small lesions usually involves **excision** or **electrodesiccation and curettage (ED&C)**. **Cryosurgery** or topical 5% imiquimod (Aldara—not approved for face, hands, or feet) can

TABLE 15–3. RE-EXCISION MARGINS FOR MALIGNANT MELANOMA

Melanoma in situ	0.5 cm
<1 mm	1 cm
1–4 mm	1–2 cm based on location/feasibility
>4 mm	2 cm, 3 cm if feasible

be used for superficial lesions with a slightly lower cure rate. Radiation therapy can be used for rare cases where a patient cannot tolerate other treatments.

a. Shave biopsy is the simplest way to confirm the diagnosis. **Small BCCs** may be removed by a primary care physician using **ED&C,** a punch or an elliptical excision to obtain clear margins around the lesion. If excised, clear margins surrounding the lesion in all directions should be verified by pathology. **ED&C** is usually performed after confirming the diagnosis by a shave biopsy, and its technique of curetting in all directions helps to detect and remove subclinical spread at the margins of the lesion.

b. Larger BCCs, recurrent BCCs, and those located on sensitive structures including the **eyes or ears** should be referred for expert surgical removal. This might include excision by a dermatologist trained in **Moh micrographic surgery** or excision by a plastic surgeon.

2. Squamous cell carcinoma. Spread most commonly occurs by local extension and, less commonly, by metastasis. Superficial squamous cell carcinomas (Bowen disease) may be treated with electrodesiccation and curettage. Excisional treatment is recommended for most lesions and Moh micrographic surgery should be used for large lesions or those near sensitive structures. Squamous cell lesions arising within chronic ulcers, burns, or scar tissue or in mucous membranes have a high metastatic potential, and patients with such lesions should be referred to a provider with experience with these.

3. Malignant melanomas have a tendency to spread rapidly and metastasize early. Prognosis, margin for re-excision, and recommendations for further treatment are based on Breslow method of measuring the depth of tumor on initial excision. See Table 15–3 for recommended re-excision margins. Melanomas greater than 1 mm in thickness warrant sentinel lymph node biopsy by an experienced surgeon, and regular follow-up for recurrent disease. (SOR **Ⓐ**) Palliative chemotherapy, debulking surgery, radiation therapy, and immunotherapy with interferon and other agents may extend life in metastatic melanoma.

4. Congenital nevi. Congenital nevi have malignant potential based on their size and composition. See Table 15–2 for treatment recommendations. For large congenital lesions referral to a plastic surgeon experienced in this area is important.

SELECTED REFERENCES

American Cancer Society Web site. www.Cancer.org. Accessed January 29, 2013.

Gupta AK, Paquet M, Villanueva E, Brintnell W. Interventions for actinic keratoses. *Cochrane Database Syst Rev.* 2012;(12):CD004415.

Habif TP. *Clinical Dermatology: A Color Guide to Diagnosis and Therapy.* 5th ed. St. Louis, MO: Mosby; 2009.

Herschorn A. Dermoscopy for melanoma detection in family practice. *Can Fam Physician.* 2012;58(7): 740–745, e372–e378.

Johnson TM, Sondak VK, Bichakjian CK, Sabel MS. The role of sentinel lymph node biopsy for melanoma: evidence assessment. *J Am Acad Dermatol.* 2006;54(1);19–27.

Kwok CS, Gibbs S, Bennett C, et al. Topical treatments for cutaneous warts. *Cochrane Database Syst Rev.* 2012;(9):CD001781.

Levine SM, Shaprio RL. Surgical treatment of malignant melanoma: paractical guidelines. *Dermatol Clin.* 2012;30(3):487–501.

Luba MC, Bangs SA, Mohler AM, Stulberg DL. Common benign skin tumors. *Am Fam Physician.* 2003; 67(4):729–738.

Morelli JG. Cutaneous nevi. In *Nelson Textbook of Pediatrics.* 19th ed. Philadelphia, PA: Elsevier; 2011: 643:2231–2236.

Scattolin MA. Neurocutaneous melanosis: follow-up and literature review. *J Neuroradiol.* 2011;38(5): 313–318.

16   Diarrhea

Michael A. Noll, MD, Jeanne M. Ferrante, MD, MPH, &
Laura Hargro, MD, MBA

KEY POINTS

- Most episodes of acute diarrhea are self-limited. (SOR ⒞)
- A thorough history is crucial to accurate patient assessment. (SOR ⒞)
- Supportive care is usually the only required treatment. (SOR ⒞)

I. **Definition and Common Causes. Diarrhea** is an increased number (three or more) or decreased consistency of stools (soft or liquid) from a person's baseline during a 24-hour period. Diarrhea is one of the most common symptoms for which patients visit their physician. In the United States, there are estimated 211 to 375 million annual episodes of diarrheal illnesses, resulting in 73 million physician visits, >900,000 hospitalizations, and 6000 deaths. Up to 55% of travelers to less developed areas of the world (e.g., Mexico, Latin America, Africa, the Middle East, and Asia) will have travelers' diarrhea (see Chapter 107).

   A. **Normal functions of the gastrointestinal (GI) tract** are assimilation of nutrients and elimination of waste. The small intestines serve most of the nutrient absorptive function while the colon prepares waste material by dehydrating the stool about 10-fold. GI motility varies by location with transit times of seconds through the esophagus, minutes to a few hours through the stomach and small intestines, and about 24 hours to move through the colon in most individuals.

   B. **Acute diarrhea** has a duration of symptoms of 14 days or less. Common causes include:

      1. **Viral infections** (e.g., rotavirus, enteric adenovirus, Norovirus/Norwalk virus, calicivirus, astrovirus, and cytomegalovirus).

      2. **Bacterial infections** are characterized as **enterotoxigenic** (e.g., *Escherichia coli, Staphylococcus aureus, Bacillus cereus, Clostridium perfringens, Clostridium difficile, Vibrio cholera* and other vibrios, *Aeromonas* spp., and *Plesiomonas* spp.) or **inflammatory** (*Salmonella* spp., *Shigella* spp., *Campylobacter* spp., *Yersinia enterocolitica*, and *Shiga* toxin-producing *E. coli* 0157:H7 [*STEC*]).

      3. **Parasitic infections** (e.g., *Giardia lamblia, Cryptosporidium, Entamoeba histolytica, Microsporidian, Isospora belli*, and *Cyclospora cayetanensis*).

      4. **Drugs** (e.g., caffeine, alcohol, other prescription, and nonprescription drugs).

      5. **Chemical contamination of water (e.g., copper, ethylene glycol, ethyl benzene).**

      6. **Miscellaneous noninfectious causes** (e.g., irritable bowel syndrome [IBS]; fecal impaction with paradoxical diarrhea; inflammatory bowel disease; or ingestions of large amounts of lactose, fructose, or artificial sweeteners).

   C. **Persistent diarrhea** is when symptoms last for more than 14 days; symptoms lasting for more than 1 month constitute **chronic diarrhea**. The prevalence of chronic diarrhea is estimated to be 5% with direct costs from medical care predicted at $524 million per year and the indirect costs from disability and lost productivity exceeding $136 million per year.

      1. **Chronic diarrhea** may be classified as:

         a. **Watery—due to** the following:

            (1) **Osmotic factors** (osmotic gap of stool >50 mOsm/kg). Osmotic diarrhea occurs when too much water is drawn into the bowel. This can occur with ingestion of Mg^{2+}, PO_4^{-3}, or SO_4^{-2}; magnesium laxatives; lactase deficiency; and carbohydrate malabsorption.

            (2) **Secretory factors** (osmotic gap of stool <50 mOsm/kg). Secretory diarrhea refers to an increase in fluid secretion or an inhibition of fluid absorption from the bowel. Secretory diarrhea can be endogenous (large volume not decreased with fasting) from neuroendocrine tumors such as carcinoid and

gastrinoma; neoplasias such as colon carcinoma, lymphoma, and villous adenoma; vasculitis; and congenital syndromes or exogenous (large volume decreased with removal of offending agent) from stimulant laxatives, medications, or toxins.

    (3) Dysmotility or rapid movement of food through the intestines can occur with IBS, diabetic autonomic neuropathy, hyperthyroidism and thyrotoxicosis, and scleroderma.

  b. Inflammatory—due to **infections** (possibly with fever, eosinophilia, e.g., parasitic, helminthic, and ulcerating viral infections); **inflammatory bowel disease** (with fever, hematochezia, e.g., ulcerative colitis); **neoplasia; ischemia;** or **radiation**.

  c. Fatty—due to malabsorption (e.g., celiac disease) or **maldigestion** (e.g., pancreatic insufficiency, bile acid deficiency).

II. Prevention

  A. The World Health Organization (WHO) has recommended **vaccination against rotavirus** in all countries since 2009. There currently are two vaccines available to immunize against rotavirus: **Rotarix** (a monovalent vaccine) and **RotaTeq** (a pentavalent vaccine). In a recent meta-analysis of randomized controlled trials (RCTs) that examined immunization against rotavirus in the first 2 years of life, both Rotarix and RotaTeq were shown to significantly reduce severe cases of rotavirus diarrhea in both low-mortality and high-mortality nations. (SOR **Ⓐ**) Adverse effects of immunization were similar to placebo.

  B. Probiotics. Diarrhea is a common side effect of antimicrobial therapy. Specifically, antibiotic-associated diarrhea (AAD) is identified in up to 39% of patients receiving antibiotic therapy. Single or multi-species **probiotics** containing at least *Lactobacillus* or *Saccharomyces boulardii* can decrease the likelihood of **antibiotic-induced diarrhea (but not traveler's diarrhea)** by 33% in children and adults. (SOR **Ⓐ**)

    1. These products (e.g., VSL#3, Florastor, Culturelle) are sold over the counter and can be found in the vitamin or diarrhea section of the pharmacy. A typical dosage is 5 to 10 billion viable organisms three to four times a day in adults (half the dosage in children) for the duration of antibiotic use. Additionally, the use of probiotics for the prevention of AAD may lead to **significant financial savings** in direct medical costs and decreased length of hospitalization. (SOR **Ⓐ**)

    2. Evidence for the use of **probiotics for the primary prevention of *C. difficile* infection is inconsistent,** but promising. More studies are required to identify whether or not probiotics are effective agents in *C. difficile* prophylaxis. (SOR **Ⓑ**)

III. Common Diagnoses. For information on sexually transmitted proctitis and colon ischemia, see sidebars.

  A. Acute diarrhea. Most acute diarrhea is caused by infections and usually occurs after the ingestion of contaminated food or water, or by direct person-to-person contact. **Underlying medical conditions** predisposing to infections include extremes of age, recent hospitalization, impaired immune system, human immunodeficiency virus, immunosuppressive therapy for organ transplant, long-term prednisone therapy, cancer chemotherapy, immunoglobulin A deficiency, or prior gastrectomy. **Other risk factors** include recent travel to developing countries, day care attendance, residence at an institution (nursing home, psychiatric facility, prison), lowered gastric acidity (patients taking H2 blockers or proton pump inhibitors), and certain occupations (farmer, food handler, health care or day care provider). The common causes include the following:

    1. Viral (70%–80% of acute infectious diarrhea). **Rotavirus,** the most frequent cause, typically presents in winter and may be transmitted by aerosol spread as well as through the fecal–oral route. Most cases occur between the ages of 3 months and 2 years. **Enteric adenoviruses** are the second most common type. Contaminated water, salads, and shellfish may transmit **Norwalk virus,** one of the noroviruses, which are the most common causes of outbreaks especially on cruise ships.

    2. Bacterial (10%–20% of acute cases). Risk factors include consumption of cooked foods that are later refrigerated such as custard, pastries, and processed meats (*S. aureus*); raw or undercooked meat (*Salmonella, Yersinia, STEC*) or seafood (*Vibrio, Plesiomonas*); improperly refrigerated foods (*B. cereus, C. perfringens*); or unpasteurized milk, juice, soft cheese, or unheated deli meats (*Listeria monocytogenes*). *Clostridium difficile* causes approximately 20% of **AAD**. The antibiotics that most commonly cause *C. difficile* infection are fluoroquinolones, clindamycin, broad-spectrum cephalosporins, and penicillin derivatives taken in the past 8 weeks.

SEXUALLY TRANSMITTED PROCTITIS

Sexually transmitted proctitis can cause rectal pain, small-volume bloody diarrhea, and tenesmus. **Herpesvirus, gonorrhea, chlamydia,** and **syphilis** are likely causes. Those at risk are homosexual men and receptive partners during anal intercourse. Diagnosis is by proctoscopy with rectal swabs sent for polymerase chain reaction (PCR) testing or cultures. Treatment consists of antiviral drugs or antibiotics for the sexually transmitted infection (see Chapter 102).

> 3. **Parasitic** (<10% of acute diarrhea). Parasitic infections (*G. lamblia, Cryptosporidium, E. histolytica*) are uncommon in the general population, but may be more prevalent in children in day care centers, residents of mental institutions or nursing homes, immunocompromised persons, or persons exposed to untreated water from a lake or stream. *Entamoeba histolytica* can be found in up to 30% of homosexual men.
> 4. **Drugs.** Common causes include laxatives, antibiotics, cardiovascular drugs, nonsteroidal anti-inflammatory drugs, antiparkinson drugs, colchicine, and excessive caffeine or alcohol. **Proton-pump inhibitors** have been shown to significantly increase the risk of *C. difficile*-associated diarrhea and should be used with prudence. (SOR **Ⓐ**) Any new drug or recent dosage change may result in diarrhea.
> 5. **Seafood ingestion syndromes** can also cause diarrhea and include diarrheic shellfish poisoning, ciguatera poisoning, and scombroid poisoning.

COLON ISCHEMIA

Colon ischemia is a rare cause of diarrhea, but it can be life-threatening. The diarrhea may be associated with mild-to-moderate abdominal pain or lower intestinal bleeding. Risk factors include history of coronary artery disease/hypertension/chronic renal failure/arrhythmia, recent aortic or cardiac bypass surgery, vasculitides (e.g., systemic lupus erythematosus), infections (e.g., STEC, cytomegalovirus), coagulopathies (e.g., protein C and S deficiencies), medications (e.g., vasoactive meds, oral contraceptives), drugs (e.g., cocaine), long-distance running, preceding major cardiovascular episode with hypotension, and obstructing lesions of the colon (e.g., carcinoma).

Diagnosis is by colonoscopy or arteriography. Most cases resolve spontaneously within 48 hours and do not require specific therapy. Patients with severe or continuing symptoms should be hospitalized and placed on bowel rest (nothing by mouth for 48–72 hours), intravenous fluids, and broad-spectrum antibiotics. Surgery is required for patients with peritoneal signs or those unresponsive to medical therapy.

> **B.** The differential diagnosis of **chronic diarrhea** is extensive.
> **1.** Most chronic diarrheas in **adults** are caused by the following:
> **a. IBS** is a complex of abnormal GI motility, altered visceral sensation, and psychological factors. IBS occurs in 20% of the US population, but only 10% to 20% of people with IBS seek medical care. In more than 50% of cases, symptoms develop before 35 years of age. Women are twice as likely to have IBS as men.
> **b. Lactose intolerance** is genetically controlled and occurs because of a normal decline in the intestinal lactase activity after childhood. It is present in 75% to 90% of US Blacks, Asians, American Indians, persons of Mediterranean origin, and Jews compared with less than 5% of descendants of Northern and Central Europeans. Secondary lactose intolerance can develop from injury to the intestinal mucosa (e.g., infectious diarrhea, celiac disease) or a decrease in mucosal surface (e.g., resection) and resolves with successful treatment of the underlying disease.
> **c. Idiopathic inflammatory bowel disease** (see Chapter 78). **Crohn disease,** characterized by transmural, focal, and asymmetric inflammation of any part of the GI tract, occurs in 4 to 20 per 10,000 individuals in North America, most frequently in people of European descent, particularly Jews. The onset is usually in adolescence and young adulthood. **Ulcerative colitis** is a diffused, continuous, superficial inflammation of the rectum and colon, occurring in 4 to 20 per 10,000 individuals in North America. Its onset is between ages 15 and 35 years,

with a second and smaller peak in the seventh decade. Ulcerative colitis is also more common in Jews, and there is a positive family history in approximately 10%. Occasionally, it develops after an acute infection.

d. Malabsorption syndrome. Celiac disease, an autoimmune inflammatory disease of the small intestine precipitated by gluten ingestion, is more common than previously thought, at approximately 1 case per 120 to 300 persons. Approximately 75% of new adult cases are in women. Celiac disease should be considered in patients at genetic risk (i.e., a family history of celiac disease or personal history of type I diabetes) and in patients with unexplained chronic diarrhea, anemia, fatigue, or weight loss.

e. Chronic infections (usually parasitic infections). Risk factors include travel to endemic areas, including Russia (*Giardia*), Peru, Haiti (*Cyclospora*), Thailand (*Campylobacter*), Nepal (*Cyclospora* and *Campylobacter*), or any developing country (*E. histolytica*), and drinking water from lakes or streams (*Giardia*). Immunosuppressed individuals and the elderly may have persistent diarrhea from *Campylobacter* and *Salmonella*. Risk factors for relapse of *C. difficile* infection (20% of patients) include intercurrent antibiotics, renal failure, and female gender. Other uncommon bacterial causes include *Aeromonas* (untreated water), *Plesiomonas* (foreign travel, raw shellfish, untreated water), *Yersinia* (contaminated stream and lake water, milk, or ice cream), *Mycobacterium tuberculosis* (travel to undeveloped country), and Brainerd diarrhea agent (unpasteurized milk and water).

2. In **children,** most chronic diarrhea is caused by the following factors:

a. Postinfectious diarrhea (intractable diarrhea of infancy). Postinfectious diarrhea is characterized by persistence of diarrhea and failure to gain weight more than 7 days after hospital admission for gastroenteritis. It appears to be due to small intestine mucosal injury with impaired disaccharidase and lactase activity. Risk factors include being a neonate or very young; being nonwhite; using antibiotics or antidiarrheal agents before admission; or having a previous history of diarrhea, a longer duration of diarrhea before hospitalization, severe diarrhea during the initial enteritis, weight below the tenth percentile, low blood urea nitrogen, and bacterial etiology of the initial enteritis.

b. Primary lactase deficiency. This deficiency starts between ages 3 and 5 years. Secondary lactose intolerance develops in 50% or more of infants with an acute or chronic diarrhea (especially with rotavirus) and is also fairly common with giardiasis, inflammatory bowel disease, and the AIDS malabsorption syndrome.

c. Cow's milk and soy protein hypersensitivity. Cow's milk hypersensitivity is the most common sensitivity in infancy, with an incidence between 0.3% and 7%. Thirty to fifty percent of infants with cow's milk protein sensitivity may also have soy protein hypersensitivity. Most patients achieve tolerance during their second year of life.

d. Celiac disease (see Section III.B.1.d).

e. Chronic nonspecific diarrhea. Chronic nonspecific diarrhea (IBS of children or toddler's diarrhea) appears between 6 months and 2 years of age. The cause is unknown, but may follow an acute infection or gastroenteritis. It is self-limited, usually resolving spontaneously before 4 years of age.

Infrequent causes of chronic diarrhea in children include immune deficiencies, AIDS, endocrine disorders (e.g., hyperthyroidism, adrenal insufficiency, diabetes), IBS, cystic fibrosis, and anatomic lesions (e.g., Hirschsprung disease). Pseudomembranous enterocolitis with *C. difficile* is rare, but severe and sometimes fatal. It is precipitated by antibiotics and causes profuse diarrhea, dehydration, abdominal pain, fever, electrolyte imbalance, hypoproteinemia, and leukocytosis.

IV. Symptoms. A thorough history is key in guiding the evaluation and management of patients with diarrhea. Important questions include **when and how the illness began** (abrupt or gradual onset, duration of diarrhea), **stool characteristics** (frequency; quantity; watery, bloody, mucus-filled, purulent, greasy), symptoms of **dehydration** (thirst, lethargy, postural lightheadedness, decreased urination), relationship to food intake, presence of dysentery (fever; tenesmus; blood, pus, or both), and associated **symptoms** (nausea, vomiting, abdominal cramps, bloating, constipation, flatus or belching, headache, myalgias).

In **chronic diarrhea,** a history of other medical conditions can be helpful in diagnosis such as seronegative spondyloarthropathies (inflammatory bowel disease), autoimmune diseases such as diabetes or thyroid disorders (chronic dysmotility diarrhea, celiac disease), and immune deficiencies (infections). Patients should be asked about **fecal incontinence,** especially with low-volume stools, because the evaluation for incontinence differs from that of diarrhea. **Previous surgery** to the GI or biliary tracts may be the cause of chronic diarrhea. Use of all **current medications** including nonprescription medicines, herbal or nutritional supplements, illicit drugs, alcohol, and caffeine should be elicited. Questions on antibiotic use in the past 8 weeks, a new or increased dose in medication, and laxative use should be specifically asked.

A. Viral diarrhea is usually self-limited, large volume, and watery, without blood, lasting from 1 to 2 days to 1 week. There may be nausea, vomiting, headache, low-grade fever, cramping, and malaise. Dehydration, especially in children, can occur.

B. Bacterial diarrhea
   1. Food poisoning by *S. aureus* and *B. cereus* cause symptoms from preformed toxins within 1 to 6 hours of exposure. *Clostridium perfringens* causes symptoms within 8 to 16 hours. These symptoms are of a sudden onset and generally last 2 to 24 hours. Nausea and vomiting are variable with some abdominal cramping. There is usually none of the following: fever, severe abdominal pain, headache, malaise, myalgia, or prolonged nausea or vomiting.
   2. Most bacterial diarrhea is more gradual in an onset, causing symptoms after 16 hours and lasting 1 to 7 days. Traveler's diarrhea typically begins 3 to 7 days after arrival in a foreign location. With invasive disease, fever, tenesmus, and gross blood, pus, or both are usually present. STEC causes bloody diarrhea without high fever or leukocytes. Severe cases may lead to hemolytic-uremic syndrome (bloody diarrhea, thrombocytopenia, hemolytic anemia, and renal failure).
      a. Reiter syndrome (arthritis, conjunctivitis, and urethritis or cervicitis) is a known complication of infections with *Campylobacter, Salmonella, Shigella,* and *Yersinia, especially* in persons who are HLA-B27 positive. *Campylobacter* has also been associated with **Guillain-Barre** (group of demyelinating diseases of peripheral nerves causing ascending progressive weakness).
      b. There is an increasing body of literature linking infectious, invasive gastroenteritis and traveler's diarrhea with chronic GI complaints and the onset of postinfectious IBS.
      c. Infection with *C. difficile* can occur several days to 8 weeks after use of antibiotics. Watery diarrhea and abdominal cramps are typical. In severe cases, bloody diarrhea, fever, and abdominal pain can be present. There is usually no nausea or vomiting.

C. Parasitic diarrhea
   1. *Giardia lamblia* causes watery diarrhea, sometimes with mucus. Nausea, anorexia, abdominal cramping, flatulence, steatorrhea, and weight loss may be present.
   2. *Cryptosporidium* causes prolonged diarrhea, associated with fatigue, flatulence, and abdominal pain. Fever is usually not present.
   3. Clinical symptoms of *E. histolytica* vary from asymptomatic carriage to severe bloody diarrhea that can be indistinguishable from ulcerative colitis. Abdominal cramping, diarrhea with blood or mucus, and malaise are common. In severe cases, massive bleeding, obstruction, dilation, or perforation may occur. Liver abscesses may result from systemic spread.

D. Chronic diarrhea. Watery stools suggest osmotic or secretory diarrhea. **Gross blood in the stool or other red flag symptoms** such as weight loss suggests inflammatory bowel or malignancy. The description of **foul-smelling,** light-colored, floating stool or undigested foods in stool suggests malabsorption.
   1. The Rome III criteria (http://www.romecriteria.org/criteria/) are helpful for differentiating **IBS** from organic pathology. The diagnosis is likely with recurrent abdominal pain or discomfort at least 3 days/month in last 3 months associated with two or more of the following: improvement with defecation, onset associated with a change in frequency of stool, or onset associated with a change in the form (appearance) of stool.
      To diagnose **IBS in a child,** abdominal discomfort or pain must be associated with two or more of the following at least 25% of the time: improvement with defecation, onset associated with a change in frequency of stool, or onset associated with

a change in form of stool. Additionally, there must be no evidence of an inflammatory, anatomic, metabolic, or neoplastic process that can account for the symptoms. Rome III criterion defines "discomfort" as any uncomfortable sensation not described as pain.

2. The severity of symptoms in **lactose intolerance** varies with the lactose load and other foods consumed at the same time and may include diarrhea, bloating, cramping, abdominal discomfort, flatulence, and rumbling (borborygmi). In children, vomiting is common and malnutrition can occur.

3. **Crohn disease** typically presents with diarrhea, abdominal pain, and weight loss. The clinical picture of **ulcerative colitis** is variable, from occasional rectal bleeding to profuse watery and bloody diarrhea with crampy lower abdominal pain and weight loss (Chapter 78).

4. **Celiac disease** may present with a range of symptoms including diarrhea, constipation, dyspepsia, gastroesophageal reflux, bloating, flatus, belching, fatigue, weight loss, depression, fibromyalgia-like symptoms, aphthous stomatitis, hair loss, and bone pain. Infants typically present with failure to thrive, diarrhea, abdominal distention, developmental delay, and, occasionally, severe malnutrition. Older children may have constitutional short stature or dental enamel defects.

V. **Signs.** The physical examination is most important in assessing volume status and nutrition. Other clinical signs may be important clues in differentiating chronic causes of diarrhea.

   A. **Vital signs.** Fever greater than 101.3°F suggests an acute inflammatory diarrhea. Postural changes in systolic blood pressure (decrease of 10 mm Hg) and pulse rate (increase of 20 beats per minute) support dehydration. In children, acute body weight changes best assess dehydration; other helpful measurements include dry mucous membranes, decreased capillary refill time, absence of tears, and alteration in mental status. In chronic cases, weight loss and failure to thrive suggest malabsorption, inflammatory bowel disease, infection, and neoplasm.

   B. **Skin.** Characteristic skin changes can be seen in less common causes of chronic diarrhea such as carcinoid syndrome (flushing, telangiectasias), celiac disease (dermatitis herpetiformis), mastocytosis (urticaria, linear telangiectasias), and Addison disease (hyperpigmentation).

   C. **Oral.** Aphthous oral ulcers and stomatitis may be present in inflammatory bowel disease or celiac disease.

   D. **Thyroid.** Nodules or mass suggests medullary carcinoma of thyroid or thyroid adenoma.

   E. **Cardiac.** Right-sided heart murmur may be present in carcinoid syndrome. Signs of severe atherosclerosis or peripheral vascular disease may be present with intestinal ischemia.

   F. **Abdominal examination.** This examination should assess for distention (IBS, infections), bruit (colon ischemia), tenderness (IBS, inflammatory bowel disease, infections, ischemia), mass (neoplasia), and hepatosplenomegaly (amyloidosis).

   G. **Rectal examination.** This examination should evaluate sphincter tone (fecal incontinence) and tenderness (proctitis). The presence of fistula, painless anal fissure, or a perirectal abscess may suggest Crohn disease. Fecal impaction in pediatric or geriatric age groups suggests overflow diarrhea.

   H. **Extremities.** Edema and clubbing suggest malabsorption. Arthritis may be noted in inflammatory bowel disease, Whipple disease, and some enteric infections.

   I. **Lymphadenopathy** may suggest lymphoma or other neoplasm.

VI. **Diagnostic Tests**

   A. **Acute diarrhea** (Figure 16–1). Testing is needed only in patients with dysentery, patients aged younger than 3 months or older than 70 years, immunocompromised patients, patients with persistent diarrhea, or those at risk for transmitting infections (e.g., food handlers in food service establishments, health care workers, attendees/residents, employees of day care, or an institutional facility such as a psychiatric hospital, prison, or nursing home). The modified 3-day rule rejects submitting routine stool cultures for low-risk patients hospitalized <3 days and dictates performing only *C. difficile* toxin tests. (SOR **Ⓐ**)

   B. **Chronic diarrhea** (Figure 16–2). Findings from the history, examination, routine laboratory tests, and quantitative stool analysis should guide specific, confirmatory testing or a trial of empiric therapy.

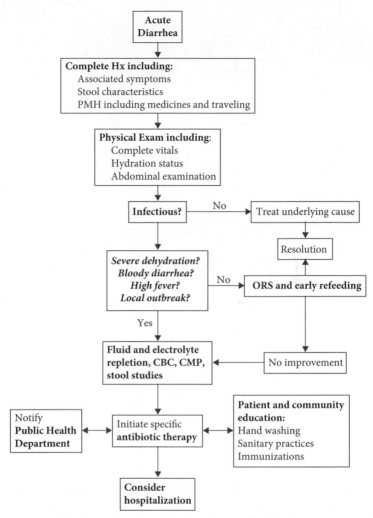

FIGURE 16–1. Approach to the patient with acute diarrhea. CBC, complete blood count; CMP, comprehensive metabolic panel; Hx, history; PMH, past medical history; ORS, oral rehydration solution.

1. **Blood tests.** A complete blood count may show anemia (blood loss, malabsorption) or leukocytosis (infection). A chemistry screen may be helpful in assessing fluid/electrolyte balance and nutritional status (malabsorption). TSH and tissue transglutaminase antibodies (for celiac disease) may also be ordered.

2. A **48-hour quantitative stool collection** on a regular diet of moderately high fat (80–100 g fat per day) can help classify diarrhea as osmotic, secretory, inflammatory, or fatty. The fecal analysis should include weight, electrolytes, calculation of osmotic gap (290 − 2[Na+ + K+]), pH, occult blood, stool leukocytes (or lactoferrin), total quantitative fecal fat (grams of fat/24 hours) and percent fat, and analysis for laxatives.

VII. Treatment for acute and chronic diarrheas should include supportive measures as well as measures directed at underlying causes determined through careful history, examination, and appropriate laboratory evaluation (Figures 16–1 and 16–2).

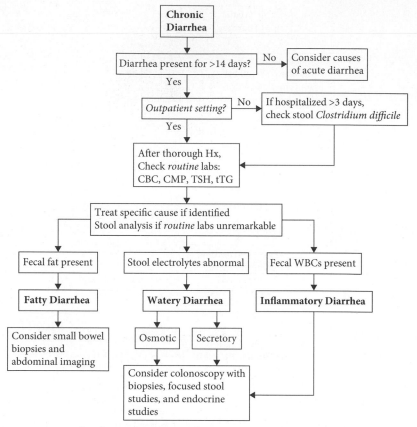

FIGURE 16–2. Approach to the patient with chronic diarrhea. CBC, complete blood count; CMP, comprehensive metabolic panel; Hx, history; TSH, thyroid stimulating hormone; tTG, tissue transglutaminase.

A. Maintenance of hydration and rehydration

1. In the **healthy adult with mild-to-moderate acute diarrhea,** oral glucose or starch containing products, for example, carbonated drinks, fruit juice, or sports drinks with saltine crackers, are adequate. (SOR **A**) These should not be used in infants and young children because of excessive carbohydrate content and inadequate sodium and potassium.

2. For **children, the elderly, or those with moderate-to-severe diarrhea,** the WHO formula or commercial oral rehydration solutions (ORSs) such as Pedialyte, Rehydralyte, Infalyte, Naturalyte, and Resol are recommended and are superior to intravenous fluids in resolving diarrhea and restoring weight. WHO's recently restructured formula reflects decreased osmolarity from 311 to 245 in response to studies noted by Cochrane that showed reduced osmolarity ORS when compared with WHO standard ORS was associated with fewer unscheduled intravenous fluid infusions, lower stool volume postrandomization, and less vomiting with no additional risk of developing hyponatremia. (SOR **A**)

   a. **Homemade ORS** can be prepared by adding seven teaspoons of sugar and one teaspoon of salt to 1 L of bottled water.

   b. **Rice-based ORS** decreases stool output compared with standard ORS and can be prepared by mixing half cup dry, precooked baby rice cereal with two cups water, and one-fourth teaspoon salt. With mild-to-moderate dehydration, 50 to

100 mL/kg should be given over 2 to 4 hours and an additional 50 to 100 mL after each stool to children younger than 2 years, 100 to 200 mL to 2- to 10-year-old children, and unlimited to children older than 10 years and adults.

3. In **severe dehydration** with obtunded mental status or when oral intake is not able to keep up with ongoing losses, intravenous fluids (0.9 N saline or Ringer solution 20–40 mL/kg per hour for children, D5 Ringer lactate or D5 0.9 N saline 1 L every 1–2 hours for adults) should be given for 4 to 6 hours until adequate rehydration (determined by weight gain in children and clinical signs in adults) is established. The patient's usual diet supplemented with ORS can then be resumed.

B. Diet

1. **Children** should be continued on their preferred, usual, and age-appropriate diet. Frequent small feedings (every 10–60 minutes) of any tolerated foods or ORS may be helpful, if vomiting occurs. Breast-feeding should be continued. Formula-fed infants should continue with their usual formula immediately upon rehydration. Additionally, supplementation with elemental zinc (typically 20 mg per day) has been shown to decrease stool output and the frequency and duration of acute infectious diarrhea in children aged 6 months and older. The efficacy of zinc supplementation is most notable in malnourished children, particularly in developing nations. In these regions, zinc supplementation has been shown to be safe, efficacious, and affordable. (SOR **Ⓐ**)

2. For children with **intractable diarrhea of infancy,** oral elemental diets appear helpful.

3. **Adults** should be encouraged to eat potatoes, rice, wheat, noodles, crackers, bananas, yogurt, boiled vegetables, and soup. Dairy products, caffeine, and alcohol should be avoided.

4. In **chronic diarrhea,** fasting can differentiate between osmotic diarrhea (which resolves with fasting) and some secretory diarrheas. Dietary measures beneficial in chronic diarrhea include eating a high-fiber diet for IBS; avoiding lactose for lactose intolerance; and avoiding wheat, barley, and rye for celiac disease. In children with postinfectious diarrhea, management with a soy-based formula, lactose-free formula, or semielemental diet is indicated.

C. Symptomatic treatment

1. **Antimotility** agents can be considered in adult patients with watery, noninflammatory diarrhea. They should be avoided in young children and patients with dysentery. (SOR **Ⓑ**) First-line therapies are usually opiate derivatives such as loperamide (Imodium [maximum dose 8 mg per day]) or diphenoxylate with atropine (Lomotil), used after each diarrheal movement, not to exceed eight tablets (20 mg of diphenoxylate) per day. (SOR **Ⓐ**)

2. In **chronic diarrhea,** bulk-forming agents (psyllium or methylcellulose) can be used to increase stool bulk and consistency, but they do not reduce stool weight. Opiates (e.g., tincture of opium [10%], six drops [0.6 mL] every 6 hours or 0.005 to 0.01 mL/kg/dose every 3 to 4 hours for children, or codeine for adults, 15–30 mg every 4–6 hours) may be necessary.

D. Antibiotic treatment (see Table 16–1).

1. **Empiric treatment**
   a. Treatment for **travelers' diarrhea** (see Chapter 107).
   b. Patients with **persistent diarrhea** can be empirically treated for presumed giardiasis, especially if there was a history of travel or exposure to untreated water (e.g., lake, stream, or well), and if other evaluations are negative.
   c. Empiric treatment can also be considered in those with dysentery, those who appear septic or toxic, and **high-risk patients** (infants younger than 3 months, persons older than 70 years, and immunocompromised patients) after a stool specimen is obtained.
   d. In **chronic diarrhea,** a therapeutic trial of broad-spectrum antibiotics may be considered for suspected small-bowel bacterial overgrowth (resulting from stasis of intestinal contents, e.g., in individuals with diabetes and slowed intestinal motility, postgastrectomy patients, or persons with partial intestinal obstruction from Crohn disease).

2. **Specific antibiotic treatment.** Other infections should be treated based on the specific causative organism. Antibiotics or antimotility agents should not be used in enterohemorrhagic *STEC,* as they may enhance toxin release and increase the risk of hemolytic-uremic syndrome.

TABLE 16–1. TREATMENT OPTIONS FOR SPECIFIC PATHOGENS

Pathogen	Drug	Dose	Major Side Effects	Contraindications	Drug Interactions with More Common Medicines
Aeromonas/Plesiomonas	Ciprofloxacin	Adult: 500 mg oral twice daily × 3 d Pediatric: 20–30 mg/kg/d oral twice daily × 3 d	*Common:* GI upset, headache *Severe:* Tendon rupture (over 60 years of age, concomitant steroid therapy)	Avoid in myasthenia gravis Caution in children and elderly	May prolong QT with cisapride, dronedone, phenothiazines, and others; theophylline (theophylline tox); antidiabetic (↑hypo- or hyperglycemia); warfarin (↑ bleeding risk); simvastatin (↑myopathy, rhabdomyolysis); methadone (↑ serum methadone, ↑ QT); clozapine (↑ clozapine exposure and risk of QT prolongation)
Campylobacter species	Azithromycin **OR** Ciprofloxacin	Adult: 500 mg oral daily × 3 d Pediatric: 10 mg/kg oral daily × 3 d, (max. 500 mg/d) Adult: 500–750 mg oral twice daily × 5 d Pediatric: 15–30 mg/kg/d every 8–12 h × 5 d	*Common:* GI upset, headache, ↑ liver enzymes *Severe:* Prolong QT GI upset (see above)	Caution in elderly, hepatic impairment, jaundice, cholestatic (see above)	May prolong QT with cisapride, phenothiazines, and others; disopyramide (↑ arrhythmial), simvastatin (↑ myalgia risk), warfarin (↑ bleed) (see above)
Clostridium difficile	Metronidazole Vancomycin[a] (for severe disease or failure to respond to metronidazole within 7 d)	Adult: 500 mg oral every 8 h for 10–14 d Elderly: 250–500 mg oral every 6–8 h for 10–14 d Pediatric: 30 mg/kg/d every 6 h × 7–10 d Adult: 125 mg orally four times daily for 10–14 d Pediatric: 40–50 mg/kg/d orally every 6 h × 7–10 d (max. 500 mg)	*Common:* GI upset, headache *Severe:* Steven-Johnson syndrome, TEN, aseptic meningitis *Common:* Fever, GI upset, eosinophilia, hypokalemia *Serious:* Nephrotoxicity	Avoid in first trimester Caution in renal impairment Caution in hearing impairment Caution in the elderly	Avoid alcohol until 72 h after treatment, amprenavir (↑ propylene glycol tox [seizure, tachycardia, lactic acidosis, renal tox, hemolysis]), disulfiram (CNS tox), amiodarone (cardiotoxicity), fluorouracil (anemia, granulocytopenia, thrombocytopenia, stomatitis, V), warfarin (↑ bleeding risk) Avoid with cidofovir and streptozocin (overlapping renal tox)
Cryptosporidium species	Nitazoxanide	Adult: 500 mg orally twice daily × 3 d Age 1–3 years: 100 mg oral twice daily × 3 d; age 4–11 years: 200 mg oral twice daily × 3 d	Abdominal pain	Caution in renal/hepatic impairment, immunodeficiency, diabetes (suspension contains 1.48 g sucrose/5 mL)	None known

Organism	Drug	Dose	Adverse Effects	Contraindications	Comments
Cyclospora species	Trimethoprim sulfamethoxazole (TMP-SMX)	Adult: DS oral twice daily × 5 d (traveler's diarrhea)[b] Pediatric: TMP 5 mg/kg, SMX 25 mg/kg/d orally in 2 doses × 7–10 d	Nausea, vomiting, anorexia, rash	Hepatic/renal insufficiency, megaloblastic anemia, or thrombocytopenia, infants <2 mo, pregnancy near-term	Contraindicated with methenamine, spironolactone (hyperkalemia), MTX (MTX tox), warfarin (↑ bleeding risk), TCA (↑ cardiotox), gemifloxacin (cardiotox), pyrimethamine (megalo-blastic anemia), Class IA antiarrhythmic agents, leucovorin (treatment failure)
Entamoeba histolytica Asymptomatic Mild-to-moderate disease	**Iodoquinol** Metronidazole	Adult: 650 mg oral three times daily × 20 d Pediatric: 30–40 mg/kg/d (max. 2 g) orally in 3 doses 20 d Adult: 500–750 mg oral three times daily × 7–10 d Pediatric: 35–50 mg/kg/d oral in 3 divided doses × 7–10 d followed by iodoquinol as above	GI upset (see above)	(see above)	(see above)
Escherichia coli (not hemor-rhagic)	Ciprofloxacin	Adult: 500 mg oral twice daily × 3 d Pediatric: 20–30 mg/kg/d oral divided every 12 h (max. 750 mg/dose)	GI upset (see above)	(see above)	(see above)
Giardia	Metronidazole or Tinidazole	Adult: 250 mg three times daily × 5–7 d Elderly: 250 mg three times daily × 5–7 d Pediatric: 35–50 mg/kg/d divided every 8 h Adult: 200 mg oral × 1 dose (with food) Elderly: 200 mg oral × 1 dose (with food) Pediatric: >3 y: 50 mg/kg/day × 1 dose max. 2000 mg/dose (with food)	GI upset (see above) Metallic taste, nausea, and vomiting; candida vaginitis *Serious:* Seizure	(see above) Avoid in first trimester	(see above) Contraindicated with disulfiram; allow 2 wk after disulfiram discontinuation

(continued)

TABLE 16–1. TREATMENT OPTIONS FOR SPECIFIC PATHOGENS (Continued)

Pathogen	Drug	Dose	Major Side Effects	Contraindications	Drug Interactions with More Common Medicines
Isospora species	TMP-SMX	Adult: TMP-SMX DS oral × 14–28 d Pediatric: 8–10 mg/kg/d TMP oral/IV divided every 12 h	(see above)	(see above)	(see above)
Listeria monocytogenes	Ampicillin or Penicillin G	Adult: 2 g IV every 6 h × 14 d Pediatric: 300 mg/kg/d IV divided doses every 6 h × 14 d Adult: 12–18 million units/d IV given in divided doses every 4–6 h × 14 d Pediatric: 20,000 units/kg/d IV given in divided doses q4–6 h × 14 d	*Common:* GI upset, urticaria, rash *Serious:* Stevens–Johnson syndrome, TEN, anaphylaxis, thrombocytopenia, agranulocytosis *Common:* Drug-induced eosinophillia *Serious:* Hyperkalemia, hemolytic anemia, decreased renal fx, seizure, interstitial nephritis	Contraindicated in mononucleosis Infection due to penicillinase-producing organism Anaphylactic reaction to penicillin	Contraindicated with chloroquine Contraindicated if anaphylactic reaction to beta-lactams MTX (↑ MTX tox), warfarin (increases risk of bleeding)
Microsporidium species	Albendazole (given with food)	Over age 13 y: 400 mg oral twice daily × 21 d Age 1 mo–12 y: 7.5 mg/kg oral twice daily × 21 d (max. 400 mg/dose)	Abnormal LFTs *Common:* nausea, V, diarrhea, abdominal pain *Serious:* Agranulocytosis, TEN, Stevens–Johnson syndrome	During pregnancy and avoid <1 mo after treatment cessation Caution in hepatic impairment	Contraindicated with cimetidine, dexamethasone, and praziquantel
Salmonella (nontyphiod species)	Ciprofloxacin or Azithromycin	Adult: 500 mg oral twice daily × 5–7 d Pediatric: 20–30 mg/kg/d oral given in two divided doses × 5–7 d Adult: 1 g oral on day 1, then 500 mg orally daily × 6 d Pediatric: 10 mg/kg/d oral (max. 500 mg/d)	GI upset (see above) (see above)	(see above) (see above)	(see above) (see above)
Shigella	Ciprofloxacin	Adults: 500 mg oral twice daily × 3 d Pediatric: 15 mg/kg oral twice daily × 3 d	(see above)	(see above)	(see above)

Vibrio cholerae	Oral rehydration with Doxycycline or Ciprofloxacin	Adult/pediatric: As much fluid as possible orally Adult: 100 mg oral twice daily × 3 d Pediatric: 2.2 mg/kg oral/IV daily × 3 d Adult: 500 mg oral twice daily × 3 d Pediatric: 20–30 mg/kg/d oral divided 8–12 h (max. 750 mg/dose)	N/A Tooth discoloration (in those <8 y), Photosensitivity (see above)	N/A Contraindicated in hepatic disease, pregnancy, and children <8 y (see above)	N/A Increase risk of pseudotumor cerebri and papilledema with acitretin, isoretinoin; MTX (↑ MTX tox) (see above)
Yersinia	Doxycycline or Ciprofloxacin	Adult: 100 mg oral twice daily × 7 d Pediatric (<45 kg): 2.2 mg/kg oral twice daily (max. 200 mg/d) Adult: 500 mg oral twice daily × 7 d Pediatric: 20 mg/kg oral twice daily (max. 1000 mg/d)	(see above) (see above)	(see above) (see above)	(see above) (see above)
Acute diarrhea in persons >6 mo with zinc deficiency and malnourishment	Zinc	Pediatric (>6 mo): 20 mg elemental zinc daily	GI upset	Caution with bleeding disorder	N/A
All diarrhea requiring treatment with antibiotics	Probiotics: VSL#3 or Florastor or Culturelle	All: One cap orally twice daily for duration of antibiotic treatment Adult: (as above) Pediatric: One sachet daily for duration of antibiotic treatment Adult: (as above) Pediatric (11–22 kg): One packet daily (>22 kg): One chewable cap daily	Bloating	N/A	N/A

tox, toxicity; CNS, central nervous system; IV, intravenous; V, vomiting; LFTs, liver function tests; MTX, methotrexate; TEN, toxic epidermal necrolysis.
[a]Vancomycin is not effective when given intravenously for *C. difficile* colitis; can give via nasogastric tube or retention enema if oral not tolerated.
[b]TMP-SMX DS is given four times daily for 7 days for patients with HIV and *Cyclospora* infection.

E. Probiotics appear to be a useful adjunct to rehydration therapy in **treating acute, infectious diarrhea,** decreasing the duration of illness by 30 to 48 hours. (SOR **A**) Efficacy is most evident in viral diarrheas and less or absent in invasive, bacterial diarrheas. In children, *Lactobacillus* GG has been shown to reduce the duration of acute diarrhea by 1 day and duration of rotavirus shedding; it is most effective when given during the first 2.5 days of illness. The dosage is at least 10 billion colony-forming units daily. (SOR **B**)

F. Other agents for chronic diarrhea. Empiric trials of cholestyramine (for bile acid diarrheas, after ileal resection, vagotomy, or cholecystectomy) and pancreatic enzymes (for pancreatic insufficiency) may be diagnostic and therapeutic. Lactase capsules can be helpful in lactose intolerance.

VIII. Patient Education

A. Acute diarrhea

1. Most episodes of acute diarrhea are self-limited. Good hygiene, including regular hand-washing with soap and water and sanitary handling of food products, helps prevent contamination and decrease transmission of disease. Compliance with local vaccination protocol and immunizing against rotavirus has proven effective in significantly reducing severe cases of rotavirus diarrhea. (SOR **A**)

2. Fluid and electrolyte imbalance are the most dangerous consequences of acute diarrhea. Left untreated, dehydration can lead to significant morbidity and mortality. If dehydration is suspected, ORS should be started immediately. Homemade solutions are as effective as commercial ORS products. Parents should be encouraged to continue breast or bottle feeding, and eating normal foods should begin as soon as possible after beginning ORS. (SOR **A**) Food should not be limited to the BRAT (banana, rice, applesauce, toast) diet. There is no harm in early refeeding after ORS has been instituted. (SOR **A**)

3. Physician consultation is warranted when there is no improvement after 24 hours of starting ORS or when there is difficulty in administering ORS. A physician should be contacted promptly for any signs of severe dehydration such as changes in mental status (e.g., marked increase in fatigue or irritability) or dry mucous membranes (dry lips and tongue, decreased tears, decreased saliva). Additionally, a physician should be called for diarrhea accompanied by high fevers (>100.4°F if <3 months and >101°F if >3 months), bloody diarrhea, or a history of prematurity or other medical problem. (SOR **A**)

B. Chronic diarrhea

1. Chronic diarrhea embodies a vast number of distinct diseases, often with multifactorial etiologies. Any diarrhea persisting for more than 14 days requires physician consultation. A detailed history is most useful for the physician during an initial encounter. Providing the physician with a detailed inventory of symptoms, ideally recorded in a journal, will be most helpful in zeroing in on a diagnosis. When and how symptoms began, stool characteristics, and associated symptoms (e.g., flatus, headache, fevers, myalgia), as well as laboratory studies, are key to making a diagnosis.

SELECTED REFERENCES

Hickson M. Probiotics in the prevention of antibiotic-associated diarrhoea and *Clostridium difficile* infection. *Therap Adv Gastroenterol.* 2011;4(3):185–197.

Kamdeu FAA, Guertin JR, LeLorier J. Savings from the use of a probiotic formula in the prophylaxis of antibiotic-associated diarrhea. *J Med Econ.* 2012;15(1):53–60.

Janarthanan S, Ditah I, Phil M, et al. Clostridium difficile-associated diarrhea and proton pump inhibitor therapy: a meta-analysis. *Am J Gastroenterol.* 2012;107(7):1001–1010.

Johnson S, Maziade PJ, McFarland LV, et al. Is primary prevention of *Clostridium difficile* infection possible with specific probiotics? *Int J Infect Dis.* 2012;16(11):e786–e792.

Rome Foundation. Rome III diagnostic criteria for functional gastrointestinal disorders. www.romecriteria.org, online version 2012.

17   Dizziness

Diane J. Madlon-Kay, MD, MS

KEY POINTS

- Peripheral vestibular disorders are the most common cause of dizziness. (SOR C)
- A directed history and physical examination can usually rule out the few serious causes of dizziness. (SOR C)
- Treatment options are limited, although symptoms resolve spontaneously in most patients. Supporting evidence is strongest for use of vestibular exercises for movement provoked dizziness (SOR B) and canalith repositioning or Epley maneuver for benign positional vertigo. (SOR A)

I. **Definition.** *Dizziness* is an imprecise term commonly used by patients to describe symptoms such as faintness, giddiness, lightheadedness, or unsteadiness as well as vertigo.

II. **Common Diagnoses.** In up to 19% of cases, a definitive cause of dizziness cannot be found. The various diagnoses of dizziness can be divided into three main categories.

   A. **Peripheral vestibular disorders,** which account for up to 44% of cases, include vestibular neuronitis, benign positional vertigo, Ménière disease, acoustic neuroma, and otitis media. These patients have a disorder at some point along the course of the vestibular nerve other than at its origin in the brain stem. Most often, the problem is at the termination of the nerve in the inner ear, known as the labyrinth.

ACOUSTIC NEUROMA

Acoustic neuroma typically presents as unilateral tinnitus and hearing loss. Few patients have vertigo initially. Symptoms are slowly progressive, and continued growth of the tumor is associated with facial weakness and ataxia.

   B. **Adverse effects from drugs or systemic diseases,** such as cardiac problems, metabolic abnormalities, anemia, infection, and psychogenic causes, can result in dizziness. About 20% to 30% of all cases of dizziness are believed to be psychogenic. Disorders in almost any organ system can cause dizziness. Spatial orientation depends on the complex interaction of adequate sensation, central integration, and the proper motor response.

   C. **Central nervous system diseases,** such as stroke, transient ischemic attack, migraines, or multiple sclerosis, are responsible for dizziness in 5% of patients. Any disease that disrupts the pathway between the vestibular apparatus and the brain may result in dizziness. Normally, impulses from this apparatus proceed through the eighth cranial nerve to the vestibular nuclei of the brain stem. From the brain stem, they are transmitted to the cerebellum and the cerebral cortex.

CENTRAL NERVOUS SYSTEM DISEASES

Central nervous system diseases, such as strokes, can cause vertigo. However, the vertigo is almost always accompanied by other central nervous system symptoms such as facial numbness, hemiparesis, and diplopia. Dysarthria, facial numbness, hemiparesis, or diplopia may be found on examination.

III. **Symptoms and Signs.** Dizziness can be divided into four basic types: vertigo, presyncope, disequilibrium, and lightheadedness. Details about the types of dizziness are shown in Table 17–1. Patient description of the type of dizziness symptom are not helpful in determining the cause. Patients are most helpful when describing the duration, triggers, and associated symptoms.

TABLE 17–1. TYPES OF DIZZINESS

	Vertigo	Presyncope	Disequilibrium	Lightheadedness
Sensation	Rotational; spinning or whirling	Lightheaded, faint feeling	Unsteadiness; loss of balance on walking	Vague; may be floating sensation
Temporal characteristics	May be episodic or continuous	Typically, episodes last seconds to hours	Usually present, although it may fluctuate in intensity	Usually present all or most of the time for days or weeks, sometimes years
Simulation tests	Dix-Hallpike maneuver	Orthostatic blood pressure measurement	Romberg test, tandem gait	Hyperventilation
Differential diagnosis	**Peripheral Causes** • Vestibular neuronitis • Benign positional vertigo • Ménière disease • Acoustic neuroma • Otitis media • Motion sickness • Drug use **Central Causes** • Stroke • Transient ischemic attack • Multiple sclerosis • Basilar artery migraine • Temporal lobe seizure	• Arrhythmias • Vasovagal reflex • Orthostatic hypotension • Anemia • Aortic stenosis • Low cardiac output states • Carotid sinus hypersensitivity • Hypoglycemia • Hypoxemia	• Multiple sensory deficits • Altered visual input • Primary disequilibrium of aging • Parkinsonism • Cerebellar disease • Frontal lobe apraxia • Drug use	• Anxiety • Depression • Hyperventilation • Panic disorder

A. Vertigo (i.e., a sensation of turning or spinning) accompanied by **nausea, vomiting, diaphoresis,** and **difficulty with balance** suggests peripheral vestibular disorders. Patients may also have **auditory symptoms** such as decreased hearing, tinnitus, and ear pain. Symptoms of particular disorders are described below.

　1. Vestibular neuronitis or acute labyrinthitis. After an acute onset of severe vertigo lasting several days, gradual improvement follows for several weeks. Symptoms frequently follow a viral illness.

　2. Benign positional vertigo. Instances of vertigo related to position are extremely brief, can be associated with nausea, and often will wake the patient from sleep when turning over in bed. Although the disorder is generally self-limited, its course is variable.

　3. Ménière disease. Patients with this disease have discrete attacks of vertigo of abrupt onset. The attacks last for several hours, not days, and are often accompanied by nausea and vomiting. The interval between attacks may be weeks to months. Between attacks, the patient is asymptomatic. Fluctuating hearing loss, typically accompanied by tinnitus and a feeling of pressure in the ear, is usually present during attacks. Irreversible hearing loss and chronic tinnitus develop in the affected ear over time.

B. Presyncope is dizziness associated with the feeling of an impending faint. Actual loss of consciousness does not occur. It is episodic.

C. Disequilibrium is a problem with balance, usually associated with an unsteady gait. If patients are asked, "Is the dizziness in your head or in your feet?" those with disequilibrium respond with the latter choice.

D. Lightheadedness is a vague or floating sensation, often imprecisely described by the patient. Such dizziness is generally present much of the time. It is often accompanied by other somatic symptoms, such as headache or abdominal pain.

TABLE 17-2. DISTINGUISHING PERIPHERAL FROM CENTRAL VERTIGO WITH POSITION TESTING

	Peripheral	Central
Latency (time to onset of vertigo or nystagmus)	3–10 s	None; begins immediately
Fatigability (lessening signs and symptoms with repetition)	Yes	No
Nystagmus direction	Fixed	Changing
Intensity of signs and symptoms	Severe	Mild

E. **Diagnostic maneuvers**
  1. The **head impulse or head thrust test** is the best bedside predictor of peripheral versus central causes of acute vestibular syndrome. The patient sits in front of the examiner while the examiner holds the patient's head. The patient is told to maintain gaze on the examiner's nose. The examiner quickly moves the head to each side, about 10 degrees, and observes if the patient is able to keep their eyes on the examiner's nose after each movement. If the patient's eyes stay on the nose, the peripheral vestibular system is working normally. If the patient's eyes move with the head so that the patient needs to make voluntary eye movements back to the nose, there is a lesion of the peripheral vestibular system. A video demonstrating this test is available at: http://www.youtube.com/watch?v=CZXDNLLGG8k.
  2. The **Dix–Hallpike (Nylen–Barany) maneuver** can be helpful in distinguishing peripheral from central vestibulopathy. The patient should sit on the edge of the examining table and lie down suddenly, with the head hanging 45 degrees backward and turned 45 degrees to one side. Then repeat the test twice, once with the head turned to the other side and once with the head in the middle position. The patient's eyes should be kept open to observe (1) the development of vertigo and (2) the time of onset, duration, and direction of nystagmus. This maneuver will reveal a central or peripheral pattern of vertigo, as shown in Table 17–2. (SOR **C**) A video demonstrating this maneuver can be seen at: http://www.youtube.com/watch?v=ZVCliBpclnw.
F. Inspection of the eardrum can reveal otitis media or serous otitis.
G. **Orthostatic blood pressure** determinations are helpful when the history suggests dizziness caused by hypovolemia from blood loss or dehydration. A drop in systolic blood pressure of as much as 20 mm Hg, a decline in diastolic pressure of up to 10 mm Hg, and a rise in pulse rate of up to 20 beats per minute can be normal findings with standing. If standing causes a greater blood pressure drop or pulse rise and reproduces the patient's symptoms, some form of hypovolemia is the most likely cause.
H. If the history suggests disequilibrium, **gait and stationary testing** should be done. Static balance can be tested with the Romberg test. The gait can be tested by asking the patient to rise from a chair, without using their arms, walk 10 feet, and then turn around. In addition, evaluation of muscle strength, coordination, reflexes, and proprioception should be conducted. The posture should be inspected. Often, patients with postural instability stand bent over, with their knees and hips flexed. A gentle tap on the chest (the nudge test) while standing behind the patient can give an indication of the patient's likelihood of falling backward. Testing visual fields and acuity can uncover visual impairment.
I. If the history suggests a psychological cause, the patient should hyperventilate by blowing vigorously for 3 minutes on a paper towel held 6 inches from the mouth. This action may cause some circumoral and digital numbness, as well as reproduce the patient's dizziness.

IV. **Laboratory Tests**
  A. A few patients with suspected peripheral vestibular disorders require laboratory testing. Patients whose symptoms are progressive or recurrent should have an **audiologic evaluation** that includes a pure tone audiogram, speech discrimination testing, and tympanometry. Such patients should also undergo vestibular examination by **electronystagmography**.
     Laboratory testing of patients whose dizziness may be caused by systemic diseases must be guided by the history and physical examination. Most "screening" laboratory tests, such as complete blood cell count and electrolyte determination, are rarely helpful.
  B. **Magnetic resonance imaging** with gadolinium enhancement is particularly useful in detecting acoustic neuromas and is the current gold standard test. (SOR **C**)

V. Treatment
   A. Peripheral vestibular disorders. The symptoms of vertigo are frightening to patients. The physician must be supportive and reassuring, since most causes of vertigo are not a serious health threat.
   1. Initial treatment of acutely vertiginous patients usually involves having them lie still in a darkened room and avoid head movement. It is important to have patients mobilized as soon as the most severe nausea and vertigo subside, to avoid protracted disability.
   2. Drug therapy can provide symptomatic relief; doses listed below are for adults.
      a. Antihistamines, the most commonly prescribed drugs for vertigo, suppress the vestibular end-organ receptors and inhibit activation of vagal responses. Patients should take the medication for a few weeks and then try discontinuing the drug. The major side effects are dry mouth and sedation. Commonly recommended drugs are meclizine, dose 25 mg orally once up to four times daily, and diphenhydramine, 25 to 50 mg orally every 4 to 6 hours. (SOR ❸)
      b. Antiemetics can be tried when nausea and vomiting are pronounced. These agents suppress central vestibular pathways, which activate a vagal response. Their major side effect is sedation. Commonly recommended antiemetic drugs are prochlorperazine, 5 to 10 mg orally three to four times daily *or* 25-mg suppository per rectum twice daily, and trimethobenzamide, 300 mg orally three to four times daily. Acute dystonic reactions occur occasionally with prochlorperazine.
   3. Vestibular exercises can reduce symptoms, disability, and handicap from movement provoked dizziness. (SOR ❸)
   4. The **canalith repositioning or Epley maneuver** eliminates symptoms of benign positional vertigo in up to 80% of patients after one treatment. (SOR ❹) A video demonstrating this maneuver can be seen at: http://www.youtube.com/watch?v=YK2Zj_TrBhE.
   5. Surgery may be indicated if other medical therapies fail to adequately relieve severe vertigo. Surgical procedures include sectioning of the vestibular nerve, repair of an inner ear fistula, labyrinthectomy, or placement of a lymphatic shunt. Unilateral deafness can result.
   B. Systemic diseases. Systemic diseases causing dizziness require treatment that is cause-specific.
   C. Central nervous system diseases. Symptomatic treatment of vertigo as described above may be helpful. Treatment of the underlying central nervous system condition is crucial.
VI. Patient Education
   A. Explain that dizziness is a feeling that is often hard to describe, but may be a feeling that you are going to fall or pass out, or that you are spinning. Dizziness can make you to feel lightheaded or giddy, or have difficulty walking. It is not usually caused by a serious condition.
   B. Patients should be encouraged to get help right away if they have any of the following in addition to dizziness: seeing double, having trouble speaking, weakness in an arm or a leg, or vomiting that will not stop.
   C. Treatment depends on the cause of the dizziness and can include medicine or head and neck exercises.

SELECTED REFERENCES

Kerber KA, Baloh RW. The evaluation of a patient with dizziness. *Neurol Clin Pract.* 2011;1:24–32.
Post RE, Dickerson LM. Dizziness: a diagnostic approach. *Am Fam Physician.* 2010;82:361–368.
Tarnutzer AA, Berkowitz AL, Robinson KA, et al. *CMAJ.* 2011;183:E571–E592.

18 Dysmenorrhea

Suzanne L. Harrison, MD, & Lisa M. Johnson, MD

KEY POINTS

- Dysmenorrhea is the most commonly reported gynecologic symptom experienced by menstruating women, with an estimated 90% of all women being affected at least once in their life. (SOR C)
- Dysmenorrhea causes significant disruption in the quality of life. It is the leading cause of short-term school absenteeism in adolescents, and a common cause of missed work for adult women. (SOR C)
- If dysmenorrhea fails to respond to first-line treatment with nonsteroidal anti-inflammatory drugs (NSAIDs) or oral contraceptives (OCs), an underlying cause should be considered. (SOR C)

I. **Definition.** Dysmenorrhea is painful menstruation, frequently described as crampy pelvic pain that may radiate to the low back and thighs. The distinction must be made between primary and secondary dysmenorrhea.
   A. **Primary dysmenorrhea** is menstrual pain in women with normal pelvic anatomy. Pain generally starts in adolescence, peaks in the second and third decades of life, and decreases in frequency with advancing age. Increased levels of prostaglandins in menstrual fluid have been identified in women with dysmenorrhea, especially on the first two days of menses. Altered levels of leukotrienes, thromboxanes, and prostacyclin have also been implicated and contribute to uterine hypercontractility and vasoconstriction seen in severe dysmenorrhea. Vasopressin is also elevated in women with dysmenorrhea and causes increased uterine contractility and ischemic pain due to vasoconstriction. Women with painful menses have increased uterine basal tone and myometrial contractile pressure. Uterine contractions are more frequent and dysrhythmic in women diagnosed with dysmenorrhea.
   B. **Secondary dysmenorrhea** is painful menses associated with underlying pelvic organ pathology.
II. **Common Diagnoses**
   A. **Primary dysmenorrhea** affects 40% to 70% of menstruating women. Prevalence is highest in teens, with estimates as high as 90%. Primary dysmenorrhea is associated with ovulatory cycles, so symptoms typically do not begin with the first menstrual cycles. Fifteen percent of adolescents report severe dysmenorrhea that causes significant disruption in activities, including school absence. Early menarche, family history, nulliparity, and heavy menses are risk factors for dysmenorrhea. Behavioral risk factors include cigarette smoking and weight loss attempts (independent of body mass index). Mental health risk factors include depression, anxiety, and disruption of social support networks.
   B. **Secondary dysmenorrhea** can be caused by several different conditions:
      1. **Endometriosis** is defined as foci of endometrial tissue outside the endometrial cavity and uterine musculature. It is the most common cause of secondary dysmenorrhea. Estimates for women of reproductive age are <10% with higher rates in women with chronic pelvic pain and infertility. The age at diagnosis is typically 25 to 35 years. Endometriosis is increasingly being diagnosed in adolescents and accounts for symptoms in 47% to 73% of teens with severe menstrual pain and no response to nonsteroidal anti-inflammatory drugs (NSAIDs) or oral contraceptives (OCs).
      2. **Adenomyosis** is observed most frequently in women after 35 years of age and is caused by foci of endometrial tissue in the myometrium. Fifteen percent of women with adenomyosis have associated endometriosis.
      3. **Leiomyomas (fibroids)** are benign uterine smooth muscle tumors. They are the most common gynecologic tumors and are more common in black women. Twenty

percent of women develop fibroids by 40 years of age; most are asymptomatic. Leiomyomas are estrogen-dependent tumors, so they resolve at menopause.

4. **Pelvic inflammatory disease (PID)** (see Chapter 50).
5. **Ovarian cysts**
6. **Nonhormonal intrauterine devices (IUDs).** Levonorgestrel-releasing IUDs
improve both dysmenorrhea and duration of menstrual bleeding.
7. **Endometrial polyps**
8. **Anatomical** causes of dysmenorrhea include congenital anomalies (bicornuate or
septate uterus), cervical stenosis, and imperforate hymen.

III. Symptoms and Signs
   A. Primary dysmenorrhea most often begins 6 to 12 months after menarche with the
   onset of ovulatory cycles. Pain is typically described as suprapubic cramping and usually begins just before or with the onset of menstrual bleeding; typically lasting from 8 to
   72 hours. Pain often radiates to the low back and inner/anterior thighs on the first and
   second days of menstruation. Discomfort is often accompanied by diarrhea, headache,
   fatigue, and nausea and vomiting. The **physical examination** is usually normal. Tenderness on uterine palpation may be present during menstruation; severe pain does not
   occur with movement of the cervix or palpation of the adnexal structures.
   B. The pain of **secondary dysmenorrhea** is a key differentiating factor as the presence of symptoms of pain and menstrual bleeding persists beyond the normal menstrual
   cycle. Secondary dysmenorrhea can present early or late in a woman's reproductive
   life, or as a change in the timing or intensity of preexisting primary dysmenorrhea.
   Causes of secondary dysmenorrhea should be evaluated if a woman describes dyspareunia, menorrhagia, dyschezia, intermenstrual bleeding, postcoital bleeding, or
   irregular cycles.
      1. Endometriosis is usually described as a deep aching pain that begins several days
      prior to menses and may last throughout the cycle. It may be associated with dyspa-
      reunia, infertility, hematuria, unilateral pain, or irregular bleeding despite ovulatory
      cycles. Not all women with endometriosis have dysmenorrhea or chronic pelvic pain.
      On physical examination, endometriosis is **classically associated with palpable
      nodules** in the posterior cul-de-sac and anterior vaginal wall, and a tender fixed
      uterus on bimanual examination. The physical examination may be normal.
      2. Adenomyosis is usually associated with severe dysmenorrhea and menorrhagia,
      although some patients are asymptomatic. On physical examination, the uterus is
      symmetrically enlarged. Mobility is usually not restricted and there is no associated
      adnexal pathology.
      3. Most **leiomyomas** (fibroids) are asymptomatic. Women may experience pelvic
      pressure, bloating, menorrhagia, or metrorrhagia, depending on the location and
      size of the tumor. Leiomyomas are suspected if the uterus is irregularly enlarged or
      nodular.
      4. PID (see Chapter 50).

IV. Diagnostic Evaluation
   A. Primary dysmenorrhea. With a suggestive history and a normal physical examination, no laboratory evaluation is indicated. Pelvic examination is not necessary in all
   women, but is indicated in those with a history of sexual activity or symptoms inconsistent
   with primary dysmenorrhea. If menorrhagia is present, it may be prudent to check hemoglobin to evaluate for microcytic anemia.
   B. Evaluation of **secondary dysmenorrhea** may include:
      1. Nucleic acid amplification tests (NAATs) for gonorrhea and chlamydia
      if signs or symptoms suggest PID or the patient is at risk for sexually transmitted infec-
      tions (see Chapter 102).
      2. Complete blood count and erythrocyte sedimentation rate if suspicious of endometritis
      or subacute PID.
      3. Transvaginal pelvic ultrasound can be used to diagnose fibroids, mass lesions,
      endometriomas, or ovarian cysts. Stage 3 or 4 endometriosis can sometimes be identi-
      fied with high-resolution ultrasonography.
      4. Hysterosalpingogram is performed if a uterine anomaly is suspected.
      5. Laparoscopy is used to diagnose endometriosis and can be helpful if other tests do
      not reveal the etiology of secondary dysmenorrhea.
      6. Urinalysis is indicated if the patient gives a history consistent with endometriosis
      and reports hematuria.

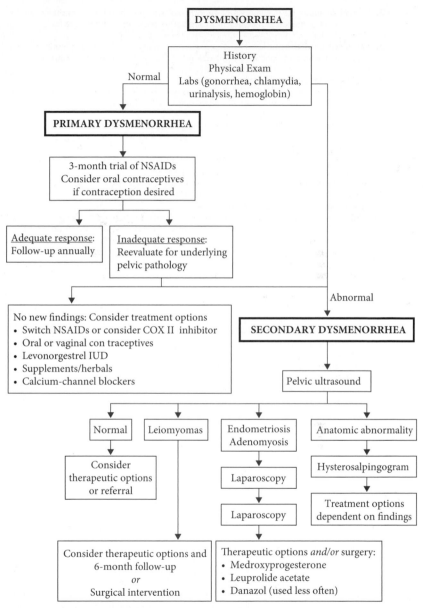

FIGURE 18–1. Evaluation and treatment of dysmenorrhea. NSAIDs, nonsteroidal anti-inflammatory drugs; COX, cyclooxygenase; IUD, intrauterine device.

V. Treatment (Figure 18–1).

A. Nonpharmacologic approaches to the treatment of dysmenorrhea.

1. Low-fat vegetarian diet is associated with decreased duration and intensity of dysmenorrhea. (SOR **B**)

2. Exercise stimulates the release of endorphins, which can act as nonspecific analgesics, but the evidence is insufficient to support exercise as a treatment for dysmenorrhea. (SOR **C**)

3. Physical treatments for dysmenorrhea may be used in combination with pharmacological treatments, and often provide relief for those women choosing not to use medications.

   a. Heating pad or patch diminishes menstrual pain. (SOR **B**) The onset of analgesia is faster than with a NSAID. These are good for women who cannot tolerate NSAIDs but can be used in combination with NSAIDs for improved symptom management. (SOR **B**)

   b. Acupuncture and acupressure have been shown to be effective in some patients. Acupressure was shown to be as effective as ibuprofen in one study. (SOR **B**)

   c. Transcutaneous electrical nerve stimulation (TENS) is effective for some patients with refractory dysmenorrhea. (SOR **B**)

   d. Manipulation has not been shown to be an effective treatment for dysmenorrhea. (SOR **C**)

B. Pharmacologic approaches (Table 18–1).

   1. NSAIDs are effective at relieving primary dysmenorrhea in 70% to 90% of cases, and should be considered first-line therapy unless there is a contraindication to use. (SOR **A**) NSAIDs inhibit endometrial prostaglandin production without affecting endometrial development. They also have direct analgesic properties at the central nervous system level. They should be started a few hours before the onset of menstrual bleeding or with the onset of pain and continued for 1 to 3 days. NSAIDs appear to be equal in efficacy, so cost, convenience, and patient preference should be used to determine the best choice for a particular woman. Contraindications to NSAIDs include gastrointestinal symptoms, bronchospasm, and fluid retention, but side effects are usually mild and occur in fewer than 5% of patients.

   2. Cyclooxygenase II inhibitors (COX II inhibitors) are also effective and have the advantage of decreased gastrointestinal side effects and once-daily dosing. (SOR **B**) Cost argues against regular use except when other NSAIDs have proven to be ineffective or are poorly tolerated.

   3. OCs suppress both menstrual fluid volume and prostaglandin release, but not synthesis; this is achieved by causing endometrial hypoplasia. OCs are effective in most patients and are best suited for those also desiring hormonal contraception. (SOR **B**) Combination, extended-cycle, and progestin-only pills can be used. Contraceptive patches are less effective than OCs in treating dysmenorrhea. If severe dysmenorrhea is not improved with combined use of NSAIDs and OCs, reevaluation for underlying pelvic pathology should be pursued. (SOR **C**)

   4. Levonorgestrel intrauterine devices (Mirena®) effectively cause amenorrhea after the first year and decrease the prevalence of dysmenorrhea by 50%. (SOR **B**) They are effective in the treatment of endometriosis (see Chapter 50).

   5. Depo-medroxyprogesterone acetate (DMPA) induces anovulation and thereby prevents dysmenorrhea. (SOR **B**) DMPA is also often used in women with endometriosis (see Chapter 50).

   6. Intravaginal administration of hormonal contraceptives such as the etonogestrel and ethinyl estradiol vaginal ring (NuvaRing®) decreases dysmenorrhea. (SOR **B**) There seem to be fewer systemic side effects when compared with administration of oral combination OCs.

   7. Both **danazol and leuprolide acetate** can effectively suppress menstruation and induce medical menopause. (SOR **B**) These agents are used only for severe and refractory dysmenorrhea. While both drugs can have significant side effects (Figure 19–1), danazol is used less often as it is associated with many drug interactions in addition to side effects.

   8. Calcium-channel blockers reduce myometrial activity and relieve dysmenorrhea by decreasing uterine contractions. (SOR **C**)

   9. Glyceryl trinitrate has been shown to be helpful with severe dysmenorrhea, especially when taken in the first 6 hours of menstruation. (SOR **C**) It is strongly associated with headache.

   10. Supplements such as thiamine, pyridoxine, vitamin E, and omega-3 fatty acids have all been used effectively to treat dysmenorrhea. (SOR **B**)

TABLE 18–1. PHARMACOLOGIC TREATMENT OF DYSMENORRHEA

Medication	Category	Dose and Frequency	Common Side Effects	Drug Interactions
Ibuprofen	NSAID	400–600 mg every 4–6 h	Nausea, heartburn, dizziness	**Multiple Interactions** Cyclosporine (cyclosporine toxicity); antiplatelet agents, anticoagulants, venlafaxine, SSRI, ginkgo (bleeding); methotrexate (methotrexate toxicity); lithium (lithium toxicity); phenytoin (phenytoin toxicity); CCBs (GI hemorrhage, loss of hypotensive effect)
Ketoprofen	NSAID	25–50 mg every 6–8 h	Nausea, constipation, diarrhea, gas, headache	See ibuprofen
Naproxen sodium Naproxen	NSAID	550 mg, then 275 mg every 6–8 h 500 mg, then 250 mg every 6–8 h	GI distress, constipation, heartburn, headache	See ibuprofen
Diclofenac potassium	NSAID	100 mg, then 50 mg every 8 h	Nausea, headache, dizziness, somnolence	See ibuprofen
Celecoxib[a]	NSAID (COX II)	400 mg, then 200 mg every 12 h	Nausea, headache, diarrhea	See ibuprofen
Oral contraceptives	Hormone	one tablet daily for 21–28 d per mo[b]	Nausea, headache, breakthrough bleeding	**Multiple Interactions** Fentanyl (fentanyl toxicity); isotretinoin, phenytoin, barbiturates, rifampin, St. John's wort (decreased contraceptive efficacy); alprazolam (alprazolam toxicity)
Danazol	Hormone	100–200 mg twice daily for dysmenorrhea	Acne, weight gain	Statins (myopathy); bupropion (seizures); warfarin (bleeding); carbamazepine (carbamazepine toxicity); cyclosporine (cyclosporine toxicity)
Leuprolide	Hormone	3.75 mg IM monthly[c]	Acne, flushing, hot flashes, increased triglycerides, nausea, asthenia, constipation, arthralgia, myalgia, dizziness, headache, insomnia	None
Thiamine	Supplement	100 mg daily	None	None
Omega-3 fatty acids	Supplement	2 g daily	IF fish oil is the source: fishy burps; antiplatelet effect (easy bruising)	Anticoagulants and antiplatelet agents (additive antiplatelet effect, bleeding)

NSAID, nonsteroidal anti-inflammatory drug; SSRIs, selective serotonin reuptake inhibitors; CCB, calcium-channel blockers; GI, gastrointestinal; IM, intramuscularly.
[a]Black box warning: Celecoxib may increase risk of serious cardiovascular thrombotic events, myocardial infarction, and stroke; risk may be increased in patients with cardiovascular disease or risk factors for cardiovascular disease.
[b]Dosage varies for extended cycle, continuous use, and varied cycle oral contraceptive products.
[c]Treatment beyond 6 months not recommended.

11. Herbal preparations have been used for treatment of menstrual pain. Toki-shakuyaku-san (Japanese herb) has been shown to be effective, although the dosage is unclear. (SOR **B**) Ovulatory function and thus fertility does not seem to be suppressed.

C. Surgical therapies should be reserved for patients unresponsive to other treatment modalities.

   1. Hysterectomy is sometimes used for refractory dysmenorrhea and is commonly used in the treatment of fibroids. (SOR **B**)

   2. Laparoscopic uterosacral nerve ablation (LUNA) and **presacral neurectomy** are used only in the most severe cases. (SOR **C**) Presacral neurectomy has more adverse effects.

   3. Endometrial ablation is sometimes used in women with severe dysmenorrhea and menorrhagia. (SOR **B**)

SELECTED REFERENCES

Davis A. *Danforth's Obstetrics & Gynecology.* 10th ed. Philadelphia, PA: Lippincott Williams & Wilkins; 2008:562–563.

French L. Dysmenorrhea. *Am Fam Physician.* 2005;71(2):285–291.

Harel Z. Dysmenorrhea in adolescents and young adults: etiology and management. *J Pediatr Adolesc Gynecol.* 2006;19(6):363–371.

Kelekci S, Kelekci KH, Yilmaz B. Effects of levonorgestrel-releasing intrauterine system and T380A intrauterine copper device on dysmenorrhea and days of bleeding in women with and without adenomyosis. *Contraception.* 2012;86(5):458–463.

Marjoribanks J, Proctor ML, Farquhar C, et al. Nonsteroidal anti-inflammatory drugs for dysmenorrhea. *Cochrane Database Syst Rev.* 2010;(1):CD001751.

Morrow C, Naumburg E. Dysmenorrhea. *Prim Care Clin Office Pract.* 2009;36(1):19–32.

Parker A, Sneddon AE, Arbon P. The Menstrual Disorders of Teenagers (MDOT) study: determining typical menstrual patterns and menstrual disturbances in a large population-based study of Australian teenagers. *BJOG.* 2010;117:185–192.

Peacock A, Alvi NS, Mushtaq T. Period problems: disorders of menstruation in adolescents. *Arch Dis Child.* 2012;97(6):554–560.

Rapkin AJ, Nathan L. *Berek & Novak's Gynecology.* 15th ed. Philadelphia, PA: Lippincott Williams & Wilkins; 2011:471–501.

Zahradnik HP, Hanjalic-Beck A, Groth K. Nonsteroidal anti-inflammatory drugs and hormonal contraceptives for pain relief from dysmenorrhea: a review. *Contraception.* 2012;81:185–196.

---

19   Dyspepsia

Kalyanakrishnan Ramakrishnan, MD, MS, FRCS

KEY POINTS

- The majority of patients with dyspepsia have no structural abnormality (nonulcer dyspepsia [NUD]). (SOR **C**)
- Patients without alarm symptoms should be tested for *Helicobacter pylori* and treated if test results are positive ("test-and-treat" strategy). (SOR **A**)
- Patients with NUD can be treated with a proton pump inhibitor (PPI), histamine-2 receptor blocking agent (H$_2$ blocker), or a prokinetic agent. (SOR **A**)

I. Definition. Dyspepsia is defined as pain or discomfort felt to arise in the upper gastrointestinal (GI) tract, with symptoms on more than 25% of the days over the past 4 weeks. It may be characterized by epigastric discomfort or pain and can be associated with epigastric heaviness or fullness, belching or regurgitation, bloating, early satiety, heartburn, food intolerance, nausea, or vomiting. Lower bowel function is usually not affected.

II. Common Diagnoses. Dyspepsia is a common complaint, occurring in 20% to 30% of the general population. It accounts for approximately 2% to 5% of family practice consultations. Common causes include the following:

A. Medications. Aspirin, nonsteroidal anti-inflammatory drugs (NSAIDs), corticosteroids, bisphosphonates, iron, erythromycin, tetracycline, alcohol, and potassium supplements can cause upper abdominal discomfort.

B. Nonulcer dyspepsia (NUD). This disorder is found in up to 60% of patients with dyspepsia. The incidence of NUD is age dependent; approximately 70% of patients younger than 40 years of age have NUD as opposed to only 40% of those older than 60 years of age. The cause of NUD is unknown. No definite link between NUD and *Helicobacter pylori* has been established.

C. Peptic ulcer disease (PUD) includes gastric and duodenal ulcers, gastritis, and duodenitis and is found in 20% to 30% of patients with dyspepsia. Both NUD and PUD account for 50% to 80% of all cases of dyspepsia. Duodenal ulcers affect men twice as often as women. The peak incidence is between ages 45 and 64 years in men and at age 55 years in women. Gastric ulcers occur much less frequently than duodenal ulcers and increase in incidence with advancing age. A past history of PUD, *H. pylori* infection, NSAID use, male gender, and cigarette smoking all are associated with an increased chance of finding gastric or duodenal ulcers on upper endoscopy.

D. Gastroesophageal reflux disease (GERD) is found in 5% to 15% of patients with dyspepsia.

E. Gastric, esophageal, or pancreatic cancer. Fewer than 2% of patients with dyspepsia have cancer. The incidence increases with advancing age. Toxins (e.g., nitrosamines or polycyclic hydrocarbons), genetic factors, pernicious anemia, and atrophic gastritis are associated with gastric cancer.

F. Cholecystitis or cholelithiasis (see Chapter 1).

G. Other causes of dyspepsia. Irritable bowel syndrome (see Chapter 1), Zollinger–Ellison syndrome, chronic pancreatitis, malabsorption, abdominal angina, and coronary artery disease are uncommon.

III. Symptoms. Although symptoms have low specificity in patients with dyspepsia, they can be helpful in excluding other diagnoses and determining the need for additional workup or treatment (Figure 19–1).

A. Heartburn. Heartburn, regurgitation, painful swallowing, and chest pain are symptoms suggestive of GERD.

B. Alarm symptoms. The presence of alarm symptoms including age older than 55 years, unexplained significant weight loss (≥10–15 lbs), persistent vomiting, melena, hematemesis, or dysphagia should prompt immediate workup, usually with endoscopy (Figure 19–1). (SOR ❸)

C. Symptoms that poorly discriminate between specific disease and NUD include relief with antacids or food, nocturnal pain, food intolerance (e.g., fatty food intolerance), duration of pain, pain that occurs within 1 hour of eating, and anorexia.

D. Symptoms that can be used to identify patients with complications of PUD or other specific causes of dyspepsia are given below:

    1. Hematemesis, melena, or both indicate GI bleeding.

    2. Dizziness, especially upon sitting or standing, or syncope may indicate significant blood loss.

    3. Persistent vomiting is a symptom of gastric outlet obstruction.

    4. Pain that radiates straight through to the back can indicate a penetrating ulcer, leaking abdominal aneurysm, pancreatitis, or pancreatic cancer.

    5. Pain radiating to the shoulder can result from diaphragmatic irritation caused by pus, blood, or free air in the peritoneum.

IV. Signs. In general, the physical examination is not helpful in determining the cause of dyspepsia. In uncomplicated cases, the examination usually reveals only mild to moderate epigastric tenderness. The following signs can be helpful in identifying patients with complications of PUD or serious systemic illness:

A. Unexplained tachycardia (pulse ≥120 beats per minute) or postural hypotension (orthostatic change in blood pressure ≥20 mm Hg) can indicate significant blood loss from GI bleeding.

B. Abdominal rebound tenderness or rigidity suggests peritoneal irritation. A perforated viscus, blood, or infection in the peritoneal cavity can cause peritoneal irritation.

C. Blood in the stool can indicate GI tract bleeding.

D. Jaundice can indicate biliary tract obstruction from pancreatic cancer or cholelithiasis.

E. Palpable mass in the upper abdomen may be a hepatic, gastric, or pancreatic malignancy.

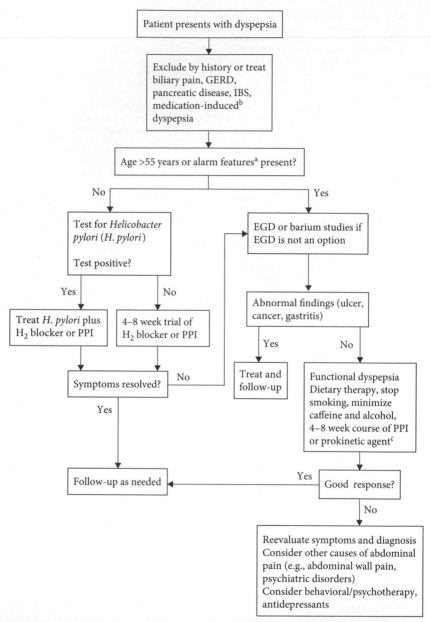

FIGURE 19–1. Approach to the patient with dyspepsia. GERD, gastroesophageal reflux disease; IBS, irritable bowel syndrome; EGD, esophagogastroduodenoscopy; PPI, proton pump inhibitor. [a]Alarm features include weight loss (>10%), persistent vomiting, upper GI bleed, dysphagia, lymphadenopathy, abdominal mass, history of esophagogastric cancer. [b]Medications causing dyspepsia include NSAIDs, potassium, iron, bisphosphonates, digoxin, antibiotics, theophylline, corticosteroids. [c]PPI/H_2 blocker if epigastric discomfort or reflux symptoms.

V. Laboratory Tests. In general, the laboratory evaluation consists of testing for *H. pylori* in those individuals without alarm symptoms. This is referred to as the "test-and-treat" strategy (see Figure 19–1).

  A. Tests that can be useful include the following:

   1. Tests for *H. pylori.* These can be either noninvasive (urea breath test, urine- or stool-based antigen tests) or invasive (rapid urease test or biopsies, obtained at the time of upper endoscopy). (SOR **G**)

   2. Upper GI series. The upper GI series is noninvasive and relatively inexpensive. It is sensitive in detecting gastric and duodenal ulcers (80%–90%). Its accuracy improves with disease severity. The double-contrast technique including spot views during vigorous compression with the barium-filled bulb improves detection of duodenal ulcers. In patients with GERD, only severe esophagitis can be detected, although reflux and motility disorders of the esophagus can be seen. The presence of a hiatal hernia does not correlate with GERD.

   3. Upper GI endoscopy. Upper GI endoscopy or esophagogastroduodenoscopy (EGD) is the gold standard for identifying esophageal or gastroduodenal pathology and is the investigation of choice for patients older than 55 years with uninvestigated dyspepsia or in the presence of alarm features (see Figure 19–1). (SOR **G**) Upper endoscopy is preferred to an upper GI series because lesions can be directly visualized and biopsy can be performed. In addition, testing for *H. pylori* can be performed.

   4. Intraesophageal pH monitoring. Most physicians consider this procedure to be the single best test for diagnosis of GERD. (SOR **B**) Coupled with a symptom diary, 24-hour monitoring has a sensitivity between 87% and 93% and a specificity of 92% to 97% for GERD.

   5. Scintigraphy is best used to detect delayed gastric emptying. GERD and delayed gastric emptying can be detected using [^{99m}Tc] sulfur colloid, although intraesophageal pH monitoring is a better test for GERD.

  B. Indications for further testing. Diagnostic testing should be started promptly in patients with severe systemic illness, bleeding, perforation, symptoms of upper GI tract obstruction, or evidence of cancer.

   1. Persistence of symptoms after empiric treatment requires further evaluation with endoscopy or upper GI series.

   2. In patients who experience a **recurrence of dyspepsia** following empiric treatment, a specific diagnosis should be made.

VI. Treatment. Figure 19–1 presents the "test-and-treat" approach to a patient with dyspepsia.

  A. A practical approach for patients with dyspepsia who are younger than 55 years and have no alarm symptoms, complications of PUD, or serious systemic illness is to treat empirically with a histamine-2 receptor blocking agent (H$_2$ blocker) or a proton pump inhibitor (PPI) (SOR **B**) (Figure 19–1) and test for *H. pylori*. Table 19–1 lists the medication options with dosing information and frequency. If a patient tests positive for *H. pylori;* treat (see Chapter 84). Helidac (bismuth subsalicylate–metronidazole–tetracycline) plus a PPI or Prevpac (amoxicillin–clarithromycin–lansoprazole) administered for 14 days are both effective in the treatment of *H. pylori* (80%–90% response). (SOR **A**) The test-and-treat option is preferable in populations with a moderate-to-high prevalence of *H. pylori* infection (≥10%), whereas empiric PPI strategy is preferable in low-prevalence situations. (SOR **A**) Patients should also be encouraged to discontinue ulcerogenic agents (e.g., alcohol or NSAIDs) and cigarette smoking. (SOR **G**) If NSAID therapy is needed, a PPI, an H$_2$ blocker, or a cytoprotective agent can be used concomitantly (see Table 19–1) or consider switching to a COX-2 inhibitor (e.g., celecoxib). (SOR **G**)

  B. For **individuals with dyspepsia who are older than 55 years,** empiric treatment should be preceded or followed by the establishment of a definitive diagnosis with EGD (see Figure 19–1). If symptoms worsen or persist despite therapy, the patient should undergo further evaluation (see Section V.B). (SOR **G**)

  C. When the cause of the patient's dyspepsia is known, the following therapeutic measures can be helpful:

   1. NUD. At present, the optimal therapy for NUD is unclear. Fortunately, for most individuals, abdominal discomfort resolves within several weeks. Treatment for *H. pylori*, if identified, sometimes resolves dyspeptic symptoms. (SOR **B**) In *H. pylori* negative patients with abdominal pain, nausea, or bloating as predominant symptoms, a 4- to 6-week course of a PPI, an H$_2$ receptor blocker, or a prokinetic agent can be tried (see Figure 19–1). (SOR **A**) Patients with prominent somatic complaints, anxiety, or

TABLE 19–1. MEDICATIONS USED IN THE TREATMENT OF DYSPEPSIA

Drug	Dose[a]	Major Side Effects	Contraindications	Drug Interactions
Proton Pump Inhibitors				
Esomeprazole	Adult: 20–40 mg daily Pediatric (age >1 mol): 2.5–40 mg daily	Diarrhea, headache With prolonged use: Hypomagnesemia, increased risk of pneumonia, C. difficile diarrhea, osteoporosis, and fractures	Hypersensitivity	Azole antifungals, cilostazol, clopidogrel[b], HIV medications, risedronate, St. John's wort, tacrolimus, methotrexate, iron, citalopram (max. dose of 20 mg/d), mesalamine, rifampin, dasatinib, dabigatran, warfarin
Lansoprazole	Adult: 15–30 mg daily Pediatric (age >1 y): 15–30 mg daily			
Omeprazole	Adult: 20–40 mg daily Pediatric (age >1 y): 5–20 mg daily			
Pantoprazole	Adult: 40 mg daily Pediatric (age 5 or more years): 20–40 mg daily			
Rabeprazole	Adult: 20 mg daily Pediatric (age 12 or more years): 20 mg daily			
Histamine-2 Receptor Blockers				
Cimetidine	Adult: 400 mg twice daily, 300 or 400 mg 4 times daily or 800 mg once or twice daily Pediatric (infants and older): 10–40 mg/kg/d divided every 6 h	Headache, dizziness, agitation, diarrhea, somnolence, gynecomastia, reversible confusion in elderly and renal impairment	Hypersensitivity	Azole antifungals, risedronate, HIV medications, mesalamine, varenicline **Cimetidine:** calcium-channel blockers (exception: amlodipine, clevidipine, nicardipine), benzodiazepines, clozapine, colchicine, beta-blockers, clopidogrel, dofetilide, phenytoin, escitalopram, eplerenone, lurasidone, metformin, ranolazine, SSRIs, warfarin **Famotidine:** QT-prolonging agents **Ranitidine:** warfarin, prasugrel, sulfonylureas
Famotidine	Adult: 20–40 mg twice daily Pediatric (infants and older): 0.5 mg/kg once or twice daily	Agitation, vomiting (in children <1 y), headache, diarrhea, reversible confusion, prolonged QT interval with renal impairment		
Nizatidine	Adult: 300 mg nightly or 150 mg twice daily Pediatric (<12 years old): 10 mg/kg/d in two divided doses	Headache, dizziness, rash, abdominal pain, flatulence, diarrhea Reported in children: fever, irritability, nasal congestion, cough		
Ranitidine	Adult: 300 mg nightly or 150 mg twice daily to 4 times daily Pediatric (>1 mo): treatment: 4–10 mg/kg/d divided twice daily, maintenance: 2–4 mg/kg/d divided twice daily	Headache, dizziness, abdominal pain, diarrhea, Rare: agranulocytosis, reversible confusion associated with renal impairment		

	Dosing	Adverse Effects	Contraindications	Drug Interactions
Cytoprotective Agents				
Sucralfate	Adult: 1 g 4 times daily or 2 g twice daily Pediatric: Dose not established, 40–80 mg/kg/d divided every 6 h have been used	Constipation	Hypersensitivity	Digoxin, furosemide, warfarin, iron, multivitamins, quinolones, tetracyclines
Misoprostol	Adult: 100–200 µg 4 times daily Pediatric: Not recommended	Diarrhea, abdominal pain, headache, vomiting	Hypersensitivity, pregnancy	Antacids, carbetocin oxytocin
Prokinetic Agent				
Metoclopramide	Adult: 10–15 mg 4 times daily Pediatric (infants and older): 0.4–0.8 mg/kg/d in four divided doses	Bradyarrhythmias, fluid retention, drowsiness (dose related), depression, extrapyramidal symptoms, dizziness, confusion, rash, hyperprolactinemia, leukopenia	Hypersensitivity, bowel obstruction, hemorrhage or perforation, seizure disorder, use of other agents that increase extrapyramidal side effects, pheochromocytoma	Antipsychotics, promethazine, antidepressants, droperidol, SSRIs, TCAs, trimetazidine

Abbreviations: HIV, human immunodeficiency virus; SSRI, selective serotonin reuptake inhibitor; TCA, tricyclic antidepressant.
[a]Dose reductions may be necessary in hepatic impairment (PPI), renal impairment (H_2 blockers and metoclopramide).
[b]This interaction may only occur in poor metabolizers of clopidogrel.

depression are more likely to have a psychologic basis for their symptoms and may benefit from behavior therapy, antidepressants, or anxiolytics. (SOR **C**)

2. **PUD** (see Chapter 84).

3. **GERD.** Patients with mild GERD symptoms can benefit from adopting antireflux measures, which include losing weight, avoiding lying down or bending over after meals, consuming few large meals and bedtime snacks, elevating the head of the bed on 4- to 8-inch blocks, modifying the diet (avoiding caffeine, chocolate, peppermint, fatty foods), and discontinuing alcohol consumption and cigarette smoking. (SOR **C**)

   a. In patients with a dominant symptom of heartburn or acid regurgitation, a PPI, an H_2 blocker, or a prokinetic agent are options (see Table 19–1). (SOR **C**)

   b. Antireflux surgery should be considered in patients with severe esophagitis with inability to tolerate medication (including noncompliance), development of Barrett esophagus, persistent reflux symptoms despite acid suppression, or severe asthma or aspiration pneumonia in association with GERD. (SOR **C**)

PEDIATRIC GERD

Gastroesophageal reflux is fairly common in infants. It is marked by regurgitation with normal weight gain. The peak incidence is at 1 to 4 months and is usually resolved by 1 year of age. "Happy spitters" can be treated conservatively by reassuring parents and using thickened feedings, change from cow's milk-based formula, use of a hypoallergenic formula, and/or upright positioning after feedings.

Infants who present with regurgitation and alarm symptoms such as respiratory problems (stridor, wheezing, cough), poor weight gain or growth, or irritability require further evaluation. GERD should be considered in the differential diagnosis of these children. In older children and adolescents, GERD usually presents with heartburn, regurgitation, or lower chest pain. Infants or children with esophageal atresia with repair, neurologic impairment/delay, bronchopulmonary dysplasia, asthma, or cystic fibrosis have an increased risk of GERD. A pediatric gastroenterologist can help guide the workup of GERD. Medical management includes H_2 blockers and PPIs. Prokinetic agents may have a role.

   4. Gastric or pancreatic cancer. The primary treatment of gastric or pancreatic cancer is surgery. At present, surgery offers the only chance for cure; chemotherapy and radiation therapy are palliative.

SELECTED REFERENCES

American Gastroenterological Association medical position statement. Evaluation of dyspepsia. *Gastroenterology.* 2005;129:1753–1755.

Conroy RT, Siddiqi B. Dyspepsia. *Prim Care Clin Office Pract.* 2007;34(1):99–108.

Harmon RC, Peura RA. Evaluation and management of dyspepsia. *Ther Adv Gastroenterol.* 2010;3(2): 87–98.

Loyd RA, McClellan DA. Update on the evaluation and management of functional dyspepsia. *Am Fam Physician.* 2011;83(5):547–552.

Management of dyspepsia in adults in primary care. NICE Clinical Guideline No. 17. http://www.nice. org.uk/CG017NICEguideline. Accessed January 16, 2013.

Manes G, Menchise A, de Nucci C, Balzano A. Empirical prescribing for dyspepsia: randomized controlled trial of test and treat versus omeprazole treatment. *BMJ.* 2003;326:1118.

Talley NJ, Vakil MB, Moayyedi P. American Gastroenterological Association technical review on the evaluation of dyspepsia. *Gastroenterology.* 2005;129:1756–1780.

Winter HS. Gastroesophageal reflux disease in infants. Uptodate 2013. www.uptodate.com. Accessed January 6, 2013.

20 Dil Dyspnea

James C. Chesnutt, MD, Mark R. Stephan, MD, Scott A. Fields, MD, &
William L. Toffler, MD

KEY POINTS

- Dyspnea is mainly caused by pulmonary or cardiac disorders. (SOR **G**)
- The history and physical examination will reveal the cause in most cases. (SOR **G**)
- The airway, breathing, and circulation (ABCs) should be used to screen for life-threatening disorders, with further diagnostic testing as indicated. (SOR **G**)

I. **Definition.** Dyspnea is an unpleasant, subjective sensation of difficult breathing (breathlessness). Respiratory physiology relies on sensory input from peripheral and central chemoreceptors (monitoring pO_2, pCO_2, and pH) and mechanoreceptors (located in the heart, lung, vessels, and chest wall) with central processing and control in the medulla, receiving additional input from higher brain centers, including the cerebral cortex. The sensation of dyspnea is related to a mismatch of sensory input, central respiratory drive, and peripheral ventilatory performance. Dyspnea can vary in quality and intensity and is affected not only by physiologic disturbances but also by psychological, social, and environmental factors.

II. **Common Diagnoses.** Dyspnea is an extremely common concern of patients presenting for acute medical care. Shortness of breath is the chief complaint for 16% to 25% of nonsurgical admissions from the emergency department, and dyspnea is present in up to 50% of acute admissions and 25% of ambulatory clinic visits. Seventy percent of patients with advanced cancer have dyspnea, of which one-quarter have moderate or severe symptoms. The most common causes of dyspnea relate to either pulmonary or cardiac disorders.

A. Pulmonary disorders

1. Those at risk for **obstructive lung disease** include pediatric patients (asthma, bronchiolitis, bronchitis), adults with asthma, and adults with a chronic cigarette smoking history (chronic bronchitis and emphysema) (see Chapters 68 and 70).

2. Dyspnea caused by **restrictive lung disease** is more likely in patients with an occupational exposure (asbestos, coal, beryllium, silica, uranium, cotton dust, grain dust, hay mold), those with severe scoliosis/kyphosis, the morbidly obese, and pregnant women (caused by uterine growth-restricting lung expansion). Chest wall trauma and smoking are associated with pneumothorax. Cancer and congestive heart failure (CHF) are more likely to be associated with a pleural effusion.

3. Severe **pneumonia** also causes dyspnea; those at risk include immunocompromised patients (e.g., *Pneumocystis carinii* pneumonia in HIV disease), the very young, the very old, and those at risk for aspiration (e.g., alcoholics or individuals with stroke or history of swallowing disorders).

B. Cardiac dyspnea. Risk factors for cardiac dyspnea include CHF (see Chapter 73), valvular heart disease, ischemic cardiovascular disease (angina, myocardial infarction, claudication, or stroke [see Chapters 79 and 88]), individuals with comorbid conditions (diabetes mellitus [see Chapter 75], dyslipidemia [see Chapter 76], or tobacco abuse), and those with a strong family history of premature coronary disease (i.e., myocardial infarction in the 40s or 50s in first-degree relatives). Arrhythmias (e.g., sick sinus syndrome, atrial fibrillation, and ventricular tachycardia [see Chapter 48]) can also cause dyspnea.

C. Mixed cardiopulmonary dyspnea. Risk factors for mixed cardiopulmonary dyspnea (most notably pulmonary embolism; see Chapter 64) include hypercoagulable states, immobilization, major surgery or trauma, malignancy, pregnancy, and oral contraceptives. Morbid obesity and a sedentary lifestyle contribute to deconditioning.

D. Noncardiopulmonary causes

1. Uncommonly, **neuromuscular diseases** (e.g., Parkinson disease, amyotrophic lateral sclerosis, and Guillain–Barré syndrome) can cause dyspnea from respiratory muscle paralysis or dysfunction.

2. In the presence of clinical findings supporting them, the following **systemic diseases** can cause dyspnea: anemia, thyrotoxicosis, diabetic ketoacidosis, metabolic acidosis, and carbon monoxide poisoning.

3. A **psychogenic cause** for dyspnea should be considered in patients with a known history of psychiatric disease, multiple life stressors, and poor coping skills or a history of ill-defined somatic complaints (see Chapter 96). Extreme pain or hyperventilation can cause dyspnea.

4. **Upper airway causes** of dyspnea are more likely in children (e.g., tonsillar hypertrophy, croup, epiglottitis, or foreign body aspiration) and in alcoholics or individuals with a history of stroke or of swallowing disorders.

LIFE-THREATENING CAUSES OF DYSPNEA

Pulmonary
Pneumonia
Status asthmaticus
Tension pneumothorax
Cardiac
Congestive heart failure
Myocardial infarction
Ventricular tachycardia
Mixed cardiopulmonary
Pulmonary embolism
Noncardiopulmonary causes
Anaphylactic laryngeal edema
Bacterial epiglottitis
Carbon monoxide poisoning
Diabetic ketoacidosis
Guillain–Barré syndrome

III. Symptoms and Signs (Table 20–1). Assessing the patient for dyspnea severity, onset (acute vs. chronic), descriptive qualities, and associated symptoms and signs can be extremely helpful in identifying the underlying cause of new or worsening dyspnea. Studies show that different descriptive qualities of dyspnea are related to distinct physiologic abnormalities and that a dyspnea scale can be helpful in monitoring severity.

In order to quickly and accurately identify severe or life-threatening causes of dyspnea, special attention should be given to a rapid assessment of the patient's general level of distress and vital signs (Figure 20–1). In addition, the cardiopulmonary examination is most helpful in identifying the underlying causes of dyspnea.

A. Vital signs. The patient's respiratory rate, temperature, pulse, and blood pressure should be determined. An increased respiratory rate ($\geq$20 breaths per minute in adults; >60 breaths per minute in infants; >35 breaths per minute in young children; >25–30 breaths per minute in school-aged children) helps quantify dyspnea, but it is a nonspecific sign. Fever ($\geq$38.5°C [101°F]) is associated with respiratory infection. An increased pulse rate ($\geq$100 beats per minute) may be associated with pulmonary embolism, dysrhythmia, or metabolic disorder.

B. Focused physical examination

1. The **pulmonary examination** should consist of auscultation and percussion of the lungs to assess for the presence of rales, rhonchi, wheezing, decreased breath sounds, egophony, or dullness to percussion. Inspection of the oral/nasal cavities, chest wall, and extremities can reveal airway obstruction, an increased thoracic anteroposterior diameter, chest wall deformity, or clubbing. Nasal flaring, sternal retractions, and accessory muscle use indicate more severe respiratory distress.

2. The **cardiac examination** should include an evaluation for rhythm, abnormal heart sounds (S_3 and S_4), murmurs, rubs, increased jugular venous distention, peripheral edema and pulses, and pulmonary rales in the lower lung fields.

3. The extent of additional **noncardiopulmonary examination** should be driven by symptoms. If a dyspneic patient has weakness, tremor, gait problems, or other muscular or neurologic complaints, a screening neurologic examination should be performed including testing gait, reflexes, sensation, motor strength, tone, and coordination.

TABLE 20–1. FINDINGS IN COMMON CAUSES OF DYSPNEA

Cause	Symptoms	Signs
Pulmonary		
OLD, RLD	"Air hunger" (hypoxemia) "Chest tightness" (bronchospasm) "Increased effort of breathing" (COPD, RLD) Exercise-induced coughing/wheezing (asthma) Daily sputum production (COPD)	Rales/rhonchi/wheezes Tachypnea/tachycardia Nasal flaring, sternal retractions, and accessory muscle use (more severe) Cyanosis or clubbing Increased A-P chest diameter Scoliosis or chest wall deformity
Pneumonia	Cough, purulent sputum (dark or rust) "Air hunger" (hypoxemia) Pleuritic chest pain Chills, rigors	Fever ≥38.5°C (101°F) Tachypnea, cyanosis Coarse rales Dullness to percussion Egophony (e to a change)
Cardiac		
Ischemic, dysrhythmic, heart failure	Anginal chest pressure/pain, palpitations Orthopnea, dyspnea on exertion, fatigue	Tachycardia, arrhythmia Abnormal heart sounds (murmur, rub, gallop) Cardiomegaly, JVD Dependent edema Basilar fine rales and decreased breath sounds
Mixed Cardiopulmonary		
PE	"Air hunger" (hypoxemia) Pleuritic chest pain, syncope, unilateral leg pain, or swelling	Tachypnea/tachycardia, cyanosis Calf tenderness, edema, positive Homan sign
Noncardiopulmonary		
Deconditioning	"Heavy breathing" "Increased effort or work of breathing"	Obesity (deconditioning) Muscle atrophy
Neuromuscular	Fatigue, weakness, tremor, motor dysfunction (neuromuscular weakness)	Abnormal muscle tone, strength, gait, or reflexes
Psychogenic	Anxiety, depression, pain	Hyperventilation
Systemic disease	Polyuria, polydipsia, polyphagia (DM) Headache, confusion, dizziness (CO poisoning)	Pale (anemia) Red skin (CO poisoning)
Upper airway	Dysphagia, gagging, drooling, sore throat, hoarseness (epiglottitis) Allergic exposure: food, cat, drug, bee sting (anaphylaxis/laryngeal edema) Snoring, sleep apnea, daytime fatigue (OSAS)	Tachypnea, distress, inspiratory stridor, high fever (epiglottitis) Cyanosis, urticaria (angioedema) Tonsil hypertrophy, nasal obstruction, obesity, large neck (OSAS)

AP, anteroposterior; CO, carbon monoxide; COPD, chronic obstructive pulmonary disease; DM, diabetes mellitus; JVD, jugular venous distention; OLD, obstructive lung disease; OSAS, obstructive sleep apnea syndrome; PE, pulmonary embolism; RLD, restrictive lung disease.

IV. Diagnostic Tests. The need for testing is based on the patient's history and physical examination and ordered only if needed to help establish the cause or illness severity. A stepwise **"ABC&D"** approach to dyspnea diagnosis and testing can simplify the diagnostic process and decrease both cost and patient discomfort. When dyspnea is severe, a rapid assessment for life-threatening medical problems should focus on the ABCs (**a**irway, **b**reathing, and **c**irculation) and special **d**iagnostic tests **(D)** focused on evaluating the common causes of dyspnea.
  A. Airway. A **peak expiratory flow rate (PEFR)** of ≤150 L/min (normal value, 400–600 L/min) predicts a pulmonary cause for dyspnea, indicating significant obstructive airway disease that may require hospitalization. The PEFR is easily measured with a handheld peak flow meter and should be compared to the patient's baseline value, and it helps guide a stepwise asthma/chronic obstructive pulmonary disease (COPD) treatment plan (see Chapters 68 and 70).

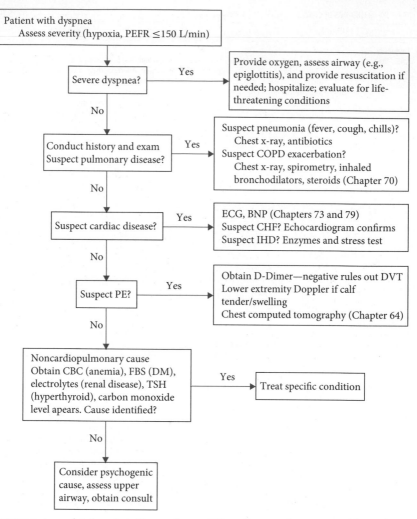

FIGURE 20–1. Approach to the patient with acute dyspnea. PEFR, peek expiratory flow rate; COPD, chronic obstructive pulmonary disease; ECG, electrocardiogram; BNP, beta-type natriuretic peptide; CHF, congestive heart failure; IHD, ischemic heart disease; DVT, deep vein thrombosis; CBC, complete blood count; FBS, fasting blood sugar; TSH, thyroid stimulating hormone.

B. Breathing

1. **Pulse oximetry** can be used as a rapid and accurate assessment of oxygenation. For hypoxemia of ≤90% pO_2 on pulse oximetry, an **arterial blood gas (ABG) analysis** profile should be considered, which provides precise levels of oxygenation, carbon dioxide, and pH (normal values: pH, 7.40; pCO_2, 40 mm Hg; pO_2, 90–100 mm Hg). An ABG can aid in the diagnosis of severe dyspnea or dyspnea of unclear origin.
2. **Chest x-ray** can demonstrate an infiltrate, effusion, pneumothorax, signs of CHF (e.g., pulmonary vascular congestion or cardiomegaly), or lung disease (e.g., fibrosis or tumor).

C. Circulation. An electrocardiogram (ECG) is essential for evaluation of cardiac arrhythmia or ischemia and can aid in the diagnosis of pulmonary embolism, pericarditis, or other cardiac problems. The ECG should be correlated with blood pressure, pulse, and an assessment of perfusion.

D. Diagnostics: special tests. Further testing can be based on likely disorders guided by the acuity and severity of symptoms, initial testing, and pertinent examination findings (Figure 20–1).

1. **Cardiac tests**
   a. **BNP (brain or b-type natriuretic peptide)** is a validated test to evaluate for the presence of CHF in patients with dyspnea. A low value (≤100 pg/mL) makes CHF unlikely. Values ≥100 and ≤500 pg/mL require clinical judgment and further diagnostic testing to confirm CHF. Levels ≥500 pg/mL make CHF the most likely diagnosis. (SOR **B**)
   b. Other useful cardiac studies can include **echocardiography, cardiac catheterization, cardiac event monitors, and exercise treadmill testing.** These tests should be reserved for evaluation of abnormal ECG or examination findings or suspicious unexplained symptoms. Exercise testing is helpful in the evaluation of cardiac abnormalities as well as in the diagnosis of exercise-induced asthma, deconditioning, and muscle metabolism disorders.

2. **Pulmonary tests.** These tests can be used to evaluate possible lung disease. **Formal spirometry** is useful in the assessment of patients with lung disease. In **restrictive disease,** forced vital capacity (FVC) is low and forced expiratory volume in 1 second (FEV_1) and the maximal midexpiratory flow ($FEV_{25\%-75\%}$) may be low. The FEV–FVC ratio may be normal or even high. In **obstructive disease,** FVC, FEV, FEV_1–FVC ratio, or $FEV_{25\%-75\%}$, or all four, may be low. In mixed disease, all these values are low.

3. **Mixed cardiopulmonary tests.** PE can cause pleuritic chest pain, dyspnea, tachycardia, and hypoxemia. For the evaluation of PE, see Chapter 64.

4. **Noncardiopulmonary tests**
   a. **A complete blood cell count** can establish the presence of anemia or a possible underlying infection. Anemia leads to decreased oxygen-carrying capacity and therefore reduced oxygen delivery.
   b. **Blood glucose, basic metabolic panel, and thyroid-stimulating hormone** can be useful in assessing metabolic status in unclear cases. High levels of glucose can cause ketoacidosis. Renal or electrolyte abnormalities can cause dyspnea. Thyrotoxicosis results in increased oxygen demand.
   c. A **carbon monoxide level** (normal value ≤2%) can be used to document a toxic exposure to smoke or exhaust from a furnace or other sources. Levels are elevated in active smokers (≤10%), thereby decreasing oxygen-carrying capacity. Carbon monoxide binds to hemoglobin with 200 times the affinity of oxygen, severely compromising oxygen delivery to tissue. Lethal levels (≥50%) can occur despite relatively normal arterial blood gas levels.
   d. Further neurologic testing or imaging should be guided by abnormal physical examination findings and is unlikely to be cost-effective if a screening neurologic examination is normal.

V. **Treatment.** Once the underlying diagnosis has been made, treatment strategies should involve increasing oxygen delivery and correcting the underlying disease process, which usually relieves the sensation of dyspnea. For treatment of specific medical problems, please see the following chapters: Cough (Chapter 13), Deep vein thrombosis and pulmonary embolism (Chapter 64), Wheezing (Chapter 65), Asthma (Chapter 68), Chronic Obstructive Pulmonary Disease (Chapter 70), Congestive Heart Failure (Chapter 73), and Ischemic Heart Disease & Acute Coronary Syndromes (Chapter 79).

Medical therapies aimed at alleviating the symptoms of dyspnea can be used while the disease process is being treated or in cases where the cause of dyspnea is uncertain or related to a terminal condition such as cancer or end-stage COPD.

A. **Oxygen.** Oxygen delivered via nasal cannula at 1 to 4 L/min can provide good relief for mild or severe hypoxemia, at rest or with exercise, regardless of initial oxygen saturation; in patients with COPD, oxygen therapy can suppress respiratory drive and cause CO_2 retention, which can present as sedation.

B. **Bronchodilators.** Both beta-agonists and anticholinergics alone or in combination provide symptomatic relief in COPD (see Chapter 70). (SOR **A**)

C. **Intravenous steroids** do not help dyspnea acutely; prolonged use of **oral steroids** can cause muscle weakness; **inhaled steroids** improve airway reactivity in asthma and COPD and are associated with decreased symptoms and hospitalizations.
D. **Pulmonary rehabilitation programs** relieve dyspnea and fatigue in patients with COPD. (SOR **Ⓐ**)
E. A Cochrane review found strong evidence that **opioids** relieve dyspnea and improve exercise tolerance in patients with cancer and severe COPD. (SOR **Ⓐ**)
  1. Immediate-release forms (e.g., oxycodone IR) are more effective than sustained-release forms (e.g., OxyContin/oxycodone SR).
  2. Constipation is a problem, but tolerance develops to other side effects.
  3. Studies show that opioids do not severely suppress respiration or cause early death in terminally ill patients.
F. **Anxiolytics.** In end-stage COPD and cancer, oral buspirone (target dose for most adults 10–15 mg twice daily) or lorazepam (2–6 mg per day in divided doses) can relieve anxiety associated with dyspnea rather than dyspnea itself.
G. **Nonpharmacologic methods.** Use of fans; open windows; cognitive behavioral therapy; stress management for patient and caregiver; and nutritional, spiritual, and emotional support have all proven useful in decreasing dyspnea.

SELECTED REFERENCES

Carpenter CR, Keim SM, Worster A, Rosen P. Brain natriuretic peptide in the evaluation of emergency department dyspnea: is there a role? *J Emerg Med.* 2012:42:197–205.
Kamal AH, Maguire JM, Wheeler JL, et al. Dyspnea review for the palliative care professional: treatment goals and therapeutic options. *J Palliat Med.* 2012:15:106–114.
McCrory DC, Brown CD. Anticholinergic bronchodilators versus beta2-sympathomimetic agents for acute exacerbations of chronic obstructive pulmonary disease. *Cochrane Database Syst Rev.* 2002; (4):CD003900.
Parshall MB, Schwartzstein RM, Adams L, et al. An official American Thoracic Society Statement: update on the mechanisms, assessment, and management of dyspnea. *Am J Respir Crit Care Med.* 2012:185:435–452.
Segal JB, Eng J, Tamariz LJ, Bass E. Review of the evidence on diagnosis of deep venous thrombosis and pulmonary embolism. *Ann Fam Med.* 2007;5:63–73.

---

21 Dysuria in Women

L. Peter Schwiebert, MD

KEY POINTS

- In women with dysuria, consideration of historic risk factors and presenting signs and symptoms should drive differential diagnosis and evaluation. (SOR **Ⓒ**)
- Hematuria or positive nitrite dipstick testing are findings most predictive for diagnosis of urinary tract infection. (SOR **Ⓒ**)
- Findings compatible with an acute uncomplicated urinary tract infection warrant empiric treatment for *Escherichia coli.* (SOR **Ⓐ**)

I. **Definition. Dysuria** is discomfort associated with micturition, commonly caused by **bacterial urinary tract infection** (UTI). Among uncomplicated UTIs, over 80% are caused by *Escherichia coli, with less frequent infections caused by Staphylococcus saprophyticus, Proteus mirabilis, and Klebsiella species.* These organisms may also cause recurrent or difficult to eradicate (i.e., complicated) UTIs; such infections can also be caused by *Serratia, Pseudomonas aeruginosa,* enterococci, and Enterobacteriaceae species.
  Other causes of dysuria include the following:
  A. **Bladder irritation** (e.g., interstitial cystitis [IC]).
  B. **Urethral trauma or irritation from bubble baths or dietary factors.**

    C. Vaginal atrophy (postmenopausal or other hypoestrogenic state) (see Chapter 80).

    D. Urethritis, often caused by sexually transmitted infections (STIs), including *Chlamydia trachomatis, Neisseria gonorrhoeae, Trichomonas vaginalis,* or herpes simplex virus (HSV) infection.

    E. Psychogenic dysuria (often a component of somatization disorder, depression, chronic pain, or sexual abuse).

II. Common Diagnoses. In the United States, UTIs account for 2% to 3% of all visits in primary care (7–8 million annual visits) and 2% of all prescriptions, resulting in an annual expenditure of 1.6 billion dollars. In one study, almost half of women with acute uncomplicated UTI reported missing work or school because of this problem.

    A. Acute bacterial cystitis (25%–35% of cases) is more likely with a past history of cystitis, sexual intercourse, diaphragm/spermicidal contraception, douching, or postponement of micturition. Risk factors for complicated UTIs include pregnancy, indwelling urinary catheter, urinary tract instrumentation within the past 2 weeks, urinary tract anomaly or stones, recent systemic antibiotic use, or immunosuppression (e.g., poorly controlled diabetes mellitus).

    B. Vulvovaginitis (21%–38% of cases) is a more frequent cause of dysuria in college-aged women than are UTIs.

    C. The likelihood of **acute or subclinical pyelonephritis** (up to 30% of cases) increases in women reporting sexual intercourse three or more times per week over the previous month, UTI or a new sex partner in the foregoing year, stress urinary incontinence in the prior month, a maternal history of UTI, recent spermicide use, or who have other risk factors for complicated UTI (see Section II.A). Approximately one-third of women with lower UTI symptoms will have unrecognized or subclinical pyelonephritis.

    D. The likelihood of **dysuria without pyuria** (15%–30% of cases) is increased in women with a history of urethral trauma, in postmenopausal women who are not receiving estrogen therapy, or in women exposed to physical or chemical irritants (e.g., douching or consumption of citrus, ethanol, caffeinated carbonated beverages, sugar, or spicy foods). Ninety percent of patients with interstitial cystitis (IC) are women (up to1.2 million US women are affected); patients with this syndrome have a median age of 40 years and often have a past history of childhood or adult UTIs.

    E. Urethritis (3%–10% of cases) should be considered in women with a recent new sex partner, multiple partners, or a partner with urethritis. Thirty to fifty percent of nongonococcal urethritis is caused by *C. trachomatis;* other organisms implicated include ureaplasmids and *T. vaginalis.*

III. Symptoms. The onset of symptoms is usually abrupt and the patient may describe suprapubic pain or stinging of the skin around their urethra.

    A. Dysuria (see Figure 21–1)

        1. In a recent meta-analysis, dysuria, urgency, nocturia, and sexual activity were weak predictors of UTI, and increase in vaginal discharge and suprapubic pain weakly predicted absence of UTI. Another meta-analysis using the threshold of >100 colony-forming units [cfu]/mL found that dysuria, urgency, frequency, hematuria, or nocturia increased the likelihood of UTI, with hematuria having the highest diagnostic utility.

        2. The dysuria accompanying urethritis often has a stuttering, gradual onset. Increased frequency and urgency of urination can indicate dysuria without pyuria.

        3. Patients who complain of a burning sensation as the urine passes the inflamed labia may have vulvovaginitis.

    B. Vaginal discharge

        1. Dysuria and an associated increase in vaginal discharge from concomitant cervicitis may indicate urethritis.

        2. Patients with vulvovaginitis can report vaginal discharge, odor, or itching.

    C. Pain. Localized pain in the flank, low back, or abdomen and systemic symptoms (e.g., fever, rigors, sweats, headaches, nausea, vomiting, malaise, and prostration) can occur with UTI, particularly pyelonephritis.

    D. Interstitial cystitis (IC) is suggested by complaints of suprapubic pain, urinary frequency/urgency/nocturia, pelvic/perineal/labial pain, or exacerbations related to menses or sexual intercourse.

IV. Signs

    A. Acute bacterial cystitis

        1. Fever almost never develops when a UTI is localized to the bladder.

        2. Suprapubic tenderness is present in only 10% of patients with cystitis. If this sign is present, however, it has a high-predictive value for cystitis.

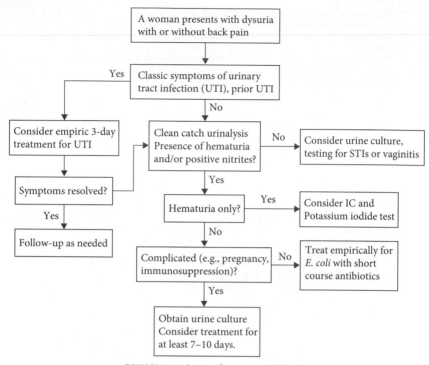

FIGURE 21-1. Evaluation of a woman with dysuria.

B. Vulvovaginitis. For signs of this condition, see Chapter 63.

C. Pyelonephritis. The patient often has a fever (temperature of 38–39°C [101–102°F]), costovertebral angle tenderness, and tachycardia.

D. Dysuria without pyuria. In this case, the physical findings just described are absent. However, the pelvic examination can show some periurethral or vulvar irritation.

E. Urethritis. Urethritis is frequently associated with mucopurulent cervicitis.

V. Laboratory Tests

   A. A **clean-catch midstream urinalysis (UA)** can be performed in most offices and is essential for evaluating patients with dysuria. Using the definition of significant bacteriuria as $\geq 10^2$ of a single uropathogenic bacterial species per milliliter in a symptomatic patient, presence of hematuria has the highest diagnostic utility, raising the post-test probability of UTI to 75.8% at ≥ 100 cfu/mL and 67.4% at ≥ 1000 cfu/mL. Probability of UTI increases to 93.3% and 90.1% at ≥ 100 cfu/mL and ≥ 1000 cfu/mL, respectively, when the presence of hematuria is combined with a positive dipstick test for nitrites.

   B. Urine culture

   1. Urine culture is indicated in the following situations:

   a. If an acute bacterial cystitis is suspected, but clinical findings and UA leave the diagnosis in question.

   b. If the patient has symptoms and signs of upper or complicated UTI (see Section II.C).

   c. Two to four days after a patient completes treatment for a complicated UTI.

   2. In women in whom **urethritis** is suspected, urethral and cervical cultures for N. gonorrhoeae and C. trachomatis should be performed.

   C. The **potassium iodide sensitivity test** involves catheter infusion first of sterile water with the patient rating pain and urgency, then draining the bladder and instilling 40 mg KCl and 100 mL water. Increased pain immediately or within 5 minutes of infusion of the potassium solution indicates damaged uroepithelium. The bladder is drained and a therapeutic solution (heparin 40,000 units/8–10 mL 2% lidocaine, and 4 mL 8.4% sodium bicarbonate) may be infused. The test is considered positive if the pain with infusion of the potassium solution is rated higher than the water infusion. False-positive tests for IC can occur with other types of cystitis (e.g., radiation or bacterial). Lack of evidence regarding the benefit of cystoscopy with hydrodistention has led to consensus that it is not needed to confirm diagnosis of IC, though it may be useful to document bladder inflammation and disease severity.

VI. Treatment of women with dysuria is based on the clinical picture, supplemented by appropriate laboratory studies. In patients with findings compatible with an acute, uncomplicated bacterial cystitis, it is reasonable to initiate treatment for *E. coli* based on UA findings alone.

A. Acute, uncomplicated bacterial cystitis

    1. Short-course antibiotics

        a. Short-course (3 days) treatment is equivalent in efficacy to treatment for 5 or more days for symptomatic cure. (SOR **Ⓐ**) However, 5% to 15% of *E. coli* are resistant to trimethoprim-sulfamethoxazole (TMP-SMX), and the likelihood of resistance increases with recent hospitalization, use of TMP-SMX during the previous 6 months, or recurrent UTIs during the past year. If resistance is likely, selection of an alternative Tier I medication (Table 21–1) is reasonable.

TELEPHONE PROTOCOL FOR UNCOMPLICATED UTI IN WOMEN

An adult, nonpregnant woman calls with symptoms consistent with UTI (dysuria, urinary frequency, urinary urgency).

1. Has she had an uncomplicated UTI in the past?
2. No other symptoms are reported (fever, vaginal discharge, back pain, hematuria)?

If answers are yes, the patient is eligible for over-the-phone treatment with first-line antibiotics. If not symptom free in 3 days, the patient needs to be seen. If the patient answers no to above questions, she should be asked to come for an office visit.

---

    2. Recurrent UTIs. Women experiencing two or more UTIs over a year benefit from continuous prophylaxis (Table 21–2). There is no difference in recurrence rate following discontinuation of continuous 6-month versus 12-month prophylaxis.

        a. Cranberry juice (150–750 mL daily) is moderately beneficial in decreasing the number of UTIs.

        b. If a postcoital regimen is not effective, long-term prophylaxis is indicated. Recommended regimens include one of the following: TMP-SMX, one single-strength tablet taken each evening or thrice weekly; TMP, 100 mg once daily at bedtime.

B. Vulvovaginitis (see Chapter 63).

C. Pyelonephritis

    1. Febrile, ill-appearing patients should be hospitalized for treatment with parenteral antibiotics; those with mild symptoms (temperature ≤38.3°C, no nausea or vomiting, good oral intake) in whom close follow-up is feasible can be treated as outpatients. Ciprofloxacin 500 mg orally twice daily for 7 days or levofloxacin 750 mg orally daily for 5 days are effective when fluoroquinolone resistance among *E. coli* isolates is <10%; if resistance exceeds 10%, inpatient management is recommended.

    2. Patients with complicated UTI are at risk for subclinical pyelonephritis and should be treated with a standard 10- to 14-day regimen (Table 21–1).

D. Dysuria without pyuria

    1. Offending agents identified through careful history should be eliminated.

    2. Postmenopausal women whose symptoms are believed due to estrogen deficiency may benefit from estrogen replacement (see Chapter 80).

    3. Other measures possibly helpful include taking warm baths, avoiding acidic foods (e.g., coffee, citrus fruits, tomato products, chocolate) and alcohol, artificial sweeteners, and carbonated beverages; increasing fluid intake (water is best) to dilute urine; or taking antispasmodics, such as phenazopyridine (e.g., Pyridium) 100 to 200 mg orally three times daily or hyoscyamine sulfate (e.g., Levsin) 0.125 to 0.250 mg orally every 4 hours.

TABLE 21–1. ANTIBIOTICS RECOMMENDED FOR AMBULATORY MANAGEMENT OF UTIs IN WOMEN

Tier	Drug	Dosage (mg)[b]	Serious Adverse Reactions (Rare)[c]	Selected Clinically Relevant Drug Interactions and Effects
1	Trimethoprim-sulfamethoxazole (TMP-SMX)[a]	160/800 twice daily	Stevens–Johnson syndrome (SJS) Toxic epidermal necrolysis (TEN) Aplastic anemia	Digoxin (↑ risk of digoxin toxicity), sulfonylureas (increased hypoglycemic effects), methotrexate (↑ risk of methotrexate toxicity)
	Nitrofurantoin (macrocrystals)	100 twice daily for 5 d	Peripheral neuropathy Hemolytic anemia Hepatitis	N/A
	Fosfomycin[d]	3000 (single dose)	Angioedema Aplastic anemia Asthma exacerbation Vaginitis	N/A
2	Ciprofloxacin	250 twice daily	Anaphylaxis SJS, TEN Phototoxicity Hypersensitivity reaction QT prolongation Tendinitis Disrupts natural flora	Simvastatin (↑ risk of myopathy); zolpidem (↑ zolpidem levels); dairy foods, calcium, zinc, iron, magnesium, aluminum supplements (↓ fluoroquinolone absorption) Consult package labeling for recommendations for each quinolone
	Ofloxacin	200 daily or 400 (single dose)	See above Insomnia	See above
	Levofloxacin	250 daily	See above	See above
3	Amoxicillin/Clavulanate	500/125 twice daily for 7 d	Anaphylaxis Serum sickness Erythema multiforme	Methotrexate (↑ risk of methotrexate toxicity)
	Cefdinir	300 twice daily for 10 d	Anaphylaxis SJS, TEN	Aluminum, magnesium, iron supplements (↓ cefdinir)[e]
	Cefpodoxime	100 twice daily for 7 d	Anaphylaxis	H₂ receptor antagonists (↓ cefpodoxime efficacy)[e]; dairy products, calcium, zinc, iron, magnesium, aluminum supplements (decrease cefpodoxime efficacy)[e]

[a]First-line option in nonsulfa-allergic patients and in populations with low resistance rates (documented resistance in region <20%).
[b]Duration: 3 days unless indicated otherwise.
[c]Most antibiotics have similar common side effects of nausea, vomiting, abdominal pain, diarrhea, and anorexia. A rash from antibiotics may demonstrate an allergy to that specific antibiotic class.
[d]Relatively expensive.
[e]Take the antibiotic 2 hours before listed drug or product.

TABLE 21–2. CONTINUOUS[a] OR POST-COITAL[b] ANTIMICROBIAL PROPHYLAXIS FOR RECURRENT UTIs

Drug	Dosage (mg)
Cephalexin	125 (continuous) or 250 (post-coital)
Ciprofloxacin	125
Nitrofurantoin	50–100
Norfloxacin	200
Trimethoprim (TMP)	100
TMP/sulfamethoxazole	40/200 or 80/400 (post-coital)

[a]Typically dosed in the evening.
[b]Taken within 2 hours of sexual intercourse (one-time dose).

4. For **IC,** oral cimetidine (300 mg twice daily) can improve suprapubic pain and nocturia (SOR **B**).

    a. The only agent approved for IC by the US Food and Drug Administration is pentosan polysulfate (e.g., Elmiron), 100 mg orally three times daily. (SOR **B**) Twenty-eight percent of women receiving pentosan (vs. 13% receiving placebo) noted improvement in pain/urgency/pressure but no appreciable improvement in frequency, nocturia, or volumes voided. Patients can take 3 to 6 months to respond and may experience side effects, including diarrhea, dyspepsia, headaches, rashes, or abdominal pain.

    b. Patients responding poorly to oral therapies and patients with severe symptoms may benefit from urologic referral for further management, such as intravesical dimethyl sulfoxide (DMSO) or combined oral and intravesical pentosan polysulfate. (SOR **B**)

E. Urethritis. Empiric therapy for *C. trachomatis* or *N. gonorrhoeae* can be instituted in high-risk individuals while one is awaiting culture results. Because of the coprevalence of *N. gonorrhoeae* and *C. trachomatis* infection, patients should be treated with ceftriaxone, 250 mg intramuscularly (1 dose), and doxycycline, 100 mg orally twice a day for 7 days. Alternatives to doxycycline for *C. trachomatis* include azithromycin, 1.0 g orally for one dose, or erythromycin base, 500 mg, or erythromycin ethylsuccinate, 800 mg orally four times daily for 7 days. **Pregnant or breast-feeding women should receive ceftriaxone plus azithromycin.**

ASYMPTOMATIC BACTERIURIA

Asymptomatic bacteriuria (ASB) is present in between 5% and 10% of pregnant women, with an increased likelihood in women who are sexually active or have diabetes, increased parity, or lower socioeconomic status. In 20% to 35% of women with ASB in pregnancy, overt UTI eventually develops. The American Congress of Obstetrics and Gynecologists recommends screening all pregnant patients with urine culture at the initial prenatal visit and in the third trimester.

Recommended antibiotics for treating UTI in pregnancy include nitrofurantoin, 100 mg orally every 12 hours for 7 days, or a cephalosporin (e.g., cephalexin), 250 to 500 mg orally four times daily for 7 days. Follow-up culture after treatment and monthly for the duration of the pregnancy is recommended with consideration of prophylactic nitrofurantoin following a bout of pyelonephritis.

The evaluation and management of **elderly women with symptomatic UTI** is as described in the main text. In a healthy, **elderly women with asymptomatic bacteriuria,** there is no evidence that treatment reduces long-term renal problems; treatment increases cost, the likelihood of drug reactions (or drug–drug interactions), and the likelihood of drug-resistant microorganisms.

SELECTED REFERENCES

Bent S, Saint S. The optimal use of diagnostic testing in women with acute uncomplicated cystitis. *Am J Med.* 2002;113(1A):20S–28S.

Bent S, Nallamouthu BK, Simel DL, et al. Does this woman have an acute uncomplicated urinary tract infection? *JAMA.* 2002;287(20):2701–2710.

Bremnor JD, Sadovsky R. Evaluation of dysuria in adults. *Am Fam Physician.* 2002;65(8):1589–1596.

Colgan R, Williams M. Diagnosis and treatment of acute uncomplicated cystitis. *Am Fam Physician.* 2011;84(7):771–776.

Katchman EA, Milo G, Paul M, et al. Three-day vs longer duration of antibiotic treatment for cystitis in women: systematic review and meta-analysis. *Am J Med.* 2005;118(11):1196–1207.

Kodner CM, Thomas-Gupton EK. Recurrent urinary tract infections in women: diagnosis and management. *Am Fam Physician.* 2010;82(6):638–643.

Nicolle LE. Urinary tract infection: traditional pharmacologic therapies. *Dis Mon.* 2003;49(2):111–128.

Rosamilia A. Painful bladder syndrome/interstitial cystitis. *Best Pract Res Clin Obstet Gynecol.* 2005; 19(6):843–859.

22   Earache

David Berkson, MD, FAAFP, Greeshma Naini, MD, & Carmelo DiSalvo, MD

KEY POINTS

- Most causes of otalgia are benign and can be diagnosed and managed in the office setting. (SOR **©**)
- Not all causes of otalgia are intrinsic to the ear itself. Referred pain can be causal and indicative of serious problems such as an underlying cancer and other non-ear diseases. (SOR **©**)
- Unexplained otalgia or otalgia not resolving with appropriate therapy should be evaluated by an otolaryngologist. (SOR **©**)

I. **Definition.** Earache (otalgia) is pain or discomfort perceived in the ear or surrounding structures. It can be primary, including pain from diseases of the auricle, external canal, middle ear, or inner ear, or referred, occurring secondary to the complex innervations of the head and neck. The ear is innervated by sensory branches of the trigeminal, facial, vagus, and glossopharyngeal cranial nerves and by the lesser occipital and great auricular cervical nerves.

II. **Common Diagnoses.** Earache most commonly originates from middle ear or external auditory canal pathology.

    A. Acute otitis media (AOM) occurs most frequently during the winter months, thus coinciding with the peak incidence of viral upper respiratory tract infections. The peak age incidence is 6 months to 7 years. Native Americans and Eskimos experience otitis media more frequently than do people of other races. Otitis media is also more prevalent in children with Down syndrome or cleft palate. The two major risk factors for AOM in children are group day care involvement and exposure to secondhand smoke. Other risk factors include a family history of AOM, bottle-feeding, Eustachian tube dysfunction, and enlarged adenoids.

    B. Otitis externa (OE) is a generalized inflammation of the external ear canal that can involve both the pinna and tympanic membrane (TM). OE requires the presence of pathogens and the breakage of skin to cause disease. It is 10 to 20 times more common in the summer than in cooler months, particularly in individuals who swim in lakes or pools. This condition is more likely to affect patients with diabetes mellitus (DM) and other immunocompromised persons, who are also more likely to develop invasive disease. Local trauma with cotton swabs and scratching are among the most frequent known causes. Other risk factors include, but are not limited to, moisture in the ear canal, canal occlusion, and conditions of abnormal keratin production (e.g., psoriasis and atopic and seborrheic dermatitis).

    C. Barotrauma most commonly occurs either after flying in an unpressurized aircraft or after scuba diving. Acute upper respiratory infections and allergies increase susceptibility to this condition.

    D. Direct trauma is seen more frequently in young men, resulting from fights or automobile accidents; in military personnel or miners, who may work near explosions; or in hikers, mountain climbers, or outdoor workers in cold climates, who may suffer frostbite.

    E. Referred otalgia

        1. Temporomandibular joint dysfunction tends to occur in patients with the following conditions: (1) dental malocclusion or poorly fitting dental prostheses, (2) bruxism (nocturnal tooth grinding), (3) trauma to the mandible, or (4) degenerative temporomandibular joint disease, especially in women in the third or fourth decade of life.

        2. Dental diseases, such as **abscesses,** are likely to develop in individuals with poor oral hygiene.

        3. Cancers of the ear, nose, and throat region have an increased risk in patients with a history of heavy tobacco or alcohol use or serous otitis (in adults), those of Chinese ancestry, and those with dysphagia or hemoptysis.

III. Symptoms and Signs. Examination of patients with otalgia should be directed by risk factors and symptoms and should include systematic evaluation of the auricle, auditory canals, and TMs, as well as sources of referred otalgia as indicated (Table 22–1).
- **A. Pain**
  1. Severe deep pain or ear pain that interferes with normal activity or sleep suggests AOM.
  2. Moderate pain, especially when lying on the affected side or movement of the jaw, can be present in OE. **Pain** with movement of the auricle or pressure on the tragus can also occur with OE.
  3. Pressure progressing to moderate-to-severe pain over a few hours can be related to **barotrauma**.
  4. Pain in the injured part of the ear is evident with **direct trauma;** frostbite of the auricle usually causes burning pain lasting several hours.
  5. Pain in **referred otalgia** depends on the cause (Table 22–1).
- **B. Tinnitus** can be present with barotrauma or can indicate more serious disease.
- **C. Hearing loss,** if unilateral, can be a sign of an effusion or other underlying pathology that warrants further investigation.
- **D. Auricle**
  1. **OE** may cause erythema or crusting if this portion of the ear is involved.
  2. **In direct trauma,** injury to the auricle is evident from inspection; frostbite can initially present with auricular pallor followed by erythema and sometimes bullae. Examination of the posterior aspect of the auricle is essential to avoid missing signs of **trauma**.
- **E. External auditory canal**
  1. The canal in OE is red and edematous, usually with purulent drainage. The presence of spores or black-colored material can signify a fungal infection. A greenish discharge can indicate *Pseudomonas*.
  2. A purulent nonmalodorous discharge in the canal can be seen with TM rupture in **AOM;** perforation often occurs near the annulus, necessitating clear view of the entire TM to detect.
  3. Canal injuries with **direct trauma** include lacerations, abrasions, or hematomas. A bloody, serous, or foul smelling discharge can indicate **trauma** with or without accompanying infection.
- **F. Tympanic membrane**
  1. A **normal** appearing TM is a pearly colored, partially translucent tissue that vibrates as it transmits sound to the inner ear (see Figure 22–1). The presence of a reddened TM alone, without pneumatic otoscopic evidence of immobility, is not sufficient to diagnose AOM, as an erythematous TM can also occur due to increased intravascular pressure (e.g., a crying infant or child). In performing pneumatic otoscopy, it is imperative that a speculum of proper shape and diameter be selected to ensure a proper seal in the external auditory canal.
  2. A diagnosis of AOM requires: (1) a history of acute onset of signs and symptoms, (2) the presence of middle-ear effusion, and (3) signs and symptoms of middle-ear inflammation. Pneumatic otoscopy is the primary method for evaluating the presence of effusion with AOM. (SOR **Ⓐ**) Positive predictive values in the 90% range compared to myringotomy have been achieved with the following findings: an opaque TM, a bulging TM, and impaired TM mobility. An air–fluid level behind the TM indicates the presence of middle-ear effusion (see Figure 22–2).
  3. A **cholesteatoma** (pearl tumor) can appear as white or yellow flecks and/or as chronic debris behind the TM. Suspicion should arise when there is a perforated or retracted TM with debris that is difficult to clear. Severe complications include central nervous system infection and thrombosis (see Figure 22–3).
  4. In **barotrauma**, the TM initially appears red, later becoming blue or yellow. With continued blockage, bubbles or air–fluid levels can be seen. Other manifestations of barotraumas include TM rupture and rupture of the inner ear membrane, ova, or round window. Barotrauma can present with otorrhea, hemotympanum, and/or vertigo.
- **G. Itching** can be present in **OE** or following minor **trauma**.
- **H. Associated symptoms**
  1. Fever, dizziness, nausea, and vomiting can occur with **AOM**.
  2. Parents of infants and small children with **AOM** sometimes observe irritability, decreased feeding, or pulling at the ears.

TABLE 22-1. CAUSES OF REFERRED OTALGIA

Cause	Mechanism	Symptoms	Signs	Laboratory Tests	Treatment	Comments
TMJ dysfunction	Internal derangement of joints, malocclusion, poorly fitting dental prostheses, bruxism	Deep pain that becomes worse with eating	Pain on palpation, crepitus, asymmetry of motion	None	NSAIDs plus jaw-opening exercises; moist heat; mechanical soft diet. Refer if not relieved in 3–4 wk	
Dental disease	Inflammation or pressure on nerves by abscessed teeth, impacted molars	Dull to lancinating pain worse with eating, tooth sensitive to cold	Carious teeth, tender teeth, red or necrotic gingiva	None	Dental referral; pain control; consider antibiotics	
Head and neck tumors	Traction on or inflammation of nerves	Hoarseness, dysphagia, lump, pain or pressure slowly increasing	Tumor in nasopharynx or larynx	CT, MRI	Refer for excision/biopsy and further treatment	
Infection of sinuses, pharynx	Nerve irritation from infection	Retro-orbital or frontal pain, sore throat	Sinus tenderness, poor transillumination, exudative pharyngitis	Strep screen, consider further sinus evaluation	See Chapters 54 and 56	
Carotodynia	Pain referred along same nerve pathways as ear	Throat pain, dysphagia	Tender bifurcation of carotid artery	Consider radiographic evaluation of carotid anatomy	Consider steroids, moist heat to affected area	Differential includes arteritis and dissection
Temporal arteritis	Collagen vascular disease with inflammation	Pain near affected arteries, weight loss, fever, jaw claudication	Tender, indurated temporal artery	Elevated ESR, temporal artery biopsy	Long-term oral steroid taper is mainstay of therapy	Treat to prevent visual loss; use ESR to monitor therapy
Trigeminal, glossopharyngeal, or sphenopalatine neuralgia	Compression of nerves	Lancinating pain triggered by chewing or swallowing cold liquids	Trigger points in nasopharynx	None	Multiple options for oral neuropathic pain; surgical therapy or ablation for nonresponders	Significant potential side effects with medications—monitoring may be necessary
Gastroesophageal reflux disease	Nerve irritation from acid stimulation	Worse at night or with stimulating foods	None	pH study, upper GI study	Diet and behavioral changes; antacids H$_2$ blockers, PPIs (see Chapters 19 and 84)	Caution of potential long-term side effects with PPIs (osteopenia)

NSAIDs, nonsteroidal anti-inflammatory drugs; ESR, erythrocyte sedimentation rate; CT, computed tomography; GI, gastrointestinal; MRI, magnetic resonance imaging; TMJ, temporomandibular joint; PPI, proton-pump inhibitor.

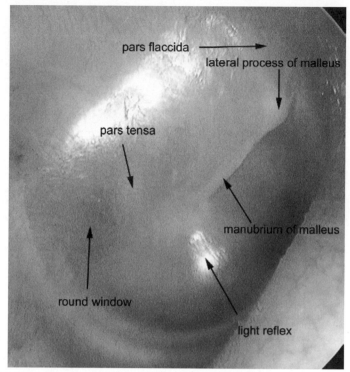

FIGURE 22-1. Normal right TM. (see color insert) (Used with permission of William Clark, MD.)

IV. Laboratory Tests. The cause of otalgia is usually evident from the history and examination. The following laboratory tests can be helpful in delineating the cause in certain situations:

   A. Tympanometry, a technique that measures admittance (how energy is transmitted) through the middle ear at various levels of air pressure, can be helpful for follow-up examination of patients treated for AOM, especially for confirming the resolution of AOM with effusion. See Chapter 34 for more information on tympanometry.

   B. The **white blood cell count** in cases of AOM is frequently elevated and left shifted, particularly in children. The complete blood count is not routinely obtained in non–toxic-appearing children with AOM.

   C. Radiography and **computerized tomography (CT)** are useful to determine the presence of other associated injury when occult fractures of the skull or intracerebral injury are suspected. When dealing with otalgia, CT is most valuable for evaluating the middle ear and the mastoid when infections of these structures are suspected. Magnetic resonance imaging with contrast is more appropriate for the evaluation of the soft tissues, lesions around the ear, diseases of the cranial nerves VII and VIII, and when evaluating the cerebellar-pontine angle.

   D. Referred pain (see Table 22–1 for details).

V. Treatment

   A. Otitis media

   1. AOM. Numerous antibacterial agents are available and clinically effective. The decision to treat with antibiotics is based on age, diagnostic certainty, and complicating factors (Figure 22–4). Once deciding to use antimicrobials, antibiotic choice is based upon the organisms most likely to be present and cost. In most cases, amoxicillin is used as a first-line therapy. In patients with severe illness (moderate-to-severe otalgia or fever ≥39.0°C) and when additional coverage to treat β-lactamase-positive organisms

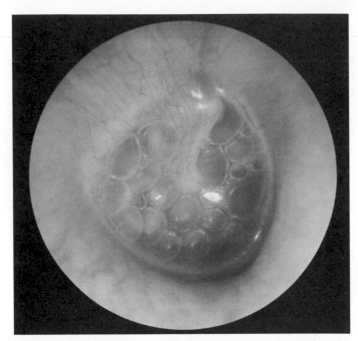

FIGURE 22–2. OME (otitis media with effusion) in the right ear. Note multiple air-fluid levels in this slightly retracted, translucent, nonerythematous TM. (see color insert) (Used with permission of Frank Miller, MD.)

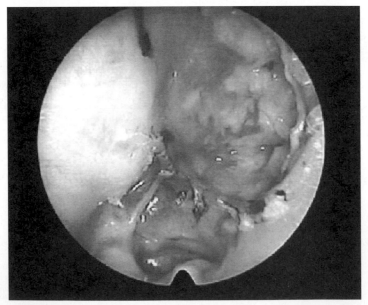

FIGURE 22–3. Cholesteatoma.(see color insert) (Used with permission of Vladimir Zlinsky, MD.)

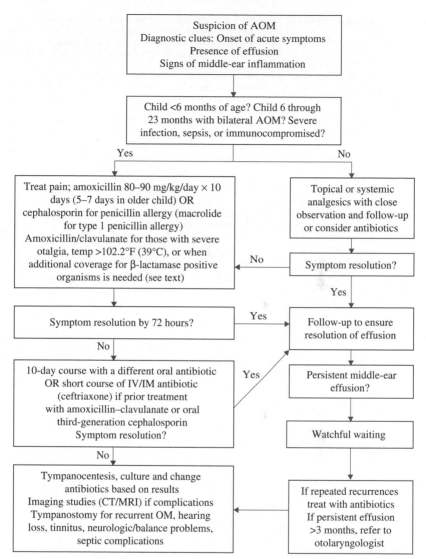

FIGURE 22–4. Approach to the patient with acute otitis media. AOM, acute otitis media; CT, computed tomography; MRI, magnetic resonance imaging.

is required (i.e., *Haemophilus influenzae* and *Moraxella catarrhalis*), therapy should be initiated with high-dose amoxicillin–clavulanate (90 mg/kg/d of amoxicillin and 6.4 mg/kg of clavulanate per day in 2 divided doses). Based on limited and controversial data, there are currently no recommendations for treatment of AOM with complementary and alternative medicine. See Figure 22–4 for an approach to the treatment of AOM.

    a. Watchful waiting. Subsequent studies support the 2004 American Academy of Pediatrics (AAP) and American Academy of Family Physicians (AAFP) clinical guideline for watchful waiting as an option for uncomplicated AOM in children aged >6 months. Since the initial publication of the guideline, it was shown that prescribing amoxicillin and analgesics increased appropriately; however, treatment of AOM with antibiotics did not decrease. Improved adherence to guidelines will help decrease antibiotic use and potentially decrease microbial antibiotic resistance.

b. Antibiotic selection. It is important to remember that the bacteria most commonly isolated with middle-ear effusions are *Streptococcus pneumoniae* (50%), *H. influenzae* (30%), and *M. catarrhalis* (25%). Of these, the most important pathogen is *S. pneumoniae*, which if left untreated can progress to more invasive disease. Drug-resistant *S. pneumoniae* is common and develops resistance by alterations in penicillin-binding proteins, not β-lactamase mechanisms. Therefore, in all but highly resistant organisms, resistance is overcome by higher doses of penicillin, not by adding β-lactam stabilizers (e.g., clavulanic acid). Check your local susceptibility patterns for resistance to recommended antibiotics. AOM caused by viruses, nontypeable *H. influenzae*, or *M. catarrhalis* is likely to resolve spontaneously and unlikely to progress to more invasive disease. See Tables 22–2 and 22–3. (SOR **B**)

c. Decongestants/antihistamines. There is no grade A or grade B evidence that suggests these products shorten the course of the illness and it is not clear that they are useful for symptomatic care (see Chapter 54 for dosage). In fact, authors of a Cochrane-based review found that in AOM with effusion, not only was no statistical or clinical benefit found but also treated subjects experienced 11% more side effects than untreated subjects.

d. Treatments for otalgia. Regardless of whether or not antibiotics are going to be prescribed, otalgia should be addressed and dealt with appropriately. (SOR **A**) Otalgia treatments include:

(1) Analgesics: Acetaminophen and ibuprofen are appropriate for mild-to-moderate pain and are the mainstay of pain management for AOM. Narcotics such as codeine can be effective for moderate or severe pain, but require a prescription and are associated with respiratory depression, altered mental status, gastrointestinal upset, and constipation.

(2) External application of heat or cold can be considered as tolerated.

(3) Topical agents such as benzocaine (Auralgan, Americaine Otic) provide short-term benefit over acetaminophen in patients aged ≥5 years. Naturopathic agents (Otikon Otic Solution) can also provide comparable benefit to amethocaine/phenazone drops (anesthetic) in patients aged ≥6 years.

(4) Other options include home remedies, homeopathic agents, and distraction for young children. None have supporting evidence on effectiveness.

(5) Tympanostomy/myringotomy can be considered for severe pain.

e. Education. The parents of young patients with AOM should be educated concerning the importance of having the child finish the course of antibiotics as well as keeping follow-up appointments. They should also be made aware of signs of possible invasive disease (i.e., extreme irritability or somnolence, worsening pain, persistent fever). Clinicians should encourage the prevention of AOM through reduction of risk factors (e.g., tobacco smoke exposure, group daycare). (SOR **B**)

f. Follow-up.

(1) The patient should be **reevaluated in 48 to 72 hours if fever or pain persists** at pretreatment levels. In this case, a 10-day course of a different oral antibiotic or possibly a short course of IV/IM antibiotics should be instituted. (SOR **B**) (See Table 22–3) If the symptoms fail to improve after this intervention, the patient should be referred to a physician who can perform tympanocentesis for further evaluation, fluid culture, and management. At this point, inpatient care and intravenous antibiotics can be necessary.

(2) The patient should **be reevaluated** at **4- to 6-week intervals** if an effusion has not resolved. An effusion can require up to 3 months to clear. Antibiotics are not indicated for persistent middle-ear effusion in the absence of AOM. Effusions persisting beyond 3 months should be evaluated by an otolaryngologist.

2. AOM in infants

a. Infants younger than 2 months of age should be hospitalized for fever even if a source (e.g., AOM) is identified. Children with fever and AOM between

TABLE 22–2. RECOMMENDED ANTIBACTERIAL AGENTS FOR AOM AT DIAGNOSIS

Temperature ≥39°C and/or Severe Otalgia	Drug or Test	Dose	Major Side Effects	Contraindication	Drug Interactions
Initial Treatment with Antibacterial Agents					
No	Recommended: Amoxicillin	80–90 mg/kg	Nausea, vomiting, diarrhea, rash, *Clostridium difficile*, SJS, TEN	PKU, concurrent mononucleosis, renal impairment, seizures	Methotrexate, OCs, chloroquine, PPI, tramadol, exenatide
	Alternative: Nontype I[a] Cefdinir, Cefuroxime, Cefpodoxime	*Cefdinir:* 14 mg/kg/d in one or two doses	Nausea, diarrhea, pruritis, SJS, *C. difficile*	PCN allergy, seizures, renal impairment	Exenatide, antacids, OCs
		Cefuroxime: 30 mg/kg/d in two divided doses	Nausea, diarrhea, diaper rash, SJS, pancytopenia, *C. difficile*	PCN allergy, seizures, renal or hepatic impairment	PPI, antacids, OCs, H₂ blockers
	Type I[a] Azithromycin, Clarithromycin	*Cefpodoxime:* 10 mg/kg	Diarrhea, nausea, thrombocytopenia, rash	PCN allergy, seizures, renal impairment	PPI, antacids, OCs, H₂ blockers
		Azithromycin: 10 mg/kg then 5 mg/kg	Diarrhea, nausea, QT prolongation, SJS	QT prolongation, renal or hepatic impairment	Quinolones, OCs, antipsychotics
		Clarithromycin: 15 mg/kg	Diarrhea, dyspepsia, QT prolongation, SJS	QT prolongation, renal impairment	Quinolones, statins, OCs, antipsychotic
Yes	Recommended: Amoxicillin-clavulanate	90 mg/kg Amoxicillin component with 6.4 mg/kg clavulanate	Diarrhea, nausea, cholestatic jaundice, agranulocytosis, SJS	PCN allergy, PKU, seizures, HIV, renal or hepatic impairment	Methotrexate, OCs, chloroquine, PPI, tramadol, exenatide
	Alternative: Ceftriaxone	50 mg/kg/d for 3 days	Thrombocytosis, SJS, diarrhea, jaundice	PCN allergy, seizures, vitamin K deficiency	OCs, probenecid, warfarin

Source: Based on information from AAP/AAFP Clinical Practice Guideline; Subcommittee on Management of Acute Otitis Media: Diagnosis and management of acute otitis media. *Pediatrics.* 2004;113(5):1451–1465.

SJS, Stevens–Johnson syndrome; TEN, toxic epidermal necrolysis; PKU, phenylketonuria; OCs, oral contraceptives; PPI, proton-pump inhibitor; PCN, penicillin; HIV, human immunodeficiency virus.

[a]Refers to nontype 1 and type 1 penicillin allergies.

TABLE 22–3. RECOMMENDED ANTIBACTERIAL AGENTS FOR AOM AFTER 48–72 HOURS OF OBSERVATION, OR TREATMENT FAILURE AFTER 48–72 HOURS

Temperature ≥39°C and/or Severe Otalgia	Drug or Test	Dose	Major Side Effects	Contraindication	Drug Interactions
Clinically Defined Treatment Failure at 48–72 h after Initial Management with Observation					
No	Recommended: Amoxicillin	80–90 mg/kg	Nausea, vomiting, diarrhea, rash, C. difficile, SJS, TEN	PKU, concurrent mononucleosis, renal impairment, seizures	Methotrexate, OCs, chloroquine, PPI, tramadol, exenatide
	Alternative: Nontype I[a] Cefdinir, Cefuroxime, Cefpodoxime	Cefdinir: 14 mg/kg/d in one or two doses	Nausea, diarrhea, pruritus, SJS, C. difficile	PCN allergy, seizure, renal impairment	Exenatide, antacids, OCs
		Cefuroxime: 30 mg/kg/d in two divided doses	Nausea, diarrhea, diaper rash, SJS, pancytopenia, C. difficile	PCN allergy, seizure, renal and hepatic impairment	PPI, antacids, OCs, H₂ blockers
		Cefpodoxime: 10 mg/kg	Diarrhea, nausea, thrombocytopenia, rash	PCN allergy, seizure, renal impairment	PPI, antacids, OCs, H₂ blockers
	Type I[a] Azithromycin Clarithromycin	Azithromycin: 10 mg/kg then 5 mg/kg	Diarrhea, nausea, QT prolongation, SJS	QT prolongation, renal or hepatic impairment	Quinolones, OCs, antipsychotics
		Clarithromycin: 15 mg/kg/d for 3 days	Diarrhea, dyspepsia, QT prolongation, SJS	QT prolongation, renal impairment	Quinolones, statins, OCs, antipsychotic
Yes	Recommended: Amoxicillin-clavulanate	90 mg/kg amoxicillin component with 6.4 mg/kg clavulanate	Diarrhea, nausea, cholestatic jaundice, agranulocytosis, SJS	PCN allergy, PKU, seizures, HIV, renal or hepatic impairment	Methotrexate, OCs, chloroquine, PPI, tramadol, exenatide
	Alternative: Ceftriaxone	50 mg/kg/d for 3 days	Thrombocytosis, SJS, diarrhea, jaundice	PCN allergy, seizures, vitamin K deficiency	OCs, probenecid, warfarin
Clinically Defined Treatment Failure at 48–72 h after Initial Management with Antibiotics					
No	Recommended: Amoxicillin-clavulanate	90 mg/kg amoxicillin component with 6.4 mg/kg clavulanate	Diarrhea, nausea, cholestatic jaundice, agranulocytosis, SJS	PCN allergy, PKU, seizures, HIV, renal or hepatic impairment	Methotrexate, OCs, chloroquine, PPI, tramadol, exenatide
	Alternative: None Type I Ceftriaxone	Ceftriaxone: 50 mg/kg/d for 3 days	Thrombocytosis, SJS, diarrhea, jaundice	PCN allergy, seizures, vitamin K deficiency	OCs, probenecid, warfarin
	Type I Clindamycin	Clindamycin: 30–40 mg/kg/d	Diarrhea, nausea, rash, C. difficile, hypotension, thrombocytopenia	Ulcerative colitis, hepatic or renal impairment	OCs, botulinum toxin, exenatide
Yes	Recommended: Ceftriaxone	50 mg/kg/d for 3 days	Thrombocytosis, SJS, diarrhea, jaundice	PCN allergy, seizures, vitamin K deficiency	OCs, probenecid, warfarin
	Alternative:[b] Clindamycin	30–40 mg/kg/d	Diarrhea, nausea, rash, C. difficile, hypotension, thrombocytopenia	Ulcerative colitis, hepatic or renal impairment	OCs, botulinum toxin, exenatide

Source: Based on information from AAP/AAFP Clinical Practice Guideline; Subcommittee on Management of Acute Otitis Media: Diagnosis and management of acute otitis media. *Pediatrics.* 2004;113(5):1451–1465.

SJS, Stevens-Johnson syndrome; TEN, toxic epidermal necrolysis; PKU, phenylketonuria; OCs, oral contraceptives; PPI, proton-pump inhibitor; PCN, penicillin; HIV, human immunodeficiency virus.

[a]Refers to nontype 1 and type 1 penicillin allergies.
[b]Consider tympanocentesis.

ages 2 and 6 months can be treated as outpatients with antibiotics after careful evaluation by a seasoned clinician. Children older than 6 months can be treated with an outpatient course of antibiotics if there is no complicating history or physical finding (TM perforation, craniofacial abnormality, recurrent or chronic infection, or immunocompromise). If the diagnosis of AOM is uncertain, observation may be appropriate in cases with nonsevere illness, when follow-up can be ensured. Controlled trials concluded that a wait-and-see prescription approach substantially reduced unnecessary use of antibiotics in children with AOM seen in an emergency department and is an alternative to routine use of antimicrobials for treatment of such children. (SOR **B**) Providing there are no further complications, follow-up examination should take place in 4 weeks.

   b. A **polyvalent pneumococcal vaccine** is available for infants and has been shown to decrease the incidence of AOM and invasive pneumococcal disease.

3. Recurrent AOM

   a. Recurrent disease is defined as three episodes of AOM in a 6-month period or four or more episodes in a 12-month period. Underlying conditions predisposing to recurrent disease should be treated when associated with recurrence. Such disorders include enlarged adenoids, allergies, immunodeficiencies, nasal septal deviation, and sinusitis.

   b. Tympanostomy tube insertion, which results in immediate improvement in hearing, has been advocated for the prevention of recurrent otitis media. However, this intervention has not been proved superior to antibiotic prophylaxis or interval treatment of recurrences for preserving hearing. The interpretation of these data is controversial. Tympanostomy tube placement for persistent effusion in children younger than 3 years has not been shown to improve multiple developmental outcomes up to 9 to 11 years. (SOR **B**)

   c. Prophylactic antibiotics for recurrent otitis media include **amoxicillin,** 25 mg/kg/d at bedtime; **sulfisoxazole,** 75 mg/kg/d at bedtime; and **trimethoprim–sulfamethoxazole,** 25 mg/kg/d at bedtime, based on the sulfamethoxazole component.

B. Otitis externa

   1. Acute OE is frequently a polymicrobial infection involving *Pseudomonas aeruginosa,* *Staphylococcus aureus,* **or both.**

   2. In 2006, the American Academy of Otolaryngology created the first, explicit, evidence-based clinical practice guidelines for **acute OE**:

   a. Assess pain and recommend analgesic treatment based on severity. (SOR **B**)

   b. Distinguish OE from other causes of otalgia. (SOR **C**)

   c. Evaluate patient for factors that modify management such as nonintact TM, tympanostomy tubes, immunocompromised, and/or prior radiotherapy. (SOR **C**)

   d. Use topical preparations for initial therapy of uncomplicated acute OE. (SOR **B**)

   e. Avoid systemic antibiotics unless there is extension of cellulitis outside of the ear canal, DM, immunodeficiency, or other factors prohibiting the delivery of topical therapy. Oral antibiotics can cause adverse reactions and be less effective than eardrops. (SOR **B**)

   f. Topical antibiotic therapy of acute OE should be based on efficacy, low incidence of adverse events, likelihood of adherence to therapy, and cost. Patients should be given proper instruction in their use. (SOR **B**)

   g. When the ear canal is obstructed, enhance delivery of topical preparations with aural toilet, placing a wick, or both. (SOR **C**)

   h. Nonototoxic topical preparations should be prescribed for patients with TM rupture or with tympanostomy tubes. Quinolone antibiotic drops are approved for this purpose and do not contribute to hearing loss. (SOR **C**)

   i. If a patient fails to respond within 48 to 72 hours after initiation of treatment, reassess for confirmation of OE and to rule out other causes; this includes but is not limited to obstructed ear canal, poor adherence to therapy, misdiagnosis, microbiologic factors, host factors, or contact sensitivity to eardrops. (SOR **C**)

   j. Ear candles are not recommended for treating acute OE because efficacy has not been demonstrated. In addition, they can cause adverse effects such as burns and TM rupture.

    k. Patients should abstain from water-related sports for a period of 7 to 10 days after the diagnosis of OE.

    l. Meta-analysis of topical treatment for acute OE found that 65% to 90% of subjects improved within 7 to 10 days of initiation of treatment, irrespective of the type of topical treatment used. No statistically significant differences in clinical outcomes of acute OE exist for antiseptic versus antimicrobial, quinolone antibiotic versus nonquinolone antibiotic(s), or steroid plus antimicrobial versus antimicrobial alone. The combination of antimicrobial and steroid appeared superior to steroid drops alone. Generally, 7 to 10 days of treatment are necessary for the resolution of acute OE.

  3. Patients with **necrotizing OE,** formerly malignant OE, a severe infection involving the deeper periauricular tissue, should be hospitalized and treated with parenteral antibiotics providing adequate pseudomonal coverage. Necrotizing OE should be suspected when there is no resolution of either the otalgia or headache despite adequate treatment. In addition, pain out of proportion to clinical findings and/or the presence of granulation tissue at the bony cartilaginous junction should prompt further investigation. High clinical suspicion for patients with DM and other immunocompromised patients is warranted.

C. Barotrauma

  1. The **acute episode** can be treated with decongestants (e.g., **pseudoephedrine,** 30–60 mg every 4–6 hours) and analgesics (**acetaminophen,** 325–650 mg every 4–6 hours, or **codeine,** 30–60 mg every 4–6 hours).

  2. Patients with multiple episodes of barotrauma should use a long-acting oral decongestant, such as timed-release **pseudoephedrine,** 120 mg once or twice daily, or a topical nasal decongestant such as **phenylephrine,** two sprays 5 minutes apart in each nostril 30 minutes prior to flying or diving. Individuals who use topical decongestants should be cautioned to limit use to 3 days and/ or apply them only intermittently to avoid rhinitis medicamentosum. To prevent future recurrences, the diver or flier should be instructed in the proper methods of equalizing middle ear and ambient pressure, such as swallowing hard or exhaling against closed nostrils.

D. Direct trauma

  1. Abrasions and small lacerations of the auricle should be treated as are other minor skin injuries (see Chapter 40).

  2. Hematomas of the auricle should be aspirated and a pressure dressing applied to prevent formation of a cauliflower ear.

  3. Traumatic perforations of the TM are treated by keeping the canal dry. If the perforations do not heal within several weeks, the patient should be referred to an otolaryngologist.

E. Referred otalgia (see Table 22–1).

SELECTED REFERENCES

American Academy of Pediatrics, Subcommittee on Management of Acute Otitis Media. Diagnosis and management of acute otitis media. *Pediatrics.* 2004;113(5):1451–1465.

Bhattacharya N, Kepnes L. Initial impact of the acute otitis externa clinical practice guideline on clinical care. *Otolaryngol Head Neck Surg.* 2011;145(3):414–417.

Coco A, Vernachio L, Horst M, Anderson A. Management of acute otitis media after publication of the 2004 AAP and AAFP clinical practice guideline. *Pediatrics.* 2010;125(2):214–220.

Griffin G, Flynn CA. Antihistamines and/or decongestants for otitis media with effusion (OME) in children. *Cochrane Database Syst Rev.* 2011;(9):CD003423.

Kaushik V, Malik T, Saeed SR. Interventions for acute otitis externa. *Cochrane Database Syst Rev.* 2010;(1):CD004740.

Rosenfeld RM, Brown L, Cannon CR, et al; American Academy of Otolaryngology–Head and Neck Surgery Foundation. Clinical practice guideline: acute otitis externa. *Otolaryngol Head Neck Surg.* 2006;134(4 Suppl):S4–S23.

Tähtinen PA, Laine MK, Ruuskanen O, Rohola A. Delayed versus immediate antimicrobial treatment for acute otitis media. *Pediatr Infect Dis J.* 2012;31(12):1227–1232.

Venekamp RP, Sanders S, Glasziou PP, Del Mar CB, Rovers MM. Antibiotics for acute otitis media in children. *Cochrane Database Sys Rev.* 2013;(1):CD000219.

23 Enuresis

Kalyanakrishnan Ramakrishnan, MD, MS, FRCS

KEY POINTS

- Primary monosymptomatic enuresis (enuresis in children without lower urinary tract symptoms other than nocturia and no evidence of bladder dysfunction) is the most common form of enuresis. (SOR **C**)
- Parents of children in whom primary monosymptomatic enuresis is not distressing should receive reassurance about their child's physical and emotional well-being and should be counseled about eliminating guilt, shame, and punishment. Pharmacotherapy and/or alarms should be used only when enuresis poses a significant problem for the child. (SOR **B**)
- Enuresis alarm is an effective treatment for monosymptomatic nocturnal enuresis in older children with motivated families. (SOR **A**)
- Desmopressin is most effective in children with monosymptomatic enuresis with nocturnal polyuria and normal bladder capacity, or when enuresis alarm is impractical or ineffective. (SOR **A**)

I. **Definition. Enuresis** (primary nocturnal urinary incontinence) is repeated spontaneous voiding of urine into the bed or clothes at least twice a week for at least three consecutive months in a child who is at least 5 years of age.
  A. **Primary monosymptomatic enuresis** is bed-wetting without a history of nocturnal continence and unassociated with other symptoms.
  B. **Secondary monosymptomatic enuresis** is recurrence of bed-wetting after at least 6 months of nocturnal continence.
  C. **Non-monosymptomatic enuresis** is bed-wetting associated with urinary urgency, frequency, straining, dribbling, pain, chronic constipation, or encopresis.
  D. Children 5 years or older with involuntary or intentional urination into clothing while awake or asleep are said to have daytime incontinence and enuresis. The term diurnal enuresis is considered obsolete.
II. **Common Diagnoses.** An estimated five to seven million children in the United States have primary enuresis; 80% are monosymptomatic and about 5% have an organic cause.
  A. Risk factors for **primary monosymptomatic enuresis** include the following:
    1. **Family history.** Five to seven times risk if one parent is affected; more than 11 times risk if both parents are affected.
    2. **Preterm birth, low birth weight, and maturational delay.** Enuresis affects 6.7% of children with this history who are between the ages of 4 and 6 years, decreasing to 2.8% by 11 to 12 years of age (15% spontaneous resolution every year). These children can manifest delay in central nervous system maturation and delay in development of language and motor skills.
    3. **Male gender.** Seen three times more often in boys.
    4. **Deep sleep.** Abnormally deep sleep patterns in children with enuresis (increased arousal threshold).
    5. **Bladder function—detrusor overactivity.** Smaller functional bladder capacity and nocturnal polyuria, with inability to hold urine.
    6. **Lower nocturnal levels of antidiuretic hormone (ADH).**
  B. Twenty percent of enuretic children experience some daytime wetting. Risk factors include constipation, urinary tract infection, psychologic stress (e.g., dysfunctional home, abuse), sickle-cell disease, obstructive sleep apnea (OSA), chronic renal failure, attention deficit hyperactivity disorder, and diabetes mellitus.
III. **Symptoms.** When evaluating a child with enuresis, responses to several key questions will assist in assessing causes and management for the problem (see Table 23–1).
IV. **Signs.** Most children presenting with enuresis in primary care settings will have a normal physical examination. A focused evaluation is important for detecting underlying or contributing causes.

TABLE 23–1. IMPORTANT HISTORY IN CHILDREN WITH ENURESIS

Question	Significance/Suggestions
Distinguishing primary from secondary enuresis:	
Has your child ever been consistently dry at night?	"Never dry" suggests primary enuresis
Distinguishing uncomplicated from complicated enuresis:	
Does your child wet his or her pants during the day?	Yes, see daytime incontinence and enuresis
Does your child appear to have pain with urination?	Urinary tract infection
How often does your child have bowel movements?	Infrequent stools: constipation
Are bowel movements ever hard to pass?	Constipation
Does your child ever soil his or her pants?	Encopresis
Distinguishing possible functional bladder disorder from nocturnal polyuria:	
How many times a day does your child void? (frequency)	More than seven times a day: functional bladder disorder
Does your child have to run to the bathroom? (urgency)	Positive response: functional bladder disorder
Does your child hold urine until the last minute?	Positive response: functional bladder disorder
How many nights a week does your child wet the bed?	Most nights: functional bladder disorder; one or two nights: nocturnal polyuria
Does your child wet more than once every night?	Positive response: functional bladder disorder
Does your child seem to wet large or small volumes?	Large volumes: nocturnal polyuria
	Small volumes: functional bladder disorder
To determine how parents have handled bed-wetting:	
How have you handled the nighttime accident?	Elicits information on interventions that have already been tried; be alert for responses suggesting that the child has been punished or shamed

Source: Adapted with permission from Thiedke CC. Nocturnal enuresis. *Am Fam Physician.* 2003;67(7): 1499–1506, 1509–1510. Copyright © 2003 American Academy of Family Physicians. All Rights Reserved.

   - A. **Blood pressure.** Elevated blood pressure suggests renal disease.
   - B. **Growth chart.** Poor growth suggests renal disease, especially with hypertension.
   - C. Abdomen/**genital examination** to detect renal and bladder enlargement, fecal masses indicating encopresis, and genital anomalies (e.g., hypospadias, meatal stenosis).
   - D. **Neurologic examination,** including gait, power, muscle tone, sensation, reflexes, and rectal tone (for underlying neurologic disease).
   - E. **Observed voiding** for stream/ability to initiate and interrupt in midstream (for neurologic disease or urethral stricture).
   - V. **Laboratory Tests.** Most children presenting in ambulatory primary care settings will have a **normal physical examination;** in these patients, the only testing indicated is **urinalysis (UA)** and **estimation of bladder capacity by ultrasound (US)**. Bladder capacity is estimated by measuring the postvoid residual (PVR). The normal bladder capacity in ounces is age plus 2; the normal PVR in children should be less than 10% of maximal bladder capacity.
      - A. **Children with normal physical examination, UA,** and a normal PVR on US require no further evaluation.
      - B. **Children with abnormal examination, UA, or both** require further evaluation.
         - 1. **Urinalysis. Specific gravity** (SG) ≤ 1.005 is seen in diabetes insipidus, acute tubular necrosis, and pyelonephritis; SG of 1.010 that remains unchanged despite fluid intake is seen in chronic renal disease; SG ≥ 1.035 is seen in dehydration, congestive heart failure, liver failure, and shock. **Glycosuria** can indicate diabetes mellitus or low renal glycemic threshold (e.g., pregnancy). **Proteinuria** can be benign or indicate underlying disease (see Chapter 52). **Hematuria** can indicate cystitis or urinary calculi and warrants further evaluation (see Chapter 35). **White blood cells** with significant pyuria on a clean-catch specimen suggest urinary tract infection, a cause of polysymptomatic enuresis (see Chapter 21); antibiotic treatment should be instituted.
         - 2. **Blood count, serum chemistry.** Useful in diagnosing chronic renal insufficiency or sickle-cell disease.

3. **Imaging studies. Renal and bladder US, voiding cystourethrogram.** Useful in evaluating renal and bladder abnormalities, PVR, and vesicoureteral reflux in children with urinary tract infection. Magnetic resonance imaging of the lumbosacral spine is considered if there is an abnormal neurologic examination (detects spinal dysraphism).
4. **Urodynamic studies.** Measurement of residual urine and cystometry. Useful in evaluating voiding dysfunction.

VI. **Treatment** should not commence until the child is approximately 7 years old, unless enuresis causes severe emotional distress. The child must comprehend and perceive the condition as a problem and be a willing participant in therapy. Parental involvement is essential to treatment success. It is important to educate or reassure parents about rates of spontaneous resolution of enuresis (see Section II.A). Secondary causes identified should be treated. (SOR Ⓒ) Encopresis-associated enuresis responds to fecal disimpaction and bowel retraining, with nearly two-thirds responding to successful treatment of constipation in one study. (SOR Ⓑ) A stool softener such as polyethylene glycol (MiraLax) facilitates bowel movements. (SOR Ⓐ)

Children with OSA respond to surgical correction of the upper airway. Psychotherapy or family therapy is indicated in psychogenic enuresis. Biofeedback is an option for motivated children with dysfunctional voiding. Enuresis associated with infection responds to antibiotics.

A. **Nonpharmacologic measures.** Tried for 3 to 6 months.
   1. **Lifestyle modifications,** effective in monosymptomatic enuresis, include the following:
      a. Goal-setting for **the child to get up at night and use the toilet**. Alarm or parent-awakening approaches can be used.
      b. Improve **access to the toilet**—provide a bedside potty.
      c. Limiting fluids before bedtime is advocated but is not effective. It is, however, reasonable to **avoid giving excessive fluids and caffeine-containing products before bedtime**.
      d. **Encourage the child to empty the bladder** at bedtime.
      e. **Discontinue diapers** or pull-ups so that the sensation of wetness is recognized.
      f. **Include the child in morning cleanup** in a nonpunitive manner; criticism and punishment can cause secondary psychologic problems.
      g. Provide a **diary or chart** with a tally of wet and dry nights to monitor progress. This helps evaluate the efficacy of other therapeutic interventions and has an independent beneficial effect. (SOR Ⓑ)
      h. Use **positive reinforcement** (have the child place a favorite sticker on the calendar for dry days).
   2. **Behavioral conditioning** can be effective in children with frequent daytime voiding, few or no dry nights, or ≥1 enuretic episode per night; these children sometimes have low functional bladder capacity and benefit from an alarm.
      a. **Enuresis alarm** (Table 23–2). Nonpharmacological treatment of choice for enuresis. Small transistorized mini-alarms are attached to the patient's bed or underwear and are activated (via sound, vibration, or both) with the release of first few drops of urine. Eventually, a conditioned response occurs. Treatment is continued until 14 or more consecutive dry nights. An alarm requires a minimum of 2–3 months trial period. It is discontinued if no response is observed after this time period. Useful in older children with motivated families. (SOR Ⓐ) Cures occur in approximately 50% of children.
      b. **Nighttime alarm** (Table 23–2). An alarm clock is set for 3 hours after going to sleep to awaken the child to get up and void.
   3. **Self-hypnosis** with posthypnotic suggestion that the child will wake up and use the bathroom. The cure rate is reported at 77% for children 5 years and older.

B. **Pharmacologic therapy** (Table 23–2).
   1. **Desmopressin (1-desamino-8-D-arginine vasopressin; DDAVP)** reduces urine volume by reabsorbing water from the distal convoluted and collecting tubules. Medication of choice for enuresis in the oral form.
      a. Sixty to seventy percent of children respond during treatment; most (80%) relapse following treatment cessation. It is available in nasal spray and tablet. It is most effective in children with monosymptomatic enuresis, nocturnal polyuria, normal bladder capacity, less-frequent bed-wetting, positive family history, and family unwilling or unable to cooperate with nonpharmacologic measures. (SOR Ⓐ)
      b. Few side effects with prolonged use. Rarely causes water intoxication, hyponatremia, or convulsions, seen more often with the nasal spray. Desmopressin Nasal

TABLE 23–2. INTERVENTIONS FOR ENURESIS

Intervention	Mechanism	Dosage/Instructions	Side Effects/Comments	Efficacy
Dry bed training program	Timed voiding to empty bladder	Parent awakens child 3 hours after bedtime	Side effects: None Safe. Does not require bedwetting to initiate alarm	Insufficient evidence if used alone; 75% efficacy when combined with alarm Relapse rate: 38%
Enuresis alarm[a]	Alarm system activated by wetness that awakens child so child can get up to void	Worn nightly for 2–3 mo	Side effects: Sleep disruption to child and family members	Most effective intervention. Initial cure rate: 66% (50% dry on continued treatment) Relapse rate: up to 50% with discontinuance
Desmopressin[a]	Synthetic analog of vasopressin; reduces urine production by increasing water retention and urine concentration in the distal tubules	One spray into each nostril of 10 µg (20 µg total) nightly Oral: 0.2–0.6 mg nightly	Common side effects: Headache, abdominal discomfort, nausea, nasal congestion, epistaxis, visual disturbances, bad taste Comments: Contraindicated in patients who have habit polydipsia, hypertension, or heart disease; caution in cystic fibrosis	Initial cure rates: 30% full response, 40% partial response Relapse rate with discontinuation: 80%. With propiverine, administered over 3 mo: 97% efficacy; desmopressin plus anticholinergic may be appropriate for children with bladder instability
Imipramine	Increases bladder capacity and tightens bladder neck sphincter	Initially 25 mg at night 7–12 years: increase to 50 mg if no response at 25 mg ≥12 years: increase to 75 mg	Common side effects: Drowsiness, lethargy, agitation, depression, sleep disturbance, gastrointestinal upsets Rare adverse effects: Seizures, cardiac arrhythmias, accidental overdose Caution in individuals with epilepsy	Efficacy 40%–60% if used for more than 4–6 months Relapse rate with discontinuation: 50% Used until child has achieved (at minimum) 14–28 consecutive dry nights then gradually tapered
Oxybutynin Oxybutynin transdermal patch[a] Tolterodine Propiverine	Anticholinergic, antispasmodic effects reduce uninhibited detrusor contractions	2.5–5 mg—two to three times daily One patch twice weekly 1–2 mg twice daily 15–20 mg daily; children: 0.2–0.4 mg/kg/d	Common side effects: Dry mouth, blurred vision, headache, nausea, dizziness, gastrointestinal upset, and tachycardia Comments: Drug of choice for polysymptomatic enuresis	Nearly half of children respond; over 80% response if combined with desmopressin Efficacy of tolterodine not established in children; see data regarding propiverine above
Indomethacin (not FDA approved for this indication)	Inhibits nitric oxide and prostaglandin synthesis, decreases urine volume, and bladder and urethral contractions	50 mg rectally every night for 2–3 wk	Nausea, vomiting, diarrhea, gastric discomfort, renal dysfunction; risk of side effects low with short courses	More effective than placebo; duration of response still under investigation

[a]Associated with greatest efficacy and likely fewer adverse drug reactions.

Spray solution should, therefore, only be used in patients when orally administered formulations are not feasible or available, and if so, should only be administered under careful medical supervision, and fluid restriction should be discussed with the patient and the caregiver.

   c. Oral desmopressin **should be held during acute illnesses** such as fever, recurrent vomiting, or diarrhea that may lead to fluid and/or electrolyte imbalances, or under conditions of extremely hot weather, vigorous exercise, or other conditions associated with increased water intake.

2. **Anticholinergics** such as the tricyclic antidepressant imipramine (Tofranil), oxybutynin (Ditropan), and tolterodine (Detrol) decrease detrusor tone, improve bladder capacity, and decrease frequency and urgency; second-line therapy for enuresis. These drugs are useful in children with urgency, restricted bladder capacity as a result of detrusor hyperactivity, day-time incontinence and enuresis, and unresponsiveness to desmopressin. (SOR ❸) Side effects include dry mouth, blurred vision, headache, nausea, dizziness, gastrointestinal disturbance (e.g., constipation), and tachycardia. Imipramine is potentially cardiotoxic and its use mandates prior exclusion of long QT syndrome by electrocardiogram, especially in a child with palpitations or syncope or a family history of sudden cardiac death.

3. **Combination therapy** with enuresis alarm and desmopressin is useful in children with both excessive urine output and reduced bladder capacity, with over 75% becoming dry.

C. **Follow-up.** Regular follow-up visits are important to address issues or concerns, answer questions, and encourage the child and parents. In children receiving medications for enuresis, follow-up is recommended 2 weeks after initiation of therapy, then monthly for 3 months.

SELECTED REFERENCES

Neveus T. Diagnosis and management of nocturnal enuresis. *Curr Opin Pediatr.* 2009;21:199–202.
Neveus T, Eggert P, Evans J, et al. Evaluation of and treatment for monosymptomatic enuresis: a standardization document from the international children's continence society. *J Urol.* 2010;183:441–447.
Robson WLM. Evaluation and management of enuresis. *N Engl J Med.* 2009;360:1429–1436.
Sureshkumar P, Jones M, Caldwell HY, Craig JC. Risk factors for nocturnal enuresis in school-age children. *J Urol.* 2009;182:2893–2899.
Vande Walle J, Rittig S, Bauer S, et al.; American Academy of Pediatrics; European Society for Paediatric Urology; European Society for Paediatric Nephrology; International Children's Continence Society. Practical consensus guidelines for the management of enuresis. *Eur J Pediatr.* 2012;171:971–983.

Additional references are available online at http://langetextbooks.com/fm6e

---

24   Failure to Thrive

Jacqueline L. Gerhart, MD, & Cathy Kamens, MD

KEY POINTS

- Growth of children should be measured over time and plotted on a standardized growth chart at every visit. (SOR ❸)
- A thorough history and physical examination and selective laboratory tests are the foundation for accurate diagnosis and management in failure to thrive (FTT). (SOR ❸)
- Provision of calories and a multidisciplinary approach are keys to treating children with FTT. (SOR ❸)

I. **Definition. Failure to thrive (FTT)** is a condition seen in infants and children who lose weight or fail to gain weight in accordance with standardized growth charts. It is a sign that a child is receiving inadequate nutrition for optimal growth and development. The cause of FTT is often multifactorial.

   A. At each office visit, all infants and children should be accurately measured for weight, length (recumbent, younger than 2 years), or height (standing, 2 years and older), and head circumference. These measurements should be plotted on standardized growth curves (http://www.cdc.gov/growthcharts/). Growth should be evaluated over time with attention to growth velocity and any change in growth percentiles. Weight should be compared to length (or height), as well as head circumference, to identify children with disproportionate growth.

   B. There is no consensus on criteria for FTT, but investigation is appropriate in any child whose:

      1. Weight, height, or body mass index (BMI) for age is below the fifth percentile.

      2. Weight deceleration crossing two major percentile lines.

      3. Weight is less than 75% of median weight for age or median weight for length.

II. Epidemiology. FTT occurs in 5% to 10% of children in primary care settings and 3% to 5% of children in hospital settings. Approximately 80% of children with FTT present prior to 18 months of age. Although the list of underlying diagnosis that lead to FTT is long (Table 24–1), the etiology of FTT can be classified into four categories:

   A. Inadequate caloric intake, as in feeding errors or mechanical feeding difficulties.

   B. Inadequate absorption, due to gastrointestinal disease.

   C. Defective utilization, as in metabolic or congenital disorders.

   D. Excess metabolic demand, as seen in metabolic, cardiopulmonary, or renal disease.

III. Differential Diagnosis. FTT must be distinguished from the following normal variants, in which growth failure is usually symmetric:

   A. Familial short stature. Genetically, the child is predisposed to a low percentile weight and height. Calculation of midparental height can be helpful in establishing a child's growth potential.

MIDPARENTAL HEIGHT

Girls:

$$\frac{\text{Father's height} + \text{Mother's height} - 13 \text{ cm [5 in]}}{2}$$

Boys:

$$\frac{\text{Father's height} + \text{Mother's height} + 13 \text{ cm [5 in]}}{2}$$

Characteristics of familial short stature include:

      1. A proportional decrease in weight and length.

      2. Bone age consistent with chronological age.

      3. A family history of short stature.

      4. A normal annual growth rate without further deceleration.

   B. Constitutional growth delay. Growth decelerates in the first 3 years of life, followed by stabilization on a new growth curve until adolescence, when a growth spurt occurs. Characteristics of constitutional growth delay include:

      1. A proportional decrease in weight and length.

      2. Bone age less than chronological age, with a 2- to 3-year delay in skeletal maturation.

      3. A family history of a parent or sibling with constitutional growth delay.

      4. An evaluation does not reveal inadequate nutrition or other cause for growth delay.

   C. Intrauterine growth restriction is failure of intrauterine growth because of prenatal factors and not genetic predisposition. Characteristics include:

      1. Birth weight below the fifth percentile, or less than 2500 g.

      2. Growth rate may be slower than the normal growth curve.

         a. Low-birth-weight infants should double their birth weight by age 4 months and triple it by 1 year.

         b. Premature infants or those weighing less than 1500 g should be followed on growth charts that are adjusted for gestational age.

TABLE 24–1. DIFFERENTIAL DIAGNOSIS, PRESENTATION, AND LABORATORY EVALUATION OF FAILURE TO THRIVE (FTT)

Cause	History	Signs	Tests
Psychosocial			
Breast-feeding problems	Sore nipples, lack of supply	Asymmetric FTT (see Chapter 100)	None
Feeding errors	Insufficient quantity offered, formula preparation error, excessive juice intake	Asymmetric FTT	None
Infant behavior/bonding	Refusal of bottle, irritability, poor understanding or response to infant cues	Apathetic, minimal smiling, decreased vocalizations	None
Abuse or neglect	Maternal depression or mental illness, parental drug use, abuse or neglect	Poor hygiene, bruises in different stages of healing, characteristic patterns of injury	None
Economic deprivation	Homelessness, public assistance, "rationing" food supplies, low-cost or low-quality foods	Asymmetric FTT, poor hygiene	None
Gastrointestinal			
Gastroesophageal reflux	Very frequent "wet burps"	Emesis, cough, wheezing	Esophageal pH probe
Craniofacial abnormalities	Nasal regurgitation, choking, unilateral rhinorrhea	Cleft or small jaw, unable to pass catheter through nose	None
Cleft lip/palate			
Choanal atresia			
Micrognathia			
Malabsorption	Diarrhea, abdominal pain, foul-smelling stools	Abdominal distention, dehydration, fatty stools	Lactose tolerance test, stool pH, electrolytes, sweat test, fecal fat, jejunal biopsy, antiendomysial antibodies
Celiac disease			
Lactose intolerance			
Milk protein intolerance			
Pancreatic Insufficiency			
Inflammatory bowel disease	Abdominal pain, diarrhea, melena	Heme-positive stool, fever Jaundice, hepatomegaly	Stool Hematest, ESR, barium enema
Biliary disease	Pale stools		LFTs, abdominal US, liver biopsy
Atresia			
Cirrhosis			
Obstruction	Vomiting, may be projectile vomiting after meals	Abdominal distension, palpable mass (olive), dehydration	Electrolytes, KUB, abdominal US
Pyloric stenosis			
Malrotation			
Hirschsprung disease			
Renal			
Renal tubular acidosis	Polyuria, vomiting	Tachypnea, muscular weakness	Renal US, electrolytes, blood gas
Chronic renal failure	Listlessness, pruritus	Pallor, edema	BUN, creatinine, US, UA, electrolytes
Diabetes insipidus	Polyuria, thirst	Dehydration, irritability	
Cardiopulmonary			
Congenital heart disease	Shortness of breath, swelling, blue lips	Cyanosis, rales, edema	CXR, echocardiogram
Asthma	Cough, shortness of breath	Tachypnea, wheezing	Pulmonary function tests
Bronchopulmonary dysplasia	History of prematurity or respiratory disease	Tachypnea, retractions	Pulse oximetry, pulmonary function tests
Cystic fibrosis	Frequent respiratory infections	Tachypnea, wheezing	Sweat test

(continued)

TABLE 24–1. DIFFERENTIAL DIAGNOSIS, PRESENTATION, AND LABORATORY EVALUATION OF
       FAILURE TO THRIVE (FTT) (*Continued*)

Cause	History	Signs	Tests
Anatomic upper airway abnormalities	Slow feeding, coughing and choking, history of pneumonia	Stridor, inability to pass a catheter into the stomach	CXR, barium esophagogram
Tracheoesophageal fistula			
Vascular slings			
Obstructive sleep apnea	Snoring, mouth breathing	Adenotonsillar hypertrophy	Sleep study
Endocrine			
Thyroid disease	Dry or moist skin, cold or heat intolerance	Irritability or slow movements, warm or cold skin	TSH, T4
Diabetes mellitus	Polydipsia, polyphagia, polyuria	Lethargy, Kussmaul respirations	Serum glucose
Adrenal disorder	Obesity, poor sleeping	Hypertension or hypotension, diabetes mellitus	Urine-free cortisol, plasma ACTH
Parathyroid disorders	Muscle pain and cramps, abdominal pain	Tetany, cataracts	Calcium, PTH
Pituitary disorders	May have none	Prominent forehead, large abdomen	Growth hormone level
Growth hormone deficiency			
Neurologic			
Developmental disorder	History of developmental delay	May be normal or with dysmorphic features	None
Hydrocephalus	Irritability, lethargy, vomiting	Increased head circumference, wide bulging fontanelle, dilated scalp veins	Head CT or MRI
Neuromuscular disorder	History of developmental motor delay	Spasticity or hypotonia, microcephaly	Head CT or MRI
Cerebral palsy			
Hypotonia			
Myopathy			
Cerebral hemorrhages	Headache, vomiting, history of trauma	Nuchal rigidity, hemiparesis	Head CT or MRI
Infectious			
UTI	Fever, irritability	Fever, suprapubic tenderness	UA and culture
Infectious diarrhea	Diarrhea, melena	Abdominal distention, pain, fever	Stool culture, ova, parasites
Thrush	Refuses bottle	White plaque on oral mucosa	None
Recurrent tonsillitis	Sore throat, bad breath, mouth breathing	Tonsillar hypertrophy, cervical lymphadenopathy	Throat culture
Tuberculosis	Travel in high-risk area or exposure to high-risk persons	Lymphadenopathy	PPD, CXR
Human immunodeficiency virus	Maternal history of high-risk behaviors	Fever, lymphadenopathy	HIV antibody test
Hepatitis	Maternal history or risk factors for hepatitis	Jaundice, hepatomegaly	LFTs, hepatitis serology
Immunologic deficiency	Frequent infections	Lymphadenopathy	CBC, quantitative serum IgG, IgM, IgA
Metabolic			
Inborn errors of metabolism	Lethargy	May be normal	Newborn screen
Congenital			
Chromosomal abnormalities	Advanced maternal age, loose neck skin, and hand puffiness	Dysmorphic features such as short/webbed neck, epicanthal folds, simian crease	Karyotyping
Turner syndrome			
Down syndrome			

TABLE 24–1. DIFFERENTIAL DIAGNOSIS, PRESENTATION, AND LABORATORY EVALUATION OF
FAILURE TO THRIVE (FTT) (*Continued*)

Cause	History	Signs	Tests
Skeletal dysplasias	Positive family history	Short extremities, trident hands	Pelvic, lumbar, extremity x-rays
Congenital syndromes Fetal alcohol syndrome	Maternal history of alcohol or drug use, delayed development	Symmetric FTT, short palpebral fissures, epicanthal folds, maxillary hypoplasia, micrognathia	None
Miscellaneous			
Malignancy	Fever, fatigue	Lymphadenopathy, tumors	CBC, ESR
Drugs or toxins Lead poisoning Accidental intake	Exposure to lead paint, medication errors	May be normal	Lead levels, toxicology screen
Nutritional deficiencies Iron deficiency Zinc deficiency	Exclusive breast-feeding, unsupplemented formula	Pallor, dermatitis	CBC
Vitamin D deficiency (rickets)	Exclusive breast-feeding, no exposure to sunlight	Large fontanelle, bony deformities	X-rays, calcium, alkaline phosphatase
Connective tissue disease	Fever, arthralgia, myalgia	Arthritis, rash, myositis	ESR, CBC, ANA
Normal Variants			
Familial short stature	Short members of family	Symmetric FTT, normal examination	Bone age x-rays
Constitutional delay of growth	Family history of late puberty	Symmetric FTT, normal examination, delayed puberty	Bone age x-rays
Intrauterine growth retardation	Small for gestational age at birth or prematurity	Hepatosplenomegaly, chorioretinitis	Viral antibody titers, urine for CMV

ACTH, adrenocorticotropic hormone; ANA, antinuclear antibody; BUN, blood urea nitrogen; CBC, complete blood count; CMV, cytomegalovirus; CT, computerized tomography; CXR, chest radiograph; ECG, electrocardiogram; ESR, erythrocyte sedimentation rate; FTT, failure to thrive; HIV, human immunodeficiency virus; KUB, kidney/ureter/bladder (abdominal plain radiograph); LFTs, liver function tests; MRI, magnetic resonance imaging; PTH, parathyroid hormone; PPD, purified protein derivative (TB test); TSH, thyroid-stimulating hormone; UA, urinalysis; US, ultrasound; UTI, urinary tract infection.

IV. Symptoms. A thorough history should be elicited in poorly growing children, including the following specific areas (Table 24–1):

A. Feeding history. Discuss breastfeeding patterns, engorgement and letdown, frequency, quantity, formula preparation, length and quality of feeding time, feeding techniques, and personal and cultural beliefs about food and feeding.

B. Dietary history. Ask the family to record all feedings and voiding/elimination for the last 72 hours. Review any food intolerances, aversions, or allergies.

C. Past medical history. Record birth weight, prenatal and birth history, illnesses, and hospitalizations.

D. Developmental history. Assess gross and fine motor milestones, language milestones, behavior, and temperament.

E. Social history. Query living situation, financial constraints, family stressors, parental employment, parental substance abuse, and domestic violence or abuse.

F. Family history. Query mental illness in the family (especially maternal depression), childhood illnesses, mental retardation, genetic abnormalities, growth delays in parents or siblings, and midparental height.

G. Review of systems. Ask about vomiting, spitting up, choking, diarrhea, dyspnea, and tachypnea.

V. Signs (Table 24–1)

A. The FTT physical examination should include:

1. Accurate measurements and plotting of weight, height, and head circumference. Measurement or plotting errors can give the appearance of FTT, or delay the diagnosis.

Therefore, the first step in the diagnosis should be to recheck the child's measurements and re-plot them on the growth curve.

2. General appearance and vital signs.
3. Dysmorphic features or structural anomalies.
4. Signs of abuse or neglect.
5. Cardiac, respiratory, and gastrointestinal findings and checking of the oropharynx and lymph nodes.
6. Neurologic examination.

B. Patterns of growth can provide helpful clues to diagnosis.

1. **Asymmetric FTT,** in which the weight falls first and the head circumference is preserved, is generally due to poor intake, psychosocial factors, or a systemic illness.
2. **Symmetric FTT,** in which weight, height, and head circumference are proportional, may represent a normal variant or a primary central nervous system disorder.
3. **Isolated short stature,** where the weight is preserved, is likely to represent an endocrine or genetic disorder.
4. **Isolated low head circumference** suggests a lack of brain growth.

VI. **Laboratory Tests** (Table 24–1). No routine laboratory tests are indicated in the child with FTT, as only approximately 1% of all laboratory tests ordered in a typical FTT workup provide useful information. (SOR ⦿) Investigations should be guided by the history and physical examination, as well as response to nutrition intervention.

VII. **Treatment.** A multidisciplinary approach (e.g., primary care provider, nurse, social worker, nutritionist, pediatric specialist) is ideal.

A. Identify and treat any underlying disorder.
B. Provide nutrition counseling:

1. High-calorie concentrated formula, or addition of rice cereal or supplements to usual diet, to provide 150% of the recommended daily calories. Calorie requirements for catch-up growth can be estimated from the following formula:

CALORIE REQUIREMENTS FOR CATCH-UP GROWTH IN kcal/kg

$$\text{RDA kcal/kg weight} = \frac{\text{Age} \times \text{Ideal (median) weight for age in kg}}{\text{Actual weight}}$$

2. Consider adding a multivitamin containing vitamin D, iron, and zinc.
3. Consider consultation with a nutritionist or dietician.

C. Institute a multidisciplinary support team to support and educate the family. A growth plan should be made. The treatment plan should be realistic and sensitive to ethnic and cultural differences and the values of the family.
D. Close follow-up either by a home health nurse or in the primary care provider's office for weight, height, and head circumference measurements.
E. Routine preventive health visits to assess developmental milestones.

VIII. **Hospitalization.** This is rarely indicated, but may be necessary if:

A. There is an evidence of, or a high risk for, physical abuse or severe neglect.
B. The child is severely malnourished or medically unstable.
C. Outpatient management has failed to demonstrate any appreciable improvement.

IX. **Prognosis.** Severe, prolonged malnutrition can negatively affect a child's future growth and cognitive development. Low-birth-weight preterm infants with FTT have shown developmental delay, lower cognitive scores, and poorer overall academic performance than those without FTT. However, with early multidisciplinary, home-based interventions, much of this discrepancy can be eliminated.

SELECTED REFERENCES

Cole SZ, Lanham JS. Failure to thrive: an update. *Am Fam Physician.* 2011;83(7):829–834.
Corbett SS, Drewett RF. To what extent is failure to thrive in infancy associated with poorer cognitive development? A review and meta-analysis. *J Child Psychol Psychiatry.* 2004;45(3):641–654.
Jaffe AC. Failure to thrive: current clinical concepts. *Pediatr Rev.* 2011;32(3);100–107.
Jolley CD. Failure to thrive. *Curr Probl Pediatr Adolesc Health Care.* 2003;33:183–206.
Rudolph CD. Gastroenterology and nutrition. In: Rudolph CD, Rudolph AM, Hostetter MK, Lister G, Siegel NJ, eds. *Rudolph's pediatrics,* 21st ed. New York: McGraw-Hill, 2003:1336–1337.

Samuels RC, Cohen LE. Understanding growth patterns in short stature. *Contemp Pediatr.* 2001;18(6): 94–112.
Shields B, Wacogne I, Wright CM. Weight faltering and failure to thrive in infancy and early childhood. *BMJ.* 2012;345:e5931.
Sullivan PB. Commentary: the epidemiology of failure-to-thrive in infants. *Int J Epidemiol.* 2004;33(4): 847–848.
Stephens MB, Gentry BC, Michener MD, et al. *J Fam Pract.* 2008;57(4):264–266.

25   Fatigue

Anthony F. Valdini, MD, MS

KEY POINTS

- The longer a person is fatigued, the more likely it is that a psychological problem is present. (SOR ❻)
- History and physical examination are more likely to reveal the cause of fatigue than blind laboratory testing. (SOR ❻)
- Fatigue can be caused by physical, psychological, physiologic (appropriate, as in lack of sleep), or mixed etiologies. The mixed category is more common than once thought and may explain the difficulty in resolving the symptom. (SOR ❻)
- Even if an abnormality is discovered, it does not mean that the problem of fatigue is "solved." There is often more than one etiology, and the abnormality discovered may be treated and resolved without changing the patient's complaint of fatigue. (SOR ❻)
- The majority of patients complaining of chronic fatigue are depressed. (SOR ❻)

 I. **Definition.** Fatigue is a subjective complaint of tiredness, weariness, or lack of energy.
II. **Common Diagnoses.** Fatigue is the seventh most common symptom in primary care and accounts for more than 10 million office visits every year. Various studies have found the prevalence of fatigue in primary care to be between 10% and 20%. One group of investigators found that 6.7% of patients presenting to a family medicine clinic had a primary complaint of fatigue. Patients identified as fatigued visit the physician and are admitted to the hospital more often, incur greater charges for prescription medications, develop more new diagnoses, and have a greater proportion of their diagnoses containing a psychological component than do their nonfatigued counterparts. Fatigue may result from virtually every physical and psychological illness. Four major classes of fatigue useful in evaluating the tired patient are listed below.

 A. **Physiologic fatigue** is due to of overwork, lack of sleep, or a defined physical stress, such as pregnancy. It can normally be expected in a mentally and physically healthy individual experiencing such stress. Females, as a group, work more hours in a day and more years in their lives than males and this may partially account for women visiting physicians more often for fatigue than men. Individuals with irregular or inadequate sleep patterns (including parents of young children), reducing diets, excessive or minimal exercise, or long hours spent commuting and working are at an increased risk for physiologic fatigue.

 B. **Physical fatigue** is caused by infections, endocrine imbalances, cardiovascular disease, anemia, and medications (prescription, nonprescription, alcohol, or other drugs of abuse); less commonly, cancer, connective tissue diseases, and other ailments cause physical fatigue.

 C. **Psychological illness,** including depression, anxiety, stress, and adjustment reaction, can cause fatigue. Children of alcoholics have an increased incidence of fatigue and depression.

 D. **"Mixed" fatigue,** which is often overlooked, involves any of the above categories occurring in combination. In persons who are fatigued for more than 6 months, classification branches.

TABLE 25–1. DIAGNOSTIC CRITERIA FOR CHRONIC FATIGUE SYNDROME (CDC)

1. The individual has had severe chronic fatigue for six or more consecutive months that is not due to ongoing exertion or other medical conditions associated with fatigue (these other conditions need to be ruled out by a doctor after diagnostic tests have been conducted)
2. The fatigue significantly interferes with daily activities and work
3. The individual concurrently has four or more of the following eight symptoms:
   - Postexertion malaise lasting more than 24 hours
   - Unrefreshing sleep
   - Significant impairment of short-term memory or concentration
   - Muscle pain
   - Pain in the joints without swelling or redness
   - Headaches of a new type, pattern, or severity
   - Tender lymph nodes in the neck or armpit
   - A sore throat that is frequent or recurring

These symptoms should have persisted or recurred during six or more consecutive months of illness and they cannot have first appeared before the fatigue.

Source: Available at http://www.cdc.gov/cfs/case-definition/index.html. Accessed April 2013.

    E. Chronic fatigue syndrome (CFS) is a distinct and infrequently occurring (0.3% prevalence) diagnostic category. The International Chronic Fatigue Syndrome Study Group revised the 1988 case definition in 1994. The new definition includes a duration of 6 months or longer, absence of an identified cause, and the presence of at least four specific symptoms (see Table 25–1). Despite the findings of "subtle and diffuse" immunologic abnormalities and possibly associated viruses—Epstein–Barr virus, enterovirus, herpes virus type 6, retrovirus, and others—the syndrome remains enigmatic. Ambiguities in the 1994 case definition were addressed in the 2003 publication wherein the study group recommended use of several standardized instruments to quantify key symptom domains and disability.

        1. Chronic idiopathic fatigue. Not all patients with chronic fatigue symptoms meet the criteria for CFS. Persons tired for 6 months or longer, with no apparent cause, who do not meet CFS criteria for severity or specific symptoms after clinical evaluation are classified as having "chronic idiopathic fatigue." Chronic idiopathic fatigue is 10 times more common than CFS.

        2. Most patients who are tired for more than 1 year have significant psychological problems.

            Because depression is the most common psychological cause of fatigue, and not all providers feel comfortable making the diagnosis, an instrument to measure depression (such as Beck's) may be useful (see Chapter 94).

III. Symptoms and Signs (Table 25–2)

    A. Fatigue lasting 1 month or less is commonly a result of physical causes; fatigue lasting 3 months or more is likely to be caused by psychological factors.

    B. Fever, chills, sweats, and **significant weight loss** are associated with infection and carcinoma.

    C. Specific historical features including endocrine and cardiovascular review of systems may indicate psychological, physical, or mixed origins of fatigue. Review of sleep, work, and travel history, in addition to physical functional capacity can help elucidate the cause of fatigue. Fatigue should be distinguished from weakness and hypersomnolence, which indicate a different origin, such as neuromuscular (e.g., myasthenia) or sleep disorder (obstructive sleep apnea, narcolepsy). The feature most solidly linked with physical versus psychological causes is the chronicity of fatigue; that is, **acute fatigue is likely to be caused by physical or physiologic events, while chronic fatigue is associated with psychological and mixed causes.** It has been reported that 69% to 80% of primary care patients with depression present with exclusive complaints related to a physical symptom, and that having five or more physical symptoms is an independent predictor of major depression.

    D. The **physical causes** of acute fatigue (e.g., rales, edema, and gallops of congestive heart failure) may be obvious.

    E. Subtle signs of infections (e.g., lymphadenopathy or temperature elevation), connective tissue disease (e.g., extra-articular manifestations), and cancer should not be overlooked.

TABLE 25–2. CHARACTERISTICS PROPOSED TO DISTINGUISH PSYCHOLOGICAL FATIGUE FROM PHYSICAL FATIGUE

Characteristic	Psychological	Physical
Duration	Chronic	Acute
Primary deficit	Desire	Ability
Onset	Stress related	Unrelated to stress
Diurnal pattern	Worse in morning	Worse in evening
Course	Fluctuates	Progressive
Effect of activity	Relieves	Worsens
Associated symptoms	Multiple and nonspecific	Few and specific
Previous problems	Functional	Organic
Family	Stressful	Supportive
Appearance	Anxious/depressed	Ill
Family history	Psychological/alcoholism	None
Placebo effect	Present	Absent
Effect of sleep	Unaffected/worsened	Relieved
Decreased ability to cope	No	Yes

Source: Adapted with permission from Katerndahl DA. Differentiation of physical and psychological fatigue. *Fam Pract Res J.* 1993;13:82.

IV. Laboratory Tests (Figure 25–1). Laboratory investigation based on signs will be more productive than screening based on the complaint of fatigue alone. (SOR Ⓐ) The patient often needs the reassurance of a laboratory investigation. The clinician should bear in mind, however, that laboratory investigations of persons fatigued for more than 1 year have been remarkably unproductive.

    A. Since the most common physical causes of fatigue are infectious (viral infections are the most common), endocrine (thyroid disease and diabetes mellitus predominate), and cardiovascular, (SOR Ⓐ) a level one laboratory evaluation would consist of the following tests (Figure 25–1).

        1. Complete blood cell count with differential, **sedimentation rate, urinalysis,** and **chemistry panel**.

        2. Thyroid panel.

        3. Pregnancy testing in females of childbearing age.

        4. Appropriate cancer screening for age/gender (USPSTF guidelines). Cancer screening tests will rarely reveal the cause of fatigue, yet they can be reassuring to the patient and physician, and should be a part of a thorough evaluation.

    B. Second-level investigation is rarely useful, but such an evaluation would include the following tests.

        1. Chest x-ray for adenopathy, signs of congestive heart failure, pulmonary infections, and tumors.

        2. Electrocardiogram to look for silent infarction or ischemia.

        3. Serologies. Rheumatoid factor, ANA, and subtypes, if positive, can be ordered to test for connective tissue diseases presenting with fatigue.

        4. A **drug screen** for unreported drug (including alcohol) use can occasionally be productive.

        5. In appropriate patients and geographic areas, **hepatitis C antibodies, human immunodeficiency virus tests, skin tests for tuberculosis** with controls, **Lyme titers,** and venereal disease research laboratory **tests** should be performed.

    C. Third-level testing for uncommon causes of fatigue prompted by specific suspicion or sign (e.g., for Addison disease, multiple sclerosis, myasthenia gravis, and poisoning) is best considered last, since these problems represent uncommon causes of fatigue.

    D. Abnormal laboratory findings. Treatment of the underlying condition until the laboratory abnormality resolves is necessary to determine whether it represented the cause of the fatigue. One should be prepared to resume the search for a cause if a particular laboratory value returns to normal but the patient's condition does not.

V. Treatment

    A. Etiology identified. Specific treatments for defined physical and psychological causes should be administered when possible.

B. Etiology undetermined

1. **Behavioral treatment.** Despite intensive investigation and follow-up, the cause of chronic fatigue remains undetermined in approximately one-third of patients. In such a case, cognitive behavioral therapy, and graded exercise programs have often been shown to be effective. (SOR Ⓐ) Additionally, group therapy may provide the patient with some solace. These modalities should be offered to all fatigued patients whose problems do not resolve with more specific treatment.

2. **Drug therapy.** A host of medications have been used with limited success to provide relief from fatigue of unknown origin. A partial list includes vitamins, thyroid supplementation (for subclinical hypothyroidism), growth hormone, amphetamines, pemoline, modafinil, and hydrocortisone. Iron has been prescribed for fatigued patients who are not anemic but have low serum ferritin levels. The use of any medication for treatment of a symptom without a specific, identified cause is problematic.

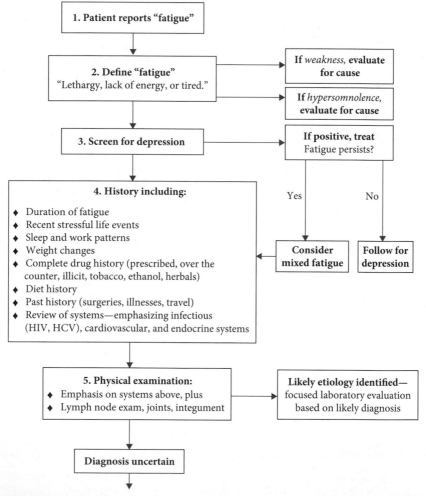

FIGURE 25–1. Evaluation of the patient with fatigue. ANA, anti-nuclear antibody; CHF, congestive heart failure; HIV, human immunodeficiency virus; HCV, hepatitis C virus; PPD, purified protein derivative; VDRL test, venereal disease research laboratory test.

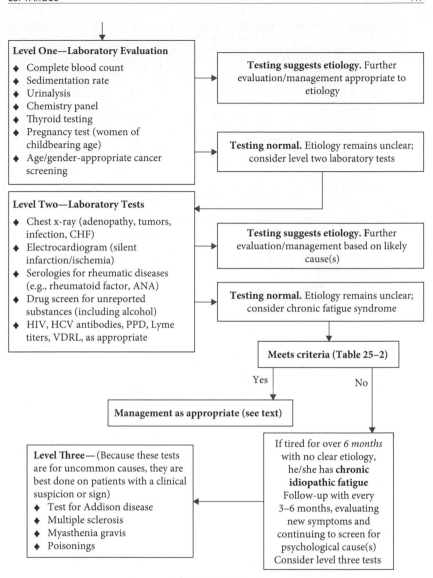

Level One—Laboratory Evaluation

- Complete blood count
- Sedimentation rate
- Urinalysis
- Chemistry panel
- Thyroid testing
- Pregnancy test (women of childbearing age)
- Age/gender-appropriate cancer screening

Testing suggests etiology. Further evaluation/management appropriate to etiology

Testing normal. Etiology remains unclear; consider level two laboratory tests

Level Two—Laboratory Tests

- Chest x-ray (adenopathy, tumors, infection, CHF)
- Electrocardiogram (silent infarction/ischemia)
- Serologies for rheumatic diseases (e.g., rheumatoid factor, ANA)
- Drug screen for unreported substances (including alcohol)
- HIV, HCV antibodies, PPD, Lyme titers, VDRL, as appropriate

Testing suggests etiology. Further evaluation/management based on likely cause(s)

Testing normal. Etiology remains unclear; consider chronic fatigue syndrome

Meets criteria (Table 25–2)

Yes   No

Management as appropriate (see text)

Level Three— (Because these tests are for uncommon causes, they are best done on patients with a clinical suspicion or sign)

- Test for Addison disease
- Multiple sclerosis
- Myasthenia gravis
- Poisonings

If tired for over *6 months* with no clear etiology, he/she has **chronic idiopathic fatigue** Follow-up with every 3–6 months, evaluating new symptoms and continuing to screen for psychological cause(s) Consider level three tests

FIGURE 25–1. (*Continued*)

However, the likelihood of depression or fibromyalgia causing fatigue in persons with no obvious cause probably warrants a full-dose therapeutic trial of antidepressants. This approach is supported by a study showing a positive response when used as part of a multidimensional treatment plan in a majority of patients with medically unexplained symptoms.

3. Diet therapy. Several unproven diets have been proposed. Although fatigue has been associated with a body mass index of 40 or greater, it is not certain that weight loss will alleviate fatigue in greatly obese persons. Nevertheless, achieving and maintaining ideal body weight through balanced nutrition is recommended for general health and may be helpful in fatigued patients.

4. **Complementary/alternative medical therapy (CAM).** While studies of CAM therapies such as herbal medicine, acupuncture, and manual medicine have not, as yet, provided significant positive benefit, there have been no reports of adverse effects on fatigued patients using CAM. The use of CAM for fatigued patients is empirical.

5. **Patient follow-up.** It is not known exactly how often the fatigued patient should return to the physician. A few bimonthly visits early in the investigation of the complaint will serve to cement the patient–physician relationship and establish good faith. Regularly scheduled visits, even as seldom as twice a year, remind the patient that they are not adrift and that changes in the patient's condition will receive serious consideration. At each visit, a review of physical, environmental, and psychological symptoms and signs should be conducted. Physician support, reassurance, and follow-up are important for the patient whose fatigue appears to have no clear cause.

VI. **Patient Education.** While patients can be somewhat reassured by scheduled follow-up and pursuit of new symptoms/signs, they also need to know that the prognosis is not always grim (i.e., that recovery is possible).

A. The **natural history** of the symptom "fatigue" was explored in a series in which 73 fatigued and 72 nonfatigued subjects were reevaluated using Rand Index of Vitality scores. After 1 year, 41% of the fatigued patients were no longer fatigued, and 15 of the 72 nonfatigued subjects had become fatigued. The difference in improvement between fatigued patients with physical diagnoses and those with psychological diagnoses was not significant.

Other series suggest a resolution of fatigue in the majority of cases, with poorer prognosis in patients with anxiety, depression, and with longer duration. When patients are classified as CFS, they can improve with therapy but their prospects for complete resolution are less than with the general population complaining of fatigue.

B. **Resources.** The CDC maintains a CFS website (www.cdc.gov/cfs) that can provide information and education to patients and providers alike. Additionally, working with physical and occupational therapists can provide useful tips on how best to manage daily activities.

SELECTED REFERENCES

Fukada K, Strauss SE, Hickie I, et al. The chronic fatigue syndrome: a comprehensive approach to its definition and study. *Ann Intern Med.* 1994;121:953–959.

Komaroff AL, Buchwald D. Symptoms and signs of chronic fatigue syndrome. *Rev Infect Dis.* 1991;13(Suppl 1):S8–S11.

Kroenke K, Wood Dr, Mangelsdorff AD, et al. Chronic fatigue in primary care. Prevalence, patient characteristics and outcome. *JAMA.* 1988;260:929–934.

Reeves WC, Lloyd A, Vernon SD, et al.; the International Chronic Fatigue Syndrome Study Group. Identification of ambiguities in the 1994 chronic fatigue syndrome research case definition and recommendations for resolution. BMC Health Serv Res. 2003;3(1):25.

Whiting P, Gagnall AM, Sowden AJ, et al. Interventions for the treatment and management of the chronic fatigue syndrome. *JAMA.* 2001;286:1360–1368.

---

26   Fluid, Electrolyte, and Acid–Base Disturbances

Mudit Gilotra, MD, Marc Altshuler, MD, & Lara Carson Weinstein, MD, MPH

KEY POINTS

• In the ambulatory care setting, fluid, electrolyte, and acid–base disturbances often present initially as abnormal chemical screening panels in patients with known chronic disease, new medications, previously undiagnosed endocrine disorders, or acute gastrointestinal illnesses. Patients are often asymptomatic. (SOR **C**)

- Disorders of salt and water balance, exceedingly common in geriatric patients, should initially be assessed by evaluating volume status. (SOR ⊙)
- When a patient presents with hypo-osmotic hypovolemic hypernatremia or hypokalemia in the outpatient setting, consider diuretic use. (SOR ⊙)
- To avoid hypokalemia, patients taking either a thiazide diuretic or a loop diuretic should be instructed to increase their dietary intake of potassium-rich foods. (SOR ⊙)
- With incidental hypercalcemia noted on routine screening, consider primary hyperparathyroidism. (SOR ⊙)
- Syndrome of inappropriate secretion of antidiuretic hormone (SIADH) is treated with free water restriction. (SOR ⊙)

I. Definition and Common Diagnoses

A. Decreases in effective circulating volume commonly occur from **gastrointestinal (GI) losses** (vomiting, diarrhea), **loss through skin** (sweating, fever), **renal losses** (diuretics, interstitial renal disease), and **third-space accumulations** (pharmaceutical excess vasodilatation, pancreatitis). **Expansion of interstitial volume** causes edema. Congestive heart failure is the most common cause of edematous conditions seen in the outpatient setting. Edema is also seen in cirrhosis, renal failure, and nephrotic syndrome.

1. **Hyponatremia,** serum sodium ≤135 mmol/L, is a state of overabundance of free water compared to sodium. It can be characterized by osmolar and volume status. In most cases, hyponatremia is hypo-osmolar.

    a. Hypo-osmolar hypervolemic hyponatremia occurs in patients with congestive heart failure, liver disease, chronic renal failure, or pregnancy.

    b. Hypo-osmolar euvolemic hyponatremia occurs with hypothyroidism, primary polydipsia, beer drinker's potomania, and adrenal insufficiency. However, the most common cause is the syndrome of inappropriate secretion of antidiuretic hormone (SIADH). SIADH can be caused by malignancy (e.g., small cell lung cancer), pulmonary disease (e.g., legionella pneumonia), CNS disease (trauma, infection, tumors), or medications (e.g., selective serotonin reuptake inhibitors [SSRIs], tricyclics, carbamazepine, metformin, theophylline).

    c. Hypo-osmolar hypovolemic hyponatremia, from decreased real or effective circulating volume, commonly occurs in the outpatient setting from diuretic use. It is also seen with other renal losses (osmotic diuresis, diabetes insipidus [DI]), GI losses (diarrhea, vomiting), severe burns, or sequestration without actual loss (e.g., intestinal obstruction, pancreatitis, peritonitis).

    d. Hyperosmolar hyponatremia is classically seen with severe hyperglycemia.

    e. Iso-osmolar hyponatremia occurs with severe hypertriglyceridemia or paraproteinemia (pseudohyponatremia), or in the posttransurethral prostatic resection syndrome when massive volumes of a sodium-free irrigant (such as glycine) are systemically absorbed intraoperatively, causing dilutional hyponatremia.

2. **Hypernatremia,** serum sodium ≥145 mmol/L, is a state of free water deficit (WD) compared to sodium. Risk factors for hypernatremia include extremes of age, impaired thirst mechanism, insensible water losses (GI tract or skin), and use of medications that can cause nephrogenic DI (e.g., lithium).

3. **Hypokalemia,** plasma potassium ≤3.5 mmol/L, most commonly occurs with diuretic use and GI losses (i.e., large-volume diarrhea, eating disorders with laxative use, and vomiting). Other medications that can cause transcellular potassium shifts include Beta-2 sympathomimetic agonists, theophylline, and insulin. Less common causes include primary and secondary hyperaldosteronism, hypothermia, and type I and II renal tubular acidosis.

4. **Hyperkalemia,** plasma potassium ≥5 mmol/L, occurs with impaired renal excretion of potassium or by a shift of potassium into the extracellular space. Hyperkalemia is commonly seen in chronic renal failure, often with medications (e.g., potassium-sparing diuretics, angiotensin-converting enzyme inhibitors, angiotensin receptor blockers, nonsteroidal anti-inflammatory drugs, beta-blockers) that interfere with potassium excretion. It can also occur in adrenal insufficiency, metabolic acidosis, uncontrolled diabetes, or ingestion of potassium supplements. Pseudohyperkalemia occurs with blood sample hemolysis.

5. Hypocalcemia, serum calcium ≤8 mg/dL (ionized calcium ≤4 mg/dL), occurs in patients with chronic renal failure, acute pancreatitis, widespread osteoblastic metastases, hypoparathyroidism, or "hungry bone syndrome" following thyroid or parathyroid surgery, vitamin D deficiency, alcoholism, and HIV infection and in premature/low-birth-weight infants. It is important to check magnesium levels because hypomagnesemia can play a role in parathyroid hormone secretion and resistance.

6. Hypercalcemia is serum calcium ≥10 mg/dL (ionized calcium ≥5.6 mg/dL). Primary hyperparathyroidism or malignancy (e.g., bone metastases, multiple myeloma, paraneoplastic syndromes) cause more than 90% of hypercalcemia. Primary hyperparathyroidism occurs in 1/500 elderly women. Rare causes of hypercalcemia include sarcoidosis, hyperthyroidism, lithium use, and the milk–alkali syndrome.

B. Common causes and mechanisms of **primary acid–base disorders** are outlined in Figure 26–1.

II. Symptoms and Signs associated with fluid, electrolyte, and acid–base disorders are subtle, nonspecific, and less sensitive than laboratory testing in detecting these disorders. Symptoms are more likely with large or rapid shifts in fluid, electrolyte, or acid–base status. The most common symptoms include **lethargy, fatigue/weakness, or irritability**. Symptoms and findings associated with particular disorders include the following:

A. Hyponatremia. Symptoms are related to cerebral overhydration including nausea, malaise, headache, lethargy, and eventually seizures, coma, and respiratory arrest.

B. Hypernatremia. Symptoms are related to decrease in brain volume, demyelinating brain lesions, and cerebral hemorrhage including lethargy, seizures, and coma.

C. Hypo- and Hyperkalemia. Both states are characterized by similar symptoms including muscle weakness and paralysis, with differing cardiac conduction abnormalities (see below).

D. Hypocalcemia. Acute hypocalcemia is characterized by mild paresthesias to more dramatic signs of neuromuscular irritability including carpopedal spasm and seizures. **Chvostek sign** (facial muscle twitching when the facial nerve is tapped anterior to the ear) and Trousseau sign (spasm of the muscles of the hand when a blood pressure cuff is applied to the arm for 3 minutes) also can occur.

E. Hypercalcemia. At low levels (<12 mg/dL), it is usually asymptomatic. At higher levels, patients may suffer from polyuria, polydipsia, anorexia, and constipation and eventually suffer from weakness, confusion, and coma. **Ectopic soft tissue calcifications** may also be seen.

F. Metabolic acidosis and alkalosis. Symptoms are similar in these two conditions and include nausea, vomiting, abdominal pain, lethargy, stupor, coma, and seizures. Anxiety and tachypnea can be seen in **respiratory alkalosis** or **respiratory acidosis**.

III. Diagnostic Tests. Focused **laboratory evaluation** should be based on risk factors/symptoms/signs and will clarify the cause of common fluid/electrolyte and acid–base disorders (Figures 26–1 to 26–4).

A. In **hyper-** or **hyponatremia,** testing includes serum and urine electrolytes, serum and urine osmolality, creatinine, blood urea nitrogen (BUN), glucose, and testing for the underlying cause.

B. In patients with **hyper-** or **hypokalemia,** testing includes serum electrolytes; creatinine; BUN; glucose; arterial blood gas; spot urine measurement of sodium, potassium, chloride, creatinine; and electrocardiography (ECG).

1. In **hypokalemia,** ECG may show flat or inverted T waves, U-wave formation, and ST-segment depression; urine potassium excretion and acid–base status should be assessed.

2. In **hyperkalemia,** ECG shows peaked T waves, progressing to QRS widening, and eventually ventricular fibrillation.

C. With **hypocalcemia and hypercalcemia,** serum ionized (free) calcium, phosphorus, magnesium, chloride, parathyroid hormone, and 25-hydroxyvitamin D levels should be checked.

D. With **respiratory alkalosis,** flattening or inversion of ECG ST-segments may occur because of hypocapnia.

IV. Treatment is directed at correcting underlying causes along with identified fluid, electrolyte, and acid–base abnormalities.

A. Hyponatremia

1. Fluid replacement in the setting of hyponatremia must be done with caution; the risk of hyponatremia-related cerebral edema must be balanced against the risk of the

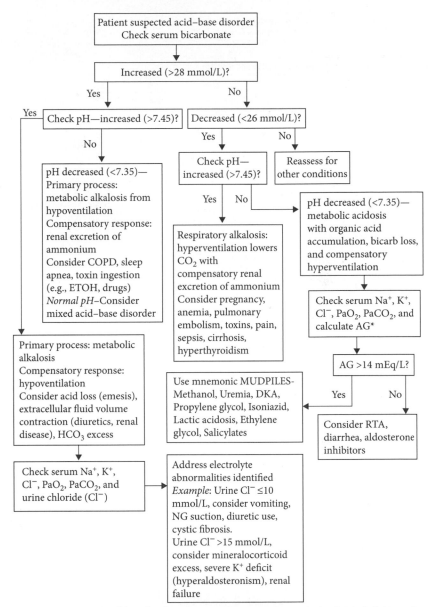

FIGURE 26–1. Overview of acid–base disorders. *AG = Na⁺-[HCO₃⁻ + Cl⁻]; Normal AG = 8–14 mEq/L. Na, sodium; K, potassium; PaO₂, partial pressure of oxygen; PaCO₂, partial pressure of carbon dioxide; COPD, chronic obstructive pulmonary disease; ETOH, alcohol; DKA, diabetic ketoacidosis; AG, anion gap; RTA, renal tubular acidosis.

osmotic demyelination syndrome (ODS) from overzealous correction (especially in the setting of chronic [≥48 hours] hyponatremia). (SOR **B**) Hypovolemic patients with mild symptoms and chronic hyponatremia can be treated in the hospital setting with 0.9% normal saline to increase the serum sodium by 0.5 mEq/L/h, with a maximum sodium increase of 10 to 12 mEq/L over 24 hours.

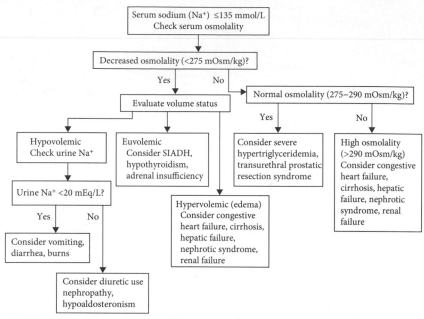

FIGURE 26–2. Evaluation of hyponatremia. SIADH, syndrome of inappropriate secretion of antidiuretic hormone.

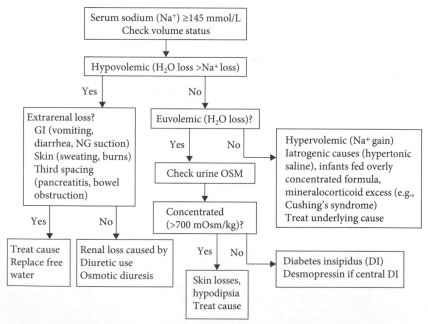

FIGURE 26–3. Evaluation of hypernatremia. GI, gastrointestinal; NG, nasogastric.

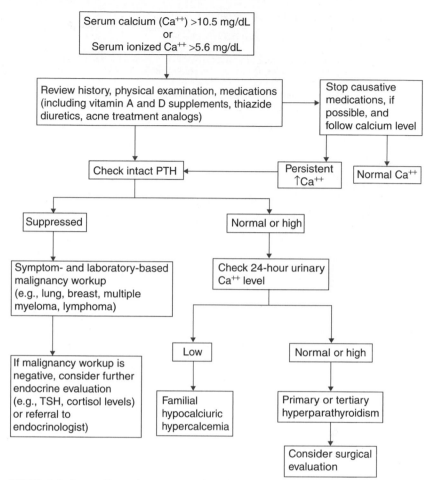

FIGURE 26–4. Evaluation of hypercalcemia. PTH, parathyroid hormone; TSH, thyroid-stimulating hormone. (Adapted with permission from Carroll MF. A practical approach to hypercalcemia. *Am Fam Physician.* 2003;67(9):1959–1966. Copyright © 2003 American Academy of Family Physicians. All Rights Reserved.)

2. **Severe acute hyponatremia with significant neurologic symptoms (i.e., seizures) requires hospitalization** with administration of 3% hypertonic saline intravenously for the first 3 to 4 hours to raise serum sodium concentration at a rate of 1 to 2 mEq/L/h to a goal of 120 mEq/L. (SOR **B**)

3. Use of an angiotensin-converting enzyme inhibitor along with fluid and sodium restriction is beneficial for the treatment of **hyponatremia associated with congestive heart failure**.

4. **SIADH** or other mild hyponatremic states are treated with free water restriction (1000–1500 mL per day) pending correction of the underlying cause.

B. **Hypernatremia**

1. **General treatment principles consist of replacing free water;** with hypovolemia, volume must be corrected in the hospital setting initially with isotonic 0.9% saline until the patient is hemodynamically stable despite possible worsening hypernatremia.

a. WD can be calculated as follows:

$$WD = TBW \times \left(\frac{Plasma\ Na}{140} - 1 \right),$$

where TBW is the total body water. TBW = 0.6 (weight in kg) in pediatrics; 0.6 (weight in kg) in males; 0.5 (weight in kg) in females; 0.5 (weight in kg) in elderly males; 0.45 (weight in kg) in elderly females.

b. In general, **no more than 50% of the WD** along with any ongoing losses should be corrected in the first 24 hours, and the remainder over the next 1 to 2 days. To avoid cerebral edema, the serum sodium should be lowered by 0.5 to 1 mEq/L/h, with a maximum decrease of 10 to 12 mEq/L in 24 hours. Initially, free water and volume can be replaced intravenously if necessary. To prevent recurrences, the patient can be given a fluid prescription quantifying recommended daily fluid ingestion.

2. **Central DI** should be treated with desmopressin, starting with 5 μg per day intranasally.
3. **Nephrogenic DI** is managed by treating the underlying disorder.

C. **Hypokalemia**
1. Patients taking a **thiazide diuretic or a loop diuretic** generally require 20 to 60 mEq per day of potassium.
   a. Patients should be encouraged to increase dietary potassium because this is the safest and least expensive means of supplementation. Potassium-rich food sources are listed in Table 26–1.
   b. If hypokalemia persists, addition of a potassium supplement (e.g., potassium chloride), starting at 20 mEq per day, or a potassium-sparing diuretic (e.g., spironolactone) can be considered. Potassium levels require regular monitoring; this should be initially done weekly, then every 2 to 4 weeks until stable. Patients with chronic renal insufficiency require closer monitoring.
   c. Moderate to **severe hypokalemia (≤3.0 mEq/L)** requires more urgent potassium replacement and management in an inpatient setting.

D. **Hyperkalemia**
1. Office management of **mild hyperkalemia (≤6 mEq/L)** involves dietary potassium restriction in renal insufficiency and reevaluation of medications.
2. **Severe hyperkalemia (≥6 mEq/L)** with ECG changes, rapid onset, decreased renal function, or acidosis requires urgent inpatient treatment. (SOR ❸) Intravenous calcium gluconate should be used to stabilize the myocardium in patients with ECG changes. (SOR ❸) Insulin and glucose, a beta-2 agonist, or loop diuretics should be used to lower the potassium level acutely. (SOR ❸) Sodium polystyrene sulfonate (Kayexalate) and loop diuretics can be used to decrease total body potassium. Hemodialysis can be used as a last resort. (SOR ❸)

E. **Hypocalcemia.** Treatment in the office of mild hypocalcemia (ionized calcium of 3.2–3.9 mg/dL) includes oral calcium supplementation (e.g., calcium carbonate, 1–2 g of elemental calcium per day).
1. **Vitamin D supplementation** with vitamin D2 (ergocalciferol) or vitamin D analog (e.g., calcitriol) is indicated, with dose depending on the underlying cause. 25-Hydroxyvitamin D levels should be maintained above 32 ng/dL to preserve bone health. (SOR ❸)

TABLE 26–1. EXAMPLES OF POTASSIUM RICH FOODS

Food Source	mEq of Potassium
Acorn squash (one cup cooked)	23
Baked potato	22
Spinach (one cup cooked)	21
Lentils (one cup cooked)	19
Kidney beans (one cup cooked)	18
Split peas (one cup cooked)	18
Orange juice (one cup)	13
Banana (medium)	12

     a. Severe vitamin D deficiency is treated with 50,000 IU vitamin D daily for 1 to 3 weeks and then 50,000 IU weekly. (SOR ❸) Once stores have been replete, maintenance therapy can be started with 800 IU vitamin D daily or 50,000 IU once or twice a month. (SOR ❸)

     b. Patients with impaired vitamin D metabolism (e.g., chronic renal insufficiency and hypoparathyroidism) may benefit from **calcitriol,** (SOR ❸) 0.25 to 2 µg daily, generally in consultation with an endocrinologist, nephrologist, or both, with close monitoring to avoid hypercalcemia.

    2. Vitamin D therapy requires close laboratory monitoring to avoid hypercalciuria, hypercalcemia, and renal toxicity.

    3. Hospitalization should be considered for management of patients with ionized calcium levels ≤3.2 mg/dL or with signs of neuromuscular irritability (Chvostek sign or carpopedal spasm).

F. Hypercalcemia

    1. Patients with **serum calcium levels ≥13 mg/dL or severe symptoms** require hospitalization for evaluation and treatment. Initial treatment includes aggressive rehydration with 0.9% normal saline to restore intravascular volume; this can be followed by IV loop diuretics and other therapies (e.g., calcitonin, bisphosphonates) as indicated.

    2. Patients with mild hypercalcemia (≤13 mg/dL) of known etiology (e.g., known cancer diagnosis) can be treated as outpatients with oral rehydration and possible addition of a loop diuretic.

    3. Asymptomatic patients with primary hyperparathyroidism, who have normal renal and bone status and only mildly elevated serum calcium, may be candidates for medical management with frequent monitoring. (SOR ❸)

    4. Referral to a neck surgeon for consideration of parathyroidectomy is appropriate in patients with primary hyperparathyroidism with nephrolithiasis, persistently increased serum calcium, hypercalciuria, osteoporosis, decreased creatinine clearance, age ≤50 years, limited medical surveillance, or patient request.

G. Metabolic acidosis and alkalosis

    1. Metabolic acidosis is managed by treating the underlying cause. This includes providing nutrition and rehydration for alcoholic or starvation ketosis (often in a hospital setting), eliminating suspect drugs, or treating underlying diabetes mellitus (see Chapter 75), diarrhea (see Chapter 16), or causes of lactic acidosis. Renal tubular acidosis should initially be evaluated and managed in consultation with a nephrologist. In addition, the body's compensatory mechanism for metabolic acidosis is to decrease PCO_2 through hyperventilation.

    2. Metabolic alkalosis management likewise depends on its cause. Suspected causative medications (e.g., diuretics) should be eliminated if possible, vomiting or nasogastric losses should be replaced (often in the inpatient setting), renal failure should be managed in consultation with nephrology, and mineralocorticoid excess (Cushing syndrome, primary aldosteronism) should be managed by treating the underlying disease. In metabolic alkalosis, the body's compensatory mechanism is to increase PCO_2 through hypoventilation.

H. Respiratory acidosis is managed by correcting or stabilizing underlying pulmonary or metabolic disorders and improving ventilation. This can include controlling bronchospasm (see Chapter 68) and congestive heart failure (see Chapter 73). The body tries to reverse the acidosis by increasing HCO_3 through increased renal excretion as ammonium. Patients may need intubation and pressure support.

I. Respiratory alkalosis treatment also focuses on underlying disorders. For example, patients with symptomatic, anxiety-related hyperventilation may respond to rebreathing (e.g., breathing into a paper bag) when symptoms develop. The compensatory mechanism in respiratory alkalosis involves decreasing HCO_3 through decreased renal excretion as ammonium.

V. Patient Education

    A. Electrolyte disturbances are often asymptomatic, especially in mild forms. When patients have symptoms they are nonspecific, often including nausea, muscle aches, weakness, and lethargy.

B. In severe cases, patients often need to be hospitalized to correct their electrolyte imbalances and acid–base disorders.
C. Acute disturbances can be corrected within a few days, but often chronic states require daily medications or nutritional supplements.

SELECTED REFERENCES

Carroll MF, Schade DS. A Practical approach to hypocalcaemia. *Am Fam Physician.* 2003;67: 1959–1966.
Dzierba AL, Abraham P. A practical approach to understanding acid-base abnormalities in critical illness. *J Pharm Practice.* 2011;24(1):17–26.
Goh KP. Management of hyponatremia. *Am Fam Physician.* 2004;69:2387–2394.
Higdon ML, Higdon JA. Treatment of oncologic emergencies. *Am Fam Physician.* 2006;74:1873–1880.
Hollander-Rodriguez JC. Hyperkalemia. *Am Fam Physician.* 2006;73:283–290.
Lin M, Liu SJ, Lim IT. Disorders of water imbalance. *Emerg Med Clin N Am.* 2005;23:749–770.
Lynman D. Undiagnosed vitamin D deficiency in the hospital patient. *Am Fam Physician.* 2005;71: 299–304.
Sarko J. Bone and mineral metabolism. *Emerg Med Clin N Am.* 2005;23:703–721.
Schaefer TJ, Wolford RW. Disorders of potassium. *Emerg Med Clin N Am.* 2005;23:723–747.
Taniergra ED. Hyperparathyroidism. *Am Fam Physician.* 2004;69:333–339.
Vaidya C, Ho W, Freda BJ. Management of hyponatremia: providing treatment and avoiding harm. *Clev Clin J Med.* 2010;77(10):715–725.
Whittier WL, Rutecki GW. Primer on clinical acid-base problem solving. *Dis Mon.* 2004;50:117–162.

---

27   Foot Conditions

James R. Barrett, MD, CAQSM

KEY POINTS

- One should look for contributing factors, such as improper footwear, when evaluating foot pain since correcting these will decrease the chance of pain recurrence. (SOR ☻)
- Stress fractures are a common cause of foot pain and may have no initial x-ray findings. A high index of suspicion should be maintained. (SOR ☻)
- Four types of injuries need to be identified early to reduce morbidity and improve successful treatment: Achilles tendon rupture, Lisfranc injury, and fractures of the fifth metatarsal and navicular bones. (SOR ☻)

I. Definition. The foot, which has 26 bones and 55 articulations, acts as a platform and shock absorber to support the weight of the body as well as a powerful lever to propel the body. Foot complaints are usually related to overuse, trauma, or degenerative changes. Contributing factors include foot type such as high arch (pes cavus) and flatfoot (pes planus); foot deformities (i.e., hallux valgus); improper footwear; excessive weight; and underlying systemic diseases (i.e., diabetes or osteoporosis). The foot and ankle can have numerous accessory ossicles that can be confused with a possible fracture.

II. Common Diagnoses. Because of the amount of weight that the foot carries every day, it is little wonder that 18% of the population each year will have foot problems, an incidence that increases with age. Diagnosis can be facilitated by considering three distinct regions of the foot: the forefoot, the midfoot, and the hindfoot (see Figures 27–1 and 27–2).

A. Forefoot. The forefoot, comprising the toes and metatarsals, is the most common site of foot complaints, with a prevalence of 2% to 10%. Most forefoot conditions are caused by poor shoe selection (tight toe boxes, high-heeled shoes); foot deformities (hallux valgus, hammer toes); overuse; or degenerative changes. Common conditions affecting the toes (followed by their prevalence) include calluses/corns (4.5%), plantar warts (2%), onychomycosis (10%), ingrown toenails (3%–5%), phalangeal fractures, and peripheral

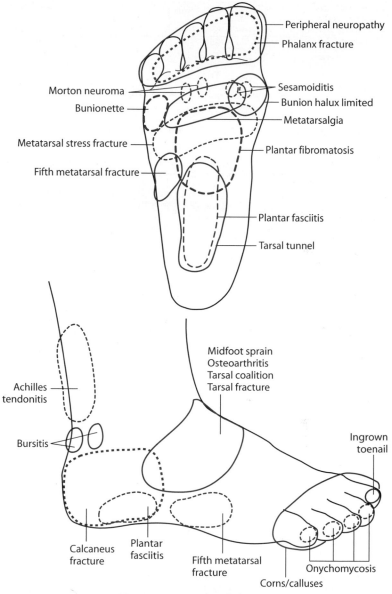

FIGURE 27–1. Foot complaints by location.

neuropathy. Common conditions affecting the metatarsals include bunions (hallux valgus) (1.8%), hallux limitus (2%), metatarsalgia, Morton (interdigital) neuromas, fractures (stress and fifth metatarsal), and sesamoiditis.

B. Midfoot. Midfoot complaints, caused by degenerative changes, trauma, or foot deformity, are relatively uncommon but can lead to significant disability. Common conditions affecting the midfoot, which comprises the cuneiforms, cuboid, and navicular bones of

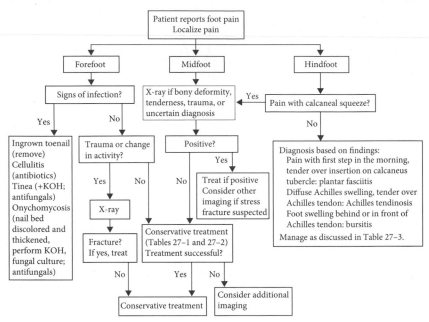

FIGURE 27–2. Approach to the patient with foot pain. KOH, potassium hydroxide.

the foot, include midfoot sprain, osteoarthritis, tarsal fractures, plantar fibromatosis, posterior tibialis dysfunction, and tarsal coalition.

LISFRANC INJURY

Lisfranc injury is a severe form of midfoot sprain to the tarsometatarsal articulation and is frequently missed. Pain and swelling over the tarsometatarsal articulation and inability to bear weight on the tiptoes are clues to the injury. Weight-bearing x-rays of the foot may show avulsed bone between the first and second metatarsals and loss of congruity between the first metatarsal and the first cuneiform, the second metatarsal and the second cuneiform, or both. Computerized tomography (CT) of the foot may be necessary for diagnosis. Patients with this injury should be placed in a nonweight-bearing cast and referred to orthopedics.

TARSAL NAVICULAR BONE FRACTURES

Tarsal navicular bone fractures are easily missed because patients may have minimal pain over the midfoot and the medial arch. These fractures are important to diagnose early because navicular fractures have a high rate of nonunion. Examination reveals tenderness over the navicular bone and increased pain with hopping on the foot. Plain x-rays of the foot are often inconclusive; therefore, bone scan, CT, or magnetic resonance imaging (MRI) may be necessary for diagnosis. Treatment of nondisplaced fractures involves a nonweight-bearing cast for 6 to 8 weeks. Displaced fractures require orthopedic consultation.

C. Hindfoot. Hindfoot conditions are the second most common type of foot complaint, with a prevalence of 1%. Common conditions affecting the hindfoot, which comprises the calcaneus and talus, include plantar fasciitis (0.4% prevalence), calcaneal stress fractures, Achilles tendinosis, and bursitis. Most hindfoot conditions are caused by overuse or excessive weight.

ACHILLES TENDON RUPTURE

Achilles tendon rupture usually causes acute pain in the posterior heel. Examination will often reveal swelling and ecchymosis over the posterior heel, a palpable defect of the Achilles tendon, inability to walk normally, and a positive Thompson test (no plantar flexion when the calf is squeezed). Treatment is usually surgical and warrants an urgent referral to orthopedics.

III. Symptom and Signs (see Tables 27–1 to 27–3 and Figure 27–1)
IV. Diagnostic Tests (see Tables 27–1 to 27–3)
    A. Laboratory tests are generally not necessary in evaluating foot concerns. Atrau-
    matic symmetric foot swelling and pain can be caused by systemic arthritis (such as

TABLE 27–1. EVALUATION AND MANAGEMENT OF COMMON FOREFOOT COMPLAINTS

Diagnosis	Symptoms	Findings	Testing	Treatment
Corn/callus	Pain with pressure on lesion	Skin thickening under bony prominence (calluses) or between the toes (corns); tenderness with direct pressure	None	Paring of calluses[a] Padding[b] Shoes with wide toe box
Plantar wart	Pain with pressure on lesion	Skin thickening or papules that interrupt skin lines and have blood vessels within core; pain on squeezing	No routine testing but can do a biopsy for diagnosis	Observation (some spontaneously resolve within 6–12 months) Wart removal[c]
Onychomycosis (fungal toenail infection)	Thickened nail, occasionally painful	Thickened discolored nail, occasionally crumbles	KOH scraping Fungal culture from scraping	Trimming/thinning of the nail Shoes with wide toe box Oral antifungals (SOR Ⓑ) Nail removal
Ingrown toenail (Onychocryptosis)	Pain, swelling, and discharge along border of the nail	Nail border swollen, erythematous, occasional discharge	None	Ingrown toenail removal[d] If surrounding cellulitis, use antibiotic
Phalanx fracture	Acute pain and swelling of digit usually after trauma	Bony tenderness, swelling, ecchymosis, pain with toe motion	X-ray	Nondisplaced fracture: buddy taping to the adjacent toe, hard-soled shoe Displaced fracture: foot specialist referral
Peripheral neuropathy	Tingling, burning, and/or pain initially in the toes, then later in a stocking distribution, usually bilateral	May have decreased light touch, vibratory, and temperature sensation over the toes; sensation abnormalities tend to progress to involve the entire foot with associated loss of motor strength in the foot and loss of Achilles tendon reflex	Electromyography and nerve conduction velocity; laboratory tests to rule out underlying condition	Identify and treat underlying condition if present; amitriptyline, gabapentin, pregabalin, or duloxetine (SOR Ⓑ)
Bunion or bunionette	Painful bony protuberance of the first or fifth MTP joint	Tender bony MTP joint prominence with valgus, first MTP deformity (bunion) or varus fifth MTP deformity (bunionette)	X-ray reveals bony angular deformity (angle between the first and second metatarsals ≥15 degrees, angle between the fourth and fifth metatarsals ≥10 degrees)	Shoes with wide toe box Bunion shield Acetaminophen or NSAID Arch support orthotic Surgical removal if continued pain despite conservative treatment for 6–12 months

(continued)

TABLE 27–1. EVALUATION AND MANAGEMENT OF COMMON FOREFOOT COMPLAINTS (*Continued*)

Diagnosis	Symptoms	Findings	Testing	Treatment
Hallux limitus or hallux rigiditus	Pain and swelling with movement, especially at toe off stage of gait	Loss of motion of first metatarsal, pain with extension of first metatarsal	X-ray may show degenerative spurs and loss of joint space of the first MTP joint	Padding[b] Acetaminophen or NSAID Hard-soled shoes Surgery if severe pain despite conservative measures 6–12 months
Metatarsalgia	Pain at metatarsal heads	Tenderness on palpation of metatarsal heads	X-ray to rule out fracture, arthritis	Relative rest Padding[b] Acetaminophen or NSAID
Morton neuroma (interdigital)	Pain between the metatarsal heads, numbness and tingling into the toes, cramping of the toes	Tenderness with squeezing the metatarsal heads— occasionally accompanied by a click, fullness, or soft tissue mass between the metatarsal heads	None	Shoes with wide toe box; Morton neuroma injection[e] If continued pain referral to foot specialist
Metatarsal stress fracture	Pain and swelling over the foot with activity, particularly during toe off stage of gait	Exquisite tenderness over metatarsal, occasional swelling and/or ecchymosis	X-ray findings may be absent; periosteal reaction, fracture line, or bony callous formation may be present; consider bone scan or MRI if negative x-ray and diagnosis in doubt	Relative rest Padding Short leg removable cast-brace, hard-soled shoe, or short leg walking cast for 4–8 weeks Orthopedic referral for the fifth metatarsal stress fractures as healing is often delayed
Fifth metatarsal fracture	Pain over the lateral foot	Tenderness to palpation of the fifth metatarsal Swelling over the lateral foot	X-ray to evaluate for avulsion fracture versus Jones fracture (Figure 27–2)	Avulsion fracture: Short leg walking cast or air stirrup for 4–6 weeks; Jones fracture: Nonweight-bearing short leg cast until callous formation (3–6 weeks), then short leg walking cast for 3–6 weeks Orthopedic referral if nonunion after 3 months, displaced fracture, stress fracture, or patient preference
Sesamoiditis	Pain in ball of foot (first MTP joint) with toe off stage of gait	Tenderness and swelling over plantar first MTP joint and just proximal to joint	X-ray to rule out sesamoid fracture	Padding[b] Relative rest NSAID

MRI, magnetic resonance imaging; NSAID, nonsteroidal anti-inflammatory drug; MPT, metatarsophalangeal.

[a]**Paring of calluses:** http://www.youtube.com/watch?v=rlEz582XNys.

[b]**Padding:** http://www.youtube.com/watch?v=Tt4DBIY6MTU.

[c]For **wart removal:** 50% salicylic acid paste method and liquid nitrogen method (SOR A): http://www.aafp.org/afp/2011/0801/p288.html.

[d]**Ingrown toenail removal:** http://www.youtube.com/watch?v=YNnsGxy1SC0.

[e]**Morton neuroma injection:** http://www.youtube.com/watch?v=ZaBNBb5pVbY.

TABLE 27–2. EVALUATION AND MANAGEMENT OF COMMON MIDFOOT COMPLAINTS

Diagnosis	Symptoms	Findings	Testing	Treatment
Midfoot sprain	Swelling and pain diffusely over the midfoot with hyperflexion	Tender midfoot diffusely	X-ray to rule out Lisfranc injury	Relative rest Acetaminophen and/or NSAID Shoes with supportive arch cushions Surgical referral if Lisfranc injury
Osteoarthritis	Midfoot pain and stiffness	Diffuse tenderness, occasional diffuse swelling, bony prominence	X-ray may show spurring, loss of joint space; laboratory tests to rule out arthritis	Acetaminophen and/or NSAID (SOR **Ⓐ**) Shoes with supportive arch cushions
Plantar fibromatosis	Painful bumps on bottom of the foot	Nodules on plantar aspect of the foot	Usually none but can do biopsy for diagnosis	No effective treatment, as there is high recurrence with excision; scars from excision can cause pain
Posterior tibialis dysfunction	History of twisting injury, sudden loss of arch, pain posterior and inferior to medial malleolus	Medial ankle swelling, asymmetric pes planus, inability to walk on the toes, poor internal rotation and inversion, tenderness posterior and inferior to medial malleolus	MRI if rupture suspected (no strength with inversion and internal rotation, tendon not palpable)	Relative rest Arch support (nonprescription or custom) Surgery if continued pain despite conservative treatment for 6–12 months
Tarsal coalition	Vague midfoot pain, frequent ankle sprains, lower leg pain with activity	Limited inversion and eversion of foot, tenderness of the midfoot and ankle	X-ray may show bony bridge between talus-navicular or talus-calcaneus, CT scan if suspicion but no x-ray findings	Custom arch support Surgery if continued pain despite conservative treatment for 6–12 months
Tarsal tunnel syndrome	Numbness or burning pain over bottom of the foot, worse with walking and sometimes awakens patient from sleep	Positive Tinel sign (tingling over bottom of the foot) on tapping over posterior tibial nerve inferior-lateral to medial malleolus	Laboratory tests for peripheral neuropathy EMG/NCV (SOR **Ⓒ**)	NSAID Arch support (nonprescription or custom) Physical therapy referral if no improvement in 1–2 months Referral to foot specialist in cases of severe pain not responsive to conservative management in 2–6 months

CT, computerized tomography; EMG, electromyography; MRI, magnetic resonance imaging; NCV, nerve conduction velocity; NSAID, nonsteroidal anti-inflammatory drug.

rheumatoid arthritis and systemic lupus erythematosus) and should be evaluated with tests for sedimentation rate, C-reactive protein (CRP), complete blood count (CBC), rheumatoid factor, antinuclear antibody, and uric acid. Pain caused by peripheral neuropathy is evaluated with a CBC (pernicious anemia, lead poisoning), complete metabolic profile (diabetes, renal disease, liver disease), thyroid-stimulating hormone (TSH), tests for vitamin B_{12}, and, depending on the history, urine heavy metal screen and serum protein electrophoresis (multiple myeloma).

B. Radiography. X-rays of the foot should be performed on initial presentation in four instances: (1) when bony deformity is present, (2) when fracture is suspected such as bony tenderness, (3) when trauma to the foot has occurred, or (4) when the diagnosis is

TABLE 27–3. EVALUATION AND MANAGEMENT OF COMMON HINDFOOT COMPLAINTS

Diagnosis	Symptoms	Findings	Testing	Treatment
Plantar fasciitis	Dull, achy pain in inferior heel, especially upon awakening	Tender calcaneal tubercle and arch	X-ray to rule out stress fracture of calcaneus; calcaneal spurs do not correlate with pain (10%–27% of asymptomatic patients have spurs)	Stretching and strengthening of plantar fascia and Achilles tendon (SOR B) NSAID Heel cup arch support and night splint (SOR B) Physical therapy referral if no improvement after 2–3 months Plantar fascia injection[a] Referral to foot specialist if no improvement in 6–12 months of conservative treatment
Calcaneus stress fracture	Heel pain and swelling with walking, ecchymosis	Squeeze tenderness of calcaneus	X-ray may reveal stress reaction Bone scan or MRI	Relative rest Short leg removable cast-brace or short leg walking cast for 4–8 weeks
Achilles tendinosis	Activity-related pain and swelling behind the heel	Swelling, tenderness over Achilles tendon (2–6 cm proximal to insertion), weak plantarflexion	None	Relative rest NSAID Heel lift Stretching of Achilles tendon Physical therapy if no improvement after 1 month of above measures
Bursitis (superficial calcaneal or retrocalcaneal)	Pain and swelling localized on the posterior ankle near Achilles tendon insertion	Tender posterior ankle, localized swelling/erythema, Haglund deformity (prominent bony deformity of posterior calcaneus)	None	See Achilles tendinosis treatment

[a]**Plantar fascia injection:** http://www.youtube.com/watch?v=WLRPQxbtPWI

in question. Typically, standing anteroposterior, oblique, and lateral views are obtained. **Technetium bone scan** can be used for identifying stress fractures if plain x-ray does not show any abnormality. Bone scan is very sensitive but not very specific in identifying stress fractures and requires a higher exposure to radiation. **MRI** is preferred in identifying stress fractures and soft tissue abnormalities (e.g., ligament/tendon pathology). (SOR Ⓒ) MRI is very sensitive and specific but is frequently more costly than a bone scan. Local expertise and procedure availability can influence the decision between performing an MRI or a bone scan. **CT** is useful in evaluating bony pathology such as tarsal fractures if initial x-ray results are negative and there is strong clinical suspicion of fracture.

    C. **Electromyography and nerve conduction velocity** are frequently ordered to evaluate neurogenic pain when an obvious source is not identifiable or for confirmation of clinical diagnosis. These tests are usually performed by a neurologist or physiatrist and help to anatomically localize the nerve involved or distinguish between mononeuropathies and polyneuropathies.

V. **General Treatment Principles.** (Also see Tables 27–1 to 27–3 and Figures 27–1 to 27–5)

    A. **Appropriate footwear** can prevent and, in some cases, resolve many problems related to the foot. Characteristics of good footwear include roomy wide toe box,

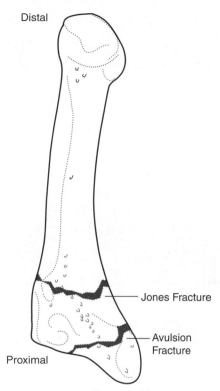

Distal

Jones Fracture

Avulsion
Fracture

Proximal

FIGURE 27–3. Fifth metatarsal fractures.

supportive arch, and low heel with a firm cushioned heel counter at the back of the shoe.

B. Treatment of pain and inflammation involves the use of relative rest, ice, and medications. **Relative rest** means decreasing pain-provoking activity to the point where there is no pain with that activity and substituting alternative minimal weight-bearing activities (i.e., swimming, biking) during healing. Acetaminophen (500–1000 mg orally four times daily) can be used for pain. Nonsteroidal anti-inflammatory medications (e.g., ibuprofen, 400–600 mg orally thrice daily, or naproxen, 250–500 mg orally twice daily) can be used for pain, inflammation, or both. Chronic neurogenic pain can be treated with amitriptyline (10–25 mg orally at bedtime; may increase at weekly intervals to a maximum dose of 100 mg per day), gabapentin (300–1800 mg per day orally in three divided doses), pregabalin (150–300 mg per day in three divided doses), or duloxetine (30 mg orally once daily for 1 week; maintenance, 60 mg orally once daily), starting with low doses and slowly titrating the doses higher to obtain pain relief and minimize side effects (see Table 27–1). (SOR **B**)

C. Stretching exercises are commonly used for foot complaints (especially plantar fasciitis and Achilles tendinosis) and involve stretching the plantar fascia and posterior heel cord muscles (gastrocnemius and soleus). Stretching for the plantar fascia is accomplished in a seated position by grasping the forefoot, dorsiflexing it for 10 seconds, then releasing and repeating this three to five times a day. The posterior heel cord is stretched by standing facing a wall with one foot placed approximately 24 inches from the wall and the other foot placed 48 to 60 inches from the wall. The patient leans toward the wall with hands on the wall in a "pushing fashion," keeping both heels on the ground.

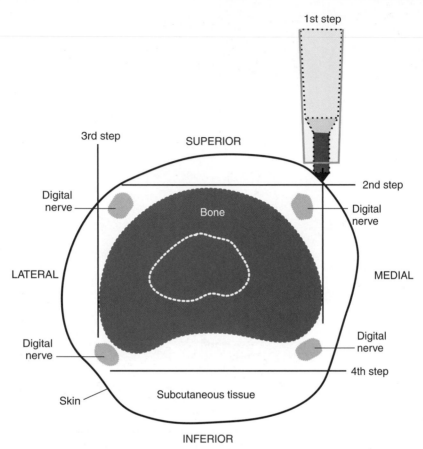

FIGURE 27–4. Digital nerve block: cross section through proximal phalanx.

The knee of the leg in back is extended, while the front knee is slightly flexed. This position is held for 10 to 20 seconds, repeated three to five times, alternating which foot is forward.

D. Orthotics are used for a wide variety of foot conditions.

   1. Nonprescription **arch cushion insoles** can be used initially for plantar fasciitis, bunions, and posterior tibialis dysfunction. Nonprescription bunion shields, made of felt or silicone, can be used to protect the medial aspect of a bunion.

   2. Heel lifts, made of cork, felt, or viscoelastic material, are commonly used for Achilles tendinosis and bursitis.

   3. A **tension night splint for plantar fasciitis** can be commercially obtained or made with fiberglass splinting material, placing the ankle in an 80- to 90-degree angle, with the splint over the plantar aspect of the foot and posterior ankle and calf. ACE bandages secure the posterior splint. (SOR ❸)

   4. If these items are not helpful, referral to a foot specialist or orthotist for custom-made arch supports is appropriate.

   5. A short leg removable cast brace (cam walker boot) can be used for most stress fractures of the foot.

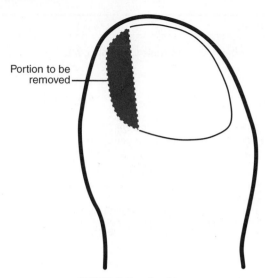

FIGURE 27–5. Toenail avulsion.

E. Systemic antifungal drugs can be used for onychomycosis (see Chapter 31 for doses). They are expensive, require treatment for 3 months, have a high rate of recurrence of infection (complete cure in ≤50%), and require monitoring of liver function tests (and CBC for terbinafine) at baseline, 6 weeks, and 3 months. Common systemic antifungal drugs given orally include terbinafine and itraconazole. (SOR Ⓐ) Topical ciclopirox 8% nail lacquer (applied daily to the nail for 48 weeks) can also be used for onychomycosis but it is seldom effective, as only 5% to 8% of patients have a complete cure (see Table 27–1).

F. Systemic antibiotics are used for foot infections such as cellulitis (see Chapter 9).

VI. Patient Education. Foot pain is frequently caused by improper footwear or overuse. Characteristics of good foot wear include a toe box that is wide enough for the toes to comfortably wiggle, an insole that provides support and cushion, and a heel that is snug. Overuse can often be prevented by gradual increases in activity over a period of several weeks, warming up prior to activities, and stopping activities that cause pain or swelling and investigating the cause.

SELECTED REFERENCES

BellSyer EMS, Khan SM, Torgerson DJ. Oral treatments for fungal infections of the skin of the foot. *Cochrane Database Syst Rev.* 2012;(10):CD003584.

Benirschke S, Meinberg E, Anderson S, et al. Fractures and dislocations of the midfoot: Lisfranc and Chopart injuries. *J Bone Joint Surg.* 2012;94(14):1326–1337.

Bril V, England J, Franklin G, et al. Evidence-based guideline: treatment of painful diabetic neuropathy: Report of the American Academy of Neurology, the American Association of Neuromuscular and Electrodiagnostic Medicine, and the American Academy of Physical Medicine and Rehabilitation. *Neurology.* 2011;76(20):1758–1765.

Cutts S, Obi N, Pasapula C, Chan W. Plantar fasciitis. *Ann R Coll Surg Engl.* 2012;94:539–542.

Mulhem E, Pinelis S. Treatment of nongenital cutaneous warts. *Am Fam Physician.* 2011;84(3):288–293.

Patel D, Roth M, Kapil N. Stress fractures: diagnosis, treatment and prevention. *Am Fam Physician.* 2011;83(1):39–46.

Sinusas K. Osteoarthritis: diagnosis and treatment. *Am Fam Physician.* 2012;85(1):49–56.

28   Fractures

Ted C. Schaffer, MD, & Melanie C. Schaffer, MD

KEY POINTS

- After trauma, one should assume a fracture has occurred and immobilize the affected region until x-rays have been obtained. (SOR ☉)
- The hallmark symptom of a new fracture is pain. Although the amount of pain correlates poorly with fracture severity, the absence of pain with an abnormal x-ray result makes it unlikely that a fracture has occurred. (SOR ☉)
- When x-ray results are negative but clinical suspicion for a fracture is high, a magnetic resonance imaging scan (high cost with high sensitivity/specificity) can provide supplemental information. (SOR ☉)
- While there is a great deal of variability depending on fracture location and individual physiologic status, a rough guide for clinical fracture healing is 3–4 weeks for pediatric patients and 4–6 weeks for adult patients. (SOR ☉)

  I. **Definition.** A fracture is a complete or incomplete break in the continuity of a bone. Fractures can be caused by direct trauma, repetitive forces to a bone (stress fracture), or abnormal bone architecture (e.g., osteoporosis or bone tumors).
 II. **Common Diagnoses.** Evaluation of musculoskeletal injuries that are potential fractures accounts for 3% to 5% of all office visits. A fracture should be differentiated from a **sprain** (joint injury to the ligaments attaching to the bone), a **strain** (injury to the musculotendinous unit that attaches to the bone), and a **contusion** (injury to the soft tissue surrounding the bone). Conditions associated with fractures include **dislocations** (complete loss of continuity between two articular surfaces) and **subluxations** (partial loss of continuity).

   As many as 1% of newborns sustain a fractured clavicle at the time of delivery. In **childhood,** the incidence of long bone fractures increases, with common areas including buckle fractures of the forearm, clavicle fractures, and growth plate injuries. Common **adult** trauma includes finger, metacarpal, and wrist fractures, as well as fractures of the ankle, metatarsals, and toes. The **elderly** are at greater risk for osteoporotic fractures such as vertebral, hip, and wrist fractures.

   Stress fractures are caused by repeated stresses that individually would not be strong enough to cause a fracture. The repeated nature of the stress causes a fracture. Stress fractures are more common in athletes and military recruits.

   A pathologic fracture is due to a loss of strength in a bone from a disease process that affects the strength of the bone. Examples include infections, tumors (either primary bone tumors or bony metastases), or bone cysts.
III. **Signs and Symptoms**
   A. **Pain** is the hallmark of new fracture occurrence. The amount of pain experienced by the patient, however, often correlates poorly with the amount of bone damage. In children, pain at an epiphyseal plate is usually a fracture, not a joint sprain, since the growth plate is often the weakest area when a joint is stressed.
   B. **Loss of motion** can occur with fractures, especially when the fracture is located near a joint surface.
   C. **Loss of function** may be noted by the patient, either because of the pain involved or because of soft tissue swelling.
   D. **Tenderness** to palpation should be present over a new fracture site. If there appears to be radiographic evidence of a fracture but the area is not tender on examination, the diagnosis of a fracture is unlikely. Such findings could represent a previously healed fracture or accessory bones.
   E. **Swelling, deformity, or ecchymosis** may be apparent when the area of injury is inspected. The deformity may appear either as an obvious angulation at the bone or as an abnormal manner in which the extremity is being held.

F. Abnormal mobility may be observed. Motion of the joint above and below the injured area should always be tested to ensure that these adjacent regions are not also affected by the injury.

IV. Imaging

A. An **x-ray** of any suspected fracture must be performed, since this is the method by which most fractures are confirmed. At least two views directed 90 degrees apart are required, since a nondisplaced fracture may not be visible if only a single view is obtained. Comparison x-rays of the opposite limb can be obtained in children to aid the physician in distinguishing a fracture line from a normal epiphyseal growth plate.

1. Ottawa Ankle Rules are well-established clinical guidelines used to determine the need for radiography in ankle injury (SOR **Ⓐ**). Ankle or foot radiography is indicated if any of the characteristics shown in Table 28–1 are observed.

B. When clinical suspicion for a fracture is great but initial x-ray results are negative, the area can be immobilized and x-rays repeated in 7 to 14 days to look for a new fracture line. If a fracture diagnosis is more urgent, then a **bone scan** or **magnetic resonance imaging (MRI)** scan can be obtained. MRI is more costly than bone scintigraphy, but its high degree of sensitivity and specificity has made it the diagnostic test of choice for many physicians when initial x-ray results are negative, suspicion of fracture remains, and an early diagnosis is important for management. Bone scans have a high degree of sensitivity but lack the specificity of MRI and do not provide information about surrounding soft tissue injuries.

V. Treatment

A. General principles for the management of a potential fracture are as follows:

1. The physician should **assume a fracture has occurred** until an x-ray has proven otherwise.

2. A **splint** should be applied to the injured area in order to decrease bone motion and hold the bone in place. This procedure will alleviate pain and prevent further tissue damage.

3. Elevation of the injured extremity will help reduce pain and swelling.

4. Ice applied immediately for 20 to 30 minutes will curtail swelling and provide pain relief. The ice should not directly touch the skin. Ice therapy may be repeated at 90-minute intervals.

5. Most **dislocations** should not be reduced until x-rays have been taken. Reduction before x-ray is advisable when there is evidence of vascular compromise to an extremity that may be relieved by immediate reduction of the dislocation or fracture. Immediate posttraumatic reduction of a dislocation is also permissible when the patient is having substantial pain and the reduction is easily accomplished, such as in an anterior shoulder or finger dislocation.

B. A period of immobilization will be necessary for most fractures, especially those of an extremity.

1. Historically, a circumferential cast has been used for most long bone fractures, including those around the wrist and ankle. However, new data suggest that a

---

TABLE 28–1. OTTAWA ANKLE AND FOOT RULES FOR DETERMINING NEED FOR X-RAY

Obtain an ankle x-ray if the following are present:
Pain in malleolar zone
Plus
Bone tenderness over areas of potential fracture (especially posterior edge or tip of lateral or medial malleolus)
Or
Inability to bear weight for four steps immediately after the injury and in the emergency department or physician's office

Obtain a foot x-ray if the following are present:
Pain in midfoot zone
Plus
Bone tenderness over areas of potential fracture (especially base of the fifth metatarsal or the navicular bone of the midfoot)
Or
Inability to bear weight for four steps immediately after the injury and in the emergency department or physician's office

fitted removable splint may improve function and reduce complications associated with casting. This has been most studied in pediatric buckle fractures of the wrist. (SOR **B**)

2. Time for immobilization will depend on several factors including the age of the patient and the fracture location. An approximate guideline is to immobilize children for 3 to 4 weeks and adults for 4 to 6 weeks.

C. The following **specific fractures** can be managed in an ambulatory setting:

1. Finger fractures

    a. Distal phalangeal fractures are usually crush injuries, which can be managed by immobilization and protection. If the extensor tendon has been involved, then a mallet finger injury has occurred (see Chapter 33).

    b. Middle and proximal phalangeal fractures can be managed if the injury is nondisplaced, without angulation or rotation. Fracture angulation is evident on x-ray and is caused by the pull of intrinsic hand muscles as they attach to the bone. Rotation is evaluated by having patients flex their fingers into the palm and observing that the fingers remain parallel and do not overlap. Nondisplaced fractures should be treated with a finger splint on the flexor surface for 2 to 4 weeks, keeping the PIP (proximal interphalangeal) joint at 30- to 50-degree flexion and the DIP (distal interphalangeal) joint at 10- to 20-degree flexion.

    c. PIP joint dislocations often occur with a hyperextension injury, causing a dorsal dislocation of the middle phalanx on the proximal phalanx (a coach's finger). These are usually easily reduced by **gentle** traction and **gentle** hyperextension, followed by a flexor surface splint for 2 to 4 weeks.

2. Metacarpal fractures

    a. Fractures of the neck of the fifth metacarpal (boxer's fracture) commonly occur after punching a person or wall. An ulnar gutter splint extending from midforearm to the fingertip is applied for 3 to 6 weeks, keeping the MCP (metacarpal phalangeal) joint at 90-degree flexion. (SOR **B**)

    b. Fractures of the shaft of the fourth and fifth metacarpals can be treated with an ulnar gutter splint if there is angulation less than 30 degrees and no rotational injury.

    c. Fractures of the first, second, and third metacarpals generally require orthopedic referral because of functional problems related to residual angulation.

3. Wrist and arm fractures

    a. The **scaphoid** is the most common wrist fracture. Those that involve the distal scaphoid (5% of fractures) or middle scaphoid (80% of fractures) have a good blood supply and can be immobilized for 8 to 12 weeks with a long-arm (extending above the elbow) or a short-arm cast (extending to the proximal forearm); the thumb must be immobilized to the level of the IP (interphalangeal) joint. Fractures of the proximal scaphoid have a poor blood supply and a high risk of nonunion and are therefore referred to an orthopedic surgeon.

    b. Nondisplaced distal radial fractures can be treated with short-arm cast immobilization for 6 weeks in adults. The cast should extend from the metacarpals to the proximal forearm, with the thumb allowed free mobility.

    c. Children more commonly sustain a nondisplaced fracture of the radius above the growth plate, which is known as a **buckle fracture**. The patient should wear a short-arm cast or fitted splint for 3 to 4 weeks. Immobilization should extend from the metacarpal heads to the proximal forearm.

    d. Proximal radial head fractures near the elbow can also occur with a fall on an outstretched hand. Unless there is x-ray evidence of a displaced radial head, these fractures can be managed with a long-arm splint extending along the ulnar surface from the metacarpals to the proximal humerus, with the elbow at 90-degree flexion. The splint should be maintained for 2 to 4 weeks with early mobilization to maintain elbow motion, especially in the elderly.

    e. Humeral head fractures are common in elderly individuals after falling on an outstretched arm or sustaining a blow to the lateral arm. Eighty percent of proximal humerus fractures are minimally displaced. Treatment, even if the shaft of the humerus is impacted, consists of providing the patient with a shoulder sling for 1 to 2 weeks and, after the sling is removed, providing the patient with range-of-motion exercises. (SOR **A**) The major risk in humeral head fractures of the elderly is loss of shoulder motion after immobilization. Orthopedic referral is needed if there is ≥1 cm fracture displacement between the proximal and distal components.

4. **Clavicle fractures**
   a. **Middle third (midclavicular) fractures** account for 80% of clavicle fractures and most are easily managed. While previous treatment utilized a "figure-of-eight" clavicular strap, more recent data suggest that a simple sling is just as effective and more comfortable. (SOR **Ⓐ**) Immobilization is usually required for 3 to 6 weeks for children and for 6 weeks for adults. A residual callus is often left, but the fracture usually heals well. If there is complete separation of the fracture fragments, surgical treatment may be warranted.
   b. **Distal fractures,** which account for 15% of all fractures, can be more complicated than midclavicular fractures. If the fracture is nondisplaced, the initial management is the same and can be performed by the family physician. However, painful acromioclavicular joint arthritis may develop, especially if the fracture is displaced, necessitating orthopedic resection of the distal clavicle.
   c. **Proximal fractures** occur in 5% of cases and should be evaluated carefully. The physician should look for signs of vascular injury owing to the close proximity of the great vessels of the neck. Orthopedic consultation should be strongly considered.

5. **Simple torso fractures**
   a. **Rib fractures** are common in the elderly only with minor trauma. In young adults and children, they are usually the result of greater traumatic force. A chest x-ray should be obtained to exclude pneumothorax or pulmonary contusion. Rib fractures are easily managed if the bones are not displaced.
      (1) **Pain relief** is the main focus of treatment. Oral systemic narcotics (e.g., hydrocodone, 5–10 mg four times daily [often given in combination with acetaminophen which should be limited to 4 g per day]) and **nonsteroidal agents** (e.g., ibuprofen, 600 mg three times daily) are usually adequate, but **intercostal nerve blocks** (usually done by an anesthesiologist) can be considered if a patient is in severe pain. Rib belts should be avoided, since they cause substantial atelectasis and increase the incidence of pneumonia.
      (2) **Hospitalization** should be considered for multiple rib fractures (three or more) because of the increased risk of pulmonary contusion and atelectasis. In the elderly, even a single rib fracture can occasionally lead to pulmonary compromise.
   b. **Vertebral compression fractures** are common in elderly patients with osteoporosis and can occur with minimal trauma. They can be seen from the T-4 through L-5 vertebrae, and neurologic compromise is extremely rare. Treatment is aimed at pain relief, with immobilization for a few days followed by ambulation with a support such as a lumbosacral garment. Calcitonin (intramuscular, subcutaneous, or via nasal spray) can be used in the immediate postfracture period to treat back pain associated with an acute vertebral compression fracture (reduces pain by 1 week); there is a controversy over the use of calcitonin for long-term treatment as reduction in fracture has not been demonstrated and concern about increased cancer risk has been raised.
   c. **Nondisplaced pelvic fractures** are another problem in the elderly, occasionally complicated by blood loss, even with minor fractures. Treatment is aimed at pain relief (see above) and ambulatory support with devices such as a walker or cane until pain resolves.

6. **Leg fractures**
   a. **Hip fracture** after a minor fall is common in the elderly and associated with a mortality rate of 15% to 20% within 6 months of the injury. While hip fractures usually present with pain, shortening, and external rotation, nondisplaced fractures can present with referred knee pain. While diagnosis on plain films is often obvious, MRI may be needed for more subtle nondisplaced fractures. Early surgical intervention will help reduce morbidity. Femoral neck fractures in the elderly are treated with total hip arthroplasty. While younger patients with a fracture due to high-velocity trauma can be treated with other surgeries, these have a high risk of avascular necrosis due to the precarious blood supply of this region. Intertrochanteric fractures are associated with significant blood loss.

    b. Special pediatric problems of the hip, including Legg–Calve–Perthes disease and slipped capital femoral epiphysis are covered elsewhere (see Chapter 41).

    c. Femoral shaft fractures, while less common, have a number of etiologies including avulsion injuries, stress fractures, pathologic fractures from primary bone tumors or metastatic cancer, and high-impact trauma. When nondisplaced, many can be managed by nonoperative means, but they generally require orthopedic consultation.

    d. Tibial fractures are the most common long-bone fracture. Because of its weight-bearing function, near-perfect alignment must be maintained for traumatic fractures, otherwise surgery will be needed. Most stress fractures of the tibia can be managed nonoperatively by the family physician, with the exception of a stress fracture of the anterior medial cortex, "the dreaded black line," which is higher risk for both nonunion and recurrence. The toddler's fracture, a spiral fracture in children aged 9 months to 3 years, requires distinction from a similar fracture related to child abuse and is managed nonoperatively by casting.

7. Ankle fractures

    a. Fibular fractures below the tibial dome are avulsion fractures caused by ligamentous pulling during sudden foot inversion. Treatment is a posterior leg splint for 5 to 7 days until the swelling has subsided, followed by a short leg walking cast for 4 to 6 weeks. A pneumatic ankle support (e.g., Aircast) can be considered as an alternative to casting, since ankle inversion/eversion will be protected. In children, tenderness over the epiphyseal plate of the distal fibula should be regarded as a Salter I fracture (see Figure 28–1), not an ankle sprain. Treatment consists of a short leg walking cast or walking boot for 3 to 4 weeks.

    b. When fibular fractures are **at or above the tibial dome,** greater ligamentous instability occurs because the syndesmotic ligaments and interosseous membrane are involved. Referral is indicated in these cases, since surgery may be required.

8. Foot and toe fractures

    a. Second, third, and fourth metatarsal fractures often occur as stress fractures from overuse. Frequently, initial x-ray results are negative, but repeat films in

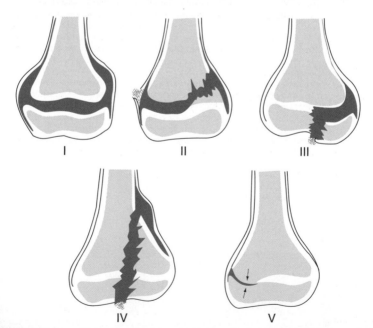

FIGURE 28–1. Salter–Harris classification of epiphyseal injuries in children. (Reproduced with permission from Doherty GM, Way LW, eds. *Current Surgical Diagnosis & Treatment.* 12th ed. Originally published by Appleton & Lange; 2006. Copyright © 2006 by the McGraw-Hill Companies, Inc.)

2 to 4 weeks show healing callus. The treatment is relative rest and use of a hard-soled shoe for 2 to 4 weeks until pain subsides. Patient education is important to prevent recurrent injury.

   b. Fifth metatarsal fractures can be treated nonoperatively if they are within 1.5 cm of the proximal styloid tip. These are avulsion injuries that respond to relative rest and a hard-soled shoe. Distal fifth metatarsal fractures have a high incidence of nonunion, often require operative intervention, and are best referred to someone with management experience.

   c. Toe fractures are common, and generally require just buddy-taping to an adjacent toe for 1 to 2 weeks to provide symptomatic relief. A small piece of gauze or tissue should be placed between the toes to prevent skin maceration.

D. Special features of **pediatric fractures** are described below.

   1. The time needed for **cast or splint immobilization** for fractures in children is generally one-half to one-third the time needed for immobilization of an adult fracture, since bone healing occurs much faster in children than in adults.

   2. The **Salter–Harris classification** of pediatric fractures should be understood (see Figure 28–1).

      a. Salter I fractures through the epiphyseal plate are a clinical diagnosis, often with normal x-ray findings. The prognosis is excellent. Salter II fractures through the metaphysis are also stable injuries. Nondisplaced Salter I and II fractures are treated like any other fracture, with cast or splint immobilization for several weeks.

      b. Salter III and IV fractures, which involve the epiphysis, and Salter V fractures, which are crush injuries to the growth plates, are more serious problems, especially when they involve long bones of the body.

      c. Parents of children with growth plate injuries should be advised of the possibility of growth abnormalities. These abnormalities are quite rare with Salter I and II fractures, except when the fractures are in the distal femur or tibia.

      d. In children, tenderness at the growth plate is assumed to be a bony injury rather than a ligamentous sprain, since the ligaments are stronger than the bone at this age. Immobilization often with casting is indicated, depending on the bone involved. Common growth plate fractures include the ankle and wrist.

E. Fractures requiring referral. In an ambulatory setting, the physician must know which injuries should be managed by an orthopedist because of the increased risk of complication. The following list serves as a guideline for situations in which consultation is advisable.

   1. Open fractures increase the risk of infection, especially osteomyelitis, and fracture nonunion.

   2. Neurovascular compromise is an orthopedic emergency necessitating immediate care by a qualified surgeon.

   3. Unstable fractures, where bone alignment cannot be maintained without external forces, usually require open reduction and internal fixation.

   4. Intra-articular fractures create a high risk for the development of long-term traumatic arthritis. Open surgical reduction is often required in order to achieve the best possible bone alignment.

   5. Growth plate injuries of long bones that involve the epiphysis (Salter III, IV, or V fractures) create a high risk of complications, and therefore, the patient may require long-term orthopedic management.

SELECTED REFERENCES

Eiff MP, Hatch RL. *Fracture Management for Primary Care*. 3rd ed. Elsevier Saunders; 2012.

Lenza M, Belloti JC, Andriolo RB, et al. Conservative interventions for treating collarbone fractures in adolescents and adults. *Cochrane Database Syst Rev.* 2009;(2):CD007121.

Knopp-Sihota JA, Newburn-Cook CV, Homik J, et al. Calcitonin for treating acute and chronic pain of recent and remote osteoporotic vertebral compression fractures: a systematic review and meta-analysis. *Osteoporos Int.* 2012;23(1):17–38.

Tiemstra JD. Update on acute ankle sprains. *Am Fam Physician.* 2012;85(12):1170–1176.

Patient Education

Safran MR, Zachazewski J, Stone DA. *Instructions for Sports Medicine Patients.* 2nd ed. Philadelphia, PA: Elsevier; 2012.

29   Gastrointestinal Bleeding

Erin C. Contratto, MD, & May S. Jennings, MD

KEY POINTS

- Initial assessment of hemodynamic status and appropriate triage of patients with gastrointestinal (GI) bleeding are strongly linked to patient outcomes. (SOR **B**)
- The majority of cases (80%) of GI bleeding will resolve spontaneously with appropriate supportive care. (SOR **C**)
- The risk of further upper GI bleeding can be minimized by changes in lifestyle and use of medications. (SOR **B**)

I. **Definition.** Gastrointestinal (GI) bleeding is blood loss from any part of the GI tract, including both symptomatic and occult blood loss.

II. **Common Diagnoses.** The incidence of GI bleeding increases with age. Each year in the United States, over 1% of adults over 80 years of age require hospitalization for GI bleeding.

   A. **Upper GI (UGI) bleeding** is defined as any GI bleeding proximal to the ligament of Treitz (duodenojejunal junction) and is approximately five times more common than lower GI (LGI) bleeding.

   1. **Peptic ulcer disease** is the most common cause of UGI bleeding, comprising >60% of cases. Risk factors include nonsteroidal anti-inflammatory drugs (NSAIDs), clopidogrel, warfarin, selective serotonin reuptake inhibitors (SSRIs), corticosteroids, alcohol, *Helicobacter pylori* infection, and excess acid production. About 25% of chronic NSAID users develop gastroduodenal ulcers and as many as 2% to 4% of patients with an NSAID ulcer will bleed or perforate. Each year, NSAIDs account for at least 100,000 hospitalizations and between 7000 and 10,000 deaths in the United States.

   2. **Gastritis** is the presence of subepithelial hemorrhages and erosions in the gastric mucosa. It is associated with NSAIDs, alcohol, corticosteroids, and critical illness.

   3. **Esophagitis** is the presence of mucosal injury to the esophagus. It is commonly associated with drug-induced injury.

   4. **Mallory–Weiss tear,** also known as gastroesophageal laceration syndrome, refers to bleeding from tears in the gastroesophageal junction usually caused by recurrent or severe retching, vomiting, or coughing. It represents 5% of UGI bleeding.

   5. **Esophageal and gastric varices** are caused by increased venous collateral flow from the portal circulation, usually as a complication of cirrhosis. Varices are only responsible for approximately 6% of UGI bleeding, but the overall mortality rate from bleeding varices is >30%.

   6. **Dieulafoy lesion** refers to a dilated submucosal artery. These lesions are more common in the gastric cardia. Rupture is rare, but can result in a severe GI bleeding.

   7. **Aortoenteric fistula** occurs in approximately 0.5% of patients with aortoiliac bypass surgery. Fistulas are most common in the duodenum but can occur anywhere throughout the GI tract.

   8. **Gastric antral vascular ectasia** (watermelon stomach) refers to dilation of small blood vessels in the gastric antrum and is associated with end-stage renal disease and cirrhosis.

   B. **LGI bleeding** is defined as any GI bleeding distal to the ligament of Treitz.

   1. **Diverticulosis** is the most common cause of significant LGI bleeding in older adults. Approximately 60% of all US adults older than 60 years have diverticula (sac-like protrusions of the colonic wall). Bleeding is arterial in origin and hemorrhage can be significant. Three to five percent of patients with diverticula develop an acute GI bleed.

   2. **Vascular ectasias** (angiodysplasias) are degenerative lesions of previously normal blood vessels, resulting in dilated and tortuous vessels that are prone to rupture. Bleeding is venous in origin. Vascular ectasias are most commonly found in the cecum and right colon and are the second most common cause of LGI bleeding in older adults.

3. **Colitis** refers to acute mucosal injury of the colonic wall caused by infection, inflammation, radiation, or ischemia. Infectious causes of colitis include viruses (e.g., norovirus, rotavirus), parasites (e.g., *Entamoeba histolytica*), and bacteria (e.g., *Clostridium difficile, Salmonella, Shigella,* and *Vibrio* organisms). Ischemic colitis is often precipitated by hypotension and is more commonly localized to watershed areas of the colon (e.g., splenic flexure, right colon, or rectosigmoid colon).
4. **Neoplasms and polyps** usually cause occult GI bleeding. Colon cancer is responsible for approximately 10% of LGI bleeding cases in patients >50 years old. The risk of post-polypectomy bleeding is increased in patients >65 years old.
5. **Hemorrhoids,** both external and internal, are associated with constipation and straining. They are the most common cause of LGI bleeding in patients <50 years old but rarely cause significant LGI bleeding.
6. **Anal fissure** is a tear in the anal dermis caused by excess stretching of the anal mucosa. It is associated with blood coating the stool after a painful bowel movement and causes minor LGI bleeding.

C. **Obscure GI bleeding** is defined as bleeding from a source not identified after upper and lower endoscopic evaluation. Likely sources include vascular ectasias and lesions in the small bowel including duodenitis, celiac sprue, and Crohn disease.

D. **UGI bleeding in children** comprises approximately 20% of GI bleeding. Etiology in Western countries is very similar to etiology of UGI bleeding in adults (see above).

E. **LGI bleeding in children.** Significant LGI bleeding is not common and etiology is dependent on age.
1. **Meckel diverticulum** is a congenital abnormality due to incomplete obliteration of the omphalomesenteric duct and is the most common cause of significant GI bleeding in children. It occurs in 2% of the population and is usually found within 2 feet of the ileocecal valve. Sixty percent of patients with Meckel diverticulum present with upper or LGI bleeding at ages 2 years or younger.
2. **Intussusception** is the second most common cause of significant LGI bleeding in children. It is caused by the involution of one segment of the bowel into another segment of the bowel.
3. **Juvenile polyps** usually present in children aged 2 to 8 years. These polyps are often benign but can be associated with familial polyposis syndromes.
4. **Colitis** is usually caused by infection, inflammation, or allergy. Milk- or soy-induced allergic colitis is more common in infants. Inflammatory bowel disease often presents in school-aged children (see Chapter 78).
5. **Mesenteric ischemia** can be acute or chronic (intestinal angina) and is associated with abdominal pain more often than rectal bleeding.
6. **Anal fissure or rectal foreign bodies** are associated with minor rectal bleeding in children.

RARE BUT SERIOUS CONDITIONS

Vomiting, pain, and blood in the stool of a young child are suggestive of intussusception.

History of an aortic aneurysm repair or aortic bypass suggests a potentially life-threatening aortoenteric fistula, usually to the duodenum, as the cause of GI bleeding.

III. **Symptoms and Signs**
A. **Bleeding history**
1. **Hematemesis** is the vomiting of blood. A careful history should be taken to exclude nasopharyngeal bleeding and hemoptysis.
2. **Melena** refers to black, tarry stools and suggests an UGI source in 80% to 90% of cases. Medications containing iron or bismuth can darken the stools and be misinterpreted as melena.
3. **Hematochezia** is passing fresh blood through the rectum. It indicates an LGI source in 85% of cases. However, a very brisk UGI bleeding can present with rectal bleeding.

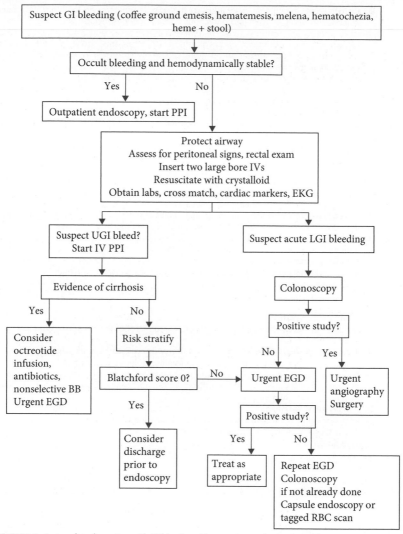

FIGURE 29–1. Approach to the patient with GI bleeding. GI, gastrointestinal; U, upper; L, lower; IV, intravenous; PPI, proton pump inhibitor; EGD, esophagogastroduodenoscopy; BB, beta-blocker.

4. **Currant jelly stool** is blood, mucus, and stool in combination. It is associated with intussusception or acute colitis.
5. Formed stool mixed with blood suggests anorectal bleeding.

B. General history
1. **Confusion, dizziness, or syncope.** Any recent history represents a hemodynamically unstable patient who requires urgent attention (see Figure 29–1).
2. **Abdominal pain.** Epigastric pain and UGI bleeding are consistent with peptic ulcer disease or gastritis. Crampy pain and LGI bleeding suggest colitis in adults. Severe abdominal pain in children suggests Meckel diverticulum or intussusception. Bowel perforation should always be considered in patients with severe pain.
3. **Coughing, vomiting, or retching.** These symptoms suggest Mallory–Weiss tear.
4. **Dysphagia or indigestion** is associated with esophagitis.

5. Number of stools. Quantifying stools may be helpful in determining the rate of the bleeding.

6. History of prior GI bleeding. Although not always accurate, a history of a prior UGI bleeding is suggestive of a current UGI source, whereas a history of LGI bleeding makes an upper source less likely.

7. Atherosclerotic disease. Atherosclerotic disease such as coronary artery disease or peripheral vascular disease increases the risk that the bleeding source is ischemic colitis.

8. Medications: NSAIDs, warfarin, clopidogrel, aspirin, SSRIs, corticosteroids, and alcohol. NSAID use increases the risk of UGI bleeding by threefold to fivefold, depending on the specific medication. (SOR **Ⓐ**) SSRIs can inhibit platelet aggregation.

9. Weight loss suggests malignancy. Colon carcinoma is suggested by weight loss plus a change in bowel habits.

C. Vital signs. Orthostasis (rise in pulse by 20 beats per minute and a fall in systolic blood pressure by 20 mmHg when standing) indicates hemodynamic instability and rapid bleeding. The presence of orthostasis represents approximately 15% blood loss and a clinical emergency. Supine hypotension represents a 40% blood loss. Beta-blockers can mask tachycardia normally associated with hemodynamic instability.

D. Mentation. Altered mental status is an ominous finding and should be considered a sign of hypovolemic shock until proven otherwise.

E. Abdominal examination

1. Peritoneal signs or severe tenderness raise suspicion for bowel perforation.

2. Pain that is disproportional to the abdominal examination suggests acute mesenteric ischemia.

F. Rectal examination should be performed in all patients with GI bleeding. This includes the following:

1. Inspection and digital examination for masses, hemorrhoids, and anal fissures.

2. Examination of retrieved stool for melena and hematochezia. Presence of melena on examination is the most useful finding to suggest an UGI bleeding source. If no obvious bleeding is noted, stool guaiac testing should be performed.

a. Stools will appear black (not tarry) after ingestion of iron or bismuth subsalicylate.

b. Ingestion of tomatoes, rare meat, and cherries can cause a false-positive stool guaiac study.

c. Guaiac-positive stools can continue for up to 3 weeks after an acute bleeding episode.

G. Sequelae of chronic liver disease including spider angiomas, ascites, caput medusa, palmar erythema, jaundice, and splenomegaly raises suspicion for variceal bleeding (see Chapter 72).

H. A **nasogastric (NG) tube** can be placed to differentiate UGI bleeding from LGI bleeding. However, NG lavage has poor sensitivity in detecting UGI bleeding in patients presenting with melena or hematochezia. (SOR **Ⓒ**) Bright red blood or "coffee ground" material in the NG tube suggests an UGI source. A clear NG or bilious NG lavage does not rule out UGI bleeding. (SOR **Ⓒ**) There is no contraindication to NG tube placement in patients with known or suspected esophageal varices. (SOR **Ⓒ**) Guaiac testing of the NG aspirate is not recommended. (SOR **Ⓒ**)

IV. Tests

A. Endoscopy (esophagogastroduodenoscopy [EGD] or colonoscopy) is the first step in further evaluation of most patients with GI bleeding. (SOR **Ⓐ**) In addition to localizing the source of bleeding, endoscopy allows therapeutic interventions including banding of varices, mucosal biopsy to diagnose *H. pylori*, sclerotherapy, cauterization, and snaring of polyps.

1. In patients with hematochezia and hemodynamic instability, EGD should precede colonoscopy (Figure 29–1). (SOR **Ⓑ**) Thirteen percent of patients presenting with hematochezia have an UGI bleeding source.

2. Pre-endoscopic treatment with promotility agents such as erythromycin and metoclopramide has been shown to decrease the need for repeat endoscopy and can be considered. (SOR **Ⓒ**) Similarly, colonic preparation with polyethylene glycol prior to colonoscopy may increase the diagnostic yield of colonoscopy in cases of LGI bleeding. (SOR **Ⓒ**)

3. In patients older than 40 years with occult GI bleeding (guaiac-positive stool with minimal or no symptoms), colonoscopy is indicated. After a negative colonoscopy, further workup may not be productive, unless iron-deficiency anemia is present (see Chapter 4).

4. In patients younger than 40 years with minor rectal bleeding, anoscopy (see Chapter 51) or sigmoidoscopy that reveals a likely cause is often a sufficient workup.

5. EGD performed within 24 hours of UGI bleeding onset improves patient outcomes and length of hospital stay. Very early endoscopy (<12 hours from bleeding onset) has not been proven to reduce recurrence of bleeding or need for surgery or to improve mortality compared to later endoscopy (within 24 hours) in patients with nonvariceal bleeding. (SOR **B**)

B. Hematologic studies

1. Hemoglobin and hematocrit will be normal early in acute bleeding. A low hematocrit and a low mean corpuscular volume without hemodynamic compromise suggests slow, chronic bleeding. A hemoglobin level of <8 g/dL increases the likelihood of severe bleeding. (SOR **B**)

2. A blood urea nitrogen (BUN) to creatine ratio ≥30 suggests UGI bleeding.

3. Prothrombin time, partial thromboplastin time, and platelet count assess possible contribution of coagulopathy or thrombocytopenia to the bleeding.

C. An electrocardiogram is recommended in adults, especially those with known coronary artery disease, especially if they are hemodynamically unstable (Figure 29–1). (SOR **C**)

D. Barium studies are contraindicated in the setting of acute bleeding because they can interfere with additional evaluation.

E. Technetium red cell scan is highly sensitive and detects bleeding at a rate of 0.1 to 0.5 mL/min. This test can identify GI bleeding anywhere throughout the GI tract, but can only localize bleeding to a generalized area. This scan is the procedure of choice in confirming Meckel diverticulum.

F. Angiography should be considered in patients with emergent GI bleeding that might not be visualized with endoscopy. Angiography can detect bleeding at a rate of 0.3 to 0.5 mL/min. It is highly sensitive and allows therapeutic intervention during the procedure. However, angiography cannot localize slow bleeds and carries the risk of radiation and contrast exposure.

G. Video capsule endoscopy (wireless capsule endoscopy) can be used to identify sources of obscure GI bleeding and has a diagnostic yield of approximately 60%. It is safe to use in patients with pacemakers and implantable defibrillators. The most common source identified by this method is angiodysplasia.

H. Double-balloon enteroscopy is used to identify and treat lesions in patients with obscure GI bleeding. This test has a diagnostic yield of approximately 65%.

V. Treatment. GI bleeding is an emergency until proven otherwise.

A. Risk stratification. A well-validated risk stratification score (Blatchford or Rockall score) should be completed on patients presenting with nonvariceal UGI bleeding to assess prognosis. Patients with a Blatchford score of 0 (BUN <18.2, hemoglobin >13 g/dL for men and >12 g/dL for women, systolic blood pressure >109 mmHg, pulse <100 beats per minute, and no history of melena, syncope, and liver or heart disease) can be considered for discharge prior to endoscopy. (SOR **B**)

B. Hospitalization is always indicated for those with signs or symptoms of hemodynamic instability and those with melena or comorbid disease. (SOR **B**) Hospitalization is also recommended for elderly patients because of poor functional reserves and frequent comorbidities. (SOR **B**) The inpatient setting allows for aggressive intravenous fluid resuscitation, transfusion (packed red blood cells, fresh frozen plasma, or platelets as indicated), efficient localization of bleeding source (see Section IV), and initiation of specific therapy (e.g., octreotide for acute variceal bleeding). **Surgery** is a last resort for bleeding that is uncontrolled with other interventions.

1. Blood products. Packed red blood cell transfusion is indicated for patients who are actively bleeding or have a hemoglobin level <7 g/dL. A restrictive transfusion strategy, with target hemoglobin of 7 g/dL, is associated with improved mortality in patients with UGI hemorrhage. (SOR **B**) Correction of coagulopathy prior to endoscopy is advised but should not delay endoscopic therapy. (SOR **B**)

2. Pharmacologic therapy. Proton pump inhibitors (PPIs) started prior to endoscopy decrease the need for endoscopic therapies but do not affect mortality, risk of rebleeding, or need for surgery. Intravenous PPIs should be started on patients with acute

TABLE 29–1. INITIAL PREDICTORS OF POOR CLINICAL OUTCOME IN GI BLEEDING[a]

Age ≥60 years
Comorbidities
  Cirrhosis
  Malignancy
  Heart disease
Medications
  Warfarin
  Corticosteroids
Examination
  Melena
  Hemodynamic instability
  Bloody nasogastric aspirate
Laboratory tests
  Elevated liver function tests
  Elevated prothrombin time
  Hypoalbuminemia
  Thrombocytopenia
  White blood cell count $>12 \times 10^9$/L
  Blood urea nitrogen >90 mg/dL
  Hemoglobin ≤8 mg/dL
  Electrocardiographic changes

[a]Poor clinical outcome is defined as risk of rebleeding and risk of death.

UGI bleeding due to confirmed peptic ulcers. (SOR ❸) Medical treatment for acute variceal hemorrhage includes intravenous somatostatin analogs to reduce splanchnic circulation and broad-spectrum antibiotics (ceftriaxone, ciprofloxacin) to reduce mortality and risk of rebleeding in addition to nonselective beta-blockers for primary and secondary prevention, when the patient is hemodynamically stable. (SOR ❸)

C. Outpatient management is appropriate for patients with occult bleeding and no high-risk features of a poor clinical outcome (see Table 29–1).

D. Preventive measures are often effective in minimizing recurrences, once the bleeding source has been identified and controlled (see Chapters 72 and 84). Patients with H. pylori confirmed peptic ulcer disease should be treated. If bleeding can be attributed to aspirin or NSAIDs, these medicines should be discontinued if possible. If NSAIDS or aspirin are continued, patients should be started on a PPI to suppress acid secretion.

E. Prognosis. In all types of GI bleeding, 80% resolve spontaneously with supportive care. (SOR ❸) Prognosis is largely dependent on compliance with preventative measures.

SELECTED REFERENCES

Barkun AN, Bardou M, Kulpers EJ, et al. International consensus recommendations on the management of patients with nonvariceal upper gastrointestinal bleeding. *Ann Intern Med.* 2010;152:101–113.

Management of acute upper and lower gastrointestinal bleeding. A national clinical guideline, 2008. http://www.guideline.gov/content.aspx?id=13167&search=gastrointestinal+bleeding. Accessed March 2013.

Srygley FD, Gerago CJ, Tran T, Fisher DA. Does this patient have a severe upper gastrointestinal bleed? *JAMA.* 2012;307(10):1072–1079.

Strate L. Approach to resuscitation and diagnosis of acute lower gastrointestinal bleeding in the adult patient. www.uptodate.com, online version 14.0. Accessed March 2013.

Strate L. Etiology of lower gastrointestinal bleeding in adults. www.uptodate.com, online version 9.0. Accessed March 2013.

Villa X. Approach to upper gastrointestinal bleeding in children. www.uptodate.com, online version 10.0. Accessed March 2013.

Villanueva C, Colomo A, Bosch A, et al. Transfusion strategies for acute upper gastrointestinal bleeding. *N Engl J Med.* 2013;368(1):11–21.

Wilkins T, Kahn N, Nabh A, Schade R. Diagnosis and management of upper gastrointestinal bleeding. *Am Fam Physician.* 2012;85(5):469–476.

Yachimski PS, Friedman LS. Gastrointestinal bleeding in the elderly. *Gastroenterol Hepatol.* 2008;5(2):80-90.

Additional references are available online at http://langetextbooks.com/fm6e

30   Genital Lesions

Tomás P. Owens, Jr., MD

KEY POINTS

- In evaluating patients with genital lesions, a history of sexual preferences/practices is important. (SOR **©**)
- Most genital lesions can be diagnosed by a careful history and examination, with minimal laboratory testing. (SOR **©**)
- Human immunodeficiency virus testing should always be considered in patients with genital lesions believed to be sexually transmitted. (SOR **©**)

I. **Definition.** Genital lesions are any acquired abnormality of the external genitalia.
II. **Common Diagnoses.** The 2010 National Ambulatory Medical Care Survey describes diseases of the skin and subcutaneous tissue as being the principal diagnosis in 4.4% of all office visits and diseases of the genitourinary system as 4.8% of all office visits.
   A. **Ulcerative lesions**
      1. **Herpes simplex virus types 1 and 2** (HSV-1 and -2). The presence of antibodies to **HSV-2** varies from 3% in nuns to 70% to 80% in prostitutes and is directly proportional to sexual activity and number of partners. **In the United States, about 17% of people are seropositive; of those, only 19% are aware of having the infection. HSV-1,** which is present in up to 90% of the population, can cause genital herpes, although less frequently.
      2. **Primary syphilis** (chancre). There has been a 90% decline in the number of cases reported in the United States from 1991 to 2000, and a slow and steady 9.5% increase has been noted since 2000. The highest incidence is reported among Blacks, Hispanics, and in the South; with the rate reaching 4.1/100,000 in 2010. There has been an upsurge in cases of men who have sex with men (MSM), along with a precipitous increase of the male-to-female ratio.
      3. **Chancroid,** caused by *Haemophilus ducreyi,* a gram-negative coccobacillary organism, is a rare condition with just eight cases reported in 2011.
   B. **Verrucous/papillomatous lesions**
      1. **Condylomata acuminata** caused by human papillomavirus, most commonly serotypes 6 and 11, are the most common sexually transmitted entity, although this condition can also be transmitted nonsexually via skin-to-skin contact or horizontal perinatal or postnatal transmission. Condylomata are most common during the reproductive years, are commonly associated with other sexually transmitted infections (STIs), and may grow dramatically with pregnancy, human immunodeficiency virus (HIV), or corticosteroid use.
      2. **Secondary syphilis** condyloma latum (see Section II.A.2).
      3. Genital lesions of **molluscum contagiosum** are associated with, but not always because of, sexual transmission. HIV infection is associated with an increased number and size of lesions.
      4. **Pearly penile papules** are present in up to 30% of men. There are no known predisposing risk factors.
   C. **Pruritic lesions**
      1. **Balanitis,** irritation of the glans penis, occurs most commonly in uncircumcised patients with diabetes and in those with poor hygiene. It can be precipitated by smegma and exogenous contact irritants.
      2. **Erythrasma** is a chronic bacterial infection that occurs more often in obese dark-skinned men.
      3. *Phthirus pubis* (pubic lice) occurs only in humans, most commonly in young adults. Public lice are highly contagious and can be transmitted sexually or by sharing clothing, towels, or bed linens. The lice prefer moist environments, seldom go into neighboring skin, and have been described rarely on facial hair.
      4. **Vulvar dystrophy/lichen sclerosus et atrophicus (LSA)** is a common process of unknown etiology that occurs in postmenopausal women but can be seen in all

age groups. In men, it is very rare and is called balanitis xerotica obliterans **(BXO)**. It is more common in middle-aged patients with diabetes, but can be seen in all age groups.

D. Cystic lesions. Bartholin gland cysts or inflammation occurs on either side of the lower vaginal vestibule. They account for 2% of all new patients in a gynecologic practice, are more common after menarche and before menopause, and are unrelated to STIs.

E. Other causes of genital lesions, discussed elsewhere, include psoriasis, seborrheic dermatitis, scabies, tinea cruris, and allergic/contact dermatitis (see Chapter 14); testicular torsion, epididymo-orchitis, and spermatocele/epididymal cyst/varicocele (see Chapter 55); folliculitis (see Chapter 9); urethritis (see Chapter 60); and vaginitis, cervicitis, and chlamydia (see Chapters 50, 63, and 102). Causes of genital lesions not discussed here because of their relative rarity include penile cancer, bowenoid papulosis of the penis/vulvar epithelial neoplasia, testicular cancer, lymphogranuloma venereum, granuloma inguinale, lichen planus, fixed drug eruption, erythroplasia of Queyrat, Peyronie disease, penile/vulvar trauma, penile prostheses, and priapism.

III. Symptoms

A. Ulcerative lesions

1. HSV-1 or -2

    a. The incubation period is 2 to 14 days. Primary infection, which is associated with viremia, may manifest as fever, generalized myalgia, malaise, headaches, and weakness, peaking 3 to 4 days after the onset of lesions. Painful inguinal or deep pelvic lymphadenopathy arises 2 to 3 weeks later. Burning pain and pruritus along with vaginal or urethral discharge and dysuria are common.

    b. There is a prodrome of burning or lancinating pain 1 to 2 days before eruption. Direct local inflammatory changes and cytolysis account for most of the syndrome in recurrences, which rarely cause systemic symptoms.

2. Chancres of syphilis are painless, unless secondarily infected. Patients present for evaluation of the lesion or accompanying lymphadenopathy. The genital lesions in **chancroid** are tender.

B. Verrucous/papillomatous lesions

1. Condylomata acuminata have an incubation period from weeks to years, are painless, and commonly recur during the first few years. Rarely, a patient may complain of hematuria from a urethral condyloma.

2. Condyloma lata from syphilis are painless lesions, although generalized myalgia, fever, chills, and arthralgia may occur in the early phase of eruption, which occurs 6 to 24 weeks after untreated primary syphilis or, rarely, synchronously with the chancre.

3. The lesions of **molluscum contagiosum** develop slowly over a 2- to 3-month period and rarely are pruritic.

4. Pearly penile papules are asymptomatic but worrisome to some patients.

C. Pruritic lesions

1. Balanitis is associated with pruritus and burning pain during or after sexual intercourse or with excessive smegma production. Dysuria and more severe pain occur with more severe disease.

2. Pruritus and long-standing rash persisting after fungicidal therapy are common presentations for **erythrasma**.

3. *Phthirus pubis* infestation manifests as pruritus, rarely severe. Some patients describe nits on their pubic hair or visible lice.

4. Patients with **vulvar dystrophy/LSA** and **BXO** present with varying degrees of pruritus and concerns about the lesion's appearance.

D. Small **Bartholin gland cysts** are usually asymptomatic. Larger lesions cause discomfort, pruritus, and sometimes dyspareunia. As the lesions become infected, there is at times very severe pain, external dysuria, and vulvar discharge. Systemic symptoms are rare.

IV. Signs

A. Ulcerative lesions

1. HSV-1 or -2 initially is an erythematous papule, which is followed by small, grouped vesicles hours to a few days later. These can occur in men on the glans, on the distal and sometimes proximal shaft of the penis, or on the scrotum. In women, lesions can occur on the pubis, labia, clitoris, vulva, buttocks, or anus; the entire vulva can be involved. Pustules, erosions, or ulceration occur, which heal by crusting in 2 to 4 weeks,

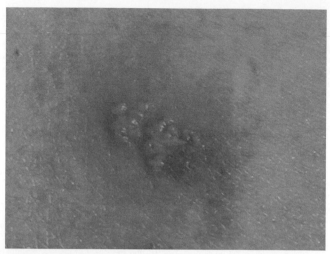

FIGURE 30–1. Tightly grouped vesicles 1 to 3 mm in diameter forming a lobulated irregular plaque over a larger erythematous base represent a herpetic lesion about 2-day-old (see color insert). (Used with permission from Tomás P. Owens, Jr., MD.)

leaving some hypomelanosis or hypermelanosis. Scarring occurs only with manipulation or secondary infection. **Primary infection** produces larger numbers of lesions than **recurrent infection (see Figure 30–1)**.

2. Primary infection with *Treponema pallidum* produces a **chancre** at the site of inoculation 10 to 90 days after direct contact with secretions of an infected person. The **chancre** is a papule that erodes into a single, round, beefy-red ulcer with hard, raised borders and yellow-green exudative material on its base **(Figure 30–2)**. Chancres occur on the inside penile foreskin, coronal sulcus, shaft, or base, or on the cervix and vagina (where patients seldom detect it), vulva, or clitoris. Extragenital

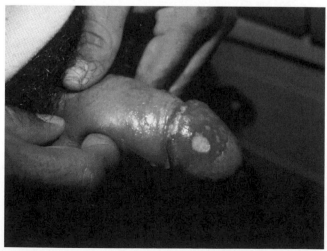

FIGURE 30–2. Primary syphilis with a large chancre on the glands of the penis. The multiple small surrounding ulcers are part of the syphilis and not a second disease (see color insert). (Used with permission from Richard P. Usatine, MD.)

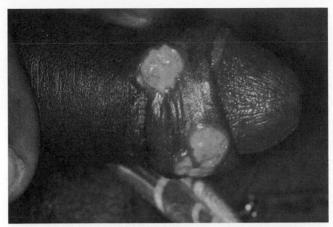

FIGURE 30–3. Culture-proven indurated beefy chancroid lesions in an HIV-positive man (see color insert). (Used with permission from Richard P. Usatine, MD.)

sites for chancres are the mouth, lips, breast, fingers, and thighs. Multiple chancres can be seen in patients with HIV infection.

3. **Chancroid** is caused by *Haemophilus ducreyi*, a gram-negative coccobacillary organism, and presents as a tender genital papule that erodes into single or multiple round, oval, or serpiginous painful ulcers with sharp, flat, and nonindurated borders along with regional lymphadenopathy **(Figure 30–3)**. As many as 10% of patients with chancroid may be coinfected with *T. pallidum* or HSV. The disease may have an important role in the transmission of HIV.

B. **Verrucous/papillomatous lesions**

1. **Condylomata acuminata** are skin-colored or pink-red tumors, which are localized, fleshy, soft, moist, elongated, and dome-shaped with filiform or conical vegetating projections in grape- to cauliflower-like clusters on moist surfaces (see **Figure 30–4**). They can be keratotic or smooth papular warts on dry surfaces or

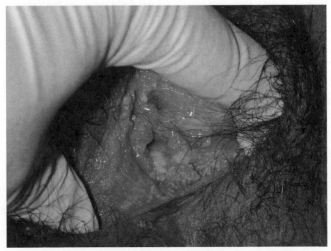

FIGURE 30–4. A peach-colored cauliflower-like lesion is noted on the comisure of the labia majora immediately caudal to the fourchette. Single coniform lighter pink lesions are also present at the R periurethral area, R superior labia majora, and L labia minora (see color insert). (Used with permission from Tomás P. Owens, Jr., MD.)

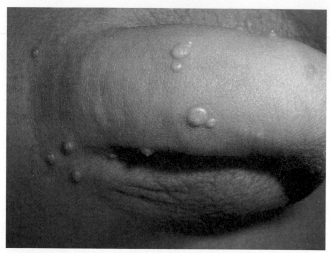

FIGURE 30–5. Molluscum contagiosum on and around the penis of a young boy. There was no evidence for sexual abuse (see color insert). (Used with permission from Richard P. Usatine, MD.)

appear as subclinical "flat" warts. Large lesions occur perianally in immunosuppressed persons.

2. **Condylomata lata** are soft, flat-topped, moist, skin-colored or pale pink papules, warts, nodules, or plaques, which may become confluent. These lesions occur on any body surface, but have a preference for the anogenital area and intertriginous sites.

3. **Molluscum contagiosum** presents as pearly white papules or nodules 2 to 8 mm in diameter, which are mostly round or oval with a classic umbilicated top (see **Figure 30–5**). The papules are localized in clusters, with preference for the genital area, neck, and trunk and may evolve to pustules and small crusts or plaques. Large size or large number of lesions, particularly on the face, suggests HIV.

4. **Pearly penile papules** histologically are angiofibromas that first appear around puberty. They are thin, conical, white, or pale pink uniformly sized groups of papules, forming multiple parallel lines mostly on the corona, but also in the balanopreputial sulcus.

C. Pruritic lesions

1. Erythema, excess amounts of smegma, and flat white-gray "empty" or erythematous papules suggest **balanitis (see Figure 30–6);** erosions and fine scaling sometimes associated with marked edema of the prepuce suggest **balanoposthitis. Phimosis** (a contraction of the distal foreskin) may be present, revealing only edema and obstructing the view of the glans. In uncircumcised males, phimosis can be a cause or a complication of balanitis (or both). Paraphimosis can occur if the foreskin has been retracted, constricting the glans or the shaft just proximal to the glans, and causing ischemia; this presents as swelling and acute pain. Any papule, plaque, or white discoloration that is not resolved by therapy (see Section VI.C.1.c) suggests possible malignancy.

2. An erythematous to brownish-red plaque with sharp borders and minimal scaling located on the inner thigh extending into the scrotum or vulva suggests **erythrasma**.

3. Minuscule white-gray nits are seen attached to hair shafts, and brownish-gray lice of similar size (1–2 mm) are seen on the perifollicular skin in **Phthirus pubis** infestation. Papules, lichenification, and excoriations from scratching can be seen.

4. **Vulvar dystrophy/LSA** varies from nonspecific thinned skin, to multiple flat, irregular pearly/ivory white, or pink/reddish (less common) papules or macules in multiple sites. They may eventually coalesce into white plaques involving the entire perineum. Hyperplastic dystrophy and leukoplakia are less common and considered premalignant; vulvar carcinoma is uncommon. In **BXO,** there is a ring of white sclerotic tissue

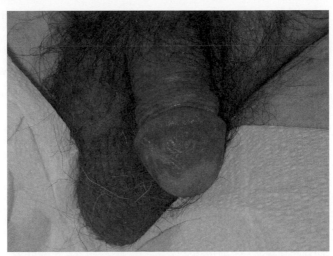

FIGURE 30-6. Irregular erythematous plaques following cleansing of smegma and debris. These lesions completely disappeared after topical antifungals, confirming the absence of Bowenoid disease (see color insert). (Used with permission from Tomás P. Owens, Jr., MD.)

at the tip of the foreskin (which causes phimosis) or meatus, but is not accompanied by inflammatory changes. Kraurosis vulvae (atrophy and shriveling of the skin or mucous membranes) with hypomelanosis, telangiectasias, and a "keyhole" vaginal opening is an old, now abandoned gynecologic term for end-stage atrophy not necessarily caused by sclerosis.

D. Cystic lesions

    1. A rubbery, soft, renitent bulge in the inner aspect of the lower vaginal vestibule (outside of the introitus) suggests **Bartholin gland cyst;** if infected, the cyst is red and extremely tender.

V. Laboratory Tests

    A. Ulcerative lesions. Testing for chlamydia, gonorrhea, and HIV (with adequate counseling) should be considered in persons with primary HSV-1 or -2, syphilis, or chancroid, with retesting in 3 to 6 months. In addition, testing for syphilis is recommended for those with primary HSV-1 or -2.

        1. Laboratory studies are rarely necessary in HSV-1 or -2; they are reserved for situations in which the diagnosis is not clear and certainty is imperative, such as a primary infection soon before parturition or when strict confirmation is necessary for medicolegal cases.

            a. In the **Tzanck test** (mostly of historical interest today), a vesicle is unroofed and its fluid is smeared on a slide, dried, and stained with Giemsa or Wright stain. Presence of giant multinucleated acanthocytes is considered a positive test result for **Herpesviridae** (simplex or zoster). This is very insensitive and nonspecific.

            b. **Polymerase chain reaction (PCR) of HSV DNA** swab has largely replaced **direct fluorescent antibody (DFA)** and **viral culture** which are expensive and require an incubation period of 7 days before being read. Positive cultures can occur in persons with nonherpetic lesions who shed the herpes virus regularly. Falsely negative cultures are common with recurrent lesions or late eruptive phase.

            c. **Enzyme-linked immunosorbent assays (ELISA HSV-2) type-specific to glycoprotein G (gG)** are highly sensitive and specific, but will not be positive for 2 weeks to 3 months after the acute infection. Thus, they are useful in combination with PCR only to assess timeline of infection.

        2. Primary syphilis

            a. Dark-field microscopic examination of the lesion's secretions is diagnostic but rarely available to the clinician. It reveals treponemes contracting and kinking, but these may not be seen if the chancre has been treated with topical antibiotics.

    b. Rapid plasma reagin (RPR) and venereal disease research labora-tory (VDRL) tests, the nontreponemal tests, become positive 1 week after the appearance of the chancre. These tests become negative up to 1 year after treat-ment, but may remain positive for life at a low titer in a small percentage of patients.

    c. Confirmatory treponemal tests such as the **fluorescent treponemal anti-body-absorption** (FTA-ABS) or *T. pallidum* **hemagglutination assay** (TPHA) may take 2 weeks to become positive. Treponemal tests remain weakly positive for life.

B. Verrucous/papillomatous lesions. Testing for chlamydia, gonorrhea, and HIV (with adequate counseling, including safe-sex information) should be considered in per-sons with condylomata acuminata, condyloma lata, or molluscum contagiosum. In addi-tion, testing for syphilis is recommended for those with condylomata acuminata.

1. The diagnosis of **condylomata acuminata** is clinical.

    a. Occasionally, a **biopsy** confirms the diagnosis.

    b. Subclinical lesions can be soaked with **5% acetic acid** (white vinegar) for 5 minutes, which results in white epithelium that can be observed with a colposcope or magnifying glass of 4x to 10x magnification. White papules may be noted, although other changes such as mosaicism and punctation are possible.

2. RPR and VDRL tests are always positive when **condyloma lata** are present. FTA confirmation is warranted.

3. Sticking a needle through a lesion releases the semisolid core of **molluscum conta-giosum,** which is considered diagnostic, but is rarely needed. Microscopic observa-tion, rarely necessary, reveals inclusion "molluscum" bodies or Lipschütz cells.

4. No laboratory test is necessary to diagnose **pearly penile papules**. A biopsy reveals an angiofibroma.

C. Pruritic lesions

1. Balanitis is a clinical diagnosis; however, biopsy of any associated glanular mass is needed. Biopsy can be done under local anesthesia using a shallow punch at the office.

2. Wood lamp examination shows a classic coral-red fluorescence in **erythrasma**. Scraping of the lesions may show gram-positive rods and do not show hyphae.

3. Lice and nits can be observed microscopically in *Phthirus pubis* infestation. Testing for chlamydia, gonorrhea, syphilis, and HIV (with adequate counseling) should be considered in those who were infested by direct sexual contact.

4. Biopsy is necessary in **vulvar dystrophy** to distinguish **LSA/BXO** from leukopla-kia, vitiligo, lichen planus, or carcinoma. This can be accomplished in the office under local anesthesia using a punch biopsy of the leading edge or a full excision, if the lesion is less than 1 cm in diameter.

D. Cystic lesions. Diagnosis of **Bartholin gland cyst** is clinical. Cultures should be considered only when cellulitis is present.

VI. Treatment

A. Ulcerative lesions

1. Maximal viral shedding in HSV-1 or -2 occurs within 24 hours of the appearance of lesions and diminishes by the fifth day; nevertheless, viral shedding occurs intermit-tently in the absence of any signs in many persons. Herpes is generally self-limited, with recurrences decreasing over years. Therapy does not eradicate **HSV-1 or -2,** nor does it affect the severity or rate of recurrences after discontinuation. Sig-nificant clinical improvement is seen when therapy is started promptly after onset of symptoms.

    a. For primary infection, oral drugs of choice include acyclovir, 400 mg, or fam-ciclovir, 250 mg three times daily, *or* valacyclovir 1 g twice daily for 7 to 10 days. (SOR **Ⓐ**) It is unclear whether higher doses (e.g., acyclovir, 400 mg five times per day) are warranted for stomatitis, pharyngitis, or proctitis.

    b. Recurrent infection

        (1) At onset, oral acyclovir, 200 mg five times daily, or 400 mg three times daily, or 800 mg twice daily for 5 days, *or* famciclovir, 125 mg, or vala-cyclovir, 500 mg twice daily or 1000 mg every day for 5 days, can be prescribed. (SOR **Ⓐ**)

        (2) Oral suppressive therapy options include acyclovir, 400 mg, or famciclovir, 250 mg twice daily, *or* valacyclovir, 500 mg or 1 g once daily (for 9 or fewer or >9 recurrences, respectively) for 1 year. (SOR **Ⓐ**) Consider a drug-free period at 1 year to assess the need for continued therapy.

c. Counseling regarding potential for recurrence, amelioration of symptoms over the years, transmission through viral shedding in the absence of lesions, and the need for condom use is important.

2. Primary syphilis is treated with benzathine penicillin G, 2.4 million units intramuscularly in a single dose. (SOR **Ⓐ**) Some experts recommend two extra doses, 1 week apart, for patients with HIV. (SOR **Ⓑ**) Persons who are allergic to penicillin should receive doxycycline, 100 mg orally twice daily for 2 weeks. (SOR **Ⓐ**) If compliance is an issue, penicillin desensitization should be considered. Dosages and effectiveness of ceftriaxone have not been defined. Azithromycin should not be used as it is commonly ineffective.

3. Persons with **chancroid** should be treated with azithromycin, 1 g orally in a single dose, *or* ceftriaxone, 250 mg intramuscularly in a single dose, *or* erythromycin base, 500 mg orally 3 times a day for 7 days; *or* ciprofloxacin, 500 mg orally twice daily for 3 days. Ciprofloxacin should not be given to children or pregnant/lactating women. There has been intermediate resistance to ciprofloxacin and erythromycin worldwide. Uncircumcised males and HIV-infected patients are more resistant to therapy and may require retreatment or longer courses if the condition is not resolved in 7 days.

B. Verrucous/papillomatous lesions

1. Condylomata acuminata resolve spontaneously in 6 to 15 months, except in immunocompromised persons. Most clinicians treat to avoid persistent growth. Treatment removes only the wart and does not eliminate the virus, which could remain for months to years. Recurrences are common during the first year, even after adequate removal. An additional Papanicolaou smear is recommended for women with warts at the time of diagnosis. Two vaccines are available, with the recombinant vaccine effective against HPV types 6, 11, 16, and 18 (Gardasil) recommended for females (2006) and males (2009) aged 9 to 26 years (see Chapter 105). The vaccines are not intended for treatment.

a. Most effective therapies include the following:

(1) For **cryotherapy** with liquid nitrogen, the cryotherapy probe, spray "gun," or cotton-tipped applicator is applied until blanching occurs no more than 1 mm around the perimeter of the lesions, which fall off in 24 to 72 hours, leaving a shallow ulcer.

(2) **Trichloroacetic acid** or **bichloroacetic acid** 80% to 90% can be applied, only to warts, which turns them white in seconds. Lesions should be powdered with talc or sodium bicarbonate immediately to remove unreacted acid. Treatment can be repeated weekly as necessary.

(3) **Imiquimod** (Aldara) 5% cream is applied by the patient's finger on each lesion at bedtime and washed off in the morning, three times a week for as long as 16 weeks. (SOR **Ⓑ**) Caution should be used in pregnancy as imiquimod is assigned a pregnancy category C and animal studies found fetal adverse effects.

(4) **Podophyllin,** 10% to 25%, in compound tincture of benzoin, is applied to warts. It is used very rarely anymore as it is unstable and thus not easy to store. The total amount applied per session should be limited to 0.5 mL or less than 10 cm2 to avoid systemic toxicity; medication should be washed off in 4 hours. Treatment may be repeated weekly and is contraindicated in pregnancy.

(5) **Podofilox** (Condylox), 0.5% solution, for self-treatment, is applied twice daily for 3 days followed by 4 days of no therapy. Treatment can be repeated up to four cycles and is contraindicated in pregnancy. The clinician should teach the patient which lesions to treat and how to apply the drug.

(6) **Salicylic acid 17% liquid** (Compound W, DuoFilm, others) can be as effective and less expensive. Apply after covering the surrounding unaffected skin with petroleum jelly.

(7) **Electrodesiccation** or **electrocautery** is contraindicated in patients with anal lesions or with a pacemaker.

(8) **Surgical tangential shave/scissor excision** or **curettage.**

    b. Other therapies include the following:

        (1) Carbon dioxide laser is necessary only with warts that are very extensive or very resistant to other therapies.

        (2) Interferon alpha-2b (Intron-A) can be injected on the base of lesions three times per week for 3 weeks and repeated as needed. (SOR **☻**) This drug is expensive and its use should be restricted to recalcitrant cases.

  2. Treatment for **secondary syphilis,** which is extremely contagious, is the same as for primary syphilis.

  3. Spontaneous remission of **molluscum contagiosum** occurs in weeks to several months. **Cryotherapy, curettage,** or **electrocautery** can be performed (see Section VI.B.1.a).

  4. Reassurance is all that is necessary for **pearly penile papules**.

C. Pruritic lesions

  1. Balanitis

    a. The foreskin should be kept retracted as much as possible.

    b. The glans should be dried thoroughly after showering and micturition. In addition, the glans and prepuce should be washed with soap and water and dried thoroughly after sexual intercourse.

    c. Candidiasis superinfection should be treated with an **imidazole** cream (butoconazole, clotrimazole, econazole, miconazole, isoconazole, tioconazole, or terconazole), ciclopirox, or **nystatin** cream, topically twice daily, *or* fluconazole, 150 mg orally in a single dose. (SOR **Ⓐ**) Ketoconazole and itraconazole might be as effective but have a higher potential for toxicity. Terbinafine should not be used as a primary agent for *Candida*.

    d. Circumcision may be needed if phimosis develops or in resistant cases, since chronic balanitis is a potential precursor of premalignant penile glanular changes.

  2. Cleaning with povidone-iodine soap can be sufficient for **erythrasma**. **Clindamycin 2%** cream or **sodium fusidate 2% ointment** twice daily for 14 days or **erythromycin base** 250 mg orally four times daily for 14 days (SOR **Ⓐ**) is also effective against the causative agent (*Corynebacterium minutissimum*). **Clarithromycin 1 g single dose orally is an alternative treatment.**

  3. Lindane 1% shampoo applied for 4 minutes *or* **permethrin** 1% creme rinse or **pyrethrin with piperonyl butoxide** applied for 10 minutes and then thoroughly washed off are effective treatments for **pubic lice.** (SOR **Ⓐ**) Lindane should be avoided in children and during gestation and lactation. It is banned in California since 2002. **Permethrin** has less potential for toxicity than lindane.

  4. Vulvar dystrophy/LSA and BXO

    a. When biopsy reveals intraepithelial neoplasia, either **laser therapy** or conventional **surgical excision** is indicated.

    b. In **LSA/BXO, topical testosterone** is no longer recommended. Highly potent **topical steroids** (e.g., clobetasol 0.05%) improve symptoms but often not appearance and should be carefully rubbed on the lesion twice daily for 1 month and then once daily for 2 to 3 weeks followed by lower-potency steroids (triamcinolone acetonide 0.1% or betamethasone valerate 0.1%) twice daily for a few weeks. (SOR **Ⓑ**) Tacrolimus ointment 0.1% and pimecrolimus cream 1% twice daily are also effective (off-label use). Leukoplakia requires close follow-up; 5-fluorouracil topically is often used instead. (SOR **☻**)

D. Cystic lesions. Bartholin gland cysts/inflammation

  1. Hot, wet dressings, or sitz baths may promote spontaneous drainage of cysts.

  2. Incision and drainage are effective in most abscesses.

  3. Marsupialization is recommended for recurrences with placement of a Word catheter (http://www.youtube.com/watch?v=BfXq0HSzlQo).

  4. Antibiotic therapy is not necessary unless there is associated cellulitis, generally caused by staphylococci, streptococci, coliforms, or anaerobes.

SELECTED REFERENCES

Gilbert DN, Moellering RC, Sande MA. *The Sanford Guide to Antimicrobial Therapy.* 43rd ed. Antimicrobial Therapy; 2013.

Guidelines for treatment of sexually transmitted diseases. *Morb Mortal Wkly Rep.* 2010;59:RR-12. http://www.cdc.gov/std/treatment/2010/STD-Treatment-2010-RR5912.pdf. Accessed September 2013.

National Center for Health Statistics. National Ambulatory Medical Care Survey (NAMCS): 2010 Summary. Advance Data from Vital and Health Statistics National Center for Health Statistics, Centers for Disease Control and Prevention. http://www.cdc.gov/nchs/data/hus/2011/044.pdf. Accessed September 2013.

Pickering LK, ed. Red Book: 2012 Report of the Committee on Infectious Diseases. 29th ed. American Academy of Pediatrics; 2012.

Wolff K, Johnson RA; Saavedra AP. Fitzpatrick's Color Atlas and Synopsis of Clinical Dermatology. 7th ed. McGraw-Hill; 2013.

31   Hair and Nail Disorders

Amy D. Crawford-Faucher, MD, FAAFP

KEY POINTS

- Ninety-five percent of alopecia cases presenting to primary care physicians are potentially treatable. (SOR ❸)
- Hirsutism associated with virilization requires hormonal evaluation. (SOR ❸)
- Only 50% of dystrophic nails are onychomycotic; accurate diagnosis is key to appropriate therapy. (SOR ❸)
- Melanoma and metastatic cancers sometimes present as nail disorders. (SOR ❸)

I. Definition. Hair follicles produce one of two types of human hair: **vellus hair** is fine, hypopigmented, and barely visible; and **terminal hair** is coarse and usually pigmented. Follicles cycle through three stages: anagen (hair growth), catagen (transition), and telogen (rest). Hair shafts mature and are shed after the telogen phase. Scalp hair follicles normally stay in anagen for 2 to 8 years, producing potentially long hairs, and then "rest" in telogen for 2 to 3 months. While abnormal hair growth or loss is usually not medically serious, it can indicate systemic disease, and often causes significant emotional distress.

   Alopecia (hair loss) can be localized, patchy, diffuse, or total. Metabolic diseases, medications, and physiologic stresses can slow or disrupt the normal hair growth cycle and result in alopecia. Hair follicles can also be damaged by chemical or physical agents, or by infectious or immunologically mediated inflammation. Alopecia is considered **noncicatricial (nonscarring)** when hair follicles are retained and there is potential for hair regrowth. If hair follicles are destroyed, the alopecia is **cicatricial (scarring)**.

   Hirsutism is excess hair growth in a typically male distribution and results from excess androgen (testosterone and its precursors dehydroepiandrosterone sulfate [DHEAs] and 17α-hydroxyprogesterone [17-OHP]) originating in the ovaries or adrenals, or exogenously from medications. These androgens act on a woman's androgen-sensitive follicles (located primarily on the face, chest, upper back, lower abdomen, and inner thighs) to produce terminal instead of vellus hair. Hirsutism can be an isolated condition or occur in conjunction with other virilizing symptoms and signs that indicate androgen excess. **Hypertrichosis** refers to excess hair growth that may be diffuse and is not sensitive to androgens.

   Normal nail anatomy includes a vascular and highly innervated nail bed that underlies the nail, which is composed of dead keratin. The proximal end of the nail bed comprises the matrix, from which new nail grows. The perionychium folds around the nail edge proximally and laterally, producing the nail folds. Abnormal nails result from trauma, infection, systemic disease, or congenital conditions or can be normal variants. Damage to the matrix can cause permanent nail-growth abnormalities. Accurate diagnosis of nail disorders is necessary for effective treatment and for prompt evaluation of potentially serious systemic disease.

II. Common Diagnoses

   A. Alopecias (Table 31–1). Many forms of hair loss are common and affect up to half of men and women. Nonscarring alopecias account for the vast majority of the hair loss seen by primary care physicians. The six causes listed below are the most common and clinically significant.

TABLE 31–1. DIAGNOSES AND ETIOLOGIC CLASSIFICATIONS OF ALOPECIA

Cicatricial (Scarring) Alopecias

Neoplastic: localized or metastatic

Nevoid: nevus sebaceous, epidermal nevus

Physical or chemical: burns, freezing, trauma, radiation, acids, alkalis

Infectious: bacterial, fungal, protozoal, viral, mycobacterial

Congenital or developmental: aplasia cutis, Darier disease, recessive X-linked ichthyosis, keratosis pilaris atrophicans

Dermatosis-related: lichen planus, necrobiosis lipoidica diabeticorum, cicatricial pemphigoid, folliculitis decalvans, sclerosing frontal alopecia

Systemic disease: lupus erythematosus, sarcoidosis, scleroderma, dermatomyositis, amyloidosis

Noncicatricial (Nonscarring) Alopecias

Drug-induced: antimetabolites, anticoagulants, beta-blockers, antidepressants, lithium, levodopa

Congenital: ectodermal dysplasias, hair shaft disorders

Infectious: secondary syphilis, tinea capitis, human immunodeficiency virus infection

Toxic: arsenic, boric acid, thallium, vitamin A

Nutritional: anorexia nervosa, marasmus, kwashiorkor, "crash" diets, iron or zinc deficiency

Traumatic: trichotillomania, traction, friction, chemical, thermal

Endocrine: hyper- or hypothyroidism, hypopituitarism, hyper- or hypoparathyroidism

Immunologic: alopecia areata

Genetic or developmental: male- and female-pattern baldness (androgenetic alopecia)

Radiation-induced: x-ray epilation

Physiologic: telogen effluvium (postpartum, postsurgical, febrile illness, severe psychological stress, puberty)

1. **Androgenetic alopecia,** commonly called male- and female-pattern baldness, is more common than all other causes of alopecia combined. It affects approximately 70% of men to some degree, and up to 40% of women. More than half of men show signs of this hair loss by 50 years of age. In genetically susceptible people, androgens gradually transform terminal follicles on the scalp to vellus-like follicles, which eventually leads to atrophy. Androgenetic alopecia is controlled by one dominant, sex-limited, autosomal gene that may be incompletely expressed because of polygenic modifying factors.

2. **Traumatic alopecia** is relatively common on the occiput of infants who sleep on their backs, and in persons with hairstyles (tight braids, curlers) that put continuous traction on the follicle (also called traction alopecia; Figure 31–1). Recurrent, compulsive hair plucking (trichotillomania) can also lead to traumatic alopecia.

3. **Infectious alopecia,** mainly due to **tinea capitis,** affects up to 4% of children; it occurs much less commonly in adults. In severe cases, intense inflammation can injure the hair follicles.

4. **Physiologic alopecia,** called **telogen effluvium,** results in diffuse hair loss and most often occurs 2 to 3 months postpartum, following the cessation of oral contraception or corticosteroids, or after serious illness or stress. This hair loss occurs when an unusually large number of follicles (25%–45%) abruptly end anagen and move through catagen and into the telogen (rest) phase. Large numbers of telogen hair then synchronously fall out.

5. **Alopecia areata** (Figure 31–2) has a prevalence of 0.1% of the general population, with lifetime risk approaching 2%. It affects men and women equally. More than half the cases arise by 40 years of age, and there is a familial tendency. Alopecia areata tends to be associated with other autoimmune diseases, such as pernicious anemia, vitiligo, Hashimoto thyroiditis, and atopic dermatitis, and with Down syndrome. While most cases eventually resolve spontaneously, those that present before puberty, are recurrent or extensive, or do not respond to treatment carry a poor prognosis for hair regrowth.

6. **Systemic processes** including thyroid disease, other endocrinopathies, and malnutrition can cause hair loss by slowing the rate of hair growth or altering the balance between the anagen and telogen phases in the hair follicles.

B. **Hirsutism** (Table 31–2) affects approximately 7% of all women.

1. **Polycystic ovarian syndrome (PCOS)** is the most common androgen-excess condition and is responsible for 72% to 82% of hirsutism cases (see Chapter 3).

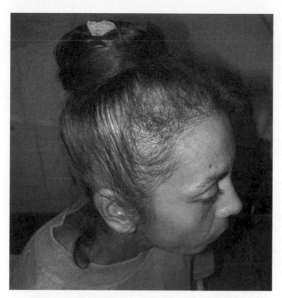

FIGURE 31-1. Traction alopecia from pulling the hair up in a tight bun (see color insert). (Used with permission from Richard P. Usatine, MD.)

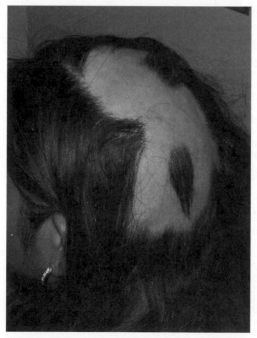

FIGURE 31-2. Extensive alopecia areata for over 6 months in an adult woman (see color insert). (Used with permission from Richard P. Usatine, MD.)

TABLE 31-2. CAUSES OF HYPERTRICHOSIS AND HIRSUTISM

Hypertrichosis	Hirsutism
Idiopathic	Polycystic ovarian syndrome (PCOS)
	Idiopathic hirsutism
Familial	Congenital adrenal hyperplasia
Puberty	Adrenal or ovarian neoplasm
Pregnancy	Rare: Cushing syndrome, hyperprolactinemia, thyroid dysfunction
Menopause	
Hypothyroidism	
Acromegaly	
Hurler syndrome	
Porphyria cutaneous tarda	
Multiple sclerosis	
Encephalitis	

2. **Idiopathic hirsutism** is most common in women of Mediterranean ancestry and is thought to represent increased follicle sensitivity to normal levels of circulating androgens. Idiopathic hirsutism is a diagnosis of exclusion.
3. Prevalence of **adult-onset congenital adrenal hyperplasia** is unclear but varies with ethnic background. The disorder is uncommon in women of Northern European ancestry and occurs with greater frequency in Ashkenazi Jews, Hispanics, and Slavs.
4. **Ovarian or adrenal tumors** are rare causes of hirsutism.
5. **Cushing syndrome** is a rare cause of hirsutism.
6. **Medications** can cause both hirsutism and hypertrichosis (Table 31–3).

C. **Nail disorders.** The most common nail disorders are listed below.
   1. **Onychomycosis** (Figure 31–3), a fungal infection of the nails, accounts for one-half of nail diagnoses, affecting up to 20% of adults and a much smaller percentage of children. Toenails are more commonly involved than fingernails. Prolonged or repeated foot dampness and locker room exposure can predispose to infection.
   2. **Paronychia** (Figure 31–4) infection of the proximal or lateral nail folds is due acutely to local trauma, such as a "hangnail," and chronically to repeated exposure to moisture, as with dishwashers or swimmers.
   3. Direct trauma to the nail and fingertip or toe can cause a **subungual hematoma,** when blood from ruptured nail bed vessels collects in the potential space between the nail bed and the plate.
   4. **Ingrown nails** are also common, occurring most commonly on the medial edge of the great toenail. Ill-fitting shoes, nail dystrophies, and onychomycosis can all predispose to this condition.
   5. **Discolored nails** can be caused by a wide variety of conditions (Table 31–4).
   6. **Systemic diseases** can manifest as nail disorders. Alopecia areata, chronic hypoxia, iron-deficiency anemia, zinc deficiency, and hypocalcemia can cause nail abnormalities.

TABLE 31-3. MEDICATIONS CAUSING HYPERTRICHOSIS OR HIRSUTISM

Hypertrichosis	Hirsutism
Acetazolamide	Aldomet
Corticosteroids	Anabolic steroids
Cyclosporine	Danazol
Diazoxide	Phenothiazines
Interferon	Progestins
Minoxidil (forearms and legs in women)	Reglan
Phenothiazines	Reserpine
Phenytoin	Testosterone
Psoralens	
Streptomycin	

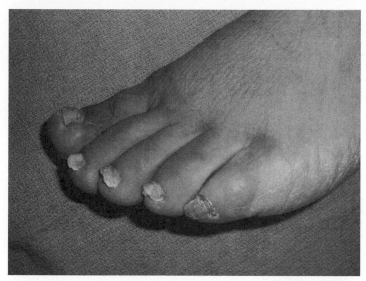

FIGURE 31–3. Onychomycosis in all toenails of a 29-year-old woman. Note the nail plate thickening and discoloration along with the subungual keratosis. She also has tinea pedis in a moccasin distribution (see color insert). (Used with permission of Richard P. Usatine, MD.)

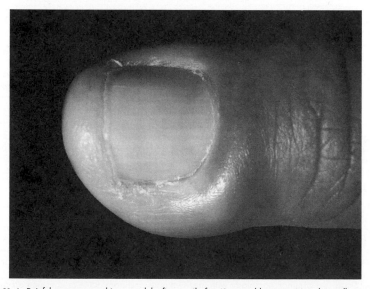

FIGURE 31–4. Painful acute paronychia around the fingernail of a 41-year-old woman. Note the swelling and erythema with as small white-yellow area suggesting purulence (see color insert). (Used with permission from Richard P. Usatine, MD.)

TABLE 31–4. CAUSES OF DISCOLORED NAILS

White (Leukonychia)
Fungus
Physical stress/mild trauma (transverse lines or spots that grow out with the nail)
Nail bed injury (transverse lines that do not move with the nail)
Heavy metal poisoning (e.g., arsenic) (transverse lines)
Liver disease (all-white nails)
Renal failure and uremia (half white, half pink nails)
Idiopathic (spots and lines)
Congenital

Brown/Black
Lines common in dark-skinned persons
Nevus (confined to nail)
Melanoma (may "run over" onto the nail fold)
Fungus
Psoriasis or alopecia areata
Chloroquine (bluish)
Quinacrine (bluish)
Several chemotherapeutic agents
Heavy metal poisoning

Yellow
Fungus
Nonpseudomonal bacteria
Psoriasis (usually not uniform)
Alopecia areata (usually not uniform)
Lymphedema
AIDS
Addison disease

Green
Pseudomonal infection

Blue
Minocycline
Doxorubicin (brownish)
Wilson disease
Ochronosis (gray–blue)

Red
Darier disease (longitudinal streaks)

III. **Symptoms.** Evaluation of patients with **alopecia** should include duration and location of hair loss, major life changes, physical trauma, medication use, and hair care habits. For **hirsutism,** the knowledge of the onset, severity (measured by the Ferriman–Gallwey scoring system [https://www.endocrine.org/~/media/endosociety/Files/Publications/Clinical%20Practice%20Guidelines/Hirsutism_Guideline.pdf; Figure 1]), associated signs and symptoms, medication use, ethnic origin, and affected family members is important.

    A. The vast majority of processes leading to alopecia, hirsutism, and hypertrichosis are generally asymptomatic. Trauma or infectious processes such as tinea capitis can cause itching and pain. Women with hirsutism and **PCOS** often give a history of oligomenorrhea and infertility. Those with **idiopathic hirsutism** report gradual onset of mild hirsutism, normal menses, and no virilizing signs. Women with **hirsutism from severe androgen excess** commonly report rapid onset of postpubertal virilization and irregular menses.

    B. Pain is a common complaint with ingrown nails and from acute or chronic paronychia. Onychomycosis and other nail infections may be painless. Significant throbbing pain at the nail is the hallmark of subungual hematoma, occurring within hours to a day of a crush injury to the fingertip and nail.

IV. **Signs.** In **alopecia,** a helpful clinical clue is the presence of follicular orifices, which implies a noncicatricial (and therefore potentially reversible) process. With **hirsutism,** signs of virilization should be sought including varying degrees of clitoromegaly, cystic acne, decreased breast size, deepened voice, increased libido, increased muscle mass, malodorous perspiration, oligomenorrhea, and temporal hair recession and balding. The following local signs will rapidly narrow the differential diagnosis in alopecia, hirsutism, and nail abnormalities:

A. Androgenetic alopecia
1. **Male-pattern baldness** is most often characterized by frontotemporal hairline recession (in an "M" pattern) with variable hair loss at the scalp vertex.
2. **Female-pattern baldness** predominantly results from diffuse or vertex hair loss. Sometimes the part becomes prominent, but the hair along the frontal hairline is spared.

B. Traumatic alopecia usually shows patchy hair loss but can also be diffuse (Figure 31–1). Localized breakage with variously shortened hair suggests mechanical damage.

C. Infectious alopecia caused by **tinea capitis** exhibits discrete patches of partial hair loss and breakage overlying scaly, inflamed skin, which is usually accompanied by tender occipital lymphadenopathy (see Chapter 14 and Figure 14–9). Less commonly, a **kerion** induced by the dermatophyte *Trichophyton tonsurans* causes a deep, purulent folliculitis. With severe fungal infections or marked cellulitis, inflammation and suppuration can cause destruction and scarring. Secondary syphilis, in contrast, leads to a diffuse, moth-eaten appearance of the scalp.

D. Physiologic alopecia is suggested by acute, diffuse, yet reversible hair thinning. When present, transverse nail depressions (Beau lines) imply a subacute physiologic injury.

E. Alopecia areata is characterized by the abrupt onset of patchy but very well demarcated hair loss (Figure 31–2). This process leaves discrete areas of smooth, hairless, noninflamed skin that is surrounded by easily plucked hairs. "Exclamation point" hairs are short, heavily pigmented shafts with wide, brush-like distal ends that taper at the skin surface and can sometimes be found at the periphery of areata patches. There can be complete loss of scalp hair **(alopecia totalis)** or of all body hair **(alopecia universalis),** although these types account for only 4.5% to 30% of all alopecia areata cases. Pitted nails are seen in up to one-third of patients.

F. Systemic diseases, such as thyroid disease (see Chapter 89), exhibit their specific associated signs in addition to diffuse hair loss and thinning.

G. PCOS can be associated with obesity.

H. Adrenal or ovarian neoplasms are associated with rapid onset of significant hair growth many years after puberty and with other virilizing signs.

MELANOMA/CARCINOMA AND NAILS

Malignant melanoma can present as a new hyperpigmented longitudinal line on a nail, especially if it "runs over" onto the proximal nail fold or takes over the entire nail.

Squamous cell carcinoma, melanoma, or, rarely, **metastatic cancer** can manifest as a paronychia that does not respond to usual treatments. Biopsy of the nail bed is necessary to diagnose these cancers.

I. Onychomycosis
1. **Distal onychomycosis** causes nails to become white, yellow, or brownish. The nail thickens and subungual debris collects at the distal tip (Figure 31–3).
2. **White superficial onychomycosis** causes soft, rough nails that crumble.
3. **Proximal onychomycosis** is least common and occurs when *Trichophyton rubrum* invades the proximal nail fold, infects the newly formed nail plate, and moves distally.

J. Acute paronychia presents with significant erythema, tenderness, and fluctuance along the proximal or lateral nail border (Figure 31–4). **Chronic paronychia** often involves many nails and is less erythematous. Affected nails become tender intermittently, especially after water exposure. The proximal nail folds become edematous but are rarely fluctuant.

K. Subungual hematoma causes an exquisitely tender nail that may appear partially or completely red–blue, purple, or black because of accumulated blood. If significant portions of the bed are affected, the nail may separate partially or completely (onycholysis).

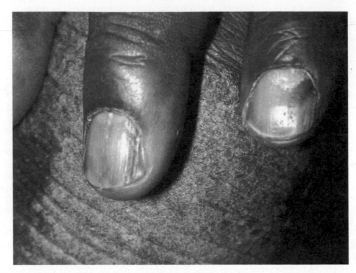

FIGURE 31–5. Nail psoriasis demonstrating nail pitting, onycholysis, oil-drop sign, and longitudinal ridging. Nails held over the silvery plaque on the knee (see color insert). (Used with permission from Richard P. Usatine, MD.)

    L. Ingrown nails act as a foreign body to cause inflammation and sometimes infection at the site where the corner of the nail grows into the adjacent lateral nail bed. With chronic inflammation, the granulation tissue grows over the affected portion of the nail. The area is extremely tender to touch and may be fluctuant.

  M. Systemic diseases can manifest specific nail abnormalities. **Psoriasis** most commonly causes deep pits in the nails, but can also cause separation (onycholysis), discoloration, and subungual thickening with nail debris accumulation (see Chapter 14; Figure 31–5). Nail bed psoriasis can produce onycholysis, which appears similar to a drop of oil on paper (oil-drop sign; Figure 31–5). These findings may be confused with onychomycosis. Usually, the nail involvement occurs in conjunction with typical skin symptoms, but it may be the sole sign of the disease. **Alopecia areata** causes shallow pitting with progressive opacification. Clubbing from **chronic hypoxemia** is a chronic and permanent convex nail curvature and swelling of the skin around the proximal nail fold. Occasionally, clubbing occurs as a normal variant. Spoon-shaped (concave) nails in adults can occur with **iron-deficiency anemia,** transverse depressions (Beau lines) may indicate **zinc deficiency** or **physiologic stress** (Figure 31–6), whereas whitish nails may occur in hypocalcemia.

  N. Nail curvature, hypertrophy, or splitting can result from repeated nail trauma such as from constricting shoes, although the etiology is not always clear.

V. Laboratory Tests

  A. Most cases of **alopecia** can be diagnosed by a thorough personal history and a careful physical examination. Ancillary tests may be helpful in certain situations.

    1. The **hair pull or pluck test** involves a moderately firm pull of 10 to 20 closely grouped hairs from an affected area. Normally, less than 20% of the shafts will be removed, but in telogen effluvium and active androgenetic alopecia, more than 40% of the shafts will be uprooted.

    2. Potassium hydroxide (KOH) preparation of hair shafts or scalp scrapings on a gently warmed slide is used primarily to diagnose tinea capitis. Rarely, fungal cultures of hair shafts are needed. Wood light examination is only helpful in 5% to 10% of the tinea capitis infections that are caused by *Microsporum* species.

    3. A **trichogram** involves the microscopic analysis of at least 50 plucked hairs to determine hair structure and the proportion of telogen follicles. These hairs are removed

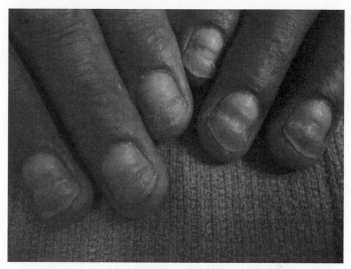

FIGURE 31-6. Beaulines most likely due to an acute cholecystitis episode before a couple of months (see color insert). (Used with permission from Richard P. Usatine, MD.)

from one area using a hemostat. Telogen hairs have small, unpigmented, ovoid bulbs and no internal root sheath. Anagen hairs have larger, elongated, pigmented bulbs shaped like the end of a broom, with a narrow internal root sheath. In telogen effluvium, between 20% and 60% of the patient's hair will be telogen hairs. Anagen hairs that show atrophied bulbs are typical in patients with androgenetic alopecia.

4. A **hair count** is the actual count of all hairs lost over several days. Up to 100 hairs per day is considered normal. Elevated counts are typical of telogen effluvium.

5. **Scalp biopsy** is usually reserved for cases of uncertain origin but may be helpful in determining the prognosis of patients with alopecia areata and lupus erythematosus based on the degree of perifollicular lymphocytic infiltration and antibody deposition, respectively.

6. **Assessment of endocrine dysfunction** may include thyroid tests (e.g., thyroid-stimulating hormone). Women with androgenetic hair loss should undergo the same evaluation as hirsute women if they also have signs and symptoms of hyperandrogenism (see Section V.B).

7. **Hematologic, serologic, rheumatologic,** and **blood chemistry tests** should be performed only when systemic disease is suspected, although iron and zinc deficiencies can contribute to hair thinning and are reasonable to assess. (SOR **C**)

B. Women with mild **hirsutism,** normal menses and fertility, and no other virilizing signs likely have idiopathic hirsutism and do not need a laboratory evaluation before a treatment trial. (SOR **C**) With more significant symptoms or signs, laboratory tests can help detect serious systemic disease; a sequential approach is best (Figure 31-7).

1. The role of testing is to determine the presence of significant hyperandrogenism and its source. For **moderate or severe hirsutism or virilization,** early-morning total testosterone should be measured first. Markedly elevated testosterone, especially in the presence of **virilization,** requires a complete hormonal evaluation including DHEAS and 17-OHP levels and imaging (computerized tomography or magnetic resonance imaging) of the adrenal glands or ovaries. (SOR **C**)

2. Normal or mildly elevated testosterone in the setting of **irregular menses** is most often associated with PCOS, but thyroid function, prolactin, and 17-OHP should be measured to exclude other causes. If these are normal, PCOS and anovulation are likely. For suspected PCOS, blood glucose and lipid screening should be obtained (see Chapter 3).

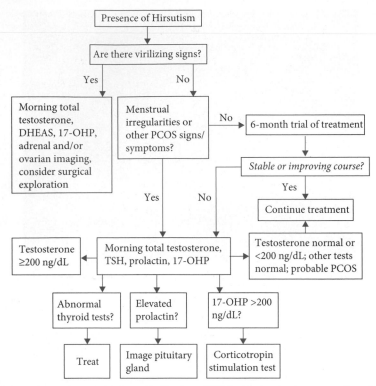

FIGURE 31–7. Approach to the patient with hirsutism. DHEAS, dehydroepiandrosterone sulfate; 17-OHP, 17α-hydroxyprogesterone; PCOS, polycystic ovary syndrome; TSH, thyroid-stimulating hormone. (Information from Bode D, Seehusen DA, Baird D. Hirsutism in women. *Am Fam Physician.* 2012;85(4):373–380; Martin KA, et al. Evaluation and treatment of hirsutism in premenopausal women: an Endocrine Society Clinical Practice Guideline. *J Clin Endocrinol Metab.* 2008;93:1105–1120.)

    C. Many **nail conditions** can be adequately diagnosed by careful history and physical examination, including search for other signs of systemic illness. Testing primarily confirms the diagnosis of onychomycosis.

        1. KOH stain and fungal cultures are necessary to diagnose onychomycosis because only 50% of dystrophic nails are actually mycotic. Although office-based tests exist, the standard remains KOH stain, culture, or both. Affected nail and nail bed should be sampled using a no. 15 blade or sharp curette to obtain debris from different locations on multiple affected nails. Testing for specific species is generally not warranted, as current treatments are effective against most fungi.

        2. Biopsy is indicated to diagnose tumors, inflammatory disease, and infections when the diagnosis is unclear. The nail bed, perionychium, or matrix can be biopsied. As nail matrix biopsy can cause permanent nail dystrophy, referral to a dermatologist is usually warranted.

VI. Treatment

    A. The goals of **alopecia** treatment are slowing hair loss and maximizing hair regrowth. No "magic pill" exists, and any gains may be subtle. Treatment may be required indefinitely to prevent further hair loss.

        1. Androgenetic alopecia

            a. Minoxidil (Rogaine) solution is a topical agent with unclear mechanism of action that can increase the number of new hairs in thinning scalp. A total of 1 mL of minoxidil solution is applied to the affected areas in the morning and at night.

(1) Minoxidil is not effective on receding temporal baldness, and is most successful in those with hair loss of ≤5 years, vertex baldness ≤10 cm, and with the presence of many indeterminate (between vellus and terminal) hairs.

(2) Approximately 40% of men report acceptable hair regrowth after 1 year of treatment.

(3) Minoxidil comes as 2% and 5% solutions. Both strengths are significantly more effective in men than placebo and are generally well tolerated, although the 5% solution can cause more local irritation. (SOR Ⓐ) Only the 2% solution is approved by the US Food and Drug Administration (FDA) for women. The main side effect in women is hypertrichosis of the face and arms that generally resolves over a year of continued use.

b. Finasteride (Propecia) is dosed at 1 mg daily and inhibits 5α-reductase in the follicle to reduce the effects of testosterone. Results can be slow, but two-thirds of men have increased hair growth by 2 years of treatment. Sometimes used in combination with minoxidil in men, and it must be used indefinitely to maintain hair growth. Sexual dysfunction including decreased libido, impotence, and ejaculation disorders occurs in 2% to 4% of men taking finasteride, although these effects often abate with continued therapy.

(1) Propecia is not effective for androgenetic alopecia in postmenopausal women.

c. Spironolactone can modestly decrease hair loss in women and can be used as an adjunct to topical therapy.

d. Oral contraceptives do not treat androgenetic alopecia in women, but progesterones with low androgen effects (e.g., norgestimate, norethindrone, desogestrel, and ethynodiol diacetate) may help prevent worsening of alopecia.

e. Other therapies may improve androgenetic alopecia. Other 5α-reductase inhibitors are being studied, but safety is a concern as higher doses are required for hair growth than for treatment of benign prostatic hypertrophy. Laser therapy is available for the treatment of alopecia, although robust studies of effectiveness are lacking. Many products, from scalp camouflaging powders, fibers or sprays, to hair extensions and wigs, can be used in conjunction with medical treatments and can be effective in minimizing the appearance of hair loss.

f. Surgical methods, including hair transplantation, remain options for men, but results are generally less satisfactory in women whose hair loss is usually more diffuse.

2. Traumatic alopecia is treated by avoidance of the causative action. Trichotillomania can be difficult to treat; a combination of psychological counseling and antidepressant medication may be effective.

3. Tinea capitis needs to be treated systemically, as topical antifungals do not penetrate the hair shaft. Griseofulvin and terbinafine (Lamisil) are approved by the FDA for children over 2 years of age, and a recent meta-analysis found no significant difference in efficacy between them (Table 31–5). (SOR Ⓐ) Although griseofulvin is less expensive, the required treatment duration is longer. Terbinafine oral granules can be sprinkled on soft non-acidic food (e.g., pudding, mashed potatoes; NOT applesauce or other fruit) and swallowed without chewing. Fluconazole is less effective for most tinea capitis infections, but is the only systemic antifungal agent approved by the FDA for this indication for infants and children aged less than 2 years. Adjunct treatment twice a week during the treatment course with selenium sulfide shampoo in patients of all ages and in household contacts may help decrease fungal shedding.

4. Telogen effluvium requires recognition of the inciting event and reassurance that hair growth will normalize.

5. Alopecia areata remains challenging to treat.

a. Intralesional steroid injection is the treatment of choice for less severe cases (≤50% of the scalp affected). **Triamcinolone (Kenalog)** 5 to 10 mg/mL is used: 0.1 mL is injected intradermally into multiple sites of each patch up to a monthly maximum of 20 to 30 mg. (SOR Ⓒ) Applying **minoxidil,** a mid-potency topical steroid, or both in between injections may hasten resolution. (SOR Ⓑ) These treatments are effective for short-term hair regrowth, but the effect on long-term outcomes and the course of the disease is unknown.

b. Strategies for more severe cases (affecting ≥50% of the scalp) can be complex and include topical immunotherapy, anthralin, and topical or systemic

TABLE 31–5. ANTIFUNGAL THERAPY FOR TINEA CAPITIS AND ONYCHOMYCOSIS

Drug	Dose	Adverse Effects and Drug Interactions	Monitoring
Oral Therapy: Tinea capitis			
Griseofulvin Ultramicro Micro	Adult: 330–375 mg/d in single or divided dose Child: 10 mg/kg/d for 8–16 wk Adult: 500 mg/d in single or divided dose xfor 4–6 wk Child: 20 mg/kg/d for 8–16 wk	Can cause rash, itching, headache, GI distress Interactions: OCs (↓ contraceptive efficacy); phenobarbital (↓ griseofulvin absorption/ efficacy); warfarin (↓ anticoagulant effect); cyclosporine (↓ cyclosporine efficacy); ethanol (disulfiram-like reaction: GI distress, flushing, tachycardia, hypotension)	None recommended
Terbinafine Oral granules	Adult: 250 mg daily for 6 wk Child: see below	Can cause nausea/GI distress, reversible taste disturbance, leukopenia, hepatotoxicity No clinically important drug interactions	AST and ALT at baseline, then during and after therapy
Continuous Therapy: Onychomycosis			
Terbinafine (Lamisil)	Adult: 250 mg/d for 6 wk (fingernails); 12 wk (toenails) Child: <20 kg—62.5 mg/d 20–40 kg—125 mg/d >40 kg—250 mg/d (duration as per adult)	As above	CBC, AST, ALT at baseline, then every 4–6 wk
Itraconazole (Sporanox)	Adults: 200 mg/d for 6 wk (fingernails); 12 wk (toenails)	Can cause nausea/GI distress, rash, itching, hypokalemia, CHF, hepatotoxicity Interactions (selective)[a]: simvastatin, lovastatin (↑ myopathy risk); alprazolam (↑ sedation); cisapride (QT prolongation); methadone (cardiovascular toxicity, QT prolongation); cyclosporine (cyclosporine toxicity); rifampin (↓ itraconazole efficacy); ergot (ergot toxicity, nausea, vasospastic ischemia)	AST and ALT at baseline, then every 4–6 wk
Pulse Therapy: Onychomycosis			
Itraconazole (Sporanox)	Adult: 200 mg twice daily for seven consecutive days per month; repeat for 2–3 mo (fingernails) and 3–4 mo (toenails) Child: 5 mg/kg/d for seven consecutive days per month; 2 pulses for fingernails; 3 pulses for toenails		None recommended
Fluconazole (Diflucan)	Adult: 150 mg once weekly for 6–9 mo (until the nail is improved) Child: 3–6 mg/kg once weekly (until the nail is improved), 12–16 wk for fingernails; 18–24 wk for toenails	Can cause nausea/GI distress, rash, itching, thrombocytopenia, hepatotoxicity Interactions (selective)[a]: citalopram (QT prolongation, serotonin syndrome); cisapride (cardiotoxicity); rifabutin (rifabutin toxicity); warfarin (↑ bleeding risk); levofloxacin (QT prolongation); clarithromycin (QT prolongation); fentanyl (↑ opioid effect); colchicine (risk of hepatic and pulmonary toxicity); nitrofurantoin (risk of hepatic and pulmonary toxicity)	None recommended

Sources: Information from Rodgers P, Bassler M. Treating onychomycosis. *Am Fam Physician.* 2001;63:663–672, 677–678; Micromedex® 2.0. www.micromedexsolutions.com. Accessed May 2013; Facts & Comparisons® eAnswers. http://online.factsandcomparisons.com. Accessed May 2013; Semla TP, Beizer JL, Higbee MD. *Geriatric Dosage Handbook.* 15th ed. Hudson, OH: Lexi-Comp Inc.; 2010.
GI, gastrointestinal; OC, oral contraceptive; N/A, not applicable; CBC, complete blood count; ALT, alanine aminotransferase; AST, aspartate aminotransferase; CHF, congestive heart failure.
[a]Selective interactions among numerous others.

steroids. Therapy for severe alopecia areata is best managed by practitioners experienced with the disorder.

B. Hirsutism can be controlled either through hair removal processes, suppression of androgens, or a combination of both.

1. Hair removal

    a. Mechanical hair removal includes shaving, plucking, and waxing. These techniques are relatively inexpensive, but the results are variably short (2–3 days for shaving, 2 weeks for plucking, up to 8 weeks for waxing), can be painful, and often are unacceptable to women. Bleaching unwanted hair, especially on the face, will not reduce hair volume but may make it less noticeable.

    b. Nonprescription **chemical depilatories** can provide a 2-week hair-free interval. Local skin irritation is common.

    c. Electrolysis is performed by specially trained technicians. While considered more effective than laser for permanent hair removal, the results are operator and technique dependent. As electrolysis works by destroying hair follicles individually, it is time-consuming and uncomfortable. Depending on the amount of unwanted hair, many electrolysis sessions may be needed over 18–24 months at a cost of up to $90 per session.

    d. Laser therapy is becoming more popular for hair removal as it is considered less painful and faster than electrolysis. Lasers direct specific wavelengths of light at the follicles; the absorbed energy damages and sometimes destroys the follicle. Advances in laser technology have made laser therapy more effective for short-term hair reduction for all skin types and all types of hair; although light-colored hair may be more difficult to remove. Supporting evidence of long-term effectiveness is lacking and hair regrowth appears to be common. Often 3 to 8 treatments several weeks apart are needed to produce significant results, at a cost of $150–$500 per treatment. Laser therapy may not result in permanent hair removal, and side effects include hyperpigmentation and hair regrowth.

    e. Eflornithine HCl (Vaniqa) is a topical hair growth modulator that can be effective against unwanted facial hair in women. Eflornithine is applied twice daily to the affected areas of the face; results are usually apparent after 4 to 8 weeks of regular use. Often prescribed by primary care physicians, eflornithine can be used indefinitely and is most effective when used in conjunction with other modalities of hair removal (such as laser therapy or hormonal treatment). Eflornithine HCL is usually not covered by medical insurance and can cost $125 for a 30-g tube.

2. Several **hormonal therapies** suppress androgens and reduce hirsutism. These anti-androgens are generally considered equally effective, although none is FDA approved for hirsutism. Because of significant teratogenic potential, reliable contraception is an important component of therapy. There are no systemic medications for hirsutism that can be safely used in women who are pregnant or trying to conceive.

    a. Oral contraceptives with low androgen effects (see Section VI.A.1.c) are considered first-line therapy for most women and can decrease hair growth by 50% to 75% after 6 months of use. (SOR ⊙) They confer other benefits to patients with PCOS and can be used in conjunction with antiandrogen medications, such as spironolactone and finasteride.

    b. Spironolactone (see Section VI.A.1.d) is an antiandrogen that suppresses testosterone production and inhibits uptake through 5α-reductase in the follicle. The usual dose is 100 mg to 200 mg daily.

    c. Finasteride is an antiandrogen; the usual daily dose is 5 mg orally although some studies suggest that the 2.5 mg dose is equally effective.

    d. Other medications **not** generally recommended include **flutamide**, an antiandrogen that has been linked to liver failure, and **glucocorticoids** that are only used in hirsute women with classic congenital adrenal hyperplasia. **GnRH agonists,** such as leuprolide, are at least as effective as the other antiandrogens, but the expense, injectable formulation, and significant side effects limit their usefulness in a woman with hirsutism.

    e. Cyproterone is a progestin that acts as a gonadotropin-releasing hormone blocker. It is not available in the United States but is commonly used in other countries for hirsutism and as a combination oral contraceptive **(Diane)** for maintenance therapy.

C. Treatment of **nail disorders** is specific to the underlying cause.

1. Oral antifungal therapy remains the mainstay of treatment for **onychomycosis,** because local agents generally cannot penetrate the nail. Some data suggest that topical ciclopirox can be effective, but needs to be applied daily for 6 months to 1 year. Authors of a metaanalysis comparing all oral therapies found terbinafine (Lamisil) to be the most effective agent for dermatophyte infections, followed by itraconazole (Sporanox), either in continuous therapy or in pulse therapy. (SOR **Ⓐ**) Fluconazole (Diflucan) had lower cure rates. The prescription medication regimens are compared in Table 31–5.

   An alternative approach is use of an inexpensive topical nonprescription product—Vicks VapoRub. In one study, application of Vicks VapoRub nightly for 48 weeks resulted in 83% of patients with improvement and 28% with a mycological and clinical cure. This compares favorably with the cure rate for prescription topical ciclopirox (8%).

2. **Subungual hematomas** respond best to immediate drainage to relieve pressure. Any heated probe, such as an electrocautery probe or even the tip of a paper clip (heated until red hot) is pressed against the nail over the hematoma to make a small puncture. The blood is expressed with gentle pressure, affording almost immediate pain relief. (YouTube video: https://www.google.com/url?sa=t&rct=j&q=&esrc=s&source=web&cd=5&cad=rja&ved=0CD8QtwIwBA&url=http%3A%2F%2Fwww.youtube.com%2Fwatch%3Fv%3DMXxCVDpS57I&ei=FQRbUaCMKtPk4AOisoH4Ag&usg=AFQjCNFu9sfhR-6LbloK7Fb8J4q5GPxQfQh)

3. **Ingrown nails** with mild inflammation can be treated conservatively with warm soaks, elevating the nail corner with cotton to avoid contact with the inflamed tissue as it grows out, and oral antibiotics if there is a superinfection. Patients should be counseled to trim the nails straight across, which prevents cutting the corners of the nail too short, and to avoid shoes with a narrow toe box. If the ingrown nail does not resolve with these methods, the medial third of the nail should be removed (see Chapter 27).

4. **Acute paronychia** usually requires incision and drainage of any fluid collection. The most fluctuant area along the nail fold can be drained by incising with a small blade (either a no. 11 blade or a no. 15 blade) or by gently separating the nail fold from the nail plate to facilitate drainage without cutting the skin. The incision is irrigated and frequent warm soaks are applied to keep the wound open. Antibiotics are usually not necessary but are appropriate if local drainage and soaks do not resolve the paronychia. Sulfamethoxazole–trimethoprim (Bactrim) or clindamycin (Cleocin) are reasonable choices, given the increasing prevalence of methicillin-resistant *Staphylococcus aureus* in some communities. (You tube video: https://www.google.com/url?sa=t&rct=j&q=&esrc=s&source=web&cd=3&cad=rja&sqi=2&ved=0CDkQtwIwAg&url=http%3A%2F%2Fwww.youtube.com%2Fwatch%3Fv%3Dt19yCFTnMrE&ei=fAJbUZreBLa84AOoh4GlBg&usg=AFQjCNFzjKDkv-xVbdojAEwDs1Qa2wozIQ)

5. **Chronic paronychia** is more difficult to treat, because several nails are affected and incision and drainage is usually not an option. Treatments include avoiding chronic exposure to moisture (or wearing cotton-lined rubber gloves when unable to prevent exposure) and using 1:1 vinegar–water soaks. A small, randomized study reported greater cure rates with the use of topical steroids than with oral antifungals, suggesting that the presence of candidal infection may not contribute significantly to the condition. (SOR **Ⓑ**) Areas of inflammation or discharge can be cultured to allow specific treatment, as *Staphylococcus* species and *Pseudomonas* have also been implicated and require oral antibiotics. Treatment failure should prompt a search for an underlying systemic disease, such as psoriasis.

6. **Nail changes of underlying systemic disorders,** such as psoriasis and alopecia areata, may improve with treatment of the disease but nail-specific treatment has not been overly successful. Clubbing is usually a permanent change.

SELECTED REFERENCES

Andrews M, Burns M. Common tinea infections in children. *Am Fam Physician.* 2008;77(10):1415–1420.

Bode D, Seehusen D, Baird D. Hirsutism in women. *Am Fam Physician.* 2012;85(4):373–380.

Martin KA, Chang RJ, Ehrmann DA, et al. Evaluation and treatment of hirsutism in premenopausal women: an Endocrine Society Clinical Practice Guideline. *J Clin Endocrinol Metab.* 2008;93:1105–1120.

Mounsey AL, Reed SW. Diagnosing and treating hair loss. *Am Fam Physician.* 2009;80(4):356–362.

Additional references are available online at http://langetextbooks.com/fm6e

32 Hand and Wrist Complaints*

Jessica T. Servey, MD, FAAFP, Col, USAF, Ted Boehm, MD, &
Nicole G. Stern, MD

KEY POINTS

- Methodical examination of the hand and wrist in combination with knowledge of the mechanism of injury can be used to diagnose most conditions. (SOR **G**)
- A normal neurovascular examination should always be documented, including two-point tactile discrimination. (SOR **G**)
- The contralateral side should be examined for comparison. (SOR **G**)
- Conditions warranting more urgent surgical consultation include intra-articular fractures and significant scaphoid fractures. (SOR **B**)

I. **Definition.** The hand and wrist consist of 28 bones, numerous articulations, and 19 intrinsic and 20 extrinsic muscles. The surface anatomy can be separated into dorsal, volar (palmar), radial, and ulnar sides. The palm is divided into thenar, midpalm, and hypothenar areas; the **thenar eminence,** containing the small thumb muscles, represents the area just proximal to the thumb, and the opposite side of the palm is the **hypothenar eminence**. Overall, the unique anatomy of the hand and wrist, with closely situated and interrelated structures, allows for extensive variability of movement necessary in functional and recreational activities.

Whether occurring acutely or chronically, injuries to the hand or wrist can be debilitating. **Common complaints involving the hand and wrist** include pain, numbness, tingling, instability, weakness, skin discoloration, coldness, swelling, and bony deformity. These are most often due to overuse, trauma, nerve compression, and underlying systemic diseases such as diabetes mellitus, hypothyroidism, and rheumatoid arthritis. This chapter provides an approach to the differential diagnosis and management of common hand and wrist disorders.

II. **Common Diagnoses.** Hand and wrist injuries are particularly common in certain occupations, hobbies, and sports. They can be particularly debilitating when affecting the dominant hand, and difficult to rest. Having a systematic approach to the hand and wrist history and examination combined with an understanding of the functional anatomy (Figure 32–1) allows a careful diagnosis and treatment plan to be made by the primary care provider in any setting.

A. **Tendon injuries,** including tendon ruptures and avulsion, or tendonitis, are common especially in sports and among industrial workers.

1. **Boutonnière deformity** (Figure 32–2) can be seen in athletes, especially those involved in contact or ball sports.

2. **Mallet deformity** (Figure 32–3) occurs in athletes, especially those who hit or catch a ball, and results from an axial blow to the terminal phalanx causing forced flexion of the distal interphalangeal joint, often rupturing the terminal extensor tendon and can cause distal phalangeal avulsion fracture.

3. **Jersey finger** occurs when an athlete attempts to tackle an opponent who is pulling away. In one study, 75% of cases of jersey finger in football and rugby players involved the ring finger. The involved structural injury is avulsion of the flexor digitorum profundus. This can occur with or without a bony avulsion fracture. All jersey fingers need to be referred for specialty consult in orthopedic or hand surgery (SOR B).

4. **Trigger finger** (Figure 32–4) (stenosing tenosynovitis) usually occurs from continuous direct pressure over the distal palm or metacarpophalangeal (MCP) flexion crease in athletes holding a racquet, golf club, or bat.

5. **de Quervain tenosynovitis** is inflammation of the extensor pollicis longus, extensor pollicis brevis, and abductor pollicis longus. It occurs in athletes and industrial

---

*The opinions herein are those of the author. They do not represent official policy of the Uniformed Services University, the Department of the Air Force or the Department of Defense.

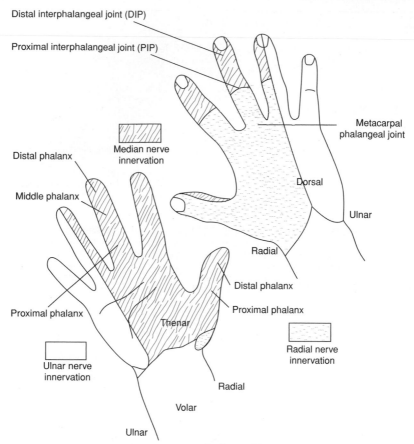

FIGURE 32–1. Sensory distribution of the hand.

workers who engage in repetitive wrist motion, which includes radial and ulnar deviation as well as flexion and extension. This is the most common tendinopathy in athletes. Sports and activities most commonly associated with de Quervain include racquet sports, golf, and fishing. It is also often seen in postpartum and breastfeeding mothers.

B. Sprains and contusions represent the most common injuries seen in sporting events (especially basketball, football, and skiing) and likely comprise a majority (incidence unknown) of the hand, finger, and wrist injuries that account for 3% to 9% of all sports-related injuries reported in the literature.

    1. Swan-neck deformity (Figure 32–5) occasionally occurs in athletes playing either contact or noncontact sports. Chronically, swan-neck deformities can also occur in patients with inflammatory arthritis, such as rheumatoid arthritis and gout. These can occur from prior mallet finger not adequately treated.

    2. Ulnar collateral ligament injury of the thumb MCP joint commonly occurs in football players, skiers, and wrestlers when athletes attempt to break their fall with their hand. The mechanism of injury generally involves forced radial deviation of the thumb at the MCP joint. The rupture of the ligament may or may not include a concomitant bony avulsion. When the ligament is forced outside of the aponeurosis, a Stener lesion may occur. This should not be missed since there can be significant long-term morbidity. Early surgery is required for any Stener lesion.

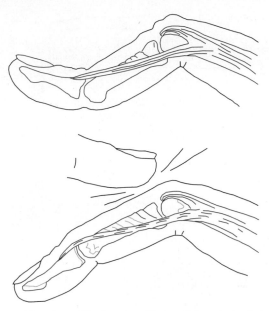

FIGURE 32–2. Boutonnière deformity caused by disruption of the central slip and volar displacement of the lateral bands. The point tenderness test elicits tenderness over the base of the middle phalanx.

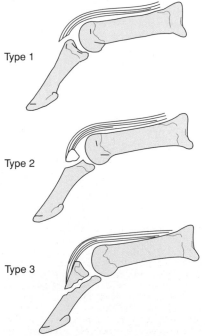

Type 1

Type 2

Type 3

FIGURE 32–3. The three types of mallet finger.

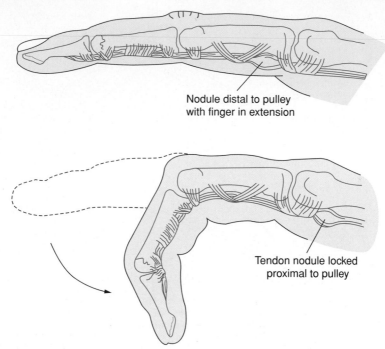

Nodule distal to pulley
with finger in extension

Tendon nodule locked
proximal to pulley

FIGURE 32–4. Trigger finger results from nodular constriction of the flexor tendon by inflammation of the fibrous sheath at the metacarpophalangeal joint. (Reproduced with permission from Greene WB (ed): *Essentials of Musculoskeletal Care,* 2nd ed. Rosemont, IL: American Academy of Orthopaedic Surgeons; 2001.)

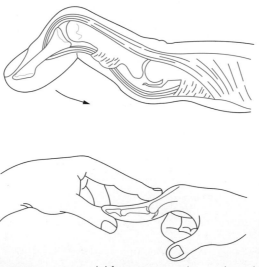

FIGURE 32–5. Volar plate rupture causes swan-neck deformity. A stress test shows an abnormal increase in extension.

3. Triangular fibrocartilage complex (TFCC) tears, often seen in sports such as baseball and gymnastics, result when the athlete suddenly, or repetitively, loads all their weight on their wrist with or without simultaneous, excessive torque. This can have an acute or insidious onset.

C. Fractures are very common in the wrist and hand. Metacarpal fractures account for up to one-third of the fractures of the hand.

1. Fractures of the first metacarpal occur most often in football players and athletes requiring a strong pinch-grip mechanism in their sport, such as in racquet sports, hockey, or bull riding. Dexterity of the hand is dependent on the thumb both in its great mobility and oppositional strength with the other fingers. There are three types of fractures to the first metacarpal, two of which require referral to an orthopedic or hand surgeon. Bennett and Rolando fractures involve the intra-articular surface, and all other fractures are extra-articular. Bennett and Rolando fractures need to have specialty referral after initial splinting and/or casting.

2. Other metacarpal fractures of the hand are common. As long as there is careful examination of the area, this can be managed by a primary care physician. The most common is the Boxer fracture, involving the fifth metacarpal. This occurs after an axial load with flexed fingers, such as when a fist hits a wall. Checking for rotation is essential. This is performed by looking at the hand with a closed fist (fingers flexed). The second through fifth fingers should all point to the scaphoid without overlapping. The contralateral hand should be used as a reference for any normal variations. The metacarpals can have varying amounts of rotation, from 10 degrees on the second metacarpal to 35 to 40 degrees on the fifth.

3. Scaphoid fractures represent about two-thirds of all carpal fractures. They are usually due to a fall onto an outstretched hand with the wrist in hyperextension. This area of the wrist has limited blood supply causing a risk of avascular necrosis. Additionally, these fractures can be missed on initial evaluation. A strong suspicion warrants splinting and reevaluation with examination and x-ray in 1 to 2 weeks; some of these fractures take 4 weeks before visualization on plain film. Computerized tomography (CT) scan has become a quick and reliable way to look for occult fractures. Any scaphoid fracture not healing should be referred to an orthopedic or hand surgeon.

4. Scapholunate dissociation (Figures 32–6 and 32–7) also occurs commonly in those sustaining a fall onto an outstretched hand.

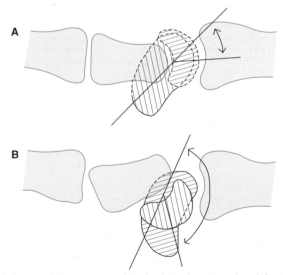

FIGURE 32–6. Scapholunate angle measurements on lateral radiograph. **A.** Normal scapholunate angle is 30 to 60 degrees. **B.** Vertical scaphoid and lunate subluxated palmarward in an abnormal scapholunate angle measured greater than 65 degrees.

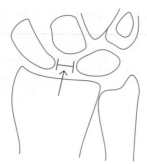

FIGURE 32–7. Distance between the scaphoid and lunate is greater than 3 mm, sometimes called the "Terry Thomas" or "David Letterman" sign.

     5. Phalangeal fractures are very common and are the second most common fracture type in children.

  D. Dislocations of the fingers are very common injuries seen acutely by a primary care physician. Dislocations are often relocated by the patient or during an x-ray. Dislocations can occur in three directions: lateral, dorsal, or volar. It is critical to note the neurovascular status before and after any reduction with two-point tactile discrimination.

  E. Among **ganglia injuries,** dorsal and volar wrist ganglion cysts are the most common soft-tissue masses of the hand and wrist. The incidence is unknown, but there may be a predilection in those with carpal tunnel syndrome, in those with previous wrist impaction injury, or in athletes such as gymnasts.

  F. Arthritis. The hands, notably the base of the thumb, are susceptible to osteoarthritis; carpometacarpal (CMC) arthritis is very common in women, especially those doing repetitive activities (e.g., professional seamstresses). CMC arthritis also occurs idiopathically in women and following trauma in men (see Chapter 82).

  G. Entrapment neuropathies are commonly seen in the workplace or other situations requiring repetitive hand movement.

    1. Carpal tunnel syndrome is considered the most common entrapment neuropathy and is seen in occupations requiring continuous typing and in athletes, but it may also occur spontaneously in pregnant women or in patients with diabetes, hypothyroidism, or acromegaly. Approximately 50% of patients have bilateral carpal tunnel syndrome. Conservative treatment can be tried followed by injections or iontophoresis if unsuccessful (see below). Refer for surgical treatment if a patient fails conservative therapy.

    2. Ulnar neuropathy of the hand, also called Guyon canal syndrome, can be seen in cyclists (often called handlebar palsy) and racquet sport athletes where repetitive power gripping is required. Injury to the ulnar nerve occurs when there is continuous pressure on the nerve, causing inflammation, or from traumatic fractures of the hamate or pisiform.

    3. Radial nerve compression, also known as "handcuff neuropathy," is commonly seen in tennis and other racquet sports in which the athlete performs repetitive ulnar flexion, pronation, and supination.

III. Symptoms and Signs (Table 32–1). An accurate history, including occupation, activities, handedness, and mechanism of injury for acute injuries, is critical in diagnosing hand and wrist complaints. An accurate diagnosis may be obtained by a detailed history in up to 70% of wrist pain cases. In addition, localizing symptoms to specific areas, such as dorsal, volar, radial, and ulnar, can assist in narrowing the differential diagnosis. Examination of individuals with hand and wrist complaints is facilitated by knowledge of relevant anatomy and a systematic approach, beginning with inspection (deformity, skin color changes, and edema), followed by palpation (tenderness), range of motion (active, passive, instability check), neurovascular examination (Figures 32–1 to 32–7), and specific provocative testing. Specifically checking pre- and postreduction neurovascular status is imperative and must be documented.

TABLE 32–1. DIFFERENTIAL DIAGNOSIS AND MANAGEMENT OF COMMON HAND AND WRIST COMPLAINTS

	Diagnosis	Symptoms	Signs	Testing	Treatment
Tendon injuries	Boutonnière deformity	Pain after sudden forced flexion of PIP	Swelling Flexion of the PIP and hyperextension of the DIP (Figure 32–2) Tenderness with pressure directly over base of the middle phalanx	X-ray anteroposterior and lateral, rule out avulsion fracture	Splint PIP full extension/leave the DIP free Immobilize 6–8 wk and athletes for 4–6 wk more Surgery if fracture
	Mallet deformity	Pain after forceful axial blow causing forced flexion of the DIP	Tenderness on the DIP Cannot actively extend distal phalanx (Figure 32–3)	X-ray to rule out fracture	Splint DIP in extension for 6–8 wk, nighttime splint for 3–4 wk, then wean depending on severity of injury
	Jersey finger (flexor digitorum profundus tendon rupture or avulsion)	Pain on flexor side from forced extension of the DIP during maximum contracture	Patient cannot flex at the DIP PIP swelling or palm tenderness from FDP retraction in these areas	X-ray to rule out fracture	All acute injuries need specialty consult for early surgical repair Conservative therapy if chronic injury can be tried
	Trigger finger (digital flexor tenosynovitis)	Nodule on the distal palm, "catching" or "triggering" of the finger	Nodular thickening of the flexor tendon within the distal palm resulting in loss of smooth extension or flexion of the finger (Figure 32–4)	X-ray not necessary unless concern for tumor	Corticosteroid injection into sheath (Table 32–2) Surgical decompression of the A-1 pulley
	de Quervain tenosynovitis	Pain, swelling near or over radial styloid, gradually or suddenly, worse with use of the hand and thumb especially gripping or twisting	Tenderness, swelling over radial styloid (inflammation in first dorsal extensor compartment); positive Finkelstein test (see Section III.A.1)	X-ray to rule out bony pathology only if suspicion of fracture or not improving with conservative treatment	Thumb/wrist immobilization in thumb spica splint NSAIDs Physical or occupational therapy Steroid injection (Table 32–2) and/or surgical decompression if conservative therapy fails
Sprains	Swan-neck deformity	Pain at the PIP, deformity often chronic and seen in RA	Tender at the PIP, deformity with hyperextension at the PIP, and flexion at the DIP (Figure 32–5)	X-ray shows deformity	Open repair of volar plate if acute, and if deformity causes disability in chronic cases

(continued)

TABLE 32–1. DIFFERENTIAL DIAGNOSIS AND MANAGEMENT OF COMMON HAND AND WRIST COMPLAINTS (Continued)

	Diagnosis	Symptoms	Signs	Testing	Treatment
	Ulnar collateral ligament (UCL) sprain of the thumb MCP (gamekeeper's or skier's thumb)	Pain at the MCP of the thumb from abduction force across the joint	Tender at the MCP of the thumb and a positive gamekeeper's test (see Section III.A.2), may also have a mass palpable if Stener lesion is present	X-ray to rule out avulsion fracture, get PA, lateral and oblique views; stress views may be necessary MRI if plain films negative	Grade I/II immobilize in thumb spica cast 2–4 wk, then thumb spica splint 2–4 wk or more Grade III treated surgically acutely
	Triangular fibrocartilage complex (TFCC) tears	Dorsal ulnar-sided pain during ulnar deviation with pronation and supination	Pain with forced passive pronation and supination of the wrist; dorsal subluxation of the ulna often with a painful "clunk," TFCC compression test positive (see Section III.A.11)	X-ray to rule out radioulnar arthritis or other bony pathology; magnetic resonance arthrogram to look at the cartilage	Neutral splint for 4–6 wk, NSAIDs, rest; surgical referral for refractory symptoms
Fractures	Fracture of the first metacarpal	Pain after blow to the distal thumb while flexed, swelling base of the thumb	Base of the thumb metacarpal displaced up and back, while tip of the thumb is held into the palm, Froment sign showing weakness of the thumb grip	X-ray to demonstrate oblique fracture of base of the thumb metacarpal and dislocation (if present)— add oblique view of the thumb to PA/lateral views	Bennett and Rolando types place in the thumb spica splint and refer to specialty evaluation; otherwise short arm thumb spica for 4 wk
	Scaphoid fracture	Radial-sided pain after fall onto the outstretched hand	Tender in anatomic snuffbox or volar side of radiocarpal area	X-ray: need longitudinal view of scaphoid. CT/MRI often needed for definitive diagnosis	Nondisplaced fracture: Short arm TS cast or splint 4–6 wk Middle/proximal fractures: Long arm TS cast 6 wk, then short arm TS cast 4–14 wk until x-ray union Displaced fractures: Long arm TS cast or splint, refer to hand surgeon
	Scapholunate dissociation	Dorsal radial wrist pain, decreased grip strength, and "clicking"	Tender in anatomic snuffbox or dorsal wrist at the scapholunate joint, "click" with pain during Watson test	X-ray (AP and lateral): scapholunate angle ≥60 degrees (Figure 32–6) or scapholunate space ≥3 mm ("Terry Thomas" or "David Letterman" sign) (Figure 32–7)	Immobilize and refer to hand surgeon

TABLE 32–1. DIFFERENTIAL DIAGNOSIS AND MANAGEMENT OF COMMON HAND AND WRIST COMPLAINTS (Continued)

	Diagnosis	Symptoms	Signs	Testing	Treatment
	Metacarpal fractures; Boxer fracture is most common (fifth metacarpal)	Blunt force axial trauma with flexed phalanges, or crush injuries, pain and swelling in the mid-hand	Tender over the area of broken bone, may have tenderness elsewhere from soft tissue swelling, check for volar angulation with closed-fist examination, note any skin lacerations and risk of open fracture	X-ray including oblique view to look for rotation and angulation	Reduction if angulated and gutter splint for 4–6 wk with periodic evaluation to check for movement
	Phalangeal fractures	Crush injury, direct blow or torsion as mechanism, pain, and swelling	Tender over the area, potential deformity from bone shortening	X-ray may include oblique view	Aluminum splint or buddy taping for mid-shaft, specialty referral for intra-articular injuries; special cases discussed in sections above
Ganglia	Ganglion cysts	Often originate on tendon sheath; pain or "bump"	Tender or non-tender mobile soft-tissue mass over radial or dorsal wrist or over flexor/extensor tendon sheath	X-ray to rule out bony pathology; arteriogram as needed to rule out radial artery aneurysm or traumatic pseudo-aneurysm	Observation if asymptomatic; neutral wrist splint, aspiration, injection (Table 32–2), or excision
Arthritis	Carpometacarpal (CMC) of thumb arthritis	Pain at base of the thumb with pinching and gripping activities; pain can radiate up the arm with "clicking" or "catching" sensation in the thumb	Tender over volar or radial sides of the CMC joint; positive grind test (see Section III.A.3)	X-ray shows loss of joint space, subchondral sclerosis, bone spurs, subluxation, or dislocation at the CMC joint	Immobilize in TS splint 3–6 wk; occupational therapy; injection (Table 32–2); referral to hand surgeon if failed conservative treatment
Neuropathies	Carpal tunnel syndrome	Numbness, tingling, pain in the palmar wrist and hand; worse overnight and in the morning, after repetitive use, and cold sensitivity, color changes	Swelling, weakness, sensation loss in nerve distribution (Figure 32–1); positive Tinel test; negative Spurling test (see Section III.A.7)	X-ray to rule out bony pathology; nerve conduction velocity studies (NCVs) show delayed terminal sensory latency; c-spine x-ray if indicated to rule out cervical neuroforaminal encroachment	Ergonomic correction, night neutral wrist splints, NSAIDs; injection (Table 32–2), and/or surgery for carpal tunnel release if conservative treatment fails

(continued)

TABLE 32–1. DIFFERENTIAL DIAGNOSIS AND MANAGEMENT OF COMMON HAND AND WRIST COMPLAINTS (Continued)

Diagnosis	Symptoms	Signs	Testing	Treatment
Ulnar neuropathy (Guyon canal syndrome)	Numbness and tingling in fourth and fifth digits, pain, and weakness (Figure 32–1)	Swelling, weakness, sensation loss; positive ulnar Tinel test (see Section III.A.4)	X-ray to rule out bony pathology (e.g., hamate fracture); NCVs and Allen test (see Section III.A.6)	Immobilize, cryotherapy, NSAIDs; surgical decompression for refractory cases
Radial nerve compression	Pain/numbness/tingling over dorsoradial aspect of wrist and thumb (Figure 32–1)	Swelling, weakness, sensation loss; positive radial Tinel test	X-ray to rule out bony pathology; NCVs, two-point discrimination test (see Section III.A.8)	Immobilize, NSAIDs, molded orthoses; surgical decompression and nerve transfer for refractory cases

DIP, distal interphalangeal joint; FDP, flexor digitorum profundus; MCP, metacarpophalangeal joint; MRI, magnetic resonance imaging; NSAIDs, nonsteroidal anti-inflammatory drugs; PIP, tendon proximal interphalangeal joint; RA, rheumatoid arthritis.

- **A. Special tests** (Table 32–2)
  1. **Finkelstein test.** This test is used to diagnose de Quervain tenosynovitis.
  2. **Gamekeeper test.** This test is used to diagnose ulnar collateral ligament (UCL) injury at the thumb–MCP joint. Prior to performing this test, an x-ray should be obtained to rule out fracture. If a fracture is seen, the test should not be performed. (SOR C)
  3. **Grind test.** This test is helpful in diagnosing thumb CMC arthritis.
  4. **Watson "click" test.** This test is performed to evaluate for scapholunate dissociation.
  5. **Tinel test.** This test is provocative for carpal tunnel syndrome or for ulnar or radial neuropathy.
  6. **Phalen test.** This is another test for carpal tunnel syndrome.
  7. **Allen test.** This test is useful to rule out vascular disorders such as hypothenar hammer syndrome (ulnar artery injury) or Raynaud disease (seen in collagen vascular diseases).
  8. **Spurling test.** This test attempts to create neural foraminal narrowing that may or may not reproduce radicular arm pain, numbness, or tingling.
  9. **Froment sign.** This test shows weakness of the adductor pollicis muscles and can be positive when the first metacarpal is fractured.
  10. **Two-point discrimination.** This test is used to assess nerve function.
  11. **TFCC compression test.** This test is used to detect tears in the TFCC.
- **IV. Laboratory Tests** (Table 32–1)
  - **A. X-rays.** When diagnosing hand and wrist complaints, initial evaluation often includes obtaining a plain radiograph following physical examination. Finger x-rays should be done with AP, lateral, and oblique views. (SOR **G**) When reviewing wrist films to evaluate a possible scaphoid or scapholunate injury, a clenched fist view or ulnar deviation view can be obtained. A gap of more than 3 mm in the scapholunate joint should alert the physician to consider scapholunate dissociation until proven otherwise ("Terry Thomas" or "David Letterman" sign). In tendon injuries, it is essential to rule out an avulsion fracture while reviewing a plain x-ray.
  - **B. Other radiographic imaging.** MRI can be very helpful to rule out other injuries to bone, muscle, and tendons. It can also be extremely helpful to evaluate the **TFCC** for a tear. The examiner should make sure to order a magnetic resonance arthrogram of the wrist if a TFCC tear is suspected. The dye helps to delineate very small injuries to the TFCC that could otherwise not be visualized. CT scan of the wrist and hand with computerized reconstructions can also be beneficial to evaluate for a small fracture that may be difficult to visualize because of overlapping of the carpal and hand bones on x-ray.

TABLE 32-2. SPECIAL TESTS

Test	Method	Result	Demonstration
Finkelstein test	The patient fully flexes the thumb into the palm, followed by passive ulnar deviation of the wrist by the examiner	Pain elicited on this maneuver suggests de Quervain tenosynovitis	http://www.youtube.com/ watch?v=RfyXClxY_E0
Game-keeper test	After a fracture has been ruled out, with one hand, the examiner holds the patient's thumb metacarpal and the other hand holds the patient's thumb proximal phalanx. A gentle radial deviation is applied to the thumb tip MCP joint to stress the UCL	A UCL sprain will show laxity, while a complete rupture (**Stener lesion**) can be diagnosed on clinical examination by not feeling an end point during stress testing in either full extension or 30 degrees of MCP flexion	http://www.youtube.com/ watch?v=ysr1AR26Snc
Grind test	The examiner holds the patient's wrist with one hand and the other hand holds the patient's thumb metacarpal. The examiner then provides an axial load to the thumb and gently rotates it side-to-side	A positive test reproduces pain and crepitus and sometimes shows instability, indicating degenerative arthritis	http://www.youtube.com/ watch?v=-6KBlJJowZs
Watson "click" test	The scaphoid is stabilized by the examiner and the patient's wrist is brought from ulnar deviation to radial deviation	Pain is elicited and a "click" is heard from subluxation of the scaphoid, demonstrating scapho-lunate instability	http://www.youtube.com/ watch?v=ZOD-4ltpTa0
Tinel test	The examiner percusses over and just distal to the distal palmar crease midline on the volar wrist or percusses the distal crease over the radial or ulnar nerve	Reproduces the patient's paresthesias (in a median, radial, or ulnar nerve distribution)	http://www.youtube.com/ watch?v=J3i1MYNDHHA
Phalen test	The patient holds the wrists in maximum flexion for 1 to 2 min	Paresthesias occur within 1 to 2 min	http://www.youtube.com/ watch?v=RpGHYujo37o
Allen test	The patient rests a hand on the knee or a table while the examiner compresses the radial artery with one thumb and the ulnar artery with the other thumb. Next, the patient clenches and opens the fist three times. Then the patient opens the palm and the radial artery is released to see how fast color returns to the palm. The test is then repeated, this time releasing the ulnar artery	Lack of return of color to the portion of the hand supplied by that artery within 7–10 s	http://www.youtube.com/ watch?v=dfQ5chcmDH0
Spurling test	With the patient sitting upright on the examination table, the examiner provides gentle axial loading on top of the head while passively extending the neck, then tilting the head to the side	Reproducing radicular arm pain, numbness, or tingling may represent cervical disk herniation or cervical spondylosis (osteoarthritis)	http://www.youtube.com/ watch?v=Fhr1yWkwwDU

(continued)

TABLE 32–2. SPECIAL TESTS (Continued)

Test	Method	Result	Demonstration
Froment sign	The test is performed by having the patient pinch a piece of paper between the thumb and second finger and attempting to pull it free	A positive test is the inability to hold the paper securely	http://www.youtube.com/watch?v=F-9fgil2r4A
Two-point discrimination	To perform this test, use two sterile pins to simultaneously prick the skin on the hand in the area of numbness. The pins are separated at different distances in order to determine when the patient perceives the pins as two points versus one	Fingertip two-point discrimination is normally 2 to 8 mm; used to detect nerve injury/compression	http://www.youtube.com/watch?v=QplcT2MjuEc
Triangular fibrocartilage compression test	To perform this test axially load the wrist then deviate to the ulnar side	A positive test is pain and often a "click" indicating a tear in the triangular fibrocartilage complex	http://www.youtube.com/watch?v=tM_O2cnlgh8

V. Treatment (Table 32–1)

A. Pharmacologic treatment. The cornerstone for the treatment of most hand and wrist injuries often involves one or more of the following: **nonsteroidal anti-inflammatory drugs (NSAIDs)** (e.g., oral ibuprofen, 600–800 mg with food three times daily, or naproxen, 500 mg with food twice daily) for 2 weeks or longer depending on the condition, with precautions for **renal and gastrointestinal toxicity, immobilization, injection** (Table 32–3), or **surgery. Some new data suggest that NSAIDs inhibit fracture healing.** Consider NSAID use only for low-risk patients and for a short time period, probably not exceeding a week after fracture.

B. Nonpharmacologic treatment. There are many potential ways to aid in pain reduction and decrease swelling after injuries of any type to the hand and wrist.

   1. Splinting controls motion and as such decreases pain. This also allows for a decrease in swelling through active compression.

   a. For **Mallet deformity,** a stacked splint must be worn 24 hours a day for the first 6 weeks. The patient should be told to keep the distal interphalangeal joint extended on a hard surface if the splint is removed. Monitoring patients for compliance as well as ensuring that the initial splint is waterproof is critical in healing. All extension splints appear to achieve similar long-term results, but data are insufficient to fully evaluate comparative effectiveness. (SOR ⦿)

   b. Phalangeal fractures. Many of these can be managed with aluminum splinting or buddy taping.

   c. Phalangeal dislocations. Dorsal dislocations can be splinted in flexion after reduction. Lateral dislocations can usually be buddy taped after reduction. Volar dislocations need more attention. After reduction, these must be placed in full extension to decrease morbidity.

   d. Entrapment neuropathies. For patients with carpal tunnel syndrome, conservative treatment with night splints and change of activities that exacerbate the symptoms should be tried first. There are limited data supporting the use of a night splint for short-term benefit (vs. no splint), but insufficient evidence regarding effectiveness or safety of a particular type of splint or wearing regimen. (SOR ⦿) A short trial of NSAIDs can also be suggested.

   2. Ice and elevation are well-known adjuncts to decreasing pain and swelling in all musculoskeletal injuries or inflammation. Hands should be elevated above the level of the heart.

   3. Physical therapy and occupational therapy are adjuncts to all injuries especially to maintain mobility and strength in the hand. Other modalities may be useful in tendinopathies.

   4. Steroid injections. For patients with **carpal tunnel syndrome,** steroid injections have strong evidence demonstrating short-term relief, (SOR ⦿) but no benefit over

TABLE 32-3. HAND AND WRIST INJECTIONS

	Diagnosis	Equipment	Anesthetic	Corticosteroid	Injection Technique
Tendon Injuries	Carpal tunnel syndrome	25–30 gauge, 1.5-inch needle with a 5-mL syringe	2–3 mL 1% lidocaine or 0.25%–0.5% bupivacaine	1 mL betamethasone (Celestone) or 40 mg/mL methylprednisolone	Insert needle at 30-degree angle on volar wrist at proximal wrist crease just ulnar to the palmaris longus tendon aiming at the fourth digit
	First CMC arthritis	25–30 gauge, 1-inch needle with a 3-mL syringe	0.5 mL 1% lidocaine or 0.25%–0.5% bupivacaine	0.25–0.5 mL Celestone or methylprednisolone	Insert needle on ulnar side of extensor pollicis brevis just proximal to first metacarpal on extensor surface
	de Quervain tenosynovitis	25–27 gauge, 1.5-inch needle with a 5-mL syringe	2 mL 1% lidocaine or 0.25%–0.5% bupivacaine	1 mL Celestone or methylprednisolone	Insert needle into first extensor compartment, direct proximally toward radial styloid (not into tendon)
	Ganglion cysts	18 gauge, 1- to 1.5-inch needle with a 20- to 30-mL syringe	1–2 mL 1% lidocaine or 0.25%–0.5% bupivacaine	1 mL Celestone or methylprednisolone	Insert needle into cyst, aspirate. Use hemostat to stabilize needle, change syringe, then inject
	Trigger finger	25–30 gauge, 1- to 1.5-inch needle with a 3-mL syringe	0.5–1 mL 1% lidocaine or 0.25%–0.5% bupivacaine	0.5 mL Celestone or methylprednisolone	Insert needle at 30-degree angle over palmar aspect distal to the metacarpal head, then direct needle proximally, almost parallel to the skin, toward the nodule

CMC, carpometacarpal joint.

either anti-inflammatory treatment and splinting after 8 weeks or Helium–Neon laser treatment after 6 months. Injections have potential risks to the nerve and overlying skin (atrophy), and two local injections do not provide added clinical benefit.

C. Patient follow-up is dependent on each injury type. If fractures and injuries are not progressing as expected, prompt referral to an orthopedic or hand surgeon is warranted.

SELECTED REFERENCES

Abraham MK, Scott S. The emergent evaluation and treatment of hand and wrist injuries. *Emerg Med Clin North Am.* 2010;28(4):789–809.

Borchers J, Best T. Common finger fractures and dislocations. *Am Fam Physician.* 2012;85(8):805–810.

Seidenberg P, Beutler A. *The Sports Medicine Resource Manual.* Philadelphia PA: Elsevier Saunders; 2008.

Tallia AF, Cardone DA. Diagnostic and therapeutic injection of the wrist and hand region. *Am Fam Physician.* 2003;67:745.

Additional references are available online at http://langetextbooks.com/fm6e

33   Headaches

Dan F. Criswell, MD

KEY POINTS

- Most headaches are benign and treatable in the primary care office setting. (SOR **C**)
- Careful attention to a focused set of symptoms and signs will alert the clinician to more serious causes of headache. (SOR **C**)
- Neuroimaging is not usually necessary in the evaluation of headaches when the history clearly suggests a primary headache disorder and a careful neurologic examination is normal. (SOR **B**)

I. **Definition.** Headache, or **cephalgia,** is pain or discomfort perceived in the head, neck, or both. **Primary headache disorders** are recurrent benign headaches whose causes are multifactorial; trigeminal serotonin receptors are felt to play a significant role in the inflammation and vasodilation contributing to pain in migraine headaches. **Secondary headaches** result from an underlying pathology caused by a distinct condition (e.g., medication overuse/withdrawal, aneurysm, infection, inflammation, or neoplasm).

II. **Primary Headache Disorders.** Most people will experience an episodic headache during their lifetime. The annual prevalence may be as high as 90%, with a minority of those sufferers pursuing medical evaluation. Still, headaches are the second most common pain syndrome seen in primary care ambulatory practice.

There are many headache classification systems. Using the International Headache Society system, **the most common primary headaches in primary care are episodic migraine, tension-type headache (TTH), and cluster.** Secondary headaches comprise fewer than 10% of headaches in primary care, but include some important treatable and life-threatening entities.

A. **Episodic migraine.** Migraine affects 18% of women and 6.5% of men each year (28–30 million individuals in the United States). The onset of symptoms is usually between adolescence and young adulthood. The peak prevalence is between 30 to 39 years of age, where it affects approximately 1 in 4 women and 1 in 10 men. Over 25% of migraineurs have more than three headache days per month. A strong correlation with family history of migraine has been observed in migraineurs. It is estimated that only 51% of women and 41% of men who experience migraine have actually been diagnosed. More than 60% of migraineurs are treated only by their primary care physicians for headache. Episodic migraine is commonly misdiagnosed as "sinus headache." In one study, 88% of patients who labeled themselves as having "sinus headaches" actually met criteria for episodic migraine headaches.

B. **TTH** is also called muscle contraction headache. The 1-year prevalence of episodic TTH is estimated at 38%. The 1-year prevalence for chronic TTH is estimated at 2.2%. TTH represents 12% of lost workdays due to headache in the United States annually. Onset varies widely and can be at any age. Fewer than half of these patients have a positive family history of headache; there is a positive association between chronic TTH and mood disorders. Once felt to be the most common headache diagnosed in the primary care office, a revised definition of migraine has identified migraines that were previously considered tension type. "Mixed headache," another common syndrome consisting of migraine and TTH in the same headache, may actually be a migraine variant or two distinct headache types.

C. **Cluster.** Although not common in the primary care office, cluster headaches are recognized as one of the more common primary headache disorders in the general population (lifetime prevalence approximately 0.1%). Men are affected more commonly than women, with onset between ages 30 and 50 years. There is a positive association with smoking.

D. **Unusual primary headache disorders:** paroxysmal hemicrania, hemicrania continua, and hypnic headaches. Although discussion is beyond the scope of the chapter, these disorders are mentioned primarily in the differential diagnosis of cluster headaches. Chronic daily headaches are usually a combination of chronic migraine/tension headache associated with medication overuse.

III. Secondary Headaches. Less than 0.4% of headaches in primary care are from serious intracranial disease. Although secondary headaches are unusual, the most common secondary headache seen in primary care is rebound or withdrawal headache.

   A. Rebound or withdrawal headaches usually develop from a preexisting primary headache disorder. Substances included in the treatment of headache such as caffeine, acetaminophen, aspirin, ergots alkaloids, opioids, butalbital, nonsteroidal anti-inflammatory drugs (NSAIDs), and Midrin are the primary agents.

   B. Other secondary headaches that are seen with regularity in primary care include those associated with neoplasm, infections (e.g., meningitis, purulent sinusitis, and abscess), temporal arteritis, acute glaucoma, and cerebral aneurysm.

IV. Symptoms. Differentiation among types of headaches is usually based on the patient's history. Emphasis should be placed on the onset, quality and intensity of pain, frequency, provoking influences, and associated symptoms. Patients frequently experience more than one headache type; to avoid misdiagnosis, it is important to define each type carefully. A headache diary can help with ongoing evaluation of episodic headaches. Using standardized inquiries, such as the five-item Migraine Disability Assessment Score (MIDAS) questionnaire, quantifies the impact of headaches on quality of life and promotes standardization of headache disability (Table 33–1).

   A. Primary headache disorder

   1. Migraine. Episodic migraine is classified as migraine with aura (classic) or without (common). Associated symptoms can include a prodrome (vague symptoms such as smells or emotions), an aura (visual or hemisensory symptoms), or even focal neurologic deficits (complicated migraine). The aura is usually stereotypical, with visual scotomata being the most common. Ninety percent of migraineurs do not exhibit aura or prodrome. The clinical features most predictive of migraine are nausea, photophobia with phonophobia, and exacerbation of headache by physical activity. Lack

TABLE 33–1. MIDAS QUESTIONNAIRE

INSTRUCTIONS: Please answer the following questions about ALL your headaches you have had over the last 3 months. Write your answer in the box next to each question. Write zero if you did not do the activity in the last 3 months. Please "tab" through all five boxes to calculate your MIDAS score.

1	On how many days in the last 3 months did you miss work or school because of your headaches?	0	days
2	How many days in the last 3 months was your productivity at work or school reduced by half or more because of your headaches? *(Do not include days you counted in question 1 where you missed work or school.)*	0	days
3	On how many days in the last 3 months did you not do household work because of your headaches?	0	days
4	How many days in the last 3 months was your productivity in household work reduced by half or more because of your headaches? *(Do not include days you counted in question 3 where you did not do household work.)*	0	days
5	On how many days in the last 3 months did you miss family, social, or leisure activities because of your headaches?	0	days
	Your rating:	**TOTAL:**	days
A	On how many days in the last 3 months did you have a headache? *(If a headache lasted more than 1 day, count each day.)*	0	days
B	On a scale of 0–10, on average how painful were these headaches? *(Where 0 = no pain at all, and 10 = pain as bad as it can be.)*	0	days

Grade	Definition	Score
I	Minimal or infrequent disability	0–5
II	Mild or infrequent disability	6–10
III	Moderate disability	11–20
IV	Severe disability	21+

Sources: http://www.uhs.berkley.edu/home/healthtopics/pdf/assessment.pdf. Accessed March 2013.
Stewart WF. Development and testing of the Migraine Disability Assessment (MIDAS) Questionnaire to assess headache-related disability. (Abstract). *Neurobiology.* 56(6 suppl 1):S20–S28.

TABLE 33–2. USE OF MNEMONIC POUNDING FOR ESTIMATING MIGRAINE PROBABILITY

Number of Clinical Features	LR	Population (Approximate Pretest Probability)		
		Male Population (6%)[a]	Female Population (18%)[a]	Primary Care, Presenting with Headache (33%)[a]
4 or 5	24	60%	81%	92%
3	3.5	18%	38%	64%
0 to 2	0.41	2.5%	6.7%	17%

Source: Reproduced with permission from Ebell MH. Diagnosis of migraine headache *Am Fam Physician.* 2006;74:2087–2088.
[a]Estimated probability of migraine in this population.

of physical impairment over the preceding 3 months along with absence of the predictive clinical symptoms effectively rules out migraine. The POUND mnemonic for diagnosis of migraine, as shown in the box, can be used as a clinical decision rule as shown in Table 33–2. The presence of four or five of these criteria has a high positive likelihood ratio (24) for migraine.

DIAGNOSTIC CRITERIA: EPISODIC MIGRAINE WITHOUT AURA

At least five attacks that include the following:

- Headache lasting 4 to 72 hours
- At least two of the following:
  Unilateral location
  Pulsating quality (throbbing)
  Moderate to severe intensity (inhibits or prohibits daily activity)
  Aggravated by climbing stairs or similar activity
- At least one of the following:
  Nausea, vomiting, or both
  Photophobia, phonophobia, or both

Mnemonic POUNDing—**P**ulsatile quality; **O**nset 4 to 72 hours ago (duration); **U**nilateral location; **N**ausea or vomiting present, **D**isabling intensity.

2. **TTH** originates with pain in the occipital or vertex regions of the skull, evolving into a "band-like" distribution. Although primarily bilateral, unilateral tension headaches also occur. The pain is usually not throbbing, but dull and not worsened by physical activity. Nausea is an occasional associated symptom. Photophobia or sonophobia may be present but not together as occurs in migraine. The duration may be hours to days. Risk factors include female gender, age 30–39 years, Caucasian, higher educational level, head and/or neck injury, and depression/anxiety.

DIAGNOSTIC CRITERIA: EPISODIC TTH

At least 10 previous headache episodes fulfill the criteria listed below. Fewer than 180 headache days. (If ≥180 days and the diagnostic criteria are present, then it is chronic TTH.)
  Headache lasting 30 minutes to 7 days.
  At least two of the following pain characteristics:
  No-pulsating quality—pressing or tightening
  Mild or moderate intensity. Not activity prohibiting
  Bilateral location
  No aggravation by routine physical activity
Both of the following:
  No nausea or vomiting
  Either photophobia or phonophobia is absent

3. **Cluster headache.** These headaches peak very quickly after onset and are "clustered" temporally over weeks to months. Pain-free intervals are variable in length. The pain is sharp, excruciating in intensity, lasting 15 to 180 minutes. The location is usually unilateral and in the orbital, supraorbital, or temporal region. Parasympathetic overactivity (lacrimation and ipsilateral rhinorrhea) is common. Risk factors for cluster headaches include sleep apnea, shift work, previous head injury, and positive family history of headache. The combination of unilateral pain plus at least 5 of 7 other key symptoms (excruciating pain, location near eye, location near temple, rhinorrhea, duration less than 3–4 hours, more than one attack in the same day, and attacks for at least seven consecutive days) was 100% sensitive and 95% specific for diagnosis of cluster headaches.

B. **Secondary headaches.** Symptoms of a "worrisome" headache that should elicit a search for an underlying cause include the following. (See below for "SNOOP" mnemonic for worrisome headache.) Symptoms shown to increase diagnostic yield when neuroimaging for secondary disorders include rapidly increasing headache frequency, history of dizziness or lack of coordination, history of numbness or tingling, and headache upon awakening from sleep.

"SNOOP" MNEMONIC FOR WORRISOME HEADACHE

S—Systemic symptoms or signs (fever, weight loss). Systemic disease (cancer, autoimmune)
N—Neurologic symptoms or signs
O—Onset sudden
O—Onset late in life
P—Pattern change

Following are the specific features that are worrisome for particular conditions:

1. **Headache that is new in onset, constant, prevents sleep, or progressively worsens over several weeks** (indicative of possible intracranial mass lesion or infection). The new headache occurring later in life is less likely to be migraine or tension.
2. **Headache that is abrupt, explosive, and extremely severe** (e.g., "the worst headache of my life" or "thunderclap") suggests intracranial hemorrhage.
3. **Headache beginning with exertion** (consider leaking aneurysm, increased intracranial pressure, or arterial dissection). Exertional headache may also be associated with primary headache types.
4. **Headache in a drowsy or confused patient** (consider sepsis, trauma, etc.).
5. **New headache in the elderly** (consider temporal arteritis, glaucoma, cerebrovascular accident).
6. **Unremitting moderate or severe headache in obese females** (consider pseudotumor cerebri).

V. **Signs.** A focused physical examination including careful neurologic, otologic, ophthalmologic, and head and neck evaluation is essential. Vital signs can reveal fever or hypertension. Although there are a few physical examination findings that are common in primary headaches, the examination is usually normal.

A. **Primary headache disorders.** Physical findings are limited but the following clues suggest a primary headache diagnosis:
1. **Migraine.** Focal neurologic deficits, such as hemiparesis or a visual field disturbance.
2. **TTH.** The physical examination can reveal muscle tightness or "trigger points" over the posterior cervical and occipital regions. The neck examination may provide clues to underlying causes of tension headache, such as cervical arthritis (e.g., stiffness, decreased range of motion, or crepitus with movement), inflammatory processes (e.g., trigger points or nodules), or infectious causes (e.g., lymphadenopathy).
3. **Cluster headaches.** Photophobia, tearing, nasal stuffiness, or Horner syndrome can be present. The patient may be unable to sit still during the interview.

B. **Secondary headaches.** Signs of a "worrisome" headache are listed below.
1. **Fever** can indicate meningitis, purulent sinusitis, otitis, dental abscess, or other infection.

    2. A **stiff neck** can indicate infection or blood in the cerebrospinal fluid.

    3. Focal neurologic deficits or **elevated blood pressure** ($\geq$200 mmHg systolic or $\geq$120 mmHg diastolic) can indicate increased intracranial pressure from mass effect, bleed, or accelerated hypertension.

    4. A **palpable, tender temporal artery** suggests temporal arteritis.

    5. Papilledema suggests increased intracranial pressure.

VI. Laboratory Tests. Diagnostic testing is unnecessary for most patients with episodic primary headaches, those with primary chronic recurring headaches, and for those at low risk (i.e., young patients, who have prior or family history of headache, are improving during their evaluation, have none of the aforementioned "worrisome" symptoms or signs, are alert and oriented, and have no focal neurologic signs). For these individuals, repeated history taking and physical examinations over time, in addition to observations of response to treatment, are the best diagnostic tools. The following tests should be considered in patients not meeting low-risk criteria.

  A. Radiologic evaluation

    1. Plain skull films are rarely useful in the evaluation of headache.

    2. Computerized tomography (CT) can assist in evaluating for midline shift, sinusitis, or diagnosing subarachnoid or intraparenchymal hemorrhage in the patient with a severe and acute headache. The acutely ill patient who requires monitoring will be most easily evaluated by CT, although a normal CT scan does not rule out an acute bleeding. If the clinical suspicion remains high, a lumbar puncture (LP) should be performed.

    3. Magnetic resonance imaging (MRI) is generally more informative than CT in patients with chronic headaches. Characteristic MRI findings have been described in patients with migraine, trigeminal neuralgia, and temporomandibular joint dysfunction. This procedure is also superior to CT in demonstrating subacute subdural hematoma in patients with a history of trauma and is useful in further characterizing lesions detected by CT. MRI has excellent resolution in the posterior fossa. Most patients with primary headache disorders will have an unremarkable study.

  B. The purposes of **LP** are (1) to establish the presence or absence of blood or inflammatory cells in the cerebrospinal fluid, (2) to detect hemorrhage or infection in the patient with a stiff neck, and (3) to determine the organism responsible for infection by fluid culture. Although LP is easy to perform and readily available, it is an invasive, uncomfortable procedure that has no role in routine headache evaluation. LP should *not* be performed when increased intracranial pressure is suspected until mass effect is ruled out. LP opening pressure may be elevated in pseudotumor cerebri.

  C. Blood analysis. A complete blood cell count is rarely useful or definitive in the evaluation of headache and has no place except, possibly, in the febrile patient. The erythrocyte sedimentation rate is indicated in an older patient with a new headache to support a diagnosis of temporal arteritis.

  D. Other studies. Radionucleotide imaging and **angiography** are usually less helpful than CT scans for identifying or ruling out significant intracranial disease and should be reserved for the few patients with normal CT scans and cerebrospinal fluid findings whose evaluations strongly suggest an intracranial lesion. MRI has largely replaced these studies. **Magnetic resonance angiography** is useful to demonstrate small aneurysms. Temporal arteritis should be confirmed by **arterial biopsy;** this procedure should not delay treatment when clinical suspicion is strong. **Electroencephalography** is not routinely helpful for the patient with a new headache, although it may be useful in ruling out seizure disorder in the chronic headache patient responding poorly to therapy.

VII. Treatment. This discussion is primarily directed to the treatment of primary episodic headache disorders.

  A. Episodic migraine (with or without aura)

    1. General measures include patient education, fatigue avoidance, and life stressor modification. Migraine frequency, duration, and severity are not increased by dietary choices. (SOR **Ⓐ**) Regular supplementation with riboflavin (400 mg per day) reduces frequency and intensity of migraines. (SOR **Ⓑ**) Alternative therapies are frequently prescribed for migraine sufferers and include aerobic exercise, biofeedback, progressive self-relaxation, meditation, manual medicine techniques, massage therapy, or acupuncture. Sham and traditional acupuncture are modestly effective over placebo in acute migraine treatment.

2. Acute therapy is appropriate when migraine attacks occur less than two to four times a month. The most effective approach is individualized and stratified, based on a given drug's ability to preserve normal function and the patient's degree of symptoms. (SOR **B**) An abortive medication with receptor-specific therapy (e.g., a triptan) should be prescribed initially in patients with moderate to severe symptoms (Table 33–4). The triptan should be administered at migraine onset or in the prodromal/aural phase, if possible. Ergot alkaloids are a good alternative to triptans; these drug classes share contraindications. If triptans or ergotamines fail or are contraindicated, rescue medications such as simple analgesics can be tried. Rescue medications also include combination products, sedatives, antiemetics, and narcotics. These are often somewhat effective, but seldom allow the patient to function normally.

The following specific agents are commonly used (Tables 33–3 and 33–4).

TABLE 33–3. MEDICATIONS FOR ACUTE MIGRAINE HEADACHES

Class	Medication	Dose	Major Side Effects	Contraindications	Drug Interactions
Triptans	Zolmitriptan	1.25–2.5 mg once orally; may repeat once at 2 h	Nausea, chest pain, fatigue, paresthesias, vasospasm, VF/VT, serotonin syndrome	CAD, uncontrolled HTN, basilar migraine	Ergot (vasospasm), SSRI, and dextromethorphan (serotonin syndrome)
	Sumatriptan	25–100 mg orallyonce; 4–6 mg SQ once; 5/20 mg/spray once. May repeat any of above one time			
	Rizatriptan[a]	5–10 mg once. May repeat twice in 2 h; MLT dispersible tablet			
	Naratriptan[b]	1–2.5 mg orally once. May repeat once in 4 h			
	Almotriptan	6.25–12.5 mg once. May repeat once in 2 h			
	Eletriptan	20–40 mg once; may repeat once in 2 h			
Ergot alkaloids	Dihydroergotamine (DHE) IM/IV and Migranal nasal spray	1 mg IM/IV to max. 3 mg/attack 0.5 mg/spray 1 spray in each nostril every 15 min twice; may repeat once in 1 h	Coronary vasospasm, hypertension, flushing, central and peripheral ischemia	Pregnancy, breastfeeding, CAD, HTN uncontrolled, basilar migraine	C/I triptans, azole antifungals, HIV protease inhibitors all increase ergot toxicity
	Ergotamine/ caffeine	1–3 tablets every 30 min—max. 6/wk			

VF/VT, ventricular fibrillation/ventricular tachycardia; CAD, coronary artery disease; HTN, hypertension; SSRI, selective serotonin reuptake inhibitor; SQ, subcutaneous; IM/IV, intramuscular/intravenous; C/I, contraindicated
[a]Concomitant use with propranolol can increase rizatriptan levels.
[b]Longer half-life.

TABLE 33-4. STRENGTH OF RECOMMENDATION FOR SELF-ADMINISTERED ACUTE TREATMENT OPTIONS IN MIGRAINE

SOR	Treatment (Route of Administration)	Comments
A	Acetaminophen + aspirin + caffeine (oral)	NNT 3.9 (3.2–4.9)
A	Aspirin (oral)	NNT 3.5–5.5
A	Aspirin + metoclopramide (oral)	NNT 3.2 (2.6–4.0)
A	Butorphanol (intranasal)	Abuse/dependence and rebound risk
A	Dihydroergotamine (intranasal)	NNT 2.5 (1.9–3.7)
A	Ibuprofen (oral)	NNT 7.5 (4.5–22)
A	Triptans (oral)	NNT 2.7–5.4
A	Sumatriptan (intranasal)	NNT 3.4 (2.9–4.1)
A	Sumatriptan (intranasal)	NNT 2.0 (1.8–2.2)
B	Acetaminophen (oral)	NNT 5.2 (3.3–13)
B	Acetaminophen + codeine (oral)	Abuse/dependence and rebound risk
B	Isometheptene compounds (oral)	Limited clinical trials
D	Butalbital compounds (oral)	No clinical trials and rebound risk
D	Ergotamine (oral)	Conflicting evidence

Source: Reproduced with permission from Polizzotto MJ. Evaluation and treatment of the adult patient with migraine. J Fam Pract. 2002;51:2. Table 3, p. 164.
All numbers needed to treat (NNT) at 95% confidence interval for headache response (reduction in headache severity from "severe" or "moderate" to "mild" or "none" at 2 h.

  a. **Triptans** are considered first-line therapy in treatment of acute migraines. Triptans are selective serotonin receptor agonists affecting primarily 5-HT 1B/1D receptors. Rizatriptan 10 mg, eletriptan 80 mg, and almotriptan 12.5 mg are associated with the highest likelihood of consistent treatment success. (SOR **A**) They have proven to be very effective in the treatment of migraines, with success rates approaching 70%. There are many triptans available, with important differences in route of administration (oral tablet, dissolving oral tablet, injectable, intranasal), onset of action, and duration of action. Triptans should be used with caution in patients with suspected coronary artery, cerebrovascular, or peripheral vascular disease, since they are associated with vasospasm. They should not be used in basilar or complicated migraine. Patients should limit use to two administrations each week and triptans should not be taken within 24 hours of an ergot alkaloid.
  b. **Ergot alkaloids** also target serotonin receptors, but are less selective. These drugs are estimated to be effective within 2 hours in ≥90% of cases when administered parenterally, 80% when given rectally, and up to 50% when given orally. They are also available in sublingual and intranasal forms. Since ergotamine preparations can result in dependency and rebound headaches, they should not be used more often than 2 days per week.
  c. **Combination products.** A combination of acetaminophen, butalbital, and caffeine (Fioricet) is commonly used for migraine; however, no studies have addressed the efficacy of butalbital.
  d. **Simple analgesics** can be effective. The best evidence exists for aspirin (ASA), ibuprofen, naproxen sodium, and tolfenamic acid. Acetaminophen (APAP) is modestly effective when NSAIDs are contraindicated. (SOR **A**)
  e. **Antiemetics** administered either by mouth, intramuscularly (IM), or by rectal suppository may be useful to offset the nausea and gastric stasis associated with migraine. Metoclopramide (5 to 10 mg orally, IM or IV), prochlorperazine, and chlorpromazine are the most commonly used agents. They can be used alone or as adjunctive therapy with narcotics.
  f. Narcotic analgesics such as **codeine** and **oxycodone** are effective during an acute attack, but their use must be carefully balanced with the risks of habituation and rebound headache.
  g. Dexamethasone (15 mg IV) reduced likelihood of recurrent headaches (NNT = 10). (SOR **A**)
3. **Prophylactic therapy** (Tables 33–5) is indicated for patients with more than three or four attacks per month or for headaches occurring on a predictable schedule (e.g.,

with menses). The most effective prophylactic agents reduce headaches by 20% to 50% compared with placebo. Effective medications include the following:

  a. Beta-blockers (propranolol [SOR **Ⓐ**, NNT 2.3–5] and timolol) are the primary drugs in this class for migraine prevention. Once- or twice-daily dosing improves compliance.

  b. Tricyclic antidepressants (amitriptyline, NNT 2.3–5) have also proven useful, probably because of serotonin effects. The higher dosages normally used for depression are unnecessary.

  c. Calcium-channel blockers are not as effective as beta-blockers for prophylaxis. Nifedipine can actually increase headaches.

  d. Reflecting the changing perception of migraine as a neurologic phenomenon perhaps propagated centrally, **antiepileptic drugs (AEDs)** have been used more frequently to suppress migraines. Experience with **divalproex sodium** (SOR **Ⓐ**, NNT 2.1–2.9) has been most encouraging. Topiramate and carbamazepine may also be effective. Anti-epileptic drugs are generally more expensive than other agents and require monitoring for adverse effects (e.g., abnormalities in liver function).

  e. Other agents. Angiotensin-converting enzyme inhibitors (Lisinopril) or angiotensin receptor blockers are reasonable second-line agents. (SOR **Ⓑ**) Selective serotonin reuptake inhibitors are similar to placebo in efficacy for prophylaxis. (SOR **Ⓐ**) Propranolol, valproic acid, and amitriptyline are effective prophylactic agents in children's migraines. (SOR **Ⓑ**) Flunarizine is efficacious, (SOR **Ⓐ**) but not available in the United States. Cyproheptadine 4 mg once or twice daily has been used for both acute and prophylaxis treatment of childhood migraine. Cyproheptadine has anticholinergic and antiserotonergic properties but the mechanism of action is uncertain. The most widely researched botanical remedy for migraine headache is a wildflower called feverfew (*Tanacetum parthenium*), which is modestly effective for acute treatment and prophylaxis (Table 33–5).

  f. Follow-up and education. Patient education during an acute headache is not very effective. The mutually cooperative, understanding relationship critical to long-term success can be established with frequent visits during medicine trials and titration. Communicating therapeutic goals clearly is essential to success. Follow-up visits to assess response to therapy, patient understanding, and frequency of attacks can be therapeutic.

B. TTH

 1. General measures. A supportive cooperative physician–patient relationship is essential. Education, insight into family and life events, consideration of environmental and emotional triggers, and counseling can help both decrease headache frequency and increase coping skills. Headache diaries, biofeedback, stress management, muscle relaxation techniques, exercise programs, and dietary changes (e.g., reducing consumption of sugar, caffeine, and red meat; increased intake of omega-three fatty acids; avoidance of dehydration) may also help. Addressing psychiatric comorbidities and substance abuse (see Chapters 90, 91, and 94) contributes to successful treatment of headaches. APAP, ASA, and NSAIDs are first-line medications. If monotherapy fails, combinations of the above with caffeine can reduce severity and duration of headaches. Third-line treatment includes combinations of caffeine, APAP/ASA, and butalbital.

  Individuals with **chronic tension headaches** may benefit from a multidisciplinary approach using both drug and nondrug treatments, including individual/family therapy and physical therapy. Treatment involves stopping all overused medications/substances; amitriptyline is useful for headache prophylaxis.

 2. Used sparingly, **muscle relaxants** (e.g., tizanidine, 2–4 mg, every 8 hours; cyclobenzaprine, 10 mg, three times daily for up to 21 days; or diazepam, 5 mg, two to three times daily) can be helpful adjunctive therapy. Narcotic analgesics generally should be avoided.

 3. Prophylactic therapy. Prophylactic therapy is recommended for patients with 15 or more headaches per month. Medications used for migraine prophylaxis (specifically, beta-blockers and tricyclic antidepressants, alone or in combination) have also proven useful in patients with frequent, recurrent, and chronic TTH. Treatment should be maintained for 8–12 weeks to achieve maximal effect. It is

TABLE 33–5. PROPHYLAXIS FOR RECURRENT MIGRAINE HEADACHES

Class	Medication	Dose	Major Side Effects	Drug Interactions
Beta-blockers	Propranolol Timolol	10–40 mg/d 10–30 mg once or twice daily	Caution in asthma, COPD, bradycardia, and the elderly	NSAID decreased anti-HTN efficacy C/I with thioridazine
Tricyclic antidepressants (TCA)	Amitriptyline Nortriptyline	25–100 mg at bedtime 25–100 mg at bedtime	Sedating, serotonergic, anticholinergic	C/I with class Ia antiarrhythmics Caution with other agents that prolong QT and in the elderly
Calcium-channel blockers	Verapamil	240 mg/d	AV block, negative inotropic	C/I with simvastatin; caution with ergots, lithium, and phenytoin
Antiepileptic drugs (AEDs)	Divalproex	250–500 mg twice daily	Drowsiness, hepatotoxicity, pancytopenia, Stevens–Johnson syndrome, SIADH	Caution with aspirin, duloxetine (SIADH), and TCAs (additive)
	Topiramate	50 mg twice daily	Drowsiness, weight loss, dizziness, Stevens–Johnson syndrome, hypokalemia	OCPs (decreased efficacy), angiotensin-converting enzyme or angiotensin receptor blockers with thiazide (hypokalemia), lithium, metformin
	Carbamazepine (Tegretol)	100–400 mg daily to twice daily	Drowsiness, hyponatremia, Stevens–Johnson syndrome, aplastic anemia	C/I azole antifungals, HIV protease inhibitors. Caution with APAP (increased APAP toxicity), OCP (decreased OCP efficacy), warfarin (increased INR)
Ergot	Dihydroergotamine (DHE 45) Ergotamine/caffeine (Cafergot)	1 mg IM/IV to max. 3 mg/attack 1–3 tabs every 30 min—max. 6/wk	Coronary vasospasm, hypertension, flushing, central and peripheral ischemia	C/I triptans, azole antifungals, HIV protease inhibitors all increase ergot toxicity
Antihistamine	Cyproheptadine (Periactin)	2–4 mg daily to twice daily	Drowsiness, xerostomia, dizziness, urinary retention	Potentiates actions of other anticholinergic agents
Herbal	Feverfew	125 mg twice daily	Indigestion, nausea, diarrhea	Potentiates warfarin
Combination products	APAP/butalbital/ caffeine (Fioricet)	1–2 tabs every 4 h—max. 6 tabs/d	Drowsiness, sedation, dependence, rebound	Avoid duloxetine. Avoid other APAP products
	Isometheptene/ dichloralphenazone/APAP	1–2 caps every 4 h not to exceed 8 caps/d	Dizziness, HTN severe, rebound	Avoid with carbamazepine (increases APAP toxicity)
Simple analgesics/ NSAIDs	Aspirin Ibuprofen	325 mg every 4 h to max. 12/d 200–800 mg 3 times daily	GI bleed, bronchospasm, pancytopenia, rebound potential	Avoid use with NSAIDs, warfarin Avoid use with ASA, warfarin
Antiemetics	Chlorpromazine	12.5 mg IM or 10–25 mg oral q 4–6 h	Sedation, hypotension	C/I class Ia antiarrhythmics, duloxetine. Caution with other sedatives
	Prochlorperazine	5–10 mg every 6–8 h	Sedation, hypotension, QT prolongation, extrapyramidal symptoms	Same as chlorpromazine
	Metoclopramide	10 mg IM/IV once	Sedation, confusion, acute dystonia	C/I carbidopa/levodopa. Caution with other anticholinergics and sedatives
Narcotic analgesics	Codeine (Tylenol #3) Hydrocodone	1 every 4 h not to exceed 8/d 5–10 mg q 6 h not to exceed 40 mg/d	Sedation, constipation, nausea, urinary retention; rebound	Other sedatives, opiates, and APAP

Source: Reproduced with permission from Polizzotto MJ. Evaluation and treatment of the adult patient with migraine. *J Fam Pract.* 2002;51(2):161–167.
C/I, contraindicated; SIADH, syndrome of inappropriate antidiuretic hormone; APAP, acetaminophen; HTN, hypertension; IM, intramuscular; IV, intravenous.

important to consider prophylaxis when patients use acute treatment medications for more than 9 days/month as this increases risk of medication-overuse headaches.

4. **Alternative therapy.** Acupuncture modestly reduced HA severity, frequency, and medication use at 3 months and 1 year. (SOR **B**) Spinal manipulation may provide improved relief after conventional treatment but appears to be inferior to amitriptyline for treating pain intensity. (SOR **C**) Both topical peppermint oil and botulinum toxin type A can be effective in acute TTH treatment and prophylaxis. (SOR **B**)

5. **Follow-up**
   a. Most **patients** with acute episodic headaches will see their primary physician only once for this complaint. Early follow-up is recommended **with new recurrent headaches** to gauge response to therapy and reconfirm history and physical findings. Review of headache diaries, precipitating factors, and life stressors may help patients identify/avoid precipitants, thereby reducing the number of headache days.
   b. Clinicians tend to underestimate the therapeutic value of **regularly scheduled follow-up,** often monthly, for chronic pain complaints like chronic TTH.

C. **Cluster headaches**
   1. **Acute therapy** during an attack includes **inhalation of 100% oxygen** by mask at a rate of 6 to 12 L/min or intranasal zolmitriptan (5–10 mg) or sumatriptan (6 mg subcutaneous (SQ) or 20 mg intranasal).
   2. **Prophylaxis** is preferable once clusters begin. Effective oral medications, alone or in combination, include (1) verapamil 240–480 mg per day; (2) lithium, 300 mg three times daily (monitoring blood levels weekly to avoid toxicity); or (3) prednisone, 40 to 60 mg per day for 5 days, followed by tapering over 10 to 14 days. Indomethacin, 25 mg orally three times a day, is a first-line treatment agent for benign paroxysmal hemicrania and hemicrania continua.

D. **Treatment of secondary headaches.** Treatment, whether medical or neurosurgical, is directed toward addressing the primary problem. When secondary headaches are due to analgesic abuse or withdrawal headaches, identification of the offending substance and withdrawing the substance is required.
   1. Those taking narcotic medication chronically may require inpatient detoxification both to treat the headache and the medication dependence. For non-narcotic agents, treating rebound headaches with ergotamine (dihydroergotamine [DHE] 1 mg SQ rescue for excruciating headaches) and stopping the offending agent(s) results in significant improvement within 3 months. (SOR **C**) Amitriptyline does not affect frequency or severity of rebound headaches, but does improve quality of life. (SOR **B**) Prednisone (tapering 60–20 mg over 6 days) or naratriptan (2.5 mg orally twice daily for 6 days) can reduce need for rescue DHE, but does not affect headache frequency or severity. (SOR **B**)
   2. **Severe chronic migraine** and **medication-associated headache requiring detoxification** are problems best managed in collaboration with a headache expert.
   3. **Continuity of care** with a single knowledgeable physician remains essential for these patients.

SELECTED REFERENCES

Beithon J, Gallenberg M, Johnson K, et al. Institute for clinical systems improvement. Diagnosis and treatment of headache. Updated January 2013. http://www.guideline.gov/content.aspx?id=25645&search=headache. Accessed March 2013.

Holland S, Silberstein SD, Freitag F, et al. Evidence-based guideline update: NSAIDs and other complementary treatments of episodic migraine prevention in adults: report of the Quality Standards subcommittee of the American Academy of Neurology and the American Headache Society. *Neurology.* 2012;78:1346–1353.

Holland S, Silberstein SD, Freitag F, et al. Evidence-based guideline update: pharmacologic treatment for episodic migraine prevention in adults: report of the Quality Standards Subcommittee of

the American Academy of Neurology and the American Headache Society. *Neurology.* 2012;78: 1337–1345.
Jackson JL, Kuriyama A, Hayashino Y. Bolulinum toxin A for prophylactic treatment of migraine and tension headaches in adults. A meta-analysis. *JAMA.* 2012;307(16):1736–1745.

34 Hearing Loss

Robert C. Salinas, MD, & Audra Fox, MD

KEY POINTS

- Hearing loss is classified as sensorineural, conductive, mixed, or central. (SOR **C**)
- Sudden deafness is a medical emergency and warrants prompt referral to an otolaryngologist. (SOR **A**)
- The treatment of hearing loss is dependent on its etiology and involves environmental alteration, assistive listening devices, active medical/surgical intervention, and hearing aids. (SOR **C**)

I. Definition. Hearing loss is a reduction in an individual's ability to perceive sound. The intensity of sound is measured with the decibel (dB), a logarithmic unit whose reference is 0 on the audiogram. Normal conversational speech occurs at frequencies of 500 Hz to 3000 Hz at 45 to 60 dB. The following classification is frequently used to describe hearing loss: normal hearing across the speech spectrum (–10 to 15 dB), slight hearing loss (16–25 dB), mild hearing loss (26–40 dB), moderate hearing loss (41–55 dB), moderate severe hearing loss (56–70 dB), severe hearing loss (71–90 dB), and profound hearing loss (above 90 dB). In assessing a patient with hearing loss, the type, degree, and configuration are all important aspects of the initial evaluation.

Hearing loss is a common problem encountered in the primary care setting and generally is classified as **sensorineural** (caused by deterioration of the cochlea or lesions to the eighth cranial nerve, which can lead to problems with converting mechanical vibrations to electrical potentials); **conductive** (caused by lesions of the external or middle ear that impede passage of sound waves to the inner ear and its conversion to mechanical vibrations); **mixed** (sensorineural and conductive); or **central** (caused by lesions of the auditory pathways proximal to the cochlea). Hearing loss may further be described as congenital or acquired. A more complete listing of etiologies of hearing loss may be found in Table 34–1.

ACOUSTIC NEUROMA

Ninety-five percent of acoustic neuromas are idiopathic; 5% occur in patients with neurofibromatosis; these tumors are more aggressive and more likely to undergo malignant transformation. The most common presenting symptoms are tinnitus and progressive hearing loss. Approximately 50% of patients also experience disequilibrium.

Audiometric findings include loss of discrimination that is disproportionate to pure-tone results and high-frequency sensorineural loss. Approximately 5% of patients have normal audiograms. Thin-section magnetic resonance imaging (MRI) with gadolinium can detect temporal bony acoustic neuromas measuring just a few millimeters. **Treatment** for acoustic neuroma is surgical excision; however, since acoustic neuromas are usually very slow growing, the elderly or those with multiple comorbid medical conditions may choose observation as an alternative to surgery.

SUDDEN DEAFNESS

Sudden deafness is a sensorineural deafness that occurs instantly or is noticed over hours or days. The degree of hearing loss ranges from mild to complete and is typically unilateral. Potential causes include **localized lesions** of the temporal bone (e.g., acoustic neuroma, aneurysm of the anteroinferior cerebellar artery), **systemic diseases** (e.g., macroglobulinemia, leukemia, polycythemia, sickle cell disease, syphilis, bacterial infection, ototoxic drugs, mumps, multiple sclerosis), **barotrauma,** and **head trauma.**

Sudden deafness should be thought of as a medical emergency, requiring prompt referral to an otolaryngologist. Prognosis is dependent on the timeliness of therapy, which may include treatment of identified causes or supportive/empiric therapies (e.g., corticosteroids, vasodilators, anticoagulants, bed rest, sedation, or a low-sodium diet).

II. **Screening and Prevention**
   A. **Screening**
      1. The United States Preventive Services Task Force (USPSTF) recommends **screening for hearing loss in all newborn infants.** (SOR ❸)
      2. Screening audiometry for **toddlers, preschoolers, and school-aged children** should be administered as requested, mandated, or when conditions place children at risk for hearing disability. (American Speech -Language -Hearing Association [ASHA]) (SOR ❸)
      3. Screening audiometry for hearing loss in **adults** is voluntary, but is recommended every 10 years until age 50 years and then every 3 years thereafter by the ASHA. (SOR ❸) The Occupational Safety and Health Administration recommends a yearly hearing test for the workers exposed to an average of 85 dB or more of noise during an 8-hour work day. (SOR ❸)
      4. The USPSTF found insufficient evidence to assess the balance of benefits and harms of screening for hearing loss in asymptomatic adults aged 50 years or older.
   B. **Prevention** of hearing loss is primarily focused on careful medication prescribing and noise-induced hearing loss.
      1. Physicians should **minimize the use of ototoxic drugs** and carefully monitor patients taking these drugs.
      2. **Individuals with exposure to noise at home or work** should receive education concerning avoidance and the use of ear protection during noise exposure; if unable to avoid noise, they should be fitted for proper ear protective devices such as earmuffs and earplugs. Authors of a Cochrane review found attenuated noise of about 20 dB with hearing protection devices, although there was variation among brands and types; the benefit of ear plugs depended almost completely on proper instruction of insertion. Overall study quality is low.
      3. **Musicians,** especially those who play violins and violas (high frequency and proximity to left ear) should be advised to use mutes during practice.
III. **Common Diagnoses** (Table 34–1). Nearly 30 million people in the United States experience some degree of hearing loss. Age-related hearing loss is also the third most prevalent chronic condition in older Americans (after hypertension and arthritis) and rises with age to a prevalence of approximately 80% by age 85 years. It is also estimated that hearing loss affects between 8% and 19% of the adolescent and young adult populations. One of every 2000 individuals is deaf or severely hearing impaired. At least 90% of these hearing problems are secondary to middle ear disorders that are potentially treatable.
   A. **Sensorineural loss.** More than 90% of hearing loss is sensorineural. Some common etiologies of sensorineural loss include presbycusis, acoustic damage, ototoxicity, and Ménière disease.
      1. **Presbycusis** is the most common type of hearing loss in the United States, is associated with aging, and may begin in middle age. Often, hearing loss is gradual, symmetrical, and predominantly of high frequencies.
      2. **Acoustic damage** (noise-induced hearing loss) can be caused by chronic exposure to excessive noise levels or from acute acoustic trauma (e.g., shotgun blast or firecracker explosion [180 dB]). Damage can occur due to increased noise intensity (over 85 dB such as shop tools and lawn mower), duration, and frequency (pitch).
         a. **As many as 30 million Americans are exposed to excessive noise levels at work.** Up to 17% of these workers have measurable hearing loss,

TABLE 34–1. COMMON ETIOLOGIES OF HEARING LOSS ENCOUNTERED IN PRIMARY CARE

Conductive	Sensorineural
Cerumen impaction	Genetic[a]
Cholesteatoma	Alport syndrome
Cysts	Usher syndrome
Eustachian tube dysfunction	Waardenburg syndrome
Exostosis	Ménière disease
Foreign body	Migraine
Hemotympanum	Multiple sclerosis
Ossicular discontinuity	Noise induced
Ossicular malformations	Ototoxicity
Otitis externa	Presbycusis
Otitis media	Sarcoidosis
Otosclerosis	Sudden idiopathic hearing loss
Perforated tympanic membrane	Syphilis
Previous ear surgery	Trauma
Temporal bone fracture	Vascular
Trauma	
Tumors	
Tympanic membrane perforation	
Tympanic membrane retraction	
Tympanosclerosis	

[a]Many genetic syndromes causing hearing loss have been identified; some of the more common examples are listed above.

making hearing loss caused by noise exposure one of the most common occupational diseases.

b. **Men are affected more frequently than women** presumably because of occupational noise exposure, military service, and recreational shooting.

c. **Noise exposure is not limited to the workplace.** Noise-induced hearing loss has been demonstrated in children and adolescents. It is estimated that 15% of school-aged children have a 16-dB hearing loss. Nonoccupational noises that exceed safe limits include car stereos (154 dB), children's toys (150 dB), rock concerts (120 dB), sports clubs (120 dB), and motorboats (115 dB).

3. **Ototoxicity** is caused primarily by exposure to certain drugs and is the most common cause of deafness in children. An increased risk of ototoxicity has been associated with decreased creatinine clearance, advanced age, certain drug classes such as aminoglycosides (especially if administered parenterally), and drug treatment longer than 14 days. However, a correlation between ototoxicity and plasma drug levels has not been observed. Environmental exposure and workplace exposure are less common causal agents. Cigarette smokers are 1.69 times as likely to have hearing loss as nonsmokers.

4. **Ménière disease,** also called endolymphatic hydrops, is the most common type of hearing loss that occurs between the fourth and sixth decades but can occur at any age (see symptoms below, Section IV.C).

5. **Congenital sensorineural hearing loss,** a form of significant hearing loss, is one of the most common major abnormalities present at birth. One in 200 children is born with some degree of congenital hearing loss, and one-third to three-fourths of these losses have a genetic component. More than 70 syndromes have been identified that involve a genetic basis for hearing loss.

Increased risk of congenital hearing loss is associated with a family history of congenital hearing loss, low birth weight; craniofacial abnormalities, syndromes known to cause hearing loss (e.g., Usher syndrome, Waardenburg syndrome), intrauterine infections (e.g., cytomegalovirus, toxoplasmosis, syphilis, and rubella), hyperbilirubinemia, prolonged stay in the neonatal intensive care unit; and low Apgar score.

B. **Conductive loss.** This type usually involves abnormalities of the middle and external ear, and generally has a mechanical cause (e.g., perforated eardrum, fluid in the middle ear, external otitis, and cerumen impaction).

1. **Obstruction.** Hearing loss often results from obstruction of the external ear canal by cerumen or foreign bodies, such as crayons, food, and toys. Cerumen sometimes accumulates in the auditory canal of individuals with either excessive production of cerumen or ineffective self-cleaning mechanisms. In the third and fourth decades of life, the hairs found in the ear canals become coarser and longer, which secondarily reduces natural clearance of cerumen. Edema associated with otitis externa can also obstruct the canal.

2. **Otosclerosis,** a progressive sclerotic fixation of the stapes in the round window dampening sound conduction to the cochlea, causes deafness in 50% of affected adults. Otosclerosis is transmitted through autosomal dominant inheritance with variable expression, typically occurs in women during the second or third decades of life, and is 10 times more common among Whites than Blacks.

3. **Otitis media** (suppurative or serous), a collection of fluid behind the tympanic membrane, most commonly causes hearing loss in children younger than 5 years with a history of recurrent ear infections (see Chapter 22).

C. **Central hearing loss.** This may be caused by demyelinating disease, ischemia, neoplasm, or hematoma.

IV. **Symptoms**
A. **Reduced hearing acuity**
1. **Presbycusis** may not cause reduced hearing acuity until late in the disease process and can manifest as difficulty in understanding conversation when ambient noise levels are relatively high, as in crowded or large areas or on the telephone. Some patients complain of sensitivity to loud noises or that people mumble.
2. Patients with **noise-induced hearing loss** first notice some muffling of sound, but they usually consult a physician only when they begin to experience difficulties in hearing speech, which is a late finding.
3. With **conductive hearing loss,** patients tend to hear conversation better in noisy rooms than in quiet rooms. Reduced hearing acuity is common in patients with impacted cerumen.

B. **Timing/onset of symptoms** suggests particular etiologies.
1. **Noise-induced hearing loss** may be most pronounced shortly after the patient leaves the workplace, and the patient's hearing may improve while away from work.
2. A temporal relationship between the **use of a toxic agent** and the symptomatology is generally present in patients with ototoxicity.
3. Symptoms of hearing loss from **impacted cerumen** frequently begin suddenly following bathing or swimming, when a drop of water closes the passageway.
4. Hearing loss associated with **presbycusis** is typically of gradual onset and bilateral.

C. **Associated symptoms**
1. **Vertigo, imbalance, nausea, and disequilibrium** can occur in patients with ototoxicity.
2. **High-pitched tinnitus** may occur in individuals with presbycusis, noise-induced hearing loss, and otosclerosis.
3. **Pain, discomfort, or itching** can occur in patients with hearing loss from impacted cerumen, otitis media, or otitis externa.
4. **Chronic cough** may be present in patients with impacted cerumen if the impaction abuts the tympanic membrane. The cough should disappear with removal of the impaction.
5. In **Ménière disease,** fluctuating unilateral hearing loss is classically associated with vertigo, tinnitus, and aural fullness.
6. **Behavioral changes** resulting from isolation and depression caused by hearing loss may include fear, anger, depression, frustration, embarrassment, or anxiety. Young children with hearing loss may experience difficulties in language acquisition and develop communication problems. Elderly people with hearing loss suffer from depression twice as often as the general population and may be at higher risk for experiencing isolation.

V. **Signs.** Physical findings may be limited.
A. **Otoscopic examination**
1. **Impacted cerumen or a foreign body** may be evident.
2. Findings consistent with **otitis externa or otitis media** (see Chapter 22) may be seen.
3. The medial wall of the middle ear promontory may appear reddish in patients with **otosclerosis**.

B. Tuning fork tests

1. **The Weber test** is performed by placing the handle of a vibrating tuning fork (512 cycles/s) against the midline of the patient's forehead. A patient with normal sensorineural function and no conductive hearing loss hears the sound equally in both ears. Lateralization of sound to one side means either a conductive loss on that side or a sensorineural loss on the opposite side.

2. The **Rinne test** assesses air and bone conduction. The handle of a vibrating tuning fork (512-cycles/s) is placed against the mastoid until the patient can no longer hear it and then the tines are held near the ear canal to assess whether the patient can still hear the sound. Air conduction persists longer than bone conduction in a patient with no hearing loss. Equal hearing levels at both positions are consistent with hearing loss of mixed cause. If air conduction is louder, either normal hearing or sensorineural loss may exist. If bone conduction is louder, conductive loss exists.

C. Developmental milestones. The primary care practitioner should be familiar with milestones associated with normal speech and hearing. Any deviation from these norms should alert the clinician to consider audiologic testing.

1. From **birth to 3 months,** infants should have a startle reflex to loud sounds. At this age, they are generally comforted by familiar voices.

2. The **ability to localize sound usually develops at around 6 months** while responding to their name and mimicking environmental sounds usually takes place around 9 months.

3. Infants usually learn to say **their first meaningful word around 12 months** and by 24 months usually have a vocabulary of approximately 20 words.

VI. Laboratory Tests

A. Audiometry measures the threshold levels (i.e., the intensity at which the patient is able to perceive sound correctly 50% of the time). This level is usually measured by presenting pure tones to the individual at preset frequencies through air conduction and occasionally through bone conduction. Often, this is done in a quiet environment, and recent exposure to loud noise may invalidate the results. Thus, before testing, patients should avoid exposure to loud noises for at least 14 hours prior to testing.

1. **Indications**

   a. Screening audiometry for toddlers, preschoolers, and school-aged children should be administered as needed, requested, mandated, or when conditions place children at risk for hearing disability. (ASHA)

   b. Screening audiometry for hearing loss in adults is voluntary, but is recommended every 10 years until age 50 years and then every 3 years thereafter. (SOR **B**) (ASHA) (SOR **C**)

   c. **Audiometry is indicated for all patients with hearing loss,** except those patients with a foreign body or an acute infection whose hearing normalizes following treatment.

   d. **Baseline audiometry should be performed within 3 days of institution of therapy with ototoxic agents** for patients who are alert enough to cooperate with the examination. Serial audiometry on an individual basis should be considered.

   e. **Follow-up should be performed annually** after treatment, if indicated by the patient's condition.

2. **Findings**

   a. **Sensorineural loss** causes lower thresholds in low frequencies than in higher frequencies.

      (1) Individuals with **presbycusis** display a pattern with a greater high-frequency loss at 8000 than at 4000 cycles, often described as a smooth, ski slope–shaped curve; the loss is generally bilateral. It is not always possible to distinguish, from an audiogram alone, whether the hearing loss is the effect of presbycusis, noise exposure, or ototoxic agents.

      (2) The classic **noise-induced pattern** on the audiogram shows high-frequency loss, greatest at 4000 cycles, with improvement at 8000 cycles. The audiogram should be measured at least 14 hours after the last significant noise exposure in order to minimize the confusion of temporary versus permanent threshold shifts.

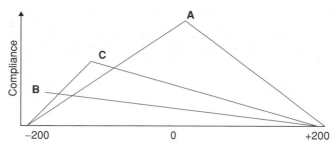

FIGURE 34–1. Tympanogram patterns: **(A)** Type A tympanogram with normal compliance of the tympanic membrane. **(B)** Type B tympanogram with no impedance peak. **(C)** Type C tympanogram with a peak in the negative range.

    b. Conductive loss causes low-frequency (i.e., 125–500 cycles) loss rather than high-frequency loss. Bone conduction testing in patients with conductive hearing loss reveals normal hearing thresholds.

    c. Mixed loss causes audiometric patterns with features of both sensorineural and conductive hearing loss.

B. Tympanometry is a simple, reliable test that takes about 5 minutes to perform in the clinic setting. This test assesses function of the tympanic membrane and Eustachian tube. A small probe is inserted into the external auditory canal and a tone of fixed characteristics is presented via the probe. The compliance of the tympanic membrane is measured electronically while the external canal pressure is artificially varied.

    1. Indications. Tympanogram is useful to confirm an otoscopic diagnosis, aid in diagnosis when otoscopy is equivocal or difficult (especially in children), and as a screening test for ear disease.

    2. Findings (Figure 34–1). In general, tympanograms provide information on presence/absence of fluid in the middle ear, mobility of the middle ear, and ear canal volume. Tympanograms are categorized as either type A, type B, or type C. Compliance is greatest when pressures are equal on both sides of the tympanic membrane. A peak will be present when the compliance is normal. **Type A tympanogram** describes normal compliance of the tympanic membrane. **Type B tympanogram** looks flat, because no impedance peak can be identified. There is little or no mobility, often because of fluid in the middle ear. Type B may also be seen with patent pressure equalization tubes and perforations. **Type C tympanogram** shows a peak in the negative range, which is consistent with a retracted tympanic membrane and Eustachian tube dysfunction.

C. Otoacoustic emission (OAE) and/or auditory brainstem response (ABR). Without screening, congenital hearing loss is often not diagnosed until as late as 2.5 years of age, and therefore could result in the delay of speech, language, and cognitive development. It has been estimated that if exclusively risk-based screening were to be used, up to 42% of profoundly hearing-impaired individuals would be missed. Those who do not pass the screen are often given a second screen to confirm findings along with referrals for follow-up medical and audiological evaluation. These evaluations should occur no later than 3 months of age. Forty-seven states and the District of Columbia have mandated newborn screening with OAE and/or ABR testing. (SOR **B**)

VII. Treatment. The treatment of hearing loss is **dependent upon its etiology** and involves environmental alteration, assistive listening devices, active medical/surgical intervention, and hearing aids.

A. Sensorineural loss

    1. Presbycusis. Patients with a presumptive diagnosis of presbycusis should be referred to an audiologist for further testing to confirm the diagnosis and for rehabilitation. Patients can increase the effectiveness of communication by cupping the hand behind the ear, reducing distractions and background noise levels, using good lighting to see the speaker and understand gestures, and learning lipreading. Amplification can be accomplished with various types of hearing aids or other assistive listening devices for which consultation with a certified audiologist may be warranted. Psychologic support, particularly for elderly patients, is very helpful. Left untreated, presbycusis can lead to social isolation and depression.

2. **Noise-induced loss.** Patients with this type of loss should be referred to an otolaryngologist for assessment of asymmetric hearing loss, rapid and progressive hearing loss, permanent threshold shift, or an occasional finding of low-frequency loss. All patients with losses presenting at threshold ≥ 25 dB are candidates for hearing aids.

   a. In a study on whether adults with hearing impairment ($N = 153$) accept intervention with either hearing aids or communication programs after informed decision-making, about one-quarter (24%) did not take up the intervention decided upon; after 6 months, 43% had obtained hearing aids, and 28 participants (18%) completed a communication program.

   b. Authors of a meta-analysis on cochlear implants concluded that unilateral implants improve hearing and quality of life; bilateral implants show greater improvement in communication-related outcomes and improve sound localization.

3. **Ototoxicity.** For patients with ototoxicity, early removal of the offending agent will reduce the likelihood of permanent hearing loss. Hearing impairment may be either permanent (e.g., when caused by drugs such as mercury, arsenic, lead, and aminoglycosides) or temporary (e.g., when caused by drugs such as aspirin, quinine, and certain diuretics). Actual recovery may be delayed and is often incomplete. Thus, follow-up with an audiologist may be necessary to evaluate for ototoxic sequelae.

B. **Conductive hearing loss**
   1. **Foreign bodies or cerumen** in the external auditory canal can almost always be removed by irrigation with or without the use of ceruminolytics, ceruminolytics alone, or manual removal with forceps, suction, or curette. Patients with objects wedged in place should be referred to an otolaryngologist because of potential risks of damage to the tympanic membrane or bony structures by attempted removal.

      a. **Hard cerumen can be softened** fairly quickly prior to irrigation with a few drops of nonprescription cerumen softener. The ear can be irrigated with water approximately 20 minutes after the softening agent is applied. The use of water at a temperature of 35 to 37.8°C (95–100°F) will prevent vertigo.

      b. **Water irrigation is contraindicated** with vegetable foreign bodies (i.e., dry beans) because it can cause swelling. Alcohol solutions should be used in such cases. A perforation in the tympanic membrane is an absolute contraindication to irrigation.

      c. **Ear candling is a home remedy that patients should be instructed to avoid** because of risks of ear wax occlusion, local burns, and tympanic membrane perforation.

   2. **Otitis externa or otitis media** should be treated with appropriate medication (see Chapter 22); hearing should normalize following treatment of infection and resolution of middle ear effusion, which can take up to 3 months.

   3. Patients with **otosclerosis** can be successfully treated with stapedectomy and should be referred to an otolaryngologist.

SELECTED REFERENCES

American Speech and Hearing Association. http://www.asha.org/public/hearing/Hearing-Loss/. Accessed March 2013.

Li-Korotky HS. Age related hearing loss: quality of care for quality of life. *Gerontologist.* 2012;52(2): 265–271.

Pacala JT, Yueh B. Hearing deficits in the older patient. *JAMA.* 2012;307(11):1185–1194.

U.S. Preventive Service Task Force. Screening for hearing loss in older adults: recommendation statement. *Am Fam Physician.* 2013;87(2):129–130.

Verbeek JH, Kateman E, Morata TC, et al. Interventions to prevent occupational noise-induced hearing loss. *Cochrane Database Syst Rev.* 2012;(10):CD006396.

Walker JJ, Cleavland LM, Davis JL, et al. Audiometry screening and interpretation. *Am Fam Physician.* 2013;87(1):41–47.

Walling AD, Dickson GM. Hearing loss in older adults. *Am Fam Physician.* 2012;85(12):1150–1156.

Additional references are available online at http://langetextbooks.com/fm6e

35   Hematuria

Cynthia M. Waickus, MD, PhD

KEY POINTS

- Hematuria is a common finding on urinalysis in both children and adults and can be a sign of a benign or serious condition; the latter, more common in patients over 40 years of age. (SOR **C**)
- Microscopic hematuria should be confirmed by repeat testing and urine microscopy. (SOR **C**)
- One of the first steps in hematuria evaluation is to distinguish between glomerular and extraglomerular bleeding. (SOR **C**)

I. **Definition.** Hematuria is defined as the presence of an abnormal quantity of red blood cells (RBCs) in the urine and is not defined merely by urine color. Hematuria may be grossly visible or microscopic (apparent only on urinalysis) and becomes clinically significant when three or more (adult) or five or more (children) RBCs are visible per high-power field (hpf) in the sediment of two of the three consecutive centrifuged, freshly voided, clean-catch, mid-stream urine specimens.

II. **Common Diagnoses.** The etiology and pathophysiology of hematuria are varied. Population-based study prevalences of microscopic hematuria vary from 0.16% to 21% in adults, with some studies reporting an even higher prevalence among women and older persons. Causes of hematuria can be classified as either nonglomerular or glomerular (Figure 35–1). This is important both prognostically and for subsequent evaluation, as evidence of glomerular involvement precludes the need for urologic workup.

   A. **Nonglomerular causes**

   1. **Infections. Cystitis, urethritis, pyelonephritis,** and **prostatitis:** infectious etiologies are the most common cause of hematuria, accounting for 30% to 35% of all cases of both gross and microscopic hematuria. Renal tuberculosis and *Schistosoma haematobium* are rare causes, but need to be considered in persons who have traveled to endemic areas.

   2. **Calculi. Nephrolithiasis** and **urolithiasis** (primarily calcium oxalate and calcium phosphate) occur in approximately 5.2% of the overall population; rates are higher in men and Whites, and increase with age. Gross hematuria occurs in most patients presenting with kidney stones.

   3. **Neoplasms**

      a. **Renal tumors. Renal cell carcinoma,** originating in the renal cortex, accounts for 80% to 85% of all primary renal tumors. **Transitional cell carcinomas,** originating in the renal pelvis, are the second most common primary renal tumor (8%). Renal tumors occur primarily after age 60 years and are unusual before age 40 years. Risk factors for renal tumors include smoking, toxin exposure (e.g., cadmium, asbestos, and petroleum by-products), obesity, male gender, acquired cystic disease of the kidney, analgesic abuse nephropathy, and genetic predisposition. The presence of hematuria indicates the tumor has invaded the collecting system. **Wilms tumor** (nephroblastoma) is the most common renal tumor in children.

      b. **Bladder carcinoma** is the most common malignancy affecting the urinary system, occurring primarily after age 60 years and in men. Exposure to environmental chemicals (aromatic amines) used in the dye, paint, aluminum, textile and rubber industries, and cigarette smoking are the primary risk factors for developing bladder cancer.

      c. **Prostate cancer** is the most common nonskin cancer and the third leading cause of deaths in American men. Age is the most important risk factor; prostate cancer rarely occurs before age 40 years. It is more common in Blacks than Whites and has a strong genetic component. Although hematuria is not a common initial presentation, its detection should prompt consideration of prostate cancer.

      d. Benign tumors and polyps. **Benign prostatic hypertrophy** (BPH) and abnormal, benign growths **(polyps)** in the bladder and ureters can cause hematuria.

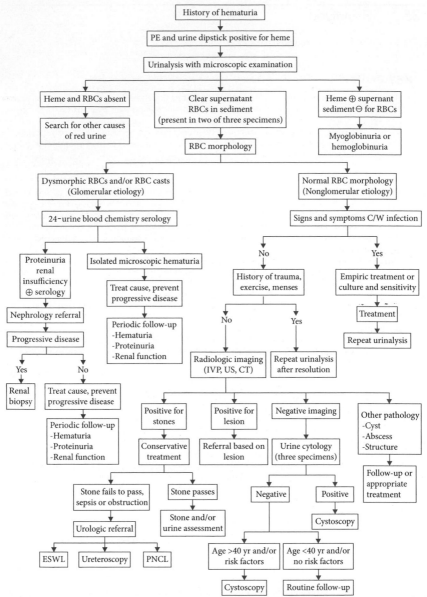

FIGURE 35–1. Algorithmic approach to the patient with hematuria. PE, physical examination; RBCs, red blood cells; C/W, compatible with; IVP, intravenous pyelogram; US, ultrasound; CT, computed tomography; ESWL, extracorporeal shockwave lithotripsy; PCNL, percutaneous nephrolithotomy.

The cellular proliferation in these conditions is associated with the formation of fragile, new blood vessels prone to bleeding.

4. **Genetically transmitted diseases. Polycystic kidney disease** (occurring in 1/400–2000 live births), **medullary cystic kidney disease** (incidence of 0.13/10,000 live births), and **sickle cell disease/trait** often include hematuria in the clinical presentation.

5. **Vascular disease. Arteriovenous malformations or fistulas** of the urologic tract typically present symptomatically as gross hematuria. **Renal infarction,** due to thrombo or atheroemboli in patients with atrial fibrillation or atherosclerotic disease, presents with the acute onset of nausea, vomiting, flank and abdominal pain, fever, and gross or microscopic hematuria (33%–50% of patients).

6. **Mechanical causes. Strictures** (ureteral and meatal), solitary renal **cysts,** and **foreign bodies** in the urinary tract can all present with hemturia.

7. **Anticoagulation therapy.** Routine use of **warfarin** should not cause either gross or microscopic hematuria unless there is an underlying abnormality; these patients should follow the same evaluative methods as other patients presenting with hematuria. The incidence of hematuria in patients taking anticoagulant therapy is the same as that of the general population unless excess dosing (e.g., unintentional overdose) occurs.

8. Hematuria due to urinary tract **trauma** is the result of direct cellular and vascular damage. **Exercise-induced hematuria** is a benign, short-term condition (resolves within 1 week) and is a diagnosis of exclusion. It occurs after noncontact sport activities and may be the result of brief renal ischemia. It is reported to occur in up to 30% of long-distance runners. It is important to differentiate exercise-induced hematuria from myoglobinuria (due to rhabdomyolysis) and hemoglobinuria.

B. **Glomerular causes** of hematuria (glomerulonephritis).

1. **IgA nephropathy** is the most common cause of primary glomerulonephritis and results from an abnormal globular deposition of IgA in the kidney. It has a peak incidence in the second and third decades of life and is more common in men, Asians, and Caucasians. Gross hematuria is a presenting symptom in 40% to 50% of cases, whereas microscopic hematuria with proteinuria is the presentation in 30% to 40% of cases.

2. **Thin basement membrane nephropathy** (benign familial hematuria) is a common cause of asymptomatic hematuria. It is characterized pathologically by diffuse thinning of the glomerular basement membrane, and clinically by persistent microscopic hematuria. It is familial, with an autosomal dominant inheritance, and has a benign prognosis as patients maintain normal renal function throughout their lives.

3. **Acute interstitial nephritis** is an important cause of acute renal failure resulting from immune-mediated tubulointerstitial injury.

   a. **Drugs** (71% of cases). Although any drug can potentially cause a hypersensitivity reaction involving the kidney, the most commonly implicated drugs are antibiotics (e.g., penicillins, cephalosporins, sulfas, quinolones, and rifampin), diuretics, nonsteroidal anti-inflammatory drugs (NSAIDs), anticonvulsants, and allopurinol.

   b. **Infection** (15% of cases) includes bacterial (e.g., streptococci, legionella, mycoplasma, syphilis), viral (e.g., cytomegalovirus [CMV], Epstein–Barr virus [EBV], human immunodeficiency virus [HIV], hepatitis B), fungal (e.g., histoplasmosis), and parasitic (e.g., toxoplasmosis, leptospirosis).

   c. **Autoimmune disorders.** Most autoimmune disorders eventually cause chronic interstitial nephritis (Sjögren syndrome, systemic lupus erythematosus [SLE], sarcoidosis, Wegeners granulomatosis).

4. **Hereditary nephritis** (Alport syndrome) is an uncommon (1 in 5000 persons), X-linked disorder that causes chronic glomerulonephritis progressing to end-stage renal disease. It presents early in life (before age 10 years) and is often associated with neural hearing loss and ocular difficulties.

III. **Symptoms**

A. Concurrent symptoms of **dysuria, frequency,** and **urgency** are classically indicative of an infectious etiology (urinary tract infection [UTI], cystitis, urethritis, prostatitis), but can also be caused by bladder cancer. The presence of **blood clots** in the urine rarely occurs with glomerular bleeding.

B. **Unilateral flank pain with radiation to the groin** typically suggests an obstructive cause in the kidney or ureter (calculi, clot, stricture, or tumor).

C. **Unilateral flank pain without radiation** but with **fever, dysuria,** and **frequency/urgency** is suggestive of pyelonephritis. **Pain** is not a symptom indicative of glomerular disease.

    D. Prostatic obstruction (BPH, prostate cancer) in older men can present as **urinary hesitancy** and **dribbling,** with or without **other symptoms of UTI**.

    E. Patient reports of **recent weight gain, edema, facial swelling,** and **decreased urine output** or **oliguria** suggest a glomerular cause.

    F. **Recent upper respiratory symptoms** or **sore throat** may suggest glomerulonephritis (poststreptococcal glomerulonephritis or IgA nephropathy); also present may be **fever, rash,** and **joint tenderness**.

    G. **Gross hematuria** can be a presenting symptom with any of the above diagnoses (benign causes to malignancies). A visible color change can be caused by as little as 1 mL/L of blood in the urine; the color change does not necessarily reflect the amount of blood loss.

    H. The most common presenting symptom for bladder cancer is **intermittent, painless, gross hematuria,** typically present **throughout micturition**.

IV. Signs. Like symptoms presented by the patient in the history, physical examination findings can be helpful in differentiating between glomerular and nonglomerular etiologies for hematuria, although clinical signs are absent in many cases.

    A. **Fever** is typically an indication of an infectious or inflammatory cause; **elevated blood pressure and weight gain** are clues to glomerular injury, whereas weight loss may be sign of a malignancy.

    B. **Costovertebral angle tenderness** may be present with pyelonephritis or renal calculi.

    C. **Digital rectal examination** revealing a firm, enlarged prostate gland is typically seen in BPH and may be present in prostate cancer. A tender, warm, enlarged, "boggy" feeling prostate adds clinical evidence for a diagnosis of prostatitis.

    D. **Examination of the external genitalia** and urethra/meatus is performed if local trauma is suspected as the cause of the hematuria.

V. Laboratory Tests

    A. **Screening.** In general, screening for hematuria (microscopic) in asymptomatic individuals is not recommended due to low prevalence of asymptomatic, undetected, early disease; lack of high-sensitivity screening tests for localized disease; and lack of ability of screening to affect prognosis. (SOR **Ⓖ**) However, certain groups of patients with microscopic hematuria who have risk factors for significant disease, especially malignancy, should undergo diagnostic workups. Those risk factors include age (>40 years), tobacco-use history, previous urologic or renal disease or history of pelvic irradiation, occupational exposure (e.g., benzenes, aromatic amines, rubber compounds/dyes), and drug exposure (previously listed).

        The principles of the diagnostic workup should pattern the clinicians' suspicion of glomerular versus nonglomerular etiologies (Figure 35–1). The identification of glomerular disease or injury as the source of hematuria is important both diagnostically and prognostically. Urologic etiologies can be ruled out, and referral to a nephrologist is typically warranted.

    B. **Urine dipstick** is a simple, fast, inexpensive, reagent-based colorimetric assay tool used in the office setting to perform screening urinalysis. The test, based on the peroxidase activity of hemoglobin, is at least as sensitive as urinalysis for the detection of microscopic **hematuria**. It can detect trace amounts of hemoglobin, equivalent to one to two RBCs per hpf, but it does not distinguish between RBCs, hemoglobin, or myoglobin, and therefore has a high false-positive rate; however, false negatives are unusual. Dipstick reagents can also detect the presence of **proteinuria** (although albumin is the only protein detected by dipstick, and a dipstick does not detect protein excretion below 300 mg per day), **leukocyte esterase,** and **nitrites**. All positive dipstick results should be confirmed by microscopic urinalysis of a properly obtained centrifuged urine specimen or by appropriate quantitative methods.

    C. **Urinalysis.** The initial evaluation of patients with a dipstick positive for heme or gross hematuria is **microscopic examination** of the **sediment** of the urine specimen (Figure 35–1). The sample should be a midstream, clean catch (foreskin retraction or labial separation followed by local disinfection of the meatus and mucosa) specimen, voided into a sterile container. Ideally, especially if infection is suspected, the specimen should be examined within 60 minutes or refrigerated for less than 24 hours. The specimen is then evaluated for:

        1. RBCs. The urine sediment is carefully examined for the presence of erythrocytes (three or more per hpf), as hematuria is only present if RBCs are present in the sediment and the supernatant remains clear. If the supernatant remains red (discolored), it should be tested for the presence of hemoglobin; red supernatant that is positive for heme is due to myoglobinuria (secondary to rhabdomyolysis) or hemoglobinuria; a red supernatant that tests negative for heme may be due to a variety of medications, certain food dyes, beets, or blackberries. **RBC morphology** by phase contrast microscopy can be helpful in distinguishing between glomerular and nonglomerular causes, as the presence of a significant number of dysmorphic RBCs suggests a renal (glomerular) source of the hematuria.

2. White blood cells (WBCs). UTI without pyuria (>10,000 WBCs/mL of uncentrifuged urine, or 2–5 WBCs per hpf in sediment) is unusual and is typically substantiated by a positive urine culture; however, sterile pyuria with hematuria may be indicative of a tuberculosis infection.

3. Urinary **casts** (tubules of precipitated or aggregated protein) are only formed in the distal convoluted tubules or the collecting ducts, and therefore are indicative of kidney involvement (except for hyaline casts). The presence of **RBC casts** is typically diagnostic of glomerulonephritis. **WBC casts** indicate an inflammatory process in the kidney and are most typical of acute pyelonephritis or glomerulonephritis.

4. Crystals can be present in the urinary sediment of patients with hematuria due to calculi, but there is no clearly defined association between crystal formation and urolithiasis.

5. Bacteria are typically present in the urine of patients with suspected UTI, but contamination is common (normal genital microbes). The diagnosis of bacteruria requires confirmation by urine culture.

D. Urine culture. A midstream, clean catch specimen should be considered for culture, colony count, and antibiotic sensitivity whenever a complicated or recurrent UTI is suspected or for suspected UTI in a child aged 3 years or younger.

E. 24-hour urine collection. The complete collection of all urine excreted in a 24-hour period by a patient with hematuria may provide important clues to the presence of glomerular disease, especially when **proteinuria** (>150 mg per day or 10 mg/dL) is present. In addition, the sample can be analyzed for creatinine clearance and a number of other compounds.

F. Blood work. The choice of a hematologic evaluation should be based on signs and symptoms, the urinalysis, and the "preliminary diagnosis" of the patient. Blood chemistry, including **electrolytes** and **renal function** (blood urea nitrogen, creatinine, **albumin/ protein levels,** and calculated glomerular filtration rate [**GFR**]), are indicated when renal disease is suspected as the cause of the hematuria. Complete blood count (**CBC**) can provide clues about the degree of blood loss and/or the presence of infection. Coagulation **studies** should be performed in patients with a history of a bleeding disorder. In certain populations, a **sickle cell prep** or **hemoglobin electrophoresis** can help establish the diagnosis of sickle cell disease or trait. Serologic testing including complement levels (complements **C3 and C4**), antinuclear antibody titers, erythrocyte sedimentation rate, and antistreptolysin (**ASO**) **titers** may support a glomerular etiology for the hematuria.

G. Imaging studies. Radiologic testing should also be based on the preliminary diagnosis. If a glomerular or infectious etiology is ruled out, the upper urinary tract should be examined radiographically to detect neoplasms, urolithiasis, cystic disease, and/or obstructive lesions. (SOR ⊙)

1. The **intravenous pyelogram (IVP),** or excretory urography, was traditionally the first imaging examination of the upper urinary tract in patients with hematuria since it defines the anatomy of the upper tract well. It is limited in its ability to identify small masses (<3 cm), and it cannot differentiate between cystic and solid lesions. In addition, IVP necessitates the use of a potentially nephrotoxic contrast dye. Except for the detection of urothelial transitional cell carcinoma, its use is often replaced by high-quality renal ultrasound (US) and/or spiral computed tomography (CT).

2. Renal US. Ultrasonography, compared with other imaging techniques of the urinary tract, is rapid, noninvasive, and readily available, does not require toxic contrast media, and causes no radiation exposure. It is therefore thought to be the safest, least expensive imaging choice for the evaluation of hematuria, especially in pregnant women. It is highly sensitive in identifying large masses (>3 cm), cysts, hydronephrosis, and hydroureter. US is not likely to detect nonobstructing ureteral stones or small urothelial masses (e.g., transitional cell carcinoma).

3. Unenhanced (no IV or oral contrast) **spiral CT** of the abdomen and pelvis is the most sensitive imaging method for detecting urinary tract calculi (96%–100% sensitive). It is also indicated in the patient with hematuria and a history of trauma. Contrast-enhanced CT of the abdomen and pelvis is superior to US or IVP for identifying small (<3 cm) masses and is typically used to further evaluate masses identified by IVP or US.

4. Abdominal plain films (kidneys, ureters, bladder [KUB]) are not typically used in the workup of hematuria, except for quick detection of radiopaque stones (calcium, struvite, or cystine stones); however, small stones, uric acid stones, or stones behind bony structures are usually not visualized. KUB also fails to detect obstruction. Plain films can be utilized to follow the progression of renal calculi down the urinary tract during passage.

H. Urine cytology. Examination of the urine for the presence of malignant cells can be used in patients with hematuria who also have risk factors for urothelial cancers. (SOR ⦿) The sensitivity of urine cytology is greatest for high-grade lesions and carcinoma in situ of the bladder (66%–79% sensitivity). Sensitivity is increased by analyzing first void specimens on three consecutive days or by obtaining a sample during cystoscopy. The utility of urine cytology is very limited for upper tract malignancies (renal cell and transitional cell carcinoma) and for low-grade bladder lesions. Positive urine cytology is routinely followed by cystoscopy.

I. Cystoscopy of the bladder, urethra, and ureteral orifices is utilized to exclude the diagnosis of bladder malignancy. It is indicated in all patients over age 40 years with hematuria, in patients less than age 40 years who present with hematuria and risk factors for bladder cancer, and in those less than age 40 years with unexplained, persistent hematuria or gross hematuria. Cystoscopy is rarely indicated in children. Cystoscopy typically requires urologic referral.

J. Renal biopsy, with subsequent microscopic examination of the tissue (light, immunofluorescence, and electron microscopy), is not routinely performed to establish a diagnosis for glomerular hematuria. It is typically considered only if there is evidence of progressive disease (increasing proteinuria, worsening blood pressure, increasing creatinine excretion, or worsening renal function).

VI. Treatment

A. Infections. UTIs (see Chapter 21) are treated with **antibiotic** therapy. The choice of drug, route of administration, and length of treatment is dictated by the patient's history, symptoms, risk factors, preferences, and culture and sensitivity results. The same principles apply to the treatment of prostatitis (see Chapter 60).

B. Calculi. The mainstay treatment for most calculi (80%–85%) is conservative—**watchful waiting**—involving hydration, analgesic medication, and often prophylactic antibiotic treatment. Stones larger than 6 mm in diameter are unlikely to pass with conservative treatment and require intervention. Urologic consultation is indicated for removal of large stones, for patients with sepsis, and for obstructive symptoms.

Urologic modalities used to manage calculi include extracorporeal shockwave lithotripsy (primarily used to break up smaller stones [0.4–2 cm] within the kidneys), percutaneous nephrolithotomy (a surgical procedure used to extract larger [>2 cm] stones from the kidney through a puncture wound in the skin), and ureteroscopy (an endoscopic procedure [through the urethra and bladder into the ureter] that can reach to the renal pelvis to break up [via laser] and/or retrieve [via a micro-basket] smaller stones [<2 cm]).

C. Neoplasms. Treatment for renal and urologic malignancies are determined by the pathology and staging of disease and include surgery, chemotherapy, and radiation therapy. Treatment modalities for BPH (see Chapter 60) include surgery and medical therapy.

D. Treatment of **glomerular causes** of hematuria is directed primarily toward slowing disease progression. For IgA nephropathy or hereditary nephritis, treatment is aimed at maintaining normal blood pressures (e.g., angiotensin-converting enzyme inhibitors and angiotensin II receptor blockers) and decreasing cardiovascular risk (statins). Poststreptococcal glomerulonephritis usually resolves gradually after treatment of the infection. Acute interstitial nephritis caused by drugs is treated by removing the causative agent, and autoimmune etiologies are typically treated with immunosuppressants under the care of nephrologists and rheumatologists.

SELECTED REFERENCES

Chou R, Dana T. Screening adults for bladder cancer: a review of the evidence for the U.S. Preventive Services Task Force. *Ann Intern Med.* 2010;153:461–468.

Davis R, Jones SJ, Barocas DA, et al. Diagnosis, evaluation and follow-up of asymptomatic microhematuria (AMH) in adults: AUA guideline. *J Urol.* 2012;188(6 Suppl):2473–2481.

Dick-Biascoechea MA, Erekson EA. Asymptomatic microscopic hematuria. *Curr Opin Obstet Gynecol.* 2012;24(5):324–330.

Grossfield GD, Litwin MS, Wolf JS, et al. Evaluation of asymptomatic microscopic hematuria in adults: the American Urological Association Best Practice Policy – part I: definition, detection, prevalence, and etiology. *Urology.* 2001;57(4):599–603.

Grossfield GD, Litwin MS, Wolf JS, et al. Evaluation of asymptomatic microscopic hematuria in adults: the American Urological Association Best Practice Policy – part II: patient evaluation, cytology, nephrology evaluation, and follow-up. *Urology.* 2001;57(4):604–610.

Kelly JD, Fawcwtt DP, Goldberg LC. Assessment and management of non-visible haematuria in primary care. *BMJ.* 2009;338:227–338.

Loo RK, Lieberman SF, Slezak JM, et al. Stratifying risk of urinary tract malignant tumors in patients with asymptomatic microscopic hematuria. *Mayo Clin Proc.* 2013;88(2):129–138.

Margulis V, Sagalowsky AI. Assessment of hematuria. *Med Clin N Am.* 2011;95:153–159.

Moreno JA, Martin-Cleary C, Gutiérrez E, et al. Haematuria: the forgotten CKD factor? *Nephrol Dial Transplant.* 2012;27(1):28–34.

O'Connor OJ, Fitzgerald E, Maher MM. Imaging of hematuria. *AJR.* 2010;195:W263–W267.

36   Insomnia

Julianne Falleroni, DO, MPH

KEY POINTS

- Insomnia is a common complaint in primary care. Symptoms are reported by 35% to 50% of the adult population. Diagnosis of an insomnia disorder ranges from 5% to 20%. (SOR **C**)
- When assessing sleep problems, clinicians should explore the role of underlying medical and psychiatric illnesses, medication use, and current sleep habits. (SOR **C**)
- Implement good sleep hygiene for all sleep disorders and consider nonpharmacologic approaches to treatment whenever possible. (SOR **B**)
- Use sleep treatment goals to determine the effectiveness of insomnia interventions. (SOR **C**)
- Use sleep aid medications at lowest dose for the shortest amount of time needed to reach sleep symptom goals. (SOR **C**)

I. **Introduction**

A. **Definition. Insomnia** is one of eight sleep disorder categories according to the *International Classification of Sleep Disorders*, 2nd edition (ICSD-2) (Table 36–1). **Insomnia is defined as the inability to fall asleep (sleep initiation) or stay asleep (sleep maintenance).**

1. **Sleep maintenance insomnia** is further divided into common symptoms such as frequent nighttime awakenings, difficulty returning to sleep after awakenings, and awakening too early and inability to fall back to sleep. These symptoms result in a lack of restorative sleep. Some individuals complain of nonrestorative sleep without the above sleep disturbances. Therefore, lack of restorative sleep is not adequate to diagnose insomnia.

2. **True insomnia** must include the above **nighttime symptoms and also have a negative effect or impairment of daytime functioning**. In addition, insomnia differs from sleep deprivation as it implies that the sleep disturbances occur despite adequate opportunity and circumstances for sleep. Sleep deprivation is caused by not spending enough time sleeping.

TABLE 36–1. ICSD-2 SLEEP DISORDER CATEGORIES

Insomnias
Sleep-related breathing disorders
Hypersomnias of central origin
Circadian rhythm disorders
Parasomnias
Sleep-related movement disorders
Isolated symptoms
Other sleep disorders

3. Insomnia can be acute/episodic or chronic. A common definition of chronic insomnia includes the presence of at least one symptom occurring three or more nights per week lasting 1 or more months.

4. Insomnia is further categorized into primary or secondary insomnia based on the likelihood that the insomnia is a symptom or result of another comorbid condition. Secondary insomnia is caused by another medical, mental health, or medication/substance use condition. It can be difficult to determine whether insomnia is a cause or effect of other conditions, and therefore, some have argued in favor of using the term "comorbid insomnia" to replace secondary insomnia.

B. Pathophysiology. Polysomnogram studies show much overlap between "good" and "bad" sleepers. Interviews demonstrate that poor sleepers tend to overestimate the length of time to fall asleep initially or after a nighttime awakening. They also tend to underestimate sleep duration. This underscores the role of perception of sleep in the diagnosis of insomnia.

1. Recent theories suggest a 24-hour hyperarousal state in individuals who are poor sleepers, which may explain why patients with insomnia complain less of daytime sleepiness compared with other daytime symptoms. They often complain of inability to nap despite poor sleep the night before. Other studies supporting the 24-hour phenomenon in insomnia include findings of elevated cortisol and adrenocorticotropic hormone in early sleep period and reduced parasympathetic tone in heart rate variability during non-rapid eye movement (REM) sleep. Functional imaging studies show fewer wake–sleep differences in brain metabolism in individuals with insomnia compared with good sleepers.

C. Prevalence, risk factors, and impact

1. The true prevalence of insomnia depends on the stringency of the definition used. Insomnia symptoms occur in 35% to 50% of the adult population at some point. Diagnosis of these symptoms with distress or impairment occurs in 10% to 15% of the adult population. Diagnosis of an insomnia disorder ranges from 5% to 20%. Insomnia can occur across cultures and races.

a. Risk factors for insomnia include depression, female gender, older age, lower socioeconomic status, shift work, concurrent medical or mental disorders, divorced/separated marital status, and African-American ethnicity.

b. Chronic insomnia occurs in 40% to 80% of individuals with insomnia. Functionally, it can result in reduced work productivity, increased work absenteeism, and increased health care costs. Patients with mental illness are at a higher risk for insomnia and patients with a history of insomnia are at an increased risk for mental illness such as depression and alcohol dependence.

II. Symptoms and Sleep History. The ICSD-2 contains criteria for diagnosing a general insomnia disorder. The criteria include nine common daytime symptoms in addition to common nighttime symptoms (Table 36–2). These symptoms can often be nonspecific and as with most conditions, diagnosing insomnia requires a thorough history (Table 36–3).

A. Primary complaint. It is important to ask the patient to characterize the sleep complaint as best they can. Many patients with insomnia have multiple and overlapping nighttime and daytime complaints. Asking about onset, duration, frequency, and

---

TABLE 36–2. ICSD-2 CRITERIA FOR GENERAL INSOMNIA DISORDER

1. A report of difficulty initiating sleep, difficulty maintaining sleep, or waking up to early or sleep that is chronically nonrestorative or poor in quality.
2. The above sleep difficulty occurs despite adequate opportunity and circumstances for sleep.
3. At least one of the following forms of daytime impairment related to the nighttime sleep difficulty:
   a. Fatigue or malaise
   b. Attention, concentration, or memory impairment
   c. Social of vocational dysfunction or poor school performance
   d. Mood disturbance or irritability
   e. Daytime sleepiness
   f. Motivation, energy, or initiative reduction
   g. Proneness for errors or accidents at work or while driving
   h. Tension, headaches, or gastrointestinal symptoms in response to sleep loss
   i. Concerns or worries about sleep

TABLE 36-3. SLEEP HISTORY

Primary insomnia complaint: Characterization of complaint(s): • Difficulty falling asleep • Awakenings • Poor or unrefreshing sleep Onset Duration Frequency Severity Course Perpetuating factors Past and current treatments and responses	**Nocturnal symptoms:** Respiratory Motor Other medical Behavioral and psychological **Daytime activities and function:** Identify sleepiness versus fatigue Napping Work Lifestyle Travel Daytime consequences (see Table 36-2)
Pre-sleep conditions: Pre-bedtime activities Bedroom environment Evening physical and mental status	• Quality of life • Mood disturbance • Cognitive dysfunction • Exacerbation of comorbid conditions
Sleep–wake schedule (average, variability): Bedtime: Time to fall asleep • Factors prolonging sleep onset • Factors shortening sleep Awakenings • Number, characterization, duration • Associated symptoms • Associated behaviors Final awakening versus time out of bed Amount of sleep obtained	

severity helps to further characterize the symptoms as well as the level of daytime disruptiveness it causes. It is helpful to ask about triggering factors and previous episodes to determine the extent to which this is a chronic condition or symptom of some other comorbid condition.

1. Pre-sleep conditions. These questions begin to address the common concept of **sleep hygiene**. Asking individuals about their home and sleep environment and pre-bedtime activities can help determine whether the environment is conducive to sleep or allows adequate opportunity for restful sleep.

    a. Patients with insomnia may develop pre-sleep **habits that can perpetuate their problem** in an attempt to combat the problem. Common examples include spending more time in bed although not sleeping, hoping to catch up on missed sleep. Others include habits in bed that perpetuate arousal and impede relaxation such as watching television, reading, and talking on the phone. In fact, devices such as cell phones and tablet computers with self-luminous backlit displays can cause decreased melatonin levels, making it much harder to fall asleep. Patients with chronic insomnia can become more anxious as bedtime approaches as they anticipate a poor night's sleep.

2. Sleep–wake schedule. These questions obtain further information regarding usual bedtime, latency or time it takes to fall asleep, number and types of awakenings through the night, and final awakening time versus time that the patient actually gets out of bed. It is important to discuss not just typical patterns but how much variation a person experiences in his/her schedule. This can be seen with insomnia related to shift work where there is so much variability in bedtime and waking time that a person cannot get accustomed to any one routine. Assessing sleep–wake schedule and variability can allow evaluation for common circadian rhythm disorders or sleep phase disorders. These disorders in the extreme can make it difficult for patients to adjust to external expectations on sleep and waking with employment or family responsibilities.

    a. Advanced sleep phase disorder: Informally known as the "early bird." Patients go to bed early and rise early.

      b. Delayed sleep phase disorder: Informally known as the "night owl." Patients go to bed late and have trouble arising in the morning.

B. Associated nocturnal symptoms. Insomnia and nighttime awakenings may be related to other comorbid conditions such as breathing-related conditions (sleep apnea, snoring, coughing), motor (restless leg syndrome) or musculoskeletal (pain) complaints, and nocturia. Often a sleeping partner, if there is one, can be a resource for reporting these symptoms as they often happen while the patient is not fully awake or awake during the night. Other examples include parasomnias such as:

    1. Nightmares: associated with limited vocalization, vivid recall, easy arousal.

    2. Night terrors: associated with loud vocalization/screams, limited recall, and difficult arousal.

    3. Somnambulism: sleep-walking.

C. Daytime activities and function. Assessing these symptoms assures that nighttime complaints of poor sleep are actually affecting daytime functioning as part of the ICSD-2 criteria. In addition, it allows the interviewer to determine whether the patient has daytime fatigue (low energy, physical tiredness, weariness) or true sleepiness (an actual tendency to fall asleep during the day). If a patient has true daytime sleepiness, it often prompts further evaluation for secondary causes or comorbid causes of insomnia.

    1. Some extreme examples of true daytime sleepiness include sleep attacks, bizarre hypnagogic hallucinations, and cataplexy, which are often components of narcolepsy.

    2. Number, duration, and timing of naps are important as these strategies are often initiated to combat insomnia but, over time, can perpetuate it.

    3. Evaluation of mood and quality of life. Often the irritability and fatigue that occurs with insomnia causes patients to avoid or restrict daytime activities such as social events, exercise, and work. This can lead to or worsen underlying mood or relationship problems, which can in turn worsen the sleep-related symptoms.

D. Additional history. An insomnia or sleep history should also include a thorough evaluation of medical, psychiatric, medication, substance, family, social, travel, and occupational histories.

    1. Many medical (Table 36–4) and psychiatric (Table 36–5) conditions can cause or result in insomnia as a condition or symptom.

    2. Many nonprescription, prescription, and recreational medications and substances can result in insomnia or poor sleep (Table 36–6).

    3. Travel history will evaluate for an obvious cause like jet lag.

    4. An occupational history will not only investigate if there is a shift work disorder but also evaluate for occupational stresses, occupational risks that can be exacerbated

TABLE 36–4. COMMON COMORBID MEDICAL DISORDERS, CONDITIONS, AND SYMPTOMS

System	Examples of Disorders, Conditions, and Symptoms
Neurological	Stroke, dementia, Parkinson disease, seizure disorders, headache disorders, traumatic brain injury, peripheral neuropathy, chronic pain disorders, neuromuscular disorders
Cardiovascular	Angina, congestive heart failure, dyspnea, dysrhythmias
Pulmonary	COPD, emphysema, asthma, laryngospasm
Digestive	Reflux, peptic ulcer disease, cholelithiasis, colitis, irritable bowel syndrome
Genitourinary	Incontinence, benign prostatic hypertrophy, nocturia, enuresis, interstitial cystitis
Endocrine	Hypothyroidism, hyperthyroidism, diabetes mellitus
Musculoskeletal	Rheumatoid arthritis, osteoarthritis, fibromyalgia, Sjögren syndrome, kyphosis
Reproductive	Pregnancy, menopause, menstrual cycle variations
Sleep disorders	Obstructive sleep apnea, central sleep apnea, restless legs syndrome, periodic limb movement disorder, circadian rhythm sleep disorders, parasomnias
Other	Allergies, rhinitis, sinusitis, bruxism, alcohol and other substance use/ dependence/ withdrawal

TABLE 36–5. COMMON COMORBID PSYCHIATRIC DISORDERS AND SYMPTOMS

Category	Examples
Mood disorders	Major depressive disorder, bipolar mood disorder, dysthymia
Anxiety disorders	Generalized anxiety disorder, panic disorder, posttraumatic stress disorder, obsessive compulsive disorder
Psychiatric disorders	Schizophrenia, schizoaffective disorder
Amnestic disorders	Alzheimer disease, other dementias
Disorders usually seen in childhood and adolescence	Attention deficit hyperactivity disorder
Other disorders and symptoms	Adjustment disorders, personality disorders, bereavement, stress, delirium

if the patient comes to work fatigued (such as operating machinery or caring for others while at work), and if there are work-related consequences from insomnia such as absenteeism.

III. Signs. There are no specific features of chronic insomnia on examination or mental status examination. However, a thorough examination can help support or refute the likelihood of comorbid or secondary causes of insomnia.

IV. Additional Tests and Studies. In most cases, a careful history and physical examination will obviate the need for additional testing and will point to underlying medical conditions. Some other helpful studies can include the following:

A. Patient reporting tools. These can include sleep logs, sleep history, and questionnaires designed to evaluate sleep quality, sleepiness, mood disorders, and quality of life. These tools can be used to further evaluate specific subtypes of insomnia. Formal neuropsychological testing can also be helpful. Clinicians should choose additional testing tools based on their own clinical expertise. These tools can also be used at subsequent follow-up evaluations to compare changes after interventions to baseline (Table 36–7). Some suggest using the following at a minimum:

1. A general medical/psychiatric/medication questionnaire to identify comorbid disorders and medication use.

2. The Epworth Sleepiness Scale.

3. A 2-week sleep log that identifies sleep–wake times, general patterns, and day-to-day variability.

B. Laboratory testing. This is often not necessary but can be used to supplement the history and physical findings especially when comorbidities are suspected. **Iron** or ferritin can be obtained in the evaluation of anemia or if a component of restless leg syndrome is suspected. **A thyroid-stimulating hormone (TSH) level** can rule out thyroid disorders if suspected. Tests for anemia, vitamin B_{12} deficiency, folate, vitamin D, and TSH should be considered for fatigue symptoms in addition to insomnia.

1. Sleep study (polysomnogram). A sleep study can be helpful to confirm or elaborate on symptoms that imply obstructive sleep apnea (OSA) (snoring, obesity, sleep

TABLE 36–6. COMMON CONTRIBUTING MEDICATIONS AND SUBSTANCES

Category	Examples
Antidepressants	Selective serotonin reuptake inhibitors, venlafaxine, duloxetine, monoamine oxidase inhibitors
Stimulants	Caffeine, methylphenidate, amphetamine derivatives, ephedrine and derivatives, cocaine
Decongestants	Pseudoephedrine, phenylephrine
Narcotic analgesics	Oxycodone, codeine, propoxyphene
Cardiovascular	Beta-blockers, alpha-receptor agonists, and antagonists, diuretics, lipid-lowering agents
Pulmonary	Theophylline, albuterol
Alcohol	

TABLE 36–7. INSOMNIA QUESTIONNAIRES USED IN BASELINE AND TREATMENT OUTCOME ASSESSMENT

Questionnaire	Description
Epworth Sleepiness Scale (http://www.stanford.edu/~dement/epworth.html)	8-item, self-report, used to assess subjective sleepiness
Insomnia Severity Index (https://www.myhealth.va.gov/mhv-portal-web/anonymous.portal?_nfpb=true&_pageLabel=healthyLiving&contentPage=healthy_living/sleep_insomnia_index.htm)	7-item, self-report, used to assess patient's perception of insomnia
Pittsburgh Sleep Quality Index (http://www.sleep.pitt.edu/includes/showFile.asp?fltype=doc&flID=2532)	24-item, self-report, used to measure sleep quality
Beck Depression Inventory (http://www.ibogaine.desk.nl/graphics/3639b1c_23.pdf)	21-item, self-report, used to measure depression
State-Trait Anxiety Inventory (http://www.google.com/url?sa=t&rct=j&q=&esrc=s&frm=1&source=web&cd=5&cad=rja&ved=0CE8QFjAE&url=http%3A%2F%2Fwww.reginfo.gov%2Fpublic%2Fdo%2FDownloadDocument%3FdocumentID%3D60884%26version%3D1&ei=qQoqUuvlNsm8yAHC14GwAw&usg=AFQjCNFZxO-gwtApmlFhnOCNRbXrXxlbrQ&sig2=9tO-Q5mMMFgPJucrE2rZSgA)	20-item, self-report, used to measure anxiety
Fatigue Severity Scale (http://www.mainedo.com/pdfs/FSS.pdf)	9-item, used to rate daytime fatigue
Short Form Health Survey (http://www.rand.org/health/surveys_tools/mos/mos_core_36item_survey.html)	36-item, self report, used to generically measure quality of life for any disorder
Dysfunctional Beliefs and Attitudes about Sleep Questionnaire (http://www.insomnomore.com/wp-content/uploads/2012/03/DBAS-16.pdf)	Self-rating of 28 statements used to assess negative cognitions or perceptions about sleep

partner reports of apneic episodes). It can also help document suspicions for periodic limb movements of sleep (restless leg syndrome) and disorders of sleep phases or parasomnias.

OBSTRUCIVE SLEEP APNEA

OSA is a condition that includes apnea events during the night and is associated with daytime fatigue and disrupted sleep. In this condition, the airway collapses or becomes blocked during sleep which causes shallow breathing or breathing pauses. Up to 20% of the adult population suffers from OSA, although many patients are unaware of it unless informed by a family member or bed partner. Risk factors include age, race (increased risk in African-Americans), obesity, smoking, craniofacial abnormalities, and upper airway soft-tissue disorders. The most common clinical presentations are a history of snoring and daytime sleepiness. Long-term consequences of OSA include resistant hypertension, heart failure, and increased all-cause mortality. Diagnosis is by nighttime sleep study that documents hypopnea and apnea episodes.

Treatment begins with smoking cessation, weight loss, avoidance of alcohol, or any other hypnotic agents. Positive pressure airways improve symptoms (SOR Ⓐ) as do some oral appliances (SOR Ⓑ); in situations where both treatments are effective, patients prefer oral appliances. Studies to date do not support use of surgery for sleep apnea.

2. **Referral to a sleep specialist.** The majority of patients with chronic insomnia are appropriately evaluated and treated in the primary care setting. Referrals to a sleep specialist can be considered in the following situations:
   a. Symptoms or high suspicion of another sleep disorder such as narcolepsy or apnea
   b. Pronounced alteration of sleep timing (or circadian rhythm sleep disorder)
   c. Unusual sleep behaviors or injuries (parasomnias, sleep eating disorder)
   d. Clinician or patient feels the problem is worsening or becoming disruptive to daily activities

V. **Treatment.** Taking an appropriate history for sleep complaints is essential prior to developing a treatment plan. Patients' symptoms, comorbidities, sleep habits, and the effects of poor sleep on daytime function all factor in to which treatments are most appropriate.

TABLE 36–8. GOALS OF INSOMNIA TREATMENT

Primary Goals

Improvements in sleep quality and/or duration

Improvement of insomnia-related daytime impairments such as energy, attention, memory, cognitive dysfunction, fatigue, somatic symptoms

Secondary and Other Goals

Improvement in an insomnia symptom such as

- Sleep onset latency less than 30 minutes and/or
- Wakening after sleep onset less than 30 minutes and/or
- Decreased frequency of awakenings or other sleep complaints
- Total sleep time (time in bed minus sleep latency and wakening after sleep onset) >6 hours
- Sleep efficiency (total sleep time divided by time in bed multiplied by 100)

Formation of a positive and clear association between the bed and sleeping

Improvement in sleep-related psychological distress

A. Early recognition of **habits that are disruptive to quality sleep** is essential. Limiting, stopping, or changing the timing of caffeine, alcohol, and other medications can provide adequate symptom improvement for many patients without requiring additional interventions. Transient or sporadic episodes of insomnia (rare to a few days per month) with minimal effects on daytime functioning, which can be linked to a specific and controllable trigger, can often be improved with simple interventions.

B. The second component of treatment is to **develop treatment goals** to set expectations for patients and providers as well as to monitor treatment responses over time (Table 36–8).

C. **Nonpharmacologic management of chronic insomnia.** These techniques are often sufficient to adequately treat chronic insomnia to an acceptable goal of improved sleep and improved daytime functioning. Even patients who need pharmacologic treatments can benefit from the addition of nonpharmacologic interventions. It is important that clinicians take time to underscore the value of these options alone or in combination with medications when outlining a treatment plan.

 1. **Cognitive behavioral therapy** includes a formal counseling plan similar to cognitive therapy employed for other conditions. It involves identifying dysfunctional beliefs about sleep, and replacing them with more valid and adaptive substitutes. It often involves setting realistic expectations about sleep requirements.

 2. **Sleep hygiene education.** Most patients with insomnia have tried some components of sleep hygiene, although many do not maintain these efforts long enough to see the effects. At times they think they are practicing sleep hygiene such as staying in bed and refusing to get out until they fall asleep which is actually counterproductive in many cases (see Section II.A). Common recommendations include avoiding caffeine, avoiding heavy meals, and limiting fluids prior to bedtime. Other interventions are to include daily exercise but to avoid it within 90 minutes of bedtime. Exposure to bright daytime light in the morning, whether natural sunlight or a light therapy box, is also helpful. Controlling outside stimuli in the room where sleep will take place is also important. Similar to teaching a newborn to fall asleep, adults become accustomed to presleep rituals. If these rituals are stimulating or counterproductive, it will impair one's ability to relax and fall asleep. For example:
    - Going to bed when a person feels tired.
    - Leaving the bed and bedroom if not asleep within 15 to 20 minutes to avoid the pattern of lying awake in bed for long periods without sleeping.
    - Avoiding napping.
    - Setting a consistent bedtime over a week as opposed to going to sleep early during week days and staying up much later during weekends.
    - Avoiding reading, watching television, using computers, and talking on the phone in the bedroom.
    - Dimming lights at night including changing your computer or iPad's screen settings to make the display dimmer or adjusting the display to remove blue hues (a free, downloadable program called F.lux will automatically adjust the hues).
    - Stop use of backlit devices several hours before bedtime.

3. Circadian rhythm adjustments. These techniques can be helpful for patients with delayed sleep phase or advanced sleep phase syndrome. It involves slowly adjusting bedtime to an earlier time (delayed sleep phase) or later (advanced sleep phase) over a period of weeks. It can be used in conjunction with a pharmacologic agent such as melatonin or other temporary sleep agent (see Section V.D).

   a. A more intense form of this therapy is sleep restriction. This involves using a sleep diary to estimate their average sleep time (no less than 5 hours) and temporarily restricting sleep to that amount. Patients then calculate their "sleep efficiency" by dividing their actual sleep time by the time they spend in bed. Once their sleep efficiency reaches 90%, they can increase their time in bed by 15 to 20 minutes. They maintain this new sleep restriction until their efficiency again reaches 90%. Over time, they increase their time in bed in 15- to 20-minute increments until they reach a time in bed that is more satisfactory.

      (1) Sleep restriction is effective and can reduce sleep latency (time to fall asleep) from 48 minutes to 19 minutes. However, it is time-consuming.

      (2) It should be avoided in patients with epilepsy (sleep deprivation lowers seizure threshold), bipolar disorder (sleep deprivation can worsen mood lability and increase risk of mania or hypomania), and parasomnias (like sleepwalking). This technique can also worsen daytime sleepiness, thus impairing driving ability or other daytime responsibilities.

4. Relaxation therapy. This is often used in conjunction with sleep hygiene techniques aimed at controlling outside stimuli. It can be thought of as controlling internal stimuli and reducing the hyperarousal state that is thought to be part of insomnia. These techniques can deactivate this hyperarousal (Table 36–9).

TABLE 36–9. COGNITIVE-BEHAVIORAL INTERVENTIONS FOR INSOMNIA

Intervention	General Description	Specific Techniques
Sleep hygiene education	Recommendations promoting behaviors that help sleep and avoiding behaviors that interfere with sleep	• Do not try to sleep • Avoid stimulants • Limit alcohol • Maintain a regular sleep schedule seven nights per week • Avoid naps • Get regular exercise at least 6 h prior to sleep • Keep the bedroom dark and quiet
Stimulus control	Based on operant conditioning: avoid nonsleep activities in the bedroom	• Go to bed only for sleep • Use the bed and bedroom for sleep only • Do not read, watch television, talk on phone, worry, or plan in the bedroom • Leave the bed and bedroom if unable to fall asleep within 10–20 min • Return only when feeling sleepy again • Set alarm and wake up at same time every day; do not use the snooze • Do not nap
Sleep restriction therapy	Based on regulating circadian and homeostatic processes; treatment reduces time in bed, maintaining a consistent wake time to reinforce circadian rhythms	• Restrict time awake in bed by setting strict bed and rising schedule • Keep fixed wake-up time, regardless of actual sleep duration • If sleep efficiency is less than 85%–90%, reduce time in bed by 15–30 min • If sleep efficiency is >85% to 90%, increase time in bed by 15–30 min
Relaxation training	Muscle tension and cognitive arousal are not compatible with sleep	• Progressive relaxation, guided imagery, paced breathing
Cognitive therapy	Identify, challenge, and replace dysfunctional beliefs and attitudes about sleep	• Challenge unhelpful beliefs and fears about sleep • Journaling to reduce rumination

5. Complementary medicine. As with many conditions, there is growing interest in complementary medicine treatments for insomnia. Acupuncture and acupressure have been shown to improve sleep quality scores but show inconsistent results on other sleep parameters such as sleep-onset latency, total sleep duration, and time to waking after sleep onset. Acupressure was found to be more beneficial than acupuncture in some studies. Other complementary medicine techniques studied include tai chi or yoga. Results for these techniques are generally supportive in their role for insomnia.

    a. Many natural and herbal preparations are reported to have positive effects on causing relaxation or drowsiness but benefits specific to treating insomnia have been mixed, unsupported, or simply not studied in controlled trials.

    b. Valerian root has been most studied as it has long been used in traditional and herbal medicines. It causes a sedative effect by inhibiting the breakdown of gamma-aminobutyric acid (GABA). The greatest benefit is usually seen in patients taking 400–900 mg of valerian extract up to 2 hours before bedtime. Randomized controlled trails and meta-analyses show mixed improvements compared with placebo. The reported decrease time to sleep onset of 14–17 minutes may not be clinically important.

    c. L-tryptophan is an amino acid found in foods such as milk, bananas, soy, whole grains, peanut butter, and turkey. It is converted into serotonin and was originally studied for its effects on depression and sleep. Studies show mixed results in producing sleepiness and decreasing sleep latency. The best results are in cases of mild insomnia with no comorbid medical or psychiatric conditions. In addition, eating heavy meals prior to bedtime can be counterproductive to sleep and the excess calories can result in weight gain.

    d. Melatonin is becoming well known as a nonprescription sleep aid. Melatonin is a hormone naturally produced as our bodies prepare for sleep; it is secreted when it is dark with peak levels occurring around a person's bedtime. Supplemental melatonin can be used to augment production. Melatonin has been shown to have a small but significant effect on sleep latency of about 12 minutes but not on other sleep parameters like sleep duration or time to waking. Melatonin is often used to slowly shift circadian rhythms toward a more effective bedtime (see Section V.C.3) or in cases of jet lag.

    e. Table 36–10 lists common foods and supplements for help in sleep but most have not been studied in true insomnia treatment.

D. Pharmacologic agents can be used in more chronic or severe cases of insomnia. They can be loosely categorized into nonprescription preparations, prescription preparations specifically designed to treat insomnia, and medications used as hypnotics but not necessarily FDA-approved for that purpose.

    1. The goals of treatment should be discussed before using a pharmacologic agent. Using an agent at as low a dose and for as short a time as possible to reach these goals is prudent. Many of these agents are habit-forming and are best used for transient or temporary episodes of insomnia. As with presleep rituals, patients can

TABLE 36–10. SUMMARY OF NATURAL, HERBAL, AND COMPLEMENTARY MEDICINE INTERVENTIONS FOR INSOMNIA

Evidence Base	Additional Information
Supportive evidence	
Tai Chi	
Yoga	
Acupressure	
Mixed evidence	**L-tryptophan containing foods:** cookies, milk, bananas, sesame seeds, whole gain,
Acupuncture	peanut butter
L-tryptophan	**Melatonin-containing foods:** tomato, rice, oranges, apples, bananas, cherries, cucumber,
Melatonin	cabbage, almonds, walnuts
Weak evidence	**Valerian:** not helpful on as needed basis
Valerian root	**Chamomile:** soothing calming effect similar to drinking other warm beverages
Chamomile	**Lavender oil:** place on cloth under pillow to inhale, do not ingest
Lavender oil	

become chemically or psychologically dependent on these agents. This can result in rebound hyperarousal and worsening insomnia when they are discontinued.

2. Pharmacologic agents have **multiple adverse reactions and side effects** and can interact with other medications. Many patients, who have insomnia severe enough to warrant pharmacologic treatment, have a high likelihood of comorbidities and therefore a high likelihood of being on multiple other medications. Special concern should be taken for the geriatric population as well since insomnia is more commonly reported in older patients. The risk of polypharmacy and adverse or paradoxical reactions to sleep medications is high. A representative list of pharmacologic sleep aids can be found in Table 36–11.

3. **Nonprescription sleep aids**. These agents primarily fall into the antihistamine category. They include diphenhydramine and doxylamine. Antihistamines cross the blood–brain barrier in differing degrees and cause drowsiness. They also antagonize muscarinic cholinergic receptors. This anticholinergic effect can result in cognitive impairment and urinary retention. Other side effects are irritability, poor sleep quality despite their sedating effect, and residual drowsiness upon awakening. These effects are often more pronounced in the geriatric population. In addition, there is little evidence to support their efficacy or safety. They are often combined with nonprescription pain medications such as acetaminophen, ibuprofen, and naproxen.

4. **Prescription sleep aids**

   a. Benzodiazepines include the earliest prescription sedatives such as triazolam, estazolam, temazepam. These medications are GABA and GABA-receptor antagonists. They increase sleep time, improve quality, and reduce latency and wakefulness after sleep onset. Those with rapid onset and shorter half-lives are preferred for insomnia but these effects are tempered by a greater potential for tolerance and dependence with prolonged use. They are most useful for short-term treatment of less than 4 weeks.

   (1) Ten to thirty percent of benzodiazepine users develop **dependence** (compulsive or chronic need) and 50% suffer from withdrawal phenomena (anxiety, depression, nausea, rebound insomnia). In addition, short-acting benzodiazepines can cause rebound insomnia on the same night they are taken which results in a state of anterograde memory impairment. This increases the risk of motor vehicle collisions, other injuries, or overdose.

   (2) These medications should be **avoided in patients with acute angle-closure glaucoma or untreated open-angle glaucoma** and avoided or used with caution concomitantly with narcotics, alcohol, or other central nervous system (CNS) depressants.

   b. Nonbenzodiazepines. These newer agents bind more specifically to CNS benzodiazepine receptors. They have little impact on sleep stages and REM sleep. They have not been directly compared to benzodiazepines but indirect comparisons have shown they are similarly effective but have fewer overall adverse effects.

   (1) These drugs can cause impaired memory and psychomotor retardation. They are also metabolized by the liver and should be used with caution in older patients and those with hepatic dysfunction.

   (2) Zolpidem, zaleplon, and eszopiclone are among these agents; all decrease sleep latency. Zaleplon can be redosed in the event of a nocturnal awakening and this can help with sleep maintenance. Zolpidem should not be redosed in the event of nocturnal awakening but has a controlled-release formula that may be better for maintaining sleep. However, the risk of next-morning impairment is highest for patients taking the extended-release forms of these drugs and the FDA recently recommended lowering the recommended dose of zolpidem to 5 mg for immediate-release products (e.g., Ambien) and 6.35 mg for extended-release products (e.g., Ambien CR). Eszopiclone is the only hypnotic with FDA approval for use longer than 35 days. Lower doses are effective for sleep latency, whereas higher doses may be needed to improve sleep maintenance.

TABLE 36–11. SUMMARY OF PHARMACOLOGIC AGENTS FOR INSOMNIA/SEDATION

Drug[a]	Dose	Comments	Side Effects
Antihistamines[b]			
Diphenhydramine[a]	25–50 mg (nonprescription)		Anticholinergic (dry mouth, blurred vision, constipation), dizziness, somnolence, CNS depression/stimulation
Doxylamine[a]	12.5–25 mg (nonprescription)		As above
Hydroxyzine	25–100 mg		As above
Antidepressants[c]			
Doxepin ([a]Only product approved is Silenor® due to its low doses)	3–6 mg	TCA, but histamine is primary mechanism of sedation	Somnolence/sedation, nausea, dry mouth
Amitriptyline	10–100 mg	TCA, often used to manage pain-related sleep issues like fibromyalgia	Anticholinergic (dry mouth, blurred vision, constipation), morning sedation, somnolence, dizziness, accidents, weight gain, serotonin syndrome when used with SSRI, worsens restless leg syndrome
Trazodone	25–100 mg (usual dose 25–50 mg)	SARI, helps with sleep latency and sleep maintenance effect, can use with SSRIs but higher doses have increasing SSRI-like action	Same as above plus priapism, nausea, headache, anxiety, hypotension
Mirtazapine	7.5–45 mg		Anticholinergic, (constipation, dry mouth) elevated liver enzymes and triglycerides, somnolence, dizziness, increased appetite, and weight gain
Sedating anticonvulsants			
Gabapentin	100–900 mg	Bedtime dosing only	Edema, hostile behavior, dizziness, nystagmus, ataxia, daytime fatigue, somnolence
Pregabalin	50–300 mg		Blurred vision, dry mouth, constipation, increased appetite and weight gain, edema, dizziness, somnolence, headache, tremor
Melatonin receptor agonist (DEA nonscheduled medication)			
Ramelteon[a]	8–16 mg	Primarily for sleep onset and early sleep maintenance, less helpful for early-morning wakening, no abuse potential	Dizziness, somnolence, nausea, exacerbated insomnia. Contraindicated with severe liver disease or those taking fluvoxamine
Benzodiazepine receptor agonistic modulators[d] (Schedule IV controlled substances)			
Benzodiazepines[e]			
Triazolam[a]	0.125–0.25 mg; max. 0.5 mg	Rapid onset, short half-life, lower dose in elderly	Anterograde amnesia, REM rebound, dizziness, headache, somnolence, ataxia

(continued)

TABLE 36–11. SUMMARY OF PHARMACOLOGIC AGENTS FOR INSOMNIA/SEDATION (*Continued*)

Drug[a]	Dose	Comments	Side Effects
Temazepam[a]	15–30 mg at bedtime (7.5 mg for elderly)	Short to intermediate acting, less effective for sleep initiation	Daytime sleepiness
Estazolam[a]	1–2 mg	Rapid onset, short to intermediate acting	Daytime sleepiness, dizziness, impaired coordination
Alprazolam	0.25–0.5 mg	Rapid onset and elimination half-life, used for insomnia from anxiety or stress	Decreased or increased appetite, weight gain, constipation, dry mouth, somnolence, cognitive and memory impairment, incoordination, irritability, reduced libido
Lorazepam[a]	2–4 mg	Medium onset and medium to long elimination half-life	Sedation, dizziness, asthenia, unsteadiness
Clonazepam	0.5–3 mg	Medium to long onset and medium to long elimination	Somnolence, ataxia, dizziness, problem behavior, depression
Nonbenzodiazepines[f]			
Zaleplon[a]	5–20 mg	Helps with sleep latency, short acting but can re-dose as long as 4 or more hours can be devoted to sleep	Drowsiness, dizziness, lightheadedness, headache, "pins and needles feeling" on skin
Zolpidem[a]	Based on gender and type[g]	Most widely prescribed hypnotic, multiple dosage forms: oral tablet, sublingual tablet, oral spray	Dizziness, headache, somnolence, nausea, diarrhea, visual disturbance
Eszopiclone[a]	1–3 mg	Helps with both sleep latency and sleep maintenance	Metallic or unpleasant taste, drowsiness, dizziness, headache, common-cold-like symptoms

CNS, central nervous system; SARI, serotonin antagonist and reuptake inhibitor; SSRI, selective serotonin reuptake inhibitor; TCA, tricyclic antidepressant.
[a]FDA-approved for insomnia.
[b]Limited data on efficacy.
[c]Antidepressants: No one class or agent is significantly better than another.
[d]FDA warning for all in this class includes risk of disruptive sleep behaviors such as sleep-walking, eating, driving, and sexual behavior. FDA warning also includes strong wording to avoid combining these medications with alcohol, other hypnotics/sedatives, or sleep restriction.
[e]The benzodiazepines flurazepam and quazempam are omitted because of their half-life >24 hours; however, they have a FDA indication for insomnia. Recommend starting and usual dose in the elderly is approximately 50% of doses listed. These drugs are contraindicated in narrow-angle glaucoma, untreated obstructive sleep apnea, and history of substance abuse.
[f]Nonbenzodiazepines: for the elderly, recommend starting and titrating usual dose 50% of those listed.
[g]5–10 mg (immediate release), 6.25–12.5 mg (extended release, Ambien CR®), 1.75 mg SL for women and 3.5 mg SL for men (Intermezzo®), 5 mg (1 spray) into mouth for women and 5–10 mg (2 sprays) into mouth for men (Zolpimist®).

   c. Melatonin receptor agonist. There is one agent available in this class, remelteon, which acts as a selective melatonin receptor agonist. It reduces sleep latency and increases sleep periods. It has not been studied in patients with depression, those with anxiety, or those with circadian disruptions like shift work or jet lag. There are a few adverse effects but mixed reports of sleep improvement. It is the only FDA-approved medication for sleep that is not a DEA-scheduled class of medication.
   d. Other hypnotics used as sleep aids. These include medications that are typically used at different doses for their varying degrees of sedating/hypnotic

effects. These agents are not FDA-approved for insomnia. Clinicians should provide informed consent when considering or recommending an off-label or non-FDA-approved treatment for insomnia.

(1) Hydroxyzine is an antihistamine available by prescription. It has the same effects and side effects as the nonprescription antihistamines listed above.

(2) Antidepressants include agents in the tricyclic class (amitriptyline and doxepin), selective serotonin reuptake inhibitors (SSRIs), or "other" class (mirtazapine and trazodone). These agents cause sedation as a side effect and thus decrease sleep-onset latency and wakefulness after sleep onset. Antidepressants improve sleep quality and sleep efficiency (percent of time sleeping compared to percent of time spent in bed) despite their tendency to suppress REM sleep stage. Trazodone is the most commonly used agent in this class for insomnia.

- Amitriptyline and trazodone have anticholinergic side effects, can cause morning sedation and serotonin syndrome when used with SSRI, and can worsen restless leg syndrome. Amitriptyline is often used when chronic pain or chronic headaches occur in conjunction with insomnia.
- Mirtazapine has anticholinergic side effects and increases appetite, but there is less concern with its interaction with other SSRIs.
- No studies have shown that one antidepressant agent or class is more effective than another. Given the common comorbidity of depression, anxiety, and sleep problems, some have argued that any agent that effectively treats underlying depression can have a positive effect on insomnia.

(3) Sedating anticonvulsant drugs include gabapentin and pregabalin. Their mechanism of action in sleep is not well understood but is likely related to being a GABA analog. They can be useful in conditions where chronic pain and insomnia coexist. Patients report improved sleep effects such as decreased latency and decreased wakefulness after sleep onset. These drugs are generally well tolerated and, in the case of gabapentin, offer a wide range of dosing options.

(4) Sedating antipsychotic drugs. These include olanzapine, quetiapine, and risperidone. These agents can be effective but have great potential for serious adverse cardiac and metabolic effects as well as weight gain. These medications are typically used as an antipsychotic choice in patients needing additional sedation. They have a limited if any role for patients with insomnia alone, even as an off-label medication.

(5) Opiates produce analgesia and subsequent sedation. However, as a sleep aid they also fragment sleep and decrease REM and stage 2 (or deeper) sleep. They may have a role in carefully selected patients with pain-associated insomnia.

(6) Barbiturates function as GABA-receptor agonists and decrease sleep-onset latency while suppressing REM sleep. They can be effective in short-term insomnia (less than 2 weeks). Beyond 2 weeks, barbiturate use is associated with tolerance, physical, psychological dependence, increased agitation, confusion, nightmares, hallucinations, lethargy, and hangover. They are included here for completeness but have a minimal role in the treatment of insomnia given safer and more effective treatments.

VI. Follow-up. Treatment plans are ideally based on a detailed history, physical findings, and clear treatment goals. As noted above, most pharmacologic and nonpharmacologic treatments are temporary or require alterations over time. Therefore, re-assessing patients after 2 to 4 weeks of interventions is reasonable. In addition, given the side effects, potential for tolerance and dependence, and DEA schedule of many pharmacologic agents, close follow-up and documentation are warranted. Reassessment of sleep goals, quality of sleep, and side effects and re-evaluation for new or worse comorbidities should be part of routine follow up. In addition, clinicians should periodically assess patients for aberrant drug behaviors such as diversion, escalating doses, concomitant use of street drugs, and excess use of other sedatives such as alcohol. Finally, clinicians should periodically assess the need to revisit sleep hygiene if initial improvements wane over time.

SELECTED REFERENCES

Buysse DJ. Insomnia. *JAMA.* 2013;309(7):706–716.

Cheuk DKL, Yeung WF, Chung KF, Wong V. Acupuncture for insomnia. *Cochrane Database Syst Rev.* 2012;(9):CD005472.

Clark MS, Smith PO, Jamieson B. FPIN's clinical inquiries: antidepressants for the treatment of insomnia in patients with depression. *Am Fam Physician.* 2011;84(9):1–2.

Giles TL, Lasserson TJ, Smith B, et al. Continuous positive airways pressure for obstructive sleep apnoea in adults. *Cochrane Database Syst Rev.* 2006;(3):CD001106.

Harsora P, Kessmann J. Nonpharmacologic management of chronic insomnia. *Am Fam Physician.* 2009;79:125–130.

Huedo-Medina TB, Kirsch I, Middlemass J, et al. Effectiveness of non-benzodiazepine hypnotics in treatment of adult insomnia: meta-analysis of data submitted to the food and drug administration. *BMJ.* 2012;345:1–13.

Kessler RC, Berglund PA, Coulouvrat C. Insomnia and the performance of US workers: results from the America insomnia a survey. *Sleep.* 2011;34(9):1161–1171.

Kierlin L, Olmstead R, Yokomizo M, et al. Diagnostic and statistical manual criteria for insomnia related impairment in daytime functioning: polysomnographic correlates in older adults. *Sleep Med.* 2012;13:958–960.

Montgomery P, Dennis JA. Cognitive behavioral interventions for sleep problems in adults aged 60+. *Cochrane Database Syst Rev.* 2003;(1):CD003161.

Montgomery P, Dennis JA. Physical exercise for sleep problems in adults aged 60+ (review). *Cochrane Database of Syst Rev.* 2002;(4):CD003404.

Morin C, LeBlanc M, Daley M, et al. Epidemiology of insomnia: prevalence, self-help treatments, consultations, and determinants of help-seeking behaviors. *Sleep Med.* 2006;7:123–130.

Neubauer DN. Chronic insomnia. *Neurology.* 2013;19:50–66.

Rakel D. Improving and maintaining a healthy sleep–wake cycle, patient handout. Integrative Medicine Program, Department of Family Medicine, University of Wisconsin-Madison. www.fammed.wisc.edu/integrative. Accessed August 2013.

Ramakrishnan K, Scheid D. Treatment options for insomnia. *Am Fam Physician.* 2007;76:517–526.

Sarris J, Byrne GJ. A systematic review of insomnia and complementary medicine. *Sleep Med Rev.* 2011;15:99–106.

Sarsour K, Kalsekar A, Swindle R, et al. The association between insomnia severity and healthcare and productivity costs in a health plan sample. *Sleep.* 2011;34(4):443–450.

Schutte-Rodin S, Broch L, Buysse D, et al. Clinical guideline for the evaluation and management of chronic insomnia in adults. *J Clin Sleep Med.* 2008;4(5):487–504.

Sundaram S, Lim J, Lasserson TJ. Surgery for obstructive sleep apnoea in adults. *Cochrane Database Syst Rev.* 2005;(4):CD001004.

Sutter JD. CNN Living with Technology. Trouble sleeping? Maybe it's your iPad. http://www.cnn.com/2010/TECH/05/13/sleep.gadgets.ipad/index.html. Accessed September 2013.

Walsh JF, Coulouvrat C, Hajak G. Nighttime insomnia symptoms and perceived health in the America insomnia survey (AIS). *Sleep.* 2011;34(8):997–1011.

---

37   Jaundice

Kalyanakrishnan Ramakrishnan, MD, MS, FRCS, & L. Peter Schwiebert, MD

KEY POINTS

- Jaundice is usually produced by one of three underlying mechanisms: excessive hemoglobin degradation/bilirubin overproduction, liver disease, and biliary obstruction. (SOR ❸)
- Most cases of jaundice in newborns result from increased red blood cell breakdown and decreased bilirubin excretion. (SOR ❸)
- Jaundice can be effectively evaluated by history (including age of onset), physical examination, and limited laboratory testing and by imaging studies. (SOR ❸)
- Jaundice in newborns can usually be managed conservatively and at home, even if phototherapy is required. Jaundiced breastfed infants should continue breastfeeding. (SOR ❸)

- Phototherapy is a low-risk, high-benefit option, especially in preterm or low-birth-weight infants, minimizing the need for exchange transfusion and preventing the development of kernicterus. (SOR **B**)
- Treatment of jaundice in adults is directed at the underlying cause. Medical management is appropriate in most instances. Surgery has a very limited role (as in extra-hepatic obstruction due to common bile duct stones or pancreatic cancer). (SOR **C**)

I. **Definition.** The major source of bilirubin is degradation of hemoglobin from senescent red blood cells. Bilirubin from the periphery is tightly bound to albumin during transport in the blood to the hepatocyte. Inside the hepatocyte, nonpolar bilirubin is enzymatically conjugated by uridine diphosphate glucuronyl transferase (UDPGT) to form water-soluble bilirubin diglucuronide. UDPGT activity is decreased in neonates, resulting in increased levels of unconjugated bilirubin. (In White and African-American neonates, bilirubin levels rise steadily, peaking at 5 to 6 mg/dL between the second and fourth days of life, then slowly declining to adult levels by days 10 to 12. In Asians and Native Americans, bilirubin levels rise more rapidly, peaking at 8 to 12 mg/dL by days 4 to 5, then declining more slowly than in White or African-American neonates.) Conjugated bilirubin is excreted and transported as bile in the biliary system to the gastrointestinal tract, with most being reabsorbed in the ileum and undergoing enterohepatic circulation.

   A. **Jaundice** is the yellow discoloration of the skin and mucous membranes caused by an elevated serum bilirubin. In adults, clinical jaundice occurs at bilirubin levels of 2 to 3 mg/dL. In newborns, the threshold is higher (5–6 mg/dL). Based on bilirubin physiology, jaundice can be categorized as being due to the following:

   1. **Excessive hemoglobin degradation/bilirubin overproduction,** as in immune hemolysis (e.g., ABO incompatibility or Rh isoimmunization), nonimmune hemolysis (e.g., glucose-6-phosphate dehydrogenase [G6PD] deficiency or hereditary spherocytosis), extravascular hemolysis (e.g., cephalohematomas in newborns), or intramarrow hemolysis (e.g., "ineffective erythropoiesis" in thalassemia or pernicious anemia).

   2. **Defective hepatic uptake/conjugation/transport** as in Gilbert disease, Crigler–Najjar or Dubin–Johnson syndrome, or hepatitis.

   3. **Impaired excretion**, as in hepatocellular disease, drug effects, primary biliary cirrhosis (PBC), or bile duct obstruction.

II. **Common Diagnoses.** Jaundice is very common in newborns, affecting 50% of full-term and 80% of preterm infants; after the neonatal period, jaundice is less prevalent, accounting for up to 4% of annual acute hospital admissions. Jaundice has myriad causes; while recognizing that more than one pathophysiologic process can be present in a single patient, it is helpful to approach jaundice based on age of onset, risk factors, and fractional elevation of bilirubin, that is, **unconjugated** (indirect fraction of bilirubin exceeds 80% of total) versus **conjugated** (indirect fraction ranges from 20% to 60% of total bilirubin).

   A. **Childhood jaundice**

   1. **Unconjugated hyperbilirubinemia**

      a. Neonatal onset.

      (1) Physiologic jaundice is present in as many as 60% of newborns.

      (2) Jaundice in breastfed infants. Breastfeeding jaundice occurs in 5% to 10% of breastfed infants and is caused by dehydration and decreased caloric intake; dietary supplementation with formula is an additional risk factor. Breast milk jaundice occurs in less than 1% of breastfed infants and is believed to be because of deconjugating enzymes in the breast milk inhibiting UDGPT.

      (3) Hemolytic anemia is the most common pathologic cause of jaundice, usually resulting from ABO or, less commonly, Rh incompatibility, hereditary spherocytosis, enzyme (G6PD) deficiency, or a hemoglobinopathy. African-Americans are prone to hemolytic anemias caused by sickle cell disease and G6PD deficiency. Patients of Mediterranean descent and Asians are at an increased risk for thalassemias.

      (4) Other causes of unconjugated neonatal hyperbilirubinemia include polycythemia, cephalohematoma reabsorption, pyloric stenosis, and congenital hypothyroidism.

b. Infancy and childhood onset. Jaundice may result from hemolytic diseases (e.g., G6PD deficiency and hereditary spherocytosis), Gilbert disease, and Crigler–Najjar or Dubin–Johnson syndrome.

2. Conjugated hyperbilirubinemia

a. Neonatal onset. Sepsis, neonatal hepatitis, ToRCHS infections (**to**xoplasmosis, **r**ubella, **c**ytomegalovirus [CMV], **h**erpes, and **s**yphilis), extrahepatic obstruction in biliary atresia or choledocholithiasis, and metabolic diseases such as galactosemia, α_1-antitrypsin deficiency, and tyrosinemia can result in jaundice.

b. Infancy and childhood onset. Viral hepatitis (see Section II.B.2.a.1) is the most common cause of jaundice in a previously healthy child. Less common causes include Wilson disease and milder forms of galactosemia.

B. Adult onset

1. Unconjugated hyperbilirubinemia may occur with **hemolytic anemia, ineffective erythropoiesis** (e.g., thalassemias, sideroblastic anemias, and pernicious anemia), **impaired uptake and conjugation of bilirubin** (e.g., Gilbert syndrome, which occurs in 3%–7% of the US population, and Crigler–Najjar syndrome type II, an uncommon disorder). In addition to risk factors already mentioned, a positive family history may be associated with Gilbert disease or hemolytic anemia.

2. Conjugated hyperbilirubinemia

a. Impaired intrahepatic excretion.

(1) Viral hepatitis accounts for 75% of jaundice in patients younger than 30 years decreasing to 5% in patients older than 60 years. Risk factors for hepatitis A include ingestion of raw shellfish, travel to countries with unsanitary water supplies, household contact with infected persons, and exposure to diapered infants in day care. Risk factors for hepatitis B include living in endemic areas (e.g., sub-Saharan Africa or Asia), fetomaternal transmission, and sexual contact with an infected patient. A history of blood transfusions (especially before 1992), intravenous drug abuse, multiple sexual partners, hemodialysis, and health care occupations are risk factors for both hepatitis B and C.

(2) Cirrhosis causes about one-third of jaundice in 30- to 60-year-old patients (see Chapter 72). PBC is more common in women; men have a higher risk for alcoholic liver disease.

(3) Congestive heart failure (CHF) accounts for 10% of jaundice after 60 years of age. Risk factors include a history of hypertension and atherosclerotic cardiovascular disease (see Chapter 73).

(4) Metastatic liver disease causes 13% of jaundice after 60 years of age.

(5) Other causes include drugs (e.g., erythromycin, nonsteroidal anti-inflammatory drugs, anabolic steroids, oral contraceptives, phenothiazines, and sulfonylureas), pregnancy, hepatoma, and Dubin–Johnson and Rotor syndromes.

b. Extrahepatic obstruction (e.g., gallstones, strictures, and tumors, especially pancreatic cancer) accounts for 60% of jaundice in patients older than 60 years. Gallstones are more common in women.

III. Symptoms

A. Onset of jaundice

1. A **rapid onset** suggests infection, drug reaction, hemolytic anemia, or acute obstruction caused by common bile duct (CBD) stones.

2. Intermittent or fluctuating jaundice occurs in Gilbert disease (typically with fasting or intercurrent illness), Crigler–Najjar syndrome, Dubin–Johnson or Rotor syndrome, recurrent CBD stones, and CHF.

3. A **gradual onset** occurs in cirrhosis, liver metastases, pregnancy, or PBC.

B. Pruritus. Severe pruritus and excoriations suggest high serum bilirubin levels and jaundice as seen in extrahepatic obstruction.

C. Abdominal pain occurs more often with obstructive jaundice than with hepatocellular disease. Colicky, right upper quadrant pain prior to the onset of jaundice suggests cholelithiasis or choledocholithiasis, especially in middle-aged and older patients.

D. Fever with chills suggests biliary obstruction and cholangitis. Charcot triad refers to the triad of pain, jaundice, and fever seen in choledocholithiasis. In Reynolds pentad (a collection of symptoms suggesting the diagnosis of obstructive ascending cholangitis), mental status changes and sepsis are also present. **Flulike symptoms** suggest viral or drug-induced hepatitis.

E. Persisting (≥2 weeks) history of acholic stools and severe jaundice is characteristic of **obstructive jaundice.**

F. Sixty to seventy percent of patients with **acute hepatitis C** are asymptomatic, 20% to 30% are jaundiced, and 10% to 20% complain only of fatigue, anorexia, nausea, arthralgia, myalgia, or abdominal pain. Chronic hepatitis C infection leads to cirrhosis in 10% to 20% of patients.

G. In neonates, historical clues include a history of premature rupture of membranes (sepsis), delay in clamping the cord (polycythemia), and a history of jaundice in a sibling (metabolic disorders or anemias). Both **breast milk** and **breastfeeding jaundice** develop in the first week of life.

IV. Signs

A. Urticaria is observed in the prodromal stage of hepatitis A, B, and C infections and is related to immune-complex deposits; it can also be associated with arthritis and headache (Caroli triad).

B. Cutaneous xanthomas are caused by hypercholesterolemia and seen in patients with chronic cholestasis (e.g., PBC).

C. Spider angiomata, palmar erythema, clubbing, bilateral parotid enlargement, gynecomastia, testicular atrophy, ascites, and signs of portal hypertension (splenomegaly, enlarged, abdominal wall venous collaterals) and pedal edema are seen in chronic hepatocellular disease or cirrhosis (see Chapter 72).

D. Kayser–Fleischer rings in the cornea are pathognomonic of Wilson disease.

E. A **palpable gallbladder** suggests malignant CBD obstruction (e.g., cancer of the head of the pancreas). Courvoisier law states that in the presence of an enlarged gallbladder, jaundice is unlikely to be caused by gallstones.

F. Large, palpable, nodular liver suggests metastatic cancer. Enlarged liver is also seen in fatty infiltration, post-hepatitic or pigment cirrhosis, and passive hepatic congestion due to CHF (all can cause jaundice).

G. Splenomegaly is found in many patients with cirrhosis, chronic active hepatitis, and alcoholic liver disease. However, it occurs in less than 5% of patients with an acute viral hepatitis, gallstones, or malignant biliary obstruction. Hepatomegaly, especially a tender enlarged liver ≥15 cm, suggests alcoholic hepatitis or malignancy; liver enlargement can also be seen in hemolysis.

H. In newborns, jaundice can be detected by examining the child in a well-lighted room and blanching the skin with digital pressure. Icterus, first seen in the face, progresses in a craniocaudal manner to the trunk and the extremities; the degree of progression correlates roughly with bilirubin levels (i.e., the face, approximately 5 mg/dL; mid-abdomen, approximately 15 mg/dL; and the soles of the feet, approximately 20 mg/dL). Visual assessment of jaundice by health care providers seems to correlate fairly well with mean total serum bilirubin levels, although babies with bilirubin levels in high-risk zones can be clinically misdiagnosed as low risk.

I. Infants should be assessed for risk factors for severe hyperbilirubinemia (Figure 37–1), sepsis, polycythemia, metabolic disorders, and biliary obstruction.

V. Laboratory tests (Figures 37–1 and 37–2). Most causes of jaundice can be determined by history, physical examination, and screening laboratory studies. (SOR ⓒ)

A. Basic tests. All patients with jaundice should have a complete blood count and total and direct bilirubin levels measured.

1. In **neonates** (Figure 37–1), Coombs testing, peripheral smear, and reticulocyte count should also be done; ill or premature infants with jaundice should also have a sepsis workup (blood count, chest x-ray, urinalysis, blood/urine cultures).

2. Liver function tests are recommended in all jaundiced **non-neonates** (Figure 37–2), with further testing based on clinical findings.

a. Liver profile.

(1) In classic hepatocellular disease, alkaline phosphatase is ≤3 times the upper limit of normal; in obstructive jaundice, values are 3 to 10 times normal.

(2) Transaminase levels (alanine aminotransferase [ALT] and aspartate aminotransferase [AST]) generally reflect the degree of hepatocellular disease. In obstructive jaundice, transaminases are typically two to three times the upper

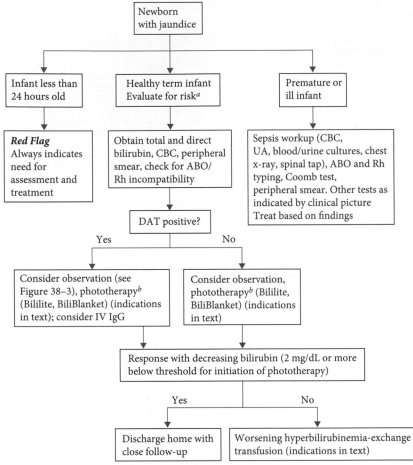

FIGURE 37–1. Evaluation of a newborn with jaundice. CBC, complete blood count; UA, urinalysis; DAT, direct antibody testing; IV IgG, intravenous immunoglobulin G. *a*Risk factors for severe hyperbilirubinemia—early onset jaundice, sibling with jaundice, East Asian background, exclusive breast feeding, bruising, cephalhematoma, large for gestational age, maternal diabetes, vacuum or forceps delivery. *b*Intensive phototherapy refers to use of both Bililite and BiliBlanket.

limit of normal, whereas higher values (≥5 times normal) are seen in hepatocellular disease.

b. A peripheral smear, reticulocyte count, and Coombs testing should be performed on all patients with unconjugated hyperbilirubinemia or anemia (checking for hemolysis). Other features suggesting hemolysis include low serum haptoglobin, urine hemosiderin, and hemoglobinuria.

c. A prothrombin time (PT) should be done if obstruction or severe liver dysfunction is suspected. In obstructive jaundice, a prolonged PT may respond dramatically to 10 mg subcutaneous vitamin K administered daily over 3 days, whereas minimal improvement is seen in hepatocellular disease.

d. Urinalysis is inexpensive and detects conjugated bilirubin and urobilinogen.

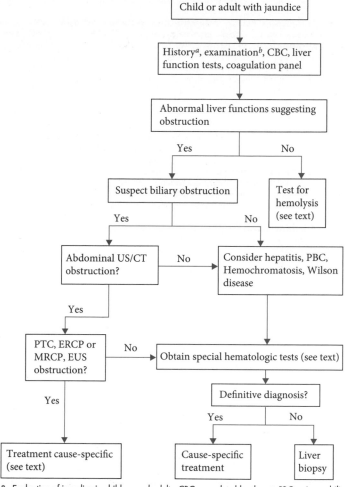

FIGURE 37–2. Evaluation of jaundice in children and adults. CBC, complete blood ount; PBC, primary biliary cirrhosis; US, ultrasound; CT, computed axial tomography; EUS, endoscopic ultrasound; PTC, percutaneous transhepatic cholangiography; ERCP, endoscopic retrograde cholangiopancreatogram; MRCP, magnetic resonance cholangiopancreatogram. [a]History of pain, anorexia, fever, weight loss, pruritus, dark urine, pale stools, alcohol/drug use, transfusions, family history, sick contacts, foreign travel, medications. [b]Fever, orthostasis, stigmata of chronic liver disease (see text), lymphadenopathy, hepatosplenomegaly, ascites, pedal edema, enlarged abdominal wall veins.

B. Additional special testing (Figure 37–2).
   1. Imaging studies
      a. In patients with extrahepatic obstruction, **ultrasonography (US)** detects dilated biliary ducts. US is non-invasive and portable, over 90% specific (71%–96%), and close to 90% sensitive (55%–95%) in detecting obstruction.
      b. Computerized tomography (CT) scan has greater specificity (90%–94%) and higher resolution than US in detecting obstruction, but has similar sensitivity (74%–96%) and is more expensive. CT scan is indicated when US is

unsatisfactory because of equivocal findings or technical limitations (e.g., overlying bowel gas).

   c. Endoscopic retrograde cholangiopancreatography (ERCP), percutaneous transhepatic cholangiography (PTC), or **magnetic resonance cholangiopancreatography (MRCP)** is indicated if extrahepatic obstruction is strongly suspected on clinical grounds (even if US is negative) or if additional anatomic information is required for diagnosis. These tests permit direct imaging of bile ducts and visualization of the periampullary region. The choice of ERCP (sensitivity 89%–98%, specificity 89%–100% in evaluating jaundice) versus PTC (sensitivity 98%–100%, specificity 89%–100%) versus MRCP (sensitivity 84%–100%, specificity 94%–98%) depends mainly on local expertise and availability. ERCP is preferred if sphincterotomy, biliary stenting, pancreatic or CBD stone removal, or biopsy is planned. MRCP is the most sensitive noninvasive method for detecting ductal pathology and is also the preferred test for evaluating anatomy because, unlike ERCP, it does not induce postprocedure pancreatitis.

   d. Endoscopic ultrasound (EUS) also can detect biliary obstruction, with a sensitivity and specificity comparable with MRCP. EUS also permits biopsy of suspected malignant lesions and may be combined with ERCP. EUS is most useful when the patient is suspected to be at a high risk for complications of ERCP or PTC.

   e. Nuclear scintigraphy of the biliary tree using radiolabeled derivatives of iminodiacetic acid (e.g., HIDA) is useful in the diagnosis of cholecystitis (sensitivity 86%). It is also useful in evaluating a potential bile leak following biliary surgery (accuracy 87%). Scintigraphy is less sensitive when the serum bilirubin exceeds 4.4 mg/dL because of impaired uptake of the agent by the liver.

   f. If biliary obstruction is suspected, US or CT is the appropriate initial test. If dilated bile ducts are seen, then ERCP or PTC is followed by therapeutic intervention. If bile ducts are not dilated and the likelihood of obstruction is low, the patient is evaluated for hepatocellular or cholestatic liver disease. If biliary obstruction is considered likely after a negative US or CT scan, MRCP or EUS is a reasonable next option.

2. Hematologic testing

   a. Viral hepatitis studies.

   (1) Immunoglobulin M (IgM) hepatitis A antibody appears at the onset of symptoms of hepatitis A infection (within 5–10 days) and clears within 6 months. The IgM hepatitis A antibody test should be used to confirm the disease in individuals with signs and symptoms suggestive of hepatitis A; sensitivity and specificity are over 95%. (SOR **C**)

   (2) Hepatitis B surface antigen (HBsAg) is the first serologic marker to appear in hepatitis B infection, starting 2 to 6 weeks before symptoms. The antigen generally clears within 6 months, but persists in patients with chronic active or persistent infection.

   (3) Hepatitis B core antibody (antiHBc) is present in virtually all patients with active hepatitis B infection. AntiHBc appears later than HBsAg, often before symptoms develop, serves to confirm infection, and persists for life.

   (4) Hepatitis C antibody becomes detectable by enzyme immunoassay (EIA) in 90% of patients by 12 weeks after infection. Because of possible transplacental transmission of maternal antibodies, EIA testing in neonates at risk is not considered reliable until 12 weeks of age. Although EIA is highly sensitive (94%–100%) and specific (97%–98%) in detecting hepatitis C, it cannot differentiate between acute, chronic, or resolved infection and should be confirmed by recombinant immunoblot assay (RIBA) testing or a test for hepatitis C RNA (polymerase chain reaction for hepatitis C RNA 96% sensitivity, 99% specificity). (SOR **C**)

   (a) Negative EIA test in low-risk populations rules out hepatitis C. A positive EIA in low-risk individuals followed by a negative RIBA indicates a false-positive antibody test (EIA) and rules out hepatitis C; these individuals require no further testing.

(b) An indeterminate RIBA should be followed by reverse transcriptase-poly-
merase chain reaction (RT-PCR) for hepatitis C RNA. (SOR ●)

(c) If both EIA and RIBA are positive, the patient has resolved or active infection and should be tested for hepatitis C RNA. Absent RNA in the serum
indicates resolved infection (complete viral clearance from the serum).

(d) Indeterminate RIBA coupled with negative RT-PCR and normal ALT rules
out hepatitis C. (SOR ●)

   (5) IgM antibody to Epstein–Barr virus and CMV should also be considered in
the appropriate clinical setting, although screening for hepatitis A and B
should usually be done first.

b. Antimitochondrial antibody to screen for PBC should be considered in patients
aged 30 to 60 years (especially women) with evidence of chronic cholestasis.
Antibodies are positive in 85% to 90% of patients with PBC.

c. Antinuclear and smooth muscle antibodies are positive in about one-third of
patients with PBC and three-fourths of patients with lupoid hepatitis (autoimmune
hepatitis) and should be considered in patients (especially women) who have
chronic liver disease without a clear cause.

d. Serum iron, transferrin saturation, and ferritin to screen for hemochromatosis
should also be considered in patients with chronic liver disease of unknown
cause. In hemochromatosis, the serum iron exceeds 200 U/dL, serum ferritin levels exceed 500 ng/mL, and transferrin saturation exceeds 70%.

e. Serum protein electrophoresis is useful to screen for α_1-antitrypsin deficiency
(decrease in α_1-globulin band).

f. Serum ceruloplasmin and urine copper levels to screen for Wilsons disease should
be considered in patients younger than 30 years of age or in patients with hepatitis and neurologic dysfunction.

g. An elevated serum secretory immunoglobulin A is more reliable than alkaline
phosphatase in differentiating mechanical from hepatocellular cholestasis.

3. Liver biopsy in hepatitis C helps determine the stage of fibrosis and degree of liver
inflammation and can help determine urgency of treatment and/or provide prognosis.
Liver biopsy is also valuable in confirming a diagnosis when the clinical, laboratory,
and imaging studies are inconclusive, especially in less-common conditions such as
autoimmune hepatitis, PBC, and primary sclerosing cholangitis. Positive diagnosis on
liver biopsy is obligatory before surgery or chemoradiation is commenced for cancer.
However, it is associated with risks (bleeding, bile leak) that entail caution and limit
its use.

VI. Treatment of jaundice is directed at its underlying cause which is diagnosed through history, examination, and appropriate selective laboratory and imaging studies.

A. Therapy for **neonatal jaundice** is directed at underlying causes and preventing kernicterus (unconjugated hyperbilirubinemia–induced neurotoxic basal ganglial/hippo-
campal damage). At least three factors determine the risk of kernicterus in neonatal
hyperbilirubinemia: (1) **gestational age**—in healthy term neonates, risk is low even
with markedly elevated total serum bilirubin (TSB), whereas lower levels are tolerated
by premature infants; (2) **age at which jaundice is evident**—clinical jaundice at
≤24 hours of life is always nonphysiologic; and (3) **maternal/neonatal** features **of
significant underlying disease**.

1. With **physiologic jaundice,** which begins between the second and fourth days
of life, TSB levels are ≤15 mg/dL, direct bilirubin is ≤1.5 mg/dL. TSB rises by ≤5
mg/dL in 24 hours and resolves by 1 week in term infants or by 2 weeks in preterm
infants.

2. Treatment of **breastfeeding jaundice**, which occurs in the first 2 to 5 days of life
and peaks by days 10 to 15, is more frequent breastfeeding. (SOR ●) Supplementing breast milk with water or dextrose water will not result in speedier resolution of
jaundice in otherwise healthy newborns.

3. Breast milk jaundice, beginning on the fourth through seventh day of life, peaking around 2 to 3 weeks, and lasting 3 to 10 weeks, can be treated by alternating
breast and formula feeding for 2 to 3 days. (SOR ●) Breast pumping should be
done at formula feedings; full-time breastfeeding can be resumed when jaundice
resolves.

4. Stopping breastfeeding in jaundiced infants does not improve clinical outcomes. Temporarily disrupting or supplementing breastfeeding is associated with premature cessation of breastfeeding. There is no significant difference in length of phototherapy, rates of exchange transfusion, or kernicterus between jaundiced breastfed term infants, and jaundiced bottle-fed term infants. (SOR **B**)

5. Exposure to sunlight will not lower serum bilirubin levels.

6. Phototherapy using blue-range lights and a BiliBlanket, which reflect the light, produce photoisomers of unconjugated bilirubin that are water soluble and can be excreted in bile or urine without conjugation. Use of both Bililite and BiliBlanket exposes as much of the infant's skin surface as possible to light and is termed **intensive phototherapy**.

    a. Phototherapy should be considered at TSB ≥15 mg/dL at 25 to 48 hours of age, ≥18 mg/dL at 49 to 72 hours of age, or ≥20 mg/dL in infants over 72 hours of age (see Figure 37–3). (SOR **C**) An online tool (http://bilitool.org/) is also available for determining risk of developing hyperbilirubinemia in newborns over 35 weeks' gestational age. A favorable response is a decrease of 1 to 2 mg/dL within 4 to 6 hours, with subsequent continued decrease. Phototherapy can be administered in the hospital or home and discontinued once the TSB is 2 mg/dL, below the threshold for initiation of therapy.

        (1) Because the efficacy of phototherapy units varies widely, the AAP's most recent technical report on phototherapy notes that to achieve device effectiveness, emission of light should be in the blue-to-green range that overlaps the in vivo plasma bilirubin absorption spectrum (460–490 nm); irradiance should be of at least 30 $\mu W/cm^2/nm^1$ (confirmed with an appropriate irradiance meter); illumination of the maximal body surface should occur; and there should be a demonstration of decreased total bilirubin concentrations during the first 4 to 6 hours of exposure.

        (2) Prophylactic phototherapy is considered for preterm (<37 weeks' gestational age) or low-birth-weight (birth weight <2500 g) infants who have a greater risk of developing jaundice compared with term or normal birth weight infants. If instituted soon after birth (within 36 hours), phototherapy will minimize the need for exchange transfusion and may reduce the risk of impairment of brain and central nervous system development. (SOR **B**)

        (3) Breastfeeding should be continued during phototherapy; supplementation with expressed breast milk or formula is appropriate if oral intake is insufficient, weight loss is excessive, or the infant appears dehydrated.

    b. The eyes of the neonate must be covered to prevent retinal damage when using Bililite. Using BiliBlanket with Bililite may allow earlier discharge. Adequate fluid intake also promotes the elimination of bilirubin and counteracts the dehydration associated with phototherapy.

7. Exchange transfusion is traditionally performed when the TSB exceeds the threshold for phototherapy by 5 mg/dL or if phototherapy fails. (SOR **C**) This threshold should be lowered by 1 to 2 mg/dL when additional risk factors for kernicterus are present such as perinatal asphyxia, respiratory distress, hypoglycemia, metabolic acidosis (pH ≤7.25), hypothermia (temperature ≤35°C [95°F]), hypoproteinemia (protein ≤5 g/dL), and signs of clinical or central nervous system deterioration.

8. Neonates with hemolytic jaundice (Rh or ABO incompatibilities) can be treated with high-dose intravenous immunoglobulins (IV IgG) to prevent anemia and hyperbilirubinemia that may develop. (SOR **B**) These infants should have hemoglobin, hematocrit, bilirubin levels, and features of hemolysis monitored serially. IV IgG reduces serum bilirubin levels, requirement for phototherapy, need for exchange transfusion, and length of hospital stay.

B. Viral hepatitis. Most patients can be treated symptomatically as outpatients. Hospital admission is indicated in patients with dehydration, evidence of severe hepatocellular failure, or ascites.

1. If liver enzymes fail to normalize within 6 months, liver biopsy is indicated.

2. Alfa-interferon can induce sustained remissions in some patients with chronic hepatitis B, C, and D. (SOR **C**) Consultation should be sought with a gastroenterologist familiar with its use.

C. Extrahepatic obstruction
  1. Surgical therapy is generally required.
  2. If fever and chills suggestive of cholangitis develop, hospitalization for intravenous antibiotics and surgical consultation is necessary. Nonoperative biliary drainage can be performed in selected patients via ERCP or transhepatically placed stents, traversing the obstruction.
D. Unconjugated hyperbilirubinemia
  1. **Hemolytic anemia,** particularly if associated with marked hyperbilirubinemia, should be managed with appropriate specialty consultation (e.g., perinatology for neonates, hematology for others).
  2. Mild, unconjugated hyperbilirubinemia (e.g., Gilbert, Dubin–Johnson, and Rotor syndromes) rarely requires treatment to lower bilirubin levels.
E. Cholestatic jaundice
  1. **Ursodeoxycholic acid** (usual dose, 13–15 mg/kg per day orally in two to four divided doses) significantly reduces ascites and jaundice and improves liver biochemistry in cholestatic jaundice and is not associated with an increase in adverse events. (SOR ⑥) In patients with PBC, ursodeoxycholic acid does not appear to delay progression of disease, enhance survival, or delay need for transplantation.
  2. Since **pruritus** can be disabling and lead to depression and even suicide, early treatment is advisable. Oral agents used to treat pruritus include **cholestyramine** 4 g orally once or twice daily initially and then 8 to 16 g daily for maintenance in two or more divided doses; **antihistamines** (e.g., diphenhydramine, 25–50 mg, three or four times a day or hydroxyzine 25 mg three times daily); **doxepin** 10 to 50 mg orally at bedtime; opioid antagonists such as naltrexone (12.5–50 mg orally daily); **rifampin** (300–600 mg orally daily); and **ondansetron** (8 mg orally or intravenously every 4 hours).
F. Underlying diseases contributing to jaundice should be treated (see Chapter 72, Cirrhosis; Chapter 73, Congestive Heart Failure; Chapter 89, Thyroid Disease; Chapter 49, Pediatric Fever); drugs contributing to jaundice should be eliminated or substituted.
G. Other hepatocellular disease. Periodic monitoring of patients is necessary with clinical examination and liver function tests (see Chapter 42). When the disease is progressive, liver biopsy may be indicated for definitive diagnosis.

SELECTED REFERENCES

Berk P, Korenblat K. Approach to the patient with jaundice or abnormal liver tests. In: Goldman L, Schafer IA, eds. *Goldman's Cecil Medicine.* 24th ed. Philadelphia, PA: WB Saunders Company; 2012;49:956–966.

Bhutani VK, Johnson L. The jaundiced newborn in the emergency department: prevention of kernicterus. *Clin Ped Emerg Med.* 2008;9:149–159.

Lidofsky SD. Jaundice. In: Feldman M, ed. *Sleisenger and Fordtran's Gastrointestinal and Liver Disease.* 9th ed. Philadelphia, PA: WB Saunders Company; 2010;20:323–335.

Rudic JS, Poropat G, Krstic MN, Bjelakovic G, Gluud C. Ursodeoxycholic acid for primary biliary cirrhosis. *Cochrane Database Syst Rev.* 2012;12:CD000551.

Winger J, Michelfelder A. Diagnostic approach to the patient with jaundice. *Prim Care Clin Office Pract.* 2011;38:469–482.

Additional references are available online at http://langetextbooks.com/fm6e

38   Joint Pain

L. Peter Schwiebert, MD

KEY POINTS

- In evaluating the complaint of joint pain, it is helpful to differentiate intra-articular from periarticular processes. (SOR **C**)
- A careful focused history, physical examination, and selective testing allow accurate diagnosis of most common causes of joint pain. (SOR **C**)
- Physicians should always consider bacterial arthritis in acute monarthritis because delayed treatment of septic arthritis risks severe joint damage. (SOR **B**)

I. **Definition.** Joint pain (arthralgia) is discomfort in one or more joints, with or without evidence of joint effusion, swelling, erythema, or tenderness. Joint pain can be due to **intra-articular** or **periarticular** processes. **Intra-articular** processes include **synovitis** (viral or bacterial infection, transient synovitis, gout/pseudogout, rheumatoid arthritis [RA], rheumatic fever, idiopathic) and **degenerative diseases** (osteoarthritis [OA], posttraumatic). **Periarticular processes** include **soft-tissue diseases** (fibromyalgia, hypermobility syndromes, viremia, primary Lyme disease) and **idiopathic diseases** (growing pains, psychogenic rheumatism).

II. **Common Diagnoses.** Surveys reveal 11% of patients visiting general and family physicians in the United States have complaints related to the back and the upper or lower extremities. Unspecified arthritis is the 14th most common principal diagnosis seen by these physicians.

A. **Intra-articular processes**

1. **Synovitis**

a. **Bacterial/viral**

(1) **Transient synovitis** occurs in children 3- to 10-year-old, related to recent (within the past week) viral infection. Males are affected more frequently than females.

(2) **Viral synovitis** can occur with a variety of infections, especially hepatitis B, mumps, and rubella.

(3) The most common causes of bacterial arthritis include *Staphylococci* (40%), *Streptococci* (28%), gram-negative bacilli (19%), and mycobacteria (8%). Risk factors for bacterial arthritis include infections of contiguous skin, intravenous drug use, recent joint surgery or intra-articular injection, damaged joint (e.g., with RA, a prosthetic joint, or degenerative joint disease), sexual activity (*Neisseria gonorrhoeae*), immune compromise (e.g., poorly controlled diabetes mellitus, human immunodeficiency virus infection, or immunosuppressive medication), and age >80 years.

b. **Crystal-induced**

(1) **Gouty arthritis,** intra-articular uric acid crystal deposition caused by enzyme deficiency/overproduction/underexcretion, occurs most commonly in men older than 40 years and postmenopausal women, especially those with obesity, ethanol abuse, diuretic therapy, or a high-purine diet (see Section VI.A.3.b). Triggers for acute attacks in predisposed individuals include infection, acidosis, rapid fluctuations in urate concentration, and intravenous contrast.

(2) **Pseudogout,** calcium pyrophosphate dihydrate deposition disease, most commonly occurs in those who are older than 60 years. Pseudogout is associated with a variety of metabolic diseases (e.g., hyperparathyroidism, hypothyroidism, diabetes mellitus, Wilson disease, gout).

c. **Immune-complex**

(1) **RA,** one of a family of autoimmune inflammatory disorders (e.g., systemic lupus erythematosus [SLE], polymyalgia rheumatica, and polymyositis/dermatomyositis), mainly affects synovial membranes. One to two percent of the US population has RA, with a female:male prevalence of 3:1 and usual age of onset between 20 and 40 years. A positive family history is a risk factor. Eighty-five percent of patients with SLE are women, Blacks are affected four times as frequently as Whites; a positive family history also plays a role. A variety of drugs can cause

a lupus-like syndrome—the most common offenders include chlorpromazine, hydralazine, isoniazid, methyldopa, procainamide, and quinidine.

   (2) Lyme disease is the most common tick-borne illness in the United States, and its incidence has steadily increased since it was first reported in 1977. Lyme disease is transmitted by the bite of a tick carrying the spirochete, *Borrelia burgdorferi*. Disease incidence is highest in 5- to 9-year-olds and 55- to 59-year-olds during summer months in the following states: Connecticut, Delaware, Maine, Massachusetts, Maryland, Minnesota, New Hampshire, New Jersey, New York, Pennsylvania, Rhode Island, and Wisconsin.

   (3) Rheumatic fever, caused by group A b-hemolytic streptococcal (GABHS)–induced immune complex synovitis, is rare ($\leq 1:10,000$), and its overall incidence is progressively declining. Rheumatic fever is most common in 5- to 15-year-old children, with a slight male predominance.

  2. Degenerative disease
    a. OA is the most common joint disease, affecting at least 20 million US adults; radiologic evidence of OA is present in weight-bearing joints of 90% of individuals by 40 years of age. Age increases the likelihood of symptomatic disease.
    b. Traumatic arthritis is more likely with a history of recent or remote trauma to the affected joint(s) (e.g., falls, motor vehicle accidents, sports injuries, and overuse).

B. Periarticular processes
  1. Soft tissue
    a. Viremia can occur at any age; influenza is commonly implicated in winter months in the Northern hemisphere.
    b. Joint hypermobility syndrome (JHS) is inherited in an autosomal dominant pattern, can be underdiagnosed, can be a common cause of widespread chronic pain, and occurs three times as commonly in women as in men.
    c. Fibromyalgia is most common in 20- to 50-year-old women, affecting 3% to 10% of the general population; it may be associated with sleep disorders, depression, heightened perception of normal stimuli, and hypothyroidism.
  2. Idiopathic
    a. Growing pains occur in up to 18% of school-aged children, peaking at age 11 years and continuing through adolescence. This problem is more common in females than in males and in those with a family history of similar symptoms.
      Psychogenic pain is more common with depression or school phobia (e.g., separation anxiety or overly dependent parent–child interaction).

III. Symptoms. A systematic history often assists in narrowing the joint pain differential diagnosis. In addition to evaluating for risk factors, history includes the following:
A. Location/number of joints involved
  1. Monarticular arthralgia
    a. Septic arthritis typically affects the knee, but can involve the shoulder, ankle, elbow, or wrist.
    b. Gout classically presents with first metatarsophalangeal (MTP) arthritis, although it may involve the midtarsal foot, ankle, or knee joints.
    c. Transient synovitis typically affects the hip.
    d. Lyme disease is typically monarticular, characteristically targeting the knee.
    e. OA affects large joints (e.g., knee, hip) and the first carpometacarpal (CMC) and distal interphalangeal (DIP) hand joints.
    f. Pseudogout also commonly affects large joints (e.g., knees, wrists) and can also affect the metacarpophalangeals (MCPs), hips, shoulders, elbows, or ankles.
  2. Polyarticular arthralgia
    a. Viremia and **growing pains** cause polyarticular arthralgia.
    b. Rheumatologic/autoimmune diseases (e.g., RA) typically present with symmetrical multiple joint involvement, often of smaller, nonweight-bearing joints (e.g., hand proximal interphalangeals [PIPs], MCPs, wrists, toes, and ankles).
    c. One criterion for **rheumatic fever** is polyarticular involvement, especially the ankles, knees, hips, wrists, elbows, and shoulders.
    d. JHS can be associated with acute or chronic pain, joint clicking, as well as history of dislocation/subluxation.
B. Chronology
  1. The pain of **trauma, gout, pseudogout,** and **septic arthritis** is typically an **acute** onset.

TABLE 38–1. JONES CRITERIA (MODIFIED) FOR DIAGNOSIS OF RHEUMATIC FEVER

Major Manifestations	Minor Manifestations	Supporting Evidence of Antecedent Group A Streptococcal Infection
Carditis	Clinical findings	Positive throat culture or rapid streptococcal antigen test
Polyarthritis	Arthralgia	Elevated or rising ASO or antiDNAse B titer
Chorea	Fever	
Erythema marginatum	Laboratory findings	
	Elevated acute phase reactants	
Subcutaneous nodules	Erythrocyte sedimentation rate	
	C-reactive protein	
	Prolonged PR interval on ECG	

If supported by evidence of preceding group A streptococcal infection, the presence of two major manifestations or one major and two minor manifestations indicates a high probability of acute rheumatic fever.
ASO, antistreptolysin-O; ECG, electrocardiogram.

    2. Arthralgias associated with growing pains, fibromyalgia, hypermobility, OA, and collagen diseases (e.g., RA) tend to follow an **insidious/chronic/recurrent** pattern.
  C. Exacerbating/alleviating factors
    1. OA, traumatic arthritis, overuse injuries, and growing pains tend to **worsen with activity**.
    2. Psychogenic pain associated with school phobia worsens before school and improves on weekends and when away from school.
    3. Nocturnal worsening is associated with growing pains; an **acute gout attack** may begin at night.
  D. Associated symptoms
    1. Complaint of an **erythema, very tender joint,** and feverishness/chills are associated with septic arthritis, gout, and RF.
    2. Stiffness following immobilization is associated with **OA** and **autoimmune arthritis** (e.g., RA); OA stiffness (gelling) typically abates within 15 minutes of activity, whereas RA stiffness persists at least 1 hour.
    3. Depending on the specific underlying disease, **autoimmune arthritis** can be associated with rashes (e.g., butterfly malar rash, sun sensitivity, alopecia, or discoid lesions with SLE).
    4. Rheumatic fever can be associated with a macular, circinate erythematous truncal rash; Sydenham chorea (choreoathetoid facial, tongue, or upper extremity movements); and subcutaneous nodules of tendon sheaths (especially in children) (see Table 38–1).
    5. Psychogenic arthralgia may be associated with symptoms of anxiety, depression, or other psychiatric disease.
    6. Fibromyalgia (FM) frequently is associated with fatigue, unrefreshing sleep, thinking or remembering disorders, chronic headaches, and irritable bowel symptoms. Proposed revised criteria for FM include a symptom severity score based on a scaled assessment of fatigue, unrefreshing sleep, cognitive disorders, and the extent of general somatic symptoms.
 IV. Signs. A careful, focused physical examination is crucial in differentiating articular from periarticular processes and, together with symptoms and risk factors, guides testing strategies.
  A. Vital signs/general appearance
    1. Fever is associated with septic arthritis, viral arthralgias, gout, and RF.
    2. Ill or toxic appearance (or both) raises suspicion of septic arthritis.
    3. Integument/mucous membranes
      a. Erythema migrans (EM) occurs in 80% of patients with early Lyme disease 3 to 30 days following a tick bite. EM begins as a red papule at the site of the bite, enlarging circumferentially over days to a month with central clearing and typical resolution over 3 to 4 weeks.
      b. A generalized evanescent, pinkish maculopapular exanthem makes **viremia** a likely cause of arthralgias.
      c. SLE lesions include malar erythema (butterfly rash), discoid macular plaque-like lesions, alopecia, or oral ulcers.

B. Joint findings. Intra-articular processes have abnormal findings of the affected joints, ranging from heat/erythema, to firm or boggy swelling, to synovial or joint line tenderness, to restricted range of motion (ROM). In **periarticular processes,** by contrast, the joint examination is often normal or minimally abnormal.

1. Intra-articular processes
   a. In **transient synovitis,** there is decreased hip ROM, especially internal rotation.
   b. **Bacterial synovitis/septic joint** presents dramatically with a warm/erythematous joint, joint effusion, and severely restricted active and passive ROM.
   c. **Viral synovitis** can show tenderness and synovial involvement, but no deformity.
   d. **Gouty arthritis** can present with swollen, red, tender-to-the-touch joint, fever, and leukocytosis or less dramatically with swollen joint, restricted ROM, and painful weight-bearing. Following multiple attacks, tophaceous invasion can grossly deform the affected sites, especially the ear helix, olecranon, and interphalangeal joints.
   e. **Pseudogout** shows less dramatic inflammation than gout; one may note firm hypertrophy caused by chronic chondrocalcinosis.
   f. **OA** findings typically include crepitus, tender joint line, firm swelling (bony hypertrophy and osteophytes, rather than synovitis), and restricted extremes of ROM.
   g. **Traumatic arthritis** findings are similar to OA; there can be deformity at the site of previous trauma or surgery.
   h. **RA** findings include symmetric, swollen, warm, tender boggy joint (especially wrists and hand PIPs and MCPs). Chronic active disease produces deformities including ulnar deviation of digits and boutonnière/"swan-neck" digit deformities. The clinical examination is considered the gold standard in the diagnosis of synovitis, (SOR **C**) although some controlled trials propose that ultrasound assessment is at least as relevant as clinical examination.
   i. A tender joint, with or without synovitis, occurs with stage 3 **Lyme disease** (late persistent infection).
   j. **Rheumatic fever** can produce tender joints/synovium (large joints) and RF can be monarticular in adults.

2. Periarticular
   a. Five criteria establish a diagnosis of **JHS;** these include (1) passive opposition of thumb to flexor forearm, (2) passive finger hyperextension parallel to forearm, (3) elbow hyperextension, (4) knee hyperextension, and (5) palms on floor with knees extended. Joint hypermobility may involve only one joint and be associated with stretchability, stretch marks, and paper-thin scars.
   b. **Fibromyalgia** is diagnosed by reproducing ≥11 of 18 mainly axial designated tender sites (occiputs, supraspinata, glutei, greater trochanters, upper trapezius borders, anterior cervical 5–7 interspaces, second anterior rib lateral to the costochondral junction, lateral epicondyles, and medial fat pads of knees) (see also Section III.D.6).
   c. There are no characteristic articular or periarticular findings with **growing pains** or **psychogenic arthralgias.**

V. Laboratory tests can be selective and based on careful history and focused physical examination as described (Figure 38–1). Because some diagnoses become apparent only over time, serial evaluation and testing is sometimes necessary to arrive at a correct diagnosis. No further testing is necessary if hypermobility syndrome is suspected or for findings consistent with growing pains in the absence of articular inflammation. If joint effusion is present and the diagnosis is uncertain, or if septic arthritis is suspected, arthrocentesis is indicated (Figure 38–1).

A. Hematologic tests
   1. In **acute rheumatic fever,** erythrocyte sedimentation rate (ESR) and antistreptolysin-O (ASO) are elevated, though these are normal in 10% of patients with other findings compatible with RF.
   2. Fifty to eighty percent of patients with **RA** have a positive **rheumatoid factor (RF), anti-citrullinated protein antibody (ACPA),** or both; ACPA is more specific for RA than for RF. The minimal laboratory panel in suspected RA includes RF, ACPA, C-reactive protein (CRP), and ESR.
   3. Hematologic abnormalities associated with **SLE** include positive ANA (in 95%–100%), antinative DNA (in 50%), antismooth muscle (in 20%), anemia (in 60%), leukopenia (in 45%), and thrombocytopenia (in 30%).

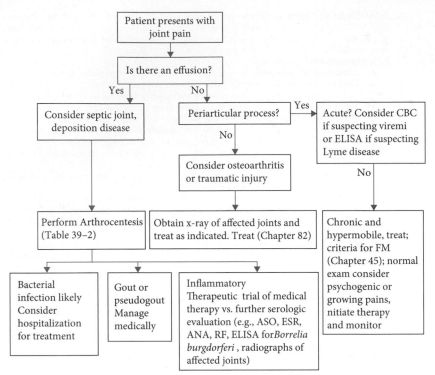

FIGURE 38–1. Approach to evaluating the patient with joint pain. ANA, antinuclear antibody; ASO, antistreptolysin-O; CBC, complete blood count; CPDD, calcium pyrophosphate deposition disease; CTD, connective tissue disease; ELISA, enzyme-linked immunosorbent assay; ESR, erythrocyte sedimentation rate; FM, fibromyalgia; OA, osteoarthritis; RF, Rheumatic fever.

4. In the appropriate clinical context, uric acid ≥ 7.5 and podagra are sufficient for diagnosis and presumptive treatment for **gout**, though uric acid levels can be normal during an acute gouty attack.

5. For suspected **Lyme disease**, current Centers for Disease Control (CDC) recommendations include confirming a positive enzyme-linked immunosorbent assay (ELISA) antibody test with a Western immunoblot test.

B. Joint fluid examination (Table 38–2). **Gouty arthritis** is definitively diagnosed by finding urate crystals (needle-like, negatively birefringent); pseudogout crystals are rhomboid shaped.

C. Radiology

1. In **OA,** plain radiographs show joint-space narrowing and irregularity, periarticular spurring, and juxta-articular sclerosis.

2. **Pseudogout** manifests with changes similar to those in OA, along with cartilage calcification.

3. In **transient synovitis,** soft-tissue periarticular swelling can be evident, but is a nonspecific finding.

4. In **RF,** one manifestation of carditis is cardiomegaly and other signs of congestive heart failure are on plain chest radiographs.

D. Other testing

1. Proteinuria occurs in 30% of **patients with SLE**.

2. Electrocardiography (ECG) in **RF** may reveal increased PR interval; **recent controlled studies document the efficacy of echocardiography in detecting subclinical rheumatic heart disease, especially in developing countries.**

TABLE 38–2. JOINT FLUID FINDINGS

	Normal	Trauma	Infection	Crystalline Disease	Inflammatory
Color	Clear to yellow	Bloody to xanthochromic	Yellow to cloudy	Yellow to cloudy	Yellow to cloudy
Cell count (cells/μL) WBC/RBC	≤200/0	≤1000/many	1000–200,000/few	1000–2000/few	1000–20,000/few
Crystals	Negative	Negative	Negative	Yes; pseudogout and gout	Negative
Culture	Negative	Negative	Positive	Negative	Negative

RBC, red blood cell; WBC, white blood cell.

VI. Treatment is directed at the underlying cause of joint pain, which can accurately be arrived at via appropriate history, focused examination, and selective testing.
  A. Intra-articular diseases
    1. Transient synovitis usually resolves on its own over a few days. Bed rest, traction with slight hip flexion, with or without age-appropriate oral nonsteroidal anti-inflammatory drugs (NSAIDs) can increase comfort. Follow-up plain hip radiographs at 1 and 3 months can detect avascular femoral head necrosis, a possible complication of transient synovitis.
    2. Septic arthritis requires treatment with systemic antibiotics and possible orthopedic consultation, which should occur in a hospital setting.
    3. Gouty arthritis
      a. Acute attack
        (1) NSAIDs (e.g., oral indomethacin, 25–50 mg every 8 hours for 5–10 days or until symptoms are controlled) showed benefit in open-label clinical trials but comorbidities (e.g. ethanol use, chronic renal insufficiency, heart disease) can increase their risk.
        (2) Alternately, **colchicine** (0.6 mg orally hourly until symptoms are controlled or diarrhea develops, with maximum of 8 mg) showed significant benefit at 48 hours versus placebo but is limited by gastrointestinal (GI) toxicity. GI symptoms can be limited using intravenous colchicine, 2 mg in 25 to 50 mL normal saline, with additional 1 mg doses every 6 hours for two more doses (maximum: 4 mg total). Colchicine should not be used in those with hepatic and renal impairment.
        (3) Intra-articular steroids (e.g., 10–40 mg of triamcinolone) can be effective for monarticular gout; an oral steroid (e.g., prednisone, 40–60 mg initially and tapered over 7 days) can be effective for polyarticular acute gout.
        (4) Analgesics (other than aspirin, which may precipitate gout) can be needed for pain control.
        (5) Bed rest during the acute attack is also helpful.
      b. Chronic management
        (1) Patient education
          (a) Patients should be advised to avoid or limit their intake of high-purine foods including meats, seafood, meat extracts and gravies, yeast and yeast extracts, alcoholic beverages (especially beer), dried beans, peas, lentils, oatmeal, spinach, asparagus, cauliflower, and mushrooms. Foods that contain meat sources of purines are more likely to trigger a gouty flare than non-meat sources.
          (b) The following medications can precipitate gouty attacks and should be avoided: thiazide and loop diuretics, low-dose aspirin (≤3 g per day), and niacin.
        (2) The decision to initiate **preventive medication** depends on the individual's risk of recurrent gouty arthritis; for example, an individual who had a single attack and is willing to avoid alcohol and lose weight is at low risk, whereas an older individual with multiple attacks, mild chronic renal insufficiency, or requiring a diuretic is considered to be at high risk. One guideline for initiating prophylaxis is to consider it in those with two or more acute gouty flares per year, presence of progressive tophi, or radiographic

changes consistent with gout. Once initiated, the target urate level is <6 mg/dL (<5 mg/dL with tophaceous gout). (SOR Ⓐ)

    (a) Oral colchicine, 0.6 mg twice daily, can be effective prophylaxis in individuals with mild hyperuricemia and few acute attacks; the risk of an acute gouty flare during initiation of prophylaxis can be significantly decreased by twice daily colchicine dosing, and continuation of colchicine for 6 months is significantly more efficacious in this regard than briefer (e.g., 8 weeks) dosing.

    (b) Urate-lowering therapy

        (i) Allopurinol and **febuxostat** are xanthine oxidase inhibitors that lower plasma urate concentrations, can mobilize tophi, and are first-line agents for gout prevention. Allopurinol dosing begins at 100 mg orally daily for the first week, with dose increases depending on serum uric acid response. Most people require 200 to 300 mg daily. Seventy-five percent of those treated with allopurinol for more than 4 months have no further gouty flares. Febuxostat dosing starts at 40 mg per day, increasing to 80 mg per day if uric acid remains above target after 2 weeks.

        (ii) Uricosurics are second-line agents indicated in those intolerant of xanthine oxidase inhibitors or in combination with xanthine oxidase inhibitors for refractory hyperuricemia. **Probenecid** is the most commonly used uricosuric and is dosed initially at 250 mg twice daily, titrating gradually up to a maximum dose of 2 g daily. Uricosurics are contraindicated with history of nephrolithiasis or creatinine clearance <50 mL/min.

  (3) Prognosis depends on age at first attack and number of attacks; destructive arthropathy is rare in those having their first attack after 50 years of age.

4. Pseudogout treatment is directed at the underlying disease. Acute symptoms can be helped with oral NSAIDs, oral colchicine (0.6 mg twice daily can benefit prophylaxis), and joint aspiration followed by intra-articular steroid injection (e.g., triamcinolone, 10–40 mg, depending on joint size).

5. RA, like other autoimmune diseases, follows a variable course with prognosis depending on disease severity; severe disease demands early aggressive treatment with disease-modifying antirheumatic drugs (DMARDs). Patients with inflammatory joint disease should be referred to a rheumatology subspecialist, especially if symptoms persist >6 weeks. (SOR Ⓒ)

  a. Supportive therapy

    (1) Patients should be educated about the disease, its variable course, and their role in self-monitoring and management.

    (2) Rest in bed is important for a severe disease flare; 2 hours' rest per day is sufficient for milder inflammation. Activity should be liberalized as tolerated by symptoms.

    (3) A supervised exercise program improves quality of life and strength in patients with RA. (SOR Ⓑ)

  b. Response to **medications** can be gauged based on the patient's stiffness, fatigue, and degree of joint swelling and changes in acute phase reactants (CRP and ESR). DMARDs are the mainstay of treatment, and methotrexate is recommended as the first-line agent. Combination therapy with two or more DMARDs is more effective than monotherapy, (SOR Ⓐ) although adverse effects can also increase. Poor response to NSAIDs warrants consideration of DMARDs. Unless the practitioner is familiar with side effects and monitoring therapy with DMARDs, rheumatology consultation for co-management is advisable.

    (1) NSAIDs (e.g., oral ibuprofen, 400–600 mg, three to four times daily, or naproxen, 550 mg twice daily) are first-line anti-inflammatory/analgesic therapy; therapy should be carefully monitored for GI toxicity.

6. Lyme disease/EM (see Chapter 7).

7. RF

  a. Bed rest is indicated until the patient is afebrile without antipyretics and has a normal pulse rate, ESR, and ECG.

  b. Acute medications

    (1) Salicylates (e.g., oral aspirin, 600–900 mg every 4 hours in adults) can markedly improve fever and joint symptoms.

    (2) An **oral steroid** (e.g., prednisone, 40–60 mg, initially and tapered over 7 days) can relieve joint symptoms poorly controlled by salicylates.

    (3) Penicillin G benzathine, 1.2 million units intramuscularly (IM) in a single dose, or **procaine penicillin,** 600,000 units IM daily for 10 days, will eradicate streptococcal infection in nonallergic patients.

    (4) Recent randomized trials have documented the efficacy of daily **amoxicillin** (1.5 g, or 750 mg for children weighing <30 kg) versus twice daily penicillin V in treating group A beta hemolytic strep.

  c. Chronic medication

    (1) Penicillin G benzathine (600,000 U IM every 3–4 weeks for those weighing <30 kg or 1.2 million units IM every 3–4 weeks for those weighing >30 kg) prophylaxis is indicated in those with RF.

    In those without carditis, prophylaxis should be continued until 5 years have elapsed since the last attack or 18 years of age, whichever is longer. With a history of carditis, prophylaxis should be continued until 10 years after the last attack or 25 years of age (whichever is longer) for mild mitral regurgitation or lifelong in the presence of severe valvular heart disease or following valvular surgery for rheumatic heart disease.

  8. Traumatic arthritis/OA (see Chapter 82).

B. Periarticular diseases

  1. Viremia-induced arthralgias should be treated symptomatically and supportively (see Chapter 46).

  2. JHS affects quality of life as it is associated with dislocations, OA, and osteonecrosis; those with hypermobility can benefit from graded conditioning to provide muscle support of affected joints.

  3. Fibromyalgia (see Chapter 46).

  4. Treatment of **growing pains** involves reassurance, symptomatic analgesics, and instructions to follow-up if the symptom pattern worsens.

  5. In **psychogenic arthralgia,** underlying stress or abnormal family dynamics should be identified and treated.

SELECTED REFERENCES

Cann MP, Sive AA, Norton RE, et al. Clinical presentation of rheumatic fever in an endemic area. *Arch Dis Child.* 2010;95(6):455–457.

Doherty M, Jansen TL, Nuki G, et al. Gout: why is this curable disease so seldom cured? *Ann Rheum Dis.* 2012;71(11):1765–1770.

Horowitz DL, Horowitz S, Barilla-LaBarca M-L. Approach to septic arthritis. *Am Fam Physician.* 2011;84(6):653–660.

Katchamart W, Johnson S, Lin HJ, et al. Predictors for remission in rheumatoid arthritis patients: a systematic review. *Arthritis Care Res.* 2010;62(8):1128–1143.

Wolfe F, Clauw DJ, Fitzcharles M-A, et al. The American College of Rheumatology preliminary diagnostic criteria for fibromyalgia and measurement of symptom severity. *Arthritis Care Res.* 2010;62(5):600–610.

---

39   Knee Complaints

Vimarie Rodriguez, MD, CAQSM, & Mitchell A. Kaminski, MD, MBA

KEY POINTS

- When evaluating a patient with knee complaints, a history including the pain characteristics, mechanism of injury, mechanical symptoms, swelling and degree of disability in conjunction with the physical examination will help narrow down the differential diagnosis list. (SOR ❸)
- In most patients, a careful history and focused examination will allow for accurate diagnosis without additional testing. (SOR ❸)

- Evidence-based application of diagnostic tests (e.g., x-ray, magnetic resonance imaging, blood work, and joint aspiration) can be used cost-effectively to establish the diagnosis. (SOR **C**)
- Knowledge of when to refer to an orthopedist is critical in acute injuries. (SOR **C**)
- Medication and an appropriate exercise program benefit the patient with chronic complaints. (SOR **B**)

I. **Definition.** The knee is the largest and most complex joint in the human body. It contains the tibiofemoral joint and the patellofemoral joint with their associated ligaments, articular cartilage, meniscus, tendons, bones, and bursa (Figures 39–1 and 39–2). Its motion characteristics (coordinated system of rotations and translations) and sudden large forces applied to it make it vulnerable to injuries.

Knee complaints can be divided into acute and chronic. **Acute complaints** are usually the result of contact and noncontact injuries but on occasion can be due to chronic problems that flare (Table 39–1). **Chronic complaints** are usually the result of overuse injuries, degenerative processes, and inflammation (Table 39–2).

II. **Common Diagnoses.** The knee joint is a frequent source of concern in primary care practice. Up to 5% of physician visits are related to knee pain. More than one million visits to US

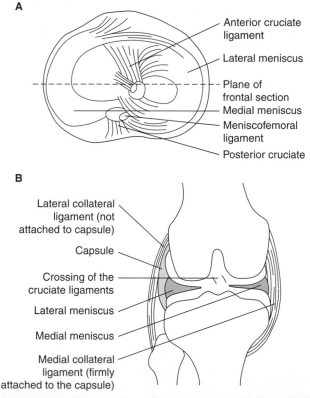

FIGURE 39–1. Relationship between the menisci, the capsule, and the ligaments of the knee. **A.** A superior view of the menisci and cruciate ligaments. **B.** A posterior view of a frontal section of the knee through the middle third. Modified with permission from Steinberg GG, Akins CM, Baran DT, et al., eds. *Orthopaedics in Primary Care*. 3rd ed. Lippincott Williams & Wilkins;1999.

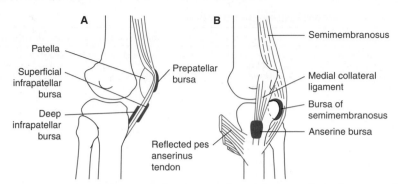

FIGURE 39-2. Bursae about the knee. **A.** The lateral view. **B.** The medial view. Modified with permission from Steinberg GG, Akins CM, Baran DT, et al., eds. *Orthopaedics in Primary Care.* 3rd ed. Lippincott Williams & Wilkins; 1999.

emergency departments occur for knee trauma and approximately 11% of patients aged 65 years and older have symptomatic osteoarthritis of the knee.

A. Ligament injuries are among the most common causes of musculoskeletal joint pain and disability encountered in primary care practice. Ligament injuries cause disruptions in the balance between joint mobility and joint stability; this imbalance can lead to abnormal transmission of forces throughout the joint and result in damage to other structures in and around the joint.

  1. The **medial collateral ligament (MCL)** can be injured as a result of a valgus force applied to the knee (e.g., blow to the lateral knee) in a contact injury or a noncontact valgus force. The MCL is the most common injured ligament structure in the knee. Table 39–3 displays the MCL injury grading system.

  2. The **anterior collateral ligament (ACL)** is most commonly injured during athletic activities by noncontact mechanisms (sudden deceleration with a directional change or rotational maneuvers). Contact injuries usually occur from a direct blow causing hyperextension or valgus stress to the knee. Women are more prone to ACL injuries than men. Sports with the greatest number of ACL tears include football, soccer, alpine skiers, and gymnastics.

  3. The **lateral collateral ligament (LCL)** is less frequently injured than the ACL or MCL. The LCL can be injured as a result of a varus force or twisting during a contact or noncontact injury.

  4. The **posterior collateral ligament (PCL)** is usually injured from a direct blow to the anterior proximal tibia.

B. Meniscal injuries can be caused by a single traumatic injury, degenerative process, or both. The prevalence of meniscal injuries increases with age. Meniscal injuries are caused when a person twists the leg while bearing weight.

C. Patellofemoral pain syndrome (PFS) can be defined as anterior knee pain involving the patella and retinaculum that excludes other intra-articular and peripatellar pathology. It is the most common diagnosis in outpatients presenting with knee pain. Its etiology is multifactorial and risk factors such as overuse (training overload),

TABLE 39–1. CAUSES OF ACUTE KNEE COMPLAINTS BY LOCATION

Anterior Knee	Medial Knee	Lateral Knee	Posterior Knee
ACL tear	MCL sprain	Lateral meniscus tear	PCL sprain
Acute flare of gouty arthritis or pseudogout	Medial meniscus tear	LCL sprain	
Patellar dislocation			
Septic arthritis			

Not-to-be missed causes include fractures of the tibial plateau, avulsion fracture of the tibial spine, osteochondritis dissecans (in children and adolescents), and quadriceps rupture.

ACL, anterior collateral ligament; LCL, lateral collateral ligament; PCL, posterior collateral ligament.

TABLE 39–2. CAUSES OF CHRONIC KNEE COMPLAINTS BY LOCATION

Anterior Knee	Medial Knee	Lateral Knee	Posterior Knee
Patellofemoral pain syndrome	Degenerative medial meniscal tear	Degenerative lateral meniscal tear	Baker cyst
Patellar tendinopathy	OA of the medial compartment	Iliotibial band syndrome	**Not to missed: Deep vein thrombosis, claudication, PCL sprain**
Osgood–Schlatter	Pes anserine bursitis	Iliotibial band syndrome	
Sinding–Larsen–Johansson	PFS	OA of the lateral compartment	
Not-to-be missed causes:	Plica syndrome	**Not-to-be missed causes: Common**	
Referred pain from the hip,	**Not-to-be missed causes:**	**peroneal nerve injury, slipped**	
osteochondritis dissecans,	**Tumor in the young, slipped**	**capital femoral epiphysis,**	
slipped capital femoral	**capital femoral epiphysis,**	**Perthes disease**	
epiphysis, Perthes disease,	**referred pain from the hip,**		
tumor in the young	**Perthes disease**		

OA, osteoarthritis; PFS, patellofemoral syndrome; PCL, posterior collateral ligament.

malalignment (abnormal patellar tracking), and trauma have been linked. PFS is commonly encountered in women, active adolescents, and adults in the second and third decades of life.

D. Patellar tendinopathy, also known as jumper's knee, is a degenerative tendinosis with a multifactorial etiology often found in recreational and top-level athletes complaining of anterior knee pain below the patella. Nine possible risk factors have been identified with limited evidence (weight, body mass index, waist-to-hip ratio, leg-length difference, arch height of the foot, quadriceps flexibility, hamstring flexibility, quadriceps strength, and vertical jump performance).

E. Patellar dislocation can occur either by a direct blow to the knee or indirectly, as the body rotates around a planted foot. **Subluxation** refers to excessive lateral movement of the patella and can occur as a result of trauma or in patients with joint laxity.

F. Bursitis
  1. Prepatellar bursitis is an inflammation of the largest knee bursa located between the patella and the overlying skin. The bursa is commonly irritated by trauma or repetitive kneeling as in housemaid's knee. The bursa can become infected, most commonly by *Staphylococcus aureus*, or become inflamed by urate crystals in patients with gout.
  2. Anserine bursitis is an inflammation of the bursa located about 6 cm below the medial joint line between the attachment of MCL at the medial tibial plateau and the conjoined tendon formed by the gracilis, sartorius, and semitendinosus.

G. Osteochondritis dissecans (OCD) is a fragment of subchondral bone and articular cartilage separated from the underlying bone that leaves either a stable or unstable fragment. This condition most commonly affects the knee medial condyle. Full-thickness focal chondral defects in the knee are more common in athletes than among the general population. More than one-half of asymptomatic athletes have a full-thickness defect.

H. Osgood–Schlatter disease is a traction apophysitis of the tibial tubercle at the insertion of the patellar tendon caused by repetitive strain and chronic avulsion of the secondary ossification center of the tibial tubercle. It is a common cause of anterior knee pain in children and adolescents between the ages of 8 and 15 years (8 and 12 years in girls, 12 and 15 years in boys) who have undergone a rapid growth spurt. The occurrence is

TABLE 39–3. MEDIAL COLLATERAL LIGAMENT INJURY GRADING SYSTEM

Grade	Definition	Physical Exam
1. Mild injury	A few fibers are torn but the **ligament is intact**, localized tenderness with no instability	Less than 5 mm of joint opening, solid endpoint
2. Moderate injury	An **incomplete tear** with some remaining ligament integrity; localized tenderness and partially torn medial collateral and posterior oblique fibers	About 5–9 mm joint opening, firm or perceptible endpoint
3. Severe injury	A **complete tear** with complete disruption of the ligament and instability with an applied valgus stress	More than 10 mm of joint opening with no perception of endpoint

more frequent in boys than in girls and it often presents bilaterally. It commonly affects children and adolescents who are active in sports that involve running, cutting, and jumping (e.g., soccer, basketball, gymnastics, volleyball, football).

  I. Sinding–Larsen–Johansson disease is a traction apophysitis of the inferior pole of the patella that affects patients between the ages of 10 and 13 years who are involved in athletic activities.

  J. Iliotibial band (ITB) syndrome is a nontraumatic overuse injury caused by friction/rubbing of the distal portion of the ITB over the lateral femoral epicondyle with repeated flexion and extension of the knee. It is the most common cause of lateral knee pain in athletes, especially with running, cycling, dancing, volleyball, tennis, football, skiing, weight lifting, and aerobics. The etiology of ITB syndrome is multifactorial with both intrinsic and extrinsic factors. Risk factors for developing this syndrome include a varus alignment of the knee, excessive running mileage, worn shoes, or continuous running on uneven terrain.

  K. Baker cyst or popliteal cyst is a cystic enlargement of synovial tissue in the popliteal space. It may be a true cyst or a posterior herniation of a chronic knee effusion. Baker cysts are associated with degenerative arthropathy and internal derangement (e.g., meniscal tears). Risk factors for the development of popliteal cysts in adults include a history of trauma (to the posterior knee) and a history of coexistent joint disease (OA, RA, meniscal tear).

  L. Arthritis (RA, OA, gout, pseudogout) (see Chapters 38 and 82).

  M. Plica syndrome. Synovial plicae are normal synovial folds within the knee joint and are remnants from the embryological development of the knee. Trauma and repetitive motion cause thickening, fibrosis, and hemorrhage, resulting in anterior knee pain.

  N. Fractures of the patella or femoral condyles follow acute trauma; compressive, rotational, or lateral stresses can result in tibial plateau fracture. Pathologic bone (e.g., osteoporosis) that is weaker than ligaments will fracture before the ligaments tear. Distal femoral Salter type fractures in adolescents may initially mask a ligament tear (see Chapter 28).

  O. Pain referred from the hip. Acute knee pain can be referred from primary pathology in the hip, such as arthritis, osteomyelitis, slipped capital femoral epiphysis (SCFE), and Legg–Calvé–Perthes disease (see Chapter 41).

III. Prevention

  A. MCL. Preventive knee braces appear to offer some protection to the MCL from a contact injury involving a valgus blow, but there may be negative effects on performance level, leg cramping, and fatigue symptoms.

  B. ACL injuries. Neuromuscular training programs that include plyometric and strengthening exercises significantly reduce noncontact ACL injuries in female soccer and handball players older than 14 years. (SOR **Ⓐ**) There is no evidence that bracing after surgery improves outcome or reduces risk of subsequent injury among patients using the brace.

IV. Symptoms and Signs. Knee complaints can be accurately diagnosed with an appropriate history and examination. The pain characteristics (onset, location, duration, severity, quality, aggravating, and alleviating factors), the mechanism of injury (contact, noncontact, twisting, hyperextension), the mechanical symptoms (locking, popping or giving way), swelling (rapid onset within 2 hours vs. delayed), medical history, and degree of disability (able to continue activity or bear weight after the injury) can help determine the likely damage structure.

  The knee examination involves **inspection, palpation** (Figure 39–3), **and special maneuvers** (Table 39–4). Knee physical examination videos can be found at http://www.youtube.com/user/BJSMVideos/videos?view=0**A**.

  A. Ligament injuries

    1. MCL sprain symptoms include pain and swelling along the medial side of the knee, giving way on valgus motion, and a sensation of instability from side to side especially for athletes when cutting and pivoting. **Signs** include localized swelling or ecchymosis along the medial side of the knee and tenderness to palpation (see Table 39–3). **Positive valgus stress test** at 30 degrees of flexion indicates injury to the superficial portion of the MCL. Laxity at 0 degrees of flexion suggests injury to the deeper structures of the MCL and possible concomitant disruption of the ACL.

    2. ACL tear is indicated by a loud pop at the time of injury with inability to continue activities, complaints of knee giving way, and acute swelling. **Signs** include a large tense effusion after the injury (hemarthrosis), positive Lachman test, positive pivot shift, and positive anterior drawer test. Videos demonstrating these tests can be found at http://www.aafp.org/afp/2010/1015/p917/videos.html.

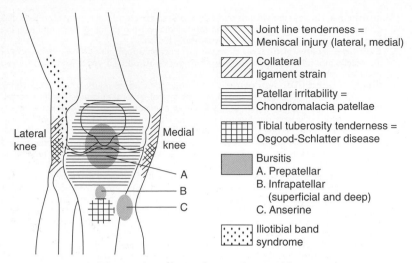

FIGURE 39-3. Sites of knee tenderness and suggested diagnoses.

   3. LCL sprain symptoms include pain over the lateral knee and give-way sensation on twisting, cutting, or pivoting. **Signs** include a positive varus stress test.

   4. PCL sprain/tear symptoms include swelling and, in chronic cases, instability of the knee on rapid deceleration or going downstairs or downhill. **Signs** include knee effusion, positive posterior drawer test, and gravity test.

B. Meniscal injuries. Mechanical symptoms may be more common than pain because only the periphery of the menisci contains nerve fibers. Mechanical symptoms include locking, popping, and catching. Other symptoms include swelling, pain with rotation or flexion (particularly at the extremes of those motions), pain along the joint line, weakness or giving way, and a generalized aching (particularly with chronic meniscal injury).

   1. MMT symptoms include swelling and medial knee pain, lack of extension, locking, slipping, and catching. **Signs** include medial joint line tenderness, effusion, and positive McMurray and Apley tests (Table 39–4).

   2. LMT symptoms include more pain than medial meniscus injury, and lateral joint line pain. **Signs** include positive McMurray and Apley tests (Table 39–4), joint-line tenderness, and effusion.

C. PFS symptoms. Anterior knee pain is worst when sitting with the knees flexed (i.e., "theater sign") and when climbing or descending stairs, squatting, running, or going downhill. Snapping, and popping around the patella, stiffness when the knee is flexed; may complain of knee giving way (due to transient inhibition of quadriceps because of pain or deconditioning). **Signs** include pain on patellofemoral compression test (Table 39–4), crepitation around the patella, and increased popliteal angle.

D. Patellar tendinopathy. Symptoms include infrapatellar pain after exercise, later during exercise, and at rest. **Signs** include tenderness at the inferior pole of the patella and knee extension weakness.

E. Patellar dislocation/subluxation

   1. Symptoms. In acute dislocation, the person will fall down or sense that something is out of place. In subluxation, the person will experience knee pain, popping or clicking, occasionally knee swelling, stiffness, or catching.

   2. Signs. In patellar dislocation, the patella may be palpable over the lateral femur, and the medial femoral condyle will appear prominent. Common signs include effusion and tenderness localized to the adductor tubercle and patellar facets (especially the lateral facet). People will often have a positive patellar apprehension test (Table 39–4).

F. Bursitis

   1. Prepatellar bursitis. Symptoms include knee swelling and pain over the anterior knee. **Signs** include presence of a ballotable collection of fluid palpable over the

TABLE 39–4. SPECIAL MANEUVERS IN THE KNEE EXAMINATION

Test	Method	Significance	URL[a]
Apley test	With the patient prone, his/her knee flexed to 90 degrees, the examiner then places his or her own knee across the posterior aspect of the patient's thigh; the *tibia* is then compressed onto the knee joint while being externally rotated	A positive test indicates pathology of the meniscus	http://www.youtube.com/watch?v=w57I1cYXICA&noredirect=1
Apprehension test (LOE C)	Apply pressure to the medial patella to push the patella laterally with quadriceps relaxed, knee extended	Pain or discomfort with lateral translation of the patella suggests patellar subluxation	http://www.youtube.com/watch?v=xXmjYVDkmVg
Collateral ligament stressing (LOE C)	Valgus varus stress of knee in full knee extension and then 30-degree flexion	Laxity with full extension suggests collateral and cruciate ligament injury. Laxity only at 30-degree flexion suggests collateral ligament tear	http://www.youtube.com/watch?v=M0KX1rxiyqM
Lachman maneuver (LOE A)	With knee flexed 20 degrees and femur supported, pull tibia anteriorly	Step-up from lower patella to tibial tuberosity indicates anterior cruciate ligament instability	http://www.fammed.wisc.edu/our-department/media/623/knee-exam-lachman-test
McMurray (LOE C)	Extend axially compressed knee with internal tibial rotation and then with external tibial rotation	Locking or popping suggests meniscal injury	http://www.youtube.com/watch?v=lwBW-X4n1fU
Medial patellar plica test	Patient supine, legs extended, apply pressure over the affected knee at the plica (inferomedial patellar border) and then flex knee to 90 degrees	Greater pain in extension than in flexion	http://www.google.ca/url?sa=i&rct=j&q=&esrc=s&frm=1&source=web&cd=2&ved=0CDgQFjAB&url=http%3A%2F%2Fmediaplayer.pearsoncmg.com%2Fmedia_flash_cc_ph_hsml_set.title.Medial_Patellar_Plica_Test_%2Fph%2Fchef%2Fhealthsci-media_library_6%2Fmedai.Patellar.Plica.m4v&ei=LQvCUfszPInwiwlyYHABQ&usg=AFGjCNG-kA749bf93jh_ysxq59g6TaaTQ&sig2=O7cp-O6rdOxAm4nnGNiPHQ&bvm=bv.48175248,d.cGE
Ober test	With the patient side-lying, unaffected leg down and flexed at hip and knee, abduct and extend the hip with knee at 90 degrees slowly lower the leg (adduct the hip)	Inability to adduct the hip, once positioned, past the neutral position indicates a tight iliotibial band	https://www.youtube.com/watch?v=A0C0WBw4l4s
Patellofemoral compression test (LOE C)	Compress patella into the trochlear grove while the leg is extended	Pain consistent with patellofemoral pain syndrome	http://www.youtube.com/watch?v=P2rYPMAZteo
Pivot shift tests (LOE B)	Patient lateral decubitus position: extend knee, internally rotate tibia, apply valgus stress and flex knee	Clunk felt at 30 degrees flexion suggests anterior cruciate ligament rupture	http://www.youtube.com/watch?v=ZWEGB0ToXZo
Thigh circumference measurement (LOE C)	Measure thigh circumference at an equal distance above both midpatellae	Decreased circumference of thigh above affected knee suggests subacute or chronic disorder with quadriceps atrophy	

[a]Video demonstrating the test can be seen on the listed websites; Accessed June 2013. For the general knee examination, see http://www.fammed.wisc.edu/our-department/media/623/knee-exam. Accessed June 2013.

patella, unimpaired range of motion (ROM) of the knee (swelling is extraarticular), cobblestone-like roughness or palpable bursal thickening, and tenderness over the bursal sac. Inflammatory signs (erythema, warmth) can also be present, especially with infection.

2. Anserine bursitis. Symptoms include an abnormal gait, pain at night, and pain in the medial knee region over the upper tibia. **Signs** include local tenderness, negative valgus stress test, and tenderness at the medial tibial plateau.

G. OCD. Symptoms are variable; people may have intermittent vague pain, swelling, and locking. **Signs** include recurrent mild effusions, quadriceps atrophy, or tenderness along the involved chondral surface.

H. Osgood–Schlatter disease. Symptoms include gradual onset of pain and swelling in the area of the tibial tubercle. The pain is exacerbated by jumping activities, kneeling, and running and relieved by rest. **Signs** include tenderness and local swelling or prominence of the tibial tubercle. Pain can be reproduced with extension of the knee against resistance.

I. Sinding–Larsen–Johansson disease. Symptoms include pain when jumping or with direct pressure over the inferior pole of the patella. **Signs** include tenderness in the inferior pole of the patella.

J. ITB: Symptoms include aching or burning pain at the site where the band courses over the lateral femoral condyle. The pain may radiate up the thigh toward the hip. **Signs** include tenderness along the ITB as it courses over the lateral femoral condyle (approximately 2–4 cm proximal to the lateral joint line) and pain with resisted hip abduction with the knee in full extension. A positive Ober test (looking for tightness of the iliotibial band) might present weakness of the knee extensors, flexors, and hip abductors.

K. Baker cyst. Symptoms include posterior knee pain, stiffness, and swelling or complaint of posterior knee mass. The pain is worse with any knee movement and the swelling softens or disappears when bending the knee. Patients frequently report discomfort with prolonged standing and with hyperflexion of the knee. **Signs** include tenderness to palpation of the popliteal fossa, significant swelling, exacerbation of pain with resisted knee flexion, decrease in ROM, and positive Foucher sign (change in pressure in the Baker cyst with extension and flexion of the knee).

L. Plica. Diagnosis of plica syndrome is suggested by a history of anterior and medial knee pain after direct trauma, twisting injury, or repetitive injury. **Symptoms** include pain and popping or snapping when rising from a seated (knee flexed) position, catching, locking, or pseudolocking. **Signs** include tenderness medial to the patella, usually slightly proximal to the inferior pole, and a positive medial patellar plica test (Table 39–4). Atrophy of the quadriceps may develop in chronic cases.

V. Diagnostic Testing. In most patients, a careful history and focused examination will allow for accurate diagnosis without additional testing. Additional studies can be ordered if a diagnosis is in doubt or if test findings will affect decisions for additional surgical or medical treatment.

The mechanism of injury, history, and physical examination provides the key elements for determining the need for radiographs. The Ottawa Knee Rules can guide the use of radiography in adults who present with isolated knee pain in which a possibility of fracture is suspected. (SOR **Ⓐ**)

Ottawa Knee Rules: An x-ray is needed in acute trauma to the knee only when:
- Age 55 years or older
- Tenderness at the head of the fibula
- Isolated tenderness of the patella
- Inability to flex to 90 degrees
- Inability to bear weight both immediately and in the emergency department (four steps)

For example, **knee trauma** (Table 39–5) does not require radiographs if the patient is able to walk without a limp, the patient had a twisting injury, or there is no effusion. Knee radiograph is needed if there is a joint effusion within 24 hours of a direct blow or fall.

A. Ligament injury

1. MCL injury. Plain x-rays are not necessary for an isolated MCL injury. Magnetic resonance imaging (MRI) can distinguish damage between the superficial and deep layers to determine the need for surgery.

2. ACL tear. Plain radiographs (AP, lateral, tunnel, and sunrise) are not necessary; they are performed to rule out fractures. The finding of a Segond fracture (avulsion fracture of the anterolateral tibial plateau at the site of attachment of the lateral capsular ligament) suggests an ACL tear. MRI is highly sensitive and specific for the diagnosis of an ACL tear.

TABLE 39–5. AMERICAN COLLEGE OF RADIOLOGY (ACR) APPROPRIATENESS CRITERIA IN ACUTE TRAUMA TO THE KNEE

1. Fall or twisting injury, no focal tenderness, no effusion, able to walk.
   - Radiologic studies usually not appropriate
2. Fall or twisting injury with one or more of the following: focal tenderness, effusion, inability to bear weight.
   First study:
   - x-ray of the knee: usually appropriate
   - MRI knee without contrast: may be appropriate
3. Fall or twisting injury with either no fracture or a Segond fracture seen on a radiograph with one or more of the following: focal tenderness, effusion, inability to bear weight. Next study:
   - MRI knee without contrast: usually appropriate
   - CT knee without contrast: may be appropriate
4. Fall or twisting injury with a tibial plateau fracture on radiograph with one or more of the following: focal tenderness, effusion, inability to bear weight. Next study:
   - CT knee without contrast: usually appropriate
   - MRI knee without contrast: usually appropriate
5. Injury to the knee 2 days ago, mechanism unknown. Focal patellar tenderness, effusion, able to walk. First study:
   - x-ray knee: usually appropriate
   - MRI knee without contrast: may be appropriate
6. Significant trauma to the knee from motor vehicle accident, suspect posterior knee dislocation. First study:
   - x-ray knee: usually appropriate
   - MRI knee without contrast: usually appropriate
   - Magnetic resonance arterogram or angiogram (MRA) knee without and with contrast: usually appropriate
   - Arteriography lower extremity: usually appropriate
   - Computed tomography angiogram (CTA) lower extremity with contrast: usually appropriate

3. **PCL.** Cross-table lateral x-ray may show sag of the tibia compared to the opposite side. An MRI is diagnostic.

4. **LCL.** An MRI is diagnostic.

B. **Meniscal injuries.** X-rays of the knee (sunrise, tunnel, posteroanterior, and lateral views) are appropriate in some patients with suspected meniscal tear. MRI can define the extent and type of meniscal tear and is the most sensitive imaging modality for detecting small tears; however, MRI is usually not necessary unless surgery is being considered.

C. **PFS.** Films are unnecessary for initial management. If symptoms fail to improve after 1 to 2 months of conservative therapy, weight-bearing PA, weight-bearing lateral, and sunrise view x-rays are useful to exclude other pathologies. MRI, computed tomography (CT) scan, musculoskeletal (MSK) ultrasound, and radionuclide scanning are not indicated.

D. **Patellar tendinopathy.** MSK ultrasound is indicated.

E. **Patellar dislocation/subluxation.** X-rays (AP, standing 45-degree flexion weight-bearing, lateral, and axial views) and MRI should be a standard practice to detect a medial patellofemoral ligament (MPFL) rupture, osteochondral lesions, or other risk factors for redislocation.

F. **Bursitis.** X-rays are not necessary. MSK ultrasound can be used for diagnosis, aspiration, and injection.

   1. **Prepatellar bursitis.** Fluid analysis for culture, gram stain, and presence of crystals and white blood cells (WBCs) (see Chapter 38 for information of joint fluid analysis).

   2. **Septic bursitis.** WBC count is normally high, over $50,000/mm^3$, but infection can be present even if the WBC count is as low as 1400 cells/mm^3.

G. **OCD.** X-rays (AP, tunnel, lateral, Merchants) are diagnostic; MRI can detect OCD. A bone scan can detect subchondral stress.

H. **Osgood–Schlatter disease.** The diagnosis is made clinically. Plain radiographs are rarely necessary for the diagnosis of Osgood–Schlatter disease. Plain radiographs of the knee are recommended only if there is suspicion of other injuries in unilateral cases (to rule out tibial apophyseal fracture, infection, or tumor in cases of atypical symptoms). Lateral view may show irregularity of the apophysis with separation from the tibial tuberosity and fragmentation.

I. **Sinding–Larsen–Johansson disease.** Radiographs can rule out other pathology. Lateral radiograph may show soft-tissue swelling and calcification of an avulsed portion of the patella.

J. **ITB.** A clinical diagnosis is based on the history and physical examination. If the diagnosis is in doubt or other joint pathology is suspected, MRI can aid in the diagnosis and provide additional information about patients considered for surgery. MRI shows a thickened ITB over the lateral femoral epicondyle and often detects a fluid collection deep to the ITB in the same region.

K. Baker cyst. The diagnosis of a popliteal (Baker) cyst can usually be based on physical examination alone. Imaging studies are performed in some patients, particularly when there is diagnostic uncertainty and when another condition is suspected. However, imaging is usually not required.

    a. Plain films can be used to assess for knee joint arthropathy and to exclude loose bodies.

    b. MRI or ultrasound demonstrates a fluid-filled cyst extending out between the medial head of the gastrocnemius muscle and the semimembranosus tendon. "Speech bubble" sign synovial thickening may be present, especially in association with inflammatory arthropathies. Loose bodies may be present within the cyst.

    c. Cyst rupture is demonstrated as superficial edema extending distally within the calf. Fluid collections are present in the calf, both superficial and deep to the gastrocnemius muscle.

L. Plica syndrome is a clinical and arthroscopic diagnosis. Imaging does not establish the diagnosis of plica syndrome but is primarily performed to exclude other knee pathology. However, imaging is frequently required to exclude other causes of knee pain. MRI shows a curvilinear high T2 signal intensity within Hoffa fat pad in the line of the infrapatellar plica.

VI. Treatment. Focused history, examination, and testing should differentiate patients likely to improve with conservative care from those in whom urgent or eventual orthopedic referral is likely.

    A. Indications for orthopedic referral are displayed in Table 39–6.

        1. For patients with ligament injuries, consult an orthopedic surgeon or transfer to the emergency room if a patient presents with **multiple knee ligament injuries or major trauma.** Patients with **ACL injury** should be referred to an orthopedic surgeon if they have recurrent giving-way episodes, a strong desire to resume high-intensity activity, or concomitant meniscal or collateral ligament damage. (SOR Ⓒ)

        2. Consultation with an orthopedic surgeon is needed if the MRI demonstrates a **large or complex meniscal tear** or the patient continues to develop joint effusions, frequent locking of the knee, or other disabling symptoms after 4 to 6 weeks of conservative management.

        3. Consultation with an orthopedic surgeon for patients with **anserine bursitis** is suggested if two consecutive aspiration and injections fail to eliminate swelling and if the patient still complains of weight-bearing pain. Bursectomy is rarely required.

    B. For **mild soft-tissue injuries**, there is insufficient evidence in the literature to support the traditional use of **RICE** (**R**est, **I**ce, **C**ompression, and **E**levation); however, it is a commonly accepted practice for the self-management of a mild soft-tissue knee injury in the first 48 to 72 hours. (SOR Ⓒ)

TABLE 39–6. INDICATIONS FOR ORTHOPEDIC REFERRAL (SOR Ⓒ)

Urgent Referral
Red flag signs and symptoms
Neurovascular damage
Extensor mechanism rupture
Infection
Bleeding disorder
Possibility of cancer
Severe knee injury
Significant fracture on x-ray

Early Referral
Injury to the anterior cruciate ligament or posterior cruciate ligament
A locked knee owing to suspected meniscal entrapment
Equivocal diagnosis

Subsequent Referral
Suspected meniscal tear if symptoms persist after a trial of rehabilitation for 6 to 8 weeks
At any stage of the rehabilitation process where symptoms persist and clinical milestones are not being achieved

C. Nonpharmacologic treatment

1. Ligament injuries. Nonoperative management with functional rehabilitation should be the first step in the treatment of **acute isolated MCL injuries**. (SOR ⊖) RICE and a brief period of immobilization (functional or hinged brace is preferable to a straight leg knee immobilizer because it results in joint stiffness) followed by functional rehabilitation (strengthening exercises: isometric quadriceps contractions followed by isotonic exercises, then a progression of activities from walking to jogging to ¾ speed to sprinting to movement in multiple directions, and finally sports-specific drills and return to competition) is usually recommended.

a. ACL tear. A trial of conservative management may be considered if the patient has a few giving-way episodes, near normal ROM on knee extension, minimal or no meniscal damage on MRI, strong quadriceps femoris, and no difficulty performing the crossover hop test. (SOR ⊖). (For an example of the crossover hop test, see http://www.youtube.com/watch?v=aHWAHmtZi0A). RICE, crutches to avoid weight bearing, a knee brace, and early referral to physical therapy (PT) is recommended to maintain ROM and develop quadriceps strength.

Patients with a partial ACL tear can be managed nonoperatively with rehabilitation and a hinged knee brace during the early rehabilitation period. Once strength and motion of the injured leg equals that of the opposite leg, the patient may return to sports. For patients who undergo surgery, there is no benefit from the use of passive-motion machines postoperatively.

b. LCL tears are treated mostly nonoperatively with RICE, crutches, a knee brace for grade 3 sprains, and functional rehabilitation.

c. PCL tears are also treated nonoperatively for patients without instability using RICE, a knee brace, and functional rehabilitation. Hamstring strengthening and open kinetic chain exercises should be avoided, because they promote posterior translation of the tibia.

2. Meniscal injuries. A degenerated meniscus or a tear that has a stable base and is without a large mobile fragment can become asymptomatic over 4 to 6 weeks with relative rest, analgesia, pain-free exercise, and a rehabilitation brace limited to 0 to 90 degrees of knee flexion.

3. PFS. The goal of treatment is to reduce pain, improve patellofemoral tracking and alignment, and return the patient previous level of function. **PT is recommended as initial treatment**. (SOR ⓐ) General quadriceps strengthening has been found to reduce pain in patients with PFS. Also recommended are icing for 15 to 20 minutes and activity modifications (e.g., avoiding activities that cause pain and activities that load the patellofemoral joint such as stairs, hills, and squatting). Patellar bracing or taping for PFS is unlikely to produce better outcomes than PT. (SOR ⓑ)

4. Patellar tendinopathy. No single treatment has proven to result in a consistent, near-complete recovery in all patients. PT (and particularly eccentric training) is the treatment of choice. Shockwave therapy, injections, and surgery all require additional research before their use can be recommended.

5. Patellar dislocation/subluxation. Nonoperative management is the initial recommended treatment for first-time **traumatic dislocation** without any osteochondral fracture and in the absence of significant risk factors for redislocation. There is insufficient high-quality evidence to confirm any significant difference in outcome between surgical and nonsurgical initial management of people following primary patellar dislocation. Patellar stabilizing orthosis is recommended in cases of **patellar subluxation** with a knee sleeve brace with a lateral buttress to prevent lateral displacement of the patella.

a. Conservative treatment consists of immobilization followed by a period of structured rehabilitation. Acutely, a patellar reduction is performed if it did not relocate by itself. RICE, immobilization with a cylinder cast, posterior splint or removable knee brace, crutches if there is pain with weight bearing, and a posterior splint might be the best therapeutic option because of the low redislocation rates and knee joint restrictions. However, this recommendation is based on only one study with significant limitations.

b. No consensus seems to exist on the most appropriate means of conservative treatment or the duration of immobilization. PT is aimed at strengthening the quadriceps, principally the vastus medialis obliquus, and minimizing knee valgus by strengthening the hip abductors and by increasing flexibility of the hip adductors.

6. Bursitis. The treatment goal is to identify the cause and reduce swelling and inflammation.
   a. Prepatellar bursitis. Treatment consists of aspiration and drainage, padding, and protection for 3 to 4 weeks. Compression dressing is used for 24 to 36 hours after aspiration and patients are instructed to avoid direct knee pressure. Neoprene pull-on brace or Velcro knee pads can be used once the compression dressing is removed. Icing may be helpful and patients are advised to limit kneeling, bending, and squatting. Straight-leg raise exercise can be started on day 4.
   b. Anserine bursitis. Activity restriction (e.g., eliminate squatting, direct pressure [pillow between the knees at night], avoid crossing legs, limit repetitious bending), knee protection, and icing can be used for acute bursitis.
7. OCD. Symptomatic, skeletally immature patients with salvageable unstable or displaced OCD lesions should be offered the option of surgery. (SOR ©) Patients who remain symptomatic after treatment for OCD should undergo a history and physical examination, x-rays, and/or MRI to assess healing. (SOR ©) Postoperatively, the patient should be offered PT. (SOR ©)
   Unstable juvenile lesions as well as symptomatic adult lesions often require operative intervention. Short-term goals focus on symptomatic relief, whereas long-term expectations include the hope of preventing early-onset arthritis.
8. Osgood–Schlatter disease is a self-limited process that responds well to activity modification, icing, and nonsteroidal anti-inflammatory drugs (NSAIDs). PT to strengthen the quadriceps and improve quadriceps and hamstrings flexibility may help reduce symptoms in recalcitrant cases. (SOR ©) Protective padding over the tibial tubercle helps reduce trauma.
9. Sinding–Larsen–Johansson disease. This is a self-limited disease for which activity modifications, knee immobilization in severe cases, and exercises to improve hamstring, quadriceps, and heel cord flexibility are recommended.
10. ITB syndrome. The treatment goal is to reduce acute discomfort using activity modification, massage, icing, and stretching and strengthening of the affected limb.
11. Baker cyst. Conservative treatment, consisting of local heat and cold, will improve symptoms in mild cases. PT, including gentle stretching, ROM exercises, and deep-heat modalities, may be beneficial in selected patients.
12. Plica syndrome. The goals of treatment are to reduce pain, strengthen the knee extensor muscles (quadriceps), mitigate mechanical factors that produce excessive knee valgus, and return the patient to as high a level of function as possible. Traditionally, the first week focuses on activity modification and icing followed by stretching (quadriceps, hip adductors, gastrocnemius, and hamstring muscles) and quadriceps strengthening. Patients with plica syndrome exacerbated by heel valgus and mid-foot pronation can benefit from an orthotic with a medial wedge.

D. Pharmacologic (Table 39–7).
1. Topical NSAIDs can provide good pain relief without the systemic adverse events associated with oral NSAIDs when used to treat acute musculoskeletal conditions. (SOR ©) Topical NSAIDs provide good pain relief likely comparable to that provided by oral NSAIDs in acute conditions such as sprains, strains, and overuse injuries.
   a. There appears to be little difference in analgesic efficacy between topical diclofenac, ibuprofen, ketoprofen, and piroxicam, but indomethacin is less effective and benzydamine is no better than placebo.
   b. Topical NSAIDs are not associated with an increased incidence of local skin reactions compared with placebo, and do not cause systemic (mainly gastrointestinal) problems commonly seen with oral NSAIDs, making them particularly useful for individuals unable to tolerate oral administration, or for whom it is contraindicated.
   c. Topical diclofenac solution is equivalent to that of oral NSAIDs in **knee and hand osteoarthritis**, but there is no supporting evidence for use in other chronic painful conditions. Formulation can influence efficacy. The incidence of local adverse events is increased with topical NSAIDs, but gastrointestinal adverse events are reduced compared with oral NSAIDs. (SOR ©)
2. Evidence does not support the use of **topical rubefacients** containing salicylates for acute injuries and suggests that, in chronic conditions, their efficacy compares poorly with topical NSAIDs. Topical salicylates seem to be relatively well tolerated in the short term, based on limited data. There is no evidence at all for topical rubefacients with other components. (SOR ©)

TABLE 39–7. PHARMACOLOGICAL OPTIONS FOR PATIENTS WITH ACUTE MUSCULOSKELETAL CONDITIONS

Drug	Dose	Major Side Effects	Contraindications	Drug Interactions
Acetaminophen	Adult: 325–1000 mg orally every 4–6 h as needed (max. 4 g/d) Infants: 75 mg/kg/d Pediatric: 10–15 mg/kg orally every 4–6 h as needed (max. 4 g/d) >12 y 325–650 mg orally every 4–6 h as needed (max. 4 g/d)	Pruritus, constipation, nausea, headache, insomnia, agitation, atelectasis Stevens–Johnson syndrome, liver failure, pneumonitis	Hepatic disease (severe and active) or hepatic impairment	Warfarin (bleeding); carbamazepine (acetaminophen toxicity); phenytoin (risk of hepatitis); zidovudine, isoniazid (hepatotoxicity)
Diclofenac 1% gel 1.5% solution 1.3% patch Diclofenac sodium Diclofenac potassium	Adult: lower extremity joints 4 g four times daily (max. 16 g/joint/d up to 32 g/d) Pediatric: no dosing available Adult: 40 drops per knee four times daily Pediatric: no dosing available Adult: 1 patch twice daily to painful area Pediatric: no dosing available Adult: 50 mg DR orally two to three times daily; 100 mg ER orally daily Adult: 50 mg orally two to three times daily (max. 200 mg/d)	Topical: pruritus, rash, dermatitis, exfoliation, paresthesia Chest pain, HTN, headache, abdominal pain, diarrhea, dyspepsia, hematuria, edema, asthma, dyspnea, increased liver enzymes or CPK Oral: edema, dizziness, headache, pruritus, rash, abdominal pain, constipation, diarrhea, heartburn, nausea, GI ulcer/bleeding, anemia, tinnitus, liver enzyme abnormalities, renal function abnormality	Asthma, urticaria to aspirin or other NSAID, aspirin triad, pregnancy third trimester, CABG surgery perioperative use, broken or inflamed skin (patch)	**Multiple drug interactions** Cyclosporine (cyclosporine nephrotoxicity); SSRIs, anticoagulants, antiplatelet agents, low-molecular-weight heparins, duloxetine, ginkgo, venlafaxine (bleeding); methotrexate (methotrexate toxicity); potassium-sparing diuretics (reduced diuretic efficacy; hyperkalemia, nephrotoxicity); antihypertensives (decreased antihypertensive effect); quinolone antibiotics (seizures)
Ibuprofen	Adult: 400–800 mg three to four times daily (max. 3200 mg/d acutely; 2400 mg/d chronic use) Pediatric: 6 mo to 12 yr: 5–10 mg/kg/d	Rash, nausea, heartburn, constipation, diarrhea, edema, dizziness, headache, tinnitus, CHF, HTN, MI, Stevens–Johnson syndrome, GI ulcer/bleeding, hepatitis, blood abnormalities (anemia, agranulocytosis, thrombocytopenia)	Asthma, urticaria to aspirin or other NSAID, aspirin triad, pregnancy third trimester, CABG surgery perioperative use	**Multiple drug interactions** Cyclosporine (cyclosporine nephrotoxicity); SSRIs, anticoagulants, antiplatelet agents, low-molecular-weight heparins, duloxetine, ginkgo, venlafaxine (bleeding); methotrexate (methotrexate toxicity); potassium-sparing diuretics (reduced diuretic efficacy; hyperkalemia, nephrotoxicity); antihypertensives (decreased antihypertensive effect); quinolone antibiotics (seizures); tacrolimus (acute renal failure); lithium (lithium toxicity); phenytoin (phenytoin toxicity)

(continued)

TABLE 39–7. PHARMACOLOGICAL OPTIONS FOR PATIENTS WITH ACUTE MUSCULOSKELETAL CONDITIONS (*Continued*)

Drug	Dose	Major Side Effects	Contraindications	Drug Interactions
Ketoprofen	Adult: 75 mg orally three times daily (max. 300 mg/d)	See ibuprofen; liver function test abnormalities	See ibuprofen	See ibuprofen
Naproxen	Adult: 250–500 mg every 12 h (max.1250 mg acute; 1000 mg chronic use)	See ketoprofen	Asthma, urticaria to aspirin or other NSAID, aspirin triad, CABG surgery perioperative use Pregnancy category C	See ibuprofen
Naproxen sodium	Pediatric: >2 y: 10–20 mg/kg/d divided two to three times daily (max. 1000 mg/d)			
	Prescription: Adult: 275–550 mg every 12 h; max. 1650 mg/24 h			
	Nonprescription: Adult: 220–440 mg, initial then 220 mg every 8–12 h; max. 440 in 8–12 h; 660 mg in 24 h			
	Pediatric: >2 y: 11–22 mg/kg/d orally divided—two to three times daily (max. 1100 mg/d)			

NSAID, nonsteroidal anti-inflammatory drug; HTN, hypertension; CABG, coronary artery bypass grafting; SSRI, selective serotonin reuptake inhibitor; CPK, creatinine phosphokinase; GI, gastrointestinal; ER, extended release; CHF, congestive heart failure; MI, myocardial infarction.

3. **Oral acetaminophen or NSAIDs** can be used as the first-line pain treatment for most injuries (Table 39–7).
4. In one study, the use of anti-inflammatory medication via phonophoresis for ITB resulted in a significant reduction in pain compared to immobilization. For cases of **ITB lasting more than 14 days,** there appears to be benefit gained from using both combined anti-inflammatory and analgesic medication over anti-inflammatories alone.
5. **Steroid injections** are effective in the **short term for patellar tendinopathy,** but show relapse in the long term. Injection should be used sparingly because of risk of tendon rupture and primarily to provide short-term windows of pain relief to allow patients to engage in rehabilitative therapy.
   a. Glucocorticoid injections are also used for patients with prepatellar bursitis if the patient has gout, recurrent nonseptic bursitis, chronic bursal thickening, or persistent post-infectious bursitis with negative culture. Steroid injection is the **preferred initial treatment for anserine bursitis;** injection can be repeated in 6 weeks if swelling persists. Corticosteroid injection also appears to be beneficial for patients with **ITB,** with patients able to return to running pain-free within 14 days of the intervention.
   b. Injection with local anesthetic and a corticosteroid will provide symptomatic relief in patients with a **Baker cyst** if conservative therapy fails or the pain limits activities of daily living.

VII. Patient Education

A. **Ligament injury.** Following an **MCL tear,** complications rarely occur. The patient can usually return to full activities within 3 to 6 weeks.
   1. After **ACL reconstruction**, most people can return to sports within 4 to 8 weeks after they have full ROM and no joint swelling. For high-level athletes, it is usually close to a year before they are able to perform at the same level as presurgery. For people who elect not to have surgery, return to activity is variable depending on recovery time and PT.
   2. After surgical reconstruction of a **PCL injury,** most people will be in their full strength 6 to 9 months after surgery. For people who elect not to have surgery, return to activity is variable.
B. **Meniscal tears.** Recovery after a meniscal tear depends on how large the tear is, and whether the treatment is surgical or supportive.
C. **PFS** is a chronic condition that is treated with exercise and rest. Most people make a full recovery.
D. **Bursitis** is usually a self-limited condition, treated conservatively, and resolves completely within a few weeks.
E. **Osgood–Schlatter disease.** Symptoms generally resolve once the growth plate is ossified; the usual course is 6 to 18 months during which symptoms may wax and wane. Tibial prominence will persist after symptoms have resolved. Surgical treatment can alleviate symptoms in patients with mature skeletons who continue to have disabling symptoms.
F. **Sinding–Larsen–Johansson disease.** Symptoms resolve within 10 to 12 months.
G. **Baker cyst.** Surgical excision is infrequently required and is reserved for cases where more conservative interventions have failed and where there is significant functional impairment that can be ascribed to the cysts. If the cyst does not resolve in a few months, patients may need further evaluation to determine what the cause of the cyst is.

SELECTED REFERENCES

Bachman LM, Haberzeth S, Steurer J, et al. The accuracy of the Ottawa knee rule to rule out knee fractures: a systematic review. *Ann Int Med.* 2004;140(2):121–124.

Ebell MH. A tool for evaluating patients with knee injury. *Am Fam Physician.* 2005;12(3):69–72.

Ellis MR, Griffin KW, Meadows S, et al. For knee pain, how predictive is physical examination for meniscal injury? *J Fam Pract.* 2004;53(11):918–921.

Harris GR, Susman JL. Managing musculoskeletal complaints with rehabilitation therapy: summary of the Philadelphia Panel evidence-based clinical practice guidelines on musculoskeletal rehabilitation interventions. *J Fam Pract.* 2002;51(12):1042–1046.

Holten KB. How should we diagnose and treat osteoarthritis of the knee? *J Fam Pract.* 2004;53(2): 134–136.

Jackson JL, O'Malley PG, Kroenke K, et al. Evaluation of acute knee pain in primary care. *Ann Int Med.* 2003;139(7):575–588.

New Zealand Guidelines Group (NZGG). *The Diagnosis and Management of Soft Tissue Knee Injuries: Internal Derangements.* Wellington, NZ: New Zealand Guidelines Group (NZGG); 2003:100.

Okazaki K, Matsuda S, Yasunaga T, et al. Assessment of anterolateral rotatory instability in the anterior cruciate ligament-deficient knee using an open magnetic resonance imaging system. *Am J Sports Med.* 2007;35(7):1091–1097.

Robb G, Reid D, Arroll B, et al. General practitioner diagnosis and management of acute knee injuries: summary of an evidence-based guideline. *N Z Med J.* 2007;120(1249):U2419.

Scholten RJ, Opstelten WI, Van der Plas CG, et al. Accuracy of physical diagnostic tests for assessing ruptures of the anterior cruciate ligament: a meta-analysis. *J Fam Pract.* 2003;52(9):689–694.

Solomon DH, Simel DL, Bates DW, et al. Does this patient have a torn meniscus or ligament of the knee? Value of the physical examination. *JAMA.* 2001;286(13):1610–2160.

Zuber TJ. Knee joint aspiration and injection. *Am Fam Physician.* 2002;66:1497–1512.

WEB RESOURCES

ACL: http://orthoinfo.aaos.org/topic.cfm?topic=A00549
http://www.aafp.org/afp/2010/1015/p923.html
PCL injury: http://orthoinfo.aaos.org/topic.cfm?topic=A00420
Meniscal tears: http://orthoinfo.aaos.org/topic.cfm?topic=A00358
PFS: http://www.aafp.org/afp/1999/1101/p2019.html
http://familydoctor.org/familydoctor/en/diseases-conditions/patellofemoral-pain-syndrome.html
Osgood-Schlatter disease: http://familydoctor.org/familydoctor/en/diseases-conditions/osgood-schlatter-disease.html http://orthoinfo.aaos.org/topic.cfm?topic=A00411
Osteochondrosis dissecans: http://familydoctor.org/familydoctor/en/diseases-conditions/osteochondritis-dissecans.html

Additional references are available online at http://langetextbooks.com/fm6e

---

40   Lacerations and Skin Biopsy

Jason Chao, MD, MS, & Rasai L. Ernst, MD

KEY POINTS

- The goals of laceration repair are to gently appose tissue so that normal healing may take place, and to minimize complications, especially infection and unsightly scars. (SOR **C**)
- Anesthesia may be accomplished using topical anesthetic or injection. (SOR **A**)
- Wound closure options include sutures, cyanoacrylate adhesive, staples, adhesive tape, and allowing healing by secondary intention. (SOR **C**)

I. Definition. A laceration is a cut or tear in the skin or mucosa that extends through the epidermis into deeper, underlying tissues. Lacerations can result in two ways: (1) from a **shearing force** that slices through the skin or (2) from **blunt trauma** that compresses or stretches the skin. Blunt trauma requires greater energy and results in more extensive tissue damage. This creates an increased inflammatory response and contributes to additional scarring and greater risk of infection.

Tensile strength of the healing wound increases most rapidly during the first 3 weeks. Sutures should be removed by 2 weeks to minimize suture scars, and dehiscence may occur at this time. Local factors that increase infection rates include poor local blood supply and the presence of any necrotic tissue, foreign bodies, hematoma, or dead space.

II. Common Diagnoses. Lacerations and open wound injuries occur in 5 to 10 of every 100 persons each year in the United States. These wounds constitute one-quarter of all injuries in this country, occurring mostly in the home environment. Lacerations are more common among males and happen more frequently during the summer. There is a bimodal age distribution, with one peak of lacerations occurring in persons younger than 5 years and a second peak occurring in persons between 18 and 24 years of age.

    A. In **superficial wounds,** the surface epidermis is left intact by contusions or bruises or is abraded, leaving underlying tissue intact.

    B. In **puncture wounds,** a small surface opening may hide a deeper, serious injury. An electrical or chemical wound with a break in the skin requires special attention since the patient may have severe soft-tissue injury that is not apparent initially.

    C. **In clean lacerations,** there is no contamination with foreign matter.

    D. **Wounds with extensive tissue loss or injury** include dirty lacerations, compound lacerations, and electrical wounds.

III. **Signs and Symptoms.** Lacerations cause **pain, bleeding,** and **swelling**.

    A. **Tissue damage**

        1. A partial or complete severing of bones, muscles, tendons, ligaments, major blood vessels, or nerves can occur in **compound lacerations**.

            a. Loss of a pulse or slow capillary refill after the application of pressure distal to wounds may indicate a vascular injury that must be treated.

            b. Sensorineural function distal to wounds should be assessed before anesthesia is administered. Loss of sensation or movement suggests a nerve injury that should be investigated. Poor finger flexion or extension indicative of a tendon injury is common in hand lacerations because the hand lacks subcutaneous fat.

        2. **Dirty lacerations** are contaminated with foreign matter. The depth and degree of contamination of lacerations and the surrounding tissue must be assessed. Full exploration of wounds is best performed after administration of anesthesia.

        3. Inflammatory reaction with surrounding erythema begins several hours after the patient sustains a laceration. Marked erythema or pus signifies wounds that are not recent and are probably infected.

IV. **Laboratory Tests**

    B. A **deep wound culture** after debridement is usually indicated if the laceration is dirty, more than 24 hours old, or obviously infected. (SOR **C**) The culture results are helpful as a guide in wound treatment if it does not improve with initial therapy.

    C. **X-rays** may be appropriate for patients with compound or deep lacerations to evaluate for associated fracture, subcutaneous air, or a foreign body. Most glass is visible on x-ray. Wood may or may not be visible on x-ray.

V. **Treatment.** The goals of treatment are to assist the healing process by approximating the wound when possible and to minimize complications, including infection and unsightly scars.

    A. **Wound preparation.** Most bleeding can be stopped by the application of direct pressure for 10 to 15 minutes. Hemostasis of active bleeders can be obtained using ligation, electrocautery, or Gelfoam.

        1. Thorough cleansing of the wound is performed to ensure that no foreign body is left in the wound.

            a. Gentle rinsing with saline solution is an adequate cleanser for many lacerations. Antiseptic solutions such as hydrogen peroxide, alcohol, Betadine, and Hibiclens should not be used because these disinfectants inhibit the wound repair process. (SOR **B**) Adding antibiotics to the lavage solution does not contribute to wound cleansing. (SOR **A**)

            b. Dirty lacerations should be forcefully irrigated with copious amounts of sterile saline. A 20- to 50-mL syringe and a 19-gauge needle should be used. Sharp debridement with a scalpel or scissor is sometimes necessary to remove the most contaminated tissue. Scrubbing the wound should be avoided if possible in order to prevent additional trauma.

            c. Areas such as the face and the neck that have a rich blood supply require less debridement than other areas.

        2. If hair removal is required, clipping with scissors is preferable to using a straight razor, to reduce tissue trauma. Eyebrows should not be shaved, since they grow slowly and a defect in the eyebrows is very noticeable.

        3. Wound edges should be perpendicular to the skin surface. If they are beveled, skin should be removed to produce a sharp perpendicular edge that will approximate with the other side. Small skin flaps with inadequate blood supply should be excised to ensure that the skin at the margins of the laceration is vascularized.

        4. If tissue is missing, preventing easy closure of the wound, consider undermining the subcutaneous layers to free the overlying skin, which will allow approximation of the skin margins.

B. Anesthesia is used for pain relief and to aid in adequate examination, debridement, and repair. Landmarks that need to be approximated should be identified and marked before local anesthesia is administered to prevent distortion.

   1. Local infiltration of the wound with anesthesia is often sufficient. A slow injection (i.e., for more than 10 seconds) of 1% **lidocaine hydrochloride** through a 27-gauge needle is commonly used. Mixing the lidocaine with **sodium bicarbonate** in a ratio of 9:1 will reduce the pain of injection. This procedure provides adequate anesthesia for as long as 2 hours.

   2. Epinephrine, a vasoconstrictor, may be included in an injection with lidocaine except in an area with reduced circulation such as the fingers, toes, tip of the nose, penis, or earlobes. Contaminated wounds should not be injected with epinephrine because these wounds become easily infected when their blood supply is reduced.

   3. Topical anesthetic avoids painful injection, and it does not distort local landmarks. LAT (4% lidocaine, 1:2000 adrenaline, and 0.5% tetracaine) or TAC (0.5% tetracaine, 1:2000 adrenaline, and 11.8% cocaine) can be used, especially in children. However, serious complications including seizures and death have been reported with improper use. Anesthesia using lidocaine and prilocaine (EMLA) cream is more effective, but can take up to an hour to become effective, compared with a half hour using LAT or TAC.

   4. A **regional block** may be suitable for wounds that are very large or involve the distal fingers or toes.

C. Skin biopsies

   1. For a diffuse skin eruption, a new or fresh lesion should be chosen. In blistering disorders, a rim of normal tissue should be included. Complete removal of a small- to moderate-sized lesion can serve both diagnostic and therapeutic purposes. If malignancy is a concern, adequate margins around the lesion should be obtained.

   2. Shave biopsy is indicated for benign exophytic lesions such as warts, seborrheic keratoses and skin tags, and superficial noduloulcerative processes. A shave biopsy should not be performed if melanoma is suspected, because they are graded on the depth of invasion. Local anesthetic infiltrated around and under the lesion makes it easier to perform the shave. A scalpel blade or flexible razor is positioned almost parallel to the skin surface, and the skin specimen is obtained in a single gentle scoop under the lesion, leaving a shallow defect with smooth borders (see https://www.youtube.com/watch?v=nbdmmukko4s). Pick-ups may be used to assist in lifting the lesion. This wound is left to heal by secondary intention. Shave biopsies heal best by using a wet healing technique, achieved by covering the biopsy site continuously with petroleum jelly. Antibiotic ointment is discouraged because many patients develop subacute allergic reactions.

   3. Punch biopsy is indicated for diagnosis in diffuse eruptions, deeper lesions, suspected vasculitis, or other inflammatory lesions requiring direct immunofluorescence. After cleansing the skin and adequate anesthesia, the skin should be stretched perpendicular to skin tension lines. The other hand is used to twist the punch into the skin down to the plastic hub of the punch. The plug of skin is gently removed and cut at the base with scissors or blade (see https://www.youtube.com/watch?v=gd7j-wYwryY). A 4-mm punch is generally adequate. Smaller punches may be useful in cosmetically important areas, but have a lower diagnostic yield. Larger lesions may require up to a 6-mm punch. Any punch biopsy 4 mm or greater should be closed with sutures as described below.

   4. Excisional or incisional biopsy is indicated for most pigmented lesions, suspected malignancies, and deep or subcutaneous lesions. After cleansing the skin and adequate anesthesia, a fusiform-shaped cut is made around the lesion. The length of the biopsy should be three times its width.

D. Wound repair

   1. Wound closure. When clean lacerations present within 12 to 24 hours, they can be closed primarily. Lacerations closed during this "golden period" are likely to heal without infection. Head wounds with good blood supply may be closed even after 24 hours and still heal well. (SOR **B**) Lacerations with extensive devitalized tissue or evidence of infection require thorough debriding, but should not be closed primarily. Delayed closure, 3 to 4 days later, may be performed if the wound appears free of infection and is adequately supplied with blood. The following techniques may also be used to close clean surgical wounds.

TABLE 40-1. WOUND CLOSURE

Site of Wound	Size of Subcutaneous Suture (Absorbable)	Size of Surface Suture (Nonabsorbable)	Time to Removal (d)
Scalp	#4-0 or #5-0	#3-0 or #4-0	5–7
Face	#5-0 or #6-0	#6-0 or #7-0	3–5
Trunk and extremities	#3-0 or #4-0	#4-0 or #5-0	7–10
Hands, feet, and skin over joints	None	#3-0 or #4-0	7–14

2. **Equipment.** The equipment required to repair a laceration includes a needle holder, smooth and toothed small forceps, scissors, small hemostats, a scalpel, sterile gauze, suture material, gloves, and drapes. Skin hooks are optional; they allow less traumatic handling of the skin. A disposable skin hook can be created by gently bending a needle with a hemostat. Adequate lighting is essential.

   The choice of suture material depends on the location and purpose of the suture (Table 40–1).

   a. **Absorbable sutures** should be used for dermal or fascial layer repair or for ligation of vessels. They lose their tensile strength by gradual degradation over days to weeks. Synthetic absorbable polymers (e.g., Dexon, Vicryl, polydioxanone (PDS), or Maxon) retain their tensile strength longer than does plain or chromic gut.

   b. **Nonabsorbable sutures** should be used for epidermal repair. Nonabsorbable sutures include silk, cotton, synthetic monofilament nylon or polypropylene (e.g., Ethilon, Dermalon, Prolene, Surgilene, or Deklene), and braided polyester. Nonabsorbable sutures remain strong, but induce a cellular reaction and increase the likelihood of infection in dirty wounds. Synthetic monofilament is the most commonly used material for the final epidermal closure.

3. **Placement of sutures.** Tissue should be handled gently to minimize additional trauma to the wound.

   a. **Dermal sutures** are used to approximate larger wounds, close dead space, and provide hemostasis and tensile strength. Sutures in fat lead to infection and should be avoided. An inverted suture will bury the knot deep in the wound.

   b. **Skin sutures** should approximate the wound edges and not be tied too tightly. Excessive tightness of sutures restricts blood flow and produces a depressed scar that is more noticeable.

   c. **Simple interrupted sutures** (Figure 40–1) are the most commonly used epidermal suture and provide good cosmetic repair. The deep portion of the suture should be wider than the surface to help evert the skin edges and prevent a depressed scar (see https://www.youtube.com/watch?v=Jix6-EF1tc0). **Vertical mattress sutures** (Figure 40–2) evert skin edges more than do simple sutures, but they are time-consuming and may lead to increased inflammatory reaction.

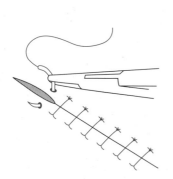
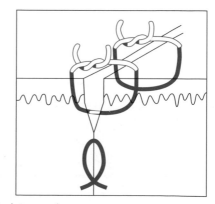

FIGURE 40–1. Simple interrupted suture.

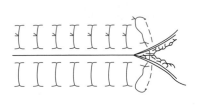

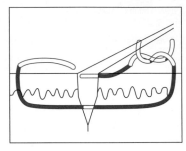

FIGURE 40-2. Vertical mattress suture.

Half-buried horizontal mattress sutures (Figure 40-3) are useful when the patient has skin flaps that appear viable. These sutures are least likely to compromise vascular supply to the flap.

d. **Running simple sutures** (Figure 40-4) provide the fastest repair; however, they are generally not used in cosmetically important areas (see https://www.youtube.com/watch?v=ol8hGoYEnTM). **Locked running sutures** (Figure 40-5) are particularly useful when the laceration is in mucosal surfaces, such as the vagina and the rectum. Absorbable suture material should be used. **Subcuticular (buried running) sutures** (see https://www.youtube.com/watch?v=sgOaBojcX-c) are time-consuming, but produce good cosmetic results without suture marks when used to close small, clean lacerations. Absorbable sutures may be used. If nonabsorbable sutures are used, the ends should be left on the outside of the skin so the suture can be easily removed.

e. In patients with facial lacerations, slight misalignments in repair of the eyebrows and the vermilion border of the lips become very noticeable even at a distance. The first sutures that are placed should align the edges of these structures. Lacerations inside the mouth do not need to be closed primarily. For through-and-through wounds, the skin and muscle should be closed, and the oral mucosa should be left alone to heal by secondary intention.

f. For patients with scalp lacerations, choosing a suture of a color different from that of the patient's hair helps the physician in repairing the laceration and during suture removal.

g. Discussion of Z-plasty and other plastic techniques is beyond the scope of this chapter. These techniques can be used on patients with long lacerations that do not follow the natural contours of the body or with lacerations over joints that are likely to involve excessive motion during the healing process.

E. **Tissue adhesive for closure**
   1. **Octylcyanoacrylate** (Dermabond) tissue adhesive has **comparable cosmetic outcome to suturing** in repair of selected traumatic lacerations. (SOR **Ⓐ**) Tissue adhesive closure is **faster** and **less painful** than suturing. Skin moisture is the catalyst for the adhesive to polymerize, generating heat.
   2. Most **facial and selected trunk and extremity lacerations** are suitable for tissue adhesive closure. It should not be used on hands or over joints.

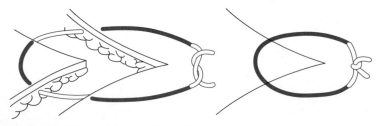

FIGURE 40-3. Half-buried horizontal mattress suture.

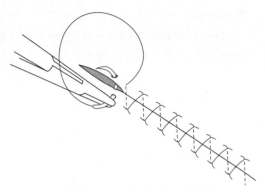

FIGURE 40-4. Running, or continuous, simple suture.

   3. When using topical tissue adhesive, care should be taken to **keep adhesive out of the wound,** which would act as a foreign body and inhibit wound healing.
   4. Wound edges should be opposed when applying the first layer of adhesive, and the adhesive should dry for 3 minutes between layers. A minimum of **three layers** of adhesive should be applied.
   5. The patient should be instructed to **avoid washing or soaking** the wound but may get it wet, as in a shower.
F. Staples. Staples can be applied quickly, but accurate placement may be difficult and they are more painful to remove than sutures. Infection rates are comparable to those of sutures.
G. Prevention of infection
   1. The physician should provide **tetanus immunization** if it is indicated (Table 40-2).
   2. Prophylactic antibiotics are not necessary except in selected cases, such as in patients with dirty compound lacerations and in patients with lacerations that involve significant tissue ischemia because of blunt trauma. Most patients with bite wounds should receive antibiotics.
H. Patient education. Patients should be given the following advices.
   1. Keep the wound clean and dry for the first 24 hours, after which the dressing should be removed, and the wound should be cleaned daily.
   2. Contact a physician if any of the following occur: (1) redness, excessive swelling, tenderness, or increased warmth of the skin around the wound; (2) pus or watery discharge; (3) tender bumps or swelling in an armpit or groin area; (4) red streaks appear in the skin near the wound; (5) a foul smell is coming from the wound; or, (6) generalized body chills or fever develop.
   3. Elevate an extremity with a laceration to reduce swelling.

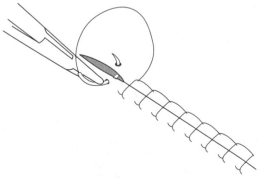

FIGURE 40-5. Locked running suture.

TABLE 40–2. GUIDE TO TETANUS PROPHYLAXIS

	Immunization Status (Doses of Tetanus Toxoid Received)	
Types of Wound	Uncertain, <3, or None Within the Last 5 y	≥3 (Booster Within 5 y)
Clean wound	Td[a]	No prophylaxis necessary
Dirty wound[b]	Td,[a] and human tetanus immune globulin, at different site	Consider human tetanus immune globulin

Source: Modified with permission from Chesnutt MS, Dewar TN, Locksley RM. *Office & Bedside Procedures.* New York:, NY: Appleton & Lange; 1992.
[a]Adult tetanus and diphtheria toxoids, 0.5 mL intramuscularly. If the patient is younger than 7 yr, diphtheria–tetanus or diphtheria–tetanus–pertussis is given intramuscularly.
[b]A wound that is grossly contaminated is more than 8-h old, contains devitalized tissue, or is of a form that prevents adequate irrigation.

4. **Limit activity** somewhat for 1 week after the sutures are removed to avoid reopening the wound. Wound healing takes several weeks.
5. **Use sunscreen** to protect the scar from sunlight in order to avoid marked pigment changes that occur in lighter-skinned patients. A scar normally appears red and slightly raised or thickened for several months after an injury.

VI. **Patient Follow-up.** See Table 40–1 concerning the timing of suture removal.

   A. The physician should see patients with contaminated wounds or deep lacerations 48 hours after sutures are placed.
   B. When lacerations are in areas of tension, every other suture may be removed initially and replaced by adhesive bandages, with tincture of benzoin applied to the normal skin to prolong bandage adhesion. The remaining sutures should be removed several days later.

SELECTED REFERENCES

Forsch RT. Essentials of skin laceration repair. *Am Fam Physician.* 2008;78(8):945–951.
Leach J. Proper handling of soft tissue in the acute phase. *Facial Plast Surg.* 2001;17:227–238.
Sheth VM, Weitzul S. Postoperative topical antimicrobial use. *Dermatitis.* 2008;19(4):181–189.
Wilson JL, Kocurek K, Doty BJ. A systematic approach to laceration repair: tricks to ensure the desired cosmetic result. *Postgrad Med.* 2000;107:77–83, 87–88.
Zuber TJ. The mattress sutures: vertical, horizontal, and corner stitch. *Am Fam Physician.* 2002;66: 2231–2236.

41   Leg and Hip Complaints

Geoffrey S. Kuhlman, MD, CAQSM, FAAFP

KEY POINTS

- Leg and hip complaints in children and adolescents often reflect serious conditions and should be treated as such until proved otherwise. (SOR **C**)
- Leg pain in athletic individuals is usually caused by overuse injuries, including stress fracture or medial tibial stress syndrome. (SOR **C**)
- The history and physical examination should guide appropriate diagnostic testing in the evaluation of hip and leg complaints. (SOR **C**)

I. **Definition. Hip complaints** arise from processes in the hip joint (e.g., transient synovitis, bacterial infection, avascular necrosis of the femoral head, slipped capital femoral epiphysis [SCFE], femoroacetabular impingement, osteoarthritis, rheumatoid arthritis), other soft tissues (e.g., bursitis), or neurovascular structures (e.g., meralgia paresthetica). **Leg complaints** arise in the lower extremity proximal to the ankle from infection (e.g., osteomyelitis of the long bones), joints (e.g., osteoarthritis), muscle (e.g., nocturnal leg cramps), vasculature

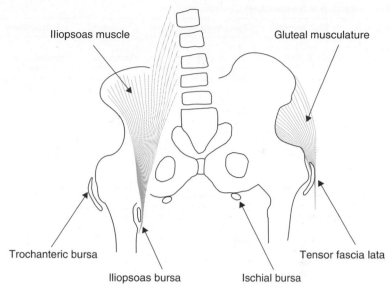

FIGURE 41-1. Bursae of the hip and pelvis.

(e.g., arterial insufficiency, deep vein thrombosis [DVT], or varicose veins), neuropathy; over-use (e.g., stress fracture, medial tibia stress syndrome, or chronic compartment syndrome), or idiopathic etiologies (e.g., growing pains).

II. Common Diagnoses (Table 41-1 and Figures 41-1 to 41-4). Hip and leg complaints are commonly seen in Family Medicine. Some causes demand urgent attention, such as

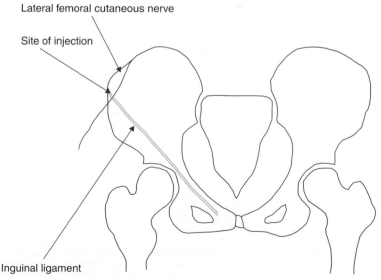

FIGURE 41-2. Meralgia paresthetica. The lateral femoral cutaneous nerve is compressed under the inguinal ligament medial to the anterior superior iliac spine (ASIS). Therapeutic injection is performed 1 cm medial to the ASIS (see text).

TABLE 41–1. EVALUATION OF COMMON HIP AND LEG COMPLAINTS

Diagnosis	Risk Factors	Symptoms and Signs	Testing	Treatment
Children				
Septic hip arthritis	Infants/toddlers	Rapid-onset, constant hip thigh/knee pain, worse with movement, failure to thrive Febrile/ill, thigh edema Flexed/abducted/externally rotated hip	Elevated WBC; plain x-rays show lateral displacement of femoral head; ESR; hip US guides needle aspiration	Hospitalization, orthopedic consultation, IV antibiotics
Transient synovitis	3- to 10-year-olds; M:F ratio, 2:1; recent upper respiratory infection	Insidious or acute painful limp Afebrile, voluntary limited hip range of motion	Hip US shows effusion CBC, ESR normal	Rest, NSAID
Perthes disease	4- to 10-year-olds M:F ratio, 5:1	Insidious pain/stiffness of groin/lateral hip/medial knee, then limp Antalgic gait, decreased hip range of motion, occasional flexion contracture	Crescent sign on x-ray (Figure 41–3), followed by progressive changes in femoral epiphysis/femoral head	Crutches, non-weight bearing on affected leg, orthopedic surgeon referral
Growing pains	15% of children 4- to 14-year-olds	Intermittent bilateral nocturnal thigh and lower leg pain Normal examination	None	Reassurance Acetaminophen
SCFE	Obese early adolescence M:F ratio 3:2	Groin/buttock/lateral hip or knee pain, simultaneous pain + limp in 50% Antalgic gait, hip externally rotated	X-ray (Figures 41–3 and 41–4)	Crutches, non-weight bearing on affected leg, orthopedic surgeon referral
Young Adults and Athletes (more common in this group)				
Chronic compartment syndromes	Late teen to early 20s, distance runners/sprinters/basketball players/soccer players	Gradual exercise-associated achiness: anterolateral (anterior compartment) calf pain/plantar paresthesia (posterior compartment), lateral lower leg achiness: lateral compartment) Involved muscle groups tender during/shortly after exercise; normal examination after adequate rest	Compartment pressure measurement immediately after exercise (by orthopedist or physiatrist)	Reduce activity Elective fasciotomy
Iliopsoas bursitis	Sports (e.g., soccer) requiring repetitive hip flexion/adduction	Deep groin pain, worse with hip extension Tender and cystic mass (30%) over bursa (Figure 41–1), limited hip extension	US detects enlarged bursa MRI if US is unavailable	NSAID Stretching psoas muscle Cortisone injection
Medial tibial stress syndrome	Adolescent/early adult runners, sudden increased training	Achy posteromedial distal tibia, initially during exercise, progressing to rest pain Tender medial edge, distal third of tibia	None MRI or bone scan have typical appearances	Ice Physical therapy Arch support
Stress fractures	Late teen to early adult athletes, increase in physical activity; oligomenorrhea/weight loss	Insidious local pain: tibia (34%), fibula (24%), metatarsal (20%), femur (14%), pelvic (6%) Focal bone tenderness, poorly resolving soft tissue symptoms	X-ray shows periosteal reaction, then fracture (2–4 wk after symptom onset) MRI or bone scan more sensitive, positive upon symptoms	Rest, limiting activity to be pain-free Avoid masking pain with analgesics Refer hip, femur shaft, and anterior tibia cortex stress fractures

TABLE 41–1. EVALUATION OF COMMON HIP AND LEG COMPLAINTS (Continued)

Diagnosis	Risk Factors	Symptoms and Signs	Testing	Treatment
Adults				
Ischial bursitis	Prolonged sitting on hard surfaces	Buttock pain, worse with sitting Tender ischial tuberosity (Figure 41–1), painful SLR	US detects enlarged bursa MRI if US is unavailable	NSAID Seat cushion Cortisone injection
Meralgia paresthetica	Abdominal obesity, middle-aged men, pregnancy	Anterolateral thigh pain, paresthesia Reproduced by pressing lateral femoral cutaneous nerve against anterior superior iliac spine (Figure 41–2)	None, NCV if diagnosis in question	Loose clothing Abdominal weight loss Cortisone injection
OA/RA	90% of adult hip pain	Stiffness after rest, insidious pain referred to groin/thigh/knee Limp, decreased hip range of motion, especially internal rotation/abduction	X-ray—spurring, narrowed joint space, periarticular sclerosis (OA)	Acetaminophen, NSAID, physical therapy for strength and flexibility Hip replacement in refractory cases
Trochanter bursitis	40- to 60-year-old women	Thigh, posterolateral hip pain Tender greater trochanter Increased with resisted abduction (Figure 41–1)	US detects enlarged bursa MRI if US is unavailable	Ice, NSAID Cortisone injection
All Ages				
DVT	Immobility, leg trauma, hypercoagulable state, major surgery, history of DVT or cancer, estrogen therapy, CHF, pregnancy, atrial arrhythmias	Variable, nonspecific unilateral swelling, pain, erythema Edema/red/warm ($\geq$50% of DVTs not clinically detectable)	Duplex US (proximal DVT), D-dimer assay, contrast venography	Anticoagulation
Nocturnal leg cramps	All ages, pregnancy, neuromuscular disease, alcoholism, diabetes, flat feet electrolyte disorders	Abrupt nocturnal calf, plantar cramps Tender affected muscles	Serum electrolytes if abnormality suspected	Treat underlying disorder Stretch calves at bedtime Magnesium, vitamin B complex, calcium channel blocker

CHF, congestive heart failure; CT, computerized tomography; DVT, deep vein thrombosis; ESR, erythrocyte sedimentation rate; M:F, male:female; MRI, magnetic resonance imaging; NCV, nerve conduction velocity; NSAID, nonsteroidal anti-inflammatory drug; OA, osteoarthritis; RA, rheumatoid arthritis; SCFE, slipped capital femoral epiphysis; SLR, straight leg raising.

osteomyelitis, septic arthritis, and SCFE. Many of the less urgent diagnoses are quite debilitating for patients causing significant pain, inability to work or exercise, or difficulty sleeping. Likely causes of hip and leg complaints depend on the patient's age and activity.

   A. Hip complaints in **children and adolescents** include transient synovitis, septic arthritis, Perthes disease, and SCFE.

   1. Transient synovitis is acute nonspecific inflammation in the hip joint and is the most common atraumatic cause of hip pain in childhood. Risk factors include antecedent upper respiratory infection, recurrent microtrauma, or allergic hypersensitivity.

   2. Septic arthritis of the hip joint can occur at any age but is most common in infants, toddlers, and the elderly. Risk factors include wounds, skin infection, hip surgery, diabetes mellitus, human immunodeficiency virus (HIV), and other immunocompromised conditions.

   3. Perthes disease, avascular necrosis of the femoral head, is bilateral 12% of the time. Low birth weight and family history are risk factors, but the cause is unknown and no consistent hereditary pattern exists.

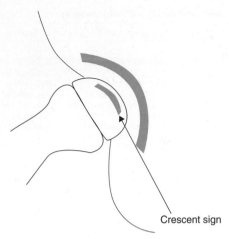

FIGURE 41–3. Crescent sign. In Perthes disease or in avascular necrosis of the hip in an adult, a radiographic finding is the crescent sign, a curvilinear lucency along the articular surface of the head of the femur.

AVASCULAR NECROSIS

Atraumatic **avascular necrosis of the femoral head** begins between ages 25 and 45 years. Predisposing factors in 75% of cases include systemic corticosteroid therapy, alcoholism, sickle cell disease, or dysbaric trauma (underground or undersea work). Avascular necrosis presents with abrupt hip pain followed by progressive, intermittent episodes in 85% of patients, worsened by movement. Rest pain is present in two-thirds of patients and night pain in 40%. Findings on examination include limp and limited abduction/internal rotation.

Plain radiographs have a 19% false-negative rate early in avascular necrosis. Initial plain radiographic findings include a crescent sign (Figure 41–3), with bone collapse and degenerative arthritic changes occurring later.

Radioisotope bone scans increase sensitivity in detecting avascular necrosis, and magnetic resonance imaging (MRI) scanning is the most sensitive, specific, and low-risk means of making this diagnosis.

Management of avascular necrosis involves orthopedic consultation for possible core decompression or, for more advanced disease, hip arthroplasty.

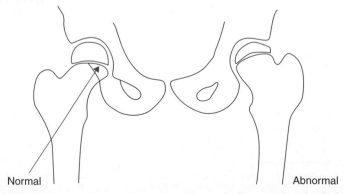

FIGURE 41–4. In SCFE, an early radiographic finding is loss of the triangle of Caper. On the right side of the picture, the entire ischium is seen (normal view). On the left side of the picture, slippage of the femoral epiphysis causes the femur metaphysis to shift medially, obscuring part of the ischium (abnormal view).

4. SCFE is slippage of the proximal femur while the epiphysis remains in its position in the acetabulum. SCFE occurs in early adolescence and is bilateral in 25% to 40% of cases. Obesity is a risk factor.

B. Hip complaints in **adults** include impingement, osteoarthritis, rheumatoid arthritis, bursitis, meralgia paresthetica, referred pain (lumbar spine or pelvis), avascular necrosis, septic arthritis, and malignancy. Hip bursitis is usually associated with trauma or overuse.

C. Leg complaints in infants and toddlers (0–3 years) include septic arthritis of the hip, osteomyelitis, and fracture.

OSTEOMYELITIS

Risk factors for osteomyelitis in children include male gender (male:female ratio of 2:1), lower socioeconomic status, immunocompromise, and the autumn season. Osteomyelitis presents with rapid-onset leg pain and refusal to walk in children. Findings include fever ≥38°C (100.4°F), ill appearance, and redness/warmth/tenderness of the involved region with limited motion of adjacent joints.

Early in osteomyelitis, plain radiographs show loss of normal fascial planes and fat shadows due to edema. Bony changes appear 7 to 10 days after symptoms and include the following: (1) destruction, with or without periosteal elevation, (2) fading cortical margins, and (3) absence of adjacent reactive new bone. Radioisotope bone scanning detects osteomyelitis before plain radiographs, and MRI is the most sensitive, specific, low-risk means of diagnosing osteomyelitis.

Suspected osteomyelitis requires hospitalization for blood cultures and prolonged parenteral antibiotics.

D. Leg complaints in children (4–14 years) include transient synovitis of the hip, Perthes disease, SCFE, growing pains, and a variety of injuries. Growing pains are idiopathic.

E. Common leg complaints in adolescents (11–16 years) are SCFE, growing pains, and knee disorders such as Osgood–Schlatter disease and Sindig–Larsen–Johansson syndrome (see Chapter 39); risk factors for which include jumping activities, weak hip muscles, and tight quadriceps muscles.

F. Leg complaints in athletic adolescents and adults

    1. Medial tibia stress syndrome, periostitis of the origin of the soleus muscle on the distal posteromedial aspect of the tibia, typically develops from repetitive dorsiflexion, as in running.

    2. Stress fractures commonly occur in the tibia or fibula of athletes who run or jump, such as in cross country, track and field, soccer, and basketball. Risk factors include increased activity, abnormal weight loss, inadequate intake of calcium or vitamin D, hyperthyroidism, and hyperparathyroidism.

    3. Chronic compartment syndrome is ischemic or neuropathic pain resulting from increased muscle mass within an unyielding compartment. **Posterior compartment syndromes** are common in cyclists; **lateral compartment syndromes** are common in football and soccer players.

    4. Other causes include patellofemoral pain, iliotibial band syndrome, muscle strain, and peripheral nerve or artery entrapment.

G. Leg complaints in adults

    1. DVT occurs in the setting of venous stasis, venous injury, or increased blood coagulability (see Chapter 64).

    2. Nocturnal leg cramps are sudden contraction of the plantar flexor muscles causing painful cramps during sleep.

    3. Other causes include patellofemoral pain (see Chapter 39), iliotibial band syndrome (see Chapter 39), peripheral neuropathy, peripheral arterial disease, acquired spinal stenosis, cancer, osteoarthritis (see Chapter 82), gout and other crystal arthropathies, and rheumatoid arthritis.

PERIPHERAL NEUROPATHIES

Peripheral neuropathies can be classified as **mononeuropathy** (a single nerve affected, usually owing to trauma, compression, or entrapment [e.g., common peroneal neuropathy at the fibular head causing dorsal foot/lateral calf sensory loss and weakened foot dorsiflexion and eversion]) or **polyneuropathy** (affecting multiple nerves simultaneously). Polyneuropathy can be classified as axonal or demyelinating. The **axonal** type involves distal sensory, burning, or tingling progressing proximally in a stocking/glove distribution and initially affecting fine touch and temperature (e.g., diabetes, vitamin B_{12} deficiency, Lyme disease, uremia, drugs, toxins, or HIV). The **demyelinating** type manifests early with diffuse loss of reflexes and strength (e.g., Guillain–Barré syndrome, multiple myeloma, or chronic inflammatory demyelinating polyneuropathy).

In approaching a patient with peripheral neuropathy, it is important to assess risk factors (e.g., history of recent viral illness, chronic systemic disease, new medications, and occupational or other exposure to toxins, such as alcohol/pesticides/heavy metals); distribution (i.e., likely mono- versus polyneuropathy); and rapidity of onset. (With regard to rapidity of onset, massive intoxications or Guillain–Barré syndrome develop over days to weeks; many toxins will develop over weeks to months; and diabetic, hereditary, or dysproteinemic neuropathies evolve over months to years.)

Examination confirms/localizes deficits (i.e., sensation, reflexes, strength, or proprioception). Further testing is based on the foregoing clinical evaluation; helpful basic testing when the cause is not clear includes blood glucose, sedimentation rate, vitamin B_{12} or methylmalonic acid levels, serum blood urea nitrogen and creatinine, and serum protein/immunoelectrophoresis. Electrodiagnostic studies (e.g., nerve conduction velocity) are also helpful in clarifying the type and location of neuropathy.

Treatment of neuropathy depends on its causes (e.g., controlling diabetes or renal failure, eliminating inciting drugs or toxins, treating vitamin B_{12} deficiency) and may involve neurologic consultation in puzzling cases.

PERIPHERAL ARTERIAL DISEASE

PAD results from endothelial injury, lipid deposits, vasoconstriction, and plaque disruption, which reduce arterial blood flow and oxygen delivery to affected muscles causing exertional calf or leg angina or nocturnal leg pain improved with walking. (This should be distinguished from neurogenic claudication, which is caused by lumbar nerve root compression from spinal stenosis.) Arterial insufficiency pain can also arise from arterial entrapment or malformation, particularly during vigorous exercise.

PAD shares risk factors (e.g., hypertension, diabetes mellitus, hypercholesterolemia, tobacco abuse) with coronary artery disease (CAD), and significant CAD coexists in 60% of patients with PAD. The best screen for leg claudication is the ankle-brachial index (ABI) and the ratio of systolic blood pressure in the posterior tibial artery/systolic blood pressure in the brachial artery and is performed supine using a Doppler ultrasound. Since ankle pressure normally is higher, a normal ABI is ≥1. Severity of PAD correlates with ABI values, such that ≤0.90 diagnoses PAD, 0.70 to 0.89 indicates mild disease, 0.5 to 0.69 indicates moderate disease, and ≤0.5 indicates severe disease.

Treatment starts with lifestyle modifications (exercise to develop collateral blood flow, smoking cessation, dietary reduction in cholesterol, glucose control, and blood pressure control) and extends to pharmacologic intervention (lipid-lowering drugs, antiplatelet agents, e.g., aspirin [325 mg daily], cilostazol [50–100 mg twice daily], clopidogrel [75 mg daily], ticlopidine [250 mg twice daily], and red-cell morphology-altering agents, e.g., pentoxifylline [400 mg three times daily]). (SOR Ⓐ) Revascularization by either angioplasty or bypass grafting is reserved for cases refractory to medical management, for rest pain, tissue loss, persistent ulcers, or gangrene. (SOR Ⓑ)

4. **Bilateral leg edema** can arise from congestive heart failure, liver failure, renal failure, anemia, lymphatic obstruction, sodium retention, medication (e.g., systemic corticosteroids, calcium channel blockers), or hypothyroidism (pretibial myxedema).
III. **Symptoms and Signs** (Table 41–1). Physical examination of hip and leg complaints begins with taking vital signs (elevated temperature can be seen with infection) and observing the patient's general appearance. The hips and legs are inspected for asymmetry, deformity, discoloration, and edema. Gait is observed for symmetry, antalgia (quick soft steps to

favor a painful area), hip circumduction (swinging one thigh outward to reduce ipsilateral hip pain), and Trendelenburg sign (dropping one side of the pelvis because of contralateral hip weakness). Palpation of bony landmarks and soft tissue should be done with precision to localize tenderness. Particularly in patients with suspected vascular or neurologic disease, quality of pulses (femoral, popliteal, posterior tibial, and dorsal pedal) and of sensation (light touch, sharp, vibration, temperature) are assessed. Range of motion (ROM) testing should include passive, active, and resisted. Hip (flexion, extension, abduction, adduction, and internal and external rotation) and knee (flexion and extension) ROM are best performed with the patient supine, whereas ankle motion (dorsiflexion, plantar flexion, inversion, and eversion) and Homan's sign (rapid passive dorsiflexion to elicit pain from DVT) are done seated. Tendon reflexes should be tested. If the examination does not clearly localize the problem, then sources of referred symptoms should be examined (e.g., pelvis, lumbar spine).

A. Transient synovitis pain occasionally will awaken children at night.

B. In **Perthes disease,** knee pain alone occurs in 15%. The patient usually tolerates symptoms for 1 to 12 months before seeing a physician. Thigh and calf circumferences are diminished due to atrophy; late in the process, leg length may decrease.

C. In **SCFE,** approximately 20% of patients present acutely with a history of a sudden twisting or falling injury. Passive hip flexion elicits external rotation and abduction of the hip; half of the patients will have thigh atrophy, and half will have shortening of the extremity up to 1 inch.

D. Hip impingement causes anterolateral hip pain worsened by hip flexion, sitting, and leaning forward, such as to tie shoes. The combination motion of flexion, adduction, and internal rotation typically causes pain.

E. Osteoarthritis and **rheumatoid arthritis** (see Chapters 38 and 82).

F. Bursitis

    1. In **trochanteric bursitis,** running or lying on the affected side worsens the pain. The greater trochanter area is tender.

    2. Iliopsoas bursitis causes pain with hip extension, as when rising from a chair or lying in bed, and patients often limp with the hip flexed and externally rotated.

G. In **meralgia paresthetica,** prolonged standing and walking may worsen the pain; sitting may relieve it. Pressure applied to the lateral femoral cutaneous nerve at the iliac crest elicits symptoms.

H. Chronic compartment syndrome gradually develops over 1 year or longer and how far the patient can walk or run before symptoms occur is usually constant; discomfort, however, can worsen over time. Examination at rest is usually normal.

    1. In **anterior compartment syndrome,** numbness in the web space between the first and second toes and dorsiflexion weakness may occur.

    2. Complaints of ankle instability are common with **lateral compartment syndrome**.

I. In **stress fractures,** pain initially occurs toward the end of exercise and usually increases over days to weeks; the pain eventually develops early in activity and finally occurs at rest if training is not decreased. The affected area of bone is tender.

IV. Imaging (Table 41–1)

    A. In **evaluating hip complaints, plain x-rays** of the involved hip in adults (anterior and lateral views) and both hips in children (often including a frog leg lateral view) are the single-most cost-effective adjunctive test. When combined with age-adjusted history and thoughtful interpretation of physical signs, radiography approaches 90% sensitivity and 90% specificity.

        1. Perthes disease shows the following sequence: crescent sign (Figure 41–3), lateral displacement of the femoral head, widening and increased density of the femoral epiphysis, flattening of the femoral head and widening of the femoral neck, demineralization and fragmentation of the femoral head, and finally, reossification of the femoral head.

        2. The **SCFE** appears widened with irregular margins. The femoral head is displaced posteriorly and medially (Figure 41–4).

        3. Findings in hip impingement can include exostosis of the superior aspect of the femoral head-neck and superior acetabulum osteophytes and overhang. MRI arthrography is often used to assess details of impingement, which can include labral tears. Hip MRI has many false positives. (SOR **A**)

V. Treatment

    A. The pain of transient synovitis is relieved with bed rest at home for 7 to 10 days and **nonsteroidal anti-inflammatory drugs (NSAIDs)** such as **ibuprofen**

(5–10 mg/kg—three to four times daily spaced every 6–8 hours) as needed. Patients may use crutches to resume weight bearing. Most children have only a single attack of transient synovitis, but it may recur. Because 6% to 15% of patients with transient synovitis develop Perthes disease, patients and their parents should be instructed to seek care if hip or leg complaints occur.

B. Losing weight and avoiding constrictive garments are key to treating **meralgia paresthetica**. Abdominal muscle strengthening is also helpful. Local corticosteroid injection at the site of lateral femoral cutaneous nerve compression may provide relief in refractory cases (e.g., triamcinolone, 10–20 mg with 1 mL lidocaine via a 27-gauge 1¼-inch needle; Figure 41–2). Patients should be reassured that this condition is benign and self-limited.

C. **Stretching** overlying muscle to reduce friction on a bursa and strengthening weak hip muscles are key to treating **bursitis**. (SOR **C**) Oral analgesics may be helpful (e.g., ibuprofen, 200–600 mg—three to four times daily spaced every 4–6 hours or naproxen, initial dose 500 mg then 500 mg twice daily or 250 mg every 6–8 hours as needed for adults). If pain persists or function is limited, the affected bursa should be injected with 20 to 40 mg of **triamcinolone** or **methylprednisolone** added to 1 to 2 mL of local anesthetic. Patients who require repeated injections should consider bursectomy.

D. Hip impingement may respond to physical therapy to improve hip strength, motion, and flexibility. Refractory cases of impingement may require arthroscopy to remove impinging bone and repair injury to the acetabular labrum.

E. **Osteoarthritis** is managed with lifestyle modification (weight reduction, moderate exercise as tolerated), topical and oral analgesia, and assistive devices (see Chapter 82).

F. **Surgical intervention**
1. A patient with **bacterial infection** of the hip should be hospitalized for **arthrotomy** to drain all purulent material and for intravenous antibiotics. (SOR **C**) Poor prognosis is correlated with delayed action. Results of ultrasound-guided aspiration can allow selection of a smaller high-risk group for operative drainage and may also shorten operative time.
2. Perthes disease requires the orthopedic use of **braces, casts,** or **surgery** in order to retain the normal spherical shape of the femoral head during the natural repair process. (SOR **B**) Under the best of circumstances (e.g., younger age or earlier diagnosis), minimal deformity and normal function will result. Premature osteoarthritis of the hip can develop.
3. **SCFE** is best treated with immediate cessation of weight bearing and **surgical stabilization**. (SOR **A**) Premature osteoarthritis of the hip is common.
4. Under ultrasound or computerized tomography guidance, diagnostic and therapeutic **aspiration and drainage** of an enlarged **iliopsoas bursa** refractory to previously described measures can be accomplished.

G. Because the cause of **growing pains** is unknown, treatment consists of supportive measures including heat, ice, massage, and acetaminophen (10–15 mg/kg per dose every 4–6 hours; if less than 60 kg, the maximum dose is the lesser of 100 mg/kg per day or 4000 mg per day in children and if 60 kg or greater, 650 to 1000 mg orally every 4 to 6 hours as needed [maximum 4000 mg per day]) or NSAIDs. If symptoms persist despite a negative work-up, referral to a rheumatologist or pediatric orthopedic surgeon should be considered. (SOR **C**)

H. **Chronic compartment syndrome** often requires surgical decompression of the affected fascial compartment. Reducing exercise or changing sports is another option. Some patients may respond to a few weeks of lower extremity musculature stretching two to four times daily to improve compliance of fascia enclosing compartments. (SOR **C**)

I. **Stress fractures**
1. Crutches or a leg brace are sometimes required. Weight-bearing exercise should be discontinued until x-ray evidence of healing is seen and there is no tenderness, after which gradual resumption of activity may proceed.
2. Use of analgesics is discouraged because of the possibility of masking pain, which reflects ongoing bone stress.
3. Stress fractures of the pelvis, femur, and anterior tibia have a high risk for complications and are best managed by a subspecialist.

J. **Medial tibia stress syndrome**
1. Initial treatment is rest and ice (15–20 minutes at a time) until pain subsides.
2. Once symptoms resolve, soleus muscle stretching should be initiated, and the patient may gradually return to running. Patients whose feet pronate excessively may benefit

from arch support and heel control, such as with off-the-shelf or custom-made orthotics. Physical therapy is sometimes needed. (SOR **Ⓒ**)

   3. In rare instances, surgical release of the involved fascia is necessary.
K. DVT (see Chapter 64).
L. Nocturnal leg cramps
   1. When cramping occurs, the calf muscles should be stretched by dorsiflexion. Calf stretching at bedtime can prevent symptoms.
   2. Magnesium supplement (mainly in pregnancy, although data on effectiveness are conflicting), vitamin B complex (three times daily in one small trial), and diltiazem (30 mg orally at bedtime) can also be used. Quinine is no longer recommended due to risks (2%–4% serious hematologic side effects).

SELECTED REFERENCES

Brewer RB, Gregory AJ. Chronic lower leg pain in athletes: a guide for the differential diagnosis, evaluation, and treatment. *Sports Health.* 2012;4(2):121–127.

Frank RM, Slabaugh MA, Grumet RC, et al. Hip pain in active patients: what you may be missing. *J Fam Pract.* 2012;61(12):736–744.

Katzberg HD, Khan AH, So YT. Assessment: symptomatic treatment for muscle cramps (an evidence-based review). *Neurology.* 2010;74:691–696.

Kuhlman GS, Domb BG. Femoroacetabular impingement: identifying and treating a common cause of hip pain. *Am Fam Physician.* 2009;80(12):1429–1434.

Sawyer JS, Kapoor M. The limping child: a systematic approach to diagnosis. *Am Fam Physician.* 2009;79(3):215-224.

---

42   Liver Function Test Abnormalities

Angie Mathai, MD, & James P. McKenna, MD

KEY POINTS

- An AST:ALT ratio ≥2:1 is highly suggestive of alcoholic hepatitis. (SOR **Ⓒ**)
- Persistent elevations of liver function tests (LFTs) for ≥6 months suggest chronic liver disease; patients should be evaluated for treatable causes and referred for liver biopsy. (SOR **Ⓒ**)
- Alcohol liver disease, hepatitis C, and nonalcoholic fatty liver disease are the most common causes of persistently abnormal LFTs. (SOR **Ⓒ**)

 I. Definition. Abnormalities in liver function tests (LFTs) are elevated levels of static biochemical tests, including aspartate aminotransferase (AST; normal range 8–48 IU/L), alanine aminotransferase (ALT; normal range: 7–55 IU/L), alkaline phosphatase (normal range 45–115 IU/L), bilirubin (normal range 0.1–1 mg/dL), and albumin (normal range 3.5–5 g/dL). Tests other than those mentioned are often included in LFT panels, but are less useful in evaluating the spectrum of liver disease and therefore are not discussed here.

   A. Cellular injury in the liver causes release of AST and ALT. ALT is a more specific indicator of liver disease, whereas AST elevations can be due to damage of other organs (heart, kidney, brain, intestine, and placenta). Truncal fat is also associated with elevated ALT.

   B. Alkaline phosphatase is associated with cellular membranes and elevated levels can be caused by injury to the liver, bone, kidneys, intestines, placenta, or leukocytes. In the liver, the enzyme is located in the bile canaliculi. Biliary obstruction, most commonly from gallstones, induces increased synthesis of alkaline phosphatase and spillage into the circulation.

   C. Hyperbilirubinemia may be caused by increased production (hemolysis, ineffective erythropoiesis), extravasation of blood (hematoma), decreased metabolism (hereditary disease, Gilbert syndrome, or acquired defects in bilirubin conjugation), or reduced bilirubin excretion caused by bile duct obstruction (see Chapter 37).

   D. Serum albumin and prothrombin time (PT) are measures of the liver's synthetic function. Albumin is produced in hepatocytes and PT is dependent on clotting factors produced by liver. However, neither test is specific for liver disease.

E. Quantitative LFTs measuring liver metabolism or clearance of caffeine, antipyrine, cholate, or galactose may be used by hepatologists to assess liver function in patients with chronic compensated liver disease, specifically to evaluate for sustained virologic response in viral hepatitis.

II. **Screening.** Abnormal LFTs in asymptomatic patients may indicate very mild hepatic dysfunction or represent a more serious illness in its presymptomatic phase.

A. Screening the general population for liver abnormalities including nonalcoholic fatty liver disease (NAFLD) is not currently advised as long-term benefits and cost effectiveness is unknown.

B. Testing for hepatitis C virus (HCV) antibodies and hepatitis B surface antigens is advisable for all patients presenting with a mild increase in aminotransferase levels.

1. The Centers for Disease Control and Prevention now recommends one-time HCV screening, independent of other risk factors, for anyone born during 1945 to 1965 based on a higher prevalence in this birth cohort.

2. Other patients who should be screened for HCV using an enzyme immunoassay (according to the American Association for the Study of Liver Disease [2009]) are:

   a. Anyone who ever injected illicit drugs.
   b. Recipients of organ transplants or transfused blood prior to July 1992.
   c. Recipients of clotting factor concentrates prior to 1987.
   d. Current sexual partners of those infected with hepatitis C.
   e. Those on chronic hemodialysis.
   f. Children born to HCV-positive mothers.
   g. Those infected with human immunodeficiency virus.
   h. Health care workers with a percutaneous or permucosal exposure to hepatitis C.
   i. Those with unexplained transaminase elevations.

III. **Common Diagnoses.** In asymptomatic populations, the prevalence of abnormal LFTs is 7.9%, with most instances either unexplained or attributed to NAFLD.

A. NAFLD is defined as evidence of steatosis (by imaging or histology) that is not due to another cause (e.g., excessive alcohol intake, medications, or hereditary disorders). It is associated with metabolic risk factors including diabetes mellitus, obesity, and dyslipidemia. Nonalcoholic steatohepatitis (NASH) is a histologic subtype with hepatocyte injury.

1. Patients with NAFLD have increased mortality; the most common cause of death is cardiovascular disease.

2. The NAFLD Fibrosis Score can help identify patients with increased likelihood of fibrosis or cirrhosis.

B. **Elevated aminotransferases (AST and ALT)** are found to some degree in almost all patients with liver disease and represent hepatocellular dysfunction (Table 42–1 and Figure 42–1). Levels up to 300 international units/L (iU/L) are nonspecific. Values >1000 iU/L are associated with acute viral hepatitis, ischemic hepatitis, or drug-induced injury (e.g., acetaminophen ingestion). Extrahepatic biliary obstruction usually has values <1000 iU/L, and alcoholic hepatitis <500 iU/L. Elevations can be seen in the absence of liver disease; examples include the setting of diabetic ketoacidosis, muscle disease, celiac sprue, and hypothyroidism.

1. In asymptomatic populations, as many as 6% of patients have abnormal values of AST.

2. Alcohol liver damage, hepatitis C, and NAFLD are the most common causes of aminotransferase abnormalities in adults. An AST:ALT ratio >2 is suggestive of alcoholic liver disease. Although statin drugs can raise transaminase levels, a meta-analysis of randomized placebo-controlled trials demonstrated that low to moderate dosages of

TABLE 42–1. CAUSES OF ELEVATED AMINOTRANSFERASES

Alcoholic hepatitis	Drug-induced hepatitis[a]
Viral hepatitis	Autoimmune hepatitis[a]
Hepatitis A	Toxic hepatitis
Hepatitis B[a]	Nonalcoholic fatty liver disease[a]
Hepatitis C[a]	Metabolic hepatitis[a]
Hepatitis D[a]	Hemochromatosis
Hepatitis E	α_1-Antitrypsin deficiency
Hepatitis G[a]	Wilson disease
Cytomegalovirus	
Epstein–Barr virus	

[a]These conditions can cause chronic active hepatitis.

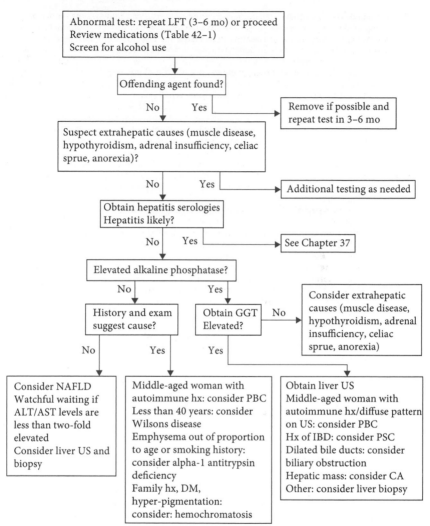

FIGURE 42–1. Evaluation of the asymptomatic patient with abnormal liver function tests. NAFLD, nonalcoholic fatty liver disease; ALT, alanine aminotransferase; AST, aspartate aminotransferase; US, ultrasound; Hx, history; PBC, primary biliary cirrhosis; DM, diabetes mellitus; IBD, inflammatory bowel disease; CA, cancer.

statins are not associated with clinically significant (i.e., greater than three times the upper limit of normal) elevations.

3. Hepatitis A virus is the most common cause of aminotransferase abnormality in children.

C. Elevated alkaline phosphatase is due to intrahepatic or extrahepatic obstruction, cholestasis from medication, or infiltrative disease (e.g., cancer, sarcoidosis). An isolated increase is also noted in the third trimester of pregnancy and during adolescence and has been found in as many as 4% of asymptomatic patients.

1. An elevated alkaline phosphatase level in patients with inflammatory bowel disease suggests primary sclerosing cholangitis.

2. In middle-aged women with pruritus and a history of autoimmune disease, consider primary biliary cirrhosis.

D. Hyperbilirubinemia is most commonly due to hemolysis and Gilbert syndrome (see Chapter 37). Jaundice is common in newborns and is most often physiologic (see Chapter 37). Mild degrees of indirect hyperbilirubinemia are found in as many as 10% of asymptomatic patients with Gilbert syndrome. Indirect bilirubin does not typically exceed 4 mg/dL in these patients.

   1. Prior to age 30 years, hepatitis causes about 75% of cases of hyperbilirubinemia.

   2. After age 60 years, extrahepatic obstruction causes about 50% of cases of hyperbilirubinemia (e.g., gallstones, pancreatic cancer).

IV. Symptoms and Signs

  A. Fatigue, nausea, malaise, pruritus, jaundice, anorexia, splenomegaly, and right upper quadrant discomfort are common complaints of patients with compensated liver disease. Patients with decompensated disease may also report weight loss, abdominal distention, and hematemesis.

  B. Pertinent examination findings include hepatomegaly, fever, jaundice, and splenomegaly. Patients with decompensated liver disease can also have ascites, spider angiomas, testicular atrophy, evidence of hepatic encephalopathy, and gynecomastia on examination.

V. Diagnostic Tests

  A. A **stepwise approach to evaluating LFT abnormalities** is recommended (Figure 42–1). (SOR **Ⓒ**)

   1. Abnormal LFTs should be repeated. If retested, more than 30% of patients with elevated AST, ALT, or bilirubin levels would be classified as normal, so retesting asymptomatic patients is recommended in about 3 to 6 months, especially after discontinuation of potentially offending agents. However, normalization does not rule out liver disease, so testing for chronic liver disease can proceed from the first abnormal test.

   2. If abnormal LFTs **persist for more than 6 months,** treatable causes of chronic hepatitis should be ruled out. Such causes include hemochromatosis; autoimmune hepatitis; α_1-antitrypsin deficiency; hepatitis B, C, and D; NAFLD; and Wilson disease (see Chapters 37 and 72).

   3. In patients with **elevated alkaline phosphatase,** liver ultrasound is a useful first step to differentiate between intra- and extrahepatic obstruction, identifying masses or liver disease. Elevated anti-mitochondrial antibodies and total IgM levels are consistent with the diagnosis of primary biliary cirrhosis (see Chapter 72).

   4. A **γ-glutamyltransferase (GGT) test** is highly sensitive for liver disease, but lacks specificity. GGT levels can be elevated up to three times the upper reference value in nearly half of patients with NAFLD and from 2 to 10 times normal in alcoholic liver disease. GGT is also increased with use of anticonvulsants and oral contraceptives.

   5. Direct and indirect **bilirubin fractions** should be obtained if total bilirubin levels are increased. If the indirect (unconjugated) fraction is elevated ($\geq$80% of the total), a reticulocyte count and a peripheral blood smear should be obtained (see Chapter 4).

   6. Serum albumin and PT. Serum albumin levels can decrease in patients with nephrotic syndrome, malabsorption, protein-losing enteropathy, or malnutrition. PT can be prolonged by warfarin treatment, vitamin K deficiency (which is needed to activate clotting factors II, VII, and X), and consumptive coagulopathy. The finding of hypoalbuminemia and no other alterations in liver tests virtually rules out a hepatic origin of this abnormality.

   7. Ultrasound is useful in identifying disease and obstruction of the bile ducts and gallbladder. It can also be used to assess liver size and consistency.

   8. Liver biopsy is the most reliable way to diagnose diffuse hepatitis disease and indications must be weighed against the small risk of complications. However, for patients with chronic viral hepatitis, the role of liver biopsy has decreased given advances in virologic testing and new noninvasive markers of fibrosis. Liver biopsy is particularly important in securing the diagnosis in autoimmune hepatitis, primary biliary cirrhosis, and primary sclerosing cholangitis. It is useful in determining the degree of inflammation and extent of fibrosis and remains essential for the diagnosis of focal lesions.

  B. Interpretation of particular abnormal LFT patterns

   1. Alcoholic liver disease results in modest elevations of the transaminases. An elevation of ALT $\geq$300 IU is not consistent with alcoholic liver damage. The ratio of AST to ALT is useful diagnostically, since a ratio of 2:1 or greater suggests a high probability of alcoholic liver disease. Elevated mean corpuscular volume and GGT suggest alcoholic liver disease.

   2. Viral hepatitis often causes significant elevations of the transaminases, with levels exceeding 1000 IU. Alkaline phosphatase is typically elevated more than AST; the AST:ALT ratio is $\leq$1.

TABLE 42–2. MEDICATIONS THAT CAN ADVERSELY AFFECT LIVER FUNCTION TESTS

Cholestatic Pattern	Cytotoxic Pattern
Amoxicillin/clavulanic acid	Acarbose
Anabolic steroids	Acetaminophen
Chlorambucil	Allopurinol
Chlorpromazine	Amiodarone
Chlorpropamide	L-Asparaginase
Clopidogrel	Aspirin and nonsteroidal anti-inflammatory drugs
Erythromycin estolate	Carbamazepine
Estrogen (oral contraceptives)	Etretinate
Methimazole	HAART drugs
Mirtazapine	Halothane
Phenobarbital	Hydralazine
Terbinafine	Imipramine
Tolbutamide	Isoniazid
Tricyclic antidepressants	Ketoconazole
	Lisinopril
	Lovastatin
	6-Mercaptopurine
	Methotrexate
	Methyldopa
	Nicotinic acid (especially sustained-release)
	Nitrofurantoin
	Omeprazole
	Paroxetine
	Phenytoin
	Propylthiouracil
	Rifampin
	Risperidone
	Statins
	Sertraline
	Sulfonamides
	Tetracycline
	Trazodone
	Valproic acid

3. **Medications** causing cholestasis (Table 42–2) can result in transaminase and alkaline phosphatase elevations that are as much as 10 times normal levels.
4. **Cytotoxic reactions** from medications can cause severe injuries resembling viral hepatitis, with transaminase values as high as 500 times normal levels.
5. **Intrahepatic or extrahepatic obstruction** cause values of alkaline phosphatase to be 5 or more times higher than normal levels. The highest values are found in primary biliary cirrhosis.
6. **Infiltrative diseases** such as neoplasm, granulomas, and amyloidosis can cause moderate to marked elevations of alkaline phosphatase. Bilirubin is minimally elevated, however.
7. **Hemolysis** causes an elevated reticulocyte count and an abnormal peripheral smear, with the bilirubin level generally ≤5 mg/dL.
8. **Gilbert syndrome** is characterized by indirect bilirubin levels of 2 to 3 mg/dL, normal LFTs, and no evidence of hemolysis.

VI. **Treatment.** For information on the management of the following causes of abnormal LFTs, refer to the chapters indicated.
   A. **NAFLD.** Weight loss reduces hepatic steatosis. (SOR **A**) Vitamin E may be helpful in patients with biopsy-proven NASH. (SOR **B**)
      1. Trials of metformin for NAFLD have shown mixed results, with only two or four studies showing some improvement in steatosis on ultrasound; no improvement was seen with metformin in NASH stages. Metformin does lead to a significant reduction in insulin resistance.
   B. **Cholelithiasis** (see Chapter 1).

C. Hemolysis (see Chapter 4).
D. Hepatitis (see Chapter 37).
E. Cirrhosis (see Chapter 72).
F. Alcohol and drug abuse (see Chapter 90).

SELECTED REFERENCES

American Gastroenterological Association. Medical position statement: evaluation of liver chemistry tests. *Gastroenterology.* 2002;123:1364–1366.

Chalasani N, Younossi Z, Lavine J, Diehl A. The diagnosis and management of non-alcoholic fatty liver disease: practice guideline by the American Association for the Study of Liver Diseases, American College of Gastroenterology, and the American Gastroenterological Association. *Hepatology.* 2012; 55(6):2005–2023.

Giannini E, Testa R, Savarino V. Liver enzyme alteration: a guide for clinicians. *CMAJ.* 2005;172(3): 367–379.

Giboney PT. Mildly elevated liver transaminase levels in the asymptomatic patient. *Am Fam Physician.* 2005;71:1105–1110.

Heidelbaugh JJ, Bruderly M. Cirrhosis and chronic liver failure: part 1. Diagnosis and evaluation. *Am Fam Physician.* 2006;74:756–762.

Hoefs JC, Chen PT, Lizotte P. Noninvasive evaluation of liver disease severity. *Clin Liver Dis.* 2006;10: 535–562.

Navarro VJ, Senior JR. Drug-related hepatotoxicity. *N Engl J Med.* 2006;254:731–739.

Scoazec JY. Liver biopsy: which role in patient management? *Annales de Pathologie.* 2010;30(6): 464–469.

Additional references are available online at http://langetextbooks.com/fm6e

---

43   Low Back Pain

Dan F. Criswell, MD

KEY POINTS

- Low back pain (LBP) is a broad category of symptomatic low back conditions organized into four distinct groups based on duration of symptoms from the initial episode: **acute,** <6 weeks duration; **subacute,** ≥6 weeks but ≤3 months duration; **chronic,** >3 months duration; and **acute imposed on chronic,** acute flares with a background of chronic back pain. (SOR **C**)
- Most of the patients seen in primary care settings for acute LBP have no evidence of serious underlying spinal pathology, and diagnostic testing should not be a routine part of their initial evaluation. Seventy percent of patients with LBP clinically improve within 2 weeks and 90% within 4 to 6 weeks. (SOR **A**)
- The clinical history and physical examination are generally effective in identifying the few patients who potentially have serious causes of LBP and need further evaluation immediately. A patient's failure to improve with 6 weeks of conservative treatment is also an indication for further evaluation. (SOR **C**)
- The treatment goal for acute or chronic LBP is for the patient to be active as soon as possible. Bed rest beyond 24 hours should be avoided. (SOR **A**)
- Pain reduction is a primary treatment goal in LBP, but attempt at restoration of function is more problematic. Patients with LBP associated with litigation or worker's compensation often have prolonged recovery times. Lack of restored function produces significant disability and costs to industry and the healthcare system. (SOR **C**)

I. Definition. LBP is pain, muscle tension, or stiffness below the costal margin and above the inferior gluteal folds, with or without pain or neuromotor deficits in the leg (sciatica). Pain can be central (midline) or referred to nonmidline structures including connective tissues and peripheral nerves innervated by the spinal cord.

Most back pain symptoms are **nonspecific** and result from overuse or injury of the ligaments and muscles that hold together the lumbosacral (LS) vertebrae, or from degenerative osteoarthritis of the articular processes of the facet joints. Nonmechanical causes of LBP account for less than 2% of all cases. Direct and indirect costs for LBP exceed $90 billion per year in the United States. Back pain accounts for 33% of all workers' compensation costs.

Specific mechanisms resulting in LBP include the following:

A. Herniation of an intervertebral disk, causing inflammation or direct pressure on nerve roots exiting from the LS spinal cord.

B. Fracture of a vertebra, which may be traumatic or pathologic.

C. Malignant neoplasm of the spine.

D. Spinal stenosis, mechanical pressure on neural structures resulting from a degenerative narrowing of the bony spinal canal.

E. A defect of the vertebral arch (spondylolysis) leading to slippage of all or part of a vertebra on another (spondylolisthesis).

F. Spinal infection.

G. Inflammatory diseases.

H. Referred visceral pain from vascular, genitourinary, or gastrointestinal diseases.

 II. Prevention and Screening. The United States Preventive Services Task Force (USPSFT) found insufficient evidence to recommend for or against routine use of interventions as primary prevention of LBP in adults in primary care settings. In general, patients should be encouraged to be as physically active as possible and to avoid aggravating factors such as bending, twisting, and lifting. (SOR **C**)

III. Diagnoses

A. Acute LBP (<6 weeks duration) is the most common form of LBP. The usual cause is mechanical. Nonspecific acute LBP affects both sexes, with men being affected at younger ages (30–50 years) than women (≥50 years). Associated risk factors include repetitive lifting, bending, stooping, or pulling, static work positions, sedentary lifestyle especially when coupled with nonaccustomed intense activity, and cigarette smoking. There is only a weak association with obesity.

Specific diagnoses presenting as acute LBP include the following:

1. Herniated nucleus pulposus (HNP), typically inducing an inflammatory response while compressing the nerve root exiting the LS cord (causing leg symptoms).

2. Vertebral fracture—traumatic or pathologic (osteoporosis or tumor).

3. LBP originating from sources other than the back (e.g., gastrointestinal or genitourinary tract or the abdominal aorta) or associated with systemic symptoms must be ruled out.

B. Subacute or **Chronic** (6 weeks to beyond 3 months) **LBP**. This can be associated with prolonged recovery of acute LBP, but may indicate more serious underlying pathology. In a 5-year study of health care claims, causes of LBP were as follows: chronic soft tissue strain (85%), HNP (4%), ankylosing spondylitis (<5%), spinal stenosis (4%), vertebral compression fracture (4%), neoplasm (0.07%), cauda equina syndrome (0.04%), and vertebral infection (0.01%). Depending upon age and other underlying factors, the following are specific causes of subacute LBP:

1. Osteoarthritis of the lumbar spine (LS) with associated conditions including spinal stenosis, osteoarthritis of the facet joints, and osteoarthritis of the sacroiliac joints.

2. HNP (also referred to as lumbar disk herniation) not spontaneously resolving by 6 weeks. As many as 75% of patients with acute disk rupture do not progress to the subacute category; those with cumulative microdiscal tears are more likely to progress to subacute or chronic LBP. About 5% of patients with HNP require surgery; 85% of these patients return to normal function after surgery.

3. Those with **intrinsic musculoskeletal defects** including spondylolysis (pars defects), spondylolisthesis (forward vertebral slippage), scoliosis of greater than 40%, limb length discrepancies of ≥1 cm are at risk of progression to subacute or chronic LBP. Spondylolysis is almost exclusively seen in adolescent athletes and should be suspected in any teen with localized lumbar pain. Idiopathic scoliosis, typically found in young women, rarely causes back pain and the USPSTF found insufficient evidence for or against routine screening of asymptomatic adolescents.

4. Patients with **osteoporosis or bony neoplasms**. Osteoporosis is age related (≥65 years in women and ≥70 years in men) and influenced by genetics and medication use (e.g., corticosteroids). Malignant neoplasms cause less than 1% of subacute or chronic LBP; metastatic lesions from breast, prostate, or lung primaries are 25 times more common than primary bone lesions.

5. **Inflammatory diseases** (including ankylosing spondylitis, rheumatoid arthritis, and Reiter syndrome) account for only 0.3% cases of chronic LBP.
6. **Infectious diseases** (osteomyelitis, diskitis, and abscesses) usually occur in patients with diabetes mellitus, sickle cell disease, immunosuppressive disorders including HIV, IV drug use, history of spinal surgery/instrumentation, or previous spinal infections.
7. In the United States, the most common causes of chronic LBP are **behavioral or psychological** issues. Patients with chronic LBP are more likely to have poor job satisfaction. Patients with compensation issues have a worse prognosis than patients without compensation issues. In children, psychosocial rather than mechanical factors are associated with LBP. Other associations include emotional problems, conduct disorders, headaches, nonspecific abdominal pain, sore throat, and daytime tiredness.

C. **Chronic with acute flares.** Any of the aforementioned chronic conditions can be associated with acute flares as well. Typically, discogenic lesions maintain a degree of chronic stability until increased activity, devolution of the underlying discal lesion, or additional trauma produces an acute flare of the chronic lesion.

IV. **Symptoms**

A. **Onset.** Back strain typically has an acute, sudden onset, as may the pain from a compression fracture. Pain caused by medical conditions (e.g., inflammation, cancer, or referred visceral pain) generally has a more gradual or insidious onset.

B. **Frequency and duration.** Most mechanical LBP occurs in intermittent episodes that last from a few days to a few months. A degenerating disk may cause low-grade, persistent discomfort that is exacerbated during acute flare-ups. Patients with osteoarthritis, inflammatory conditions, or cancer usually develop chronic persistent symptoms.

C. **Time of day.** Inflammatory conditions produce greater back pain and stiffness in the morning; mechanical disorders typically cause pain that increases with the day's activities. Most individuals with spinal cancer complain of back pain that is worse during the night.

D. **Location of pain.** Most mechanical and medical disorders result in pain localized to the LS and surrounding areas. Nerve root irritation (e.g., from a herniated disk, spinal stenosis, or spondylolisthesis) is signaled by pain that radiates from the back to the lower leg or is felt exclusively in the lower leg. Poorly localized pain along nonanatomic routes is more often seen in patients with social or psychological distress.

E. **Aggravating and alleviating factors.** Pain caused by mechanical disorders typically improves with recumbency and worsens with activity, whereas patients with back pain caused by inflammatory diseases or tumor often feel worse with bed rest. Relief of pain only with absolute immobility is often a sign of acute infection or a compression fracture.

V. **Signs.** The purpose of the physical examination of a patient with LBP is to supplement information obtained in the medical history in searching for serious underlying spinal pathology (e.g., cancer) or possible neurologic compromise. The basic elements of the examination are the following:

A. **Vital signs.** The presence of fever or weight loss may indicate infection or cancer.

B. **Inspection.** An **antalgic** gait, resulting from avoidance of weight bearing on the involved leg, can be a sign of nerve root irritation.

C. **Spinal range of motion.** Very limited range of motion is most common in patients with symptom magnification. However, in patients with fever or systemic findings, a significantly reduced range of motion suggests the possibility of a spinal infection.

D. **Palpation.** Most patients with back strain will exhibit **local tenderness** or **muscle spasm.** These signs, however, are neither highly sensitive nor specific. **Point tenderness** over bony landmarks is a sensitive but nonspecific sign of infection. It is also commonly seen in patients with arthritis or cancer. Pain from percussion of the sacroiliac joints is suggestive but not diagnostic of ankylosing spondylitis.

E. **Neurologic evaluation.** This examination emphasizes ankle and knee reflexes, ankle and great toe dorsiflexion strength, and distribution of sensory complaints.

1. **Diminished or absent ankle reflex, calf weakness or atrophy,** and **sensory loss along the lateral aspect of the foot** are caused by compression of the first sacral nerve root (S1).

2. **Weakness of dorsiflexors of the ankle or great toe** and **sensory loss along the medial foot** are caused by compression of the fifth lumbar root (L5).

3. **Diminished knee jerk** is caused by compression of the fourth lumbar nerve root (L4). This is a relatively uncommon finding.

4. Pain during a **straight leg-raising (SLR) test** indicates nerve root irritation or compression. The examiner raises the affected leg of the supine patient by the heel while keeping the knee fully extended. In a positive test, pain below the knee occurs when the leg is raised 30 to 60 degrees. SLR has a sensitivity of 92% with a highly variable specificity (0%–100%).

F. Abdominal, rectal, and pelvic examination. A mass detected on abdominal examination may indicate cancer or aortic aneurysm. A rectal and pelvic examination is especially important if cancer or infection is suspected.

G. Anatomically "inappropriate" signs. These signs elicited on examination often identify psychological distress as a result, or as an amplifier, of LBP. Such signs include back pain from downward pressure applied to the skull, patient overreaction during the examination, or marked discrepancy between the examination and the patient's ability to dress or move about.

H. Extremities. An often neglected but very important physical finding is limb length discrepancy. A greater than 1 cm discrepancy (measured from the anterosuperior iliac spine to the lateral malleolus) can cause LBP. In patients with buttock pain, the Patrick test (patient supine, thigh and knee flexed, lateral malleolus over the opposite patella, and pain produced by abducting the bent knee) indicates hip pathology instead of neurologic referred pain.

VI. Diagnostic Testing. For most patients with acute LBP, x-rays, imaging studies, and laboratory tests are unnecessary. Table 43–1 lists the signs/symptoms on the initial history and physical examination that suggest a need for immediate testing. Testing is also indicated if significant improvement of LBP is not seen after 2 to 4 weeks of conservative treatment.

A. Radiologic evaluation should be used selectively and the results interpreted with care and clinical correlation.

1. Plain films of the back do not rule out significant LS disease and may give false-negative results in as many as 40% of patients with known vertebral cancer. Moreover, conditions such as degenerative arthritis, narrowed disk space, mild scoliosis, facet subluxation, and minor congenital abnormalities (e.g., spina bifida occulta) detected radiographically may be unrelated to back pain, since these conditions are noted with the same frequency in symptomatic and asymptomatic individuals.

    a. The Agency for Healthcare Research and Quality (AHCPR) guidelines recommend plain film radiography only with major trauma, age ≤20 years or ≥70 years, history of cancer, constitutional symptoms, or back pain worse when supine or resting. (SOR **B**) However, adherence to these guidelines still overutilizes plain film radiography. Therefore, the clinical recommendation is not to use the age criterion, but to defer x-rays for 2 to 3 weeks unless there is a high risk of other serious disease. (SOR **B**)

    b. Lumber x-rays for patients with LBP for ≥6 weeks may increase patient satisfaction (at 9 months but not 3 months), but do not improve patient function, severity of pain, or overall health status. (SOR **A**)

2. Bone scan should be considered for patients with signs or symptoms suggestive of cancer, infection, or occult fractures of the vertebrae—conditions for which bone scans are more sensitive than plain films. However, positive scan results almost always need to be confirmed using other tests. For suspected spondylolysis in an adolescent, bone scintigraphy with single-photon emission computed tomography is the best diagnostic test.

3. For patients at risk for more serious conditions (Table 43–1), whose symptoms persist despite normal plain films, or who fail to improve within 6 weeks of conservative

TABLE 43–1. SIGNS/SYMPTOMS THAT SUGGEST A NEED FOR EARLY IMAGING IN ADULT PATIENTS WITH ACUTE LOW BACK PAIN

Finding	Rationale for Early Imaging
Major trauma (e.g., fall, MVA)	Possible fracture
Age ≥50 yr	Greater risk of cancer, compression fracture
History of cancer	Greater risk of underlying malignancy
Unexplained weight loss	Greater risk of cancer or infection
Fever, immunosuppression, human immunodeficiency virus, IV or injection drug use	Risk for spinal infection
Saddle anesthesia, bladder or bowel incontinence	Possible cauda equina syndrome
Severe or progressive neurologic deficit	Possible cauda equina syndrome or severe nerve root compression

IV, intravenous; MVA, motor vehicle accident.

treatment, **magnetic resonance imaging (MRI)** is a logical next imaging step. An MRI is inappropriate as a screening test unless neurologic deficits are present or strong suspicions of cancer or cauda equina syndrome are present.

4. Even in the presence of simple radiculopathy, the American Academy of Neurology recommends no MRIs until after 7 weeks of conservative therapy. (SOR **B**)

5. The sensitivity of the MRI may produce false-positive results as bulging disks, focal disk protrusions, and annular tears are common in patients without LBP. Fear may be more disabling for some patients with LBP than any organic condition, and irrelevant radiographic findings probably contribute to this fear.

B. **Simple clinical screening tests** such as the **erythrocyte sedimentation rate** and **serum alkaline phosphatase** can be used to evaluate patients with LBP at risk of having malignancy or an acute infectious or inflammatory process (Table 43–1). Abnormalities on **urinalysis** can help diagnose patients suspected of having referred back pain of urinary origin. However, **serologic tests** (e.g., antinuclear antibodies, rheumatoid factor, and HLA-B27) should not be used for routine screening of patients with LBP since the common spondyloarthropathies affecting the back are seronegative conditions.

C. **Electromyography** is occasionally useful in assessing a patient with leg symptoms that are possibly back-related and of more than 3- to 4-week duration. Test results are not reliable before this time.

VII. Treatment (Table 43–2). When back pain is found to result from medical conditions such as cancer or infection, specific treatment should be directed at the underlying disease. Treatment for almost all other causes of acute LBP (including early treatment of minor neural compression) should be conservative, aimed at relieving pain, maintaining or restoring function, and reassuring the patient that the acute symptoms are self-limited.

A. **Activity.** Staying active, within the limits permitted by the acute pain, leads to a more rapid recovery than either bed rest or specific back-mobilizing exercises. Prolonged periods of sitting and activities stressful to the back (e.g., lifting) may need to be limited temporarily. The goal, however, is for the patient to be back to normal activities as soon as possible. Neither prolonged bed rest (i.e., more than a few days) nor spinal traction has any proven efficacy in the treatment of acute LBP. In chronic back pain, most good quality studies indicate that graded activity does not significantly improve pain or long-term function. (SOR **A**)

B. **Medication**

1. **Nonsteroidal anti-inflammatory drugs** (NSAIDs), such as ibuprofen (1600 mg/d, divided four times daily), are effective for short-term symptomatic relief in patients with acute symptoms. There is no evidence that any particular NSAID has superior efficacy.

2. **Acetaminophen** (3–4 g per day, divided every 4–6 hours) is a reasonably safe and effective alternative for patients who are intolerant of NSAIDs. If the patient is at risk for hepatotoxicity (e.g., medical problem, use of other hepatotoxic drugs, ingesting three or more alcohol-containing drinks per day, or poor nutritional intake), then up to 2 g/day is suggested.

3. **Muscle relaxants do not exhibit any direct action on skeletal muscle and owe their efficacy to sedation. Such agents,** e.g., cyclobenzaprine (15–30 mg every 24 hours for several days), appear to be as effective as NSAIDs in relieving back symptoms, although drowsiness (which occurs in up to 30% of patients) may limit the patient's ability to ambulate or participate in other activities. There is no added benefit when muscle relaxants are used in combination with NSAIDs.

4. **Opioids.** Patients with severe pain not relieved with other conservative treatment may require opioids. Short-acting agents (hydrocodone 5 mg, 7.5 mg, or 10 mg in combination with acetaminophen [325–500 mg] or ibuprofen [200 mg]) are only indicated for treatment of acute LBP and uncontrolled acute flares in chronic LBP. These opioid agents have an effective half-life of only 4 to 6 hours and can be abused if used other than acutely.

5. In patients with **chronic LBP** who are only able to maintain functional capacity with opioids, long-acting opioids (methadone 10–40 mg every 12 hours or sustained release morphine or oxycodone 10–160 mg every 12 hours) can provide steady-state analgesia and avoid peaks and valleys of therapeutic effect seen with short-acting opioids. It is important to establish pain contracts in treating patients with potent long-acting opioids and help patients realize the goal of preservation of function and tolerable pain.

TABLE 43–2. MAJOR EVIDENCE-BASED RECOMMENDATIONS FOR TREATMENT OF LOW BACK PAIN

Treatment	Type of Pain[a]	SOR[b]	Effectiveness	Comments
Pharmacological Therapy (traditional)				
Acetaminophen	A–C	Ⓐ	+	Safer than NSAIDs in elderly Avoid total daily doses >4 g due to potential toxicity, particularly with use of multiple medications containing acetaminophen
Cox 2	A–C	Ⓐ	+/–	No more effective or safer than NSAIDS
Corticosteroids	A	Ⓐ	– Acute nonsciatic +/– Sciatica	Oral or epidural
NSAIDS	A–C	Ⓐ	++ Nonsciatic – Sciatic pain	No one NSAID is better than another
Opiates	A	Ⓐ	+ Nonsciatic ++ Sciatic	In comparison to NSAID alone
Tramadol	C	Ⓐ	+	Modest pain improvement, no functional improvement
TCAs	A–C	Ⓑ	– Acute +/– Chronic	More helpful with neuropathic pain
SSRI	A–C	Ⓑ	–	Only use if treating depression
Muscle relaxers	A–C	Ⓑ	+/–	No improvement added to NSAIDS. Primarily sedative effect
Pharmacological (CAM)				
Capsicum frutescens (Cayenne, capsaicin)	A–C	Ⓐ	+/–	Topical; inferior to NSAIDS—more favorable than placebo
Harpagophytum procumbens (Devils claw)	A–C	Ⓐ	–	Inferior to NSAIDS—more favorable than placebo
Salix alba (White willow bark)	A–C	Ⓐ	+/–	Inferior to NSAIDS—more favorable than placebo
Glucosamine	A–C	Ⓒ	–	Study limited to lumbar osteoarthritis
Nonpharmacological Therapy				
Alexander technique	A	Ⓐ	+ Sciatica	Combination mindfulness and stretches
Botulinum toxin injections	C	Ⓐ	+	Compared to placebo, acupuncture or epidural steroid Improved pain and function scores
Acupuncture	C	Ⓑ	+	10 sessions over 12 wk
Acupressure	C	Ⓑ	+	More effective than standard PT with improved disability and pain scores
Cognitive therapy	C	Ⓑ	+	Compared to NSAIDS
Diskectomy	C	Ⓑ	+	Greater improvement at 1 yr (NNT = 3), but no difference beyond year 4
Early mobilization	A–S	Ⓑ	+	More rapid functional return
Exercise therapy	A	Ⓑ	+/–	Compared to NSAIDS
Fusion surgery	C	Ⓑ	+	Spondylolisthesis/spinal stenosis but no better than intensive rehabilitation in functional disability scores
Ice/stretching	A	Ⓑ	+/–	Minimal cohort studies
Intensive physical and psychological therapy	C	Ⓑ	+	Recommended if failed primary treatment and high disability/psychological distress Expensive, but less so than surgery
Manipulation	A	Ⓑ	+	More rapid function return, fewer medications (nine treatments over 12 wk)
Massage	S/C	Ⓑ	+	Functional improvement to 1 yr
Neuroreflexotherapy	C	Ⓑ	+	Developed and practiced in Spain
Vertebroplasty	Osteoporotic	Ⓑ	+/–	Initially more rapid pain control but no difference in outcomes beyond 3 mo
Yoga	C	Ⓑ	+	Improved functional disability compared to usual care

(continued)

TABLE 43–2. MAJOR EVIDENCE-BASED RECOMMENDATIONS FOR TREATMENT OF LOW BACK PAIN (*Continued*)

Treatment	Type of Pain[a]	SOR[b]	Effectiveness	Comments
Balneotherapy (spa)	C	⊙	+	Effective when compared to wait list control
Insoles	A	⊙	+/−	Limited cohort studies only
Stand alone formal education (back school)	C	⊙	−	Not effective without additional treatment

[a]A, acute pain; S, subacute pain; C, chronic pain.
[b]SOR: A, consistent-good quality patient-oriented evidence; B, inconsistent or limited quality patient-oriented evidence; C, consensus, disease-oriented evidence or expert opinion.
Effectiveness: ++, highly effective; +, effective; +/−, inconclusive; −, ineffective.
NSAIDs, nonsteroidal anti-inflammatory drugs; TCA, tricyclic antidepressant; SSRI, selective serotonin receptor inhibitor; CAM, complementary and alternative medicine; PT, physical therapy; NNT, number needed to treat.

6. **Antidepressants.** Low-dose **tricyclic antidepressants** (e.g., nortriptyline 10–25 mg at bedtime, increasing if needed and tolerated by 25 mg per day on a weekly basis to a maximum of 75 mg per day as a single bedtime dose or two divided doses) in the absence of clinical depression can be useful in the treatment of subacute and chronic LBP by likely improving sleep and serving as adjuvants to other analgesics. Although these can improve pain, there is no improvement in functional status. (SOR **A**) Selective serotonin reuptake inhibitor antidepressants improve neither pain nor function compared to placebo. (SOR **A**)

7. **Willow bark extract** (standardized to 120 mg to 240 mg of salicin) for 4 weeks in the treatment of acute LBP results in statistically significant pain relief compared to placebo (number needed to treat: 3–7). (SOR **A**) The higher dose is likely more effective and can take up to 1 week before benefit is seen.

8. Systemic **corticosteroids** (e.g., prednisone 20–30 mg per day for 5–7 days) significantly improve acute pain associated with acute lumbar disk herniations.

9. **Botulinum toxin A** has been demonstrated to be safe and effective in the treatment of some patients with chronic LBP. (SOR **B**)

10. **Epidural corticosteroid injections** (in consultation with a pain management specialist) may be useful in the treatment of leg pain and sensory deficits early in the course of sciatica secondary to a herniated lumbar disk. Their use should be based on clinical findings rather than imaging results. There is no evidence that injections into facet joints or trigger points improve pain relief or function.

C. **Physical modalities. Spinal manipulation** has been shown in some studies to be effective in reducing acute LBP (and perhaps in speeding recovery) within the first month of symptoms. Patients with symptoms <16 days and no radiculopathy are most likely to benefit from manipulation.

1. **Osteopathic manipulation treatment (OMT)** and standard care have similar clinical results but medication use is less in patients undergoing OMT. (SOR **A**)

2. Other modalities such as diathermy, ultrasonography, or massage treatments have no proven effect on longer-term outcomes.

3. When compared to control injections alone, prolotherapy, injection of an irritant solution into connective tissue theoretically to strengthen tissue through scarification, demonstrates no clinical superiority in the treatment of chronic LBP. (SOR **A**)

4. There is limited evidence that lumbar supports offer no benefit compared to no treatment for nonspecific LBP and may actually risk worsening pain. (SOR **B**)

D. **Exercise.** Patients with back pain should be encouraged to begin low-impact aerobic exercise (e.g., short walks, swimming, or cycling) as soon as possible. More rigorous exercise programs to improve abdominal and paraspinal muscle tone should be delayed for at least 2 weeks following the onset of symptoms. (SOR **C**) Attainment of aerobic exercise capacity is critical in maintaining functional capacity for patients with subacute and chronic LBP. (SOR **A**) **Yoga** was found to be more effective than either exercise (stretching exercises in one trial) or a self-care book in improving functional capacity in patients with chronic LBP at 12 weeks and better than the book at 26 weeks (but not better than exercise/stretching). (SOR **B**)

E. **Patient education.** In addition to assuring the patient that, in more than 80% of cases, acute LBP will resolve or improve significantly within 4 to 6 weeks, the clinician should focus on the patient's general physical condition.

TABLE 43–3. NONRECOMMENDED THERAPY[a]

• Bedrest	• Percutaneous radiofrequency facet joint denervation
• Bipolar magnets	• Prolotherapy
• Facet join injection	• Therapeutic ultrasound
• Inferential	• Traction
• Laser	• Transcutaneous electrical nerve stimulation
• Lumbar supports	

[a]Based on the lack of effectiveness in acute and chronic low back studies.

1. A program of weight loss, exercise, and smoking cessation can help prevent recurrence of symptoms, which occurs in as many as 75% of patients with occupationally related acute episodes of LBP.
2. For **patients with work-related injuries,** instruction in body mechanics (appropriate work stance, lifting, and carrying) with follow-up can reduce incidence of recurrent injury. Job design/redesign to avoid pain-inducing movements may also help prevent recurrences.
3. Patients who are taught that they can function normally despite the LBP return to work faster than usual care (58 vs. 87 days).
4. For patients with subacute or chronic LBP, exploration of psychosocial or behavioral issues can help identify elements that may be contributing to delayed or prolonged recovery.

F. **Surgery.** The only **absolute indication** for early lumbar disk surgery is an acute disk herniation associated with either a cauda equina compression or progressive neurologic deficits.

1. Patients with significant pain and unequivocal, disk-related neurologic signs and symptoms can be treated either medically or surgically, depending on individual patient preferences. Surgical diskectomy may substantially improve the short-term symptoms and quality of life for carefully selected patients with painful herniated lumbar disks, although long-term outcomes do not appear to be superior to medical treatment.
2. Surgical consultation is not needed, however, for patients with acute LBP alone who have neither sciatica nor evidence of cancer, infection, or fracture.
3. Surgical treatment of **spinal stenosis or spondylolisthesis** should be considered only after an adequate trial of conservative therapy as recommended above for treatment of subacute and chronic LBP. There are a few randomized controlled trails indicating superiority of surgery to long-term conservative management in terms of pain or function. Outcomes for pain but not disability or walking distance are better in patients with spinal stenosis who undergo surgery compared to conservative management. (SOR **A**)

G. **Nonrecommended therapies.** Table 43–3 lists therapies for LBP that, when studied in randomized controlled trials or high-quality cohort studies, do not appear to be more effective than placebo in the treatment of pain or disability.

SELECTED REFERENCES

Chou R, Qaseem A, Owens D, et al. Clinical Guidelines Committee of the American College of Physicians Diagnostic Imaging for low back pain; advice for high-value health care from the American College of Physicians. *Ann Intern Med.* 2011;154:181–189.

Goertz M, Thorson D, Bonsell J, et al. Adult acute and subacute low back pain, Bloomington (MN). Institute for Clinical System Improvement (ICSI), updated November 2012. http://www.guideline.gov/content.aspx?id=39319&search=low+back+pain. Accessed May 2013.

Pinto RZ, Maher CG, Ferreira ML, et al. Epidural corticosteroid injections in the management of sciatica. A systematic review and meta-analysis. *Ann Intern Med.* 2012;157(12):865–877.

Roelots PDDM, Deyo R, Koes BW, et al. Non-steroidal anti-inflammatory drugs for low back pain. *Cochrane Database Syst Rev.* 2008;(1):CD000396.

Rubinstein S, van Middelkoop M, Assendelft WJJ, et al. Spinal manipulative therapy for chronic low-back pain. *Cochrane Database Syst Rev.* 2011;(2):CD008112.

Walker BF, French SD, Grant W, Green S. Combined chiropractic interventions for low-back pain. *Cochrane Database Syst Rev.* 2010;(4):CD005427.

Additional references are available online at http://langetextbooks.com/fm6e

44 Lymphadenopathy

Jo Marie Reilly, MD, FAAFP, & Fred Kobylarz, MD, MPH

KEY POINTS

- The majority of patients who present to primary care physicians with lymphadenopathy have benign, easily identifiable causes. The prevalence of malignancy in these patients is as low as 1.1%. (SOR ❸)
- Risk factors for malignancy include age >50 years, hard texture, fixed lymph nodes, weight loss, and supraclavicular location. Lymph nodes >1 cm in diameter are considered abnormal. (SOR ❸)
- Localized lymphadenopathy involves a single anatomic area and can be observed for up to 1 month. Seventy-five percent of patients with lymphadenopathy will present with localized findings. (SOR ❸)
- Generalized lymphadenopathy involves two or more noncontiguous anatomic areas, is present in 25% of patients with lymphadenopathy, usually implies a systemic disorder, and should prompt investigation. (SOR ❸)

I. **Definition.** Lymph nodes are found throughout the body except the central nervous system and serve as filtering sites of lymphatic fluid for microorganisms, malignant cells, particulate debris, or other substances. The normal immune response to acute, chronic, infectious, or noninfectious substances can lead to lymph node hardening and enlargement. **Lymphadenopathy** is defined as lymph nodes that are abnormal in size, consistency, or number.

II. **Common Diagnoses** (Table 44–1). Lymphadenopathy is common in primary care practice and occurs due to a vast array of conditions. Unexplained lymphadenopathy, however, is rare, occurring in only 0.6% of the general population in one study. Of these patients, 3.2% required a lymph node biopsy and only 1.1% were found to have a malignancy. Few additional studies have supported this low prevalence of malignancy. In contrast, in specialized clinics, the prevalence of malignancy on lymph node biopsy is 40% to 60%.

III. **Symptoms.** The patient's history often guides clinical evaluation and includes the following:
   A. **Age** is an important predictor of diagnosis. The most common causes of lymphadenopathy in children are infectious or benign. The majority of healthy children have palpable cervical, axillary, and inguinal lymph nodes. In patients older than 50 years, malignant causes of lymphadenopathy are more likely.

TABLE 44–1. COMMON CAUSES OF LYMPHADENOPATHY IN PRIMARY CARE

Diagnosis	Etiologies
Infectious	Viral infections: infectious mononucleosis, cytomegalovirus (CMV), rubella, herpes simplex, infectious hepatitis, adenovirus, rubeola, and human immunodeficiency virus (HIV) Nonviral infections: scarlet fever, cat-scratch disease, brucellosis, tuberculosis, atypical mycobacterial syphilis, histoplasmosis, leptospirosis, tularemia, malaria, toxoplasmosis, typhoid fever, and pyogenic bacterial infections
Autoimmune	Connective tissue disorders (e.g., systemic lupus erythematosus and rheumatoid arthritis, dermatomyositis, Sjögren syndrome) Benign reactive hyperplasia
Iatrogenic	Serum sickness Medications: allopurinol, atenolol, captopril, carbamazepine, cephalosporins, gold, hydralazine, penicillin, phenytoin, primidone, quinidine, sulfonamides, sulindac
Metabolic	Gaucher disease, Niemann–Pick disease, hyperthyroidism
Malignant	Leukemia, Hodgkin and non-Hodgkin lymphomas, skin neoplasms, Kaposi sarcoma, metastatic cancers, malignant histiocytosis, metastases
Miscellaneous	Kawasaki disease, sarcoidosis, and chronic pseudolymphomatous lymphadenopathy

Source: Data from Bazemore AW, Smucker DR. Lymphadenopathy and malignancy. *Am Fam Physician.* 2002;66: 2103–2110.

B. Duration. Lymphadenopathy lasting less than 1 month is usually infectious. Lymphadenopathy persisting for more than 1 month in the absence of an obvious explanation is usually abnormal and more likely due to a collagen vascular disease, malignancy, or chronic infection. The presence of supra- or infraclavicular nodes, however, is of concern.

C. Constitutional symptoms (e.g., fatigue, fever, unexplained weight loss >10% of body weight over 6 months, unusual rashes, night sweats, myalgias, or arthralgias) suggest infection, autoimmune diseases, malignancy, or serum sickness-like syndrome (e.g., medications).

D. Localized symptoms can suggest the cause of lymphadenopathy (e.g., sore throat and cervical lymphadenopathy).

E. Personal/social or family history such as travel, exposure to animals, occupation, dietary habits, hobbies, sexual history and orientation, drug use, infectious contacts, and environmental and family history can help in the diagnosis.

1. Exposures. Travelers to tropical areas have an increased risk of tuberculosis, scrub typhus, and leishmaniasis. Patients exposed to cats may have an increased risk of cat-scratch disease or toxoplasmosis. Those exposed to lacerations from gardening are at an increased risk for sporotrichosis. Hunters exposed to wild rodents have an increased risk of tularemia.

2. High-risk sexual behavior increases the likelihood of an infection due to gonorrhea, syphilis, genital herpes, or human immunodeficiency virus (HIV).

3. Patients with a personal history of dysplastic nevus syndrome may have lymphadenopathy from melanoma.

F. A **medication history** may assist diagnosis. Some medications are known to cause lymphadenopathy (e.g., phenytoin) and others (e.g., penicillins or sulfonamides) are more likely to cause a serum sickness-like syndrome with lymphadenopathy.

IV. Signs. The patient's physical examination further guides clinical diagnosis. Assessment of lymph nodes should include the following:

A. Localized versus generalized. Lymphadenopathy can be localized (enlarged lymph nodes in one region), regional (enlarged lymph nodes in two or more contiguous regions), or generalized (enlarged lymph nodes in two or more noncontiguous regions). When lymphadenopathy is localized, examination should focus on the region drained by the lymph nodes. Because most localized lymphadenopathy is in the head and neck region, physical examination should include ears, nose, throat, and neck examination. When generalized lymphadenopathy is noted, systemic disease must be considered. In a primary care setting, 75% present with localized lymphadenopathy and 25% present with generalized lymphadenopathy.

B. Size. Lymph nodes greater than 1 cm in diameter are considered abnormal. Exceptions are epitrochlear nodes, which are abnormal if greater than 0.5 cm, and inguinal nodes, which are abnormal if greater than 1.5 cm. There is little information supporting diagnosis based on size alone.

C. Consistency. Softer or fluctuant lymph nodes suggest infectious or inflammatory causes; harder nodes suggest malignancy.

D. Pain. Although nonspecific, tenderness on palpation of lymph nodes suggests an inflammatory cause; absence of pain makes a more serious condition or malignancy more likely.

E. Location. Location of lymphadenopathy can be helpful in diagnosis (Table 44–2). Of patients in the primary care setting with localized lymphadenopathy, most (55%) occur in the head and neck region, 14% in the inguinal region, 5% in the axillary region, and 1% in the supraclavicular region.

F. Mobility. Freely mobile nodes are less likely associated with malignancy. In contrast, fixed, matted nodes are more suggestive of metastatic carcinoma.

G. Generalized lymphadenopathy with splenomegaly is usually a sign of systemic disease and suggests infectious mononucleosis, lymphoma, leukemia, or sarcoidosis.

V. Diagnostic Testing and Imaging

A. Laboratory tests (Figure 44–1). A careful history and physical examination should allow the clinician to determine whether careful observation, treatment, or additional testing is needed. The critical task is to determine which patients with lymphadenopathy have benign, self-limited conditions and which patients have malignancy or other serious conditions requiring further evaluation and specific treatment.

1. A complete blood cell count with a WBC differential and a peripheral smear can provide useful diagnostic information in uncertain cases.

2. Studies based on clinical presentation can include a throat culture, a monospot, an HIV test, hepatitis serologies, antinuclear antibody, rapid plasma reagin, and purified protein derivative.

TABLE 44-2. DIFFERENTIAL DIAGNOSIS OF LYMPHADENOPATHY BY LOCATION

Location	Diagnosis
Cervical	
The most common area of lymphadenopathy and most cases are caused by infections	*Infections:* Viral upper respiratory infections, bacterial pharyngitis, infectious mononucleosis, cytomegalovirus, toxoplasmosis, mycobacterial diseases, dental abscess, tuberculosis, and rubella *Malignancy:* Non-Hodgkin lymphoma, Hodgkin disease, thyroid cancer, head and neck malignancy (older patients with a history of smoking) *Others:* Kawasaki syndrome, sarcoidosis, Kikuchi disease, oral injuries, and dental lesions
Supraclavicular	
This location has the highest risk of malignancy; 90% of patients older than 50 yr will have a malignancy when lymphadenopathy is localized here	*Infections:* Chronic fungal (histoplasmosis) and mycobacterial infections *Malignancy:* Left supraclavicular node (Virchow node) drains the abdomen or thorax and is associated with breast cancer, lymphoma, and other malignancies Right supraclavicular node drains the mediastinum, lungs, and esophagus and is associated with pathology in these areas
Axillary	
Usually secondary to infection or malignancy	*Infections: Staphylococcus* and *Streptococcus* infections of the arm, tularemia, cat-scratch disease, and toxoplasmosis *Malignancy:* Metastatic breast cancer, lymphoma, and metastatic melanoma
Epitrochlear	
Rare in healthy patients	*Infections:* Infectious mononucleosis, HIV, secondary syphilis, leprosy, rubella, tularemia, sarcoidosis, and leishmaniasis *Malignancy:* Lymphoma and leukemia (CLL)
Inguinal	
Most adults will normally have some degree of inguinal enlargement, and there is a low suspicion of malignancy.	*Infections:* Sexually transmitted diseases, cellulitis, bubonic plague *Malignancies:* Squamous cell carcinoma of the penis/vulva, lymphoma, Hodgkin and Non-Hodgkin lymphomas, or melanoma
Generalized	
Lymphadenopathy found in two or more distinct anatomic regions and needs prompt investigation.	It is more likely to result from serious infections (e.g., HIV), autoimmune disease (e.g., systemic lupus erythematosus), hematologic malignancies (e.g., leukemia), and metastatic cancers

Source: Data from Ferrer R. Lymphadenopathy: differential diagnosis and evaluation. *Am Fam Physician.* 1998;58: 1313-1320 and BMJ Best-practices.

B. **Imaging studies** such as ultrasonography, chest x-ray, computerized tomography (CT) scan, and magnetic resonance imaging (MRI) of the involved area may differentiate lymphadenopathy from nonlymphatic causes. (SOR **G**) In the diagnosis of cervical lymphadenopathy, ultrasonography can offer additional information to a fine-needle aspiration (FNA) and help avoid the need for more invasive testing such as a lymph node biopsy. CT scan and MRI are useful to demonstrate the presence of mediastinal, mesenteric, or retroperitoneal lymph nodes.

1. **FNA** of the affected lymph node(s) can be useful in obtaining a histological diagnosis in a patient with a recurrent malignancy or in the diagnosis of a patient with an underlying carcinoma.

2. **Lymph node excisional biopsy** and histological testing should be considered as first-line testing if a malignancy is suspected, if the initial studies in a patient with generalized lymphadenopathy are nondiagnostic, or if a patient presents with persistent localized lymphadenopathy and has nondiagnostic testing. Biopsies should be obtained from the largest lymph node or the area with the greatest lymph node involvement.

   a. Clinical features that suggest **the need for an early biopsy** include a diameter of greater than 2 cm, hard and fixed consistency, lack of pain or tenderness on palpation, age older than 50 years, an abnormal chest x-ray result (e.g.,

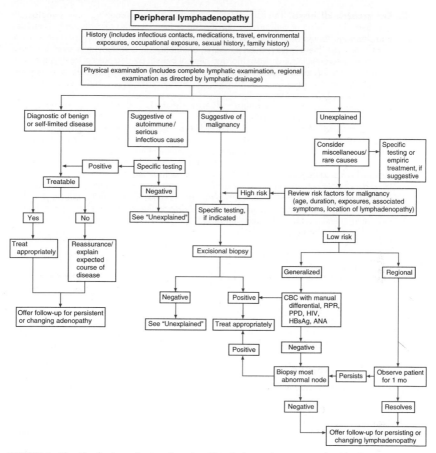

FIGURE 44–1. Algorithm for the evaluation of peripheral lymphadenopathy. CBC, complete blood count; RPR, rapid plasma reagin; PPD, purified protein derivative; HIV, human immunodeficiency virus; HBsAg, hepatitis B surface antigen; ANA, antinuclear antibody. Adapted with permission from Ferrer R. Lymphadenopathy: differential diagnosis and evaluation. *Am Fam Physician.* 1998;58(6):1313–1320.

adenopathy or infiltrate), associated worrisome signs and symptoms (e.g., weight loss or hepatosplenomegaly), an absence of upper respiratory tract symptoms, an enlargement of a supraclavicular node, or a cervical node in a smoker. Endoscopic ultrasound-guided FNA is the procedure of choice for evaluation of posterior mediastinal lymphadenopathy. (SOR **⊙**)

    b. Supraclavicular nodes have the highest yield from biopsy and inguinal nodes the lowest.

    c. During follow-up for undiagnosed lymphadenopathy, nodes that remain constant in size for 4 to 8 weeks or fail to resolve in 8 to 12 weeks should be biopsied. Up to 25% of patients with nondiagnostic initial biopsy and persistent lymphadenopathy who undergo a second biopsy have cancer.

    3. Bone marrow examination is indicated for patients with severe anemia, neutropenia, thrombocytopenia, or a peripheral smear with malignant blast cells.

VI. Treatment for Select Conditions

    A. Viral infections. Treatment of lymphadenopathy associated with viral infections is limited to symptomatic treatment such as warm compresses, analgesics, and the avoidance of trauma to the swollen node.

C. Cat-scratch disease. This disease is usually self-limited, requiring only symptomatic treatment. Aspiration of suppurative glands can reduce swelling and discomfort. Incision and drainage should be avoided to prevent sinus tract formation. For typical cases of cat-scratch disease, there is no proven benefit to antibiotics. In one study, however, treatment with oral azithromycin for 5 days afforded clinical benefit by decreasing total lymph node size. Antibiotics (azithromycin, clarithromycin, rifampin, trimethoprim-sulfamethoxazole, or ciprofloxacin) should be administered for severe cases or for immunocompromised patients (e.g., HIV). (SOR **C**)

D. Neoplasm. Patients with neoplastic disease should be referred to an oncologist for histologic diagnosis and treatment.

E. Mycobacterial disease. Nodes affected with atypical mycobacteria are treated by surgical excision. (SOR **A**) A positive culture result or the demonstration of acid-fast bacilli is the most direct method of diagnosis, although treatment of *Mycobacterium tuberculosis* can be initiated on the basis of the clinical presentation and a positive tuberculosis skin test.

F. Acute lymphadenitis. Initial therapy should be directed toward staphylococcal and streptococcal infections. First-line treatment recommendations include oral cephalexin (25–50 mg/kg in divided doses up to 500 mg four times a day) and erythromycin (30–50 mg/kg up to 500 mg four times a day). Additionally, a semisynthetic penicillinase-resistant penicillin such as dicloxacillin (25–50 mg/kg up to 500 mg four times a day for 7–10 days) can be useful.

VII. Patient Education

A. Travelers should be counseled to avoid risky behaviors that can lead to infectious sources of lymphadenopathy.

B. Primary care cancer screening and well child care visits offer ideal opportunities to counsel patients on sexual behavior and viral/bacterial syndromes likely to cause lymphadenopathy. These visits are also opportune times to counsel patients on factors that increase the risk of cancer (which can present with lymphadenopathy) such as smoking, diet and exercise, and excessive alcohol consumption.

C. In order to diagnosis and treat cancer as early as possible, patients should be reminded of the importance of cancer surveillance and the appropriate intervals for screening.

SELECTED REFERENCES

Assessment of Lymphadenopathy. http://bestpractice.bmj.com/best-practice/monograph/838/diagnosis.html. Last updated December 6, 2012. Accessed April 24, 2013.

Bazemore AW, Smucker DR. Lymphadenopathy and malignancy. *Am Fam Physician*. 2002;66:2103–2110.

Ferrer R. Lymphadenopathy: differential diagnosis and evaluation. *Am Fam Physician*. 1998;58:1313–1320.

Fletcher R, Boxer C, Tirnacew J. Evaluation of peripheral lymphadenopathy in adults. www.uptodate.com. Last updated June 19, 2012. Accessed April 24, 2013.

Khanna R, Sharma AD, Khanna S, et al. Usefulness of ultrasonography for the evaluation of cervical lymphadenopathy. *World J Surg Oncol*. 2011;9:29.

Mcgee SR. Peripheral lymphadenopathy. In: Mcgee SR, ed. *Evidence-Based Physical Diagnosis*. 2nd ed. Philadelphia, PA: Saunders Elsevier; 2007.

Richner S, Laifer G. Peripheral lymphadenopathy in immunocompetent adults. *Swiss Med Weekly*. 2010; 140(7-8):98–104.

---

45   Myalgia

Tomás P. Owens, Jr., MD

KEY POINTS

- Most common causes of myalgia can be diagnosed through careful history and examination, without laboratory testing. (SOR **C**)
- Ischemia should be considered in localized myalgia, especially with suggestive risk factors and normal muscle examination. (SOR **C**)
- Drug-induced rhabdomyolysis should be considered as a potential cause of myalgia. (SOR **C**)

I. Definition. Myalgia is defined as generalized or localized pain perceived as originating in the skeletal muscle tissue, usually characterized as a deep, aching sensation but sometimes as a burning or electric sensation. Myalgia can be classified as acute (lasting <1 month) or chronic (lasting >3–6 months), as localized (one or a few muscle groups) or generalized (involving more than four areas), and as symmetric or asymmetric.

II. Common Diagnoses. As many as one-third of patients presenting in an ambulatory primary care setting complain of muscle pain in an extremity or the back. In the general population, as many as 60% of adults have musculoskeletal pain lasting more than 1 month or caused by identified trauma. In one study, 9% of primary care visits were for myofascial pain syndrome.

A. Viral syndromes (and other infectious causes). Most **viral syndromes** have seasonal variations, with a winter peak in temperate climates; prototypical is influenza and in the tropics dengue fever. Arbovirus myalgic syndromes such as West Nile virus predominate between June and October, paralleling the mosquito vectors. Children are particularly at risk for viral syndromes, but myalgia is less common in children than in adults. Rocky Mountain spotted fever, Lyme disease, malaria, toxoplasmosis, trichinosis, malaria, and hemorrhagic fevers can all cause profound myalgia. A rare form of localized myalgia is staphylococcal myositis, which can accompany cellulitis or an abscess.

B. Major or minor trauma/exertional. Accumulated metabolic waste products cause myalgia with strenuous exercise. This occurs more so in a deconditioned patient but also in trained individuals. Direct blunt, crush injuries, or minor repetitive trauma that occurs with occupational hazards (faulty ergonomics, repetitive acts of a monotonous nature), recreational pursuits ("weekend warrior syndrome" with poor conditioning or inappropriate training), or substance abuse (repetitive accidental or self-inflicted trauma) results in hemorrhage within the muscle tissue and muscle fiber or fascial tears. Trauma also causes muscle spasm or cramping.

C. Fibromyalgia and myofascial pain (8%–10% of all visits to a primary care outpatient practice).

1. Fibromyalgia syndrome (FMS—former name: fibrositis) affects 5% to 10% of the US population during their lifetime. It is more common in women than in men (10:1), particularly in women aged 20 to 50 years (with a peak incidence at age 35 years). **FMS** is the second most common disorder in American rheumatology practices. It has been associated with a history of sexual abuse during childhood, drug use, and eating disorders, but no causal relationship has been established. Depression, personality disorders, and anxiety are also strongly associated. In FMS, there is clear evidence of regional blood flow abnormalities in the thalamus and caudate nucleus. These abnormalities are associated with low pain-threshold levels (hyperalgesia) and allodynia (pain due to a stimulus that normally does not cause pain) occurring spontaneously or as a neuroimmune response to viral, physical, or psychological trauma. Biochemical abnormalities are inconsistent and muscle biopsies are unrevealing.

2. Less generalized **myofascial pain syndromes** (not fulfilling **FMS** diagnostic criteria) are seen in up to 50% of the population, are equally common in men and women, and have a much better prognosis with appropriate therapy.

D. Collagen vascular diseases affect approximately 15% in the general population and more than 1 million newly afflicted patients each year. **Inflammatory articular diseases** such as rheumatoid arthritis and lupus occur primarily in women between ages 20 and 50 years. **Inflammatory nonarticular diseases** such as **polymyositis** and **dermatomyositis** are more common in children and occur equally in men and women, but a particular form occurs in men older than 40 years in association with malignancy of other organ systems. **Polymyositis** may be postviral; it is especially common following enteroviral infections (particularly Coxsackie) or parasitic infection such as trichinosis. **Polymyalgia rheumatica (PMR)** occurs equally in men and women, usually older than 65 years. Myalgia from these conditions is caused by immune-mediated inflammation of periarticular structures or muscles.

E. Ischemia

1. Vascular insufficiency (≤1% of patients with myalgia) has a strong association with older age, smoking, hypertension, hyperlipidemia, and diabetes mellitus and occurs due to insufficient arterial perfusion.

2. Compression due to immobility, coma, depressant (alcohol, opioid, sedatives) overdose and compartment syndromes from injury, tight splints, or casting can result in hypoperfusion.

F. Primary muscle malignancy is an extremely rare cause of myalgia in primary care, has no specific risk factors, and causes pain from rapid tumor growth with compression of surrounding structures.

G. Nontraumatic nonexertional rhabdomyolysis

   1. Substance/toxin induced. The **"statin"** class of lipid-lowering agents has been associated with generalized myalgia and rarely as **statin-induced myalgia (SIM)** due to direct muscle toxicity (rhabdomyolysis) (see Chapter 76). The synchronous use of gemfibrozil, macrolides, imidazoles, protease inhibitors, and cyclosporine and the ingestion of grapefruit potentiate the effect, as does preexisting renal insufficiency. It is believed that lipid-soluble statins are more likely to produce the syndrome.

     a. Other drugs causing myopathy or myalgia but not discussed further here include amphotericin B, colchicine, chloroquine, cimetidine, clofibrate, glucocorticoids, oral contraceptives, zidovudine, and neuroleptics via neuroleptic malignant syndrome.

     b. In the 1990s, some batches of l-tryptophan (e.g., "peak X") produced a complex immunologic response called **eosinophilia-myalgia syndrome (EMS)**. More recently, there have been reports of myalgia/rhabdomyolysis in association with intake of supplements (Hydroxycut, Diet Fuel, and Gluta-MASS). It is not clear which of the declared or, if any, undeclared components is at fault.

   2. Hyperthermia produces rhabdomyolysis through rigor.

III. Symptoms and Signs

  A. Myalgia from **most viral syndromes** is relatively mild; the time course parallels the course of the illness and is often accompanied by other systemic viral infection symptoms (malaise, weakness, and any combination of the following: headache, nausea, vomiting, diarrhea, and upper respiratory symptoms, including fever). Influenza and dengue fever are known particularly for severe myalgia. Viral myalgia is usually generalized, but many patients complain of pain in larger, proximal muscle groups and in the back (particularly the upper back, trapezius, neck, and shoulders). Many experts believe that acute viral infection can precipitate progression to chronic fibromyalgia, in which case patients report a deep, aching discomfort, an inability to be comfortable in any position, and localized, palpable pain. **Well-localized inflammation in relation to cellulitis** is the hallmark of staphylococcal myositis or abscesses.

  B. Myalgia caused by **trauma** is localized and specific to the trauma history.

   1. Patients sometimes report the **relatively acute onset of localized pain** without associated illness or obvious trauma, but further probing usually reveals some new activity or minor repetitive act (e.g., lifting furniture, gardening, painting, or new work responsibility).

   2. The **pain of major trauma** (e.g., a motor vehicle accident) or overuse usually starts several hours after the event and reaches a peak at 48 hours. The pain may persist for days or weeks, particularly if the offending activity is not identified and stopped. The patient may report some loss of function or pain with a specific movement or position, which sometimes reminds the patient of the precipitating event.

   3. Tenderness on palpation of the specific muscle, sometimes with crepitus, decreased active range of motion, and erythema, is a common finding. Blunt trauma may cause ecchymosis, hematoma (following minimal trauma in patients receiving anticoagulants or antiplatelet agents), superficial abrasions, pain on palpation, or decreased active and passive range of motion of the involved muscle.

  C. FMS and myofascial pain syndrome

   1. With **FMS,** pain is worse after even minimal activity and may include generalized symptoms such as diffuse myalgia, fatigue, a low-grade fever, muscle tension, headache, and skin sensitivity. Sleep disturbance is a particularly prominent and nearly universal complaint. The 2011 revision of the American College of Rheumatology 2010 diagnostic criteria require the patient to have a widespread pain index (WPI) of 7 or more of 19 possible areas and a symptom severity (SS) score of 5 or more out of 12 or a WPI of 3 to 6 and an SS score 9 or more (Figure 45–1).

   2. Myofascial pain syndrome includes localized muscle pain in such common areas as the paraspinous regions of the upper and middle back, trapezius, levator scapulae, neck, shoulders, arms, glutei, and legs, often manifesting as **trigger points** (excruciatingly painful foci of muscle from which diffused pain and spasm emanate).

  D. The myalgia associated with a **collagen vascular disease** parallels the course of the primary disease and is increased with muscle palpation.

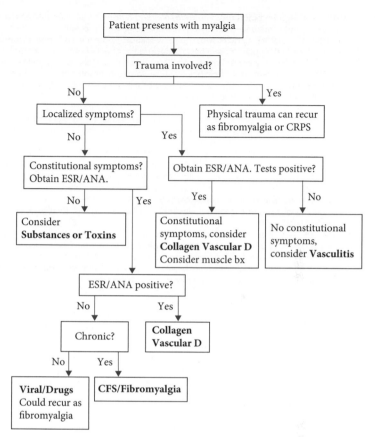

FIGURE 45–1. Approach to the patient with myalgia. ANA, antinuclear antibody; CFS, chronic fatigue syndrome; CRPS, complex regional pain syndrome; ESR, erythrocyte sedimentation rate.

1. Signs of the primary rheumatic disease dominate, including joint erythema and swelling or effusion, Raynaud's phenomenon, vasculitis, conjunctivitis, urethritis, or uveitis.
2. The onset of **polymyositis** may be acute, particularly in children, and may include fever. In polymyositis of any cause, the patient reports loss of muscle function from either pain or loss of functioning neuromuscular units. A common complaint is inability to stand up from a chair without using arms or assistance. Primary idiopathic **dermatomyositis** can present with multiple abdominal complaints (e.g., pain or dysphagia) and a classic lilac-colored (heliotrope) rash.
3. The pain and stiffness of inflammatory articular disorders such as **rheumatoid arthritis** or lupus are more severe in the morning upon arising.
4. Patients with **PMR** complain of stiffness, weakness, and pain, particularly in the hip and shoulder girdle, along with systemic symptoms such as malaise and fatigue. Headache could be a symptom of **temporal (giant cell) arteritis**.
E. **Vascular insufficiency** causes the most severe myalgia and is intermittent, and physical examination of the muscle is often normal.
   1. The pain associated with **arterial insufficiency** (intermittent claudication) occurs with exercise of a predictable type and intensity, is almost always in the lower extremity, and can be described precisely by the patient. It resolves shortly after cessation of the activity. With severe ischemia, rest pain may be present. Peripheral pulses are delayed, decreased, or absent, and extremity blood pressures are asymmetric, with a

decreased leg:arm blood pressure ratio. Marked hair loss, dry skin, decreased capillary refill, and pronounced pachyonychia are commonly present.

2. In **thoracic outlet syndrome,** pain, weakness, paresthesias, and claudication occur in one of the upper extremities. Abducting the affected arm and externally rotating the shoulder may precipitate pain with or without cyanosis and pulselessness.

3. The pain of **venous insufficiency** is more vague in onset, nature, and cessation, but is often related to a dependent position of the affected extremity (almost always the leg). Signs may include increased circumference, edema, erythema, brawny hyperpigmentation, and ulceration of dependent areas, particularly the lower legs and ankles ("venous stasis"). Rarely, a **superior vena cava syndrome** will produce symptoms in the upper extremities. These findings are accompanied by facial swelling, cyanosis, and neck vein distention.

4. Compressive ischemia can be extremely painful at first, but commonly the patient is unconscious from the original insult. The process can develop enough nerve damage to produce decreased sensation after some time has elapsed. Significant edema, decreased pulses, and paleness or cyanosis of the skin are noted.

F. The pain of **primary muscle malignancy** is gradual in onset and vague in nature, but patients usually report associated weakness and an enlarging, localized mass in the body of the muscle.

G. Generalized, slowly progressive pain, asthenia, and weakness/tenderness of major muscle groups are characteristic of **SIM.** In hyperthermia, it would be acute.

IV. Laboratory tests (Figure 45–1). An erythrocyte sedimentation rate (ESR) and antinuclear antibody can be helpful in distinguishing between types of disorders producing myalgia. Additional laboratory evaluation is not usually indicated in cases of viral syndrome, trauma, or clearcut myofascial pain or **FMS,** but may be indicated in patients with rheumatic symptoms or who have impressive systemic symptoms; whose symptoms have persisted despite conservative, nonspecific therapy for several weeks; who have joint effusions; or whose disease has caused significant disability (see polymyositis above).

A. Complete blood cell count. The white blood cell count may show a neutropenic or inflammatory (leukocytosis) reaction with a viral syndrome, although the **ESR** is usually normal. The ESR helps differentiate fibromyalgia (normal) from collagen vascular diseases (ESR ≥50 mm/h). A high ESR may prompt further testing (e.g., antinuclear antibody, rheumatoid factor, and more comprehensive rheumatologic panels) (see Chapter 38). Parasitic infection may cause eosinophilia. Mild anemia and thrombocytosis are common in rheumatic diseases.

B. Culture of specific infectious lesions (e.g., primary herpes simplex) should be performed only in appropriate clinical situations. Routine throat swabs and blood cultures are usually unrevealing with viral syndromes.

C. Imaging may be required to rule out bony pathology as a result of known or unknown trauma (particularly relating to the hip or pelvis in older persons) or may be helpful in patients with localized muscle or tendon pain that is difficult to differentiate from bone pain (e.g., lateral epicondylitis).

D. An empiric trial of a low, daily dose (10–20 mg orally) of prednisone usually has a dramatic positive effect on almost all collagen vascular diseases and thus has some diagnostic value pending more definitive studies. Unfortunately, corticosteroid use can produce a sense of well-being in patients with almost any pathology. Therefore, empiric corticosteroid use must be adapted to each clinical situation and only rarely considered. Prompt treatment of **giant cell arteritis** accompanying PMR is indicated and would not qualify as empiric therapy.

E. Creatine phosphokinase (CPK) is markedly elevated in ischemia. **Impedance Doppler studies** are diagnostic in patients with evidence of vascular insufficiency (see Chapter 41). These may be followed or, in some instances, supplanted by **arteriography** or **venography**.

F. Muscle biopsy should be arranged for any enlarging painful muscle mass not explainable by specific trauma and in patients with findings of myositis (see above). Abnormal histology on muscle biopsy is the only specific laboratory abnormality in patients with primary muscle tumors.

G. In **SIM and hyperthermia,** marked elevations of CPK and myoglobinuria are noted. In **EMS,** the eosinophil count is higher than $1000/mm^3$ and biopsy results show eosinophilic fasciitis.

V. Treatment

A. Myalgia caused by **viral syndromes** is relieved by treatment with nonsteroidal anti-inflammatory drugs (NSAIDs). **Aspirin,** 650 to 1000 mg orally every 4 hours, is as effective as a prescription NSAID, but should be avoided for treatment of fever in children when a viral syndrome occurs due to the risk of Reye syndrome. **Ibuprofen,** 600 mg orally every 6 hours, and **naproxen sodium,** 375 to 500 mg orally every 8 to 12 hours, are excellent substitutes for the anti-inflammatory effect of aspirin, but may be less effective as antipyretic agents. **Acetaminophen,** 650 to 1000 mg orally every 4 hours (maximum 4 g per day in adults, 3 g per day in the elderly, with strict alcohol avoidance), can be used for severe myalgia, particularly when associated with severe headache. Acetaminophen can be combined with **codeine,** 15 to 30 mg (e.g., Tylenol no. 2 or no. 3), or **hydrocodone,** 5 to 10 mg (e.g., Norco), one to two tablets orally every 4 hours if needed. So-called muscle *relaxants* exert their effects primarily as sedatives and have no true direct muscle action, yet they can be used with caution in selected patients where the risk/benefit ratio is favorable.

B. Myalgia caused by **blunt trauma** or repetitive minor trauma is best treated with rest of the affected muscle, ice and cold therapy (particularly after use of a muscle injured by overactivity or inappropriate athletic training), heat therapy (particularly for generalized myalgia or for localized myalgia with muscle weakness or dysfunction), and immobilization (for localized myalgia caused by trauma with significant dysfunction).

  1. Immobilization can be accomplished with either soft (e.g., felt) or rigid (e.g., commercial plastic or metal) splints for only a few days to prevent atrophy and weakness.

  2. A more specific diagnosis of the cause of **repetitive overuse injuries** (recreational or occupational) may lead to specific exercises, strengthening, or avoidance/modification of certain activities in the workplace (ergonomics evaluation) or during leisure time.

C. For myalgia caused by **fibromyalgia,** prescribed reading may give the patient encouragement by naming the problem and informing the patient that the problem is manageable, and it may help in controlling health care-seeking behavior for the multitude of associated symptoms. Support groups may have similar benefit. Multidisciplinary outpatient treatment programs, even as brief as 1.5 days, can have a significant effect on the impact of illness.

  1. An **exercise and stretching program** should be similar to that for rehabilitation following myocardial infarction, with specific submaximal heart rate targets (70%–80% of maximum heart rate), frequency (three to five times weekly), and duration (30–40 minutes with appropriate warm-up and cool down). (SOR 🄰) Physical therapy may not have significant efficacy in improving pain. (SOR 🄱)

  2. Cognitive behavioral therapy is very useful for many patients. Minimal intervention (paradoxical approach) has also been effective, particularly in the outpatient setting. (SOR 🄰) Disability claims, with legal and financial repercussions and tremendous secondary gain, make the management of this syndrome complicated in some patients.

  3. Analgesics. NSAIDs are not recommended for FMS pain. (SOR 🄰) Tramadol (50–100 mg—two to three times daily) can improve pain. Opioids should only be used after every possible alternative approach has failed.

  4. Antidepressants. Amitriptyline, 25 to 50 mg orally 1 to 2 hours before bedtime, has the strongest data support. Cyclobenzaprine 10 to 30 mg nightly can also reduce pain and improve sleep. Selective serotonin reuptake inhibitors (specifically paroxetine 10–60 mg daily and fluoxetine 10–80 mg nightly [mean effective dose 40 mg], alone or added to amitriptyline) can improve global symptom scores. Duloxetine (FDA approved) 60 to 120 mg daily can decrease pain severity and milnacipran (an FDA-approved serotonin–norepinephrine reuptake inhibitor) 50 mg twice daily after 1 week of titration may improve mood and quality of life.

  5. Other oral medications. Pregabalin (FDA approved) 300 to 450 mg daily can reduce pain, but is not well-tolerated. Gabapentin 600 to 2400 mg daily in divided doses, if tolerated, can improve well-being. Naltrexone, sodium oxybate, and pramipexole have also been used with moderate success. Sleep medications such as heterocyclics (trazodone 50–300 mg nightly) and sedatives such as benzodiazepines can be used in a moderate dosage, primarily for regulation of sleep rather than in the full dosage used for major depressive or anxiety disorder (SOR 🄰) (see Chapters 91 and

94). Guaifenesin, topical capsaicin, S-Adenosyl-L-methionine (SAM-e), magnesium malate, and growth hormone lack sufficient data to be recommended.

6. **Trigger point injection** can be performed as often as necessary with local anesthetic, (SOR **B**) but preferably no more than four or five injections per year should be given if corticosteroids are used. The trigger point should be carefully palpated to determine the point of most exquisite pain. This point is injected intramuscularly using a long 25- or 27-gauge needle that contains 0.5 to 1.0 mL of a long-acting local anesthetic such as bupivacaine 0.25%. There is some evidence of benefit from moving the needle around and pulling back into different parts of the trigger point ("needling"). A corticosteroid, such as 0.5 mL of **triamcinolone,** 40 mg/mL, can be added to the injection, but no evidence exists that the injection will be more effective than any of the local anesthetics or even normal saline.

7. **Alternative, integrative, complementary,** or **balanced medicine** approaches, including biofeedback, qi gong, spray-and-stretch techniques, acupuncture, and acupressure, can be helpful, but strong research supporting their efficacy is scarce. (SOR **B**) Data suggest yoga, meditation, tai chi, hypnosis, pleasant imagery, and electroacupuncture can reduce symptoms. (SOR **B**) Massage therapy, osteopathic manipulation, and chiropractic may also help some patients. (SOR **B**)

D. Myalgia caused by **collagen vascular diseases** is managed according to the underlying disease, usually with rheumatologic consultation (see Chapter 38).

1. **PMR,** though self-limited, is treated with low-dose (10–20 mg) oral prednisone daily for symptomatic relief. (SOR **A**) If the patient is not nearly asymptomatic in a few days, the diagnosis should be reconsidered. Treatment should continue for 1 year and the disease can be followed clinically, without regard to ESR, tapering off the prednisone over a few weeks and restarting if the pain recurs. Most people are asymptomatic in 24 months, rarely 36 months. Some patients have recurrences early or in a few years, and they respond well to retreatment.

2. If the patient has symptoms of **giant cell arteritis,** treatment with 60 mg of prednisone daily should start immediately to prevent ischemic events, which occur in 20% of all nontreated patients. If the diagnosis is uncertain, a biopsy of the affected arterial segment should be done within a few days. Response to prednisone is rapid and complete in approximately 3 to 4 days. In 4 to 6 weeks the ESR should be normal. Prednisone dose is decreased by 10% per month while continuing a monthly check of the ESR, until a dose of 10 mg per day is reached. That dose is continued for at least 2 years. Approximately 10% of patients may require 3 or more years of therapy. Some patients have recurrences or may require very long or permanent low-dose therapy. Side effects of prednisone include weight gain, worsening of glucose intolerance, and cushingoid features.

E. Myalgia caused by **ischemia** (see Chapter 41).

F. Myalgia resulting from **primary muscle malignancy** is relieved by excision of the malignant tumor, in consultation with a surgeon and oncologist.

G. In **SIM,** full resolution of symptoms and normalization of laboratory tests can be expected within days of drug withdrawal. Intense hydration and loop diuretics are recommended with CPKs higher than 2000. Chronic renal insufficiency can occur secondary to the myoglobinuria. **EMS** has been successfully treated during the acute phase with oral prednisone, 1 to 2 mg/kg per day, for days to weeks. (SOR **C**) In the late phase of the illness, no treatment has been helpful. Most symptoms and signs of the illness are resolved in 2 to 3 years, except for cognitive impairment and peripheral neuropathy.

SELECTED REFERENCES

Carville SF, Arendt-Nielsen S, Bliddal H, et al. EULAR evidence-based recommendations for the management of fibromyalgia syndrome. *Ann Rheumat Dis.* 2008;67(4):536–541.

Gilron I, Shum B, Moore RA, Wiffen PJ. Combination pharmacotherapy for the treatment of fibromyalgia. *Cochrane Pain Palliative and Supportive Care Group* [published online ahead of print June 13, 2013]. DOI: 10.1002/14651858.CD010585.

Goldenberg DL, Burckhardt C, Crofford L. Management of fibromyalgia syndrome. *JAMA.* 2004;292: 2388–2395.

Klippel JH, ed. *Primer on the Rheumatic Diseases.* 13th ed. Atlanta, GA: Arthritis Foundation; 2008.

Wolfe F, Clauw DJ, Fitzcharles MA, et al. Fibromyalgia criteria and severity scales for clinical and epidemiological studies: a modification of the ACR preliminary diagnostic criteria for fibromyalgia. *J Rheumatol.* 2011;38:1113–1122.

46 Nausea and Vomiting

Nipa R. Shah, MD, & George R. Wilson, MD

KEY POINTS

- Nausea and vomiting are common complaints that are usually self-limited. (SOR **C**)
- Serious etiologies can be ruled out with a thorough history and a directed examination. (SOR **C**)
- Once any necessary tests show negative results, treatment can be directed toward symptom control and dehydration precautions. (SOR **C**)
- Complementary and alternative medical therapies provide additional, nonpharmacologic treatment of nausea and vomiting. (SOR **B**; acupuncture, SOR **A**)

I. **Definition. Nausea** is a discomfort or an unpleasant sensation of impending vomiting, usually felt in the upper abdominal and chest areas. **Retching** is a strong, involuntary effort to vomit without bringing up emesis. **Regurgitation** is the return of gas or small amounts of food from the stomach. It is often, but not always, caused by an incompetent lower esophageal sphincter. **Eructation** is the voiding of gas or, on occasion, small quantities of acidic fluid from the stomach through the mouth. It involves a process similar to regurgitation and is roughly equivalent to belching. **Vomiting** is the forceful expulsion of stomach contents in a series of involuntary, spastic movements. Vomiting occurs when the neuroreceptors in the emetic center are stimulated. The emetic center is located in the reticular formation of the medulla oblongata and is rich in histamine (H_1) receptors, muscarinic (M) cholinergic receptors, and serotonin (5-HT_3) receptors. The emetic center can be stimulated through the following:
   - **Stomach** or **biliary duct distention** via vagal afferents
   - **Vestibular dysfunction** via H_1 and M receptors
   - **Metabolic derangements, toxins, and some medications** (cardiac glycosides, chemotherapy, and opiates) via the chemoreceptor trigger zone, which is rich in 5-HT_3 and dopamine (D_2) receptors
   - **Inflammation or ischemia** of the heart, pericardium, liver, pancreas, gallbladder, or peritoneum.
II. **Common Diagnoses.** Nausea and vomiting are common presenting symptoms in a variety of ailments found in most age and gender groups. Because of loss of function, nausea and vomiting inflict significant costs on the patient, their employers, and society. Common etiologies of nausea and vomiting generally fall into one (or more) of a number of groups, irrespective of age or gender (Table 46–1), but there are a few unique patient groups requiring special mention.
   A. **Vomiting in infants** may be associated with acute gastroenteritis or any acute illness (e.g., urinary tract infections, otitis media, or asthma), feeding disorders, hypertrophic pyloric stenosis, or intussusception.
      1. **Hypertrophic pyloric stenosis** is the most common surgical condition encountered in the first 2 to 8 weeks of life. Risk factors include firstborn, male gender (5:1), and a positive family history.
      2. **Intussusception** usually occurs later, between 6 and 18 months of life, but a small percentage occurs after 3 years of age.
      3. **Regurgitation** (spitting up) often is a normal variant and should be distinguished from vomiting. Simple regurgitation usually resolves by 6 to 12 months of age. Faulty feeding technique can lead to excessive regurgitation and vomiting, and this should be considered when confronted with an infant with failure to thrive (see Chapter 24).
   B. **Vomiting in children,** in addition to the above diagnoses, may be from abdominal migraines (cyclic vomiting syndrome). They occur in as much as 2% of all children, at the mean age of 9.6 years (range 5–13); male incidence is higher in younger children, but male–female incidence equalizes as children grow older. Cyclic vomiting has a familial component and may be associated with migraine headaches.
   C. **Vomiting in women** is common during the first trimester of normal pregnancy and, while discomforting, rarely is of much clinical significance (see Chapter 99). However,

TABLE 46–1. DIFFERENTIAL DIAGNOSIS OF NAUSEA AND VOMITING

Toxic Etiologies	Infectious Causes	Disorders of the Gut and Peritoneum	CNS Causes	Endocrinologic and Metabolic Causes
Cancer chemotherapy	Bacterial	Functional	Anorexia nervosa	Diabetic ketoacidosis
Hypervitaminosis A, D	Gastroenteritis	gastrointestinal disorders	Bulimia nervosa	Pregnancy
Jamaican vomiting sickness	Non-GI infections	Gastric outlet obstruction	Depression	Starvation
Nicotine	Other viral	Mechanical obstruction	Fluorescein angiography	Uremia
Radiation Therapy		Mesenteric ischemia	Hemorrhage	
		Mucosal metastases	Increased intracranial pressure	
		Retroperitoneal fibrosis	Labyrinthine disorders	
		Small-bowel obstruction	Malignancy	
			Migraine	
			Motion sickness	
			Pain	
			Tumors	

Source: Reproduced with permission from Quigley EM, Hasler WL, Parkman HP. AGA technical review on nausea and vomiting. Gastroenterology. 2001;120(1):263–286.

when the vomiting is excessive and leads to poor weight gain, weight loss, or dehydration, other etiologies must be considered. These would include **hyperemesis gravidarum, hydatidiform molar pregnancy,** and **extrauterine pregnancy** (with and without abdominal pain).

D. **Vomiting in adolescents and adults** is usually caused by common and benign disorders, which are listed in the approximate order of frequency:

1. **Acute gastroenteritis,** usually viral (rotavirus, norovirus) and self-limited. Most common between the ages of 20 and 29 years and occurs most often in autumn and winter. Bacterial etiologies include *Escherichia coli, Campylobacter* spp., *Staphylococcus aureus, Salmonella, Bacillus cereus, and Clostridium, Streptococcus,* and others.

2. **Reaction to drugs** (Table 46–2), **toxins** (environmental exposures, alcohol, illicit drugs), or **tumor-produced peptides**.

3. **Gastrointestinal tract inflammation.** Gastroesophageal reflux disease **(GERD)** and **peptic ulcer disease** are more common with excessive caffeine, alcohol, or nicotine use (see Chapter 19).

4. **Pancreatitis** occurs with alcohol, hypertriglyceridemia, cholelithiasis, or idiopathic. Risk factors for **cholelithiasis** include obesity, rapid weight loss, pregnancy, female gender, and age more than 40 years. It may also be seen in women taking oral contraceptives.

5. **Hepatitis, appendicitis, pyelonephritis, Reye syndrome** (a complication of aspirin use in children with viral illnesses, especially with influenza or varicella), and **postgastrectomy states** (often associated with bile reflux or the inability to digest and clear foods normally).

6. **Motility disorders** including diabetic gastroparesis and postvagotomy states, as well as intestinal pseudo-obstruction (gastroduodenal motor dysfunction occurring in patients with neuromuscular disorders).

7. **Gastrointestinal obstruction** such as gastric outlet obstruction, small-bowel obstruction, incarcerated hernia (femoral or inguinal), volvulus, and achalasia. Risk factors and related diagnoses include prior abdominal surgeries (including bariatric surgery), being elderly, or having hernias or cancer. Bariatric surgery is a new surgical cause for nausea and vomiting.

8. **Vestibular disorders,** to include motion sickness, Ménière disease, perilymphatic fistula, or labyrinthitis (either viral or toxic).

9. **Increased intracranial pressure** associated with meningitis or space-occupying lesions (e.g., tumor or subdural hematoma).

10. **Metabolic disorders** including severe electrolyte derangements, uremia, diabetic ketoacidosis, hypercalcemia, adrenal insufficiency, and thyrotoxicosis.

TABLE 46–2. MEDICATIONS ASSOCIATED WITH NAUSEA AND VOMITING

Antidepressants	SSRIs (fluoxetine, paroxetine, sertraline)
	Venlafaxine
Cardiac medications	Antiarrhythmics
	Antihypertensive medications (diuretics, beta-blockers, calcium channel blockers)
	Cholesterol lowering agents (statins, gemfibrozil, niacin)
	Digoxin
Chemotherapy agents	Mild-fluorouracil, vinblastine, tamoxifen
	Moderate-etoposide, methotrexate, cytarabine, carboplatin, cyclophosphamide (doses <1500 mg/m^2), daunorubicin, doxorubicin, epirubicin, idarubicin, ifosfamide, irinotecan, oxaliplatin, procarbazine
	Severe-cisplatinum, dacarbazine, nitrogen mustard, carmustine, cyclophospha-mide (doses ≥1500 mg/m^2), dactinomycin, mechlorethamine, streptozotocin
Gastrointestinal medications	Sulfasalazine
	Azathioprine
Infectious disease treatments	Acyclovir
	Antifungal agents
	Erythromycin, tetracycline, penicillins
	Nitrofurantoin
	Sulfa drugs
	Tuberculosis medications
Pain medications	Antigout drugs
	Aspirin
	Nonsteroidal anti-inflammatory drugs
	Opioid analgesics (codeine, morphine, hydrocodone, oxycodone etc.)
Other medications	Lithium
	Metformin
	Oral contraceptives
	Quinidine
	Lithium

    11. Psychogenic vomiting associated with syndromes of physical or sexual abuse, posttraumatic stress, and eating disorders.

    12. Other causes include exposure to unpleasant smells.

III. Symptoms (Table 46–3). Because there are many diagnoses associated with nausea and vomiting, an accurate history is essential to determining the underlying cause. Details about the **timing** of symptoms (time of day and any association with eating), **characteristics of the vomitus** (digested chyme, bilious, etc.), any **associated symptoms** (abdominal pain or other symptoms), **associated past history,** and **duration of symptoms** are important.

    A. Timing and relationship to eating. For example, symptoms before the first meal of the day are often seen in pregnancy. Symptoms immediately after eating can be seen in bulimia or peptic ulcer disease, while symptoms that are delayed for several hours after a meal could be due to a small bowel obstruction or gastroparesis.

    B. Duration of symptoms. Acute nausea and vomiting usually lasts for a few days. Acute symptoms are most often caused by drugs, toxins, infections (e.g., gastroenteritis, systemic), inflammation (e.g., cardiac, gastrointestinal), or obstruction. Chronic nausea and vomiting, defined as persistence of symptoms for longer than 1 month, poses a more challenging diagnostic dilemma.

    C. Past medical history. Abdominal surgery, previous central nervous system (CNS) tumor, or eating disorder (bulimia, anorexia nervosa), regardless of whenever in past, must be explored.

    D. Specific symptoms

        1. Diffuse abdominal pain and distention are common findings in mechanical bowel obstruction. Distention without pain is consistent with ileus. Periumbilical pain moving toward the right lower quadrant is associated with acute appendicitis. Right upper quadrant pain is consistent with acute cholelithiasis and acute alcoholic hepatitis. Upper abdominal pain is seen with gastritis. Epigastric pain can be consistent with acute pancreatitis or peptic ulcer disease. Severe flank pain, radiating to the groin, is a common complaint in renal colic.

TABLE 46–3. DIAGNOSIS USING SYMPTOMS OF NAUSEA AND VOMITING IN ADULTS

Timing	Characteristics of Vomitus	± Associated Symptoms	± Associated Medical History	Possible Diagnoses
Before breakfast	Projectile	Breast tenderness, fatigue		Pregnancy
		Headache, dizziness		Increased intracranial pressure
		Headache, shakiness	Kidney disease	Alcohol Uremia
Delayed (≥1 h after meal)	Digested food	Early satiety, nonpainful	Diabetes	Gastroparesis
	Nonbilious, undigested	Painless or colicky pain		Achalasia, Zenker's diverticula, or gastric outlet obstruction
	Bilious, feculent	Colicky pain		Small-bowel obstruction
After meals		Abdominal pain		Ulcerative disease
		Abdominal or back pain		Pancreatitis
		Right upper quadrant abdominal pain		Cholecystitis
Immediately after meals (but can make it to the toilet)		No dysphagia	Psychiatric disorders	Bulimia, anorexia, nervosa, or psycho-neurotic vomiting
Intermittent attacks			Migraine headache	Cyclic vomiting syndrome (usually initially diagnosed in childhood)

2. **Diaphoresis** may be related to syncope, vagal stimulation, vestibular dysfunction, dysrhythmia, and CNS events.
3. **Sialorrhea** (excessive salivary secretion) is related to toxins, drugs, and acute gastritis. Associated diarrhea is usual in acute food poisoning (*Staphylococcus*).
4. **Chills,** fever, cough, and rhinorrhea are consistent with a concomitant viral infection.
IV. **Signs.** The physical examination is unremarkable in many cases of nausea and vomiting, especially when associated with motility disorders, metabolic disorders, drugs, and toxins.
   A. **Vomiting (infants and children).**
      1. If there is no fever, weight loss, or abdominal distention, and the child does not appear ill, the cause may be a **feeding disorder** or **normal regurgitation**.
      2. **Hypertrophic pyloric stenosis is associated with** weight loss, dehydration, occasionally a palpable "olive" mass in the epigastric area in male infants younger than 8 weeks, and usually occurs after a feeding. Careful observation can identify the peristaltic wave progressing across the abdominal wall that precedes a vomiting episode.
      3. Children with **intussusception have** significant abdominal pain, possible palpable sausage-shaped mass located anywhere in the abdomen but most commonly on the left side, and Hemoccult positive loose stools described as "currant jelly."
   B. **Gastrointestinal tract obstruction (all ages).**
      1. **Small-bowel obstruction** is associated with high-pitched bowel sounds with occasional visible peristalsis.
      2. **Incarcerated hernia** is painful and represents a medical emergency. The two most common hernias are inguinal and umbilical. Hernias can occasionally be diagnosed by auscultating bowel sounds in the hernia sac. Transillumination in a darkened room can be helpful.
      3. **Volvulus** is associated with acute abdominal distention and periumbilical tenderness.
      4. **Gastric outlet obstruction** may cause distention. An epigastric succussion splash can be demonstrated more than 4 hours postprandial.

TABLE 46–4. RELATIVE BENEFITS AND RISKS OF COMMON DIAGNOSTIC TESTS FOR NAUSEA AND VOMITING

Test	Benefit	Risk
Abdominal x-ray	May suggest obstruction, CIIP; may be performed on day of clinical evaluation	Radiation exposure (minimal)
Abdominal CT with oral and IV contrast	Arguably the optimal technique to detect and diagnose cause of obstruction; also examines other intra-abdominal organs	Radiation exposure (modest); possible reaction to IV contrast; high cost
Esophagogastroduode-noscopy	Optimal examination of esophageal, gastric and duodenal mucosa; biopsies possible	Minimal risk of GI bleeding, perforation, and sepsis; risks of sedation, if used; high cost
Ultrasound	Used in the evaluation of abdominal pain when accompanied with nausea and vomiting	None

GI, gastrointestinal; IV, intravenous; CIIP, chronic idiopathic intestinal pseudo-obstruction; CT, computed tomography. *Source:* Adapted with permission from Quigley EM, Hasler WL, Parkman HP. AGA technical review on nausea and vomiting. *Gastroenterology.* 2001;120(1):263–286.

C. Increased intracranial pressure (all ages).
   1. Focal neurologic signs are usually present with **space-occupying CNS lesions**. Neurologic signs and changes in mental status are associated with embolic or hemorrhagic stroke (cerebral or cerebellar).
   2. A change in mental status, fever, and neck stiffness can be signs of **meningitis** or other CNS infections. A positive Brudzinski sign (hip and knees flex when the neck is actively flexed), when present and not appreciated, can lead to a false assumption of no neck stiffness.
V. Diagnostic Testing. This is directed by the history and physical examination. Common tests and studies that aid in the evaluation of nausea and vomiting are listed in Table 46–4. The history will guide the examiner toward one or more broad classes of diagnoses. Specific testing can then be directed toward likely etiologies. Pregnancy must be considered and excluded in all female patients capable of childbearing, regardless of age. When symptoms are severe, diagnostic tests should be done to determine the patient's renal function, electrolyte, and hydration status before definitive studies to determine etiology. When infection is likely, a complete blood count with differential and urinalysis is required. Further urgent diagnostics may be needed if symptoms, risk profiling, and examination suggest life-threatening etiologies such as increased intracranial pressure, obstruction, meningitis, or drug overdosing. When the cause remains cryptic or symptoms persist or worsen, more complex diagnostic testing or gastroenterology referral may be necessary. Following are additional points:
   A. Ultrasound use is noninvasive and used to evaluate causes of abdominal pain, which often accompany nausea and vomiting, such as pyloric stenosis and gallstones.
   B. Supine and upright abdominal x-ray series (KUB) are appropriate when pain is present. These are inexpensive, easy to obtain, and helpful when obstruction, incarcerated hernia, perforation, or ileus are considered.
   C. Air-contrast barium enema may have a place in evaluation of the gut but has largely been replaced in many situations by **computerized tomographic (CT) scan** without and with contrast. In children, it may be effective in reducing volvulus.
   D. Endoscopy is not usually a first-line test, but is useful for evaluating anatomic lesions, especially if biopsy is required. Included is sigmoidoscopy, colonoscopy, or esophagogastroduodenoscopy. Endoscopy is not reliable in diagnosing physiologic gastrointestinal motility disorders, although it can be helpful in diagnoses such as GERD, hiatal hernia, gastric outlet obstruction, and gastroparesis or delayed gastric emptying. Endoscopy of the biliary tract, endoscopic retrograde cholangiopancreatography, can assist in diagnosing biliary tract obstruction.
   E. Nasogastric tube aspiration that returns significant residual gastric content following an overnight fast suggests gastric outlet obstruction or gastroparesis and should be followed by endoscopic evaluation.
   F. Upper gastrointestinal series and **small-bowel follow-through** can help detect obstruction, masses, and large ulcers. Low-grade obstruction and smaller mucosal lesions may not be seen. Enteroclysis (small-bowel enema) may also be necessary.

G. Formal **psychiatric assessment** should be considered for patients with unexplained chronic nausea and vomiting, especially when there is no associated weight loss, dehydration, or electrolyte abnormalities. Psychogenic vomiting **(bulimia)** can result in severe weight loss and metabolic derangement. This etiology must be considered when a reasonable clinical evaluation has not determined a physiologic cause.

H. Specialized testing is required when a definitive diagnosis is not found and there is clinical evidence to support presence of physiologic dysfunction. These studies are generally entertained on referral to a gastroenterologist.

1. Radionuclide testing measures gastric emptying rate.

2. Antroduodenal manometry and **electrogastrography** measure gastric motility and rhythmic functions.

VI. Treatment. Given the various causative etiologies responsible for nausea and vomiting, choosing the optimal therapeutic approach is of utmost importance. When choosing, take into consideration the following: (1) underlying cause, (2) ability of the patient to follow recommendations, (3) route of drug administration, (4) potential side effects of therapy, and (5) patient's ability to afford medication or alternative therapeutic intervention. During diagnostic testing, management is usually symptomatic and must include electrolyte and fluid replacement if needed. If gastrointestinal obstruction is evident, hospitalization for skilled nursing, close monitoring, and surgical consultation are required. If appropriate testing has been done and a definitive diagnosis is still uncertain, symptoms, in a stable patient, may be controlled with a combination of nonpharmacologic measures and antiemetics.

A. Nonpharmacologic treatment is appropriate for acute illness when history and physical examination are consistent with a benign process. This can be initiated prior to or in conjunction with pharmaceutical management. In clinically stable adults and older children, limiting oral intake for a period of several hours can be beneficial. This approach can also be used in small children and infants but, because of their small size, careful monitoring is necessary to prevent dehydration and electrolyte problems. Once the patient has been free of symptoms for several hours, reintroducing clear liquids in small quantities and bland foods served cool are helpful. (SOR **C**)

B. Complementary and alternative medicine is an evolving field in medicine but use of alternative therapies is already widespread. It is important to inquire about use of these types of therapies because patients are often reluctant to share this information.

1. Acupuncture has some effect in preventing nausea and vomiting. Stimulation of the P6 acupuncture point has been shown to prevent postoperative nausea and vomiting (PONV) at levels similar to medications. (SOR **A**) Acupressure is effective in reducing chemotherapy-related nausea and vomiting, but acupuncture combined with antiemetics and electroacupuncture have been shown to be more beneficial. (SOR **A**)

2. Ginger extract. One gram of ginger is more effective than placebo in preventing postoperative nausea and vomiting. (SOR **B**)

3. Psychological techniques. Progressive muscle relaxation and guided mental imagery can be used with good effect during chemotherapy treatment. (SOR **C**)

4. Wrist banding. Acupressure bands improve nausea on the day of chemotherapy treatment, but generally not beyond. Emesis is not reduced. (SOR **A**) These may be effective for reducing motion sickness and nausea associated with pregnancy, but data are inconsistent; the former topic is currently under review by Cochrane authors.

5. Cannabinoids (nabilone, dronabinol, and levonantradol) are slightly superior to conventional antiemetics (prochlorperazine, metoclopramide, chlorpromazine, haloperidol, domperidone, thiethylperazine, or alizapride), and many patients prefer them. (SOR **A**) Significant side effects such as dizziness, hallucinations, and dysphoria may limit their use.

C. Pharmacologic therapies are the mainstay of primary care treatment of nausea and vomiting (Table 46–5). Multiple classes of drugs have been found useful and their efficacy has been demonstrated over time. The limiting factors to use of these drugs tend to be route of administration and side-effect profiles. There is a tendency to use these drugs in a linear fashion; however, use of these drugs in combination can often improve efficacy and provide faster relief of symptoms. Drugs useful in treating nausea and vomiting are classified by drug type (e.g., antipsychotics, antihistamines, prokinetic agents) or clinical situation (e.g., bowel obstruction, chemotherapy-induced nausea and vomiting (CINV), and postanesthesia).

1. Drug type

a. Antipsychotics. The phenothiazines and butyrophenones are useful treatments of acute nausea and vomiting although their side effect profile generally limits long-term therapy. Table 46–5 lists the drugs in this category. Haloperidol and

TABLE 46–5. PHARMACOLOGIC TREATMENT FOR NAUSEA AND VOMITING

Drug	Adult Dose	Common Class Side Effects	Contraindications	Drug Interactions (Commonly Used Drugs)
Phenothiazines—D₂ Prochlorperazine (Compazine)	Oral: 5–10 mg every 6–8 h IM: 5–10 mg every 3–4 h IV: 2.5–5 mg slow IV or infusion (max rate 5 mg/min) PR: 25 mg every 12 h	Drowsiness, blurred vision Amenorrhea, dizziness, hypotension, dry mouth, rash, tinnitus, weight gain, impotence GI (xerostomia, nausea), cholestasis, extrapyramidal reactions (more in children) Rare: agranulocytosis, neuroleptic malignant syndrome	Children <2 yr or <9 kg weight Comatose state or severe CNS depression	**Multiple Drug Interactions** Agents that prolong QT interval (e.g., cisapride, fluoroquinolones, ziprasidone, dronedarone, octreotide, metoclopramide, fluoxetine, TCAs, TMP-SMX) Oxycodone, fentanyl, and other CNS depressants Lithium (increased extrapyramidal side effects) Tramadol (increased seizure risk)
Promethazine (Phenergan)	12.5–25 mg oral/IM/IV/PR every 4–6 h as needed (deep IM preferred to IV)		Children <2 yr Treatment of lower respiratory tract symptoms or asthma	
Butyrophenones—D₂ Haloperidol (Haldol)	**Off-label chemo-induced nausea: 1–2 mg orally every 4–6 h**	Sedation/somnolence, hypotension, anticholinergic side effects (xerostomia, blurred vision), extrapyramidal symptoms, prolonged QT interval	Parkinson's disease Severe CNS depression or comatose state	**Multiple Drug Interactions** Agents that prolong QT interval (e.g., cisapride, quetiapine, fluoroquinolones, ziprasidone, dronedarone, octreotide, metoclopramide, fluoxetine, TCAs, TMP-SMX, and many others) Propranolol (risk of hypotension, cardiac arrest) Fluoxetine (risk of haloperidol toxicity and cardiotoxicity) Venlafaxine Ketoconazole Lithium Tacrolimus

(continued)

TABLE 46–5. PHARMACOLOGIC TREATMENT FOR NAUSEA AND VOMITING *(Continued)*

Drug	Adult Dose	Common Class Side Effects	Contraindications	Drug Interactions (Commonly Used Drugs)
Serotonin receptor antagonists—5-HT$_3$				
Ondansetron (Zofran)	*Chemo prophylaxis:* IV: 0.15 mg/kg/dose, 3 times daily **OR** 0.45 mg/kg once daily **OR** 8–10 mg 1–2 times per day **OR** 24 mg or 32 mg once daily[1,4] Oral: variable dose depending on emetogenic potential of regimen	GI (constipation, diarrhea, xerostomia), headache, weakness Fever, dizziness, drowsiness, rash, blurred vision, QT prolongation	Concomitant use of apomorphine	**Multiple Drug Interactions** Agents that prolong QT interval (e.g., cisapride, fluoroquinolones, ziprasidone, dronedarone, octreotide, azithromycin, metoclopramide, fluoxetine, TCAs, citalopram, TMP-SMX, many others) CYP3A4 inhibitors (e.g., fluconazole, many others) Apomorphine
Dolasetron (Anzemet)	*Nausea with chemo:* 1.8 mg/kg **OR** 100 mg single dose *Postoperative nausea:* Adults: 12.5 mg IV, Peds: 0.35 mg/kg IV (max 12.5 mg/dose)			
Granisetron (Kytril, Sancuso)	Transdermal patch (34.3 mg) every 24 h. Max 7 days		Concomitant use of apomorphine	
Palonosetron (Aloxi) *Not effective in terminating nausea/vomiting once it occurs	*Chemo prophylaxis:* 0.25 mg IV 30 min prior to start of chemo **OR** 0.5 mg orally 1 hour prior to chemo *Postoperative prophylaxis:* 0.075 mg immediately prior to anesthesia induction			

	Dose	Adverse Effects	Contraindications	Multiple Drug Interactions
Prokinetic Agents — D$_2$				
Metoclopramide (Reglan)	*Gastroparesis:* 10–20 mg orally 4 times daily, before meals and bedtime *Postoperative:* 10–20 mg IV/IM every 4–6 h as needed	Drowsiness, fatigue, extrapyramidal symptoms/dystonic reactions, GI (nausea, vomiting), cardiac abnormalities (AV block, bradycardia, hypertension, hypotension), urinary retention/incontinence, vision changes Rare: hallucinations, neuroleptic malignant syndrome	Concomitant use with drugs likely to cause extrapyramidal reactions Epilepsy GI hemorrhage, obstruction, or perforation Pheochromocytoma	Anticholinergics, narcotic analgesics (antagonism of motility effects) CNS depressants (additive sedative effects) Cabergoline Cimetidine Cyclosporine Digoxin Linezolid, SSRIs (risks serotonin syndrome) Venlafaxine, bupropion, rivastigmine, nefazodone, mirtazapine, promethazine, trimethobenzamide, TCAs, antipsychotics, (increased risk of extrapyramidal reactions)
Antihistamines — H$_1$				
Dimenhydrinate (Dramamine)	*Motion sickness:* 50–100 mg oral/IM every 4–6 (max 400 mg per 24 h) **OR** 50 mg IV over 2 min	Fatigue/somnolence, headache, Xerostomia, palpitations, GI, blurred vision		Procarbazine (risk of CNS depression) CNS depressants (additive effect)
Meclizine (Antivert, Bonine)	*Motion sickness:* 12.5–50 mg orally 1 h before departure, repeat at 24-h intervals if necessary *Radiation-induced:* 50 mg orally, 2–12 h prior to therapy *Vertigo:* 25–100 mg daily in divided doses			CNS depressants (additive effect)
Anticholinergics — M				
Scopolamine (Transderm Scop)	*Postoperative nausea:* apply 1 patch the night before surgery **OR** 1 h prior to cesarean section, remove within 24 h of surgery *Motion sickness:* apply 1 patch at least 4 h prior to exposure and every 3 days as needed (best if applied 12 h prior to exposure)	Rash, dry mouth, urinary retention, drowsiness, blurred vision	Narrow-angle glaucoma Concurrent use of potassium	Potassium (risk of GI lesions) Belladonna

(continued)

TABLE 46–5. PHARMACOLOGIC TREATMENT FOR NAUSEA AND VOMITING (Continued)

Drug	Adult Dose	Common Class Side Effects	Contraindications	Drug Interactions (Commonly Used Drugs)
Others				
Trimethobenzamide (Tigan)	*Postoperative or gastroenteritis-related nausea:* Oral: 300 mg every 6–8 h IM: 200 mg every 6–8 h	Dizziness, drowsiness, headache, diarrhea, extrapyramidal symptoms, depression, hypotension		Metoclopramide (risk of extrapyramidal side effects)
Dronabinol (Marinol)—Cannabinoid	*Chemo-induced:* 5 mg/m² every 1–3 h before chemo then every 2–4 h for 4–6 doses per day (max 15 mg/m² per dose)	Amnesia, confusion, hallucinations, euphoria, paranoia, somnolence, palpitations, vasodilation, weakness, GI (abdominal pain, nausea, vomiting)	Hypersensitivity to any cannabinoid or sesame oil	Ritonavir (increased dronabinol concentrations)
Aprepitant (Emend)—Substance P/neurokinin 1	*Postoperative nausea:* 40 mg orally w/in 3 h prior to induction of anesthesia *Chemo-induced:* 125 mg orally day 1 of chemo, then 80 mg daily on days 2 and 3. Use with other antiemetics	Alopecia, fatigue, dizziness, fever, headache, GI (constipation, diarrhea, loss of appetite), hiccoughs, anorexia, tinnitus, weakness, Stevens–Johnson syndrome	Concomitant use of pimozide, terfenadine, astemizole, or cisapride	Agents metabolized via CYP3A4 (e.g., docetaxel, paclitaxel, etoposide, irinotecan, ifosfamide, imatinib, vinorelbine, vinblastine, vincristine, and many others) Warfarin (reduced warfarin levels) Clozapine (increased clozapine exposure) Colchicine (increased colchicine exposure)

IM, intramuscular; IV, intravenous; PR, per rectum; GI, gastrointestinal; CNS, central nervous system; TCA, tricyclic antidepressant; TMP-SMX, trimethoprim-sulfamethoxazole; SSRI, selective serotonin receptor inhibitor.

risperidone are butyrophenones that have been used successfully in controlling postoperative (former) and opioid-induced (latter) nausea and vomiting. Their site of action is different from that of the phenothiazines, acting centrally by binding to the dopamine receptors DA_2 and, to a lesser degree, DA_1.

b. Antihistamines are useful in treatment of acute and chronic nausea and vomiting. They are efficacious in treating motion sickness. Examples include dimenhydrinate and meclizine.

c. Prokinetic agents are useful in treating motility disorder, such as diabetic gastroparesis and postvagotomy states. They act centrally, blocking dopaminergic receptors, specifically the D_2 subtype, in the chemoreceptor trigger zone. They improve gastric motility through direct stimulation of gastrointestinal smooth muscle. The only prokinetic agent currently available in the United States is metoclopramide. In addition to its central activity, it augments cholinergic activity peripherally by causing release of acetylcholine from postganglionic nerve endings or by sensitizing muscarinic receptors on smooth muscle. Care must be taken to avoid idiopathic extrapyramidal side effects.

d. Serotonin-receptor antagonists are relative newcomers to the treatment of nausea and vomiting. They include the anti-CINV medications such as ondansetron, dolasetron, and granisetron. There has been a recent Food and Drug Administration (FDA) warning about the risk of QT prolongation and development of potentially fatal arrhythmia with higher dose intravenous (IV) ondansetron. See http://www.fda.gov/Drugs/DrugSafety/ucm310190.htm for more information. At this time, no single IV dose should exceed 16 mg.

e. Anticholinergic agents include scopolamine and trimethobenzamide. Trimethobenzamide (Tigan®) should not be used in children when the diagnosis is not clearly defined, since it may worsen Reye syndrome. In addition, the FDA has withdrawn approval of trimethobenzamide suppository products due to the lack of evidence of safety or effectiveness; the oral and injectable forms of this drug are not affected by this approval withdrawal.

f. Vitamin B_6 alone or combined with doxylamine has some efficacy in treating nausea of pregnancy based on limited evidence. (SOR **Ⓑ**)

2. Clinical situation

a. Bowel obstruction. Treatment of bowel obstruction-induced nausea and vomiting should start with conservative management. Restoring and maintaining adequate hydration, restricting oral intake, and management of pain should be initiated immediately when this diagnosis is considered. In nonsurgical candidates, octreotide is effective. IV haloperidol, at 1 to 2 mg, is effective in treating nausea and vomiting associated with obstruction.

b. Vestibular dysfunction. Agents to prevent motion sickness and vertigo (Table 46–5) affect the vestibular system and probably the emetic center through antagonism of H_1 and M (muscarinic cholinergic) receptors. These agents are most effective if administered prior to the onset of nausea and vomiting. Because acetylcholine mediates impulses from the inner ear, **scopolamine** is an effective motion sickness antiemetic. Side effects include dry mouth and blurred vision. Meclizine is a widely used nonprescription medication for the prevention of nausea and vomiting caused by motion sickness. It exerts its antiemetic effect via depression of labyrinthine excitability and vestibular stimulation.

c. Infection, toxin, and drug induced. Treatment of the underlying etiology is paramount. Removal of causative factors (e.g., toxins) and discontinuing or decreasing the dose of drugs suspected of inducing nausea and vomiting should be considered. Infections causing nausea and vomiting are usually viral and only require maintenance of adequate hydration and electrolytes until resolved. If bacterial infection is suspected, use of appropriate antibiotics is indicated.

d. Pregnancy-induced nausea and vomiting. On the basis of the American Congress of Obstetricians and Gynecologists guidelines, prevention and treatment of pregnancy-related nausea and vomiting should include taking a **multivitamin** at the time of conception and taking **vitamin B_6** alone or with doxylamine. (SOR **Ⓒ**) The U.S. Food and Drug Administration recently approved the drug Diclegis (doxylamine succinate and pyridoxine hydrochloride), a delayed release tablet taken twice daily, to treat pregnant women experiencing nausea and vomiting. (SOR **Ⓑ**) Diclegis can cause drowsiness. **Ginger extract** will reduce nausea and, to a lesser degree, retching. (SOR **Ⓐ**) Trials using combination therapy (pyridoxine and metoclopramide) have been shown to be superior to monotherapy with either drug in the treatment of pregnancy-induced nausea and vomiting. (SOR **Ⓑ**) Trials of nerve stimulation have been effective in treating pregnancy-induced emesis. (SOR **Ⓐ**) Corticosteroids used to treat hyperemesis gravidarum are not harmful to the pregnancy or fetus, but have not been shown to be beneficial. (SOR **Ⓐ**)

D. CINV is an area where new antiemetics are **being developed. Ondansetron** (Zofran®), **dolasetron** (Anzemet®) granisetron (Sancuso), and palonosetron (Aloxi) are 5-HT$_3$ receptor serotonin antagonist antiemetics used primarily for the prevention of nausea and vomiting associated with chemotherapy. They are generally superior in antiemetic relief compared to prochlorperazine and metoclopramide. (SOR **Ⓑ**) This may also be true with the combination of a 5-HT$_3$ receptor serotonin antagonist (e.g., ondansetron) plus dexamethasone compared to metoclopramide plus dexamethasone. (SOR **Ⓑ**)

   1. The use of **steroids** in treating nausea and vomiting should be considered more often for CINV, radiation-induced nausea and vomiting (RINV), and postoperative nausea and vomiting. The 2011 American Society of Clinical Oncology's updated guidelines for treating CINV in high emetic-risk patients are the **three-drug combination**: aprepitant or fosaprepitant, dexamethasone, and a 5-HT$_3$ serotonin receptor antagonist. Moderate-risk patients should be treated with dexamethasone and palonosetron. Dexamethasone can be offered to low-risk patients before beginning chemotherapy. (SOR **Ⓑ**)

E. RINV is quite similar to CINV in etiology and treatment. Dopamine receptor antagonists, including metoclopramide, prochlorperazine, and haloperidol, have proven to be effective in treating RINV. 5-HT$_3$ serotonin receptor antagonists are also effective RINV antiemetics. Dexamethasone has been the most widely used corticosteroid in preventing and treating radiation-induced nausea and vomiting. The American Society of Clinical Oncologists recommends antiemetic therapy be instituted before each fraction for patients undergoing high emetic risk radiation therapy and continued for at least 24 hours post-therapy. Patients can receive a 5-day course of dexamethasone prior to fractions 1 to 5.

F. PONV therapy is another area where new treatments are being developed. The following are recommendations for managing PONV:

   1. Serotonin receptor (5-HT$_3$) antagonists are more effective when given at the end of surgery. They have a favorable side effect (headache, constipation, increased liver enzymes) profile and are considered equally safe to conventional therapies. Ondansetron is one most studied of this group, and there appears to be some difference in efficacy, but overall their efficacy appears to be equivalent.

   2. Corticosteroids are most effective when given prior to anesthesia induction.

   3. Droperidol, dosed below 1 mg and administered at the end of surgery, is effective in controlling PONV. (SOR **Ⓒ**) It is effective when used in concert with patient-controlled analgesia devices delivering morphine. Droperidol has an FDA warning for induced torsades de pointes, as well as QT prolongation and death, but there are no documented cases of dysrhythmia or cardiac death reported at the doses used in managing PONV. (SOR **Ⓒ**)

SELECTED REFERENCES

Abu-Arafeh I, Russel G. Cyclic vomiting syndrome in children: a population based study. *J Pediatr Gastroenterol Nutr.* 1995;21:454–458.

American Gastroenterological Association. American Gastroenterological Association medical position statement: nausea and vomiting. *Gastroenterology.* 2001;120(1):261–262.

Basch E, Prestud AA, Hesketh PJ, et al. Antiemetics: ASCO Clinical Practice Guideline Update. *J Clin Onc.* 2011;29(31):4189–4198.

Bsat FA, Hoffman DE, Seubert DE. Comparison of three outpatient regimens in the management of nausea and vomiting in pregnancy. *J Perinatol.* 2003;23(7):531–535.

FDA Drug Safety Communication: New information regarding QT prolongation with ondansetron (Zofran). http://www.fda.gov/Drugs/DrugSafety/ucm310190.htm. Accessed April 2013.

FDA approves Diclegis for pregnant women experiencing nausea and vomiting. http://www.fda.gov/NewsEvents/Newsroom/PressAnnouncements/ucm347087.htm. Accessed April 2013.

Kris MG, Hesketh PJ, Somerfield MR, et al. American society of clinical oncology guideline for antiemetics in oncology: update 2006. *J Clin Onc.* 2006;24(18):2932–2947, 5341–5342.

Li Buk, Lefevre F, Chelimsky GG, et al. North American Society for Pediatric Gastroenterolgy, Hepatology and Nutrition consensus statement on the diagnosis and management of cyclic vomiting syndrome. *J Ped Gastroenterol Nutr.* 2008;47:379–393.

Longstreth GF. Approach to the patient with nausea and vomiting. UpToDate online, version 15.1, current through December 2006. www.uptodate.com. Accessed April 2013.

Longstreth GF, Hesketh PJ. Characteristics of antiemetic drugs. UpToDate online, version 15.1, current through December 2006. www.uptodate.com. Accessed April 2013.

Matthews A, Dowswell T, Haas DM, et al. Interventions for nausea and vomiting in early pregnancy. *Cochrane Database Syst Rev.* 2010;(9):CD007575.

Quigley EM, Hasler WL, Parkman HP. AGA Technical review on nausea and vomiting. *Gastroenterol.* 2001;120(1):263–286.

Yost NP, McIntire DD, Wians FH, Ramin SM, Balko JA, Leveno KJ. A randomized, placebo-controlled trial of corticosteroids for hyperemesis due to pregnancy. *Obstet Gynecol.* 2003;102(6):1250–1254.

---

47   Neck Pain

Michael P. Rowane, DO, MS, FAAFP, FAAO

KEY POINTS

- Nearly two-thirds of individuals experience uncomplicated neck pain primarily occurring during midlife. (SOR ⊙)
- A careful history and physical examination are usually sufficient to establish a diagnosis; however, in most cases, no definable pathology is found. (SOR ⊙)
- Laboratory investigations play a minor role in most cases of neck pain, but they may help confirm a diagnosis. (SOR ⊙)
- Treatment of problems arising primarily from neck joints and associated ligaments and muscles successfully alleviates symptoms, whereas treatment of problems involving the cervical nerve roots or spinal cord often does not achieve complete pain relief. (SOR ⊙)
- A full recovery occurs in 40% of patients with acute neck pain, whereas 80% completely recover within 1 year of a whiplash injury. (SOR ⊙)

I. **Introduction**
  A. **Definition.** Neck pain is perceived as posterior cervical discomfort, from the superior nuchal line to the first thoracic spinal process, not equivalent to cervical radicular pain, and may present as referred pain to the region. Neck pain can be classified as:
   - **Mechanical,** including nontraumatic (neck strain/torticollis, spondylosis, and myelopathy) and traumatic (whiplash, disk herniation, cervical fracture, neck sprain, and stinger).
   - **Nonmechanical** (rheumatologic/inflammatory, neoplastic, infectious, neurologic, and referred).
   - **Miscellaneous** (e.g., sarcoidosis and Paget disease).
  B. **Epidemiology.** The lifetime prevalence of at least one episode of significant neck pain is estimated at 40% to 70%, whereas nonspecific neck pain over the last 6 months is reported by 40% of adults.
II. **Diagnosis.** Neck pain is most commonly mechanical or due to age-related changes in the cervical spine.
  A. **Symptoms** (Table 47–1)
   1. **Pain. Acute torticollis** is a recent, sudden onset of unilateral, muscular pain, whereas **cervical sprain/whiplash** is a severe generalized discomfort in the neck and upper back after an acute trauma. When pain is aggravated by movement, worse after activities, and there is a dull ache in the base of the neck or interscapular region, **osteoarthritis (cervical spondylosis)** should be considered.
   2. **Loss of motion.** Mechanical pain is typically worse on movement and relieved by rest.

TABLE 47–1. DIFFERENTIAL DIAGNOSIS OF COMMON CAUSES OF NECK PAIN

Condition	Risk Factors	Symptoms	Signs	Evidenced-Based Testing
Acute nonspecific neck pain	Young adults under some stress	Typically, unilateral neck pain that radiates to the top of the shoulder and periscapular area	Limited ROM; widespread tender/trigger points suggest fibromyalgia	C-spine radiographs are only indicated with positive red flags and by Canadian C-spine rules. CT scan is only used when plain films reveal possible fracture
Chronic mechanical neck pain	Older individuals	Intermittent acute attacks superimposed on chronic pain; pain often radiates to scapular region and top of the arms	Limited ROM, tenderness to palpation	Radiographic and CT scans are not indicated. MRI is indicated for work-up of an occult lesion
Spondylosis or osteoarthritis	Individuals ≥50 years, history of OA (osteophytes)	Neck stiffness after rest, possible paresthesias, or numbness	Limited ROM, neurologic changes with progression	Cervical spondylosis is the single most common finding on C-spine radiographs, but poorly correlated with symptoms
Cervical nerve root irritation	History of spondylosis, osteophytes	Discomfort worsening when turning head toward the side of neck pain; paresthesias, weakness	Abnormal Spurling maneuver	**CT** scan can assess for spinal stenosis (older individual with axial stiffness and paresthesias over several dermatomes) **MRI** provides the best anatomic assessment of disk herniation and soft tissue/spinal cord abnormalities **EMG** is helpful in localizing radiculopathy/myelopathy
Acceleration injury/whiplash	Rear-end or side-impact motor vehicle accidents	Acute pain and stiffness within hours, headache	Limited ROM	**C-spine radiographs** may be indicated by Canadian C-spine rules (Table 47–4)
Torticollis (cervical dystonia)	History of congenital or acquired fixed head or C-spine rotation	Usually painless if congenital; usually painful if acquired	Limited ROM; neck is laterally flexed and rotated	No definitive diagnostic test. Consider laboratory tests and neuroimaging to rule out metabolic or structural causes

CT, computerized tomography; EMG, electromyogram; MRI, magnetic resonance imagery; OA, osteoarthritis; ROM, range of motion.

3. **Headache.** Patients with **whiplash** (cervical flexion-extension injuries) frequently have headaches, along with associated nausea, blurred vision, or vertigo.
4. **Radiating symptoms. Mechanical pain** frequently radiates to the shoulder blades or the top of the arm, even without any nerve root or spinal cord involvement. **Cervical root irritation** should be considered with radiation of symptoms down the arms, or weakness, numbness, or paresthesias in the arms along the involved nerve root dermatomes. With bilateral, radicular symptoms, a **cervical cord compression syndrome** should be considered.
5. **Precipitating factors.** Tension and stress, along with frequent bouts of pain and depression, may suggest an underlying behavioral or psychiatric diagnosis.
6. **Difficulty walking** can be the presenting symptom of **cervical myelopathy**.
7. **Other.** A **whiplash injury** especially may be accompanied by anxiety, loss of sleep, dizziness, paresthesias, or nerve root pain. Table 47–2 lists findings suggesting significant underlying disease.

TABLE 47–2. RED FLAGS IN NECK PAIN (THINK "RIFT": CLUES TO POTENTIAL SERIOUS UNDERLYING DISEASE)

Radiculopathy (lower extremity sensory/motor changes/spasticity, bowel/bladder incontinence)
Infection (fever/chills; immunocompromised population-alcohol/drug abuse, elderly)
Fracture (significant trauma; osteoporosis history)
Tumor (history of cancer; unexplained weight loss; age $\leq 20/\geq 50$ yr, failure to improve with treatment)

B. **Signs (Table 47–1).** A focused examination of the patient presenting with neck pain should include **inspection** (for posture, asymmetry, and deformity), **palpation** (for localized tenderness), passive/active/resisted **range of motion (ROM)** (for restrictions and severity of disease), and **provocative maneuvers/neurologic testing** (for radiculopathy).
1. **Tenderness to palpation. Tender points** are common in nonspecific, acute neck pain. Associated widespread tender points, which are sometimes referred to as trigger points, may be indicative of fibromyalgia (see Chapters 38 and 45). Muscle spasm occurs in acute, nonspecific neck pain, whiplash injury, and torticollis.
2. **ROM.** Normal neck ROM includes rotation 60 to 90 degrees, flexion 60 to 90 degrees, extension 60 to 90 degrees, and lateral flexion (side-bending) 30 to 60 degrees. ROM normally decreases with age. Loss of motion is common in an acute, nonspecific, and chronic mechanical neck pain.
3. **Neurologic testing/provocative maneuvers (Table 47–3).** Evaluation for possible levels of sensory and motor involvement, including weakness of the upper extremities, suggests lesions of the nerve roots, brachial plexus, or muscles. A **Spurling test or maneuver,** or the neck compression test, requires side-bending and rotating the patient's head toward the side of radicular pain and exerting downward pressure (http://www.youtube.com/watch?v=09bG1EtPhis). This maneuver reproduces symptoms in the affected upper extremity. The Spurling test has a high specificity but a low sensitivity for cervical radiculopathy. Nonspecific mechanical pain should be considered when a Spurling test or contralateral neck motion results only in neck discomfort.
C. **Laboratory tests and imaging** are usually not necessary. Testing should be considered if a careful history and physical examination do not clearly suggest a diagnosis or to guide management (e.g., surgical consultation).
1. **Blood tests** are rarely indicated. Erythrocyte sedimentation rate and complete blood count with differential may help evaluate for suspected serious disorders including tumor, infection, and inflammatory arthritis, especially with a "Red Flag" history or physical examination (Table 47–2).
2. **Plain C-spine radiographs (Table 47–1).** A cervical spine injury is unlikely in the absence of neck pain/tenderness, neurologic signs/symptoms, loss of consciousness, and distracting injury, and with a normal mental status examination. **The Canadian Cervical Spine Rules (Table 47–4)** are a validated tool to determine which patients with neck pain require radiographic evaluation.
3. In the presence of neurologic abnormalities, **other imaging techniques** should be used to characterize lesion anatomy (Table 47–1).
   a. A **bone scan** can be used to appraise osseous pathology, including osteomyelitis and neoplastic lesions in bone.
   b. **Bone densitometry** diagnoses suspected osteoporosis.

TABLE 47–3. EVALUATION FOR CERVICAL NERVE ROOT LESIONS

Nerve Root	Disk Level	Muscle Weakness/ Movement Affected	Reflex	Paresthesia	Site of Pain
C-5	C-4/5	Shoulder abduction, elbow flexion	Biceps	Shoulder	Shoulder, lateral arm
C-6	C-5/6	Wrist extension/ pronation	Brachioradialis and biceps	Thumb	Deltoid, rhomboid muscle areas
C-7	C-6/7	Elbow/finger extension	Triceps	Middle finger	Dorsolateral upper arm, superomedial angle of scapula
C-8	C-7/T-1	Wrist/finger extension	Triceps and finger	Ring and little finger	Scapula, ulnar side of upper arm

TABLE 47–4. CANADIAN CERVICAL SPINE RULES

Is there **one high-risk factor that mandates immobilization?**
  Age ≥65 yr, or
  Dangerous mechanism (fall from 1 m or greater, axial load to head, motorized recreational vehicles, bicycle collision, or motor vehicle collision (MVC) with high speed, rollover, or ejection), or
  Numbness/tingling in extremities
Is there one low-risk factor to allow safe assessment of range of motion?
  Simple rear-end MVC, or
  Ambulatory at any time at scene, or
  No neck pain at scene, or
  Absence of midline C-spine tenderness
Is patient **able to voluntarily actively rotate neck 45 degrees** to the left and right when requested, regardless of pain?

An answer "yes" to the first question or "no" to the second or third question requires radiography.

III. Treatment. The management of neck pain is aimed at relieving symptoms and maintaining good function.
  A. Uncomplicated neck pain without severe neurologic deficit, including acute, nonspecific neck pain and chronic mechanical neck pain.
    1. Manual manipulation/mobilization, active physiotherapy, pulsed electromagnetic field treatment, and exercise are likely to be beneficial. Therapeutic exercises, initiated either in the office or in consultation with a physical therapist, include ROM, isometrics, dynamic exercises, postural training, and general fitness programs. (SOR **B**)
    2. Pharmacologic treatments include analgesics, nonsteroidal anti-inflammatory drugs (NSAIDs), antidepressants, and muscle relaxants. Mild to moderate pain is primarily managed with acetaminophen (1 g four times daily) and NSAIDs (e.g., ibuprofen 400–600 mg four times daily).
    3. Additional non-pharmacological treatments. Behavioral interventions/biofeedback, patient education, application of heat/cold, home or office cervical traction, acupuncture, spray and stretch, laser treatment, and soft collars/special pillows have unknown effectiveness, yet are common conservative treatments. (SOR **C**)
  B. Spondylosis/osteoarthritis. Treatment must involve reducing pain and stiffness, while minimizing risk. Complementary techniques include transcutaneous electrical nerve stimulation (TENS) units, acupuncture, and a variety of heat, light, or magnetic therapies, but there is little data to support their efficacy.
  C. Cervical nerve root irritation/radiculopathy. In patients followed up for over a year, there are currently no data supporting surgery compared to conservative treatment. Conservative modalities include local heat, analgesics, cervical collar in the acute phase, and consideration of cervical traction. Pharmacologic treatment, including oral medications and referral for epidural steroid injections, has unknown effectiveness. (SOR **C**)
  D. Acute whiplash injury. Likely beneficial interventions include early mobilization and return to normal activity, electrotherapy (diathermy and TENS units), and multimodal treatment. (SOR **B**) Multimodal or combined therapy typically refers to intensive programs incorporating exercise as well as pharmacologic, behavioral, and psychosocial interventions. (SOR **C**)
  E. Chronic whiplash injury. Outcomes are no different comparing physiotherapy alone and multimodal treatment. One study showed significant numbers of pain-free patients 6 months after undergoing percutaneous radiofrequency neurotomy. Another demonstrated significant pain reduction in those undergoing percutaneous radiofrequency neurotomy combined with other modalities, compared to those treated with single modalities. (SOR **C**)
  F. Torticollis (cervical dystonia) in adults has been typically managed with physical therapy, stretching techniques, gentle manual manipulation, judicious use of a soft cervical collar, and ice/heat. (SOR **C**) Evidence-based studies have demonstrated benefit of botulinum A and B toxin. (SOR **A**) Medications have unknown effectiveness. (SOR **C**) Physiotherapy in children is likely to be beneficial. (SOR **B**) There is unknown **effectiveness** with surgical treatments, acupuncture, biofeedback, manipulation, and occupational therapy. (SOR **C**)
IV. Management Strategies. Clinicians commonly offer advice and education for their patients with neck pain. There is no strong evidence that educational interventions, such as methods to deal with pain and stress-coping skills, along with workplace ergonomics and self-care strategies are effective. Exercise therapy for neck pain is a commonly used treatment

for neck pain and is safe. Exercise is effective for the treatment of chronic neck pain and cervicogenic headache when stretching and strengthening exercises are focused on the neck and scapular region. (SOR ❸) In the event that neck pain persists beyond six weeks, radiologic studies are recommended to determine the etiology of the symptoms.

V. Prognosis. Neck pain usually resolves within days or weeks. Approximately 10% of acute neck pain becomes chronic and 5% of patients experience severe disability.

SELECTED REFERENCES

Anderson B, Zacharia I. Treatment of neck pain. www.uptodate.com, online version 17.0. July 2013.
Eubanks JD. Cervical radiculopathy: nonoperative management of neck pain and radicular sysmptoms. *Am Fam Physician.* 2010;81(1):33–40.
Gross A, Forget M, St George K, et al. Patient education for neck pain. *Cochrane Database of Systematic Reviews.* 2012;(4):CD005106.
Kay TM, Gross A, Goldsmith CH, et al. Exercises for mechanical neck disorders. *Cochrane Database Syst Rev.* 2012;(8):CD004250.
Nikolaidis I, Fouyas IP, Sandercock PAG, Statham PF. Surgery for cervical radiculopathy or myelopathy. *Cochrane Database Syst Rev.* 2010;(1):CD001466.
Zacharia I, Anderson BC. Evaluation of the patient with neck pain and cervical spine disorders. www.uptodate.com, online version 17.0. July 2013.

---

48   Palpitations

Jose E. Rodríguez, MD, & Mike D. Hardin, Jr., MD

KEY POINTS

- Most causes of palpitations are benign and do not require extensive work-up or treatment. (SOR ❸)
- Palpitations that are sustained or associated with syncope or presyncope require further work-up, electrophysiologic evaluation, or both. (SOR ❸)
- In general, palpitations are insensitive indicators of arrhythmias. (SOR ❸)

I. Definition. Palpitations are an awareness of the heartbeat, are usually benign, and are caused either by intrinsic cardiac conditions or by noncardiac conditions influencing cardiac rate, rhythm, or force (Table 48–1).

II. Common Diagnoses. Palpitations are a common chief complaint, accounting for up to 16% of outpatient visits. Relative incidence and risk factors for common causes of palpitations follow:

A. Cardiac (43% of cases). Factors increasing the likelihood of a cardiac etiology of palpitations include (1) male gender, (2) description of an irregular heartbeat, (3) history of heart disease, and (4) event duration 5 minutes or more. Patients with three predictors have a 71% chance of a cardiac etiology; those with two predictors, a 48% chance; those with one predictor, a 26% chance; and those with zero predictor, a 0% chance of cardiac etiology. The most common cardiac cause is benign supraventricular or ventricular ectopy.

B. Psychiatric (31% of cases). Palpitations can be a feature of panic attacks, generalized anxiety disorder, somatization, and depression. Because these disorders are common, they may coexist with other causes of palpitations.

C. Ten percent of palpitations are due to a **variety of defined causes** such as endocrine disorders (e.g., hyperthyroidism), cardiac stimulants (e.g., caffeine, nonprescription sympathomimetics, illicit drugs), and anemia.

D. In 16% of cases, the cause of palpitations is **unknown**.

TABLE 48–1. ETIOLOGIES OF PALPITATIONS

Cardiac	*Habits*
Arrhythmia	Cocaine
Sinus tachycardia	Amphetamines
Ventricular premature contractions	Caffeine
Atrial premature contractions	Nicotine
Re-entrant atrial tachycardias	*Metabolic disorders*
Atrial fibrillation or flutter	Thyrotoxicosis
Sinus bradycardia	Hypoglycemia
Sick sinus syndrome	Pheochromocytoma
Atrioventricular nodal block	Mastocytosis
Conduction defects	Scombroid food poisoning (e.g., tuna fish)
Ventricular tachycardia	
Ventricular fibrillation	*High-output states*
Cardiac and extracardiac shunts	Anemia
Valvular heart disease	Pregnancy
Pacemaker	Paget disease
Atrial myxoma	Fever
Cardiomyopathy	*Catecholamine excess*
Psychiatric disease	Stress
Panic attack and disorder	Exercise
Generalized anxiety disorder	
Somatization	
Depression	
Medications[a]	
Sympathomimetic agents	
Vasodilators	
Anticholinergic drugs	
Beta-blocker withdrawal	

[a]Be aware that combination medications may contain caffeine. In addition, amphetamines are used for conditions such as attention deficit hyperactivity disorder and nicotine is also a drug product.
Source: Data from Weber BE and Kapoor WN. Evaluation and outcomes of patients with palpitations. *Am J Med.* 1996;100(2):138–148.

III. Symptoms. Because palpitations can be difficult to characterize, it may be helpful for the patient to tap out the rhythm or for the physician to tap out examples of different rhythms. Important historical features of the palpitations include the following:
  A. Description
  1. Rate and rhythm. A **rapid and regular** rhythm suggests paroxysmal supraventricular tachycardia (PSVT) or ventricular tachycardia (VT) and also suggests atrial fibrillation or atrial flutter with a variable block.
  2. A **"flip-flopping"** sensation suggests **ventricular premature contractions (VPCs) or atrial premature contractions** (APCs) with a pause followed by a forceful contraction (post extra systolic potentiation of ventricular inotropy).
  3. A description of "rapid fluttering in the chest" may represent a sustained, ventricular or supraventricular rhythm, including sinus tachycardia.
  4. A **"pounding in the neck"** sensation is caused by A waves resulting from atrial contractions against a closed tricuspid or mitral valve in **atrioventricular dissociation**. Irregular neck palpitations are seen in VPCs, complete heart block, or VT. **Rapid and regular neck pulsations** are typical of atrioventricular re-entrant tachycardia (AVNRT).
  B. Onset and offset
  1. Random, episodic, and last an instant: premature beats.
  2. Gradual onset and offset: sinus tachycardia.
  3. Abrupt onset/termination: PSVT or VT.
  4. Patient able to **terminate with vagal maneuver:** PSVT (especially AVNRT).
  C. Positional
  1. Initiated by **standing up straight after bending over,** aborted by lying down: AVNRT.

2. Augmented by supine or left lateral decubitus position: VPC or APC, due to greater awareness of heart activity while relaxed or because of the proximity of the heart to the chest wall.

D. Syncope or presyncope (from diminished cerebral perfusion).

   1. VT. Syncope is more common in association with structural heart disease.

   2. PSVT, secondary to vasodilation at the onset of the arrhythmia.

E. Reliability of reported palpitations. Although the classic descriptions noted above can be helpful, a recent review of the literature suggests the following:

   1. The vast majority of arrhythmias are unrecognized by patients as symptoms. In one study of 2099 asymptomatic adult subjects undergoing exercise treadmill tests, 3.7% had exercise-induced episodes of nonsustained VT and in another, exercise-induced SVT occurred during at least one test in 51/843 men (6.0%) and 34/540 women (6.3%).

   2. Of those reporting palpitations, patients with psychiatric disease (e.g., somatization, hypochondriasis) are less accurate historians.

   3. Palpitations are insensitive indicators of arrhythmias.

IV. Signs. During the physical examination, the clinician should search, through auscultation and observation, for the following:

A. Cardiovascular abnormalities that could serve as a substrate for arrhythmias (go to http://www.wilkes.med.ucla.edu/inex.htm for examples of heart sounds).

   1. Mitral valve prolapse: midsystolic click (associated with many arrhythmias).

   2. Hypertrophic obstructive cardiomyopathy: harsh, holosystolic murmur along the left sternal border that increases with Valsalva maneuver (associated with atrial fibrillation, VT).

   3. Dilated cardiomyopathy and heart failure: diffuse and laterally displaced apical impulse, ventricular (S_3) and atrial (S_4) gallops (associated with VT, atrial fibrillation).

B. Signs of other medical disorders such as hyperthyroidism and pheochromocytoma.

V. Diagnostic Tests (Figure 48–1). Most palpitations have a benign etiology and extensive evaluation is usually unnecessary. The history, physical examination, electrocardiogram (ECG), and limited laboratory tests will yield a diagnosis in over one-third of patients; only a small portion of the remaining cases will require further testing (see Sections V.C and V.D).

A. Laboratory. Limited laboratory tests to rule out hyperthyroidism (thyroid-stimulating hormone), anemia (hemoglobin/hematocrit), and electrolyte disturbances (potassium, magnesium) are sufficient.

B. ECG. An episode of palpitations is rarely captured on a routine ECG. Certain ECG findings, however, can suggest the etiology of the palpitations (Table 48–2).

C. Ambulatory ECG monitoring (AECG). Further AECG testing is used to rule out a serious condition, identify treatable causes of arrhythmias, or reassure a patient.

   1. A **Holter (24-hour) monitor** is useful only if a patient has daily palpitations.

   2. The preferred study for investigating palpitations is the **continuous loop event recorder,** which is activated by the patient at time of symptoms. Two weeks of monitoring is usually adequate and more cost-effective than the traditional 4 weeks.

   3. An **exercise stress test** is useful only for exertional arrhythmias.

D. Electrophysiologic testing is reserved for patients with a high pretest likelihood of serious arrhythmia (e.g., structural heart disease or sustained or poorly tolerated arrhythmia).

VI. Treatment

A. Patients with **sustained supraventricular tachycardia (SVT) or VT** should be referred to an electrophysiologist (a cardiologist specializing in the pharmacologic and invasive management of arrhythmias) for consideration of radiofrequency ablation (SVT), medical therapy, or implantable defibrillator.

B. Nonsustained ventricular tachycardia (NSVT) is defined as three or more consecutive beats at a rate of 100 beats per minute or more, with a duration of less than 30 seconds. In patients without underlying structural heart disease, NSVT is a benign finding and no treatment is necessary. Patients with structural heart disease diagnosed through echocardiography, exercise stress testing, cardiac computed tomography, or magnetic resonance imaging should be referred to electrophysiology for treatment recommendations.

C. Benign supraventricular or ventricular ectopy. Reassure the patient and remove precipitating causes (e.g., caffeine, alcohol, tobacco, or drugs such as digoxin, pseudoephedrine, aminophylline, tricyclic antidepressants, cocaine, and amphetamines). If symptoms are incapacitating, consider treatment with a beta-blocker to relieve symptoms. (Treatment, however, may not necessarily suppress the arrhythmia, just its symptoms.)

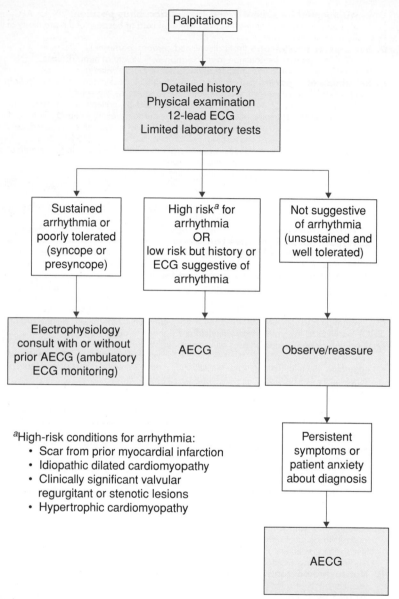

FIGURE 48–1. Decision tree for the evaluation of palpitations. AECG, ambulatory electrocardiogram; ECG, electrocardiogram.

D. Atrial fibrillation (AF). There are four principal issues regarding the treatment of AF:

1. **Reversion to normal sinus rhythm**

   a. Urgent electrical cardioversion is indicated in **unstable patients** (those with active ischemia, hypotension, or a preexcitation syndrome with an extremely rapid ventricular rate).

TABLE 48–2. ELECTROCARDIOGRAPHIC CLUES TO THE CAUSE OF PALPITATIONS

ECG Findings	Condition	Suggested Etiology
Short PR interval, delta waves	Wolff–Parkinson–White syndrome	Atrioventricular re-entrant tachycardia
P mitrale, left ventricular hypertrophy (LVH), atrial premature depolarizations	Left atrial abnormality	Atrial fibrillation
Marked LVH, deep septal Q waves in I, aVL, and V4–6	Hypertrophic obstructive cardiomyopathy	Atrial fibrillation
Ventricular premature depolarizations, left bundle-branch block with positive axis (in patients without structural heart disease)		Idiopathic VT, right ventricular outflow tract type
Ventricular premature depolarizations, right bundle-branch block with positive axis (in patients without structural heart disease)		Idiopathic VT, left ventricular type
Q waves	Prior myocardial infarction	VPCs, nonsustained or sustained VT
Complete heart block	Complete heart block	VPCs, polymorphic VT (torsade de pointes)
Long QT interval	Long QT syndrome	Polymorphic VT
Inverted T wave in V_2, with or without epsilon wave	Arrhythmogenic right ventricular dysplasia	Arrhythmogenic right ventricular dysplasia

VT, ventricular tachycardia; VPCs, ventricular premature contractions.
Source: Data from Weber BE, Kapoor WN. Evaluation and outcomes of patients with palpitations. *Am J Med.* 1996;100(2):138–148.

    b. In the **stable patient,** rate control is first attained with a calcium channel blocker, beta-blocker, or digoxin (Table 48–3).
    c. Factors that guide drug selection include the patient's medical condition, the presence of concomitant heart failure, the characteristics of the medicine, and the physician's experience with specific drugs. Digoxin is currently recommended as a second-line treatment for rate control, except in patients with heart failure. (SOR **Ⓒ**)
    d. There is no evidence that pharmacologic cardioversion of AF to sinus rhythm is superior to rate control. Rhythm control is associated with more adverse effects, increased hospitalization, and no reduction in the risk of stroke in older patients with significant cardiovascular risk factors (SOR **Ⓐ**) Thus, the decision to perform **elective pharmacologic or electrical cardioversion** should be made in consultation with a cardiologist after consideration of the risks and benefits. Successful reversion to and maintenance of normal sinus rhythm (NSR) are more likely if:
      (1) The AF has been present less than 1 year.
      (2) The left atrium is not enlarged (diameter ≤4.0 cm).
      (3) A reversible etiologic factor of the AF is present.
2. Maintenance of NSR
    a. After successful cardioversion, only 20% to 30% of patients maintain NSR without therapy.
    b. Class IA (quinidine, procainamide, disopyramide), IC (flecainide, propafenone), and III (amiodarone, sotalol, ibutilide, dofetilide, dronedarone) drugs are moderately effective in maintaining NSR after conversion of AF. However, they increase adverse events, including proarrhythmia, and some of them (disopyramide, quinidine, and sotalol) may increase mortality. (SOR **Ⓐ**) Although a cardiologist may initiate this therapy, family physicians are often involved in its maintenance and should be familiar with the **numerous drug interactions** of antiarrhythmics. Dronedarone can be initiated during outpatient therapy. (SOR **Ⓑ**)
    c. Catheter ablation performed in experienced centers is useful in maintaining sinus rhythm in selected patients with significantly symptomatic, paroxysmal AF who have failed treatment with an antiarrhythmic drug and have normal or mildly dilated left atria, normal or mildly reduced LV function, and absence of severe pulmonary disease. (SOR **Ⓐ**)
3. Rate control in chronic AF is achieved using calcium channel blockers, beta-blockers, or digoxin (Table 48–3). Treatment to achieve strict rate control of heart

TABLE 48–3. DRUGS USED FOR RATE CONTROL IN PATIENTS WITH ATRIAL FIBRILLATION

Drug[a]	Dose	Major Side effects	Contraindications	Multiple Drug Interactions
Digoxin	*Loading* **IV:** 0.25 mg IV every 2 h, up to 1.5 mg; **oral:** 0.25 mg every 2 h, up to 1.5 mg *Maintenance* **IV:** 0.125–0.25 mg daily; **oral:** 0.125–0.375 mg daily	Dizziness, mental disturbances, diarrhea, headache, nausea, vomiting, cardiac dysrhythmia, rash	Ventricular fibrillation	Amiodarone, macrolide and tetracycline antibiotics, verapamil, alprazolam, ulipristal, diphenoxylate (↑ risk of digoxin toxicity); St. John's wort (↓ digoxin efficacy)
Calcium Chanel Blockers				
Diltiazem	*Loading* **IV:** 0.25 mg/kg IV over 2 min *Maintenance* **IV:** 5–15 mg/h infusion for ≤24 h	Edema, headache, dizziness, block, peripheral edema, bradyarrhythmia, hypotension, nausea, CHF, syncope, gingival hyperplasia	2–3 degree heart block, sick sinus syndrome, Wolff–Parkinson–White syndrome, acute MI, Lown–Ganong–Levine syndrome, symptomatic hypotension, cardiogenic shock, ventricular tachyarrhythmia	Erythromycin, cisapride (QT prolongation); colchicine (colchicine toxicity); statins (myopathy); clopidogrel (↓ anti-platelet effect); aminodarone (bradycardia, AV block)
Verapamil	*Loading* **IV:** 0.075–0.15 mg/kg over 2 min *Maintenance* **Oral:** 120–360 mg/24 h (divided doses or slow-release forms available)	Headache (common), gingival hyperplasia, constipation, dizziness, hypotension, nausea, Dyspepsia, edema, rash, increased liver enzymes, sleep Disturbance, dyspnea	Cardiogenic shock, CHF, symptomatic hypotension, sick sinus syndrome without pacemaker, 2–3 degree AV block without pacemaker	Digoxin (digoxin toxicity); statins (myopathy); erythromycin (QT prolongation); amiodarone (bradycardia, AV block); clopidogrel (↓ anti-platelet effect)
Beta-Blockers[b]				
Metoprolol	*Loading* **IV:** 2.5–5 mg IV bolus over 2 min; up to three doses *Maintenance* **Oral:** 25–100 mg/24 h (divided doses or SR forms available)	Dizziness, headache, fatigue, depression (all common), diarrhea, pruritus, bradycardia, dyspnea, cold extremities, constipation, dyspepsia, heart failure, hypotension, nausea, wheezing	**Black Box Warning:** abrupt withdrawal can exacerbate ischemic heart disease, angina, and MI. Can also cause catecholamine hypersensitivity. Must be withdrawn slowly. Sinus bradycardia 2–3 degree heart block, cardiogenic shock, sick sinus syndrome, severe peripheral vascular disease, acute MI with HR <45 bpm, systolic BP <100 mm Hg, asthma, COPD, pheochromocytoma Tartarate form contraindicated in patients with CHF	Amiodarone (bradycardia, cardiac arrest, heart block); calcium channel blockers (bradycardia, AV conduction disturbances); beta-2-agonists (bronchospasm); antidiabetic agents (hypo- or hyperglycemia)

TABLE 48-3. DRUGS USED FOR RATE CONTROL IN PATIENTS WITH ATRIAL FIBRILLATION (*Continued*)

Drug[a]	Dose	Major Side effects	Contraindications	Multiple Drug Interactions
Propranolol	*Loading* **IV:** 0.15 mg/kg (typically 1–3 mg) *Maintenance* **Oral:** 80–240 mg/24 h (divided doses or SR forms available)	Aggravated CHF, bradyarrhythmia, hypotension, decrease exercise tolerance, Raynaud phenomenon, potential increase in insulin resistance, depression, fatigue, insomnia, paresthesia, psychotic disorder, pruritus, nausea, vomiting, decreased HDL, increased triglycerides, masked symptoms of hypoglycemia, bronchospasm, dyspnea	**Black Box Warning:** abrupt withdrawal can exacerbate ischemic heart disease, angina, and MI. Can also cause catecholamine hypersensitivity. Must be withdrawn slowly Asthma, COPD, sinus bradycardia, 2–3 degree heart block, cardiogenic shock, overt heart failure, sick sinus syndrome without pacemaker	Thioridazine (QT prolongation, cardiac arrest); fluoxetine, amiodarone (bradycardia, cardiac arrest, heart block); calcium channel blockers (bradycardia, AV conduction disturbances); beta-2-agonists (bronchospasm); antidiabetic agents (hypo- or hyperglycemia)

[a]Available as generic
[b]Only two representative members of the class are listed here—others may also be used.
IV, intravenous; BP, blood pressure; CHF, congestive heart failure; COPD, chronic obstructive pulmonary disease; HR, heart rate; MI, myocardial infarction.

rate (80 beats per minute [bpm] at rest or >110 bpm during a 6-minute walk) is not beneficial compared to achieving a resting heart rate of <110 bpm in patients with persistent AF who have stable ventricular function (left ventricular ejection fraction >0.40) and no or acceptable symptoms related to the arrhythmia. (SOR ❸) However, uncontrolled tachycardia, over time, is associated with a reversible decline in ventricular performance.

4. **Anticoagulation** for prevention of systemic embolization.

   a. **While restoring NSR.** If AF is present for more than 48 hours, patients should receive 3 to 4 weeks of warfarin therapy (target international normalized ratio 2.5, range 2.0–3.0) prior to cardioversion and continued for 4 weeks after cardioversion. Recent trials have suggested that long-term anticoagulation can be recommended even after cardioversion due to a 50% risk of recurrent AF. (SOR ❹) Contraindications to warfarin therapy include systemic or intracranial bleeding, noncompliance, or a significant risk of falls.

   b. **Chronic AF.** Determination of a patient's risk for an embolic event guides the selection of anticoagulant therapy (Table 48–4) (see Chapter 88). Among patients with chronic AF, the absolute stroke risk varies by 20-fold according to age and associated vascular comorbidities.

      (1) Current American Heart Association guidelines use the CHADS$_2$ stratification scheme. CHADS$_2$ is an acronym for **C**ongestive heart failure, **H**ypertension, **A**ge ≥75 years, **D**iabetes mellitus, and prior **S**troke or TIA. The score assigns one point to each risk factor except stroke or TIA which are assigned two points.

      (2) **Options include** aspirin (ASA) for low- to moderate-risk patients, ASA plus clopitogrel for high-risk patients unable to take oral anticoagulants, and warfarin (a vitamin K antagonist), dabigatran (a direct, competitive inhibitor of factor IIa [thrombin]), rivaroxaban (a direct factor IIa inhibitor), or apixaban (a direct and competitive factor Xa inhibitor) for moderate-to-high-risk patients. There are no data showing that one oral anticoagulant is superior to the other as head-to-head trials are lacking. Drug selection, therefore should be based on risk factors, cost, tolerability, patient preference, potential for drug interactions, and other clinical characteristics. Combinations of anticoagulants have not been tested.

TABLE 48–4. RISK-BASED APPROACH TO ANTITHROMBOTIC THERAPY IN NONVALVULAR ATRIAL FIBRILLATION (AF)

CHAD$_2$ Score[a]	Antithrombotic Therapy
Prevention of First Stroke	
0	ASA 325 mg daily or no therapy (SOR **Ⓐ**)
1	ASA 325 mg daily or anticoagulation as below (SOR **Ⓐ**)
2 or more	Anticoagulation:
	Warfarin (INR 2.0–3.0) (SOR **Ⓐ**)
	Dabigatran (75–150 mg twice daily)[b] (SOR **Ⓑ**)
	Rivaroxaban (15–20 mg/d)[b] (SOR **Ⓑ**)
1 as an alternative to warfarin or in those deemed unsuitable for vitamin-K-antagonist therapy and who have no more than one of the following characteristics: age >79 yr, weight ≤60 kg, or serum creatinine ≥1.5 mg/dL.	Apixaban 5 mg twice daily (not FDA-approved)[c] (SOR **Ⓑ**)
1 as an alternative to warfarin or but deemed unsuitable for vitamin-K-antagonist therapy and who have two or more of the above characteristics	Apixaban 2.5 mg twice daily (not FDA-approved)[c] (SOR **Ⓒ**)
2 or more but unable to take oral anticoagulants	ASA plus clopidogrel (SOR **Ⓑ**)[d]
Prevention of Stroke in Patients with a History of Stroke or TIA	
Prior stroke or TIA	Warfarin (INR 2.0–3.0) (SOR **Ⓐ**)
Prior stroke or TIA but unable to take oral anticoagulants	ASA 325 mg daily (SOR **Ⓐ**)[d]

[a]CHADS$_2$ stands for Congestive heart failure, Hypertension, Age ≥75 yr, Diabetes mellitus, and prior Stroke or TIA. The score assigns one point to each risk factor except stroke or TIA which are assigned two points.
[b]Dabigatran dose for patients who have creatinine clearance (CrCl) >30 mL/min is 150 mg, dose for patients who have CrCl in the range of 15–30 mL/min is 75 mg; dabigatran is not recommended in patients with more severe renal failure (CrCl < 15 mL/min). Similarly, rivaroxaban dose is lowered to 15 mg/d if the CrCl is 15 to 50 mL/min although its safety has not been established; rivaroxaban should not be used in patients with CrCL <15 mL/min.
[c]Apixaban should not be used if the CrCl is <25 mL/min.
[d]The combination of clopidogrel plus aspirin carries a risk of bleeding similar to that of warfarin and is not recommended for patients with a hemorrhagic contraindication to warfarin over ASA alone.
Source: Data from Furie KL, Goldstein LB, Albers GW, et al. Oral anti fibrillation: a science advisory for healthcare professionals from the American Heart Association/American Stroke Association. *Stroke.* 2012;43:3442–3453.

SELECTED REFERENCES

Barsky AJ. Investigating selected symptoms: palpitations, arrhythmias, and awareness of cardiac activity. *Ann Intern Med.* 2001;134:832.
Cheng A, Kumar K. Overview of atrial fibrillation. www.uptodate.com, online version 30.0. Accessed on August 21, 2013.
Cordina J, Mead GE. Pharmacological cardioversion for atrial fibrillation and flutter. *Cochrane Database Syst Rev.* 2005;(2):CD003713.
Furie KL, Goldstein LB, Albers GW, et al. Oral anti fibrillation: a science advisory for healthcare professionals from the American Heart Association/American Stroke Association. *Stroke.* 2012;43:3442–3453.
Fuster V, Rydén LE, Cannom DS, et al. ACC/AHA/ESC guidelines for the management of patients with atrial fibrillation: Executive summary. *J Am Coll Cardiol.* 2006;48:854–906.
King DE, Dickerson LM, Sack JL. Acute management of atrial fibrillation: part I. Rate and rhythm control. *Am Fam Physician.* 2002;66:249–256.
Lafuente-Lafuente C, Longas-Tejero MA, Bergmann JF, Belmin J. Antiarrythmics for maintaining sinus rhythm after cardioversion of atrial fibrillation. *Cochrane Database Syst Rev.* 2012;(5):CD005049.
Phang R. Nonsustained VT in the absence of apparent structural heart disease. www.uptodate.com, online version 10.0. Accessed August 21, 2013.
Wann LS, Curtis AB, January CT, et al. ACCF/AHA/HRS focused update on the management of patients with atrial fibrillation (updating the 2006 guideline): a report of the American College of Cardiology Foundation/American Heart Association Task Force on Practice Guidelines. *Circulation.* 2011;123:104–123.
Zimetbaum P. Overview of palpitations in adults. www.uptodate.com, online version 10.0. Accessed August 21, 2013.

Additional references are available online at http://langetextbooks.com/fm6e

49 Pediatric Fever

Joanne Dempster, MD, & Urmi A. Desai, MD

KEY POINTS

- Temperature should be taken rectally to confirm core temperature and is considered clinically significant if >38°C or 100.4°F. (SOR ⓒ)
- Infants <1 month of age with fever should be managed as inpatients. (SOR ⓒ)
- Chest x-ray is indicated only for febrile children with clinical signs of respiratory infection. (SOR ⓒ)
- Urinalysis and urine culture is recommended for all children <24 months with fever. (SOR ⓒ)
- Lumbar puncture is recommended for all infants <30 days, ill-appearing infants 1 to 3 months of age, and children 3 to 36 months of age if neurologic or meningeal signs are present. (SOR ⓒ)

I. **Introduction.** This chapter will focus on the etiology, evaluation, and treatment of fever of less than 7 days in previously healthy infants and young children up to 36 months of age. Young children average four to six acute infections per year. Febrile illness is common and has potentially serious consequences in infants and young children. It is therefore important to identify and treat infants and children with serious infections. Although the majority of children with fever have self-limiting viral infections, the goal of the evaluation is to identify sources of infection that require further evaluation and definitive treatment; these are usually bacterial causes.

   A. The evaluation of fever in children depends on the age of the child. Evaluation and treatment have been traditionally categorized into three groups—neonates and infants less than 1 month of age, infants 1 to 3 months of age, and children 3 months to 3 years of age.

   B. Infants and children with significant preexisting conditions should be managed on a case-by-case basis (e.g., neutropenic children, premature infants, or children with human immunodeficiency virus).

II. **Definitions**

   A. In this chapter, fever is defined as a **core temperature** best represented by a rectal temperature of **38°C** (100.4°F) or higher. The definition of high fever is arbitrary; however, a temperature of >40.5°C (105°F) is considered a high fever by most. Fever is not a disease, it is only a symptom. Fevers that children experience are usually not harmful unless the temperature reaches at least 41.7°C (107°F).

   B. **Fever of Unknown Origin** (FUO). Although there is no agreed-upon definition for FUO, it is often referred to as fever for >8 days without a diagnosis after initial evaluation. The range in duration of FUO has been from 5 days to 3 weeks. The assessment of broad categories of FUO is useful and includes conditions such as connective tissue diseases, malignancy, and infectious diseases. This chapter will not focus on management of FUO.

III. **Common Diagnoses.** Serious bacterial illnesses include meningitis, bacteremia, pneumonia, bacterial diarrhea, urinary tract infections (UTIs), cellulitis, mastoiditis, and osteomyelitis. Noninfectious causes of fever include immunization reactions, drug fever, malignancy, chronic inflammatory conditions (e.g., juvenile idiopathic arthritis), and central nervous system dysfunction.

   A. In **infants less than 1 month of age,** the most common infectious organisms are **Group B Streptococcus and Escherichia coli**. Less common organisms are Listeria monocytogenes, Enterococcus, Staphylococcus aureus, gram-negative organisms, and herpes simplex virus (HSV).

   B. In **infants 1 to 3 months of age,** the most common organisms are **Streptococcus pneumoniae, Haemophilus influenzae, and Neisseria meningitidis**. Less common organisms are Group B Streptococcus, E. coli, Staphylococcus aureus, Enterococcus, L. monocytogenes, Pseudomonas sp., and other gram-negative organisms.

TABLE 49–1. PROTOCOLS FOR IDENTIFYING CHILDREN 3 MONTHS OF AGE OR YOUNGER WHO CAN BE TREATED CONSERVATIVELY

	Rochester Protocol	Philadelphia Protocol	Boston Protocol
Number of Patients		747	503
Statistics	Sens 92% (83%–97%) Spec 50% (47%–53%) PPV 12.3% (10%–16%) NPV 98.9% (97%–100%)	Sens 98% (92%–100%) Spec 42% (38%–46%) PPV 14% (11%–17%) NPV 99.7% (98%–100%)	Spec 94.6%
Age	<60 d	29–60 d	28–89 d
Temperature	≥38.0°C	≥38.2°C	≥38.0°C
Criteria	• 37 or more weeks' gestation and hospitalized no longer than the mother • Infant was previously healthy • Infant is well-appearing, with no ear, soft-tissue, or bone infections • WBC 5,000–15,000/μL with an absolute band count <1,500/μL • UA with <10 WBC/hpf if obtained	• Well-appearing • WBC <15,000/mL • Band–neutrophil ratio <0.2 • UA <10 WBC/hpf and a negative urine gram stain • CSF <8 WBC/μL and a negative CSF gram stain • Chest radiograph lacking an infiltrate if one was obtained • Stool without blood and few or no WBCs on the smear in infants with diarrhea	• No immunizations or antimicrobials within the preceding 48 h • No evidence of dehydration, ear, soft-tissue, or bone infections • Overall well appearance • Caretaker available by telephone • WBC count <20,000/μL • CSF with WBC <10 μL • UA <10 WBC/hpf • No infiltrate on chest radiograph if one was obtained
Treatment if criteria met	• Follow-up required • Discharge home • No antibiotics	• Follow-up required within 24 h • Discharge home • No antibiotics	• Follow-up required 24 h later • Discharge home • Empiric antibiotics with ceftriaxone IM 50 mg/kg

Sens, sensitivity; Spec, specificity; PPV, positive predictive value; NPV, negative predictive value; WBC, white blood count; hpf, high-power field; UA, urinalysis; IM, intramuscular.
Source: Data from Jhaveri R, Byington CL, et al. Management of the non-toxic-appearing acutely febrile child: a 21st century approach. *J Pediatr.* 2011;159(2):181–185.

IV. Signs and Symptoms

A. General Considerations. There are three commonly used sets of criteria for identifying children 3 months of age or younger who can be treated conservatively and they are the Rochester Criteria, Philadelphia Protocol, and Boston Criteria (Table 49–1). They all include well-appearing children. Most clinicians, however, believe that infants younger than 1 month with fever should be hospitalized and tested due to their immature immune systems, unreliability of the physical examination, and higher proportion of serious bacterial illness (including those that are hospital-acquired and perinatal).

B. For **infants younger than 1 month,** the history should include **birth history and perinatal factors** that increase the possibility of vertically transmitted infections such as maternal history of Group B strep, maternal fever, maternal history of sexually transmitted infections (HSV, gonorrhea, and chlamydia), and prolonged rupture of membranes. Ask about exposure to sick contacts in the nursery, family members, caretakers, and day care and any previous illness in the child or antibiotic use.

1. Associated symptoms and behaviors should be reviewed such as changes in crying patterns, drowsiness, inconsolability, moaning, oral intake, cough, and vomiting.

2. Physical examination includes level of consciousness and assessment for lethargy; petechial rash; meningeal irritation; respiratory signs including tachypnea, crackles, decreased breath sounds, and cyanosis; and hypotension which are all red flags of serious illness. Signs of meningeal irritation include a positive Kernig sign (inability or reluctance to fully extend the knee when the hip is flexed at 90 degrees) or a positive Brudzinski sign (spontaneous flexion of the hip during attempted flexion of the neck). It should be noted that meningeal irritation in neonates can present as labile temperature; classic findings of nuchal rigidity may not be present.

C. For infants **older than 1 month and for young children,** the history should include the information listed above as well as functional status and travel history. Teething should not influence evaluation decisions.

1. The **immunization status** of a child is important. Children less than 6 months of age are considered to be incompletely immunized since the child has not yet received the primary booster series for Hib and PCV7 or PCV 13.

2. Physical examination should include the components listed above as well as a thorough soft tissue, bony, and articular examination. Findings on articular examination can include swelling, tenderness, limited range of movement of the joint, and refusal to bear weight. Note that in older children, signs of meningeal irritation include nuchal rigidity and positive Kernig and Brudzinski signs.

V. Diagnostic Testing (see Table 49–2).

A. Cell count. A white blood cell (WBC) count with differential is recommended for all neonates and children less than 3 months of age. In children 3 to 36 months of age, this test is not routinely recommended unless the child has signs of serious illness.

B. Blood cultures are recommended in all infants <1 month of age and for infants and children with signs of serious illness.

TABLE 49–2. SUMMARY OF MANAGEMENT OF CHILDREN WITH FEVER BY AGE GROUP

Age	<1 mo	<3 mo	3–36 mo
Fever Cutoff	>100.4°F rectal	>100.4°F rectal	>100.4°F rectal
Etiologies to Consider	• Viral infections • Serious bacterial infections (e.g., UTI, pneumonia, bacteremia, meningitis) • Herpes simplex infection • Other: bundling/excessive clothing, incorrect temperature measurement	• Viral infections • Serious bacterial infections (e.g., UTI, pneumonia, bacteremia, meningitis) • Postimmunization	• Viral infections • Otitis media (commonly viral) • UTI • Pneumonia • Soft-tissue infection • Osteomyelitis • Serious bacterial infection (bacteremia, meningitis) • Other: postimmunization, teething (usually temperature <102°F), drug fever, malignancy, chronic inflammatory conditions
Work Up	UA and culture Blood culture Lumbar puncture CBC Chest x-ray[a] Stool culture[a]	UA and culture Blood culture Lumbar puncture[a] CBC Chest x-ray[a] Stool culture[a]	Determine immunization status UA and culture for children <24 months of age with unexplained fever Lumbar puncture[a] CBC Stool culture Rapid viral testing if appropriate to symptoms and season
Management Setting	Inpatient management	Inpatient vs. outpatient management	Inpatient vs. outpatient management
Treatment	Empiric enteral antibiotic therapy while awaiting cultures: ampicillin + cefotaxime (avoid ceftriaxone) with acyclovir when HSV is suspected	Determine risk status; if high risk: third generation cephalosporin (cefotaxime or Ceftriaxone)	Localize source of infection: ceftriaxone for generalized infections, cefixime (UTI), amoxicillin/azithromycin for pneumonia, amoxicillin for OM
Most Common Pathogens Covered by Empiric Antibiotics	*Escherichia coli,* Group B *Streptococcus,* gram-negative organisms, *Listeria monocytogenes,* herpes simplex virus	*Streptococcus pneumoniae, Haemophilus influenzae, Neisseria meningitidis*	Specific to presumed etiology, consider empiric therapy for incompletely immunized children. Can give oral antibiotic therapy if clinically well-appearing

[a]If clinically indicated.

CBC, complete blood count; HSV, herpes simplex virus; OM, otitis media; UA, urinalysis, UTI, urinary tract infection.

C. **Lumbar puncture** is recommended for all infants aged <1 month, infants aged 1 to 3 months if signs of serious illness are present, and young children aged 3 to 36 months if neurologic or meningeal signs (e.g., nuchal rigidity or petechiae) are observed. A video of this procedures can be found at http://www.youtube.com/watch?v=xvVlhFZeUnY or https://www.mededportal.org/publication/8339.

D. **Urinalysis (UA) and urine culture** are recommended for all children less than 24 months of age; UA and culture should be considered in children less than 36 months of age. Urine for culture should be collected by urethral catheterization or suprapubic aspiration. In children who are toilet trained, a clean catch specimen can be obtained.

E. **Chest radiography** is recommended for all infants <1 month of age and all children with fever ≥39°C with an elevated WBC count (≥20,000 per mm) OR if respiratory signs are present.

F. **Stool tests.** Stool culture and fecal WBC count should be done if diarrhea is present in all children <36 months of age (see Chapter 16).

G. **Rapid viral testing.** There is insufficient evidence for routine rapid viral testing in children <36 months of age for influenza or respiratory syncytial virus. Influenza testing, however, is an option for children >3 months of age during influenza season.

H. **Inflammatory markers.** C-reactive protein levels, procalcitonin, and erythrocyte sedimentation rate can indicate inflammation and the need for further evaluation, however, are not routinely recommended.

VI. **Treatment.** Ultimately, treatment should target specific infections once identified. For hospitalized patients, infection control precautions (droplet, contact, or standard) should be implemented as is appropriate to the presumptive diagnosis.

A. All infants <1 month of age should be hospitalized for further evaluation and treatment. All children older than 1 month with signs of serious illness should also be hospitalized for further evaluation and treatment. Children older than 1 month who have no signs or symptoms of serious illness can be managed in an outpatient setting if good outpatient follow-up is available (Table 49–2).

B. **Antipyretics.** A high fever by itself is not harmful and reduction of fever has not been shown to reduce the overall duration of illness or recurrence of febrile seizures. However, antipyretics are useful in increasing comfort, activity, feeding, and fluid intake. Antipyretic administration should be considered for temperatures >38.9°C (102°F).

    1. Acetaminophen 10 to 15 mg/kg can be given every 4 hours as needed for up to a maximum of five doses per day. Dose should be adjusted in patients with hepatic or renal impairment.

    2. For children older than 6 months, ibuprofen 5 to 10 mg/kg can be given every 6 hours as needed for a maximum dose of 40 mg/kg/day. Ibuprofen is not recommended for use in children with renal or hepatic impairment. Ibuprofen has been shown to be a more effective antipyretic than acetaminophen and both medications have similar levels of adverse outcomes.

    3. For children with refractory fever, acetaminophen can be alternated with ibuprofen every 3 hours. If this approach is recommended, caution parents to track times and doses to avoid giving too much of one drug or forgetting where they are in the sequence.

C. **Empiric antibiotic treatment** is recommended for **all hospitalized children after cultures are obtained**. Local resistance patterns should be considered when choosing an antibiotic.

    1. **For infants <1 month of age,** empiric antibiotics options include the following:

        a. Ampicillin 100 to 150 mg/kg/day intravenous (IV) or intramuscular (IM) divided every 6 hours with a maximum daily dose of 4 g per day for mild to moderate infections **OR** 200 to 400 mg/kg/day divided every 6 hours with a maximum daily dose of 12 g per day **with or without** gentamicin 2.5 mg/kg/dose IV or IM every 8 hours.

        b. Cefotaxime 50 to 180 mg/kg/day IV divided every 6 to 8 hours with a maximum daily dose of 6 g per day for mild to moderate infections **OR** 200 to 225 mg/kg/day divided every 4 to 6 hours with a maximum daily dose of 12 g per day for severe infections.

    2. **For children 1 to 3 months of age,** ceftriaxone (50–75 mg/kg/day for mild infection **OR** 100 mg/kg/day divided every 12 hours with a maximum dose of 1 g per day for severe infections) **OR** cefotaxime (dosed as listed above) is given for UTIs.

3. For children older than 3 months, ceftriaxone (dosed as listed above) is administered for general infections, cefixime for urinary infections, and amoxicillin and azithromycin for respiratory infections. Cefixime is dosed at 16 mg/kg/day divided every 12 hours for day one, then 8 mg/kg/day given every 24 hours on days 2 to 14. Amoxicillin for respiratory infections is dosed at 25 to 50 mg/kg/day divided every 8 hours for mild infection **OR** 80 to 100 mg/kg/day divided every 8 hours for severe infection with a maximum of 500 mg/dose. Azithromycin (Zithromax) is dosed at 10 mg/kg orally on day 1 then, 5 mg/kg daily for the next 4 days, maximum dose 500 mg, for respiratory infections.

D. Empiric treatment with acyclovir, 180 mg/kg/day divided every 8 hours, is indicated for neonates with ill-appearance, mucocutaneous vesicles, seizures, or cerebrospinal fluid pleocytosis.

VII. Febrile seizures are defined as a convulsion associated with a temperature >38°C in a child less than 6 years of age with no metabolic or central nervous system infections or inflammatory causes of convulsions present and no history of previous afebrile seizure. Febrile seizures occur in about 2% to 4% of children younger than 5 years.

A. Febrile seizures are associated with bacterial infections, viral infections, and immunizations (particularly the measles, mumps, rubella vaccine and diphtheria, tetanus, pertussis vaccine). Risk factors include a family history of febrile seizures and genetic factors.

B. Evaluation. Unless other symptoms are present, imaging is not recommended. Consider a lumbar puncture if meningeal signs are present or meningitis or intracranial infection is suspected.

C. Treatment. For seizures lasting more than 5 minutes, monitor airway, respiratory status, and circulation and start with a short-acting benzodiazepine (e.g., lorazepam 0.05–0.1 mg/kg IV over 1–2 minutes or 0.1 mg/kg rectally diluted 1:1 with water; maximum 4 mg/dose in any form). After managing the seizure, control the temperature for patient comfort (antipyretics do not seem to decrease recurrence).

D. Recurrence. Risk factors for recurrent febrile seizures include young age at onset, history of febrile seizure in a first-degree relative, low degree of fever in the emergency department, and brief duration between onset of fever and the febrile seizure. About 30% of children with febrile seizures have at least one recurrence. For patients with recurrence, consider giving rectal lorazepam gel for home use. Prophylaxis with antiepileptic agents is not routinely recommended.

E. Risk of Epilepsy. About 7% of children who have a history of febrile seizures develop epilepsy, compared to 2% in the general population.

VIII. Patient Education

A. Counseling should include education on proper measurement of rectal temperature, red flag signs and symptoms for serious bacterial infections, and anticipatory guidance for when to seek medical attention.

B. For those patients who experience **febrile seizures,** parents should be counseled that there are usually no long-term neurological sequelae following febrile seizure. In addition, there is a risk of recurrence, particularly if child has risk factors as noted above. Antiepileptic drugs are not necessary for treating simple febrile seizures and antipyretics are NOT recommended for seizure prophylaxis.

SELECTED REFERENCES

Allen CH. Fever without a source in children 3 to 36 months of age. UpToDate. Updated December 17, 2012. http://www.uptodate.com/contents/fever-without-a-source-in-children-3-to-36-months-of-age. Accessed April 2013.

Fishman A. Febrile seizures. UpToDate. Updated November 16, 2012. http://www.uptodate.com/contents/febrile-seizures. Accessed April 2013.

Hamilton JL, John SP. Evaluation of fever in infants and young children. *Am Fam Physician.* 2013; 87(4):254–260.

Jhaveri R, Byington CL, Klein JO, Shapiro ED. Management of the non-toxic-appearing acutely febrile child: a 21st century approach. *J Pediatrics.* 2011;159(2):181–185.

Neligan A, Bell GS, Giavasi C, et al. Long-term risk of developing epilepsy after febrile seizures: a prospective cohort study. *Neurology.* 2012;78(15):1166–1170.

Smitherman HF, Macias CG. Evaluation and management of fever in the neonate and young infant (less than three months of age). UpToDate. Updated January 3, 2013. http://www.uptodate.com/contents/evaluation-and-management-of-fever-in-the-neonate-and-young-infant. Accessed April 2013.

Additional references are available online at http://langetextbooks.com/fm6e

50   Pelvic Pain

Guido Grasso-Knight, MD, MPH, Meredith A. Goodwin, MD, &
Niharika Khanna, MBBS, MD, DGO

KEY POINTS

- Pelvic pain originates below the umbilicus of the adult female and may be acute (<6 months' duration) or chronic (6 or more months' duration). (SOR ⑥)
- Pelvic inflammatory disease, ectopic pregnancy, appendicitis, urinary tract infection, and adnexal mass rupture/torsion/hemorrhage are the most common causes of acute pelvic pain. (SOR ⑥)
- Treatment of chronic pelvic pain should be multidisciplinary. A single etiology is often not found. Empiric therapy may be attempted. (SOR ⑥)

I. **Definition.** Pelvic pain (PP) is localized in the abdomen below the umbilicus. **Acute pelvic pain** (APP) describes pain for <6 months. **Chronic pelvic pain** (CPP) is present for 6 months or more. The pain may also involve the buttocks or lumbosacral areas. Rarely, a single cause is identified as the source of pain.

The clinician must carefully consider the patient's perception of pain, investigate underlying etiologies, and develop a comprehensive plan that includes acute therapies as well as psychosocial care for chronic conditions. Pain can be present in the absence of acute or lasting pathology. Previous experiences or events may initially trigger pain. Maladaptive physiologic and psychological processes may allow perception of pain to continue even with resolution of the precipitating condition.

   A. **Epidemiology.** Fifteen to twenty percent of women aged 18 to 50 years experience CPP lasting more than 1 year during their lifetime. Risk of CPP is not affected by race, income, or socioeconomic status. PP is the most common reason for referral to a gynecologist and accounts for up to 40% of all laparoscopies and more than 10% of hysterectomies performed in the United States.

   B. **Etiology** (Tables 50–1 and 50–2). APP may be caused by inflammation, infections, pregnancy, and trauma including psychosocial trauma. Differential diagnosis varies based on age. CPP has a wide differential diagnosis that includes neoplasia, inflammation, trauma, and infection. CPP can affect multiple systems simultaneously (e.g., gynecologic, musculoskeletal, gastrointestinal, and urologic). The four most common causes of CPP are irritable bowel syndrome (IBS), endometriosis, interstitial cystitis, and adhesions. Comorbid psychiatric illnesses are common. Depression, somatization, and substance abuse may influence the course and prognosis of PP.

II. **Common Diagnoses**

   A. **APP** accounts for 5% of all ambulatory primary care visits. Ten percent of these patients require urgent surgery. APP may present with nonspecific signs and symptoms. Among these women, hospitalization yields a diagnosis in less than 50% of cases. Recognition of signs and symptoms, associated positive predictive values of findings, and an evidence-based approach to diagnostic testing offers a greater potential for cost-effective management.

   1. **Pelvic inflammatory disease (PID)** is characterized by infection and inflammation of the upper female genital tract. Possible presentations include tubo-ovarian abscess (TOA), peritonitis, salpingitis, and endometritis. Variations in diagnostic criteria and subclinical infections confound data collection. PID requires a high degree of clinical suspicion. Empiric diagnosis in a sexually active woman with PP can be made if there is pelvic organ tenderness (cervical, uterine, or adnexal) and no other more likely diagnosis.

      a. PID is typically diagnosed based on a report of risk factors for or evidence of a sexually transmitted infection (STI) in combination with physical findings (cervical motion, uterine or adnexal tenderness). Notably, women at highest risk for chlamydia and PID include those with multiple sexual partners, between the ages of 15 and 24 years, with new or multiple sexual partners, and of African–American

TABLE 50–1. FINDINGS IN COMMON CAUSES OF ACUTE PELVIC PAIN

Diagnosis	Location/Quality/Chronology of Pain	Other Symptoms	Signs
Ovarian cyst	Unilateral dull, pressure-like; severe/diffuse low abdominal (postrupture). Within 7 days of menses, worse with strenuous physical activity	Delayed/scanty menses if lutein cyst	Smooth mobile adnexal mass/fullness; peritoneal signs if ruptured
Pelvic inflammatory disease	Lower abdominal with gradual onset, usually bilateral, worse perimenstrual	Fever, vaginal discharge, dysuria, abnormal vaginal bleeding, backache, rectal pressure, adnexal tenderness/thickening, cervical motion tenderness	See Table 50–3
Adnexal torsion	Unilateral moderate/severe pain; sudden onset, within 24–48 h of presentation	Nausea/vomiting	Adnexal mass and tenderness on the affected side, rebound, guarding may be present
Ectopic pregnancy	Diffuse or localized, colicky or dull lower abdominal, radiating to the shoulder if hemoperitoneum	Abnormal vaginal bleeding (metrorrhagia, menorrhagia, amenorrhea), nausea/breast tenderness	Adnexal tenderness/mass, uterus slightly enlarged, peritoneal signs, abdominal distention and shock if significant hemorrhage
Uterine leiomyomas	Low midline pressure, back pain; moderate to severe pain with torsion/degeneration	Menorrhagia, metrorrhagia, nausea/vomiting with torsion, dysuria (if large), dyspareunia, infertility	Enlarged, nodular uterus, tender if degeneration/torsion; possible anemia

TABLE 50–2. FINDINGS IN GYNECOLOGIC CAUSES OF CHRONIC PELVIC PAIN

Diagnosis	Location/Quality/Chronology of Pain	Other Symptoms	Signs
Endometriosis	Variable midline suprapubic, cyclic premenstrual/menstrual	Dyspareunia, painful defecation, infertility, hematuria	Often none; palpable cysts and nodules on uterosacral ligament
Mittelschmerz	Suprapubic, dull to sharp midcycle; hours to 3 days	None	None
Psychogenic	Variable	Depression, anxiety, back pain, fatigue, nausea	Signs of depression or anxiety, normal pelvic examination, occasional pelvic tenderness
Dysmenorrhea	Low abdominal starting prior/with menses, dyspareunia, pain radiates to the rectum	Painful defecation, nausea/vomiting, anorexia, headache, occasional diarrhea	None
Uterine leiomyoma	Constant mild or no ongoing pain	Menorrhagia, metrorrhagia, pelvic fullness	Enlarged or irregular uterus on examination or transvaginal ultrasound
Dyspareunia	Dull pain on vaginal entry or deep pelvic pain during sexual intercourse	Anxiety, depression, sexual dysfunction, vaginal dryness or infection	Anxiety, depression, posttraumatic stress disorder
Adhesions	Colicky, typically unilateral and focal	Bloating, nausea	Diffuse abdominal tenderness without masses; may have decreased mobility of pelvic organs

race. There is also a slightly increased risk of PID around the time of insertion of an intrauterine device (IUD), if an infection is not recognized and treated.

   b. Screening for and treatment of chlamydia and gonorrhea can decrease the incidence of PID by 60% (see Chapter 102).

2. **Adnexal mass torsion or rupture.** Ovarian cysts and ovarian torsion can be the causes of APP. Clinical suspicion must remain high among women with new onset of unilateral pain that is progressive or intermittent/colicky. Physical examination findings of an adnexal mass and pain may be absent. Ultrasonography is useful to confirm the diagnosis.

   a. Ovarian torsion is more common among pediatric patients, but the risk also increases significantly during pregnancy, accounting for 25% cases of ovarian torsion. This is likely due to the higher frequency of larger corpus luteal cysts during the first trimester. Adnexal torsion is more common among women of reproductive age and with a history of prior pelvic surgery, ovarian cysts, ovarian tumors, PID, pedunculated uterine leiomyomas, or tubal ligation.

   b. Adnexal masses in premenopausal women that are less than 5 cm in size and are cystic on transvaginal ultrasound (TVU) have >90% likelihood of being benign. Typically, **masses that are greater than 5 cm in size and are solid or complex have a greater probability of being malignant**. Postmenopausal women with similar masses have an increased likelihood of malignancy.

3. **Ectopic pregnancies** comprise approximately 1% to 2% of pregnancies in the United States, but contribute to 3% to 4% of maternal deaths (0.2 deaths/1000 ectopic pregnancies). Risks for ectopic pregnancy include age over 35 years, history of PID, use of assisted reproductive technology (ART), evidence of tubal injury, and history of tubal ligation. Similarly, other processes that confer an increased risk of an ectopic pregnancy through changes in the fallopian and uterine structures include endometriosis, obstructive uterine leiomyomas, and in utero diethylstilbestrol exposure.

4. **Uterine leiomyomas** (fibroids) occur in 20% to 40% of reproductive-age women, more commonly among African–American women. Acute degeneration or torsion of pedunculated leiomyoma may cause APP. Reports of moderate or severe dyspareunia and severe noncyclical PP are more common among women with fibroids.

B. CPP is present in more than 1 of every 10 women seeking medical care. In 61% of the cases, the cause is not identified. Screening for trauma and posttraumatic stress disorder in these women is important.

1. **Endometriosis** is found in 45% to 50% of women with CPP. Prevalence ranges from 20 to 100/1000 women of reproductive age and 250 to 350/1000 infertile women. Risk factors for endometriosis include family history (sevenfold increased risk in first-degree relatives), genetic abnormalities, immune disorders, Asian ancestry, cigarette smoking, alcohol consumption, lack of exercise, vaginal or cervical stenosis, and uterine anomalies (noncommunicating uterine horn, coelomic metaplasia).

2. **Mittelschmerz** is midcycle pain associated with ovulation. It may be accompanied by a small amount of bleeding. It is experienced by 25% of ovulating women.

3. **Dysmenorrhea** is reported by 30% to 50% of all women, and 15% are incapacitated for 1 to 3 days of each month because of severe symptoms (see Chapter 18).

4. **Dyspareunia** or pain during vaginal intercourse is common. Greater than 60% of women experience it at some time in their lives. Risk factors for dyspareunia include a history of diabetes, alcohol or marijuana use, PID, medroxyprogesterone use, fatigue, anxiety, stress, depression, sexual abuse, vulvar and perineal surgeries, scarring with immobility or stricture of the vaginal walls, vaginal dryness with friction from inadequate genital sexual arousal, and vaginismus.

5. **Adhesions** are diagnosed in 25% of women with CPP, but their causative role remains controversial. Pain caused by adhesions is experienced by nearly 3% of women undergoing operations. The risk varies by surgical site—the colon and rectum have the highest incidence, followed by the ovaries.

6. **Uterine leiomyomas** are most often asymptomatic, but can be a source of CPP (see Section II.A.4).

7. **Psychogenic pain.** Women with a history of somatization disorder, sexual abuse, posttraumatic stress disorder, and depression frequently experience CPP. The prevalence of sexual abuse history in CPP is 50%. Depression coexists with CPP in 50% and anxiety in 31% of women.

TABLE 50-3. DIAGNOSTIC CRITERIA FOR PELVIC INFLAMMATORY DISEASE

Minimum diagnostic criteria: Uterine or adnexal or cervical motion tenderness and risk for sexually transmitted infection. **Additional diagnostic criteria:** Oral temperature ≥38.3°C, cervical sampling positive for *Chlamydia trachomatis* or *Neisseria gonorrhoeae*, saline microscopy of vaginal secretions showing white blood cells, elevated erythrocyte sedimentation rate, elevated C-reactive protein, and abnormal cervical or vaginal mucopurulent discharge. **Definitive diagnostic criteria:** Endometrial biopsy with histopathologic evidence of endometritis, transvaginal ultrasonography or magnetic resonance imaging scan showing thick fluid-filled fallopian tubes, and laparoscopic abnormalities consistent with pelvic inflammatory disease.

Source: Reproduced with permission from the Centers for Disease Control and Prevention Recommendations, 2010.

     8. Chronic postoperative pain is present after hysterectomy in 17% to 32% of women. Postoperative pain is thought to be related to nerve irritation during surgery, preoperative perception of pain, and somatization.

III. Symptoms (Tables 50-1 to 50-3)
  A. Location and quality
    1. APP
      a. Unilateral sharp, moderate/severe pain can occur with ovarian torsion, hemorrhagic ovarian cyst, subserosal pedunculated leiomyomas torsion, ruptured ectopic pregnancy, PID, urethral colic, diverticulitis, and pelvic fracture. Vascular pain can reflect common iliac arterial aneurysms or mesenteric venous thrombosis.
      b. Bilateral or midline diffuse pain can occur with PID, intra-abdominal hemorrhage, and intestinal obstruction.
      c. Dull, pressure pain commonly occurs with mesenteric lymphadenitis, mesenteric ischemia, and diverticulitis.
      d. Fever occurs frequently with appendicitis and pyelonephritis and sometimes with PID.
      e. Vaginal discharge is expected among patients with PID.
      f. Dysuria is a characteristic of urinary tract infections, but may also be seen with PID.
    2. CPP
      a. Dull and deep pain characterizes interstitial cystitis, IBS, and endometriosis. Leiomyomas can create pressure on the nerves and veins, sometimes resulting in chronic venous stasis in the lower extremities.
      b. Reproducible sharp pain may occur on the pelvic floor caused by pudendal, ilioinguinal, and iliohypogastric nerve entrapment and myofascial and coccygeal pain syndromes.
      c. Dyspareunia is the genital pain during sexual intercourse, which can be caused by endometriosis, uterine fibroids, PID, estrogen deficiency, pelvic organ prolapse, interstitial cystitis, female genital mutilation, cancer therapies including radiation, and malformations.
      d. Trigger point-associated pain is often reproducible. Among patients with myofascial syndrome, it is usually restricted to an anatomical region involving the abdomen and back.
  B. Onset/chronology
    1. APP. Sudden onset of pain suggests acute perforation of hollow viscus or intraperitoneal hemorrhage. Gradual onset is more typical of inflammatory or obstructive pathology.
    2. CPP may be dull or sharp, intermittent or constant. Onset is often very gradual and may be cyclical.
  C. Associated symptoms
    1. Sexual dysfunction is a prominent feature in more than 25% of women with APP and CPP. Women with endometriosis, dyspareunia, and IBS report higher rates of sexual dysfunction.
    2. There is a high incidence of fatigue, substance abuse, somatization, anxiety, depression, and posttraumatic stress disorder in women with CPP. Up to 25% of these women have a history of physical abuse, sexual harassment, and violence.

IV. Signs (see Tables 50–1 to 50–3). Review signs of chronic endometritis, adnexal mass, pelvic congestion syndrome, and ovarian remnant syndrome.

CHRONIC ENDOMETRITIS

Chronic endometritis in nonpregnant women is usually due to infections (PID, tuberculosis), IUD, submucosal leiomyoma, or radiation therapy. CPP, menorrhagia or metrorrhagia, mucopurulent vaginal discharge, and tender enlarged uterus are characteristic findings. An endometrial biopsy may be needed for diagnosis. Chronic endometritis in recently postpartum women may be due to retained products of conception.

Recommended treatment includes removal of an IUD if present and use of azithromycin or doxycycline (for *Chlamydia trachomatis* or unknown etiology); *Mycobacterium tuberculosis* should be treated with combination drug therapy for 9 to 12 months.

ADNEXAL MASS

A family history of reproductive malignancy (uterine, breast, ovarian), presence of the BRCA gene, nulliparity, early menarche, and late menopause are all risk factors for ovarian tumors.

Eighty percent of ovarian masses in girls younger than 15 years are malignant. About 30% to 60% of adnexal masses in postmenopausal women are malignant as well. Adnexal masses can cause APP through torsion or ovarian cyst rupture or hemorrhage. Rupture of small (≤4 cm) cysts is usually asymptomatic.

The approach to an adnexal mass depends on the patient's age and cyst size. Due to high oncogenic potential (germ cell tumors) in premenarcheal patients, adnexal masses in these individuals should be evaluated by TVU and referred for surgical removal. In reproductive-age women, adnexal masses are commonly follicular or lutein cysts or complications of PID (hydrosalpinx and TOA). If pain is not acute or recurrent, palpable cysts ≤6 cm in women of childbearing age can be monitored with repeat pelvic examination in 6 weeks. Any persistent or increasing mass on serial observation or a mass initially ≥6 cm should be evaluated by TVU. Adnexal masses in postmenopausal women have a high risk of malignancy (surface epithelial or stromal tumors) and should be evaluated with TVU, tumor markers (CA-125), and possibly computerized tomography (CT) scanning.

Management of adnexal masses includes referral to a gynecologist for further evaluation and removal, unless a mass in a reproductive-age woman is cystic, small (≤6 cm), and does not persist or increase in size.

PELVIC CONGESTION SYNDROME

Pelvic congestion syndrome is caused by autonomic nervous system dysfunction manifesting as smooth muscle spasm and pelvic vasculature congestion. It is commonly associated with pelvic, vulvar, and thigh varicosities, and psychogenic disorders (depression, anxiety, and posttraumatic stress disorder). Typical symptoms include lower abdominal and back pain, dysmenorrhea, dyspareunia, abnormal uterine bleeding, chronic fatigue, and IBS. Pain usually begins with ovulation and lasts through menses. Examination reveals an enlarged, tender uterus and ovaries with multiple ovarian cysts and tender uterosacral ligaments. Evaluation for suspected pelvic congestion includes TVU with Doppler flow study and pelvic venography (the gold standard for the evaluation of pelvic congestion) demonstrating delayed disappearance of contrast medium from the uterine and ovarian veins.

Management should be based on related symptoms rather than the presence of varicosities alone. First-line treatment includes hormonal suppression with continuous progestins. Transcatheter embolization of the pelvic veins or hysterectomy with possible oophorectomy is an option in women who have completed childbearing.

TABLE 50–4. DIAGNOSTIC TESTING IN ACUTE PELVIC PAIN

Suspected Diagnosis	Tests
PID	β-hCG, CBC, cervical sampling for *Neisseria gonorrhoeae* and *Chlamydia trachomatis*, ESR, vaginal wet prep, endometrial biopsy, TVU, laparoscopy, LFTs if perihepatitis
Ectopic pregnancy	Serum β-hCG, CBC, TVU, laparoscopy
Adnexal mass torsion	TVU with Doppler flow study, CT
Uterine Leiomyomas	TVU, MRI

CBC, complete blood count; CT, computerized tomography; ESR, erythrocyte sedimentation rate; hCG, human chorionic gonadotropin; LFTs, liver function tests; PID, pelvic inflammatory disease; TVU, transvaginal ultrasound.

OVARIAN REMNANT SYNDROME

Ovarian remnant syndrome is a rare condition that develops when functional ovarian tissue is left after intended bilateral oophorectomy. Symptoms usually arise 2 to 5 years after intended oophorectomy and include cyclic (often with the luteal phase) or constant lateralizing CPP and dyspareunia, with or without adnexal mass. Patients deny menopausal symptoms. Follicle-stimulating hormone (FSH) and luteinizing hormone (LH) typically are in premenopausal range, although occasionally the remaining ovarian tissue may not be active enough to suppress FSH levels. TVU or CT scanning helps identify an adnexal mass.

Gonadotropin-releasing hormone (GnRH) agonists often provide relief, but are impractical for long-term use. Patients who achieve relief with GnRH agonists will likely respond to surgical removal of the remnant tissue.

V. Laboratory Tests (Tables 50–4 and 50–5).
    A. Pregnancy test (urine or serum) must be performed in all patients with PP, who are of reproductive age.
        1. Most currently available **urine pregnancy tests** can detect human chorionic gonadotropin (hCG) levels of 10 to 100 U/mL at 3 to 4 days after conception. Dilute urine can decrease sensitivity. Most current urine pregnancy tests are 84% to 94% sensitive by the first day of the expected period. By 1 week after the first day of the missed period, sensitivity for urinary hCG is 97%.
        2. Quantitative serum β-hCG is detected at the level of 2 to 25 mIU at 7 days after conception and doubles every 2 days during the first 4 weeks after implantation. If the serum β-hCG level increases by less than 53% in 48 hours, the pregnancy is abnormal. When β-hCG levels fail to increase as expected or plateaus, ectopic pregnancy must be considered. Although rare, a heterotopic pregnancy (intrauterine and ectopic) can also occur.
    B. Complete blood cell count. Fifty-six percent of patients with PID and 36% of patients with acute appendicitis have a normal white blood cell (WBC) count. A WBC >10.5 K has a positive likelihood ratio (LR) of only 1.3, and a negative LR of only 0.9 in the diagnosis of PID. Leukocytosis alone should not be used to determine clinical management.

TABLE 50–5. DIAGNOSTIC TESTING IN CHRONIC PELVIC PAIN

Suspected Diagnosis	Tests
Adhesions	Laparoscopy
Chronic endometritis	Endometrial biopsy
Dyspareunia	*Neisseria gonorrhoeae* and *Chlamydia trachomatis* study, vaginal wet preparation, vaginal pH, UA, urine culture
Endometriosis	TVU, MRI, laparoscopy
Mittelschmerz	None

CT, computerized tomography; MRI, magnetic resonance imaging; TVU, transvaginal ultrasound; UA, urinalysis.

C. The cervical DNA probe has a specificity of 99% and a sensitivity of 86% for *Neisseria gonorrhoeae* and a specificity of 98% and a sensitivity of 93% for *C. trachomatis*. It is useful for ruling in an infectious etiology, but may miss true positives.

D. TVU still reigns in the diagnosis of APP. For a suspicious isolated ovarian mass, TVU is preferred. Further workup with ultrasound (transvaginal plus color Doppler) can discriminate benign from malignant lesions with a sensitivity of 99.1% and a specificity of 85.9%

E. Magnetic resonance imaging (MRI) improves visualization of small cystic lesions that are undetectable on TVU (e.g., endometriomas). Increasingly, MRI is used in patients after ultrasound to further elucidate findings in the pelvis. MRI is recommended in patients with solid ovarian masses to differentiate ovarian malignancy from an exophytic leiomyoma. MRI may also be able to clarify a diagnosis of adenomyosis.

F. The sensitivity of CT is 92% for the diagnosis of peritoneal lesions (e.g., endometriosis or ovarian metastasis). MRI and CT are equally accurate and more sensitive than TVU for staging ovarian cancer and localization of endometriosis. Ultrasound is less accurate for appendicitis with a mean sensitivity of 78% and a specificity of 83% compared to pelvic CT (sensitivity of 91% and specificity of 90%).

G. Laparoscopy is the gold standard for the evaluation of CPP. CPP is the diagnosis associated with more than 40% of all laparoscopies performed each year. The decision to perform a laparoscopy should be based on the patient's history, physical examination, and findings of noninvasive tests. About 65% of women with CPP have at least one diagnosis detectable by laparoscopy. Endometriosis is found in one-third of all laparoscopies performed for CPP and adhesions are diagnosed in about one-quarter of laparoscopies. Ovarian cysts, hernias, pelvic congestion syndrome, ovarian remnant syndrome, ovarian retention syndrome, postoperative peritoneal cysts, and endosalpingiosis are other diagnoses that can be made laparoscopically.

VI. Treatment
A. APP
1. Treatment of PID. PID treatment regimens must provide empiric, broad spectrum coverage of likely pathogens including effectiveness against *N. gonorrhoeae*, *C. trachomatis*, and anaerobes such as *Bacteroides fragilis*. Early and effective treatment may prevent life-threatening complications such as sepsis, TOA, peritonitis, and Fitz-Hugh–Curtis syndrome. Long-term sequelae such as infertility, tubal scarring, and PID are less common when treatment is initiated early.

a. Inpatient treatment of PID with parenteral antibiotics is recommended for TOA, patients with severe illness with inability to tolerate oral medications, cases where surgical emergencies (appendicitis, TOA) cannot be excluded, or when there is intolerance or poor response to outpatient antimicrobial regimens. Pregnant women should receive inpatient parenteral treatment followed by oral treatment upon clinical improvement.

Parenteral therapy includes cefotetan 2 g intravenously (IV) every 12 hours **OR** cefoxitin 2 g IV every 6 hours **PLUS** doxycycline 100 mg orally or IV every 12 hours. IV antibiotics can be discontinued 24 hours after clinical improvement. Oral therapy should continue for a total of 14 days.

(1) If **TOA** is identified, oral clindamycin or metronidazole can be added to doxycycline for more effective continued coverage of anaerobes.

(2) Other parenteral regimens for PID include clindamycin 900 mg IV every 8 hours in combination with gentamicin (2 mg/kg loading dose with dosing every 8 hours at 1.5 mg/kg or once daily at 3–5 mg/kg). Failure to improve within 72 hours warrants additional investigation and hospitalization, if therapy was previously initiated to an outpatient.

b. Outpatient treatment (Table 50–6) may start presumptively while awaiting culture results.

2. Ectopic pregnancy
a. Gynecologic consultation and surgery (laparotomy or laparoscopy) are indicated for ruptured ectopic pregnancy, especially in hemodynamically unstable patients, women unable to comply with monitoring after medical treatment, and failure of medical treatment (tubal size ≥3 cm, serum β-hCG greater than 5000 mIU, or fetal cardiac activity on TVU).

b. Otherwise, women with ectopic pregnancy are managed either with methotrexate or expectantly. In comparing systemic methotrexate with tube-sparing laparoscopic surgery, randomized trials have shown no difference in overall tubal

TABLE 50–6. OUTPATIENT THERAPY FOR PID

CDC Recommended Outpatient Regimen
Ceftriaxone 250 mg IM in a single dose
OR
Cefoxitin 2 g IM in a single dose, and probenecid 1 g orally administered concurrently in a single dose
OR
Other parenteral third-generation cephalosporin (e.g., ceftizoxime or cefotaxime)
PLUS
Doxycycline 100 mg orally twice a day for 14 days
WITH OR WITHOUT
Metronidazole 500 mg twice a day for 14 days

Source: Reproduced with permission from the Centers for Disease Control and Prevention Recommendations, 2010 Update.

preservation, tubal patency, repeat ectopic pregnancy, or future pregnancies. Methotrexate is effective in 86% to 94% of patients.

(1) Prior to initiation of methotrexate therapy, the following studies are recommended: complete blood cell count with differential, aspartate aminotransferase, creatinine, blood type, and Rhesus (Rh).

(2) Typical regimens for therapy are described in Table 50–7. Particular attention is given to β-hCG levels on days 4 and 7. An appropriate response to therapy requires a 15% decline or greater between these measurements. Weekly monitoring of serum β-hCG is required. A second IM dose of methotrexate (50 mg/m^2) is recommended, if the β-hCG titer decreases by less than 15% during the 4 days after the first injection.

2. Urgent gynecologic referral is indicated for adnexal torsion and necrosis of pedunculated leiomyoma. A torsed ovary may be salvaged by detorsion

TABLE 50–7. METHOTREXATE PROTOCOLS FOR ECTOPIC PREGNANCY

Day	Single Dose Therapy	Two Dose Therapy	Multidose Therapy
0	Labs: hCG, CBC, AST, Cr, type, and Rh	Labs: hCG, CBC, AST, Cr, type, and Rh	Labs: hCG, CBC, AST, Cr, type, and Rh
1	MTX: 50 mg/m^2 IM	MTX: 50 mg/m^2 IM	MTX: 1 mg/kg IM (days 1,3,5, 7)
2	—		Leucovorin: 0.1 mg/kg IM (days 2, 4,6,8)
3	—		Labs: hCG (on days 1,3,5,7); if ≤15% decline then repeat dose cycle on day 3; if ≥15% decline, follow weekly until undetected; max: 4 MTX/Leucovorin cycles total, levels may rise initially
4	Labs: hCG	MTX: 50 mg/m^2 IM Labs: hCG	—
5	—		—
6	—		—
7	Labs: hCG; if ≤15% decline at days 4–7 then repeat dose; if ≥15% decline, measure weekly until undetected	Labs: hCG; if ≤15% decline at days 4–7 then repeat dose; if ≥15% decline, measure weekly until undetected	—
11		Labs: hCG, if ≤15% at days 7 to 11, consider repeat dose, or surgical management	

MTX, methotrexate; hCG, human chorionic gonadotropin; CBC, complete blood count; AST, aspartate aminotransferase; Cr, serum creatinine.
Source: Reproduced with permission from ACP PIER 2007. Ectopic Pregnancy. Drug Therapy: Consider drug therapy with methotrexate to treat ectopic pregnancy. Retrieved from http://pier.acponline.org/physicians/diseases/d050/tables/d050-t3.html and adapted from ACOG Committee on Practice Bulletins–Gynecology. ACOG Practice Bulletin No. 94: Medical management of ectopic pregnancy. *Obstet Gynecol.* 2008;111(6):1479–1485.

if pedunculated. Myomectomy and hysterectomy are optional treatments for necrotic pedunculated leiomyoma.

   3. Uterine leiomyomas. Stable leiomyomas can be managed medically with non-steroidal anti-inflammatory drugs (NSAIDs) such as oral ibuprofen 600 mg every 6 hours. Women unresponsive to medical therapy may require gynecologic referral for surgery (myomectomy or hysterectomy). Preoperative GnRH agonists, such as leuprolide, may be given to increase hemoglobin, reduce uterine size, and decrease intraoperative blood loss. Long-term (≥6 months) treatment with GnRH agonists is not recommended because of the risk of significant bone loss. Another option for leiomyoma treatment is interventional radiology referral for **uterine artery embolization**.

B. CPP. Specific causes of **CPP** should be identified and treated. An interdisciplinary approach with a pain management specialist is potentially helpful. NSAIDs are offered first, or hormonal therapy if a cyclical pattern is apparent. There is less evidence to support the routine use of selective serotonin reuptake inhibitors (SSRIs) and tricyclic antidepressants (TCAs). Opioid therapy is reserved as a third-line agent. If an etiology is identified, specific modalities should be offered.

   Laparoscopic nerve ablation should be limited to treatment of midline pain. Specifically, laparoscopic uterosacral nerve ablation (LUNA) has low efficacy for pain relief when compared with diagnostic laparoscopy. While 60% to 95% of women will experience relief of CPP with hysterectomy and with oophorectomy, this treatment is less effective for women <30 years of age or with comorbid psychiatric illness. There are limited data supporting use of exercise for CPP or the efficacy of physical therapy interventions.

   1. Dysmenorrhea (see Chapter 18).

   2. Uterine leiomyomas are a rare cause of CPP and patients should be treated only if symptomatic. See above for specific recommendations.

   3. Endometriosis-associated CPP can be treated medically or surgically (via laparoscopic ablation). Medications include oral contraceptives as first-line therapy if the patient is not trying to conceive, with consideration of a GnRH agonist or danazol as second-line therapy. Low-dose estrogen–progestin therapy ("add back") can help mitigate menopausal symptoms and bone loss.

   (1) Laparoscopy is often used for a diagnosis of endometriosis, but is not required before a treatment trial with a GnRH agonist. The androgenic impact and side effect profile of danazol limit its acceptability, often to only 6 months.

   (2) Third-line or maintenance therapy with the levonorgestrel intrauterine system (LNG-IUD) has also been effective in reducing both bleeding and pain although its use is not FDA-approved.

   (3) Patients with endometriosis may require therapeutic laparoscopy for electrocoagulation or laser ablation of lesions. These patients have a 66% to 80% response rate following ablation in clinical trials.

   4. Patients with **IBS** benefit from antispasmodic therapies in addition to non-pharmacologic interventions. Patients may benefit from stress management and dietary modifications (avoidance of lactose, sorbitol, caffeine, fructose, tobacco, and chewing gum). Some studies support trials of peppermint oil and fiber supplementation.

   5. Interstitial cystitis has only one FDA-approved therapeutic medication, sodium pentosan polysulfate. However, an effect may become apparent in some cases only after 6 months of continued therapy. Other modalities with less evidence include hydrodistension of the bladder, and intravesicular administration of bacille Calmette-Guerin (BCG) to decrease pain.

   6. Adhesions may be a cause of CPP. Adhesiolysis for dense adhesions with bowel involvement may provide relief. The success rate for adhesiolysis ranges from 0% to 65%.

   7. Dyspareunia treatment is driven by the suspected etiology. Estrogen deficiency with inadequate lubrication, progressing to loss of elasticity and thinning of the epithelium from vaginal atrophy, is treated with local estrogen therapy. Other causes of dyspareunia are managed as indicated by the identified underlying medical or psychological condition. Studies of the role for hysterectomy have found significant decreases in self-report of dyspareunia at 12 and 24 months after surgery.

8. **Mittelschmerz** usually requires only patient education and reassurance. It is an uncommon cause of CPP. Oral NSAIDs can be prescribed for symptoms. OCs can also be helpful.

9. **Hysterectomy.** Hysterectomy is effective in some cases of CPP; however, 40% of women continue to experience CPP after hysterectomy. Comparative effectiveness studies highlight the lack of high-quality evidence supporting surgical interventions in the diagnosis and treatment of CPP.

10. **CPP with unknown etiology**
   a. Pharmacologic methods.
   (1) Oral NSAIDs (e.g., ibuprofen) act peripherally to create analgesia. Individuals vary widely in their response to different NSAIDs. Therefore, at least three unique medications should be tried.
   (2) Oral opioids that block pain perception centrally (e.g., hydrocodone with acetaminophen 5/500 mg, one to two tablets orally every 4–6 hours) have a well-recognized role in acute pain management. Their use in the treatment of chronic pain is controversial with limited evidence to support inclusion. Careful patient selection with standard discussion of risks and benefits, purpose of opioid therapy, functional activity goals, target levels of tolerable pain, and side effects, including addiction, are all components of effective opioid implementation.
   (3) Antidepressants such as SSRIs and TCAs have been used to treat a number of chronic pain syndromes. They are thought to improve pain tolerance, restore sleep patterns, and reduce depressive symptoms. However, there is limited evidence to support their use and efficacy for CPP.
   (4) Continuous oral progestin may lead to pain relief among women with endometriosis and pelvic congestion syndrome.
   (5) Combined OCs have multiple effects, including suppressed ovulation, decreased uterine activity/contractions, decreased menstrual pain, and suppressed prostaglandin release during menses. Combined OCs, especially extended-cycle products, will also decrease fluctuations in estrogen and progestin levels.
   (6) Scheduled dosing of GnRH agonists will suppress endogenous GnRH release (pulsatile). This response will decrease the release of LH and FSH, triggering a significant decline in estradiol levels.
   b. Nonpharmacologic approaches include counseling, acupuncture, behavioral and relaxation feedback therapies, and social interventions, as well as neuroablative treatments. Neuroablative therapies employed in consultation with a pain management specialist or surgeon include presacral neurectomy, uterosacral neurectomy, paracervical denervation, uterovaginal ganglion excision, injection of neurotoxic chemicals, laser treatment, cryotherapy, or thermocoagulation. However, evidence is of poor quality with limited uncontrolled studies supporting these modalities.

SELECTED REFERENCES

ACOG Committee on Practice Bulletins–Gynecology. ACOG Practice Bulletin No. 51. Chronic pelvic pain. *Obstet Gynecol.* 2004;103(3):589–605.

ACOG Committee on Practice Bulletins–Gynecology. ACOG Practice Bulletin No. 94: Medical management of ectopic pregnancy. *Obstet Gynecol.* 2008;111(6):1479–1485.

Bordman R, Jackson B. Below the belt—approach to chronic pelvic pain. *Can Fam Physician.* 2006; 52:1556–1562.

Holzer RA, Persons RK, Jamieson B. Clinical Inquiry: evaluation of ovarian cysts. *Am Fam Physician.* 2011;84(3):online.

Kruszka PS, Kruszka SJ. Evaluation of acute pelvic pain in women. *Am Fam Physician.* 2010;82(2): 141–147.

Ortiz DD. Chronic pelvic pain in women. *Am Fam Physician.* 2008;77(11):1535–1542.

Sheth S. Acute Pelvic Pain in Women: Ultrasonography Still Reigns. *Ultrasound Clinics.* 2011;6(2):163–176.

Soper DE. Pelvic inflammatory disease. *Obstet Gynecol.* 2010;116:419–428.

Stones W, Cheong YC, Howard FM, Singh S. Interventions for treating chronic pelvic pain in women. *Cochrane Database Sys Rev.* 2000;(4):CD000387.

Additional references are available online at http://langetextbooks.com/fm6e

51   Perianal Complaints

Kalyanakrishnan Ramakrishnan, MD, MS, FRCS

KEY POINTS

- In young individuals with bleeding-associated defecation and no family history, anoscopy and flexible sigmoidoscopy are sufficient testing. (SOR **C**)
- In people older than 50 years, especially in the presence of fatigue, weight loss, or anemia, colon pathology (e.g., cancer) should be ruled out by a double-contrast barium enema or colonoscopy. (SOR **C**)
- Most treatment measures for perianal pathology (e.g., banding of hemorrhoids, sphincter-otomy for fissures, and drainage of perianal and pilonidal infections) can be performed as office procedures under local or no anesthesia. (SOR **B**)

I. Definition (Figure 51–1). The **musculature of the anal canal** consists of the **internal sphincter**, the downward continuation of the involuntary circular smooth muscle of the rectum, and the **external sphincter**, an elliptical cylinder of the voluntary skeletal muscle that surrounds the anal canal and is continuous with the **levator ani**, which forms the greater part of the pelvic floor. Sympathetic and parasympathetic nerves, both of which are inhibitory, supply the internal sphincter.

The anal mucosa is lined by the columnar epithelium above the undulating **dentate line** and supplied by sympathetic nerves (L-1–L-3); the squamous epithelium below the dentate line is supplied by somatic nerves. Above the dentate line are longitudinal folds, 6 to 14 in number, the **columns of Morgagni**. The anal glands, 3 to 10 in number, open directly into an anal crypt at the dentate line.

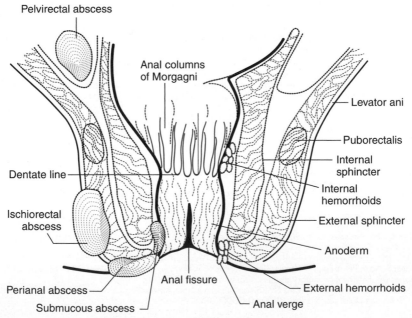

FIGURE 51-1. Anatomy and pathology of the anal canal.

Perianal complaints include irritation, soreness, and discomfort in the region surrounding the anal canal. Hemorrhoids, fissures, anorectal and pilonidal infections, and pruritus ani are all common causes.

A. Hemorrhoids are fibrovascular cushions with arteriovenous connections that bulge into the lumen of the anal canal. Their anchoring and supporting connective tissue system deteriorates with aging. Chronic straining from constipation leads to prolapse, thinning, and friability of the overlying mucosa, and results in bright-red rectal bleeding. **Perianal hematoma** is a painful swelling due to thrombosis within a saccule of the hemorrhoidal venous plexus.

B. Anal fissure is a laceration in the vertical axis of the anal canal caused by repeated trauma by hard stool. Relative ischemia at the posterior midline anoderm can also contribute. Internal sphincter spasm impairs healing.

C. Anorectal abscesses can arise from blockage of the anal glands by inspissated (thickened or dried) debris (e.g., fecal matter) followed by superimposed polymicrobial aerobic and anaerobic infections. It can also result from infection of an anal fissure or from sexually transmitted infections.

D. Fistula-in-ano is a tract lined with granulation tissue connecting a primary opening inside the anal canal to a secondary opening in the perianal skin. Fistula-in-ano is most often caused by rupture or drainage of an anorectal abscess.

E. Pilonidal cysts develop through ingrowth of hair in the natal cleft causing a foreign body reaction aggravated by repeated friction and superimposed bacterial infection.

F. The pain of **proctalgia fugax** results from puborectalis muscle spasm. Suggested causes include laxity of the anal sphincter, levator muscle tension resulting in spasm, and increased contractile activity of the sigmoid colon.

G. Proctitis arises from rectal inflammation (within 15 cm of the dentate line) and can be caused by inflammatory bowel disease (IBD), sexually transmitted infections (i.e., *Neisseria gonorrhoeae,* syphilis, *Chlamydia trachomatis, Herpes simplex* virus, or cytomegalovirus) or from bacterial infections. It can also develop as a result of prior antibiotic use (*Clostridium difficile* proctitis), radiotherapy, or diversion colostomy or ileostomy in patients with an intact rectum.

H. Pruritus ani can be caused by benign anorectal diseases producing a discharge, premalignant lesions (e.g., Paget and Bowen disease), and non-primary anal diseases (contact dermatitis, fungal infections, diabetes, pinworm infestations, psoriasis, and seborrhea).

II. Common Diagnoses

A. The incidence of hemorrhoids is high (approximately 5% of the general population), with equal prevalence for men and women, and peak incidence between 45 and 65 years of age. Symptomatic hemorrhoids are associated with aging (50% of patients over 50 years of age become symptomatic at some time), pregnancy, pelvic tumors, prolonged sitting and straining, and chronic diarrhea or constipation.

B. Anal fissures affect both genders equally; risk factors include the passage of hard stool, chronic diarrhea, habitual use of laxatives, and anal trauma during intercourse or examination.

C. Anorectal infections

  1. Anorectal abscess. The peak incidence is in the third to fourth decades. Male-to-female predominance is 2:1 to 3:1. One-third of patients report similar past episodes. Risk factors include immunosuppression, diabetes mellitus, IBD (predisposes to recurrent/multiple abscesses), and pregnancy.

  2. The incidence of **fistula-in-ano** is 8.6 cases per 100,000, and the mean age of occurrence is 38.3 years. Risk factors include trauma, Crohn disease (see Chapter 78), fissures, carcinoma, radiation, actinomycoses, tuberculosis, and chlamydial infections.

  3. Incidence of **pilonidal disease** is approximately 70,000 new cases every year and it is twice as common in men as in women. Precipitants include hyperhidrosis associated with sitting and buttock friction, poor personal hygiene, obesity, and local trauma, and buttock hair characteristics such as kinking, coarseness, and rapid growth rate.

D. Levator ani syndrome (spasm of the levator ani muscle) occurs in 6% to 7% of the general population, slightly more often in women than in men.

E. Proctalgia fugax (severe, brief, episodic rectal/sacrococcygeal pain possibly due to muscle spasm) occurs in approximately 13% of adults and is two to three times more common among women. Stress and anxiety are precipitants. Many patients have other functional bowel symptoms.

    F. Proctitis occurs predominantly in adults, more in men. Risk factors include high-risk sexual behavior (anal sex, homosexuality, multiple partners), autoimmune disorders, radiation therapy, immunocompromised state, and fecal diversion. Following radiation, 5% to 20% of patients develop proctitis within 3 to 24 months.

    G. Idiopathic **pruritus ani** (the second most common perianal complaint after hemorrhoids) is seen more often in men and is typically worse at night. Skin conditions, dietary or topical irritants, fecal incontinence, infections, and parasitic infestations (pinworms) are common causes. Less common causes include benign anorectal diseases, premalignant lesions, and non-primary anal diseases.

III. Symptoms. The common symptoms of perianal pathology include pain, bleeding, perianal mass, prolapse, pruritus, and discharge.

    A. The most common lesions causing **anorectal pain** are **fissure, abscess, and thrombosed external hemorrhoid**. Anal pain of any etiology may be aggravated by bowel movements.

        1. In **anal fissure,** pain occurs during and after defecation and feels like passing razor blades or cut glass. Pain is most acute over the first 2 to 3 days, resolving over a 7- to 10-day period.

        2. Anorectal abscess is suggested by a dull ache or throbbing pain in the perianal area worsened by coughing, sneezing, sitting, and relieved by defecation. Pain intensifies as the abscess increases in size and becomes more superficial.

        3. Perianal hematoma (external hemorrhoid) appears as a painful swelling soon after straining. **Strangulation** of internal hemorrhoids also causes severe pain, bleeding, and occasionally signs of systemic illness.

        4. Proctalgia fugax is characterized by the sudden onset of severe pain in the anus lasting several seconds or minutes which then disappears completely. Approximately one-third of patients suffer attacks following defecation and some following sexual activity.

        5. Tenesmus, an uncomfortable desire to defecate, is associated with inflammatory conditions. Tenesmus with urgency of evacuation suggests **proctitis**.

        6. The **levator ani syndrome** is associated with chronic or recurrent episodes of rectal pain or aching lasting 20 minutes or longer occurring for at least 3 months, precipitated by prolonged sitting or by defecation. Some patients have dyschezia or a sense of incomplete evacuation.

    B. Bleeding

        1. Hemorrhoids and **fissures** cause bright red blood on stool, toilet paper, or in the toilet bowl with, or following, bowel movements. Dark or clotted blood mixed with the stool suggests sources proximal to the anus. Hemorrhoids cause painless bleeding; bleeding with painful defecation suggests a fissure.

        2. Drainage of blood or pus with associated pruritus and pain suggests a **fistula**.

        3. Bleeding with a painful lump not exclusively related to defecation suggests a thrombosed external hemorrhoid; bleeding with tenesmus suggests **proctitis**.

    C. Prolapse occurs in second- and third-degree hemorrhoids, usually with a bowel movement, or during walking or heavy lifting, and is associated with an uncomfortable lower abdominal or perianal fullness, which resolves on spontaneous or manual reduction.

    D. Perianal mass. A painful perianal lump may be an abscess, a thrombosed external hemorrhoid, or a strangulated prolapsed internal hemorrhoid. **Pilonidal abscess** presents with a painful swelling overlying the coccyx, purulent drainage, fever, and constitutional symptoms.

    E. Discharge. Blood-stained discharge mixed with mucus, pus, or both is a feature of proctitis, thrombosed or prolapsed hemorrhoids, perianal or pilonidal abscess, fistula, or neoplasm.

    F. Miscellaneous. Fever and other constitutional symptoms (anorexia, nausea, vomiting, or diarrhea) can accompany strangulated hemorrhoids, perirectal and pilonidal abscesses, IBD, and proctitis.

IV. Signs

    A. Inspection. Skin changes suggestive of psoriasis, seborrhea, ulcerations, or lichenification can indicate the existence of **pruritus ani**. In **pilonidal infections,** a sinus, swelling, and redness overlying the coccyx or purulent drainage may be seen.

Perianal hematoma presents as a bluish mass at the anal verge and **anorectal abscess,** with localized erythema, purulent drainage, or perianal edema. In **anal fistulas,** external (secondary) openings are seen. Findings in **proctitis** can range from a mild mucoid exudate to marked infection with spontaneous bleeding, purulent discharge, and erosions (in patients with human immunodeficiency virus). Papules, vesicles, shallow ulcerations, and crusts around the anal and genital areas can be seen in **herpetic infections.**

B. **Palpation (including digital rectal examination)**

1. A tender fluctuant mass may be palpated at the anal verge (perianal abscess), sacrum (pilonidal abscess), or through the rectal wall (ischiorectal abscess) (Figure 51–1).

2. Most **fissures** (≥90%) are posterior (Figure 51–1) and can be observed with gentle lateral retraction around the anus or on anoscopy. Anterior fissures have an incidence of 1% in men and 10% in women. **Acute fissures** appear as a fresh laceration, whereas **chronic fissures** have raised edges, exposing the white horizontally oriented fibers of the internal sphincter. The sphincter tone is markedly increased and digital examination or anoscopy reproduces the extreme pain associated with defecation. When fissures are lateral, infections such as syphilis, tuberculosis, occult abscesses, herpes, acquired immunodeficiency syndrome, carcinoma, and IBD should be considered. Secondary changes such as a sentinel pile, induration of the fissure edge, and anal stenosis, because of spasm or a fibrotic internal sphincter, may be seen.

3. Palpable tenderness of overly contracted levator ani muscles may be noticed in the **levator ani syndrome,** as the examining finger moves from the coccyx posteriorly to the pubis anteriorly.

4. Uncomplicated internal hemorrhoids are not palpable. **Prolapsed internal hemorrhoids** may be differentiated from full-thickness rectal prolapse by the concentric mucosal folds and a sulcus between the anal canal and the proximal bowel (seen in rectal prolapse and absent in prolapsed hemorrhoids).

C. **Anoscopy.** This procedure is performed with the patient in the left lateral position. The instrument is well lubricated to ease insertion. A side-viewing anoscope is inserted with the open portion in the right anterior, then right posterior, and finally the left lateral position to look for hemorrhoidal masses, which will bulge into the anoscope.

1. **Hemorrhoids** are classified as internal, external, or combined intero-external. **External hemorrhoids** originate below the dentate line; **internal hemorrhoids** originate above it (Figure 51–1). Internal hemorrhoids are found in the right anterior, right posterior, and left lateral positions within the anal canal, and graded as first-degree (bleeding without prolapse), second-degree (prolapse on straining, reducing spontaneously), third-degree (prolapse requiring manual reduction), and fourth-degree (strangulated, irreducible, prolapsed hemorrhoid) hemorrhoids.

2. **Fissures** may also be seen, with the characteristics as stated above.

3. Internal openings may be identified in **fistulas.** The **Goodsall rule** states that fistulas with an external opening anterior to a plane passing transversely through the center of the anus will follow a straight radial course to the dentate line. Fistulas with their openings posterior to this line will follow a curved course to the posterior midline.

4. Proctitis following *Chlamydia trachomatis* and *N. gonorrhoeae* infection causes erythema, discharge, and swelling in the anal canal.

V. **Diagnostic Tests**

A. **Tests for pruritus ani and proctitis**

1. In **pruritus ani,** skin scrapings (potassium hydroxide preparation) are useful in detecting tinea cruris and yeast infections. Pinworms can be identified by microscopic examination of eggs or adult worms picked up by a transparent adhesive tape (scotch-tape test) applied to the perianal region in the morning or on scrapings under fingernails. The scotch-tape test has high sensitivity (90%) when performed on three consecutive days; negative examination on five consecutive days rules out pinworm infestation.

2. In **proctitis,** diagnosis is confirmed in most patients by anoscopic smears and culture for bacterial, fungal, and viral pathogens, Tzanck testing for multinucleate giant cells, and stool testing for *Clostridium difficile* toxin. Syphilis can be confirmed by finding spirochetes on dark-field examination of rectal discharge, and *N. gonorrhoeae* through appearance of gram-negative diplococci on Gram staining. If

warranted, cultures for *Clostridium difficile, N. gonorrhoeae, Chlamydia trachomatis,* and herpes simplex, and serologic testing for syphilis (rapid plasma regain test) should be obtained.

B. Skin biopsy. Visible abnormalities in the perianal skin may necessitate a skin biopsy (excision or punch biopsy) to rule out Paget or Bowen disease or cancer.

C. Endoscopy
   1. Rectal bleeding in people older than 50 years warrants a **colonoscopy** to rule out colorectal neoplasm. (SOR **B**)
   2. Younger individuals with bleeding-associated defecation, and no family history of colon cancer, should undergo a **flexible sigmoidoscopy**.
   3. **Flexible sigmoidoscopy or colonoscopy** is performed to exclude more proximally located inflammatory disorders with which **anal fistulas** or **perianal pruritus** may be associated. Endoscopy may show crypt abscesses or other features of IBD.

D. Miscellaneous
   1. **Endoanal ultrasound** or **magnetic resonance imaging** is useful before surgery to determine the existence, extent, and location of **anorectal abscesses**.
   2. **Ultrasound, fistulography, computerized tomography, and magnetic resonance imaging** can be helpful in identifying an occult cause of **recurrent fistula**.
   3. **Electromyography** studies can be used to differentiate the **levator ani syndrome** from pelvic floor dyssynergia, a relaxation abnormality associated with dyschezia and straining.

VI. Treatment
   A. Hemorrhoids causing minor bleeding can be managed with dietary and lifestyle modifications to minimize constipation and straining (see Chapter 12). (SOR **B**) Fiber supplementation (e.g., psyllium, unprocessed bran) can decrease bleeding, pain, prolapse, and itching. Although nonprescription topical preparations containing steroids, anesthetics, astringents, and/or antiseptics are often recommended, no clinical trials support their use. Sitz baths have not been found to be of benefit. More symptomatic hemorrhoids (e.g., third- or fourth-degree) are likely to require operative intervention. (SOR **B**)
   1. Office procedures
      a. Rubber band ligation is indicated in first-, second-, and third-degree hemorrhoids. (SOR **A**) After rectal examination, the anoscope is inserted and the hemorrhoid to be banded is identified (the largest hemorrhoid is banded first) and grasped with a modified Allis forceps placed through the ligator. In the absence of discomfort, the band is applied by depressing the trigger on the hemorrhoid ligator. Multiple hemorrhoids can be banded at one sitting, or sequentially. A dull persistent ache is common following banding. Significant anal pain owing to band placement below or close to the dentate line requires removal and reapplication. An **anoscope/ligator,** attached to wall suction, is an alternative to traditional banding methods. Complications with both methods are rare (<1%) and include urinary retention, bleeding, band slippage, pain, ulceration, thrombosis, and perineal sepsis. Bleeds are self-limited and occur immediately after banding, or 7 to 10 days later. Rubber band ligation is associated with a 65%–85% success rate. Up to 25% of patients require repeat banding over 5 years. Banding is contraindicated in patients on anticoagulants; patients on aspirin or other antiplatelet agents should stop these medications for 5 to 7 days before the procedure.
      b. Infrared coagulation is most beneficial in first- and second-degree hemorrhoids. (SOR **B**) The coagulator is applied through the anoscope for 1.5 seconds, thrice to the apex of each hemorrhoid. **Direct and bipolar cautery,** in which the current is applied in 1-second pulses of 20 watts at the base of the hemorrhoid until the underlying tissue coagulates, is useful in first-, second-, and third-degree hemorrhoids, with treatment being effective in nearly all patients. Both are associated with a minor complication rate under 10% and recurrence rates between 25% and 35%.
      c. Sclerotherapy involves the injection of a sclerosant (sodium morrhuate, 5% phenol, and hypertonic saline) through the anoscope into the submucosa at the apex of the hemorrhoid. This causes ischemia, induces fibrosis, and fixes the hemorrhoid to the rectal wall, decreasing bleeding and prolapse. It is performed

as an office procedure and requires no special training or equipment. Most patients experience a dull ache after the procedure. Complications are rare and include pain, urinary retention, and sepsis. The procedure is effective in the majority of patients (75%–89%) with first-, second-, and third-degree hemorrhoids, though recurrence is noticed in over one-fourth of patients over 4 years. (SOR **Ⓑ**) Misplacement of the sclerosant may result in perianal infection, anal ulceration, and fibrosis.

   d. Most patients with **perianal hematoma** respond to conservative measures (sitz baths twice a day, stool softeners, and analgesics). Surgical excision under local anesthesia is an office procedure that is considered for patients presenting during the first 2 to 3 days, if ulceration or rupture occurs, or if conservative treatment fails. (SOR **Ⓑ**) The anoderm overlying the swelling is infiltrated with plain lidocaine and incised with a no.15 blade, evacuating the clot. Bleeding is controlled with sutures or packing, and conservative measures are continued.

   e. Doppler-guided transanal hemorrhoidal ligation involves suture-ligation of the vessels supplying the hemorrhoids after localization with Doppler ultrasound. Post-procedure pain is less than that experienced with other procedures. It also has a high success (nearly 90%) and low complication rates (pain, bleeding, thrombosis, fissure 6%). (SOR **Ⓑ**)

2. Hemorrhoidectomy is required in 5% to 10% of patients and is reserved for large third- and fourth-degree hemorrhoids. (SOR **Ⓑ**) It has a success rate approaching 90%. This is usually performed by a surgeon as a day-case under local anesthesia; patients are generally able to return to work within 2 weeks. In **open hemorrhoidectomy,** the internal and external components of the hemorrhoid are excised after ligating the pedicle and the raw area is left to granulate. In **closed hemorrhoidectomy,** after suture ligation of the pedicle and excision of the hemorrhoid, the raw area in the anal verge is closed primarily. In **"stapled hemorrhoidectomy,"** the redundant anal mucosa with the fibrovascular cushions is removed using a modified, circular anastomotic stapler, disrupting the submucosal blood flow and effectively eliminating the hemorrhoids. Stapled hemorrhoidectomy results in less postoperative morbidity and earlier return to normal activity.

B. Anal fissures

   1. Acute (superficial) fissures can be managed with fiber supplementation, bulk laxatives, sitz baths, and topical corticosteroid or local anesthetic creams (e.g., Anusol H, Proctosedyl, or 5% lidocaine ointment applied twice daily). (SOR **Ⓑ**) Almost half of all patients with acute fissures respond to this approach, with resolution of pain and bleeding and virtually no side-effects.

   2. Other successful topical therapies are nifedipine 0.3% with lidocaine ointment 1.5%, every 12 hours for 6 weeks, topical nitroglycerin ointment 0.2% twice daily for 8 weeks, and diltiazem gel 2% three times a day for 8 weeks (over 50% healing with topical nitrates and 65%–95% with calcium channel blockers). Authors of a Cochrane review, however, concluded that these topical therapies are only marginally better than placebo and far less effective than surgery.

   3. Botulinum toxin A, a potent inhibitor of acetylcholine release from nerve endings, injected into the anal sphincter as an outpatient procedure, improves healing in 60%–80% of chronic fissures. (SOR **Ⓑ**) Temporary incontinence to flatus and less commonly to feces can occur; the fissure may recur in nearly half of patients, who generally respond to retreatment.

   4. If medical measures fail, a lateral sphincterotomy, performed as an office procedure by a surgeon or a family physician with requisite training, is usually successful. (SOR **Ⓐ**)

C. Anorectal abscess

   1. Outpatient incision and drainage under local anesthesia is reasonable in a healthy patient with a localized abscess. (SOR **Ⓑ**) The skin over the abscess is cleaned with Betadine and infiltrated with anesthetic, and a no.11 blade is used to enter the cavity. The skin edges are debrided and the cavity is syringed with saline or hydrogen peroxide and then packed with iodoform gauze. Conscious sedation is useful in the presence of excessive pain or anxiety. Analgesics, sitz baths, and stool softeners are continued. Frequent dressing changes may be necessary, until granulation is well advanced. Complications of drainage include perianal fistula (most common), sepsis, Fournier gangrene, and rarely death owing to sepsis.

2. Drainage in the operating room is advisable in poorly localized infection or for patients who are septic or immunocompromised (e.g., diabetes).

3. The need for routine use of antibiotics has not been established; routine antibiotic use does not improve healing times nor reduce recurrences. (SOR **Ⓐ**) Intravenous antibiotics may be needed in patients who are immunocompromised, septic, have heart valve abnormalities, or following valve replacements or prostheses.

D. Initial management of **perianal fistulas** should be directed at resolving acute infection (including proctitis in IBD). Surgical options include fistulotomy for simple fistulas, seton placement and staged fistulotomy, or endorectal advancement flap closure for more complex fistulas. (SOR **Ⓑ**) Asymptomatic fistulas associated with Crohn disease require no treatment. (SOR **Ⓑ**).

E. Pilonidal sinus disease

1. Conservative, nonexcisional therapy (shaving the gluteal cleft, improving perineal hygiene, incision, and drainage of localized abscesses) minimizes local infection and recurrence. This requires minimal equipment and leads to early recovery. Abscesses are drained under lidocaine infiltration anesthesia after skin preparation with Betadine, with a no.15 blade. The wound is then syringed and packed as described earlier.

2. Injecting 1 to 2 mL of **80% phenol or fibrin glue** into the sinus tract destroys the granulation tissue/epithelium lining the sinus and improves healing in chronic/recurrent sinuses (60%–95% for phenol and 90%–100% for fibrin glue). Phenol injection causes intense pain that needs to be managed.

3. Antibiotics have limited use for acute or chronic fistulas except in patients with cellulitis, underlying immunosuppression, or concurrent systemic illness.

4. Excisional therapy (simple excision, marsupialization, excision followed by flap closure) should be considered for more extensive or recurrent disease and requires a surgical referral.

F. Treatment options for the **levator ani syndrome** include digital massage of the levator ani muscles three to four times a week, sitz baths at 40°C, use of muscle relaxants (such as diazepam and methocarbamol), and biofeedback. Recalcitrant cases may benefit from a referral to a gastroenterologist for electrogalvanic stimulation through a rectal probe. (SOR **Ⓒ**) Surgical division of the puborectalis muscle is associated with a high rate of fecal incontinence and hence is not recommended.

G. Reassurance of the benign nature of **proctalgia fugax,** warm baths, and massage are often all that is necessary. In severe cases, inhaled albuterol, one or two puffs every 3 hours, or oral diltiazem, 2.5 to 5 mg every 6 hours as necessary, may help. (SOR **Ⓒ**) Coexistent behavioral and psychological issues are managed with counseling or pharmacotherapy.

H. Proctitis

1. In suspected sexually transmitted infection, oral doxycycline (100 mg twice daily for 7 days) *plus* ceftriaxone (250 mg IM once) covers chlamydia and gonococcal proctitis.

    a. Treatment options for **chancroid** include azithromycin (1 g orally once) *or* ceftriaxone (250 mg IM once) *or* ciprofloxacin (500 mg orally twice daily for 3 days) or erythromycin base (500 mg orally three times daily for 7 days).

    b. Lymphogranuloma venereum requires prolonged treatment with doxycycline (100 mg orally twice daily for 21 days) *or* erythromycin (500 mg four times daily in pregnant women or if sensitivity to tetracyclines for 21 days).

    c. Proctitis due to **herpes simplex** should be treated with acyclovir (400 mg orally three times daily for 7–10 days *or* 200 mg orally five times daily for 7–10 days) *or* famciclovir (250 mg three times daily for 7–10 days) *or* valacyclovir (1 g twice daily for 7–10 days); recurrent infections can be treated with shorter courses of acyclovir (400 mg orally three times daily or 800 mg twice daily for 5 days), famciclovir (125 mg twice daily for 5 days), or valacyclovir (1 g once daily for 5 days or 500 mg twice daily for 3 days).

2. *Clostridium difficile* **proctitis** is treated with oral metronidazole (500 mg orally three times a day) for 10 to 14 days for mild cases *or* vancomycin (125 mg four times a day) for 10 to 14 days for severe cases. The inciting antimicrobial should be stopped as soon as possible. For severe or complicated *Clostridium difficile* **diarrhea, vancomycin** 500 mg orally four times daily in combination with IV metronidazole 500 mg every 8 hours is recommended. For patients not responding to vancomycin, consider fidaxomicin (Dificid) 200 mg orally twice daily for 10 days.

3. In **radiation proctitis,** rectal corticosteroids as foam (hydrocortisone 90 mg) or enema (hydrocortisone 100 mg or methylprednisolone 20 mg) twice daily for 3 weeks, *or* mesalamine 4 g enema at bedtime or as suppositories 500 mg once or twice a day for 3 to 6 weeks, *or* sucralfate 2 g twice daily for 4 weeks are useful. Oral mesalamine (800 mg three times a day) *or* sulfasalazine (500–1000 mg four times a day) for ~3 weeks alone or in combination with topical therapy can also be effective. Systemic steroids are reserved for patients unresponsive to these forms of therapy. Bleeding caused by radiation proctitis responds well to local instillation of 10% formalin to the anorectal mucosa through an anoscope or a proctoscope or endoscopic laser photocoagulation. Surgical options include diverting loop colostomy and resection of the diseased segment of bowel.

I. Treatment of pruritus ani depends on recognizing the cause, ruling out other potential diagnoses, addressing precipitating or exacerbating conditions, and relieving the itch/scratch cycle. (SOR **C**)

1. Excessive cleaning, and particularly the use of brushes and caustic soaps, should be avoided.

2. The perianal region should be washed liberally with water to remove any soap after bathing. Following defecation, water-moistened cloths or toilet paper should be used. In between defecation, cotton balls placed next to the anal orifice may help to absorb sweat. Moisture barriers, such as zinc oxide, may ameliorate symptoms.

3. Dietary modifications (restriction of caffeinated or carbonated beverages, dairy products, alcohol, tomato-based food products, cheese, and chocolate) may be useful.

4. A short course of topical steroids (hydrocortisone 1%) can also provide symptom relief, though long-term use should be avoided because of skin atrophy. Anesthetic ointments should be avoided. A sedating antihistamine (hydroxyzine 25 mg orally) helps reduce scratching while asleep. Dilute capsaicin cream (0.006%) can relieve chronic anal pruritus.

5. ***Tinea*** and ***Candida*** respond well to 1% clotrimazole cream applied twice daily for up to 4 weeks.

6. **Pinworm infection** (enterobiasis) is treated with a single 100 mg dose of mebendazole or one 11 mg/kg dose (to a maximum of 1 g) of pyrantel pamoate for adults and children. Another single dose can be given 2 weeks later to prevent recurrences from reinfection.

7. **Condyloma acuminata** can be treated effectively with liquid nitrogen or 10% podophyllin. Podofilox applied by the patient every 12 hours for three consecutive days is an alternative. Application can be repeated after 4 days.

8. Improvement in symptoms in refractory pruritus ani has been noted with the subcutaneous injection of 30 cc of 0.5% methylene blue. Methylene blue is toxic to the nerves causing pruritus. Intradermal injection of 10 mL of 1% methylene blue appears to be extremely effective with most (96%) patients experiencing improvement and resolution in over half (57%) of patients.

SELECTED REFERENCES

Barleben A, Mills S. Anorectal anatomy and physiology. *Surg Clin N Am.* 2010;90:1–15.

Bharucha AE, Trabuco E. Functional and chronic anorectal and pelvic pain disorders. *Gastroenterol Clin N Am.* 2008;37:685–696.

Coates WC. Disorders of the anorectum. In Marx: *Rosen's Emergency Medicine.* 7th ed. 2009; Ch 94, P1243–P1256.

Perry WB, Dykes SL, Buie WD, Rafferty JF. Standards Practice Task Force of the American Society of Colon and Rectal Surgeons. Practice parameters for the management of anal fissures (3rd revision). *Dis Colon Rectum.* 2010;53:1110–1115.

Rivadeneira DE, Steele SR, Ternent C, Chalasani S, Buie WD, Rafferty JL. Standards Practice Task Force of the American Society of Colon and Rectal Surgeons. Practice parameters for the management of hemorrhoids (revised 2010). *Dis Colon Rectum.* 2011;54:1059–1064.

Steele SR, Kumar R, Feingold DL, Rafferty JL, Buie WD. Standards Practice Task Force of the American Society of Colon and Rectal Surgeons. Practice parameters for the management of perianal abscess and fistula-in-ano. *Dis Colon Rectum.* 2011;54:1465–1474.

Additional references are available online at http://langetextbooks.com/fm6e

52   Proteinuria

Aamir Siddiqi, MD

KEY POINTS

- Asymptomatic persistent proteinuria on dipstick test needs further evaluation and possible referral to nephrology. (SOR ⊙)
- Urine dipsticks are usually sensitive only to albuminuria and give false-negative results with other urinary proteins. (SOR ⊙)
- Transient proteinuria is a nonpathologic condition. (SOR ⊙)
- Routine screening for proteinuria in children and adults is not recommended. Prenatal care usually includes a urine dipstick examination on a random urine sample for proteinuria; this practice is controversial. (SOR ⊙)

I. **Definition.** Proteinuria is the presence of urinary protein in concentrations ≥150 mg per day in adults and ≥0.1 mg/m^2/day in children. Since pregnancy results in a combination of increased glomerular filtration rate and increased permeability of the glomerular basement membrane, total protein excretion is considered abnormal in pregnant women when it exceeds 300 mg/day.

Nephrotic syndrome is defined as protein excretion of 3.5 g per day or more in adults and 1 g/m^2/d or more in children along with hypoalbuminemia, edema, and hypercholesterolemia. **Microalbuminuria** is defined as excretion of 30 to 150 mg of protein per day.

II. **Screening**

   A. **Annual Screening** for proteinuria in asymptomatic adults is **not** cost effective. Although suggested by some recent studies, routine screening in children is also not recommended. The **U.S. Preventive Services Task Force has no recommendations for or against routine testing for chronic kidney disease.**

   B. **Pregnancy.** Traditionally, prenatal care included dipstick protein testing of a random voided urine sample at each prenatal visit to detect preeclampsia. However, routine dipstick testing is unreliable in detecting the moderate or variable albumin elevations that occur with preeclampsia; this test is still recommended by some guidelines but discouraged by others.

III. **Common Diagnoses**

   A. **Transient proteinuria,** defined as isolated, self-limited proteinuria, is by far the most common, occurring in 4% of males and 7% of females on a single examination. Stressors such as fever and exercise have been considered potential causes.

   B. **Orthostatic proteinuria** appears when a person is upright and accounts for up to 60% of all proteinuria seen in children and adolescents.

   C. **Persistent proteinuria** occurs in 5% to 10% of patients with isolated proteinuria. This is commonly associated with underlying extrarenal causes, such as diabetes and hypertension. After the development of proteinuria, as many as 50% of these patients develop hypertension during the next 5 years, and as many as 20% develop renal insufficiency during the next 10 years.

   D. **Primary renal diseases** including acute glomerulonephritis, acute renal failure, acute tubular necrosis, and anomalies, such as polycystic kidneys, can cause proteinuria.

   E. **Drugs** and **toxins** including antibiotics, analgesics, anticonvulsants, antihypertensives, and heavy metals can lead to proteinuria (Table 52–1).

   F. **Systemic illnesses** (Table 52–2). Approximately 33% of patients with type 1 and 25% of patients with type 2 diabetes develop persistent proteinuria. **Overload proteinuria** occurs in systemic diseases, which cause production of abnormal and excessive low-molecular-weight proteins, as in multiple myeloma.

   G. **Nephrotic syndrome** is primarily caused by minimal change disease, focal segmental glomerulosclerosis, membranous glomerulonephritis, membranoproliferative glomerulonephritis, and mesangial proliferative glomerulonephritis. The most common cause in children is minimal change disease, accounting for approximately 75% of cases; membranous glomerulonephritis is the most common cause in adults. In children, it is most

TABLE 52-1. DRUGS AND TOXINS CAUSING PROTEINURIA

Acute Interstitial Nephritis	Cyclosporine Toxicity
Cephalosporins	**Heavy metals**
Penicillins	Gold
Sulfonamides	Lead
Aminoglycoside toxicity	Mercury
Analgesic nephropathy	Heroin
Nonsteroidal anti-inflammatory drugs	Lithium
Anticonvulsants	Penicillamine
Phenytoin	Probenecid
Trimethadione	**Sulfonylureas**
Antihypertensive agents	Tolbutamide
Angiotensin-converting enzyme inhibitors	

common from age 2 to 6 years. The ratio of males to females is 2:1 in childhood and becomes 1:1 in adolescents and adults.

IV. Symptoms. It is rare to find any symptoms of proteinuria except in patients with the nephrotic syndrome, in whom swelling may be prominent. Characteristic symptoms of primary renal disease or systemic illness may appear in a patient with proteinuria caused by the pathologic process of an underlying disease.

   A. Red- or cola-colored urine can be a presenting symptom of acute glomerulonephritis.

   B. Polydipsia or polyuria can indicate uncontrolled diabetes.

   C. Joint stiffness or pain may be the presenting complaint of lupus erythematosus.

   D. Fatigue, weakness, anorexia, and malaise may be associated with chronic renal insufficiency.

   E. Bone pain, especially in the back or chest, may be associated with multiple myeloma.

V. Signs. If the patient excretes ≤2 g of protein daily, signs will usually be absent.

   A. Periorbital edema, peripheral edema, ascites, or **pleural effusions** can result from a decrease in serum albumin because of decreased plasma oncotic pressure.

   B. Elevated blood pressure can occur in patients with primary renal disease.

   C. A **toxic neuropathy** may indicate heavy metal poisoning.

   D. Fever may be present with infection.

   E. A **heart murmur** may accompany bacterial endocarditis.

   F. Characteristic signs of systemic illness may appear in patients whose proteinuria is caused by such illness.

      1. Adenopathy, organomegaly, and **masses** can occur with cancer.

      2. Malar rash and **joint inflammation** are usually present with lupus erythematosus.

      3. Diabetic retinopathy is strongly associated with proteinuria in patients with diabetes.

VI. Laboratory tests (Figure 52-1).

   A. The **initial screen** for proteinuria is a **dipstick** performed on a random clean-catch urine sample. This is a colorimetric test (quantitative chemical analysis using color)

TABLE 52-2. SYSTEMIC ILLNESSES CAUSING PROTEINURIA

Infections	Cancers	Multisystem Diseases
Acute poststreptococcal glomerulonephritis	Carcinoma	Amyloidosis
Bacterial	Leukemia	Cryoglobulinemia
Endocarditis	Lymphoma—Hodgkin disease	Diabetes mellitus
Syphilis	Multiple myeloma	Goodpasture syndrome
Tuberculosis		Henoch–Schönlein syndrome
Parasitic		Polyarteritis
Malaria		Preeclampsia
Toxoplasmosis		Sarcoidosis
Viral		Systemic lupus erythematosus
Cytomegalovirus		Transplant rejection
Epstein–Barr virus		
Hepatitis B		
Human immunodeficiency virus		

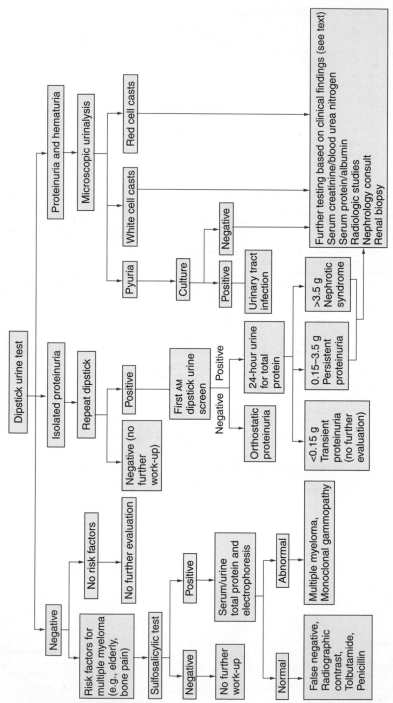

FIGURE 52-1. Algorithm for evaluation of proteinuria.

detecting urine protein concentration of ≥10 to 30 mg/dL, giving positive results if used in relatively concentrated samples.

1. False-positive dipstick test results can occur with highly concentrated urine, gross hematuria, contamination with antiseptics, or highly alkaline urine (pH ≥8.0). Radiographic contrast media, analogs of cephalosporin or penicillin, or metabolites of tolbutamide or sulfonamide can also result in false-positive tests.

2. False-negative qualitative test results may occur with dilute urine. Dipstick qualitative urine tests are relatively insensitive to proteins other than albumin and may give a false-negative result for non-albumin proteins such as Bence Jones proteins.

3. Sulfosalicylic acid test is a turbidimetric test in which one part of supernatant urine is mixed with sulfosalicylic acid. The turbidity is then graded according to a scale. The advantage of this test is detection of proteins besides albumin. This is especially helpful if multiple myeloma is suspected.

4. A negative qualitative test result on a first morning specimen (recumbent) followed 2 hours later by a positive test on second sample (upright) indicates **orthostatic proteinuria**. This can be confirmed by a split urine test in which a 16-hour upright collection is obtained between 7 AM and 11 PM, with the patient performing normal activities and finishing the collection by voiding just before 11 PM. A separate overnight 8-hour collection is obtained between 11 PM and 7 AM. The diagnosis of orthostatic proteinuria is made if urinary protein excretion is normal in the supine collection (≤50 mg/8 h).

B. A **24-hour urine test** for protein and creatinine levels will verify a repeated positive qualitative test result.

1. Urinary creatinine validates an adequate urinary collection; normal creatinine range is 16 to 26 mg/kg per day for males and 12 to 24 mg/kg per day for females. A 24-hour urine creatinine allows calculation of creatinine clearance, which is a good measure of renal function. An alternative to measuring 24-hour urine protein is to measure spot urinary protein-to-creatinine ratio. In a healthy person, the ratio seldom exceeds 0.1 (100 mg protein per 1 g creatinine).

2. A normal 24-hour **urinary protein** level indicates a false-positive qualitative test result or transient proteinuria.

C. Urinalysis of a clean-catch midstream specimen is needed to diagnose primary renal disease.

1. Positive urine culture indicates infection.

2. Red blood cell casts indicate glomerulonephritis.

3. White blood cell casts indicate an inflammatory process such as pyelonephritis and interstitial nephritis.

4. Epithelial cell casts may be seen due to acute tubular necrosis or toxin ingestion.

D. Blood tests should be performed when systemic disease is suspected.

1. Serum creatinine and **blood urea nitrogen** levels should be determined in order to evaluate renal function. Creatinine clearance is more accurate, especially in elderly patients with decreased muscle mass.

2. Blood glucose or a **glycosylated hemoglobin test** (hemoglobin A1c) is helpful in the detection of diabetes mellitus. Risk factors for these patients include symptoms of polydipsia, polyuria, and a strong family history of diabetes (see Chapter 75).

3. Protein electrophoresis or **immunoelectrophoresis** of urine and serum may assist in the diagnosis of multiple myeloma or other monoclonal gammopathies. These patients are usually elderly and may complain of bone pain and fatigue.

4. Complement studies may be helpful in the diagnosis of immune complex diseases. These include autoimmune diseases such as rheumatoid arthritis, systemic lupus erythematosus, and dermatomyositis.

5. Antistreptococcal enzyme titers can help the physician diagnose poststreptococcal glomerulonephritis. This is most common in children younger than 7 years and may be preceded by a skin infection or pharyngitis.

6. Fluorescent antinuclear antibody tests may indicate the presence of systemic lupus erythematosus. Patients usually have arthritis and fatigue and may present with the classic malar rash.

7. Serum albumin levels will be decreased in patients with nephrotic syndrome. These patients usually have significant facial and pedal edema and may have hypertension.

    8. Complete blood cell count will help in determining infection or the anemia of renal insufficiency. Systemic infections will cause an elevation of the white cell count. Anemia, if present, is usually characterized by normocytic and normochromic red blood cells.

  E. Radiographic evaluation can be used to detect congenital, obstructive, or malignant disease. This should be considered in patients complaining of abdominal pain and hematuria.

    1. Intravenous pyelography or **computerized tomographic scans** of the kidney can show structural or obstructive pathology. Caution should be observed when using contrast media in patients with diabetes, renal insufficiency, or multiple myeloma because of the risk of renal failure.

    2. Renal ultrasonography can be of value in determining renal size, obstruction, and congenital cysts. This should be considered if abdominal examination reveals a mass.

    3. Voiding cystourethrogram is useful in documenting reflux. This is usually performed in children who present with recurrent urinary tract infections.

  F. Renal biopsy is reserved for diagnosing and differentiating the glomerulonephropathies and is also performed on most patients with nephrotic-range proteinuria.

VII. Treatment of proteinuria is directed at the underlying cause.

  A. Transient proteinuria requires no further evaluation or follow-up, as no harmful sequelae have been documented.

  B. Orthostatic proteinuria is mostly a benign condition. Patients with this problem have a 50% chance of remission over 10 years. Follow-up of this problem should occur every 1 to 2 years if proteinuria persists, and should involve a blood pressure check as well as urinalysis.

  C. Removal of toxins or medications (Table 52–1) can reverse or at least prevent progression of proteinuria.

  D. Appropriate antibiotics can resolve proteinuria associated with urinary tract infections (see Chapter 21).

  E. Primary renal disease

    1. Supportive therapy, including **sodium** and **fluid restriction** (2 g per day and 1 L per day, respectively) may help relieve fluid retention.

    2. Loop diuretics such as **furosemide,** 20 to 400 mg per day, can be used to treat circulatory congestion, edema, and hypertension. These agents have not been shown to alter the course of acute renal failure or to improve the patient's chance of survival.

    3. Dietary protein restriction may prevent progression of renal disease and usually comprises 20 to 40 g (0.6–0.8 g/kg) of protein per day if chronic kidney disease is present. (SOR **A**)

    4. Corticosteroids such as **prednisone,** 1 to 1.5 mg/kg/d, and cytotoxic drugs such as **cyclophosphamide,** 1 to 2 mg/kg/d, may be of benefit to adult patients with certain types of nephrotic syndrome and primary glomerulonephritis. These should be prescribed in consultation with a nephrologist. (SOR **C**)

    5. Renal dialysis is indicated for patients with progressive renal failure and should be initiated when any of the following conditions exist: volume overload refractory to diuretics, pericarditis, or uremia (blood urea nitrogen ≥80–100 mg/dL or creatinine ≥8–10 mg/dL).

    6. Renal transplantation should be considered when a poor quality of life or health exists despite dialysis with end-stage renal disease.

  F. Specific treatment of underlying systemic illness (see Table 52–2 and Chapters 75, 77, and 86) may resolve or improve proteinuria.

    1. Persistent proteinuria is associated with a high mortality and risk of death from renal disease. Patients with persistent proteinuria from any cause should be referred to a nephrologist. Persistent proteinuria should be followed-up every 6 months to 1 year with urinalysis, blood pressure, and renal function studies.

    2. Antihypertensive therapy in a patient with nephropathy characterized by proteinuria can delay progression of renal failure. Drugs that most consistently reduce proteinuria in patients with diabetes and nondiabetic kidney disease are angiotensin-converting enzyme (ACE) inhibitors and angiotensin receptor blockers (ARBs). These drugs, in combination with dietary salt restriction, can reduce urinary protein by an average of 40% to 50%. Data support use of these agents to prevent kidney disease in patients with diabetes although data are conflicting about a reduction in all-cause mortality in patients with diabetes and kidney disease. Evidence to date does not demonstrate improvement in all-cause mortality or cardiovascular outcomes in patients with early kidney disease without diabetes.

3. **Corticosteroids** and cytotoxic drugs may improve proteinuria from lupus nephritis.
4. **Patients with diabetes and proteinuria** should be started on an ACE inhibitor or ARB to prevent progressive decline in renal function. (SOR **Ⓐ**)

SELECTED REFERENCES

ACOG Committee on Practice Bulletins–Obstetrics. ACOG practice bulletin. Diagnosis and management of preeclampsia and eclampsia. Number 33, January 2002. *Obstet Gynecol.* 2002;99(1): 159–167.

American Dietetic Association. *Chronic kidney disease evidence-based nutrition practice guideline.* Chicago, IL: American Dietetic Association http://www.guideline.gov/content.aspx?id=23924&search=renal+diet. Published 2010. Accessed June 2013.

Hajar F, Taleb M, Aoun B, Shatila A. Dipstick urine analysis screening among asymptomatic school children. *N Am J Med Sci.* 2011;3(4):179–184.

Hogg RJ, Furth S, Lemley KV, et al. National kidney foundation's kidney disease outcomes quality initiative clinical practice guidelines for chronic kidney disease in children and adolescents: evaluation, classification, and stratification. *Pediatrics.* 2003;111:1416–1421.

House AA, Cattran DC. Nephrology: 2. Evaluation of asymptomatic hematuria and proteinuria in adult primary care. *CMAJ Can Med Ass J.* 2002;166:348–353.

Johnson DW, Jones GR, Mathew TH, et al. Australasian Proteinuria Consensus Working Group. Chronic kidney disease and measurement of albuminuria or proteinuria: a position statement. *Med J Aust.* 2012;197(4):224–225.

Kim SM, Lee CH, Lee JP, et al. The association between albumin to creatinine ratio and total protein to creatinine ratio in patients with chronic kidney disease. *Clin Nephrol.* 2012;78(5):346–352.

Kirkham C, Harris S, Grzybowski S. Evidence-based prenatal care: Part I. General prenatal care and counseling issues. *Am Fam Physician.* 2005;71(7):1307–1316.

Kuritzky L, Toto R, Van Buren P. Identification and management of albuminuria in the primary care setting. *J Clin Hypertens (Greenwich).* 2011;13(6):438–449.

Roth KS, Amaker BH, Chan JC. Nephrotic syndrome: pathogenesis and management. *Pediatr Rev.* 2002;23:237–248.

Schieppati A, Perna A, Zamora J, et al. Immunosuppressive treatment for idiopathic membranous nephropathy in adults with nephrotic syndrome. *Cochrane Database Syst Rev.* 2004;(4):CD004293.

Sharma P, Blackburn RC, Parke CL, McCullough K, Marks A, Black C. Angiotensin-converting enzyme inhibitors and angiotensin receptor blockers for adults with early (stage 1 to 3) non-diabetic chronic kidney disease. *Cochrane Database Syst Rev.* 2011;(10):CD007751.

Strippoli GF, Craig M, Deeks JJ, et al. Effects of angiotensin converting enzyme inhibitors and angiotensin receptor antagonists on mortality and renal outcomes in diabetic nephropathy: systematic review. *BMJ.* 2004;329:828–839.

53 The Red Eye

Heidi S. Chumley, MD, Victor A. Diaz, Jr., MD, & Deborah K. Witt, MD

KEY POINTS

- Conjunctivitis is the most common cause of red eyes seen in the ambulatory primary care setting. (SOR **Ⓒ**)
- Bacterial conjunctivitis is more common in children aged 6 years and younger and should also be considered in patients over the age of 6 years when discharge is purulent, or when both eyes are matted shut in the morning. (SOR **Ⓒ**)
- Eye pain, vision loss, pupillary changes, and clouding of the cornea indicate more serious causes of red eye and require expedient evaluation. (SOR **Ⓑ**)
- Acute angle closure glaucoma, iritis (anterior uveitis), scleritis, and keratitis require urgent ophthalmologic referral. (SOR **Ⓑ**)

I. Definition. *Red eye* describes a group of distinct inflammatory or infectious diseases involving one or more ocular structures, that is, conjunctivae (viral/bacterial/chlamydial/allergic conjunctivitis, pterygium, pingueculum), cornea (abrasion, keratitis), sclera/episclera (scleritis, episcleritis), lids (blepharitis), uveal tract (iritis, uveitis), and anterior chamber (acute angle-closure glaucoma).

II. Common Diagnoses. The most likely source of red eye is the anterior segment, which consists of conjunctiva, cornea, anterior chamber, and iris. Conjunctivitis is the most common eye disease worldwide.

    A. Conjunctivitis, inflammation of the mucous membranes lining the eyelid or eyeball, can occur because of the following causes: .

        1. Infectious (common etiologies vary by age).

            a. Neonates with conjunctivitis most commonly have *Chlamydia trachomatis* and *Neisseria gonorrhoeae* pathogens contracted through exposure in the birth canal.

            b. Children aged 6 years and younger more commonly have bacterial than viral causes of infectious conjunctivitis. *Haemophilus* species or *Streptococcus pneumonia* account for nearly 90% of bacterial conjunctivitis cases in young children in the United States.

            c. Adults and children over the age of 6 years more commonly have viral than bacterial causes of infectious conjunctivitis. Adenovirus accounts for 85% of viral conjunctivitis infections and spreads quickly via respiratory secretions and ocular discharge. The most common bacterial cause is *Staphylococcal aureus*.

            d. Worldwide, *Chlamydia trachomatis* is the leading cause of preventable blindness and is a major public health concern in developing countries. Inclusion conjunctivitis is usually bilateral and spreads by direct contact with other family members. Spread is often associated with epidemics of bacterial conjunctivitis. Chronic conjunctivitis that resists multiple eye-drop regimens and/or the presence of associated urethritis or salpingitis should raise suspicion for chlamydial infection in sexually active teens and adults.

        2. Noninfectious or allergic conjunctivitis occurs in individuals with seasonal, environmental, (e.g., dust pollen, animal dander), or chemical (e.g., drugs, chemicals, and/or cosmetics) sensitivities.

    B. Corneal abrasion, loss of a portion of the superficial epithelium, likely the most common corneal cause of red eye, typically occurs in individuals who frequently participate in outdoor activities or certain occupations (e.g., tree trimmers, metal shop workers).

    C. Blepharitis is a common inflammatory lesion that affects the eyelid margins.

    D. Subconjunctival hemorrhage, spontaneous rupture of small conjunctival vessels, usually results from a sudden increase in intrathoracic pressure (e.g., sneezing, coughing, defecating), especially in the elderly. It also occurs with minor trauma, hypertension, and blood dyscrasias and is common in neonates following vaginal delivery.

    E. Inflamed pingueculum. Extremely common in adults, pingueculae are conjunctival areas of epithelial hyperplasia that become irritated by excessive sun and wind exposure and occasionally become inflamed for periods of weeks. At-risk individuals include farmers, lifeguards, fishermen, and welders.

    F. Pterygium, a fibrovascular proliferation of the conjunctiva, typically affects individuals in hot, dusty, or windy environments who are exposed to prolonged periods of outdoor ultraviolet light such as farmers, fishermen, and people living near the equator (Figure 53–1). Rarely seen in children.

    G. Acute angle-closure glaucoma, a rare ophthalmic emergency associated with suddenly elevated intraocular pressure (IOP), is most common in middle-aged or older patients with anatomically small anterior chambers or altered iris structure, especially in Asians, Eskimos, and hyperopic (farsighted) persons. Comprises 10% to 15% of glaucoma cases in Caucasians and approximately 5% to 10% of all glaucoma cases. Patients may reveal a recent history of topical or oral mydriatic use or eye surgery and may have a positive family history for glaucoma.

    H. Episcleritis, segmental or diffuse inflammation of the episclera, is thought to be more common in women and typically presents between the ages of 20 and 50 years (Figure 53–2). If nodular or recurrent, episcleritis may be associated with an underlying systemic condition, most commonly rheumatologic or infectious.

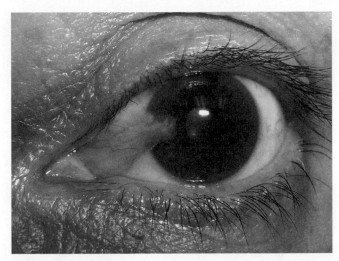

FIGURE 53–1. Pterygium that has grown into the cornea but not covering the visual axis. This fibrovascular tissue has the shape of a bird's wing (literal definition of pterygium). The small vessels are prominent in this view (see color insert) (see color insert). (Used with permission from Richard P. Usatine, MD.)

    I. **Scleritis,** inflammation of the deeper eye layers that gives a blue hue often accompanied by overlying episcleritis (which makes the eye red), is more common in women and often associated with an underlying systemic condition, most commonly rheumatologic or infectious (Figure 53–3).

    J. **Uveitis,** inflammation of any part of the uveal tract, includes anterior (iritis) (Figure 53–4), which accounts for 90% of uveitis seen in primary care, intermediate (ciliary body), and posterior (choroid) uveitis. Trauma, inflammation, infection, and idiopathic

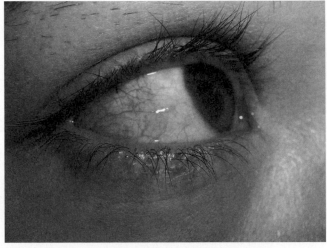

FIGURE 53–2. Episcleritis showing inflammation of only the conjunctival and episcleral tissues. Note the absence of violaceous color that is seen in scleritis (see color insert). (Used with permission from Richard P. Usatine, MD.)

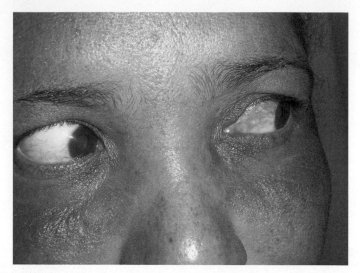

FIGURE 53–3. Scleritis in a young woman with systematic lupus erythematosus. Note the malar rash that is also present (see color insert). (Used with permission from Richard P. Usatine, MD.)

are the most common causes. Eighty percent of uveitis seen in children is due to juvenile rheumatoid arthritis. Panuveitis affects all layers and is often idiopathic, but can be due to sarcoidosis or syphilis.

K. Keratitis is an uncommon but important cause of red eye (Figure 53–5). Herpes simplex virus ocular disease presents most commonly as dendritic epithelial keratitis, but can present as another type of keratitis or in a milder form, causing blepharitis or conjunctivitis. Contact lens wearers are at risk for microbial keratitis, most commonly due to *Pseudomonas aeruginosa*.

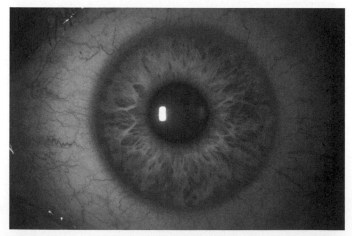

FIGURE 53–4. Iritis (anterior uveitis) with a limbal flush, red to purple perilimbal ring. This patient has eye pain and vision loss, which are absent in conjunctivitis (see color insert). (Used with permission from Paul D. Comeau.)

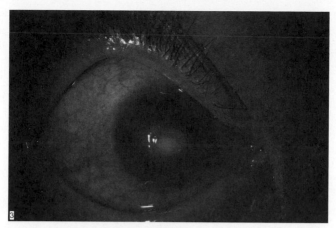

FIGURE 53–5. Diffuse ciliary injection and cloudy cornea demonstrating keratitis with corneal ulcer formation and a leukocyte infiltration (see color insert). (Used with permission from Paul D. Comeau.)

III. Symptoms/Signs (Table 53–1).

A. Conjunctivitis can be distinguished from more serious causes of red eye by the absence of both severe pain and vision loss. Patients who have severe pain and/or vision loss need further evaluation.

    a. Viral conjunctivitis presents with injected sclera, watery discharge, and burning/itching or foreign body sensation, has an incubation period of 7 to 10 days, and resolves within 10 to 14 days. Upper respiratory tract symptoms, sore throat, preauricular lymphadenopathy, and fever may also be present.

    b. Bacterial conjunctivitis presents with a beefy red appearance and matted eyelids. Copious and continuous purulent discharge is its distinguishing feature. Patients complain of a gritty sensation.

    c. Chlamydial conjunctivitis.

1. Trachoma. Symptoms are similar to bacterial conjunctivitis (e.g., tearing, photophobia, pain, and exudates). *Herbert pits*, small pathognomonic depressions in the connective tissue covered by the epithelium, develop over time. Infant/child infection is insidious and may resolve without complications. Adult infection may be clinically subacute or acute. Complications develop early in the disease course.

2. Inclusion conjunctivitis. Adults present with burning, general irritation, redness, and mucopurulent discharge primarily. Neonates develop tearing, discharge, and swollen eyelids during the first 10 days of life.

B. Allergic conjunctivitis. Symptoms include itching, burning, and watery discharge with some conjunctival swelling. Typically bilateral.

C. Corneal abrasion is associated with immediate discomfort, photophobia, blurred vision, tearing, and foreign body sensation as a result of exposed nerve endings. Fluorescein dye, which accumulates in areas where the corneal epithelium has been abraded and fluoresces bright green under magnified blue light (Wood lamp), is the diagnostic tool of choice in the office setting.

D. Blepharitis. Chronic, bilateral itching and burning with foreign body sensation. There is inflammation and crusting of lid margins, usually without discharge.

E. Subconjunctival hemorrhage is usually unilateral, painless, localized, bright red, and sharply circumscribed. Extravascular blood is seen underneath the conjunctiva obstructing the view of the sclera; the adjacent sclera is unaffected. Blood pressure should be measured for possible elevation.

F. Inflamed pingueculum. Lesions present as raised, hyperemic, yellowish nodules on the bulbar conjunctiva at the 3- and/or 9-o'clock position. Nasal lesions are more common than temporal ones. Patients report mild ocular discomfort.

TABLE 53-1. CLINICAL FEATURES IN THE DIAGNOSIS OF RED EYE

	Conjunctivitis	Episcleritis	Scleritis	Uveitis	Keratitis	Closed-Angle Glaucoma	Subconjunctival Hemorrhage	Ocular Rosacea
Redness	Diffuse	Segmental; pink	Segmental or diffuse; dark red, purple, or blue	360-degree perilimbal (worse at limbus)	Diffuse, ciliary injection	Diffuse, scleral	Blotchy, outside vessels	Diffuse
Eye pain	No	Mild, may be tender to touch	Severe, boring	Sometimes	Usually	Yes	No, unless caused by trauma	No
Vision loss	No	No	Sometimes	Sometimes	Maybe, depending on location	Yes	No	In severe cases
Discharge	Usually	No	No	No	Maybe	No	No	No
Photophobia[a]	No	No	Yes	Yes, if anterior	Yes	Yes	No	Sometimes
Pupil	Normal	Normal	Normal	Constricted	Normal to constricted	Mild dilation, less responsive	Normal; unless affected by trauma	Normal
Cornea	Clear	Clear	Clear	Clear to hazy	Hazy	Usually hazy	Clear	Clear or neovascularization, cloudy
Associated diseases	URI, allergy, exposure	Occasional systemic disease	Systemic disease	Systemic disease, idiopathic	Contact lenses, HSV or varicella, rosacea	Causes headaches, nausea, vomiting, gastrointestinal (GI) symptoms	HTN, trauma, Valsalva, cough, blood thinners	Acne rosacea (can exist without also), blepharitis

HSV, Herpes simplex virus; HTN, hypertension; URI, upper respiratory infection.

[a]For identifying serious causes of red eye, the presence of photophobia elicited with a penlight in a general practice had a positive predictive value of 60% and a negative predictive value of 90%.

(Source: Reproduced with permission from Usatine RP, Smith MA, Mayeaux EJ, Chumley HS (Eds). Color Atlas of Family Medicine. 2nd ed. New York, NY: McGraw-Hill; 2013. Table 25-1, p.164.)

G. Pterygium is usually painless, with normal or blurred vision. However, changes in vision may occur if the cornea becomes distorted. The conjunctival tissue is triangular, yellowish, fleshy, and injected. It may extend from either canthus and encroach upon or partially cover the cornea (Figure 53-1).

H. Acute angle-closure glaucoma occurs spontaneously, generally in the evening or in darkened settings when reduced light induces mydriasis, causing the iris to block the narrow anterior-chamber angle in these individuals. It is typically unilateral and presents with an acute, periocular pain and congestion, acute photophobia, rapidly progressive loss of vision, ciliary flush, and corneal haziness. Patients often describe the classic symptom of seeing colored halos around lights. Nausea, vomiting, and frontal headache occur in severe cases. Severe cases have been known to prompt abdominal exploration in an attempt to make the diagnosis.

The involved pupil is often moderately dilated and unreactive to light, whereas the other pupil is normal. Elevated IOP of the affected eye can be crudely tested by digitally palpating for a hardened globe.

I. Episcleritis
   1. *Simple* episcleritis presents with mild eye pain or eye tenderness, and focal, bright-red injection of the bulbar conjunctiva (Figure 53-2).
   2. *Nodular* episcleritis appears as a painful, hyperemic raised nodule that can be moved slightly over the underlying sclera.

J. Scleritis may manifest as *diffuse, nodular,* or *necrotizing*. Severe pain is common to all presentations and is characteristically described as a deep, boring, radiating ache, which interrupts sleep. Onset of redness and decrease in vision may be sudden or gradual and recurring episodes are common. It may be unilateral or bilateral with tenderness to palpation of the globe, photophobia, and lacrimation. Thinning of the cornea or sclera may allow the dark purple/blue color of the underlying uvea to show through.

K. Uveitis presents with 360-degree perilimbal injection, worse at the limbus, vision loss or distortion, ciliary flush, pupil constriction, and clear to hazy cornea (Figure 53-4). Iritis (anterior uveitis) is typically unilateral and associated with eye pain and photophobia. Patients with intermediate or posterior uveitis may not have eye pain or photophobia. Sarcoidosis panuveitis is typically bilateral.

L. Keratitis is characterized by diffuse erythema, blurred vision, photophobia, periocular pain, foreign body sensation (grittiness), and ciliary flush (Figure 53-5). Fragmented, corneal light reflection and corneal opacification may sometimes also be noted on inspection.

IV. Laboratory Tests/Diagnostics. Differentiating among common and serious causes of red eye generally relies upon history and physical examination. See Table 53-1.

A. Conjunctivitis is diagnosed clinically and usually does not require special testing.
   1. Viral conjunctivitis. Viruses can be grown and identified; however, clinical diagnosis is more practical.
   2. Bacterial conjunctivitis. Most cases are self-limited; however, for severe infections, can include the following tests:
      a. Culture of eye discharge for identification of bacteria and sensitivity to antibiotics.
      b. Conjunctival scrapings require local anesthesia to obtain a sample for cytologic evaluation.
         (1) Gram stain can also aid in quick identification of the bacterial organism.
         (2) Giemsa stain identifies the cell type and morphology of the microbe.
            (a) Polymorphonuclear leukocytes imply bacterial etiology.
            (b) Lymphocytes suggest viral etiology.
   3. Chlamydial conjunctivitis. Nonculture tests are now available using DNA amplification testing.

B. Corneal abrasion. Corneal reflection can be observed with a penlight. Fluorescein dye illuminated by a Wood lamp is used to detect a denuded cornea or ulcerations. A short-acting topical anesthetic (e.g., tetracaine 0.5%) is often used to facilitate the examination.

C. Blepharitis. Culturing of the conjunctiva and eyelid margins may yield the bacterial pathogen in patients in whom ulcerative blepharitis is suspected.

D. Subconjunctival hemorrhage. Coagulation studies, complete blood count with platelets, and protein C and S levels should be considered if hemorrhages are recurrent or there is a history of bleeding problems.

E. Inflamed pingueculum. No testing is required.

F. Pterygium. No tests are necessary; the diagnosis is clinical.

G. Acute angle-closure glaucoma. Tonometry measures intraocular fluid pressure using calibrated instruments that can be used in any clinic or emergency department setting; pressures between 10 to 20 mm Hg are considered normal. Slit-lamp examination and gonioscopy are the preferred diagnostic methods. Markedly elevated IOP (50–100 mm Hg), a shallow anterior chamber, and corneal edema are hallmark findings.

H. Episcleritis. Placement of phenylephrine 2.5% drops in the affected eye followed by re-examination of the vascular pattern 10 to 15 minutes later will reveal blanched episcleral vessels. Appropriate laboratory studies should be done when the history suggests an underlying etiology.

I. Scleritis. Scleral vessels do not blanch on application of topical phenylephrine 2.5%. A complete physical examination with a focus on rheumatologic findings should be performed. Appropriate laboratory tests include a complete blood count (CBC), urinalysis, erythrocyte sedimentation rate (ESR), uric acid, rapid plasma reagin (RPR), fluorescent treponemal antibody-absorption (FTA-ABS), rheumatoid factor (RF), anticyclic citrullinated peptide antibodies, antinuclear antibody (ANA), fasting blood glucose (FBG), antineutrophil cytoplasmic antibody (ANCA), and Lyme antibody in Lyme-infested regions. Other tests to consider, if suspicious, include purified protein derivative of tuberculin (PPD) with anergy panel, angiotensin-converting enzyme (ACE), a viral hepatitis panel, and cultures of scleral exudates for bacteria, virus, and fungi.

J. Iritis/anterior uveitis. If there is clinical suspicion, patients should be referred to an ophthalmologist for further work-up. The ophthalmologist can visualize a proteinaceous *flare* and cellular debris of the aqueous humor on slit-lamp biomicroscopy. Cellular deposits on the corneal endothelium are also a common finding. If pus settles in the anterior chamber, it forms a *hypopion*, a white or yellow-white, flat-surfaced accumulation that is generally visible to the naked eye. IOP may be either markedly elevated or depressed. Adhesions between the iris and the anterior lens surface form *posterior synechiae*, which may lead to decreased vision. Studies can include CBC, ESR, human leukocyte antigen B27 (HLA-B27), ACE level, ANA, RPR, FTA-ABS, PPD and anergy panel, chest x-rays, and Lyme titer.

K. Keratitis. Fluorescein dye staining will often reveal multiple punctuate lesions when the epithelium is disrupted; however, diagnosis requires a slit-lamp examination by an ophthalmologist who may also culture, scrape, and/or biopsy the cornea when the cause is uncertain. Appropriate studies (e.g., RPR, FTA-ABS, PPD, ESR, ANA, RF, and chest x-rays) should be ordered to work-up the underlying cause.

V. Treatment

A. Conjunctivitis

1. **Viral conjunctivitis** is treated with supportive measures including cold compresses and lubricating drops (e.g., artificial tears one to two drops as needed). Preventive measures include frequent handwashing (especially in environments such as medical offices and day care centers), washing of all bedding and towels, not sharing towels, and avoiding eye rubbing to prevent transmission from one eye to the other. (SOR **Ⓐ**) Because of serious ocular side effects (increased duration of viral shedding, risk of corneal ulcerations and perforation), topical ophthalmic corticosteroids are contraindicated in conjunctivitis. (SOR **Ⓑ**) Schools may require treatment with antibiotic drops prior to return to school; this issue should be discussed with the parent and the school as these drops will not improve viral conjunctivitis and may give a false sense of safety with respect to transmission to other children.

2. **Bacterial conjunctivitis** is usually self-limited, resolving within 7 to 10 days.

   a. Broad-spectrum topical ophthalmic antibiotics can be used for severe infections (eye drops are preferred for all patients except infants and young children, for whom ointment is preferable). Examples include bacitracin-polymyxin B (Polysporin ophthalmic ointment, 0.5 in every 3–4 hours for 7–10 days), polymyxin B-trimethoprim (Polytrim ophthalmic solution, one drop every 3 hours for 7–10 days), aminoglycosides (gentamicin or tobramycin, 0.3%, two drops or 0.5 in ointment every 1 hour for 24–72 hours around the clock, then a slow reduction to three to four times daily as the condition improves), or quinolones (ciprofloxin or ofloxacin, 0.3%, one to two drops every 2–4 hours for 2 days, then four times daily for 5 more days). (SOR **Ⓐ**) Antibiotics may speed resolution of symptoms and can be considered for that purpose. (SOR **Ⓐ**)

   b. Ophthalmologic referral is indicated for persistent symptoms beyond 10 days or immediately if there is diminished visual acuity or loss of vision. (SOR **Ⓐ**)

    c. Infection by *Neisseria gonorrhoeae* is a medical emergency that requires ophthalmologic referral. If untreated it can lead to corneal ulceration, perforation, and blindness within 24 hours.

  3. Chlamydial conjunctivitis is treated with oral erythromycin 250 mg 4 times daily or doxycycline 100 mg twice daily for 14 to 21 days. Sexual partner must be treated. Since coexisting infection with gonorrhea is high in sexually-active patients, intramuscular ceftriaxone should be added to the treatment regimen. Neonatal chlamydial infection is best treated with a 2-week course of oral erythromycin.

  4. Allergic conjunctivitis. Avoidance of the offending allergen, application of artificial tears (one to two drops as needed) or administration of a topical vasoconstrictor, topical antihistamines, or topical mast cell stabilizer (e.g., naphazoline, 0.025%, one to two drops four times daily; olopatadine HCl, 0.1%, one drop twice daily at 6–8-hour intervals or cromolyn sodium, 4%, one to two drops four to six times daily, respectively) until asymptomatic.

B. Corneal abrasion. Primary treatment goals are to restore patient comfort, assist in rapid healing, and prevent secondary infections. The corneal epithelium regenerates rapidly, and healing is usually complete within 24 to 48 hours.

  1. Topical cycloplegic drops (atropine ophthalmic solution) can be used to relieve pain caused by reflex spasm of the ciliary body muscles.

  2. Oral analgesics with codeine (Tylenol #3, 1–2 tabs every 3–4 hours as needed for pain) can occasionally be prescribed if needed.

  3. A topical ophthalmic antibiotic (see topical aminoglycosides or quinolones above) can also be applied. Although soft pressure patches are often used; they are usually not necessary. Contact lens wearers should not receive eye patches at all as this can promote serious corneal/conjunctival infections (e.g., Pseudomonas).

C. Blepharitis. Washing with baby shampoo once daily is an effective way of treating the seborrheic form. An antistaphylococcal antibiotic or topical sulfacetamide, 10% (Bleph-10 ointment, 0.5 inch every 3–4 hours and at bedtime for 7–10 days) can be used in the ulcerative form. Demodex (mite) infestation can be treated with tea tree oil eyelid scrubs. Most cases are chronic and require long-term therapy.

D. Subconjunctival hemorrhage. No treatment is usually required, as hemorrhage spontaneously clears in 2 to 3 weeks. Treat underlying high blood pressure or bleeding disorder and discontinue any elective aspirin or NSAID use if episodes are recurrent. Artificial tear drops (one to two drops as needed) may help for mild irritation. If the diagnosis is in doubt or some other abnormality becomes evident on examination, referral to an ophthalmologist is appropriate.

E. Inflamed pingueculum. Topical vasoconstrictors (naphazoline, 0.025%, one to two drops four times daily) work well. Non-urgent referrals to ophthalmology are appropriate if the lesion is unresponsive in 1 week. Surgical removal is not necessary.

F. Pterygia. No medical treatment is necessary for a long-standing, unchanging, asymptomatic growth. Protective glasses are recommended for at-risk individuals to prevent recurrences. If the cornea is involved and the patient is experiencing altered vision, a non-urgent referral to an ophthalmologist for possible surgical excision is indicated.

G. Acute angle-closure glaucoma is an ophthalmic emergency and patients with this condition should be referred. The key to treatment is lowering intraocular pressure. Optic nerve atrophy and irreversible loss of vision can occur within hours after onset of the disorder. The patient should alert relatives about the occurrence of these attacks since it is a highly inheritable condition.

H. Episcleritis is usually self-limited, resolving after 1 to 2 weeks. Artificial tears (one to two drops as needed) can be used in mild cases. Oral NSAIDs (e.g., naproxen 250–500 mg twice daily, or ketoprofen 200 mg daily) or mild topical steroids (prednisolone acetate, 0.12%, ophthalmic suspension, initially two drops every 1 hour for 24–48 hours, then one to two drops two to four times daily until resolved) are often successful in moderate to severe cases. Despite its benign nature, an ophthalmologist best manages these cases, as recurrences may torment the patient for years.

I. Scleritis demands urgent referral to an ophthalmologist. Recurring episodes are common. Patients with RA-associated scleritis seem to have more widespread systemic disease and a higher mortality rate than those without scleritis.

J. Iritis/Anterior uveitis. Urgent referral to an ophthalmologist is recommended to prevent permanently-impaired vision. Recurrent episodes are not uncommon. Management of the underlying systemic disorder may also require consultation with a rheumatologist.

K. Keratitis. Refer emergently to ophthalmology to prevent permanent visual loss.

VI. Patient Education
 A. Advise patients presenting with conjunctivitis about the importance of hand-washing to prevent spread, and the importance of returning if any vision loss or eye pain occur or if symptoms do not resolve in 7 days.
 B. Advise any patient with a red eye to remove contact lenses and wear glasses until the episode has resolved.
 C. Advise pregnant women about the recommendations for screening for Chlaymdia and gonorrhea during pregnancy. Advise parents about recommendations regarding prophylactic eye drops at birth to prevent neonatal eye infections that can be acquired in the birth canal.

SELECTED REFERENCES

Cronau H, Kankanala RR, Mauger T. Diagnosis and management of red eye in primary care. *Am Fam Physician.* 2010;81(2):137–144.
Deibel JP, Cowling K. Ocular inflammation and infection. *Emerg Med Clin North Am.* 2013;31(2): 387–397.
Sheikh A, Hurwitz B, van Schayck CP, et al. Antibiotics versus placebo for acute bacterial conjunctivitis. *Cochrane Database Syst Rev.* 2012;(9):CD001211.

---

54   Rhinitis and Sinus Pain

Jensena M. Carlson, MD, Melissa Stiles, MD, Robert G. Quattlebaum, MD, Vanessa A. Diaz, MD, MS, & Arch G. Mainous III, PhD

KEY POINTS

- Allergic rhinitis is a common condition that can be managed in the primary care setting with medications and lifestyle interventions. (SOR **C**)
- Acute sinusitis should be diagnosed using specific criteria in order to decrease overdiagnosis and inappropriate use of antibiotics. (SOR **C**)
- Most patients with acute sinusitis or rhinitis do not benefit from laboratory tests or imaging studies. (SOR **C**)
- Initial treatment for acute sinusitis should both analgesics and decongestants. Antibiotics for acute sinusitis should be reserved for patients with persistent symptoms after initial treatment or with severe illness. (SOR **A**)

I. Definition. Rhinitis is an inflammation of the nasal mucous membrane frequently resulting in edema, vasodilatation, and rhinorrhea. **Common causes** include viruses and other infectious agents; type I hypersensitivity reactions to antigens such as pollens, molds, and animal dander; autonomic hyper-responsiveness; rebound congestion from intranasal or certain systemic medications; or atrophy of the nasal mucosa.
 A. Five main groups of paranasal sinuses drain through sinus ostia into the nasal cavity: the maxillary, frontal, anterior ethmoid, posterior ethmoid, and sphenoid. The maxillary and ethmoid sinuses are present at birth, whereas the sphenoid sinuses develop by age 3 years and the frontal sinuses appear by age 5 years. Maxillary sinuses are noted radiographically by age 4 years, sphenoid sinuses by age 6 years, and frontal sinuses by age 7 years. However, the sinuses are often asymmetric and may not be fully developed in as many as 5% of adults.
 B. Sinusitis is an inflammatory process in one or more of the paranasal sinuses, associated with obstruction of the sinus ostia. It is usually caused by **infection**. Viral infections are the most common cause, accounting for 90% to 98% of cases of sinusitis. Bacterial infections are usually caused by *Streptoccocus pneumoniae*, *Haemophilus influenzae*, and in children *Moraxella catarrhalis* as well. Fungal infections are rarely seen except in patients with poorly controlled diabetes or in immunocompromised patients. Infection of the sphenoid sinus can lead to serious complications because of its proximity to the apex of the orbital cavity, optic nerve, hypophysis, and cavernous sinus.
  1. Based on the time course of symptoms, sinusitis is divided into four categories. **Acute sinusitis** is characterized by symptoms lasting 4 weeks. **Subacute sinusitis** is

characterized by symptoms lasting 4 to 12 weeks. **Recurrent acute sinusitis** is more than four episodes of acute sinusitis per year lasting at least 7 days with complete resolution of symptoms between bouts. **Chronic sinusitis** persists for 3 months or more.

C. **Predisposing factors** to sinusitis include **allergies, anatomic abnormalities** (e.g., nasal polyps, septal deviation, foreign bodies, or adenoidal hypertrophy), **irritants** (e.g., tobacco, smog, chemicals), **low humidity,** and **systemic diseases** such as cystic fibrosis (abnormally thick mucus), Kartagener syndrome (immobile cilia within the respiratory tract), and congenital or acquired immunodeficiency syndrome.

II. **Common Diagnoses**

A. **Common cold or viral upper respiratory infection (URI).** There are nearly 62 million cases of viral URIs annually, resulting in 22 million school days lost. Common colds peak in the winter and occur more commonly in families with children aged 2 to 7 years. The average preschool child has six to ten colds per year; the average adult, two to four. The virus is spread by hand-to-hand contact, as well as contact with wet fomites.

B. **Allergic rhinitis** is the most common cause of chronic rhinitis. Twenty to forty million Americans are affected and, annually, nine million visits to office-based physicians are attributed to allergic rhinitis. The peak incidence occurs in the late teenage years, with another peak between the ages of 30 and 40 years. Allergic rhinitis is more common in those with a family history of allergies and is often associated with atopy. It may be seasonal or perennial, depending on the types of allergens involved. The seasonal allergens are mostly encountered outdoors and include pollens and, less commonly, mold spores. The perennial allergens are more likely to be encountered indoors and include dust mites, many mold spores, cockroach feces, and animal dander.

C. **Vasomotor rhinitis** occurs most commonly in the third to fifth decades but is occasionally seen in childhood and adolescence. Vasomotor rhinitis of pregnancy occurs most frequently from the second trimester on and resolves spontaneously by the fifth postpartum day.

D. **Atrophic rhinitis** occurs mainly in elderly adults. Risk factors for its development include chronic granulomatous nasal infections (including sarcoidosis, Wegener granulomatosis, Churg–Strauss syndrome, and tuberculosis), chronic sinusitis, irradiation, trauma, or radical nasal surgery.

E. **Rhinitis medicamentosa** (rebound congestion) usually affects young to middle-aged adults, although cases have been reported in children as young as 4 years. Overusers of topical nasal decongestants are at risk (decongestant used more frequently than every 3 hours or for longer than 10 days). In some individuals, a form of rhinitis medicamentosa occurs with the use of certain antihypertensive agents (e.g., beta-blockers, guanethidine, methyldopa, or reserpine); aspirin; and oral contraceptives.

F. **Sinusitis** is commonly overdiagnosed, so its overall incidence is unclear. Approximately 32 million adults are diagnosed with sinusitis annually. Chronic sinusitis leads to 11.6 million office-based physician visits annually. The incidence peaks in winter, when viral URIs are common.

G. **Conditions that can mimic sinus pain** include migraine headaches and temporal arteritis (see Chapter 33), periapical dental abscesses of the maxillary teeth, and nasal polyps. **Other causes** of rhinitis not discussed in this chapter include pregnancy (see Chapter 99), endocrine disorders including hypothyroidism (see Chapter 89), nonallergic rhinitis with eosinophilia syndrome (NARES), nasal foreign bodies, cocaine snorting, nasal neoplasms, and menstruation-induced rhinitis.

III. **Symptoms and Signs**

A. **Overview**

1. **History.** Symptoms of rhinitis and sinusitis frequently overlap but history can help distinguish the cause of disease. History should include inquiry about duration of symptoms to help differentiate acute from chronic conditions, as well as to guide treatment if there is concern for sinusitis. Associated symptoms including fatigue, headache, ear pain, cough, sneezing, rhinorrhea and congestion, nasal and conjunctival itching, hyposmia/anosmia, halitosis, sinus pain/pressure, and dental pain should also be discussed.

2. **Physical examination**

a. **Examination of the nose** begins with inspection of the anterior and inferior surfaces, which is aided by a nasal speculum and a strong light source. Abnormalities of the nasal mucosa and septum and presence of exudates can help diagnose common causes of rhinitis. A **nasopharyngeal mirror** is required for detection of posterior abnormalities.

    b. Examination of the paranasal sinuses begins with inspection of the overlying skin for erythema, which can be associated with infection, followed by palpation for tenderness of the maxillary and frontal sinuses.

    c. Transillumination of the sinuses should be performed in a darkened room. A strong, narrow light source is placed snugly under each brow, close to the nose. A dim red glow should be seen as the light is transmitted through the air-filled frontal sinus to the forehead (http://www.youtube.com/watch?v=8Lo3bENDqzs). The maxillary sinuses are transilluminated by shining light downward from just below the inner aspect of each eye while asking the patient to tilt his head back with the mouth wide open (http://www.youtube.com/watch?v=Z-CYWdc73IQ). A reddish glow seen at the hard palate indicates a normal air-filled sinus. Asymmetrical or poor transillumination is consistent with, but not diagnostic of, sinusitis as it may also be caused by nonpathologic hypoplastic or aplastic sinuses.

    d. Physical examination of children should include evaluation of several key components. The child's **general appearance** should be assessed for lethargy and respiratory distress, which are worrisome signs. The **skin** should be examined for atopic dermatitis, often associated with allergic rhinitis. The **nasal cavity** and **oropharynx** should also be examined for mucosa and anatomy, specifically for nasal obstruction and discharge.

B. Symptoms of **cold or viral URI** are typically 7 to 10 days in duration and include sneezing, mucoid rhinorrhea that may become mucopurulent at 1 to 3 days, and cough. Fever is uncommon in adults, but frequently occurs in children. Often, these symptoms are accompanied by fatigue, headache, and ear pain/pressure. Patients with viral URI will often have sick contacts, especially for children who attend daycare or school.

    1. On general examination, patients with viral URIs will appear fatigued. The nasal examination will reveal erythematous nasal mucosa and mucoid or mucopurulent discharge. Examination of the throat will reveal erythematous mucosa. Ear examination will occasionally reveal effusions. Cervical lymph nodes may also be present, along with a fever.

C. Key symptoms of **allergic rhinitis** include sneezing, watery or mucoid rhinorrhea, and **nasal/conjunctival itching**. Symptoms of allergic rhinitis typically last greater than 2 weeks without improvement. Patients may note worsening symptoms with exposure to specific allergens, though exposures are not always easy to discern.

    1. External examination of the face in patients with allergic rhinitis often reveals a **nasal crease** (a horizontal line across the bridge of the nose caused by repeated upward rubbing of the nose—also known as the **allergic salute**) and **allergic "shiners"** (dark rings under the eyes). The nasal examination will often reveal boggy, pale, bluish-gray mucosa; but erythematous mucosa can also be present. Clear rhinorrhea and nasal polyps may also be present. On the ocular examination, the **conjunctiva** are frequently inflamed, the palpebral conjunctiva may have an edematous and cobblestone appearance, and Dennie–Morgan lines (deep creases below the inferior eyelid) may also be present.

D. The primary symptoms of **vasomotor rhinitis** are very watery rhinorrhea and unrelenting congestion, typically with a few associated symptoms. Symptoms occur with exposure to certain odors, alcohol, spicy foods, intense emotions, pregnancy, and extreme temperatures.

    1. The physical examination for vasomotor rhinitis is varied, as the nasal examination of this condition can present similarly to infectious, allergic, or atrophic rhinitis.

E. Patients with **atrophic rhinitis** will complain of rhinorrhea, nasal congestion, and obstruction, which last from weeks to months. Patients may also have **epistaxis,** but have a few other associated symptoms.

    1. The nasal examination in patients with atrophic rhinitis will reveal **nasal crusting,** a shrunken-appearing nasal mucosa, and enlarged nasal cavities. Despite the sensation of nasal congestion, there is no increase in airflow resistance in most cases.

F. Rhinitis medicamentosa presents with nasal congestion and obstruction without significant rhinorrhea, in the setting of exposure. The nasal examination of patients with this condition reveals **marked erythema** or even a hemorrhagic appearance and swelling of the nasal mucosa.

G. Sinusitis typically presents as a syndrome of "double sickening." **Double sickening** refers to patients who start out with symptoms of a viral URI, begin to improve only to have the original symptoms return and also develop sinus pain/pressure, maxillary toothaches (painful mastication), nasal obstruction, high fever, headache, halitosis, hyposmia/anosmia, nausea, and vomiting.

1. **The most common cause of sinus pain is sinusitis.** Numerous other conditions, however, can mimic this symptom (see Section II.G). Sinus pain may present as vague, tension-type headaches or may specifically localize as pain or pressure over the affected sinuses. Pain beneath the eyes suggests **maxillary sinusitis,** pain between the eyes suggests **ethmoid sinusitis,** frontal headache suggests **frontal sinusitis,** and vertex headache suggests **sphenoid sinusitis**. Headache, facial pain, and sinus pressure in sinusitis is often worse in the morning and with head movement.

2. In general, the patient is typically febrile and fatigued. **External signs** of sinusitis include erythema overlying the sinuses. The bony structures overlying the maxillary, frontal, or ethmoid sinuses may be tender to palpation, and eyelid puffiness (chemosis) may be present, especially with maxillary and ethmoid sinusitis. **Sinus transillumination** has very low sensitivity and specificity because of the great variability in sinus anatomy, including asymmetry and underdevelopment. Only normal findings are useful in ruling out maxillary or frontal sinusitis.

3. **In acute sinusitis,** infectious rhinitis is also commonly present, and therefore, the nasal examination will appear similar to those with viral URIs. When the sinus ostia are visible, purulent discharge may be seen exuding from them. In chronic sinusitis, the appearance of the mucous membranes depends on the underlying cause—pale or bluish and edematous in allergic rhinitis or even relatively normal with anatomic causes, such as choanal atresia or septal deviation.

4. **Symptoms of complications** of sinusitis include orbital swelling or redness, severe swelling over the affected sinus, proptosis, vision changes, and altered mental status. Signs of periorbital erythema, proptosis, and cranial nerve deficits, especially an abducens nerve palsy, can indicate invasive infection. Meningitis should be considered in patients with signs of severe acute sinusitis. If these findings are present, prompt surgical consultation is required.

5. Signs and symptoms of sinusitis may mimic and overlap those of other diseases, ranging from common cold to allergic rhinitis. It is therefore recommended to consider the use of major and minor criteria in making a diagnosis. **Sinusitis can be diagnosed by the presence of at least 2 major or 1 major and at least 2 minor criteria:**
   a. **Major criteria** include purulent anterior nasal discharge, purulent or discolored postnasal discharge, nasal congestion or obstruction, facial congestion or fullness, facial pain or pressure, hyposmia/anosmia, and fever.
   b. **Minor criteria** include headache, ear pain/pressure, halitosis, dental pain, cough, and fatigue.

IV. **Diagnostic Tests**
   A. **Laboratory tests** (Table 54–1) are usually indicated only if medical therapy fails, if there are symptoms and signs of complications, or if there is a serious underlying condition. (SOR ⓖ)
      1. **Study of nasal secretions** is not necessary for diagnosis but may help identify the etiology of rhinitis. Nasal secretions are obtained and placed on a glass slide, stained with Hansel, Wright, or Giemsa stain and examined microscopically. Eosinophils are seen in allergic rhinitis, NARES, and nasal polyposis; large numbers of neutrophils are seen with infection.
      2. **Cultures of nasal secretions** from nasal swabs are of limited value because they do not correlate well with bacteria aspirated directly from the sinuses. Endoscopically guided microswab cultures from the middle meatus correlate 80% to 85% with central puncture cultures. Cultures are indicated when acute sinusitis is resistant to one or two courses of antibiotic therapy and in immunocompromised individuals. Cultures are also obtained during most surgical procedures on the sinuses if persistent sinus infection is suspected. Aerobic and anaerobic cultures should be obtained, and fungal cultures should be added if a fungal origin is suspected.
   B. **Fiberoptic rhinoscopy** can reveal the presence of nasal polyps, septal deviation, or mucopurulent secretions, and can be used to obtain microswab cultures.
   C. **Allergy tests**
      1. **Allergen skin testing** is helpful in diagnosing allergic rhinitis and identifying specific allergens for which avoidance measures, allergen immunotherapy, or both are warranted. It should be considered in patients who fail medical therapy or have

TABLE 54-1. INDICATIONS FOR LABORATORY AND IMAGING IN RHINOSINUSITIS (SOR Ⓒ)

Laboratory/Imaging Modality	Indications
Microscopic nasal secretion analysis	Only necessary if unable to distinguish allergic vs. infectious rhinitis based on history and physical examination
Cultures of nasal secretions	Only beneficial in conjunction with fiberoptic rhinoscopy, especially if fungal etiology is suspected
Fiberoptic rhinoscopy	Patients with recurrent sinusitis or if polyps are suspected
Allergen skin testing	Patients (not less than 3 yr old) who fail medical therapy or have moderate to severe perennial rhinitis
Radioallergosorbent testing (RAST)	Young children (≤3 yr old), or other patients unable to have skin testing performed
Sinus films	Patients with uncertain or recurrent sinusitis
Computed tomography scan of sinus	Patients with uncertain, chronic or recurrent sinusitis; or any patient with red flag symptoms
Magnetic resonance imaging	Patients suspected of having fungal sinusitis or tumors

perennial rhinitis that is moderate to severe. These tests are relatively inexpensive and fairly reliable. They are not useful in children younger than 3 years because very young children produce inadequate amounts of histamine.

    a. Groups of allergens or single allergens are selected for testing based on the most likely causes of the patient's allergy.

    b. Allergens are introduced into the skin by intradermal injection (which is most accurate but carries a greater risk of anaphylaxis), skin prick test (the easiest, most widely used, and reasonably accurate), or scratch test. (*Note:* Methylxanthines and antihistamines should be discontinued before skin testing.)

  2. Radioallergosorbent testing is the determination of serum allergen-specific IgE levels by immunoassay. This test is useful in young children, who might not tolerate multiple skin pricks; those with skin conditions such as dermatographia and severe eczema; and those receiving medications that might affect the reliability of skin testing (e.g., antihistamines). However, it is relatively more expensive, is less sensitive, and can test for fewer antigens than skin testing.

D. Imaging studies (Table 54-1) may be helpful in uncertain cases, with recurrent symptoms despite appropriate treatment, and when symptoms of complications are present. (SOR Ⓒ)

  1. Sinus films may be helpful in uncertain or recurrent cases, but not for initial evaluation, since up to 40% of sinus films may be abnormal in viral rhinosinusitis if obtained within 7 days of symptom onset. Four views constitute the sinus series: Waters view (maxillary sinuses), the Caldwell view (ethmoid and frontal sinuses), the submental vertex view (sphenoid sinuses), and the lateral view. A single Waters view has a high level of agreement with the complete sinus series. A normal series has a negative predictive value of 90% to 100%, particularly for the maxillary and frontal sinuses. A sinus film is read as abnormal if there is mucosal thickening ≥6 mm, air–fluid levels, ≥33% loss of air space volume, or opacification of one or more sinuses on one or more views. The positive predictive value is 80% to 100%, but sensitivity is only 60%.

  2. The computed tomography (CT) scan has superior sensitivity (95% to 98%) and specificity compared to sinus films. The CT scan is particularly valuable in assessing obstruction of the sinus ostia. CT scanning is indicated when medical therapy has failed to establish the diagnosis of chronic sinusitis, in equivocal cases before starting long-term antibiotic therapy, or when complications are suspected. A complete series sinus CT scan is required prior to sinus surgery. More than 80% of scan results may be abnormal in cases of viral rhinosinusitis if obtained within 7 days of illness onset.

  3. Magnetic resonance imaging is used when fungal sinusitis and tumors are suspected. It is not used for routine evaluation of sinusitis.

V. Treatment

  A. Treatment of **common colds** is largely palliative and may include the following strategies:

    1. For **fever and headache, acetaminophen** (e.g., Tylenol), 325 mg, one or two tablets orally every 4 to 6 hours for adults (maximum 3 g/day) or 10–15 mg/kg every 4 to 6 hours for children younger than 12 years (maximum 75 mg/kg/day), or **ibuprofen** (e.g., Advil), 200 mg, one or two tablets every 4 to 6 hours for adults (maximum 1200 mg/24 h), or 5–10 mg/kg every 6 to 8 hours for children (maximum 50 mg/kg/d) may be used.

2. For **nasal congestion and rhinorrhea,** oral decongestants such as **pseudo-ephedrine** (e.g., Sudafed), 30 mg, one or two tablets every 4 to 6 hours for adults and children older than 12 years, or 2.5 to 5 mL every 4 to 6 hours of the liquid for children younger than 12 years, may be used. (SOR ⓒ) Short-term use (up to a maximum of 3–4 days) of topical decongestants such as oxymetazoline (e.g., Afrin), 0.05%, two to three sprays in each nostril every 10 to 12 hours (maximum of two doses per day) for adults and children over age 6 years; for children 2 to 6 years of age, two to three sprays of a 0.025% concentration can be used every 10 to 12 hours (maximum of two doses per day). These medications can cause insomnia, nervousness, loss of appetite, and urinary retention in males. They should be used with caution in patients with certain conditions, such as arrhythmias, hypertension, and hyperthyroidism.

3. For **acute cough,** syrups containing **dextromethorphan** (e.g., Robitussin DM) or **codeine** (e.g., Robitussin AC), 5 mL every 6 hours or **benzonatate** (e.g., Tessalon Perles) 100 mg three times daily can be prescribed for adults only, can be prescribed. (SOR ⓒ) In children under the age of 4 years, cough syrup should not be used and only single ingredient preparations should be used for children under age 6 years. Cochrane authors found insufficient evidence to support the use of non-prescription cough suppressants in adults; in children, antitussives, antihistamines, antihistamine decongestants, and antitussive/bronchodilator combinations were no more effective than placebo. (SOR ⓑ) **Honey** has been shown to be more effective than no treatment in reducing the frequency of cough in children and is about as effective in reducing cough as dextromethorphan. (SOR ⓑ) Honey should be avoided in children under age 1 year.

4. **Watery rhinorrhea** can be treated with the anticholinergic nasal spray **ipratro-pium bromide** (e.g., Atrovent 0.06%). (SOR ⓑ)

5. **Antihistamines** have not been shown to be beneficial, nor are **antibiotics** indicated or helpful in these patients.

6. **Other therapies**
   a. **General supportive measures** in the treatment of **common colds** and **allergies** include adequate sleep, increased fluids, cool vapor steam, and rest. Adequate fluids (especially water and soups) improve mucous membrane and ciliary function and may also enhance immune function. Nasal saline irrigation may be helpful; however, more research is needed.
   b. The use of other complementary therapies, such as **homeopathic medicines, vitamins, acupuncture,** and **herbs,** is controversial. Although **vitamin C** in high doses (up to 1 g daily) does not seem to prevent illness, it does reduce the duration of symptoms. (SOR ⓑ) **Zinc** may also be effective in shortening the duration of symptoms when taken within 24 to 48 hours of their onset. (SOR ⓒ) The dose is 9 to 24 mg of elemental zinc per dose administered via lozenges of zinc gluconate or acetate every 2 hours. There is some evidence that **Echinacea** preparations containing the aerial component of the plant may stimulate the immune system, thereby reducing the severity and duration of infection; however, studies do not seem to show significant efficacy over placebo. (SOR ⓑ)

B. **Allergic rhinitis**
   1. **Environmental control.** Avoidance of inciting factors is fundamental.
      a. For **pollen allergy,** patients should keep doors and windows closed, limit the amount of time spent outdoors, and use air conditioners and a high-efficiency particulate air (HEPA) filter. (SOR ⓒ)
      b. For **dust mite allergy,** patients should cover bedding (including pillows) with plastic covers, eliminate wall-to-wall carpets (especially in bedrooms), use acaricides such as tannic acid solutions regularly to kill dust mites, avoid or regularly wash stuffed animals in hot water, keep home humidity below 40%, and use HEPA filters. (SOR ⓒ)
      c. Patients with **mold allergies** should decrease mold exposure by wiping vulnerable surfaces (e.g., those in the bathroom) with household bleach, keeping indoor humidity below 40%, using air filters, avoiding piles of leaves in the fall, and cutting grass to reduce exposure outside.

    d. Cat dander (saliva) is by far the most frequent cause of allergies to animals. If sensitivity develops, contact with the animal should be minimized. The cat should be washed at least once every 2 weeks to remove the antigen-containing cat saliva from its coat.

    e. Elimination of **food allergens** may be beneficial. However, ingested allergens rarely cause isolated rhinitis without involvement of other organ systems. Relatively common food allergens include dairy products, chocolate, wheat, citrus fruits, and food additives such as artificial dyes and preservatives.

2. Pharmacologic therapy includes the following:

    a. Steroid nasal sprays are more effective than antihistamines in the treatment of allergic rhinitis in adults; however, the evidence for efficacy in children is lacking. (SOR **Ⓐ**) Available preparations include **beclomethasone** (e.g., Beconase AQ(R)), one or two sprays (42 mcg/inhalation) in each nostril two times daily (usual dose 168–336 mcg/day); **budesonide** (e.g., Rhinocort), two to four sprays per nostril daily; **flunisolide** (e.g., Nasalide), two sprays per nostril twice daily; **fluticasone** (e.g., Flonase), one or two sprays per nostril daily; and **triamcinolone acetonide** (e.g., Nasacort), two 2-metered sprays (55 mcg/spray) in each nostril once a day (110–220 mcg/day).

        (1) Steroid nasal sprays have good long-term safety records. Local side effects are minimal with proper use, although nasal irritation, bleeding, mucosal erosions, and perforation may occur. If nasal corticosteroid preparations are used in children growth should be monitored as they have been reported to reduce linear growth (at least temporarily).

        (2) Oral steroids should be avoided, except in severe cases of refractory allergic rhinitis, in rhinitis medicamentosa while topical decongestants are discontinued, and in obstructive nasal polyposis. If used in these situations, short-acting steroids should be used (e.g., in adults, prednisone, 30 mg orally for 3–7 days).

    b. Antihistamines (Table 54–2) reduce sneezing, rhinorrhea, and nasal and ocular pruritus associated with allergic rhinitis, but are less effective for nasal congestion. (SOR **Ⓐ**) They are effective when used occasionally for episodic symptoms, but work best when administered on a regular basis. These medications have a paucity of evidence for use in children.

        (1) The newer-generation antihistamines are usually preferred, because they have fewer anticholinergic side effects and especially cause less sedation. These agents include **cetirizine** (Zyrtec), **desloratadine** (Clarinex), **fexofenadine** (Allegra), and **loratadine** (Claritin). **First-generation antihistamines** are effective and less expensive than newer agents, but tend to cause more side effects, such as sedation, dry mouth, and fatigue. Even more serious side effects can occur, such as urinary obstruction and slowed reaction times, which can potentially lead to accidents.

        (2) Levocabastine (Livostin 0.05%), one drop into each affected eye four times daily, or **Patanol (olopatadine 0.1%),** one to two drops in each affected eye twice a day, can be very helpful in the treatment of allergic conjunctivitis. **Intranasal antihistamines** (e.g., azelastine) offer no therapeutic benefit over conventional treatment.

    c. Antihistamine–decongestant combinations such as **Claritin-D 12 Hour, Claritin-D 24 Hour, Tavist-D,** and **Allegra-D** can be useful, especially if nasal congestion is a prominent symptom. The dose is one tablet twice daily for all except Claritin-D 24 hour, which is taken once daily. (SOR **Ⓒ**)

    d. Mast cell–stabilizing agents such as **cromolyn sodium** (e.g., Nasalcrom), one spray per nostril three to six times per day, can be useful. Ideally, these agents should be started before major symptoms develop because they can take several weeks to be effective. (SOR **Ⓑ**)

    e. Leukotriene inhibitors, such as montelukast (Singulair) 10 mg daily in adults and 5 mg daily in children can also decrease mucosal edema and inflammation as well as mucous production. It has been shown to be at least as effective as nasal steroids in reducing symptoms. (SOR **Ⓑ**)

    f. Anticholinergic agents such as **ipratropium bromide** (e.g., Atrovent 0.03% nasal spray), one or two sprays in each nostril every 6 hours, may reduce rhinorrhea.

TABLE 54-2. ANTIHISTAMINES USEFUL IN THE TREATMENT OF ALLERGIC RHINITIS

Class	Generic Name	Sample Trade Name	Dose[a]	Sedative Effects	Anticholin-ergic Effects
First-generation					
Ethanolamines	Diphenhydr-amine	Benadryl[b]		Marked	Mild
		Allergy tablets	A: 25–50 mg four times daily		
		Elixir, solution, and syrup	C: 12.5 mg/5 mL 2.5–10 mL every 4–6 h, based on age;[c] not for infants		
	Clemastine	Tavist			
		Tablets	A: 1.32–2.68 mg one to three times daily; max. 8.04 mg/d		
		Syrup	C: 0.5 mg/5 mL 5–10 mL twice daily; max. 3 mg/d age 6–12 yr and 6 mg/d >12 yr		
Alkylamines	Chlorpheni-ramine	Chlor-Trimeton tablets	A: 4 mg every 4–6 h; max. 24 mg/d for both regular and SR	Mild	Mild
		SR	A: 8–12 mg every 8–12 h		
		Syrup (generic)[b]	C: 2 mg/5 mL Ages 6–11 yr, 5 mL every 4–6 h; max. 12 mg/d		
Phenothiazines	Promethazine	Phenergan		Marked	Mild
		Tablets	A: 25 mg at bedtime or 6.25–12.5 mg three times daily (oral or rectal)		
		Syrup	C: 6.25 mg/5 mL over age 2 yr, 5–10 mL three times daily		
Piperidines	Cyprohepta-dine	Periactin tablets	A: 4 mg three times daily; max. 0.5 mg/kg/d C: 2 mg/5 mL; 5–10 mL two to three times daily, based on age[d]	Moderate	Mild
	Azatadine	Trinalin tablets	A: 1–2 mg twice daily (Contains pseudoephedrine)		
Piperazine	Hydroxyzine	Atarax		Moderate	Mild
		Tablets	A: 10–50 mg three to four times daily		
		Syrup	C: 10 mg/5 mL 5–15 mL three to four times daily		
Second generation					
	Cetirizine	Zyrtec		Mild	None
		Tablets	A: 5–10 mg once daily		
		Syrup	C: 1 mg/mL; 2.5–10 mL daily, based on age[e]		
	Fexofenadine	Allegra tablets	A: 60 mg twice daily or 180 mg once daily with water	None	None
	Loratadine	Claritin (OTC)		None	None
		Tablets	A or over age 6 yr: 10 mg once daily		
		Syrup	C: 1 mg/mL; ages 2 to 5 yr, 5 mg once daily		
	Desloratadine	Clarinex		None	None
		Tablets	A: 5 mg once daily		
		Syrup	C: 0.5 mg/5 mL, 1.25–5 mg once daily, based on age[f]		

Children's dosages are listed for those medications with available pediatric liquid formulations. Be aware that a range of dosages are listed. Look up the exact dosages by age before prescribing these medications for children.
[a]A, adults' dose (mg); C, children's dose (mL).
[b]A decongestant is often added; not recommended for children under age 6 yr.
[c]Dose every 4–6 h—for children up to 6 yr of age, 6.25–12.5 mg; ages 6–12 yr, 12.5–25 mg (maximum dose: 150 mg/d); 12 yr and older, 25–50 mg (maximum dose: 300 mg/d).
[d]Dose two to three times daily; for children aged 2–6 yr, 2 mg dose (maximum dose: 12 mg/d); ages 7–14 yr, 4 mg dose (maximum dose: 16 mg/d).
[e]Dose for children 2–5 yr, 2.5–5 mg once daily or 2.5 mg twice daily; ages 6–11 yr, 5–10 mg once daily; ages 12 or older, 5–10 mg once daily
[f]Dose once daily for children aged 2–5 yr, 1.25 mg; 6–11 yr, 2.5 mg; 12 yr and older, 5 mg.

3. **Immunotherapy** is useful especially in severe or refractory cases and in those patients with year-round symptoms (perennial allergic rhinitis). (SOR **Ⓐ**) It is the only method demonstrated to favorably modify the long-term course of allergic rhinitis.

   a. **Criteria for treatment** include a history of at least moderate symptoms of allergic rhinitis for ≥2 years or severe symptoms for at least 6 months responding poorly to symptomatic treatment. Other considerations in choosing immunotherapy include comorbidities and failure or unacceptability of alternative treatments. Selection of antigen injection is based on the presence of specific IgE antibodies (see Section V.D) and the patient's history.

   b. The patient receives weekly injections of antigen(s), with increasing doses at weekly intervals until a maintenance dose is achieved; injections are then given every 3 to 6 weeks for 3 to 5 years. Sublingual immunotherapy, given as a daily dose by either tablet or drops, has been shown to be a viable alternative to injection immunotherapy in adults and children and carries less risk of morbidity than injection. (SOR **Ⓐ**) If therapy does not significantly relieve symptoms within 12 months, immunotherapy should be terminated.

4. **Patient education** should include information about environmental controls to minimize antigen exposure, management options, and complications.

5. **Alternative therapies**

   a. For more information on **common supportive measures,** see Section V.A.6.a.

   b. **Other alternative therapies,** such as vitamin C, quercetin, homeopathy, acupuncture, helminthic therapy, and hypnosis, require further study.

C. **Treatment of vasomotor rhinitis** consists mainly of symptomatic therapy with oral decongestants such as **pseudoephedrine** (e.g., Sudafed), 30–60 mg three or four times a day. Anti-cholinergic agents such as **ipratropium bromide** (e.g., Atrovent nasal spray) (see Section V.B.2.f) can be very helpful in alleviating profuse watery rhinorrhea. (SOR **Ⓑ**) **Intranasal steroids** (see Section V.B.2.a) may be helpful in treating troublesome exacerbations unresponsive to the therapies listed above. (SOR **Ⓑ**) **Intranasal antihistamines** (e.g., azelastine, two sprays per nostril twice daily) are also effective. (SOR **Ⓑ**)

   1. Severe nonresponsive cases may require **surgical resection** of the inferior turbinate.

   2. Patients should be educated to **avoid irritants** that may exacerbate this condition; these include tobacco and fireplace smoke, strong perfumes, chemical and gasoline fumes, and wood dust. Sudden changes in temperature or humidity should also be avoided when possible.

D. For **rhinitis medicamentosa,** topical decongestants should be slowly withdrawn, one nostril at a time. Oral decongestants or a short course of a topical nasal steroid may be helpful (see Section V.B.2.a). A short course of systemic steroids (e.g., **prednisone,** 40 mg orally initially, tapered over 7–10 days) may be required if other methods are ineffective. The problem usually resolves in 2 to 3 weeks without long-term sequelae. Patients should be educated about the causes of the condition and discouraged from further use of topical decongestants.

E. **Treatment of atrophic rhinitis** is directed toward moistening the nasal mucosa, though there is no good evidence with regards to the treatment of atrophic rhinitis. A mucolytic such as **guaifenesin,** 600 to 1200 mg twice daily, can be used in conjunction with nasal preparations such as **Alkalol liquid,** an OTC oral or intranasal mucolytic, **or intranasal saline** (e.g., Ocean Saline Nasal Spray), two to six sprays in each nostril every 2 hours. (SOR **Ⓒ**) **Pulsed irrigators** can also be helpful to cleanse and moisten areas deeper within the nasal cavity. (SOR **Ⓒ**)

   1. **Systemic estrogens** in menopausal women may alleviate rhinitis symptoms.

   2. **Surgical reductions** of nasal cavity patency are used only as a last resort.

   3. It is important to educate patients that treatment is directed at relieving symptoms and is sometimes only partially successful.

F. **Sinusitis** can usually be managed in the outpatient setting. Initial treatment should be 10 to 14 days of conservative measures (see Section V.A) and decongestants as most cases of sinusitis are viral in nature. Antibiotics for acute sinusitis should be reserved for patients with signs or symptoms associated with sinusitis lasting more than 10 to 14 days without improvement after initial treatment, worsening signs or symptoms in 5 to 6 days after initial improvement from viral URI (double sickening), or with severe illness (severe facial pain, fever with purulent nasal discharge, periorbital swelling), regardless of duration. (SOR **B**)

1. **Hospital admission** is necessary for complicated sinusitis (sinusitis associated with serious complications such as otitis media, asthma, bronchiectasis, fungal infection, multiple antibiotic allergies, or sinusitis that compromises quality of life) or when there is a high risk of complications from a serious underlying disease and close outpatient monitoring is not feasible. (SOR **C**)

2. **Nonpharmacologic measures. Humidification** with cool steam and increased oral intake of water helps thin nasal secretions. **Nasal irrigation** with a normal saline solution is recommended to liquefy secretions. It is especially helpful in infants and young children, though data are limited. (SOR **B**)

3. **Phamacotherapy**

   a. **Oral decongestants** or short-term use (3–5 days) of **topical nasal decongestants** (see Section V.A.2) decrease nasal congestion and mucosal edema that can block the sinus ostia in adults, though evidence is lacking in children.

   b. **Oral decongestant–antihistamine combinations** (Section V.B.2.c) may be helpful in patients with underlying allergic rhinitis.

   c. **Guaifenesin** in high doses (1200 mg twice daily) may thin tenacious secretions and therefore promote sinus drainage. (SOR **C**)

   d. **Nasal corticosteroids** are as effective as antibiotic therapy and are also effective adjuncts to antibiotic therapy. (SOR **B**) The short-term use of **oral corticosteroids** is reasonable in patients with nasal polyps or severe mucosal edema though data are limited and side effects may be significant.

   e. **Antibiotics** (Table 54–3).

      (1) The decision to treat adults or children for sinusitis is based on the diagnosis of bacterial sinusitis with a history of worsening course, prolonged illness (more than 10 days with no improvement), or severe initial presentation (fever, mucopurulent nasal discharge, etc.). The standard has been to treat adults and children with uncomplicated acute sinusitis for a minimum of 7 to 10 days. However, it should be noted that 80% of patients have improvement in symptoms without antibiotics versus 90% with antibiotic treatment; there is also little difference in response to various antibiotic regimens demonstrated in RCTs. It is therefore appropriate to target antibiotic treatment based on local resistance patterns. (SOR **C**)

TABLE 54–3. AMBULATORY ANTIBIOTIC REGIMENS IN THE TREATMENT OF UNCOMPLICATED SINUSITIS

Antibiotic	Dose	Common side effects
Amoxicillin (Amoxil)	Adult: 500 mg three times daily OR 875 mg twice daily for 10 d Child: 45–90 mg/kg/d divided twice daily for 10–14 d	Nausea, diarrhea
Amoxicillin-clavulanate (Augmentin)[a]	Adult: 500/125 mg three times daily OR 875/125 mg twice daily for 5–7 d Child: 45–90 mg/kg/d amoxicillin component divided twice daily for 10–14 d	Nausea, diarrhea, diaper rash
Cefuroxime axetil (Ceftin)[b]	Adult: 250 mg twice daily for 10 d Child: 30 mg/kg/d twice daily (maximum 1 g/d) for 10 d	Nausea, diarrhea
Cefpodoxime proxetil (Vantin)[b]	Adult or over age 12 yr: 200 mg twice daily for 10 d Child: 2 mo to 12 yr, 5 mg/kg twice daily for 10 d (maximum 200 mg/dose)	Nausea, diarrhea, diaper rash
Doxycycline (Vibramycin)[c]	Adult: 100 mg twice daily or 200 mg daily for 5–7 d	Diarrhea, nasopharyngitis, photosensitivity
Levofloxacin (Levaquin)[c]	Adult: 500–750 mg once daily for 10–14 d	Nausea, diarrhea, dizziness, headache, insomnia

[a]First-line treatment.
[b]Should be used in combination with clindamycin (Cleocin) as second-line treatment. Adult: 300 mg twice daily, child: 30–40 mg/kg/d divided every 8 h.
[c]Second-line treatment.

(2) For **initial treatment,** the most narrow-spectrum agent active against the likely pathogens, *S. pneumoniae* and *H. influenzae* in adults and as well as *M. caterrhalis* in children, should be used. (SOR ❸) Appropriate first-line therapy in otherwise healthy patients with both uncomplicated and complicated acute sinusitis is amoxicillin-clavulanate (Augmentin) for adults and high dose amoxicillin-clavulanate (80–90 mg/kg/d of amoxicillin component in two divided doses) for children due to the high rate of β-lactamase producing *H. influenzae* in the United States. The American Academy of Pediatrics published updated guidelines on treating **sinusitis in children** and recommends that amoxicillin be the first choice of antibiotic in children with suspected sinusitis. Second-line therapy includes amoxicillin-clavulanate. In children allergic to penicillin, a second-generation cephalosporin should be used. (SOR ❸)

(3) If **penicillin allergy** is present, second-line therapy includes doxycycline (Vibramycin) or levofloxacin (Levaquin) for adults and third-generation cephalosporin (cefpodoxime or cefixime) plus clindamycin for children. In children who have type 1 hypersensitivity to penicillin or cephalosporin allergy, consider use of a fluoroquinolone; however, this class of antibiotics must be used with caution due to risk of tendinopathy in children. Macrolides and trimethoprim-sulfamethoxazole (TMP-SMX) are no longer recommended as there is a high rate of resistance of *S. pneumoniae* (30%) to both classes and *H. influenzae* (30–40%) to TMP-SMX.

(4) If the response to first-line therapy is poor or if the patient is immunocompromised, reasonable alternative antimicrobials include **fluoroquinolones in adults**.

(5) **For chronic sinusitis,** antibiotic therapy should continue for at least 3 weeks and until the patient is well for 7 days. (SOR ❸) Antibiotics with good staphylococcal coverage are often preferred; these include **amoxicillin-clavulanate but may also include cloxacillin, dicloxacillin, cephalexin, cefadroxil monohydrate,** and **cefuroxime axetil**. With complicated sinusitis, hospital admission for parenteral antibiotics is indicated. If mucormycosis is suspected, parenteral **amphotericin B** should be used.

4. Surgery should be considered for patients who have frequent recurrences of sinusitis (i.e., three or more attacks in 1 year) despite adequate medical treatment, who have chronic sinusitis responding inadequately to medical therapy alone, or who have an anatomic obstruction amenable to surgery. Functional endoscopic sinus surgery (FESS) has supplanted older surgical techniques. FESS leads to a significant improvement of symptoms in 80% to 90% of patients. It is typically directed at the removal of locally diseased ethmoid tissue to improve ventilation and drainage. When polyps are present and cause marked mechanical obstruction, polypectomy may be indicated. Adenoidectomy may be indicated primarily in younger children with moderate to severe nasal obstruction secondary to adenoidal hyperplasia and may decrease recurrence of sinusitis.

5. Dental referral is indicated in patients in whom a tooth abscess is suspected as the underlying cause of maxillary sinusitis.

6. Patient follow-up

   a. There are no clear recommendations for follow-up of acute sinusitis; however, it is reasonable to see a patient 10 to 14 days after therapy is initiated to establish whether symptoms and signs of sinusitis have completely resolved.

   b. Complications of sinusitis are uncommon. They occur more frequently in children and in patients with immunodeficiency disorders. Patients should be instructed to return to the physician immediately if symptoms worsen or if new symptoms such as visual disturbance, neck stiffness, or lethargy develop. Complications of sinusitis can be **local, orbital,** or **intracranial**. Prompt surgical consultation should be obtained if any of these complications arise.

   (1) Local complications include mucoceles or mucopyoceles. Mucoceles occur most frequently in the frontal sinus, and patients often present complaining of diplopia because the affected eye is displaced.

   (2) Orbital complications are the most common, and children with acute ethmoid sinusitis are the most prone to this complication. Preseptal or orbital cellulitis can occur; the latter is more severe because it involves orbital structures. Signs of orbital cellulitis include swelling and inflammation of the eyelids and proptosis of the affected eye. Complete ophthalmoplegia, impairment of vision, and chemosis indicate likely orbital abscess.

(3) Intracranial complications include cavernous sinus thrombosis (signs include bilateral orbital involvement, ophthalmoplegia, progressive and severe chemosis, retinal engorgement, fever, and prostration), meningitis, subdural empyema, and brain abscess.

SELECTED REFERENCES

Ahovuo-Saloranta A, Rautakorpi UM, Borisenko OV, et al. Antibiotics for acute maxillary sinusitis. *Cochrane Database Syst Rev.* 2008;(2):CD000243.

Chow AW, Benniger MS, Brook I, et al. IDSA clinical practice guideline for acute bacterial rhinosinusitis in children and adults. *Clin Infect Dis.* 2012;54(8):e72–e112.

Committee on Drugs. Use of codeine- and dextromethorphan-containing cough remedies in children. *Pediatrics.* 1997;(99):918.

Glacy J, Putnam K, Godfrey S, et al. *Treatment for seasonal allergic rhinitis.* Agency for Healthcare Research and Quality; 2013. Effective Health Care Program/Comparative Effectiveness Review 120. AHRQ Publication No. 13-EHC098-EF.

Khalil H, Nunez DA. Functional endoscopic sinus surgery for chronic rhinosinusitis. *Cochrane Database Syst Rev.* 2006;(3):CD004458.

Linde K, Barrett B, Bauer R, et al. Echinacea for preventing and treating the common cold. *Cochrane Database Syst Rev.* 2006;(1):CD000530.

Mishra A, Kawatra R, Gola M. Interventions for atrophic rhinitis. *Cochrane Database Syst Rev.* 2012;(2):CD008280.

Oduwole O, Meremikwu MM, Oyo-Ita A, Udoh EE. Honey for acute cough in children. *Cochrane Database Syst Rev.* 2012;(3):CD007094.

Radulovic S, Calderon MA, Wilson D, Durham S. Sublingual immunotherapy for allergic rhinitis. *Cochrane Database Syst Rev.* 2010;(12):CD002893.

Shaikh N, Wald ER, Pi M. Decongestants, antihistamines and nasal irrigation for acute sinusitis in children. *Cochrane Database Syst Rev.* 2012;(9):CD007909.

Smith SM, Schroeder K, Fahey T. Over-the-counter (OTC) medications for acute cough in children and adults in ambulatory settings. *Cochrane Database Syst Rev.* 2012;(8):CD001831.

Wald ER, Applegate KE, Bordley C, et al. Clinical practice guideline for the diagnosis and management of acute bacterial sinusitis in children aged 1 to 18 years. *Pediatrics.* 2013;132(1):e262–e280.

Zalmanovici Trestioreanu A, Yaphe J. Intranasal steroids for acute sinusitis. *Cochrane Database Syst Rev.* 2009;(4):CD005149.

---

55 Scrotal Complaints

Michael N. Nduati, MD, MBA, MPH, & John A. Heydt, MD

KEY POINTS

- A firm grounding in scrotal anatomy is helpful in approaching the patient with scrotal complaints. (SOR **C**)
- Scrotal complaints affect 0.1% to 0.3% of the male population each year; most causes can be determined by history and limited testing. (SOR **C**)
- Scrotal pain can have an insidious (≥48 hours) or acute (≤48 hours) onset; it is important to identify acute scrotal emergencies quickly. (SOR **C**)

I. Definition. Scrotal pain refers to discomfort and pain originating from or referred to the scrotum. Knowledge of **scrotal anatomy** (Figure 55–1) is fundamental to diagnosing scrotal complaints. For example, the **tunica vaginalis** is a potential space where fluids (such

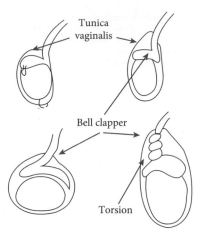

FIGURE 55–1. Normal testicular anatomy and the bell clapper deformity.

as water [hydrocele], blood [hematocele], and pus [pyocele]) can accumulate, whereas the **epididymis** houses the vas deferens and the testicular blood vessels. It is essential that a provider be able to differentiate between common benign diagnoses and **scrotal emergencies** (e.g., testicular torsion, incarcerated hernia, and Fournier gangrene) that require immediate intervention.

II. Common Diagnoses

A. Testicular causes

1. **Epididymitis** is the most common cause of scrotal pain in adults in the outpatient setting. It most commonly occurs in sexually active men from retrograde spread of prostatitis or urethral secretions through the vas deferens, but may also occur in prepubertal boys with urologic abnormalities such as ectopic ureters or congenital/acquired urethral strictures.

   a. In **sexually active men younger than 35 years,** epididymitis is usually associated with urethritis and caused by *Neisseria gonorrhoeae* or *Chlamydia trachomatis,* but it may be due to *Ureaplasma* or *Mycoplasma* infections.

   b. In **sexually monogamous men older than 35 years,** epididymitis is usually caused by urinary tract pathogens such as *Escherichia coli* and other enteric coliform bacteria, and it may occur in association with cystitis or prostatitis.

2. In cases of **orchitis,** viral infection, particularly mumps, is the most frequent culprit. Approximately 20% to 30% of males who contract mumps develop orchitis, and 30% of those affected have involvement of both testes. Other rare viral causes include varicella, coxsackievirus, and echovirus. Orchitis is usually associated with epididymitis, known as epididymo-orchitis.

3. **Testicular torsion** occurs most frequently in neonates and adolescent boys (Figure 55–1). The annual incidence in men younger than 25 years is 1 in 4000, with a peak age of 14 years. Occurrence is rare among those older than 30 years. The overall risk of having either testicular torsion or torsion of the testicular appendix by 25 years of age is 1 in 160.

   a. Predisposing conditions include the **"bell clapper deformity"** (in which the testicle lacks attachment to the tunica vaginalis and hangs freely; Figure 55–1), which occurs in 12% of males, as well as small testicles, excessive exercise, straining, cremasteric spasm, sexual activity, a sudden scare, immersion in cold water, attempted reduction of an inguinal hernia, or trauma.

   b. The incidence of **torsion of the testicular appendix** peaks at 10 years of age, and it is the leading cause of acute scrotal pathology in childhood. This condition almost always occurs prior to puberty and shares risk factors with testicular torsion.

4. With **traumatic injuries,** severe scrotal trauma is uncommon and results either from the testicle being compressed against the pubic bone or from straddle injury.

5. Testicular tumors are the most common malignant tumors in men between 25 and 35 years of age (lifetime risk of 1 in 250, or 0.4%). A history of cryptorchidism (undescended testicle[s]) greatly increases the risk of testicular neoplasm. Testicular malignancy frequently leads to testicular torsion.

CRYPTORCHIDISM

Undescended testicle(s) (cryptorchidism) occurs in 3% to 5% of term newborns and up to 30% of premature infants. Most testicles descend spontaneously, so the prevalence is 1% for boys by 1 year of age. Because of the associated risk of testicular neoplasms and decreased fertility, urologic consultation for orchiopexy is indicated between 6 months and 1 year of age.

B. **Extratesticular causes** can produce scrotal pain and swelling.
   1. **Inguinal hernias** can be direct or indirect and are common at all ages. Congenital defects and straining are predisposing factors.
   2. **Prostatitis** (see Section II.A.1.b) can refer to pain to the scrotum via the same sensory nerve fibers innervating the testicles.
   3. **Renal colic** from urinary tract lithiases also causes referred scrotal pain. Risk factors include a positive family history, decreased fluid intake, and residency in the southeastern United States.
   4. **Hydrocele,** a fluid-filled mass in the scrotal sac, is usually an idiopathic congenital condition; new-onset hydrocele in young men may be associated with testicular tumor.
   5. **Varicocele,** dilatation and tortuosity of the pampiniform plexus, rarely occurs before 10 years of age and is the main cause of male infertility. It is found in approximately 15% of older men.
   6. **Spermatocele** is a small cystic mass just above the testis.
   7. **Fournier gangrene** represents a surgical emergency. It is a necrotizing fasciitis of the perineum due to a mixed aerobic/anaerobic bacterial infection and frequently involves the scrotum.
III. **Signs and Symptoms** (see Table 55–1).
A. **Testicular causes**
   1. **Acute epididymitis** can be difficult to distinguish from testicular torsion. It may present with epididymal swelling and gradual onset of pain with fever, dysuria, and urinary frequency.
      a. The **cremasteric reflex** (elicited by stroking or pinching the inner thigh, causing the ipsilateral testicle to retract toward the inguinal canal) is present in epididymitis but not in testicular torsion.
      b. **Prehn sign** is relief of pain on elevation of the testicle when the patient is in the supine position. This may occur with epididymitis but not with testicular torsion (where elevation of the testis usually worsens pain). This maneuver is not specific to epididymitis.
   2. **Testicular torsion**
      a. Bell clapper deformity may be noted in older children at risk for testicular torsion (Figure 55–1). With torsion, the testicle rapidly becomes firm and tender and enlarges, with the epididymis, into a solitary mass. The scrotum can become erythematous and edematous, similar to the presentation in epididymitis.
      b. A small bluish discoloration (the **"blue dot sign"**) may be seen through scrotal skin near the upper testicular pole. Coupled with pain, this finding is pathognomonic for torsion of the testicular appendix.
      c. Males with torsion commonly will have experienced similar transient pain in the past, which is caused by intermittent torsion with spontaneous resolution. Complete torsion occurs when the testicle twists ≥360 degrees. Torsion rarely occurs after trauma (4%–8% of cases), but a history of trauma does not exclude the possibility of torsion. The presence of pain of less than 24 hours' duration, nausea/vomiting, high position of the testicle (on the affected side), and abnormal cremasteric reflex makes torsion more likely.

TABLE 55–1. DIFFERENTIAL DIAGNOSIS OF SCROTAL COMPLAINTS

Diagnosis	History	Examination	Tests
Testicular			
Testicular torsion	**Acute onset,** unilateral swelling and pain, nausea and vomiting, with or without previous symptoms; no constitutional symptoms	Unilateral testicular swelling; bell clapper deformity; no testicular cremasteric reflex or Prehn sign	Color Doppler US
Torsion of the testicular appendix	Moderate pain, **acute onset,** swelling; no constitutional symptoms	Firm tender nodule in the upper pole of epididymis; blue dot sign	No tests needed; color Doppler US if diagnosis unclear
Orchitis	Unilateral/bilateral testicular pain/swelling; if mumps, occurs 4–7 d after parotitis	Unilateral or bilateral testicular swelling/tenderness	No tests needed
Testicular hematomas/hematocele	**Trauma,** pain, swelling, nausea, and vomiting	Ecchymosis and enlargement of the affected testicle	Color Doppler US
Testicular rupture	**Trauma** history, pain, swelling, nausea, and vomiting	Ecchymosis and enlargement of the affected testicle	Color Doppler US
Testicular neoplasms	**Enlarging scrotal mass**/testicular nodule; occasional pain, if hemorrhage	Palpable nodule or enlarged testicle; gynecomastia, left supraclavicular node	Scrotal US, tumor markers, biopsy
Hydrocele	Painless testicular swelling	Minimally tender **transilluminating** swelling around the testicle	Scrotal US
Epididymis			
Epididymitis	Fevers, chills, rigors, unilateral scrotal swelling, and pain	**Swollen/tender** upper posterior testicle, presence of cremasteric reflex, Prehn sign	UA, urethral smear, color Doppler US if diagnosis unclear; VCUG and renal/bladder US in prepubertal boys
Spermatocele	Asymptomatic	**Painless nodule** above the testicle (spermatic cord)	No tests needed
Traumatic epididymitis	**Trauma** a few days prior; pain and swelling	Possible ecchymosis, unilateral or bilateral edema; cremasteric reflex and Prehn sign present	No tests needed; color Doppler US if diagnosis unclear
Spermatic Cord (and above)			
Inguinal hernia	Variable pain, enlargement in scrotum or bulge of the abdominal wall	Palpable swelling **on abdominal wall or extends through inguinal ring;** increases with Valsalva maneuver	No tests needed, but CT scan of the abdomen and pelvis may be helpful
Varicocele	Swelling and dull scrotal heaviness, worse with exercise	Supratesticular **"bag of worms,"** collapsing with the supine position	No tests needed; color Doppler US if uncertain
Skin Involvement			
Fournier gangrene	**Severe pain, fever,** tachycardia, hypotension	Tense skin edema, blisters/bullae, crepitus, or subcutaneous gas	No tests needed prior to surgical debridement; CT or MRI may be helpful
Sebaceous cyst (epidermoid cyst)	Slow growing, movable lump, can become painful, red, and drain cheesy, foul-smelling material	**Smooth, round mass in epidermis,** size varies up to several centimeters, contains keratin and/or purulent material	No tests needed

CT, computerized tomogram; MRI, magnetic resonance imaging; UA, urinalysis; US, ultrasound; VCUG, voiding cystourethrogram.

B. Extratesticular causes

1. **Renal colic** can produce severe, intermittent flank pain, but the pain can radiate to the abdomen, pubic area, or scrotum. Nausea, vomiting, fevers, chills, and urinary frequency may be present. Renal colic can present with hematuria, flank tenderness, and hyperparesthesias of the abdominal skin, but examination of the scrotum is unremarkable.

2. **Prostatitis** presents with fever, chills, dysuria, urinary frequency, or myalgias. Pain may be located in the scrotal, perineal, or back region. Patients may also experience pain with ejaculation and defecation. A warm, tender, spongy, enlarged prostate can be palpated on digital rectal examination.

3. **Fournier gangrene** causes severe pain and can be associated with tense edema of the skin, blisters, crepitus, and systemic signs such as fever, tachycardia, and hypotension.

4. A patient with a **strangulated inguinal hernia** often presents with severe pain, and bowel sounds can be audible in the scrotum if there is herniated bowel.

IV. **Diagnostic Tests** (see Table 55–1). Scrotal complaints can often be diagnosed with a careful history and physical examination, maintaining a high index of suspicion for serious conditions such as testicular torsion, acute infectious epididymitis, and acute incarcerated inguinal hernia.

   A. A **urinalysis** can be used to detect pyuria and bacteriuria with epididymitis or prostatitis, and microscopic hematuria in urinary lithiasis. Urinalysis is normal in testicular torsion and torsion of the testicular appendix. Urine culture should be performed if epididymitis is suspected.

   B. **Urethral smear,** produced by inserting a small, sterile cotton-tipped probe into the urethra for one 360-degree turn and then layering the secretions on a microscope slide for Gram stain and microscopic examination, is helpful in evaluation of epididymitis in sexually active men younger than 35 years or older men with suspected sexually transmitted epididymitis. The smear can demonstrate white blood cells (WBCs) and bacteria.

   C. An elevated **WBC count** and **erythrocyte sedimentation rate** or **C-reactive protein** can occur in febrile patients and those with infection; an elevated WBC count can also occur in torsion, usually as a stress reaction.

   D. **Doppler studies** can be used to measure testicular blood flow.

      1. For evaluation of scrotal masses, **color Doppler ultrasonography** is the preferred diagnostic test, with a sensitivity of approximately 90% and a specificity of 100% in testicular torsion. (SOR **B**) It is indicated for scrotal swelling and severe scrotal pain, when the diagnosis of testicular torsion is uncertain. Color Doppler ultrasonography can also be used for the diagnosis of incarcerated hernia, varicocele, hematoma, and testicular rupture and can differentiate testicular appendiceal torsion (increased blood flow) from testicular torsion (decreased/absent blood flow).

      2. **Doppler stethoscope** and **conventional grayscale ultrasonography** are not as accurate as color ultrasonography and should not be used.

   E. **Radionuclide scintigraphy** demonstrates decreased blood flow to the affected testicle within a few hours in torsion (sensitivity/specificity ≥90% for an acute torsion when performed by an experienced physician) and increased blood flow in patients with epididymitis. The main limitation with scintigraphy is the delay in results compared to color Doppler ultrasonography.

   F. **Scrotal ultrasound** is extremely accurate in distinguishing between solid and fluid-filled masses.

   G. In prepubertal boys with epididymitis/urinary tract infection, **renal/bladder ultrasound and voiding cystourethrogram** are indicated to evaluate for urinary tract anomalies.

   H. **Magnetic resonance imaging (MRI)** or **computerized tomography (CT)** may be helpful in identifying cancers or showing air along the fascial planes and deep tissue involvement in Fournier gangrene.

V. **Treatment**

   A. **Testicular conditions**

      1. In **acute epididymitis,** treatment goals include pain relief and addressing the underlying infection. In most cases, this is feasible in the outpatient setting.

         a. **Pain relief** is best accomplished by ice packs for 24 to 48 hours, bed rest, scrotal support, and oral medications, such as ibuprofen (600–800 mg, three to four times daily) as needed for mild/moderate pain, acetaminophen with codeine (325/30 mg), or hydrocodone (5 mg, four times daily) as needed for severe pain. A cord block with 5 to 8 mL of a 50:50 mixture of 1% lidocaine and 0.5% bupivacaine can be helpful if administered by an experienced physician.

         b. **Antibiotic** selection is based on age and sexual history. As a general rule, in sexually active men younger than 35 years, the treatment of choice is a single 250-mg intramuscular dose of ceftriaxone plus doxycycline (100 mg orally twice daily for 10 days). In men older than 35 years who are at a low risk for sexually transmitted infections, treatment options include fluoroquinolones (e.g., ofloxacin, 300 mg orally twice daily, or levofloxacin, 500 mg orally once daily, either for 10 days). (SOR **G**)

    c. Hospitalization may be required for men with high fevers, intractable pain, toxic appearance, or suspicion of scrotal abscess.

    d. Surgical drainage, orchiectomy, or both is warranted when severe epididymo-orchitis results in abscess formation.

    e. Urologic consultation and **surgical exploration** are indicated when the diagnosis is unclear or if testicular torsion is suspected (see Section V.A.3).

  2. The pain of **orchitis** can be managed similarly to that of epididymitis (see Section V.A.1.a).

  3. Torsion

    a. If **testicular torsion** is confirmed or high clinical suspicion is present, immediate urologic referral should be made, since the torsed spermatic cord cuts off the blood flow in the testicular vessels. Surgery should be performed within 6 hours of onset of testicular pain to maximize the odds of salvaging the testis. (SOR **B**) If detorsion is accomplished within 6 hours, 90% of testicles remain viable; after 12 hours, viability drops to 50%; and at 24 to 48 hours, only 10% of testicles are viable. No testicle is viable after 48 hours. Manual detorsion is successful in approximately 30% to 70% of cases and is performed by rotating the affected testicle away from the midline, like opening a book. In patients with torsion, bilateral orchiopexy (fixation of the testes to the scrotal wall) is recommended, because the bell clapper deformity exists in both testicles approximately 40% of the time.

    b. Testicular appendix torsion is managed conservatively with analgesics, ice, and scrotal elevation. Activity may worsen symptoms, so it should be restricted. If pain and swelling are severe and the diagnosis is clear, urologic consultation for local nerve block can control pain. If the diagnosis is unclear, prompt diagnostic testing (see Section IV.D.1), referral for exploration, or both should be done.

  4. Trauma

    a. For **testis rupture,** emergent referral should be made for repair; **testicular hematoma** and hematocele also require surgical consultation.

    b. Traumatic epididymitis, which occurs a few days after trauma, is managed conservatively with anti-inflammatory medications, elevation, and ice.

  5. Testicular neoplasms should be managed in consultation with a urologic oncologist.

B. Extratesticular causes

  1. Inguinal hernias require urgent surgical consultation if incarcerated or strangulated, and elective repair if reducible.

  2. Renal colic (see Chapter 35).

  3. Prostatitis is generally managed with antibiotics (see Chapter 60).

  4. Hydroceles in infants usually spontaneously resolve during the first 1 to 2 years of life. Hydroceles persisting beyond 1 to 2 years of age, accompanied by hernia, or occurring beyond infancy require surgical consultation for repair.

  5. Because **varicoceles** can affect testicular growth and fertility, consultation with a urologist for elective spermatic vein ligation is prudent. A noncollapsible varicocele raises suspicion for retroperitoneal tumor and requires appropriate imaging (e.g., abdominal MRI or CT scan) and specialist consultation based on findings.

  6. Only large **spermatoceles** require urologic consultation for excision.

  7. Emergent urologic consultation for surgical exploration and debridement of necrotic tissue is necessary for **Fournier gangrene.** Intravenous antibiotics and hemodynamic support should also be provided, but there is near 100% mortality if surgical debridement is not performed.

SELECTED REFERENCES

Eyre RC. Evaluation of the acute scrotum in adults. www.uptodate.com, literature review current through February 2013.

Ogunyemi OI. Testicular torsion. http://emedicine.medscape.com/article/2036003-overview. Updated August 25, 2011. Accessed April 2013.

Tiemstra JD, Kapoor S. Evaluation of scrotal masses. *Am Fam Physician.* 2008;78(10):1165–1170.

Trojian TH, Lishnak TS, Heiman D. Epididymitis and orchitis: an overview. *Am Fam Physician.* 2009; 79(7):583–587.

56 Sore Throat

L. Peter Schwiebert, MD

KEY POINTS

- Most sore throats encountered in ambulatory family medicine are caused by viruses or irritants. (SOR ❸)
- Clues to a diagnosis of strep throat include a temperature ≥38°C, absence of cough, tender anterior cervical adenopathy, or tonsillar exudate/swelling. (SOR ❸)
- Antibiotics are not indicated in most patients with sore throat. (SOR ❹)

I. **Definition.** Sore throat is a pharyngeal sensation of scratchiness or pain due to a wide spectrum of causes, including endogenous/exogenous irritants (e.g., gastroesophageal reflux, allergens, tobacco smoke, low humidity) and infections (viral or bacterial).

II. **Common Diagnoses.** In ambulatory primary care, up to 8% of patient visits per year are for a sore throat. Common causes are as follows:

   A. **Irritants.** Thirty to sixty-five percent of individuals with sore throat have no specific causative pathogen. Irritants are causative in an undetermined number of these cases. Patients at risk include smokers (tobacco is the most common environmental irritant), those whose clinical picture is compatible with allergies or gastroesophageal reflux disease (GERD) (see later), or those who are exposed to environmental irritants (e.g., dust, low humidity, animals, textiles, solvents).

   B. **Viral infections** (up to 90% of adults and 70% of children) including common cold viruses (rhinovirus, coronavirus, respiratory syncytial virus, parainfluenza virus), herpesvirus, adenovirus, coxsackievirus, and infectious mononucleosis (IM) viruses (cytomegalovirus and Epstein-Barr virus [EBV]). Sore throat is more likely caused by common cold viruses during community outbreaks in colder months of the year. Adenoviral infections are frequent (up to 19%) causes of exudative pharyngitis in children younger than 6 years, and coxsackievirus infections are also most common in young children during the summer and fall. IM is most common in upper-socioeconomic-class adolescents and young adults (industrialized societies) living in close contact with one another (e.g., students living in college dormitories).

   C. **Group A β-hemolytic streptococcal (GABHS) infection** (5%–17% of cases in adults and 15%–36% of cases in children). GABHS infection is most common in 5- to 15-year olds during the winter/spring months and can, like other infections, occur as an epidemic.

III. **Symptoms**

   A. **Sore throat**

   1. Scratchy, dry throat is most common with irritants or common cold viruses.

   2. Painful sore throat with dysphagia is typical of streptococcal infection, IM, coxsackievirus, herpesvirus, or adenovirus.

   B. **Other symptoms**

   1. Patients with **allergies** classically present with paroxysms of sneezing, watery, itchy eyes, and rhinorrhea associated with exposure to the allergen, although these symptoms may be absent (see Chapters 53 and 54).

   2. Individuals with sore throat due to **GERD** often provide a history of heartburn/sour eructations, worsening symptoms after a large meal or with recumbency, associated nonproductive cough, and relief with nonprescription histamine-2 blockers, antacids, or proton pump inhibitors (see Chapter 19).

   3. The presence of cough, rhinorrhea, conjunctivitis, or diarrhea decreases the likelihood of streptococcal infection and increases the likelihood of irritants, allergies, or viral infection.

   4. Individuals with **streptococcal infection** may complain of associated symptoms of chills, malaise, headache, mild neck stiffness, and some gastrointestinal symptoms, though these symptoms are not specific for this diagnosis.

IV. **Signs.** Since GABHS pharyngitis is the only common cause of sore throat for which antibiotics are indicated and since sore throat and patient requests for antibiotic treatment are common, researchers have investigated clinical scoring systems to predict the likelihood of streptococcal infection. The best-known system is the Centor Strep Score; McIsaac et al. validated this scoring system in a family medicine population of children and adults (Table 56–1). The Centor and McIsaac criteria can identify those with a low risk of GABHS pharyngitis in settings of no

TABLE 56-1. McISAAC MODIFICATION OF THE CENTOR STREP SCORE

1. Add Points for Patient

Symptoms or Signs	Points
History of fever or measured body temperature ≥38°C (100.4°F)	1
Absence of cough	1
Tender anterior cervical adenopathy	1
Tonsillar swelling or exudates	1
Age ≤15 yr	1
Age ≥45 yr	-1

2. Find Risk of Strep

Points	Estimated Likelihood of Streptococcal Infection (%)
-1 or 0	1-2.5
1	5-10
2	11-17
3	28-35
4 or 5	51-53

GABHS epidemics and/or low prevalence of rheumatic fever. Patients with a score of 0 or 1 do not require antibiotics or further testing for GABHS. (SOR **Ⓐ**) Because the presentation of sore throat in children younger than 3 years is different from that in older children and adults, Centor–McIsaac scoring has limited utility in a very young population. (Also see epiglottitis, retropharyngeal abscess, peritonsillar abscess, and carotidynia.)

A. The ability of an individual symptom or sign to predict a diagnosis of strep throat is limited. For example,

   1. Exudative pharyngitis also occurs with viral infections (53% of children younger than 6 years with this sign had adenoviral infection, as do 50% of patients with IM).

   2. Fifty-six percent of pediatric patients with adenoviral infection present with fever and temperature ≥40°C (104°F); moderate to high fever is also associated with coxsackievirus and initial outbreaks of herpesvirus infections.

   3. More than 90% of patients with IM have **cervical lymphadenopathy** (posterior chain).

B. Other signs characteristic of common causes of sore throat. Coxsackievirus infections are associated with erythematous-based small vesicles or ulcers in the pharynx and may be associated with similar papulovesicles on the palms and soles. The shallow, erythematous-based vesicles and ulcers of herpesvirus can occur anywhere on the pharynx, gingiva, or vermilion border.

EPIGLOTTITIS

Epiglottitis should be considered when there is a rapidly worsening sore throat, fever, muffled voice, and dysphagia. Epiglottitis is usually caused by *Haemophilus influenzae* (but pediatric incidence of this organism has decreased because of Hib immunization such that the incidence now peaks between 20 and 45 years of age); *Streptococcus pyogenes, Staphylococcus aureus,* or viruses can also be causative. Lateral neck radiographs are 90% sensitive and show an enlarged epiglottis ("thumb sign") with hypopharyngeal distention. Because of the danger of critical airway obstruction, suspected epiglottitis requires parenteral antibiotics in an intensive care setting where immediate intubation is available.

RETROPHARYNGEAL ABSCESS

Retropharyngeal abscess is a complication of infected retropharyngeal lymph nodes (usually caused by GABHS infection) and is more common in pediatric than adult populations. Presenting symptoms of dysphagia and a lateral neck radiograph showing an increased prevertebral space are characteristic.

PERITONSILLAR ABSCESS

Peritonsillar abscess (quinsy), a suppurative complication of superficial tonsillitis, is most common in 14- to 20-year olds and presents with worsening sore throat, fever, and dysphagia/odynophagia. Likely agents include *Streptococcus pyogenes, Staphylococcus aureus, H. influenzae*, or anaerobes. Examination reveals a muffled "hot potato" voice, trismus (difficulty opening the mouth), and an erythematous, swollen tonsil pushing the uvula to the opposite side. The gold standard for diagnosis is needle aspiration of pus from the abscess (should only be performed with proper training), and the currently recommended treatment is twice-daily clindamycin or a second- or third-generation cephalosporin.

CAROTIDYNIA

Carotidynia is an idiopathic inflammation of the carotid sheath and is a common cause of "sore throat," which, on examination, is actually tenderness over the common carotid sheath. Carotidynia responds rapidly to nonsteroidal drugs (e.g., indomethacin, 25–50 mg, three times daily with food, continued for 5–7 days or until symptoms resolve, whichever occurs first).

V. **Laboratory Tests.** On the basis of clinical findings alone, one can arrive at a presumptive diagnosis in many patients presenting with sore throat. In those with irritant exposure or Centor–McIsaac score of 0 to 1, no further laboratory workup of sore throat is indicated and one can proceed with symptomatic treatment. Diagnostic studies for GABHS infection are not indicated in children <3 years of age because these infections are uncommon in this age group.

A. **Streptococcal testing.** A decision on which patients with pharyngitis should have a streptococcal screen depends on the physician's goals—minimizing total cost, minimizing risks associated with a missed diagnosis, or minimizing the cost of a missed diagnosis and unnecessary use of antibiotics. The following strategy, which is more cost-effective than mass screening but minimizes chances of missing a case of streptococcal pharyngitis, is recommended. A rapid streptococcal screen should be performed on patients with a sore throat and an intermediate pretest likelihood of streptococcal pharyngitis. In patients with intermediate or higher likelihood of GABHS pharyngitis (Centor–McIsaac score of 3 or more), rapid antigen testing is recommended by the Infectious Disease Society of America to confirm the diagnosis. In children and adolescents, a negative test should be backed up by culture.

1. **Rapid streptococcal screen** is a 10-minute test with a sensitivity of 86% to 94.8% and a specificity of >95% for detection of streptococcal pharyngitis. Proper collection requires that the swab must vigorously contact both tonsils or tonsillar fossae and the posterior pharyngeal wall. It is the test of choice in confirming suspected streptococcal pharyngitis. With appropriate test selection, therapeutic decisions can confidently be based on a positive result. However, a negative screen result in the context of clinical suspicion of streptococcal pharyngitis should be followed up with blood agar plate (BAP) culture.

2. **Throat culture.** The BAP culture is 95% sensitive and has a low false-positive rate in diagnosing streptococcal pharyngitis, but it requires 24 hours' incubation.

3. A **follow-up screen** to test for cure is not recommended or indicated in patients who respond clinically to antibiotic therapy within 5 days. However, in patients with a history of rheumatic fever, post-treatment cultures should be done to ensure eradication of GABHS infection.

4. The **carrier state** (positive rapid strep screen or BAP culture with low pretest likelihood or without GABHS antigenemia) usually represents low infectivity or risk for developing rheumatic fever.

B. **Heterophile antibody latex agglutination test** has a sensitivity of 87% (79%–90%) and a specificity of 91% (82%–99%) in patients >16 years old for diagnosing IM. False-negative testing approaches 25% in the first week of illness and decreases to 5% by third week of illness. A complete blood cell count with differential smear showing relative or absolute lymphocytosis and typically >10% atypical lymphocytes, at least 50% lymphocytes, and at least 10% atypical lymphocytes also supports this diagnosis.

C. Other tests

1. Although not common, *Neisseria gonorrhoeae* infection is possible in patients with pharyngitis and a history of oral-genital sexual relations; in cases where suspicion is high (e.g., associated penile discharge), pharyngeal, endocervical, and urethral cultures for gonorrhea and chlamydia should be done.

2. **Viral capsid antigen (VCA) immunoglobulin (Ig)** M and G antibodies are highly sensitive and specific for diagnosing IM (sensitivity 97%, specificity 94%) and slightly better than a positive heterophile test (likelihood ratio 16 vs. 9.7–28), but negative VCA IgG and IgM tests are superior to heterophile testing in ruling out IM due to EBV.

3. **Abdominal ultrasound** can assess splenic size, but because of individual variability in splenic size, a single ultrasound assessment of splenic size during illness may not accurately reflect splenomegaly.

VI. Treatment. Because 80% to 90% of cases of pharyngitis are caused by viruses or irritants, antibiotics are not indicated for most patients with this complaint. Despite this finding, studies have shown that antibiotics are prescribed for 73% of adults with acute pharyngitis. Dangers of this practice include unnecessary cost, possible allergic reaction, and development of resistant bacterial strains. To avoid these drawbacks, it is important to base antibiotic use on strict criteria and use nonantibiotic treatment in cases not meeting these criteria.

A. Environmental irritants should be avoided if possible. In particular, patients should be encouraged to stop smoking, avoid allergens or dusty environments, and humidify low-humidity environments. Treatment of allergies is discussed in Chapter 54, and management of GERD is discussed in Chapter 19.

B. Viral infections (see also Chapter 54) (e.g., common cold, adenovirus, coxsackievirus, and herpesvirus) are self-limited, lasting from a few days to 2 weeks. Patients can obtain symptomatic relief with the following regimens:

1. **Adequate hydration should be encouraged and topical pain relief** can be provided by as-needed lozenges (e.g., Cepastat or Chloraseptic) or saline nasal spray or gargles, made by mixing one-fourth tsp of salt in 4 oz of warm water.

   a. Patients with oropharyngeal lesions of coxsackievirus or herpes simplex virus may benefit from viscous Xylocaine 2% or benzocaine 15%, applied to lesions every 3 to 4 hours with a cotton-tipped applicator; soothing rinses (one-fourth tsp of baking soda in 4 oz of warm water or saline, swished orally and then expectorated three or four times daily).

2. **Analgesic drugs** include either aspirin, 650 mg every 4 to 6 hours orally in adults, or acetaminophen, 5 to 10 mg/kg/d every 4 to 6 hours orally in adolescents and children (aspirin avoidance due to concern for Reye syndrome). Alternate nonprescription drugs include ibuprofen (200–400 mg every 4–6 hours) or naproxen sodium (220–440 mg initially, followed by 220 mg every 8–12 hours for those older than 11 years). Codeine relieves more severe discomfort; the dosage is 30 to 60 mg orally every 4 to 6 hours in adults or 3 mg/kg/d orally every 4 to 6 hours in children. Systematic reviews and several randomized trials confirm the superiority of analgesics to placebo in alleviating sore throat in adults. (SOR **Ⓐ**)

3. **Zinc gluconate** is not recommended (SOR **Ⓑ**), and evidence for benefit of various herbal remedies is inconsistent from well-controlled studies. (SOR **Ⓒ**)

C. Streptococcal infections. Antibiotic therapy instituted within 2 to 3 days of onset of symptoms hastens symptomatic improvement in patients with positive culture results or a high likelihood of streptococcal infection, as well as decreasing contagion (especially if the patient lives in close contact with others). The incidence of suppurative complications (e.g., peritonsillar abscess) and immune complications (e.g., glomerulonephritis) is low, regardless of whether antibiotics are used or not. For every 100 patients treated with antibiotics rather than placebo in Cochrane-reviewed trials, there was one less case of acute rheumatic fever, two fewer cases of acute otitis media, and three fewer cases of quinsy. (SOR **Ⓐ**)

1. **Indications**

   b. Intermediate or higher Centor–McIsaac score and positive rapid antigen testing (Table 56–1).

   c. Studies have demonstrated that delaying therapy for 48 hours does not interfere with antibiotic efficacy in reducing the risk of complications.

2. **Regimens**

   a. **Penicillin** is the drug of choice (in nonpenicillin-allergic patients); there is no evidence of resistance (e.g., resurgence of rheumatic fever caused by lower rates of GABHS elimination by penicillin). (SOR **Ⓐ**)

    (1) Oral penicillin V potassium, 500 mg, two to three times daily for 10 days, is the treatment for those over 60 lb (27 kg); those weighing less should receive 30 to 50 mg/kg/d in two or three divided doses, also for 10 days.

    (2) Penicillin G benzathine may be preferred for patients in whom compliance with the oral regimen or follow-up is questionable. Adults and children weighing over 27 kg (60 lb) should receive 1.2 million units (U) intramuscularly (IM) and those weighing 27 kg or less should receive 600,000 U IM. **Bicillin C-R** is also effective and causes less local reaction than penicillin G benzathine alone; dosing is 2.4 million U IM for those weighing over 60 lb, 900,000 to 1.2 million U IM for children weighing between 30 and 60 lb, and 600,000 U IM for children weighing less than 30 lb.

  b. Erythromycin (e.g., Ery-Tab, Eryc, or E-Mycin) is the drug of choice for penicillin-allergic patients. Adults should receive 500 mg orally twice daily for 10 days. The pediatric dosage is 30 to 50 mg/kg/d, given in two or four divided doses. Another macrolide, **azithromycin** (e.g., Zithromax), 500 mg orally on day 1 and 250 mg on days 2 to 5, is also effective for adults; the dosage for pediatric patients older than 2 years is 12 mg/kg/d for 5 days.

  c. In addition to azithromycin, the following 5-day regimens are effective for the treatment of GABHS infection: cefaclor 40 mg/kg/d in two doses, cefuroxime axetil 20 to 30 mg/kg/d in two doses, or cefprozil 15 to 30 mg/kg/d in two doses. Shorter regimens can improve compliance; disadvantages include higher cost and broader spectrum, which may foster bacterial resistance. Of interest, a meta-analysis of 35 studies showed superior bacteriologic and clinical cure with cephalosporins than with penicillin. (SOR **Ⓐ**)

3. Follow-up

  a. Failure to improve. Antibiotic therapy should improve symptoms within 12 to 24 hours; persistence of symptoms for a week after initiation of antibiotics may be due to poor adherence with the drug regimen or an undiagnosed second cause of pharyngitis, particularly IM, mycoplasma pneumonia, or adenovirus. In addition to evaluating for noncompliance, it may be helpful to test for other causes (see Sections V.B and V.C).

  b. Recurrent episodes of acute pharyngitis raise the issue of whether **acute streptococcal pharyngitis** or **acute viral pharyngitis with streptococcal carrier state** is occurring. **Viral pharyngitis** is suggested by clinical or epidemiologic findings consistent with viral infection, failure to improve on antistreptococcal antibiotics, no rise in antistreptolysin-O (ASO) titers, or positive streptococcal testing (rapid antigen test or culture) between episodes of pharyngitis. **Acute, recurrent streptococcal infection** is suggested by appropriate clinical or epidemiologic findings, dramatic response to antibiotic therapy, a rise in ASO titers, or negative streptococcal testing between episodes of acute pharyngitis.

  c. Based mainly on expert opinion, eradication of the carrier state may be beneficial in the following circumstances: children with a personal or family history of rheumatic fever or acute post-streptococcal glomerulonephritis, contacts of a patient with invasive streptococcal disease, GABHS epidemics in closed or semi-closed communities, or repeated documented symptomatic GABHS pharyngitis occurring in a family over several weeks despite appropriate treatment.

    (1) When eradication of the carrier state is appropriate (see Section V.A.4), the following **regimens** are effective based on evidence from a few randomized controlled trials: clindamycin, 20 mg/kg/d orally in three doses for 10 days (maximum of 1.8 g/d), or rifampin, 20 mg/kg/d orally in two doses for 4 days (up to 300 mg twice daily), *plus* the standard regimen of phenoxymethyl or penicillin G benzathine. Two other randomized controlled trials found oral cephalosporins effective in eradicating the carrier state compared with penicillin and rifampin.

4. Infectious mononucleosis

  a. Ninety-five percent of patients with **IM** recover uneventfully, and supportive treatment will suffice. Such therapy includes avoidance of contact sports or heavy lifting in the first 2 to 3 weeks of illness (especially if the patient has splenomegaly), adequate rest, and analgesics (see Section VI.B.3). Individuals evaluated a month or more after diagnosis should be afebrile, well hydrated, and asymptomatic with normal energy level without hepatomegaly or splenomegaly before gradual return to practice or competition is allowed (SOR **⊖**)

b. Corticosteroids may be necessary in the following circumstances: impending airway obstruction, severe thrombocytopenia, hemolytic anemia, or myocarditis. (SOR **❸**) Treatment should be initiated with prednisone (or any equivalent), 60 to 80 mg/d orally in divided doses, tapered over 1 to 2 weeks.

SELECTED REFERENCES

Aalbers J, O'Brien KK, Chan W-S, et al. Predicting streptococcal pharyngitis in adults in primary care: a systematic review of the diagnostic accuracy of symptoms and signs and validation of the Centor score. *BMC Med.* 2011;9:67.

Centor RM, Samlowski R. Avoiding sore throat morbidity and mortality: when is it not "just a sore throat?" *Am Fam Physician.* 2011;83:26, 28.

Chiappini D, Principi N, Mansi N, et al. Management of acute pharyngitis in children: summary of the Italian National Institute of Health guidelines. *Clin Ther.* 2012;34:1442–1458.

ESCMID Sore Throat Guideline Group, Pelucchi C, Grigoryan L, Galeone C, et al. Guideline for the management of acute sore throat. *Clin Microbiol Infect.* 2012;18(Suppl 1):1–28.

Gerber MA, Baltimore RS, et al. Prevention of rheumatic fever and diagnosis and treatment of acute streptococcal pharyngitis: a scientific statement from the American Heart Association Rheumatic Fever, Endocarditis, and Kawasaki Disease Committee of the Council on Cardiovascular Disease in the Young, the Interdisciplinary Council on Functional Genomics and Translational Biology, and the Interdisciplinary Council on Quality of Care and Outcomes Research: endorsed by the American Academy of Pediatrics. *Circulation.* 2009;119(11):1541–1551.

Putukian M, O'Connor FG, Stricker P, et al. Mononucleosis and athletic participation: an evidence-based subject review. *Clin J Sport Med.* 2008;18(4):309–315.

Shulman ST, Bisno AL, Clegg HW, et al. Clinical practice guideline for the diagnosis and management of group A streptococcal pharyngitis: 2012 update by the Infectious Diseases Society of America. *Clin Infect Dis.* 2012;55(10):1279–1282.

---

57 Syncope

Brian H. Halstater, MD, John Ragsdale III, MD, LeRoy C. White, MD, JD, & Felix Horng, MD, MBA

KEY POINTS

- A thorough history and physical examination will reveal a diagnosis in 45% of cases. (SOR **❸**)
- An electrocardiogram will be diagnostic in only 5% to 10% of cases, but should be done initially because it may reveal clues to underlying cardiac disease. (SOR **❸**)
- Most syncope is from neurally mediated reflex mechanisms (e.g., vasovagal or situational) or will be found to be idiopathic and can be effectively managed by the primary care physician. (SOR **❸**)
- Cardiac syncope is associated with a much higher 2-year mortality rate than all other types, and its detection is the primary focus of evaluation. (SOR **❸**)

I. Definition. Syncope is rapid-onset transient loss of consciousness caused by cerebral hypoperfusion followed by prompt complete recovery without intervention. Syncope is a symptom, not a disease, and must be differentiated from conditions that may at first appear as syncope. The task of the investigating physician is to determine whether the patient has syncope, rather than a condition mimicking syncope, and then to determine whether that condition is life-threatening.

  A. Syncope can be due to neurally mediated reflexes, decreased cardiac output, or cerebrovascular disease. **Neurally mediated syncope (also called neurocardiogenic syncope)** results from a reflex decrease in heart rate, blood pressure, or both. **Decreased cardiac output** can result from hypovolemia, structural heart disease, or arrhythmias.

B. Nonsyncopal disorders that may present with real or apparent loss of consciousness include seizure disorders, psychogenic "syncope," and metabolic disorders such as hypoglycemia or hyponatremia.

II. Common Diagnoses (Table 57–1). At least 10.5% of the population will have a syncopal event within a 17-year period. Based on the Framingham study, there is a 42% prevalence of syncope during the life of a 70-year-old person. Thirty-five percent of patients will have recurrences within 3 years. Eighty-two percent of recurrences occur in the first 2 years. Age older than 45 years is associated with a higher recurrence rate. Recurrences are not associated with increased mortality or sudden death.

The prevalence of syncope increases with age and is highest in the older institutionalized population. In the United States, syncope accounts for approximately 3% to 10% of emergency department visits and 6% of hospital admissions annually. Approximately 1 million patients are evaluated for syncope each year, at a cost of $750 million.

A. Syncope can be classified as **neurally mediated, cardiac, cerebrovascular, orthostatic, miscellaneous differentiated causes,** and **idiopathic** (unknown cause). Two-thirds of cases of syncope are either neurally mediated or cardiac. Multiple causes can coexist. A Mayo Clinic study of 987 patients with syncope who were referred for electrophysiological studies revealed multiple causes in 18.4%. The likelihood of multiple causes increased with age and in those with atrial fibrillation, those taking cardiac medications, or those in New York Heart Association classes II to IV.

1. Neurally mediated syncope (23% of all cases of syncope) refers to a reflex response that when triggered gives rise to vasodilation and/or bradycardia.

  a. Classic vasovagal syncope (18%) is mediated by emotional or orthostatic stress.

  b. Situational syncope (5%) is neurally mediated syncope associated with specific inciting factors such as urinating, coughing, or defecating.

2. Cardiac syncope (18%) has a higher mortality rate than all other etiologies (30% at 2 years, compared with 6% for all other etiologies).

  a. Arrhythmia underlies most cases of cardiac syncope. Risk factors for **bradyarrhythmia** include use of medications that delay atrioventricular (A-V) conduction (commonly beta- and calcium channel blockers). Risk factors for **tachyarrhythmia** include use of medications that increase A-V conduction (e.g., pseudoephedrine and other stimulants, both legal and illicit). A family history may reveal dysrhythmias such as prolonged QT interval and Wolff–Parkinson–White (WPW) syndrome.

  b. Structural heart disease. Circulatory demands outpace the heart's ability to increase its output. In patients with no known **structural heart disease,** a family history of unexplained sudden cardiac death increases the likelihood of hypertrophic obstructive cardiomyopathy or infiltrative disease such as sarcoid cardiomyopathy.

3. Cerebrovascular syncope (10%) most commonly results from vertebrobasilar artery insufficiency, transient ischemic attack (TIA), stroke (cerebrovascular accident [CVA]), or subclavian steal syndrome. Risk factors for **subclavian steal syndrome** are the same as those for CVA and TIA, but also include vigorous use of an upper extremity; when it occurs in younger individuals, a congenital anatomic variant is suspected.

4. Orthostatic syncope (8%) refers to syncope in which the upright position causes arterial hypotension. The autonomic system fails to compensate when the upright position is assumed. Medications are commonly implicated. When volume depletion is present, the autonomic system cannot maintain blood pressure due to insufficient volume. Note that similar symptoms may occur in vasovagal syncope.

5. Miscellaneous syncope (2%) most commonly includes psychiatric disorders.

6. Idiopathic syncope (34%) is when no underlying cause is identified. Interestingly, patients with idiopathic syncope have a slightly higher death rate than the general population.

III. Symptoms/pertinent history (Table 57–1). A careful history is essential to accurately assess syncope. This should include the patient's age, details of the syncopal event (timing and onset, association with activity or exercise, and associated symptoms including prodrome, palpitations, or chest pain), and previous occurrences with circumstances surrounding prior events. Additional history should include chronic diseases, family history, and medication use/substance abuse.

Differentiating between syncope and nonsyncope can be difficult. **Prodromal symptoms are common in syncope.** One notable exception is ventricular tachycardia, which can occur without a prodrome.

TABLE 57–1. DIFFERENTIAL DIAGNOSIS OF SYNCOPE

Category	Risk Factors	Signs and Symptoms
Neurally mediated vasovagal	Young women; exposure to stress, pain, enclosed space	Unpleasant stimulus Prodrome: nausea, lightheadedness, palpitations, tunnel vision, warmth Normal physical examination
Neurally mediated situational	Elderly	Preceded by micturition, cough, swallow, defecation Physical examination reveals orthostatic hypotension
Neurally mediated carotid sinus	Elderly, atherosclerotic disease	Syncope after head rotation/neck extension, wearing tight collar, shaving Carotid sinus massage causes hypotension or ventricular asystole
Orthostatic	Elderly, autonomic dysfunction, dehydration, prolonged recumbency, certain medications	Prodrome of nausea, lightheadedness, palpitations, tunnel vision, warmth Changing positions or rising to standing from sitting/lying position may reproduce symptoms
Cardiac arrhythmia	Sick sinus, A-V block medications, pacemaker malfunction; recent MI, supra- or ventricular tachycardia, WPW syndrome	No prodrome, occurrence while supine Physical examination may be normal or an abnormal heart rhythm may be found Abnormal ECG may be found
Cardiac structural	VHD, FHx sudden unexplained cardiac death	Occurrence with exertion, change in position, acute shortness of breath Cardiac examination may reveal a heart murmur Physical examination may show signs of CHF
Cerebrovascular	HTN, dyslipidemia, diabetes mellitus, old age, cigarette use	Vertigo, dysarthria, diplopia; excessive arm exercise Physical examination may reveal carotid bruit, focal neurologic deficit, or asymmetric upper extremity BPs
Miscellaneous differentiated	20- to 40-yr olds with frequent "fainting," alcohol abuse	Anxiety or depression; multiple somatic complaints Physical examination is normal Positive screen for depression or anxiety
Idiopathic		Absence of classic symptoms of other types of syncope

A-V, atrioventricular; BP, blood pressure; CHF, congestive heart failure; ECG, electrocardiogram; FHx, family history; HTN, hypertension; MI, myocardial infarction; VHD, valvular heart disease; WPW syndrome, Wolff-Parkinson–White syndrome.

A. Neurally mediated reflex syncope. Vasovagal syncope typically occurs after a prodrome of nausea, diaphoresis, or pallor following a sudden unexpected, usually unpleasant sight, smell, or sound, or with pain or fear. Vasovagal syncope also occurs with prolonged standing.

B. Cardiac syncope. Underlying arrhythmias causing syncope may not be present when the patient is evaluated, especially if it is a tachyarrhythmia. The patient may describe a prodrome of palpitations or slow heartbeat. The history commonly reveals a prodrome of acute shortness of breath or chest pain (pulmonary embolism, myocardial infarction [MI]). Cardiac syncope can also be precipitated by **exertion** (aortic stenosis, pulmonary hypertension, mitral stenosis, hypertrophic obstructive cardiomyopathy, coronary artery disease) or with **change of position** such as lying down/bending over/turning over in bed (atrial myxoma or thrombus). Pericardial disease may be related to cancer or chest trauma and may be exacerbated by positional changes.

1. Young athletes with exertional syncope are at risk for sudden death from hypertrophic cardiomyopathy or an anomalous coronary artery.

C. Orthostatic syncope. Standing up generally precipitates symptoms in this type of syncope. The history may reveal new or change in medication, polypharmacy, dehydration, alcohol, or diabetes.

D. Cerebrovascular syncope. Turning the head or flexing the neck may precipitate symptoms in a patient with vertebrobasilar insufficiency or carotid stenosis. Overhead work or activity may precipitate symptoms in subclavian steal syndrome.

IV. Signs (Table 57–1). Physical examination should focus on the **cardiovascular** and **neurologic** systems. **The physical examination is second only to the history in terms of importance in evaluating a patient with syncope.** Vital signs should be recorded, including bilateral supine and standing blood pressures and pulses. Cyanosis or pallor should be noted. Cardiopulmonary auscultation should be performed and carotid/peripheral pulses palpated. Neurologic examination should include orientation and cranial nerves, motor, sensory, and cerebellar testing (gait and Romberg testing).

A. Neurally mediated syncope

1. In **vasovagal syncope,** the patient may manifest hypotension. In patients with **orthostatic hypotension,** standing in place for 3 minutes after 5 minutes of recumbency decreases systolic blood pressure 20 mm Hg or more, diastolic blood pressure 10 mm Hg or more, or both. Volume-depleted patients may also manifest a postural increase in heart rate of 30 beats per minute or more. Patients often are diaphoretic.

2. Situational syncope. The signs are similar to vasovagal syncope. The history is diagnostic.

3. In **carotid sinus hypersensitivity,** the symptoms typically occur after head turning or wearing a tight collar. Symptoms may be reproduced by carotid sinus massage. This maneuver should not be done if carotid bruits or stenosis is present, if the patient has a history of ventricular tachycardia, or following recent TIA, stroke, or MI. Carotid sinus massage is done by vigorously massaging one side only for 5 to 10 seconds. This will produce a ventricular asystole for 3 or more seconds or fall in systolic pressure of 50 mm Hg or more. A false-positive test may occur in the absence of historical risk factors for carotid sinus hypersensitivity.

B. Cardiac syncope. With **structural heart disease**, cardiac examination is less likely to be normal than with arrhythmia-induced syncope. Auscultation may reveal murmurs of mitral regurgitation/aortic stenosis/hypertrophic obstructive cardiomyopathy, or murmurs with change in position such as lying down/bending over/turning over in bed (suggestive of atrial myxoma, thrombus, or hypertrophy), or findings of pulmonary hypertension (right ventricular lift, loud P2, prominent A-wave in jugular venous pulse).

C. In **cerebrovascular syncope,** a carotid bruit may be noted (indicating significant generalized atherosclerosis), **a focal neurologic deficit** may be uncovered (after a CVA), or an **asymmetric blood pressure or pulse** between upper extremities may be noted (suggesting subclavian steal syndrome or aortic dissection). In patients at risk, upper extremity activity could reveal pulse discrepancy between extremities (subclavian steal syndrome).

V. Laboratory Tests. A systematic history and physical examination alone can elucidate the cause of syncope in up to 45% of cases. Since **cardiac syncope** has a 2-year mortality rate of 30% compared with 6% for all other causes, testing is directed at differentiating cardiac from noncardiac causes.

A. In addition to a thorough history and physical examination, initial testing should include an **electrocardiogram (ECG)** (Figure 57-1). **Unless the history and physical**

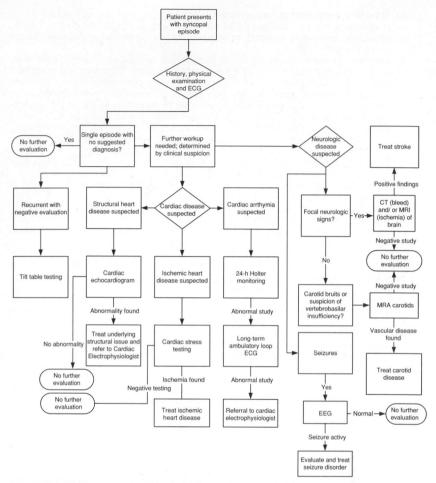

FIGURE 57–1. Algorithm for treatment of syncope. CT, computed tomography; EEG, electroencephalography; ECG, electrocardiogram; MRA, magnetic resonance angiography; MRI, magnetic resonance imaging.

examination and ECG suggest a diagnosis, no further testing should be undertaken unless patient has recurrent syncope. (SOR **Ⓒ**) All patients with syncope should have an **ECG** (Figure 57-1). Although the diagnostic yield is low (5%), half of patients with syncope will have an abnormal ECG, but most will not be diagnostic. In addition to revealing certain structural heart diseases (e.g., previous MI or left ventricular hypertrophy), the ECG is primarily helpful in uncovering arrhythmogenic causes of syncope, including **long QT interval, conduction delay/block, bundle branch block, fascicle block** (possible bradycardia); atrial and ventricular **ectopy** (nonspecific indicator of arrhythmogenic substrate); **bradycardia** (nonspecific indicator of conduction system disease); and **ventricular preexcitation/delta wave** (WPW syndrome).

B. An **echocardiogram** is recommended in all patients whose evaluation is suggestive of structural cardiac disease. This includes patients with exercise-induced syncope, as this may suggest a hypertrophic cardiomyopathy or an anomalous coronary artery in young adults.

C. Stress testing (e.g., exercise treadmill testing or stress echocardiography) is indicated in patients with syncope whose history and risk factors suggest ischemic heart disease.

D. 24-hour Holter monitoring is recommended for patients with suspected arrhythmogenic syncope (e.g., syncope without prodrome or syncope preceded by palpitations) and with suspected structural heart disease or abnormal ECG.

E. Long-term ambulatory loop ECG is a noninvasive method of cardiac monitoring indicated in patients with syncope and a structurally normal heart but abnormal ECG or 24-hour Holter monitoring.

F. Referral to a cardiac electrophysiologist for **intracardiac electrophysiologic studies** is indicated in patients with syncope and structural heart disease (e.g., history of MI, congestive heart failure, cardiomyopathy, coronary artery anomaly), identified arrhythmogenic syncope (e.g., WPW or long QT syndrome, ventricular tachycardia, refractory sinus bradycardia/A-V block, or supraventricular tachycardia), and exertional syncope.

G. Tilt-table testing is recommended in patients with unexplained recurrent syncope in whom cardiac causes of syncope, including arrhythmias, have been excluded. An abnormal result suggests vasovagal syncope, but reproducibility and yield are highly variable.

H. Neurologic testing should be reserved for patients with neurologic signs or symptoms or carotid bruits.

I. Imaging. Magnetic resonance angiography of carotid arteries is indicated for patients with bruits or possible vertebrobasilar insufficiency (prolonged loss of consciousness, diplopia, nausea, or hemiparesis). Focal neurologic signs mandate brain imaging, usually with **computerized tomography** for bleeding or **magnetic resonance imaging** for ischemia.

J. With evidence of seizure activity, **electroencephalography (EEG)** may be useful. Cardiac syncope evaluation should be obtained in patients with seizure activity, normal EEG, and no postictal symptoms, as well as for patients with seizures unresponsive to anticonvulsants.

VI. Treatment for syncope is directed at the underlying cause (Figure 57–1). The prognosis is very good (6% 1-year mortality) even without intervention in those with noncardiac syncope. In cardiac syncope, identification of and treatment for underlying causes can reduce the 30% 2-year mortality.

A. Hospitalization is indicated for patients with syncope who have known or suspected cardiac ischemia or arrhythmia, structural heart disease, cardiopulmonary circulatory disease (pulmonary embolus, pulmonary hypertension, atrial myxoma), or stroke. Hospitalization should be considered for diagnostic evaluation of syncope with known or suspected significant heart disease and ECG abnormalities, suggesting arrhythmogenic syncope.

B. Cardiology consultation is indicated for syncope with underlying structural, valvular heart disease, or underlying coronary artery disease.

C. Neurologic consultation is indicated for those suspected of a seizure disorder or TIA.

D. Vascular surgery consultation for carotid endarterectomy is clearly beneficial in symptomatic patients with 70% or more carotid artery stenosis and may also benefit those symptomatic with 50% to 65% stenosis. (SOR Ⓐ) Benefits of endarterectomy versus aspirin therapy are unclear in asymptomatic individuals with significant ($\geq$60%) stenosis; such patients have a 10% to 15% CVA risk over the ensuing 3 to 5 years. Risk of operative stroke or death in treatment trials was 7.0% (95% CI, 6.2–8.0).

E. Psychiatric evaluation should be considered in young, otherwise healthy patients who faint frequently without any associated injury and in patients presenting with many unassociated nonspecific symptoms such as nausea, lightheadedness, numbness, fear, and dread.

F. Neurally mediated reflex syncope (situational, vasovagal, or carotid sinus hypersensitivity).
  1. Patients should be counseled to:
    a. Avoid situations and stressful events that may trigger fainting, such as hot, crowded rooms or prolonged standing.
    b. Avoid dehydration and ensure adequate fluid and salt intake (SOR Ⓑ) and proper attire (possibly compression hose or season-appropriate attire).
    c. Minimize situations that trigger syncope, such as coughing excessively or wearing tight collars.
    d. Be aware of warning signs, such as feeling nauseated, sweaty, dizzy, or lightheaded, and sit or lie down to prevent loss of consciousness.

TABLE 57–2. PHARMACOLOGIC TREATMENT OPTIONS FOR PATIENTS WITH RESISTANT SYNCOPE

Drug	Dose	Major Side Effects	Contraindications	Drug Interactions
Metoprolol[a]	50 mg twice daily	Hypotension, bradycardia, dizziness, fatigue, sexual dysfunction, diarrhea, depression, shortness of breath	Sinus bradycardia, second- or third-degree A-V block, uncompensated heart failure, cardiogenic shock, severe peripheral vascular disease	Beta-agonists (severe bronchospasm); amiodarone, clonidine, calcium channel blockers (hypotension, bradycardia); venlafaxine (decreased beta-blocker efficacy); digoxin (bradycardia, digoxin toxicity); antidiabetic agents (hyper- or hypoglycemia); alpha-blockers (exaggerated hypotensive response to first dose of alpha-blocker)
Midodrine[a]	2.5–10 mg three times daily	Bradycardia, hypertension, urinary retention	Acute renal failure, urinary retention, thyrotoxicosis, pheochromocytoma, persistent and significant supine hypertension	Dihydroergotamine (extreme hypertension), sympathomimetics (enhanced pressor effect), TCAs (hypertension, arrhythmia), risperidone (dystonia)
Paroxetine[a]	10–40 mg daily	Nausea, diarrhea, constipation, loss of appetite, tremor, sweating, dizziness, headache, insomnia, somnolence, sexual dysfunction, asthenia		**Multiple interactions,** MAOI, triptans, dextromethorphan, trazodone, duloxetine, lithium (serotonin syndrome); thioridazine (cardiotoxicity); metoclopramide (extrapyramidal reactions/neuromalignant syndrome); tamoxifen (decreased efficacy of tamoxifen); anticoagulants/antiplatelet agents/apixaban (bleeding); tramadol (seizures, serotonin syndrome)

[a]Available as generic drugs.
A-V, atrioventricular; MAOI, monoamine oxidase inhibitors; SIADH, syndrome of inappropriate antidiuretic hormone; TCAs, tricyclic antidepressants.

2. Additional helpful measures include the following:
   a. Discontinue or modify medications (e.g., vasodilating antihypertensive drugs) that increase susceptibility to syncope. (SOR **A**)
   b. Although authors of a Cochrane review found insufficient evidence to support the use of any pharmacological or pacemaker treatments for vasovagal syncope and carotid sinus syncope, the following can be considered for resistant syncope (Table 57–2):
      (1) Beta-blockers (e.g., metoprolol starting at 50 mg orally twice daily) that increase catecholamine response. (SOR **B**)
      (2) Alpha adrenergic receptor agonist (midodrine, 2.5–10 mg orally three times daily) that increases peripheral vascular tone. (SOR **B**)
      (3) Selective serotonin reuptake inhibitors (paroxetine, 20 mg once daily) that alter central serotonergic regulation of sympathetic neural transmitters. (SOR **B**)
3. In **orthostatic hypotension,** treatment is directed at the underlying disorder (e.g., dehydration, medications, endocrine disorders, or neuropathies). In many cases, rising slowly and crossing the legs while standing, combined with the use of compression stockings, is helpful.
   G. If a thorough history, physical examination, and ECG fail to suggest a cause, the patient should be counseled to return for further evaluation if syncope recurs. (SOR **C**)

SELECTED REFERENCES

Blatt CM, Graboys TB. Evaluation of the patient with syncope. In: Alpert JS, ed. *Cardiology for the Primary Care Physician.* 4th ed. Philadelphia, PA: Current Medicine LLC; 2005:85–91.

Brignole M, Alboni P, Benditt D, et al. Task Force on Syncope, European Society of Cardiology. Guidelines on management (diagnosis and treatment) of syncope—update 2004. *Europace.* 2004;6:467–537.

Miller TH, Kruse JE. Evaluation of syncope. *Am Fam Physician.* 2005;72:1492–1500.

Rerkasem K, Rothwell PM. Carotid endarterectomy for symptomatic carotid stenosis. *Cochrane Database Syst Rev.* 2011;(4):CD001081.

Strickberger SA, Benson DW, Biaggioni I, et al. AHA/ACCF Scientific statement on the evaluation of syncope. *J Am Coll Cardiol.* 2006;47(2):473–484.

58   Tremors and Other Movement Disorders

Aylin Yaman, MD, Hakan Yaman, MD, MS, & Goutham Rao, MD

KEY POINTS

- Tremor is the most common movement disorder in the world. Tremors are basically classified as rest and action tremors. (SOR **C**)
- Diagnosis is based on history and physical examination. (SOR **C**)
- Selection of drugs in the treatment of Parkinson disease is based on the age of onset, duration of disease, and existence of complications related to treatment. (SOR **C**)
- Propranolol and primidone are both effective and first-line treatments for essential tremor. (SOR **A**) Recent evidence also supports the use of topiramate. (SOR **B**)

I. **Definition.** A **movement disorder** is any condition that disrupts normal voluntary movements of the body or one that consists of one or more abnormal movements. Movement disorders characterized by overall slowness of movement are classified as **hypokinesias;** those characterized by extra or exaggerated movements are classified as **hyperkinesias**. Tremors are the most common hyperkinesias.

  A. **Tremor** can be defined as a rhythmical, involuntary oscillatory movement of one or more body parts. A practical classification system divides tremors into rest tremors and action tremors.

  1. **Rest tremors** occur in a body part that is not voluntarily activated and is fully supported by gravity.

  2. **Action tremors** appear when muscles are voluntarily contracted. Action tremors can be further divided into **postural tremors** (tremor that occurs while maintaining a position against gravity) and **kinetic tremors** (tremor occurring during voluntary movement). The four principal types of kinetic tremors are as follows:

    a. Simple kinetic tremor occurs during voluntary movements that are not target-directed.

    b. Intention tremor is tremor that increases in amplitude during visually guided movements (e.g., finger-to-nose test).

    c. Task-specific kinetic is tremor that appears or is exacerbated by specific tasks (e.g., writing).

    d. Isometric tremor occurs during voluntary muscle contraction against a rigid stationary object (e.g., squeezing examiner's hand).

II. **Screening and Prevention.** Since the treatment of tremor is considered only when functional disability begins, there is no evidence supporting the usefulness of screening. Prevention is possible for the conditions of enhanced physiologic tremor and essential tremor by avoiding the use of drugs and comorbid situations that cause and augment tremor as mentioned later.

III. **Common Diagnoses.** Tremor may be associated with many conditions. The list of causes of tremor is very long. A useful starting point is to be able to distinguish among common causes of tremor (Table 58–1). (Also see at the end of this chapter on tic disorders, chorea, myoclonus, dystonia, Wilson disease, and ataxia).

  A. **Essential tremor, a visible postural tremor of the hands and forearms that may have a kinetic component,** is the most common of all movement disorders; the overall prevalence for all ages is 0.9% (95% CI, 0.5–1.5). The prevalence ranges between 2.3% and 14.3% at the age of 70 years and increases to 20% in the oldest old. A slight male predominance is observed. A family history of tremor is common (up to 60%), sometimes inherited as an autosomal dominant, and it can be exacerbated by stress, fatigue, or certain medications. Alcohol may temporarily attenuate symptoms in 50% to 70% of people.

  B. **Parkinson disease** (PD) is a chronic, progressive, neurodegenerative disorder with several characteristic features; the mean onset is 65 years (1%–1.6%), and the prevalence increases to 4% to 5% in those older than 85 years. It appears to be caused by a combination of genetic and environmental factors. First-degree relatives develop PD twice more (17% lifetime chance) than the general population. Rural residence, use of

TABLE 58–1. DIFFERENTIAL DIAGNOSIS OF TREMOR

Essential tremor	Postural or kinetic tremor of bilateral hands and arms (usually 6–12 Hz) or isolated head tremor without dystonia. No other neurologic symptom.
Physiologic tremor	Enhanced physiologic tremor of 10–12 Hz, an underlying cause exists
Parkinson disease	Mixed rest and action tremor of 4–6 Hz, rarely only action tremor. Leg and foot tremor is frequent. Usually, other parkinsonism symptoms are present.
Orthostatic tremor	Postural tremor of legs while standing, may also be seen in arms with high frequency (14–18 Hz). Disappears with walking.
Cerebellar tremor	Postural, intentional, or action tremor, low frequency (3–4 Hz). Ataxia and dysmetria exist.
Neuropathic tremor	Postural and kinetic tremor of involved extremities with other signs of peripheral neuropathy.
Rubral or midbrain tremor	Mixture of rest, postural, and intentional tremor with 2–5 Hz. Brainstem or cerebellar damage signs exist.

Source: Adapted with permission from Emre M. *Nöroloji Temel Kitabı (Book of Basic Neurology).* Ankara, Turkey: Günes Publishing; 2013.

well water, living on a farm, exposure to farm animals, and pesticide and herbicides are reported risk factors.

C. Physiologic tremor, typically a postural tremor with a frequency of 8 to 12 Hz, is present in all subjects to differing degrees. Enhanced physiologic tremor may appear at any age and does not progress in severity. It can be enhanced by stimulants such as caffeine, nicotine, and some illicit drugs as well as medications such as amiodarone, atorvastatin, beta-adrenergic agonists, caffeine, carbamazepine, corticosteroids, cyclosporine, epinephrine, fluoxetine, haloperidol, hypoglycemic agents, lithium, metoclopramide, methylphenidate, pseudoephedrine, terbutaline, theophylline, thyroid hormones, tricyclic antidepressants, valproic acid, and verapamil. Other conditions that can augment physiologic tremor include thyrotoxicosis, pheochromocytoma, hypoglycemia, and withdrawal from opioids and sedatives. The cause is usually reversible.

IV. Diagnosis. The evaluation of a patient with first presentation of tremor begins with a thorough history that includes age at onset, rate of progression, and family history of tremor, medication history, and history of neurologic symptoms other than tremor. Diagnosis mostly relies on the clinical evaluation.

A. Signs and symptoms. An approach to the patient with new-onset tremor is shown in Figure 58–1.

1. Review of medications. A review of recently prescribed and nonprescription medications may suggest the cause of tremor.

2. Age of onset. Both essential tremor and the tremor of PD usually begin after 50 years of age and are progressive in severity. Tremor before 40 years of age should raise suspicion for other neurologic pathologies such as primary dystonia or Wilson disease. Tremor in children should be taken seriously including referral to a neurologist.

3. Family history suggests essential tremor

4. Physical examination. The goal of the physical examination is to identify the key features of the tremor and to identify features other than the tremor that can help establish the diagnosis. A useful first step is to determine whether the tremor occurs at rest or during action (Figure 58–1). A **rest tremor** can be observed by having the patient position his or her hands on his or her lap. Postural tremor can be elicited by holding up an arm against gravity. A **kinetic tremor** may be apparent during purposeful movements such as using a spoon, writing, performing a finger-to-nose test, or squeezing an examiner's hand.

5. Associated symptoms. In addition to distal resting tremor, patients with PD may present with the following:

a. Asymmetrical onset is typical for PD. Such patients may complain of loss of balance and difficulty with tasks such as turning in bed, rising from a chair, and opening jars.

b. Rigidity can be detected by passively flexing and extending the patient's elbow several times. Resistance to movement can be smooth or interrupted (cog wheeling).

c. Bradykinesia can be detected by asking the patient to perform any one of a number of repetitive movements such as tapping the fingers or pinching the index finger and thumb repetitively. Obvious slowness in performing such maneuvers increases the likelihood of PD.

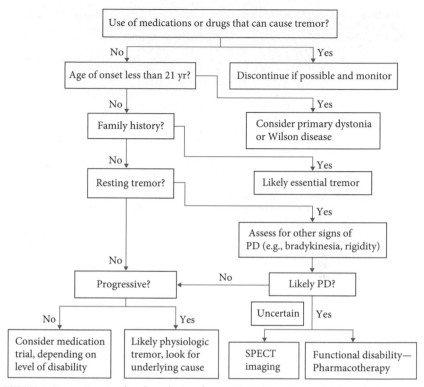

FIGURE 58–1. Systematic approach to the evaluation of tremor. PD, Parkinson disease; SPECT, single-photon emission computed tomography.

    d. The **glabella tap reflex** is tested by percussing the patient's forehead. The orbicularis oculi muscle reflexively contracts, causing both eyes to blink (http://www.youtube.com/watch?v=yexMkXq5miE). The blinking normally stops after 5 to 10 repeated taps. Persistence of blinking is a positive test (Myerson sign) and is more common among patients with PD.

    e. A sample of writing in a patient with PD may reveal **micrographia** (writing that becomes smaller across a page).

    f. Late in the course of disease, many patients with PD develop **postural instability**. It becomes difficult for patients to maintain a particular posture. Asking a patient to walk may reveal a tendency to fall or involuntary acceleration forward or backward (festination; http://www.youtube.com/watch?v=sf1N0Zf5IqA).

    g. During the evaluation of a patient with postural tremor, which suggests essential tremor, the possibility of early PD must be excluded since tremors of PD may also be of a postural and kinetic nature.

  6. The possibility of Wilson disease should always be considered in any patient with an action tremor who is younger than 40 years.

B. Specific tests. Some laboratory tests may be obtained when needed, such as thyroid function tests, drug serum levels, or renal and hepatic functions. Imaging is not usually recommended.

  1. PD. Magnetic resonance imaging (MRI) may be useful in distinguishing PD from other parkinsonian syndromes such as multisystem atrophy. Single-photon emission computed tomography is thought to be possibly useful in distinguishing PD from essential tremor and PD from vascular parkinsonism.

  2. Computed tomography and MRI may be useful for ruling out other secondary causes of tremor such as vascular parkinsonism.

V. Treatment. Therapy for most forms of tremor should target the underlying cause. Specific treatment for PD and essential tremor is discussed below.

- **A. PD** (Table 58–3). Pharmacological therapy has been shown to reduce morbidity and mortality, but it requires careful monitoring to determine the optimal dosage. The time of initiating treatment in PD is still controversial, but it has been shown that dopaminergic drugs improve quality of life for 18 months. For initial treatment of PD, carbidopa/levodopa, monoamine oxidase-B (MAO-B) inhibitors, or nonergot dopamine agonists should be considered. (SOR **A**) Antipsychotics (except quetiapine and clozapine), tricyclic antidepressants, antiemetics (except domperidone), and some antihypertensives (e.g., reserpine) are contraindicated. Use of alpha-methyldopa, buspirone, phenytoin, lithium, papaverine, risperidone, and meperidine should be weighed according to benefit and hazard.

  1. **Neuroprotective therapy** is designed to slow or stop disease progression. The MAO-B inhibitor selegiline has been shown to delay functional impairment and disease progression. Selegiline is well-tolerated and recommended as the first-line treatment in mild forms of PD. It is unclear, however, whether improvement is secondary to its neuroprotective effect or its effect on symptoms, which may mask disease progression. In randomized controlled trials, selegiline delayed the need for levodopa for up to 9 to 12 months compared with placebo. (SOR **A**) Rasagiline, another MAO-B inhibitor, is now being studied as a neuroprotective agent.

  2. **Symptomatic treatment.** Most patients with PD are treated with symptomatic therapy when they begin to experience functional impairment. Factors to consider before instituting symptomatic therapy include whether the patient's symptoms affect the patient's dominant hand, whether symptoms interfere with work or other activities, which features of PD are present, and whether quality of life is affected. Bradykinesia, for example, is usually more disabling than tremor. Levodopa is the most effective drug for PD symptoms, especially for bradykinesia. Treatment of PD with either selegiline, dopamine agonists, or the combination of levodopa and carbidopa or levodopa and carbidopa with entacapone improves symptoms and quality of life, but all these drugs have significant side effects. Dopamine agonists and anticholinergics are effective in early PD as symptomatic monotherapy (Figure 58–2), but bromocriptine, cabergoline, and pergolide are avoided because of serious side effects. (SOR **B**) Treatment should be individualized.

     There are currently six commonly used types of symptomatic therapy:

     a. The dopamine precursor **levodopa** is the most widely used and effective drug. (SOR **B**) To prevent its conversion to dopamine outside the blood–brain barrier, it is combined with the decarboxylase inhibitor, carbidopa. Dietary amino acids may interfere with levodopa absorption; therefore, protein restriction may be necessary for patients with decreased levodopa response. Levodopa is associated with serious adverse effects (e.g., cardiac arrhythmias, psychosis) that increase in severity with prolonged use (Table 58–2). Some serious disadvantages of levodopa

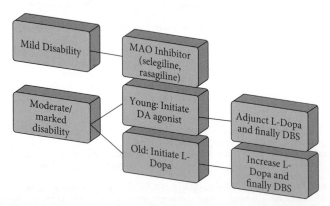

FIGURE 58–2. Treatment of Parkinson disease—initiate pharmacotherapy. DA, dopamine; DBS, deep brain stimualtion; L-Dopa, levodopa; MAO, monoamine oxidase. (*Source:* Reproduced with permission from Jankovic J, Poewe W. Therapies in Parkinson's disease. *Curr Opin Neurol.* 2012;25:433–447.)

TABLE 58–2. AVAILABLE PHARMACOTHERAPY FOR PD

Drug	Dose	Major Side Effects	Contraindications	Drug Interactions
MAO-B Inhibitors				
Selegiline	5 mg orally in the morning; can increase to twice daily, requires no titration	Dyskinesias, orthostatic hypotension, hallucinations		Meperidine, methadone, (severe hyper- or hypotension, malignant hyperpyrexia, coma); amphetamine (hypertensive crisis); TCA, SSRI, MAO-B inhibitor (CNS toxicity, serotonin S); dextromethorphan, trazodone (serotonin S); tramadol, cyclobenzaprine (seizures, serotonin S); pseudoephedrine, diphenoxylate (severe hypertension)
Rasagiline	1 mg once daily, requires no titration	Weight loss, anorexia, ataxia, orthostatic hypotension	None	See selegiline
Levodopa				
Levodopa/carbidopa (or benserazide)	Carbidopa (or benserazide) 25 mg/levodopa 100 mg two to four times daily	Dyskinesias, dystonia, akathisia, ballism, tremor, arrhythmias, orthostatic hypotension, hallucination, psychosis, wearing off, neuroleptic malignant S Long-term treatment causes vitamin B_{12} and folate deficiencies	Narrow angle glaucoma, melanoma	Multiple interactions MAO-B inhibitor (hypertension); isoniazid (deterioration of PD); phenytoin, iron (decreased levodopa effect); bupropion (nausea and vomiting, restlessness, tremor)
Levodopa/carbidopa/entacapone	100/25/200 mg two to six times daily	Dyskinesias, nausea, psychosis, cardiac arrhythmias, postural hypotension, somnolence, gastrointestinal side effects	See levodopa/carbidopa	See levodopa/carbidopa
Dopamine Agonists				
Bromocriptine	1.25 mg orally twice daily; increase by 2.5 mg/d every 2–4 wk to maximum 100 mg/d	Hypotension, hallucination, dyskinesia	Uncontrolled hypertension; caution in hepatic disease	Multiple interactions MAO-B inhibitor, ergots, nefazodone (serotonin S); triptans (prolonged vasospastic reaction)
Ropinirole	0.25 mg orally three times daily; increase 0.75 or 1.5 mg weekly until optimal therapeutic response; maximum dose 24 mg/d	Syncope, sudden episodes of sleep attack, dyskinesias, hallucinations, psychosis	None	Dopamine antagonists such as neuroleptics may diminish its efficacy
Pramipexole	0.125 mg orally three times daily; increase by 0.375 mg/d every 5–7 d until optimal response; maximum dose 5 mg/d	Orthostatic hypotension, dyskinesia, dizziness, hallucinations	Elderly patients with advanced PD and patients with kidney disease should use with caution	Cimetidine (increased pramipexole side effects)
Amantadine				
Amantadine	100 mg once or twice daily	Insomnia, anxiety, orthostatic hypotension, peripheral edema	Dose should be adjusted in renal disease	

CNS, central nervous system; MAO-B, monoamine oxidase B; PD, Parkinson disease; S, syndrome; SSRI, selective serotonin reuptake inhibitors; TCA, tricyclic antidepressants.

treatment are drug-induced dyskinesias and fluctuations in motor response, which are related to long-term treatment. These complications are irreversible. Sustained-release preparations of levodopa showed no added benefit for reducing motor complications.

b. Even when combined with carbidopa, only 10% of levodopa reaches the brain. Much of it is converted to an inert metabolite by the enzyme catechol-O-methyl-transferase (COMT). The COMT inhibitors **tolcapone** and **entacapone** can be administered with levodopa to increase its effectiveness. These drugs are also useful for managing motor fluctuations. (SOR **B**) However, COMT inhibitors are not recommended as initial agents because of their higher cost and lack of proven benefit in patients with early PD. MAO-B inhibitors, COMT inhibitors, and nonergot dopamine agonists are recommended in combination with levodopa in patients with PD with complications (e.g., motor complications such as motor fluctuations and dyskinesias) or to spare levodopa for patients older than 65 years, if possible. (SOR **A**)

c. The third class of available pharmacotherapy is **dopamine agonists such as bromocriptine, ropinirole,** and **pramipexole**. These drugs stimulate dopamine receptors. Dopamine agonists are found to reduce dyskinesia and motor fluctuations more effectively than levodopa, but they are associated with increased treatment withdrawal and poorer motor scores. Also, dopamine agonists are more likely to be associated with hallucinations, somnolence, and edema than levodopa. These agents are used to delay the complications associated with levodopa treatment, primarily in younger patients.

  (1) The dopamine agonist pergolide should be avoided because of its association with restrictive valvular heart disease and serosal fibrosis.

  (2) A powerful dopamine agonist, apomorphine, not only can be tried in complicated patients who experience sudden, resistant "off" periods but also must be used cautiously because of severe side effects.

  (3) Dopamine agonists can be used for initial symptomatic therapy or as adjuncts to therapy with levodopa. (SOR **B**) Administration of combination therapy with levodopa and dopamine agonists early in the course of the disease does not delay the development of motor complications.

d. MAO-B inhibitors selegiline and rasagiline are useful for symptomatic control of disease and as adjuvant therapy for patients with motor fluctuations. (SOR **A**)

e. Anticholinergics, mainly benztropine and trihexyphenidyl, are useful for symptomatic control, (SOR **C**) but associated with more neuropsychiatric and cognitive adverse effects than other drugs. Treatment with these agents, especially in the elderly, should be avoided.

f. Amantadine may be effective especially in managing severe dyskinesias in advanced PD. (SOR **B**) However, effectiveness in the long term is questionable. Rotigotine is a promising drug for this condition.

g. **Treatment of nonmotor symptoms in patients with PD is usually a major challenge for clinicians,** and supporting evidence is limited. For symptoms/conditions such as depression, psychosis, and sialorrhea, treatments with pramipexole, clozapine, and botulinum toxin, respectively, are effective; for depression and constipation, nortriptyline + desipramine and polyethylene glycol 3350 (MiraLAX), respectively, are likely to be effective, and continuous dopaminergic drug administration may be of benefit for sleep and other nonmotor symptoms. In cognitive impairment, drugs must be adjusted and a cholinesterase inhibitor should be considered. Anticholinergic side effects of tricyclic antidepressants could worsen cognitive status. Although clozapine is the most effective antipsychotic agent in these patients, adverse effects such as agranulocytosis make quetiapine the first-line agent in PD.

3. Surgical treatment of PD is emerging as an effective option for patients in whom pharmacotherapy fails (Figure 58–2).

  a. **Ablation** of tissue in specific areas of the brain including the ventral intermediate nucleus of the thalamus and globus pallidus pars interna with radio waves, heat, or chemicals is associated with significant improvement. Unilateral pallidotomy improved motor examination and activities of daily living better than medical treatment in one systematic review, but it was associated with a high incidence of adverse effects. (SOR **B**)

b. **Deep brain stimulation** of the ventral intermediate nucleus, globus pallidus pars interna, or subthalamic nucleus with an electrode connected to a pulse generator placed subcutaneously over the chest wall is also effective. Controlled trials comparing pallidal deep brain stimulation versus medical treatment are lacking. Cognitive and psychiatric adverse effects are observed. Adverse effects are probably less frequent with deep brain stimulation than with ablative surgery. (SOR **C**) Deep brain stimulation is recommended in patients with functional disability despite optimal medical treatment. This procedure should be performed in experienced centers. (SOR **B**)

c. **Transplantation of fetal dopaminergic neurons** into the substantia nigra has shown some promise, but it remains a controversial and experimental procedure.

4. **Physical, occupational, and speech therapies** are shown to be effective for balance, muscle strength, walking speed, and speech and depressive symptoms and should be considered. (SOR **B**) Tai chi effectively improves functional abilities and decreases falls in patients with PD. (SOR **B**)

5. **Supportive care** is an important component of management. The clinical manifestations of the disease itself are frequently accompanied by a profound psychological and social impact. Stress among caregivers is a significant concern. Health care providers should be sensitive to these problems. Patients with PD and their families should also receive counseling about the clinical features, prognosis, and impact of the disease. Treatment options, risks and benefits of each group of medications, and long-term complications should be discussed with the patient before initiating the therapy. Management should be individualized, and a number of support groups are helpful in this regard. Family, social, and work roles need to be supported to preserve mobility and independence in daily life. (SOR **C**) Access to palliative care services is needed.

B. **Essential tremor**

1. Mild essential tremor need not be treated if it causes no functional impairment. Functional impairment as assessed by the severity of symptoms and ability to perform daily tasks (e.g., writing, buttoning) should always be used as a guide to initiate or adjust therapy. Careful monitoring for side effects of medications is essential.

2. **Pharmacological therapy** (Table 58–3).

a. The beta-blocker **propranolol** and the anticonvulsant **primidone** are used as first-line treatments for more severe tremor (SOR **B**). They are roughly equally effective. Propranolol is initiated at a dose of 20 to 40 mg orally twice daily. Maintenance doses are usually 240 to 320 mg per day. It is usually well tolerated. Patients taking propranolol should be carefully monitored for side effects (Table 58–3). In general, 50% to 70% of patients obtain symptomatic relief from propranolol, but dramatic improvement occurs in a much smaller percentage of patients. Primidone dosing is shown in Table 58–3. Primidone should be started at a dose of 25 mg orally once daily and slowly increased as needed to a maximum of 750 mg per day, given in three divided doses. Long-term treatment with primidone is well-tolerated, but some patients will experience an acute reaction consisting of nausea, vomiting, or ataxia. (SOR **A**)

b. Topiramate has been shown to be effective. It improved tremor scores after 2 weeks' treatment, but it was associated with appetite suppression, weight loss, and paresthesia. (SOR **B**) Studies addressing long-term outcomes are lacking.

c. Other classes of medications include benzodiazepines, calcium channel blockers, and theophylline; these have been used with variable success. Evidence on the efficacy of olanzapine is inconclusive, and parkinsonism is a reported adverse effect. (SOR **C**)

3. Stereotaxic thalamotomy and thalamic deep brain stimulation may be considered in drug-resistant essential tremor or in patients with serious functional restriction.

VI. **Prognosis.** PD has no definitive treatment and is a disabling disease with high mortality. Treatment can slow progression and improve symptoms, but it has a limited effect on

TABLE 58–3. AVAILABLE PHARMACOTHERAPY FOR ESSENTIAL TREMOR

Drug	Dose	Major Side Effects	Contraindications	Drug Interactions
Propranolol	Initial 40 mg twice daily; maintenance 120–320 mg daily in divided doses	Bradycardia, congestive heart failure, fatigue	Heart failure, asthma, A-V block.	Thioridazine (QT prolongation); amiodarone (bradycardia, cardiac arrest); calcium channel blockers, cimetidine, disopyramide (hypotension, bradycardia)
Primidone	Starting dose is 25 mg/d, may be increased to 50–350 mg/d	Ataxia, vertigo, visual disturbance, granulocytopenia, thrombocytopenia	Porphyria	Multiple interactions Quetiapine (decreased quetiapine levels); benzodiazepines (respiratory depression); valproic acid (severe CNS depression)
Topiramate	Starting dose 25 mg once daily titrated to 50 mg twice daily over 4 wk to 300 mg/d (usual effective dose); maximum dose 400 mg/d	Paresthesia, somnolence, anorexia, confusion, dizziness, impaired cognition and/or memory, metabolic acidosis, glaucoma, hepatotoxicity	Urolithiasis, ethanol use 6 h before the first dose or after the last dose	Acetazolamide (increases risk of kidney stone), metformin (increased risk of lactic acidosis), citalopram (QT prolongation), phenytoin (altered phenytoin or topiramate levels), oral contraceptives (decreased contraceptive effectiveness

A-V, atrioventricular; CNS, central nervous system.

prolonging life. The mean duration until death is 9.1 years. The age of diagnosis is the main predictor of outcome. The older, the shorter life duration. After 10 years, 25% of patients with PD require nursing home care. In addition, the risk of melanoma is increased in patients with PD.

VII. Patient Education

A. PD is a chronic, progressive disease and full recovery is not possible in most cases. Most cases are sporadic. Time schedule and dosing of medications are important in treatment success. Levodopa and dopamine agonists should be taken before meals; protein restriction helps absorption of drugs. Periodic skin monitoring for melanoma is encouraged.

B. Essential tremor is a chronic disorder that requires long-term treatment. Tremor usually worsens with increasing age and functional disability may be prominent. Treatment options are symptomatic and combination therapies may be needed in time. A positive family history in first-degree relatives increases the risk of having the disease 5 to 10 times.

TIC DISORDERS

A tic is a brief, intermittent, repetitive, nonrhythmic, unpredictable, purposeless movement or sound. Tics are preceded by a conscious urge to execute them. Stress results when a tic is suppressed. Stress is relieved upon executing the tic. Voluntary suppression, which is more typical in tics than in other involuntary movements, is a helpful distinguishing feature. Tics are usually intermittent, but they may be repetitive and are frequently stereotypical. Motor and phonic tics may persist during all stages of sleep, unlike most other hyperkinesias. Tics have a number of causes. Tourette syndrome, which is the combination of motor and phonic tics occurring before the age of 21 years, is the most common tic disorder, affecting roughly 5 to 10 of every 10,000 children. Boys are disproportionately affected. Tourette syndrome is frequently accompanied by attention-deficit/hyperactivity disorder. Dopamine receptor blockers, such as pimozide, fluphenazine, and haloperidol, and alpha-receptor agonists, such as clonidine, provide effective treatment for the tics. (SOR **❸**) Behavioral approaches have also shown some success.

CHOREA

Chorea is an unpredictable, irregular, nonrhythmic, brief, jerky flowing, or writhing movement. Chorea can be consciously incorporated into voluntary movements, such that patients exhibit "semipurposeful" movements known as parakinesias. Chorea has several causes, including Wilson disease, stroke, and as part of an immunologic reaction after streptococcal infection (Sydenham chorea). Chorea may also be drug related, most commonly associated with dopaminergic agents, lithium, phenytoin, and rarely valproate. Huntington disease is a hereditary form inherited in an autosomal dominant pattern. Symptoms typically appear between 35 and 50 years of age.

Haloperidol (Haldol) and fluphenazine (Prolixin) are effective in treating chorea, but they can impair voluntary movements. (SOR **❸**) Both are initiated at a dose of 0.5 or 1.0 mg orally once daily and can gradually be increased to a maximum daily dose of 6 to 8 mg per day. The dopamine-depleting drugs reserpine (Serpalan) and tetrabenazine (Nitoman) and the benzodiazepine clonazepam (Klonopin) are also effective. (SOR **❸**) Reserpine is initiated at a dose of 0.1 mg orally once daily (maximum dose, 3 mg per day). Tetrabenazine is started at 25 mg orally once daily (maximum dose, 100 mg per day). Klonopin is started at a dose of 0.5 mg orally once daily (maximum dose, 4 mg per day). Wrist weights can improve function by decreasing the amplitude of chorea.

MYOCLONUS

Myoclonus is a brief, sudden movement caused by involuntary muscle contractions or lapse of muscle contraction (*asterixis*). **Generalized myoclonus** refers to synchronous "jerks" in many body parts; **focal myoclonus** affects a single body part. Physiologic myoclonus is benign and includes "sleep jerks" that occur while falling asleep. Rhythmic myoclonus may be confused with tremor and is typically characterized by brief muscle twitches, confined to one limb or to adjacent body region, associated with spike–wave complexes on the electroencephalogram or spinal lesions. Essential myoclonus is disabling and can be treated with clonazepam (starting dose of 0.25 mg orally twice daily, increasing over 3 days to 1 mg per day). (SOR **❸**) Most causes of myoclonus are secondary and include drugs such as lithium, toxins, advanced liver disease, infections including HIV infection, dementia, and brain lesions. Treatment should target the underlying disorder.

DYSTONIA

Dystonia is a syndrome that includes sustained contractions of opposing muscles that cause twisting, repetitive movements, and abnormal postures. Progressively severe tremor is also common. Primary dystonia is an inherited form that appears before 21 years of age. Dystonic movements are involuntary, but they can be diminished by specific maneuvers. In spasmodic torticollis that affects the neck, for example, placing a hand on the chin or side of the face reduces the severity of dystonia. Primary dystonia is generally hereditary and can be treated successfully with high doses of trihexyphenidyl (Artane) alone (starting dose of 1 mg orally per day, increasing gradually to 6–80 mg per day until symptoms are well controlled), or in combination with baclofen (Lioresal) (starting dose of 10 mg orally once daily, maximum dose of 30–120 mg per day). (SOR ⓒ) The list of secondary causes includes Wilson disease, metachromatic leukodystrophy, Lesch–Nyhan syndrome, stroke, and encephalitis.

WILSON DISEASE

Wilson disease is a rare inherited disorder of copper metabolism that, in addition to hepatic manifestations, often also presents with neuropsychiatric features including progressive tremor, dysarthria, parkinsonism, and dystonia. Very rarely, this disease presents with isolated action tremor. Symptoms and signs of Wilson disease usually appear at a young age. Tremor in a young patient, therefore, should raise suspicion of primary dystonia or Wilson disease. A low serum ceruloplasmin level is a useful screening test, although not diagnostic. A slit-lamp examination for Kayser–Fleischer rings should also be considered.

ATAXIA

Ataxia is a wide-based, unsteady gait associated with cerebellar dysfunction, proprioceptive defects, or both. Inherited forms include Friedreich ataxia and spinocerebellar ataxia. Ataxia can occur secondary to stroke, trauma, alcoholic degeneration, multiple sclerosis, vitamin B_{12} deficiency, and hydrocephalus. Treatment, when possible, should target the underlying cause.

SELECTED REFERENCES

Crawford P, Zimmermann EE. Differentiation and diagnosis of tremor. *Am Fam Physician*. 2011; 83(6):697–702.

Fritsch T, Smyth KA, Wallendal MS, et al. Parkinson disease: research update and clinical management. *South Med J*. 2012;105(12):650–656.

Gazewood JD, Richards DR, Clebak K. Parkinson disease: an update. *Am Fam Physician*. 2013; 87(4): 267–273.

Jankovic J, Poewe W. Therapies in Parkinson's disease. *Curr Opin Neurol*. 2012;25:433–447.

Rao SS, Hofmann LA, Shakil A. Parkinson's disease: diagnosis and treatment. *Am Fam Physician*. 2006;74: 2046–2054, 2055–2056.

Worth PF. How to treat Parkinson's disease in 2013. *Clin Med*. 2013;13(1):93–96.

Yaman A, Yaman H. How best to address these common movement disorders. *J Fam Pract*. 2011; 60(12):721–725.

Zesiewicz TA, Elble RJ, Louis ED, et al. Evidence-based guideline update: treatment of essential tremor: report of Quality Standards Subcommittee of the American Neurology. *Neurology*. 2011;77: 1752–1755.

Additional references are available online at http://langetextbooks.com/fm6e

59 Urinary Incontinence

Annette Sandretto, MSN, ANP-BC, RN, Karen D. Novielli, MD, & Barry D. Weiss, MD

KEY POINTS

- Urinary incontinence is extremely common in older patients, particularly older women. (SOR Ⓒ)
- Middle-aged and older patients should be asked routinely about urinary incontinence, because they are unlikely to spontaneously mention the condition. (SOR Ⓒ)
- Treatment is based on the cause of urinary incontinence, and behavioral management is a critical management tool. (SOR Ⓒ)

I. **Definition.** Urinary incontinence is the complaint of any involuntary leakage of urine. Since micturition is controlled by the central and peripheral nervous systems as well as by local anatomic support, incontinence can be caused by numerous conditions affecting the brain, spine, and pelvis. Among ambulatory, community-dwelling persons older than 65 years, urinary incontinence occurs in 17% to 55% of females and 11% to 34% of males. Approximately 14% of older women and 4% of older men are incontinent on a daily basis. Although this is not a life-shortening physical dysfunction, quality of life is significantly impacted for both men and women due to embarrassment, fear of going out, social isolation, and cost of products.

A. **Transient incontinence** is more likely when incontinence is defined as being less than 6 weeks from onset to evaluation and spontaneously resolves when the underlying condition is treated. The mnemonic DIAPERS may be useful in recalling the causes of transient incontinence—**D**rugs, **I**nfection, **A**trophic vaginitis, **P**sychological (e.g., depression, delirium, dementia), **E**ndocrine (hyperglycemia, hypercalcemia), **R**estricted mobility, and **S**tool impaction.

B. **Urge incontinence** is the most common cause of persistent incontinence in older individuals. In urge incontinence, involuntary leakage is accompanied by or immediately preceded by urgency and results from uncontrolled contractions of the detrusor muscle. Although most cases are idiopathic, patients with neurologic disorders (including dementia) are particularly at high risk.

C. **Stress incontinence** is usually present when involuntary leakage occurs from effort or exertion or from sneezing, going from sitting to standing, or coughing and is related to increased urethral mobility and/or poor intrinsic sphincter function.

D. **Overflow incontinence** accounts for ≤5% of incontinence in women but, because of the prevalence of prostate disorders, accounts for 30% to 50% of incontinence in older men. Overflow incontinence is caused either by obstruction of urinary outflow or by impaired detrusor contractility.

E. **Mixed incontinence** occurs when two or more of the above causes are present simultaneously, most often urge incontinence in combination with another cause. Mixed incontinence is very common and may occur in as many as 50% of patients with incontinence.

F. **Functional incontinence** is the inability or unwillingness to toilet because of physical, cognitive, psychological, or environmental factors (e.g., a patient with severe depression or who is physically restrained). Functional incontinence is common in the hospital and nursing home settings.

G. **Overactive bladder** refers to frequency and urgency without urinary incontinence.

H. **Risk factors.** Common to both women and men are cognitive and mobility impairment, bladder irritation from multiple causes, medications, diabetes, obesity, age >50 years, and neurologic loss due to Parkinson disease or multiple sclerosis.

1. **Women.** Increases with age, childbirth (vaginal delivery, age at pregnancy, fetal birth weight), oral contraceptive or hormone therapy, hysterectomy, pelvic organ prolapse, and menopause.

2. **Men.** Benign prostatic hypertrophy and prostatectomy.

II. Diagnosis

A. Initial Assessment. An assessment of the patient with urinary incontinence should include a general medical history and specific questioning for symptoms related to the lower urinary tract, bowel and sexual function, and pelvic organ prolapse. Basic elements of the history of the lower urinary tract include duration, frequency, and severity of urine loss; precipitating factors (such as coughing, change in position); and associated symptoms. Caffeine and alcohol intake can influence bladder function. A medication review can be used to assess drug–drug and other interactions or side effects that can contribute to urinary incontinence. The degree to which urinary incontinence is affecting the patient's life should also be evaluated. This can be done through direct questions or the use of assessment tools such as the Urogenital Distress Inventory Short Form and the Incontinence Impact Questionnaire Short Form (http://consultgerirn .org/uploads/File/trythis/try_this_11_2.pdf). Voiding diaries can also be useful (http://www.uwmedicine.org/services/gynecology/documents/Patient%20Ed%20 Handouts/Voiding-Diary.pdf).

B. Symptoms

1. **Urgency** is the primary symptom of uncontrolled bladder contractions (i.e., urge incontinence). The sensitivity of this symptom in identifying patients with true urge incontinence, in comparison to formal urodynamic testing, is approximately 60%.

2. **Loss of urine with coughing,** descending stairs, sneezing, and so on is a classic symptom of stress incontinence. The positive predictive value of these symptoms exceeds 85% for identifying patients with true stress incontinence and exceeds 95% when accompanied by physical examination findings typical of stress incontinence. However, symptoms similar to those of stress incontinence can occur in patients with urge incontinence, where an "irritable" bladder may contract when stimulated by repetitive increases in intra-abdominal pressure such as repetitive coughing.

3. **Dribbling** is a symptom of overflow incontinence. It may occur with sphincter weakness, especially when it is caused by sphincter denervation. It usually increases with postural change or with Valsalva maneuver.

4. **Abdominal discomfort** may be present in patients with overflow incontinence because of bladder distention, particularly if urinary retention and overflow are of recent onset.

5. **Red flags** include gross hematuria that is persistent, pelvic pain that is constant or worsening, and of sudden onset. These require urgent referral to urology or urogynecology. Neurologic symptoms such as abnormal motor or sensory function (see later) should also prompt referral.

C. Physical examination should include an evaluation of functional and cognitive status in addition to a thorough neurologic, abdominal, and pelvic evaluation. For women this should include an external genitalia, vaginal speculum, bimanual, and rectal examination. For men this should include a prostate and rectal examination.

1. **A cough stress test** should be performed on all women. With the patient in the lithotomy position and with a full bladder, the patient coughs while gauze or a menstrual pad is held over the perineum. Instantaneous leakage onto the pad during coughing suggests stress incontinence. Delayed leakage suggests urge incontinence. If there is no leakage, the test should be repeated with the patient in the standing position.

2. **Abnormal mental status** (e.g., dementia) indicates decreased function of cerebral inhibitory centers associated with urge incontinence.

3. **Abnormal reflex, motor, or sensory function** suggests the presence of a neurologic disorder that leads to neuropathic sphincter, detrusor denervation, or cerebral dysfunction and associated urge incontinence.

4. **Abdominal distention** or **palpable bladder** is suggestive of urinary retention and associated overflow incontinence.

5. **Atrophic vaginitis** indicates the possibility of urge incontinence because of estrogen-responsive irritable bladder.

6. **Prolapse of pelvic organs** is frequently associated with stress incontinence.

7. **Prostate enlargement or masses** suggest the possibility of overflow incontinence due to bladder outflow obstruction.

8. **Impacted rectal stool** suggests overflow incontinence from obstruction of urethral outflow by the fecal impaction.

D. Laboratory tests. Some patients may have preexisting conditions warranting specialized evaluations not discussed in this chapter.

   1. Urinalysis. *Pyuria* or *bacteriuria* suggests infection, and a culture can confirm the diagnosis. *Hematuria* may indicate neoplasm or calculi, necessitating further evaluation with cystoscopy, renal ultrasound, or radiography. Urine culture can be ordered at the discretion of the provider.

E. Additional office testing. These additional tests can be performed in the office by a provider.

   1. Postvoid residual (PVR) urine volume should be measured to exclude overflow incontinence. Normal PVR urine is ≤50 mL; PVR urine of 200 mL or more is abnormal and indicates outflow obstruction or diminished detrusor contractility. PVR volumes between 50 and 200 mL are equivocal, and the test should be repeated on another occasion.

      a. Postvoid catheterization is the most common method for determining PVR. A sterile catheter is inserted into the patient's bladder immediately after the patient voids, and the volume of collected urine is recorded. Inability to pass the catheter suggests obstruction from causes such as urethral stricture and prostate enlargement.

      b. Ultrasound measurement of bladder volume is a noninvasive method for determining the presence of residual urine. Where it is available, ultrasonography may be preferable to catheterization, especially in men with suspected prostate enlargement; ultrasound involves no risk of infection or urethral trauma, both of which can occur with catheterization.

F. Supplemental tests can be performed if a presumptive diagnosis cannot be reached with a history, physical examination, and the aforementioned tests. Providers not trained in these tests should consider referral to a urologist. There is currently no strong evidence, however, that testing improves outcome or changes management planning long term.

   1. Office cystometrography is a simple office procedure that is useful for detecting the presence of uncontrolled bladder contractions associated with urge incontinence.

   2. Urinary flow determination can be useful in men suspected of having prostate enlargement causing outflow obstruction.

G. Specialized tests can be performed in selected patients with specific indications or in those for whom a presumptive diagnosis cannot be reached after history, physical examination, and basic and supplemental tests. These tests are usually obtained after referral to a specialist such as a urologist or urogynecologist and include video-cystourethrography, videourodynamics, ultrasound, and magnetic resonance imaging.

III. Treatment. After the basic and supplemental evaluations described above, in most cases a presumptive diagnosis can be made as to the cause and type of incontinence. Treatment, as outlined below, can be administered based on the presumptive diagnosis (Figure 59–1). If treatment is unsuccessful after 4-8 weeks of therapy for chronic incontinence, the diagnosis should be reevaluated, and more specialized tests may be indicated to better define the cause of incontinence. The patient can keep a **voiding diary,** in which symptoms and information on the frequency and circumstances of incontinent episodes are recorded. A baseline diary is useful for defining the patient's symptoms and determining the baseline frequency of incontinence to judge subsequent effectiveness of therapy.

A. Transient causes of urinary incontinence are managed by treating the identified cause. If incontinence does not resolve, other causes should be considered. If none are found, the patient is then treated for the type of persistent incontinence (e.g., urge or stress) presumptively diagnosed based on the testing described above. (SOR ⊕)

B. Urge incontinence

   1. Behavioral therapies are first-line treatment because they are safe and often effective. In the event that pharmacotherapy is needed, behavioral therapy is important as adjunctive therapy. Principles that underlie behavioral treatments for urge incontinence are: (1) keep the bladder volume low by frequent voiding, (2) inhibit detrusor contractions by retraining cerebral and pelvic continence mechanisms, and (3) avoid bladder irritants (e.g., alcohol, caffeine, spicy foods). (SOR ⊕)

      a. Bladder training is the treatment of choice for urge incontinence. It involves encouraging the patient to postpone voiding for increasing lengths of time. Limited data suggest that bladder training is effective and that most patients experience improvement in their incontinence symptoms. At least one study found it superior to drug therapy in cognitively intact women. (SOR ⊕)

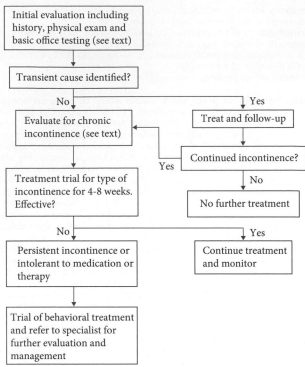

FIGURE 59–1. Approach to the patient with urinary incontinence. Note that patients with certain conditions may need specialized evaluation and should not be diagnosed and managed exclusively according to this algorithm. Such patients are those with (1) hematuria or pyuria in the absence of infection, (2) recent (within 2 months) onset of irritative voiding symptoms, (3) previous anti-incontinence surgery or radical pelvic surgery, (4) severe pelvic prolapse, (5) suspicion of prostate cancer, or (6) neurologic abnormalities.

    b. Pelvic muscle exercises (Kegel exercises) can improve symptoms of urge incontinence (see Section III.C.1.a), especially when supplemented with biofeedback. (SOR ❸) Pelvic muscle exercise can take up to 6 months to work.

  2. Medications are often added as adjunct therapy for the treatment of urge incontinence.

    a. Oral medications for urge incontinence act by diminishing bladder contractions. These include darifenacin, fesoterodine, oxybutynin, solifenacin, tolterodine, and trospium. See Table 59–1 for dosing, side effects, and contraindications. A trial of 4 to 8 weeks is recommended to evaluate effectiveness and patient tolerance. (SOR ❸) Medications need to be used with caution in older patients due to their side effect profile.

  3. Other treatments

    a. Electrical stimulation with both implantable and nonimplantable electrodes may improve urge incontinence in some patients. This therapy is used in many centers but is considered investigational. (SOR ❸)

    b. Surgical treatment of urge incontinence with procedures such as augmentation cystoplasty is likely effective, but is used only in selected patients. Bladder denervation, which reduces detrusor contractility, can be accomplished with subtrigonal phenol injections and a variety of other methods. Cure rates with bladder denervation are low. (SOR ❸)

    c. Intradetrusor injection of botulinum toxin is a new and promising treatment for patients who are refractory to pharmacotherapy. (SOR ❸)

TABLE 59-1. URINARY INCONTINENCE ORAL AND TOPICAL MEDICATIONS

Generic Name	Brand Name	Dosing	Type of Incontinence	Adverse Effects	Drug Interactions
Anti-Muscarinic					
Darifenacin	Enablex	7.5–15 mg daily	Urge or Mixed	Constipation, xerostomia	Oral potassium (GI lesions); TCA (TCA toxicity); flecainide (arrhythmias)
Fesoterodine	Toviaz	4–8 mg daily	Urge or Mixed	Constipation, xerostomia, dry eye, dysuria, urinary retention	Oral potassium (GI lesions)
Mirabegron	Mybetiq	25–50 mg daily	Mixed	Hypertension, urinary tract infection, nasopharyngitis	Thioridazine, propafenone (prolonged QT, torsades de pointes); tramadol (serotonin S); beta-blockers (orthostatic hypotension); digoxin (digoxin toxicity); atypical antipsychotics (↑ antipsychotic adverse effects)
Oxybutynin	Ditropan, Ditropan XL, Gelnique, Oxytrol	Ditropan 2.5–5 mg every 8–12 h Ditropan XL 5–30 mg daily Gelnique 1 g topical daily Oxytrol 3.9 mg transdermal patch daily	Urge or Mixed	Constipation, gastroenteritis, xerostomia, dizziness, UTI, nasopharyngitis Transdermal patch: application site itching, erythema	Oral potassium (GI lesions); cholinesterase inhibitors (↓ efficacy of cholinesterase inhibitors)
Solifenacin	Vesicare	5–10 mg daily	Urge or Mixed	Constipation, xerostomia, QT prolongation	QT prolonging agents (additive QT prolongation, torsades de pointes); oral potassium (GI lesions)
Tolterodine	Detrol, Detrol LA	Detrol 2 mg every 12 h Detrol LA 2–4 mg daily	Urge or Mixed	Constipation, xerostomia, abdominal pain, headache	Oral potassium (GI lesions); warfarin (bleeding); amiodarone, (QT prolongation); cholinesterase inhibitors (↓ efficacy of inhibitors)
Trospium	Sanctura, Sanctura XR	Sanctura 20 mg twice daily Sanctura XR 60 mg daily	Urge or Mixed	Constipation, xerostomia	Oral potassium (GI lesions); metformin (↓ trospium efficacy)
Alpha-Adrenergic Agonist					
Pseudo-ephedrine		30–60 mg three times daily	Stress	Insomnia, anxiety	MAO-I, ergots, dopamine agonists (severe hypertension)

(continued)

TABLE 59–1. URINARY INCONTINENCE ORAL AND TOPICAL MEDICATIONS (*Continued*)

Generic Name	Brand Name	Dosing	Type of Incontinence	Adverse Effects	Drug Interactions
Estrogen					
Topical cream	Premarin and others	0.5–1 g daily for 2 wk then twice weekly	Urge or Stress related to vaginal atrophy	Backache, bloating, vasodilation, abdominal pain, breast pain, asthenia, pruritus	Levothyroxine (↓ serum thyroxine)
Vaginal estradiol ring	Estring	1 ring every 3 months	Stress	Headache, vaginal discomfort, ↑ vaginal secretions	Unlikely
Vaginal tablets	Vagifem	10–25 mcg tablet daily for 2 weeks, then twice weekly	Stress	Headache, vaginal discomfort, genital itching	Unlikely
Alpha-Adrenergic Antagonists					
Alfuzosin	Uroxatral	10 mg daily	Urge associated with BPH	Xerostomia, vertigo, dizziness, fatigue, malaise	Azole antifungals, fluoroquinolones, (QT prolongation); boceprevir, tadalafil (hypotension)
Doxazosin	Cardura	IR: 1–8 mg daily XR: 4–8 mg daily	Urge associated with BPH	Edema, dizziness, somnolence, fatigue, hypotension	PDE5 inhibitors (hypotension)
Silodosin	Rapaflo	8 mg daily	Urge associated with BPH	Orthostatic hypotension, nasopharyngitis, dizziness, retroactive ejaculation	See doxazosin
Tamsulosin	Flomax	0.4–0.8 mg daily	Urge associated with BPH	Infectious disease, backache, asthenia, dizziness, rhinitis somnolence, abnormal ejaculation	See doxazosin
Terazosin	Hytrin	1–10 mg at bedtime	Urge associated with BPH	Orthostatic hypotension, palpitations, peripheral edema, asthenia, dizziness, somnolence, rhinitis	See doxazosin

BPH, benign prostatic hypertrophy; MAOI, monoamine oxidase inhibitor; S, syndrome; TCA, tricyclic antidepressant; UTI, urinary tract infection.

C. Stress incontinence
   1. Behavioral therapies are effective in some patients with stress incontinence.
   a. Pelvic muscle exercises (Kegel exercises) can lessen the severity of sphincter weakness in stress incontinence. Patients are instructed to contract the pelvic muscles for 10 seconds at a time, 30 to 80 times per day, and continue the exercises indefinitely. On average, incontinence is improved in approximately 75% to 85% of patients and eliminated in approximately 10% to 15%. Instruction in proper technique for pelvic muscle exercises is important to improve patient outcomes. (SOR **B**)
   b. Adjuncts to pelvic muscle exercises include **biofeedback** and **vaginal cones.** Each may further improve the effectiveness of treatment, although further research is necessary to quantitate the additional benefit. (SOR **C**)
   c. Bladder training (for urge incontinence as described in Section III.B.1.a) can result in additional improvement in symptoms of stress incontinence. (SOR **C**)
   2. Medications
   a. Alpha-adrenergic agonists, such as pseudoephedrine, are not recommended at this time due to limited evidence to support their efficacy. (SOR **B**)
   b. Estrogen, oral, vaginal, or transdermal, can be administered in conjunction with alpha-adrenergic agonists and may result in more improvement than alpha-adrenergic agonists alone. Vaginal estrogen alone may improve symptoms of urge or stress incontinence in women with atrophic vaginitis; however, studies to date have not shown a beneficial effect on stress incontinence. (SOR **C**) In fact, women taking hormone therapy for menopausal symptoms have a higher risk of urinary incontinence (see Chapter 80). Concerns about the risk–benefit ratio of estrogen should feature prominently in any decision about its use and if a decision is made to try hormone therapy, the lowest effective dose should be used. Low-dose vaginal estrogen (cream, suppositories or Estring®) does not require coadministration of a progestin.
   c. Duloxetine is a selective serotonin-noradrenaline receptor inhibitor that has been shown to improve quality of life and reduce episodes of stress incontinence by 50% over placebo. (SOR **B**) Duloxetine is not FDA-approved for the treatment of urinary incontinence. Nausea is a common side effect of treatment. The dose of duloxetine to treat urinary incontinence is 40 mg twice daily.
   3. Surgical options, including injections of urethral bulking agents, retropubic colposuspension, and suburethral sling, are often effective for women with stress incontinence. The appropriate surgical treatment is dictated by whether the patient's symptoms are caused by hypermobility (i.e., descent) of the urethra or by intrinsic weakness of the sphincter muscle (intrinsic sphincter deficiency). Surgery can eliminate incontinence in 70% to 85% of women with stress incontinence, though older women may have less satisfactory results. (SOR **A**) For men with stress incontinence, such as occurs after prostatectomy, injections of periurethral bulking agents (e.g., collagen) or surgical implantation of an artificial urethral sphincter can improve or eliminate incontinence. When men are treated with periurethral bulking injections and artificial sphincters, cure (i.e., complete elimination of incontinence) occurs in 20% and 50%, respectively. (SOR **C**)
   4. Devices are also available for treating stress incontinence. For women, these include pessaries, suction devices that occlude urethral outflow, and ballooned inserts that lie within the urethral orifice. For men, penile clamps are sometimes used on a temporary basis; clamps sometimes result in injury to the urethra or penile skin. There is little evidence regarding the effectiveness of these treatments. (SOR **C**)
D. Overflow incontinence must be treated by draining the bladder. Failure to drain retained urine can result in hydronephrosis and subsequent kidney damage.
   1. Intermittent catheterization, performed by patients or their caretakers, is the treatment of choice. The catheter must be clean, but not necessarily sterile, although sterile catheters are recommended for immunocompromised patients. The interval between catheterization varies, depending on how often the patient's bladder becomes distended. (SOR **C**)
   2. Chronic indwelling catheterization (i.e., Foley catheter) is generally used if intermittent catheterization is not possible. (SOR **C**)
   a. Urinary tract infection. Bacterial colonization is universal among chronically catheterized patients. Antibiotic treatment results in selection of antibiotic-resistant

organisms; therefore, only symptomatic urinary tract infections (UTIs) should be treated.

b. **Leakage around the catheter** is generally caused by encrustation of the catheter lumen and orifice with calculo-proteinaceous debris, with subsequent drainage of urine around the sides of the catheter. A larger catheter should not be used in an attempt to prevent leakage. Instead, the catheter should be replaced at a frequency dictated by the development of encrustation and leakage. **Acidification of urine** decreases buildup of encrusted material and lengthens the interval between catheter changes. Several medications can acidify urine, for example, **methenamine hippurate** (1 g orally twice daily), **ascorbic acid** (500 mg orally daily), and **acetic acid** (0.25% or less) lavage of the catheter and bladder, performed anywhere from once per week to every other day as needed to prevent encrustation.

c. **Mortality** from septic complications is increased among patients who require chronic bladder catheterization.

3. **Suprapubic catheterization** is useful in selected patients for whom neither intermittent nor chronic urethral catheterization is appropriate. (SOR ●)

E. **Intractable incontinence** exists when incontinence from any cause cannot be adequately controlled by the above measures. As noted above, irreversible overflow incontinence always requires catheter drainage. When other forms of incontinence are intractable, the following treatment options are available:

1. **Behavioral techniques** may be sufficient to decrease incontinence episodes and improve hygiene in some patients.

a. **Habit training** involves identification of the patient's natural voiding schedule and development of an individualized toileting schedule designed to preempt involuntary bladder emptying. This technique is used at nursing homes, and limited data suggest that it may improve outcomes associated with urinary incontinence. (SOR ●)

b. **Prompted voiding** involves asking patients whether they need to void and providing them with toilet facilities if they answer affirmatively. It is also used for institutionalized patients and is effective at reducing the frequency of incontinence. (SOR ●)

c. **Timed voiding** involves bringing the patient to the toilet on a fixed schedule. Limited data are available to evaluate the effectiveness of this treatment. (SOR ●)

2. **Incontinence underpants** and absorbent pads are useful for collecting and absorbing incontinent urine. The absorbent garment or pad is changed at intervals dictated by the frequency of incontinence. (SOR ●)

3. **Condom catheters** may sometimes be useful in men, especially on a short-term basis. Condom catheters increase the risk of skin problems and UTIs. (SOR ●)

4. **Intermittent catheterization,** if logistically feasible, can be used to control intractable incontinence from any cause. (SOR ●)

5. **Chronic bladder catheterization** may be used in patients whose incontinence cannot be managed by other means. (SOR ●)

6. **Diversion ureteroileostomy** may be appropriate for controlling incontinence in carefully selected patients. (SOR ●)

IV. **Management Strategies**

A. **Patient education and self-monitoring.** Patients need to be educated about the nature of their urinary incontinence and what the long- and short-term outcomes may be. Individual care planning including exercises, pharmacologic treatments, and procedures need to be carefully explained and demonstrated if possible. Providers need to be open to discussion with patients and be prepared to provide support and guidance. The following websites and handouts are available free of charge and can help lead discussions, plan treatments, and provide at-home guidance for therapies.

• For general information, PubMed provides an easy to follow explanation of urinary incontinence and helps patients identify their concerns and questions at http://www.ncbi.nlm.nih.gov/pubmedhealth/PMH0003629/ or the Urology Foundation provides multiple handouts at http://www.urologyhealth.org/urology/.

• For women, the NIDDK of the National Institute of Health provides information, exercises and diaries, as well as pre- and post-appointment information. It is publically available and providers can pick and choose the sections they would like to use at http://kidney.niddk.nih.gov/KUDiseases/pubs/bcw_ez/bcw_508.pdf.

- For men, a printable webpage is available from the NIDDK at http://kidney.niddk.nih.gov/KUDiseases/pubs/uimen/index.aspx#info.
- For bladder training, an up to date handout is publically available at http://www.nafc.org/uploads/pdf/educational%20brochures/BladderRetraining10.11.pdf.
- Information on pelvic floor exercises can be found at http://www.urologyhealth.org/_media/_pdf/Kegel%20Brochure%202009.pdf.

B. Follow-up tests. There are no specific tests to follow unless the patient has specific issues being followed by a urologist. UA with culture should be ordered when UTI is suspected.

V. Prognosis. Urinary incontinence is a long-term issue for many patients that influences their quality of life. Incontinence may worsen with age and debility. Patients need to be informed of realistic expectations for treatment and the long-term potential for treatment failure.

SELECTED REFERENCES

Gibbs CF, Johnson TM, Ouslander JG. Office management of geriatric urinary incontinence. *Am J Med.* 2007;120(3):211–220.

Glazner CMA, Lapitan MCM. Urodynamic studies (tests) for the management of urinary incontinence in children and adults. *Cochrane Database Syst Rev.* 2012;(1):CD003195.

Gormley EA, Lightner DJ, Burgio KL, et al. Diagnosis and treatment of overactive bladder (non-neurogenic) in adults: AUA/SUFU guideline. *J Urology.* 2012;188(12):2455–2463.

Goode PS, Burgio KL, Richter HE, Markland AD. Incontinence in older women. *JAMA.* 2010; 303(21):2172–2181.

Hersh L, Salzman B. Clinincal management of urinary incontinence in women. *Am Fam Physician.* 2013; 87(9):634–640.

Khandelwal C, Kistler C. Diagnosis of urinary incontinence. *Am Fam Physician.* 2013;87(8):543–550.

Ostaszkiewicz J, Chestney T, Roe B. Habit retraining for the management of urinary incontinence in adults. *Cochrane Database Syst Rew.* 2004;(2):CD002801.

Rai BP, Cody JD, Alhasso A, Stewart L. Anticholinergic drugs versus non-drug active therapies for non-neurogenic overactive bladder syndrome in adults. *Cochrane Database Syst Rev.* 2012;(12):CD003193.

Reuben DB, Herr KA, Pacala JT, et al. Incontinence-urinary and fecal. In: Reuben DB, Herr KA, Pacala JT, et al. eds. *Geriatrics at Your Fingertips.* 15th ed. New York, NY: The American Geriatrics Society; 2013:136–142.

Staskin DR, MacDiarmid SA. Pharmacological management of overactive bladder: practical options for the primary care physician. *Am J Med.* 2006;119(3A):24S–28S.

---

60 Urinary Symptoms in Men

Karl T. Rew, MD, & Linda L. Walker, MD, FAAFP

KEY POINTS

- Younger men are more likely to present with infectious processes such as **urethritis** and **acute prostatitis**. (SOR ⊙)
- Older men are prone to more insidious conditions such as **benign prostatic hypertrophy, chronic prostatitis,** and **cancers of the prostate and bladder**. Simple cystitis is not the norm in men; underlying causes of urinary tract symptoms should be sought. (SOR ⊙)

I. Definition and Key Diseases. Common urinary symptoms in men include voiding pain or discomfort, abnormal urine flow, hematuria, and urethral discharge. Pain is generally caused by infection or inflammation (e.g., urethritis or acute or chronic prostatitis). Flow is influenced by abnormal tone and physical obstruction (e.g., benign prostatic hyperplasia [BPH], prostate cancer, or urethral strictures). Hematuria may be caused by bladder or other cancers, urinary tract stones, BPH, or infections. Urethral discharge is typically caused by infections.

II. Common Diagnoses

A. Urethritis and other sexually transmitted infections (see Chapter 102).

B. Prostatitis/chronic pelvic pain syndromes (CPPS). At any time between 2% and 10% of adult males have some form of **prostatitis,** and about 15% of all men experience prostatitis in their lifetime. Risk factors for prostatitis include reflux of urine because of bladder, prostate, or urethral abnormalities; anal intercourse; epididymitis; urinary catheters; and urinary tract surgery.

The National Institutes of Health (NIH) has classified prostatitis into four categories:

1. Acute bacterial prostatitis is fairly uncommon and primarily affects men aged 30 to 50 years; it makes up 5% or fewer of all prostatitis cases.

2. Chronic bacterial prostatitis is also uncommon, making up 7% of cases and typically affecting men older than 50 years.

3. CPPS is subdivided into two categories, both of which most commonly occur in men aged 30 to 50 years.

    a. Inflammatory CPPS, also known as **nonbacterial prostatitis,** is the largest category of the prostatitis syndromes, comprising 40% to 65% of cases overall. The cause is unknown.

    b. Noninflammatory CPPS, known previously as **prostatodynia,** is also very frequently seen, occurring in 20% to 40% of cases. It also has an uncertain etiology, but may be related to internal sphincter failure and pelvic floor relaxation.

4. Asymptomatic inflammatory prostatitis is an incidental laboratory finding.

C. BPH is the most common urologic disorder of older men, leading to nearly 4.5 million patient visits each year. BPH is characterized by proliferation of the cellular elements of the prostate and can result in chronic bladder outlet, urinary retention, renal insufficiency, and recurrent urinary tract infections (UTIs) or bladder calculi. The prevalence of symptomatic BPH increases with age and is 26% in the fifth decade, 33% in the sixth decade, 41% in the seventh decade, and 46% in the eighth and older decades of life. This reflects a probable cumulative androgen effect on the prostate. Medications that may exacerbate BPH obstructive symptoms include antihistamines, anticholinergics, and decongestants.

D. The most common non-cutaneous malignancy in men is **prostate cancer,** affecting 10% of all men. As of 2013, an estimated 238,590 new cases of prostate cancer will be diagnosed annually in the United States, and approximately 29,720 men will die of prostate cancer. This makes prostate cancer the second most common cause of cancer death in men after lung cancer. However, most men with prostate cancer die of other causes including cardiovascular disease and other cancers. Rates of prostate cancer causing death vary from 16% (United States) to 49.8% (United Kingdom) in men diagnosed with prostate cancer, likely due to differences in screening protocols.

1. Risk factors. Age over 50 years is the strongest risk factor, and other risk factors include family history and being African-American. Having one, two, or three first-degree relatives with prostate cancer confers a twofold, fivefold, or 11-fold increased risk, respectively. African-Americans have the highest lifetime risk of developing prostate cancer worldwide. At an incidence rate of 229 cases per 100,000, their risk is 1.6 times greater than Caucasians for acquiring the disease and 2.4 times greater for dying from it. Asian Americans have a lower risk than Caucasians. A diet high in fat or red meat may increase risk.

E. Bladder cancer is also age-dependent; the median age at diagnosis is about 70 years, and the peak age is 85 years. It is the fourth most commonly diagnosed non-cutaneous cancer in men and the second most prevalent. As of 2013, an estimated 72,570 people in the United States will be diagnosed with bladder cancer, and approximately 15,210 will die of it; 10,820 of these deaths will be in men. The greatest risk factor is tobacco use. Other risk factors include exposure to dyes and chemicals in metal- and leather-working occupations, long-term urinary catheter use, chronic UTI, bladder calculi, and pelvic irradiation.

III. Symptoms and Signs

A. Mucopurulent urethral discharge is seen in gonococcal urethritis; in non-gonococcal urethritis, the discharge is scantier and more mucoid (see Chapter 102).

TABLE 60–1. INTERNATIONAL PROSTATE SYMPTOM SCORE (IPSS)

Over the Past Month, How Often Have You:	Scoring (0–5 Points Per Question)
1. Had a sensation of not emptying your bladder completely after you finished urinating?	Not at all = 0
2. Had to urinate again in less than 2 h after you had finished urinating?	Less than 1 time in 5 = 1
3. Found you stopped and started again several times when you urinated?	Less than half the time = 2 About half the time = 3 Greater than half the time = 4
4. Found it difficult to postpone urination?	Almost always = 5
5. Had a weak urinary stream?	
6. Had to push or strain to begin urination?	
7. Over the past month, how many times did you most typically get up to urinate from the time you went to bed at night until the time you got up in the morning?	0–5 times

Quality of Life due to Urinary Symptoms:	Score
If you were to spend the rest of your life with your urinary condition just the way it is now, how would you feel about that?	0–6 points (0 = delighted, 1 = pleased, 2 = mostly satisfied, 3 = mixed, 4 = mostly dissatisfied, 5 = unhappy, 6 = terrible)

Score 0–7: mild symptoms; Score 8–19: moderate symptoms; Score 20–35: severe symptoms.

B. Symptoms of **urinary flow abnormalities** in an older man without other complaints most commonly suggest **BPH. Lower urinary tract symptoms (LUTS)** are divided into obstructive and irritative symptoms, and most men with BPH have both.
  1. Obstructive symptoms include **hesitant or interrupted stream, decreased stream force/caliber, straining, terminal dribbling, incomplete emptying,** or **frank urinary retention** with possible **overflow incontinence** of small volumes of urine.
  2. Irritative symptoms include **frequency, urgency, urge incontinence,** and **nocturia**. These occur in BPH, prostatitis, UTIs, and malignancies, and with polyuria in systemic diseases (e.g., diabetes mellitus, congestive heart failure, or nephritic syndrome).
    a. The **International Prostate Symptom Score (IPSS)** (Table 60–1) can be used to quantify symptoms in patients who may need medication for BPH. Since these symptoms are not unique to BPH, the IPSS is most useful as a monitoring tool and should not be the sole basis for diagnosis.
  3. When **pain** is present along with flow abnormalities, **infectious, inflammatory, and malignant conditions** are higher in the differential diagnosis.
C. Pain and discomfort characterize inflammatory and infectious conditions of the prostate.
  1. Acute prostatitis usually has an unambiguous appearance when a younger man presents who is **febrile, acutely ill,** and **reports dysuria, urinary frequency and urgency, and moderate-to-severe pelvic, perineal, and low back pain.**
  2. Chronic prostatitis and CPPS typically cause gradual onset of **vague pelvic pain** or fullness, **ejaculatory or penile pain** (or both), and perhaps **testicular or scrotal aching,** along with irritative voiding and occasionally obstructive symptoms. A key component in diagnosing chronic prostatitis is a history of **recurrent UTIs** or previous bouts of prostatitis. These individuals may have **anxious or depressive symptoms** when CPPS impairs their quality of life.
D. Gross or microscopic hematuria (see Chapter 35) can be caused by **BPH** or **bladder cancer.** Urolithiasis and kidney cancer are less common causes. Patients presenting with more advanced bladder cancer may have **irritative voiding symptoms, flank pain,** or **leg edema.**
E. Acute urinary retention is most common in men who have **BPH** exacerbated by medications that precipitate sudden obstruction, or who have **acute prostatitis. Abdominal examination** or ultrasound will reveal **suprapubic tenderness,** and a **distended bladder** that may hold ≥1 L of urine; in these cases, the bladder may be percussable or palpable nearly to the umbilicus. **Chronic urinary retention** may

be asymptomatic, or may be characterized by **LUTS,** particularly **slow stream** and a **sense of incomplete emptying.**

F. Digital rectal examination of the prostate should be done in all men with urinary symptoms to evaluate for prostate size, consistency, symmetry, and masses.

1. In **acute prostatitis,** the gland is often **swollen, boggy, and tender.** To decrease the risk of bacteremia and sepsis, the examination should be done gently, particularly in the toxic, ill-appearing patient.

2. **Mild tenderness, sponginess,** or **induration** may be noted in **chronic prostatitis/CPPS.** To collect expressed prostatic secretions at the meatus for analysis and culture, the gland is massaged firmly. The examiner uses a rolling motion of the fingerpad from the lateral margins of the prostate to the midline.

3. The prostate gland may be normal in **BPH,** or it may be rubbery and enlarged.

4. Carcinoma of the prostate may be palpable as lobular asymmetry, induration, or a nodule or mass.

G. The anus, penis, testes, scrotum, and inguinal region should be evaluated for tenderness, masses, lymphadenopathy, or lesions that could be the source of the patient's genital, urinary, or pelvic complaints (e.g., anal fissure, genital ulcer, inguinal hernia, phimosis).

H. Neurologic examination should focus on anal sphincter tone (may correlate with bladder sphincter tone) and on any neurologic deficits (e.g., sudden onset of urinary or fecal incontinence, urinary retention, back pain, extremity weakness, or symmetric extremity or trunk sensory deficits) indicative of spinal cord compression if metastatic prostate cancer is suspected.

IV. Diagnostic Tests. Most common nonmalignant urologic conditions in men can be diagnosed using symptoms, physical findings, and laboratory testing available in the primary care setting. Typical patient presentations with clinical strategies for evaluation follow:

A. A sexually active man with a urethral discharge should be tested and treated for chlamydia and gonorrhea (see Chapter 102).

B. A toxic-appearing man with the acute onset of fever and chills, dysuria, severe perineal pain, obstructive symptoms, and a swollen, boggy, tender prostate has acute prostatitis; prostatic massage is contraindicated, and testing should include a **urinalysis (UA)** and **urine culture.** Tests for chlamydia and gonorrhea should be performed on urine or urethral swabs for men at risk for sexually transmitted infections (see Chapter 102). Marked pyuria will be present, and the tests are typically positive for urethritis organisms in younger men and coliform bacteria in older men.

1. **Blood cultures** should be done in hospitalized or septic-appearing patients.

2. Suspected acute urinary retention is assessed with **bladder ultrasound;** catheterization to measure residual urine is painful in men with acute prostatitis and could cause bacteremia, so it should only be done with urologic consultation.

C. A middle-aged or older man with insidious complaints of mixed irritative and obstructive voiding symptoms along with numerous genitourinary pain complaints and a mildly tender or spongy prostate gland may have chronic bacterial prostatitis or one of the two types of CPPS. All such patients should have a **UA** and **urine culture** performed. **Expressed prostatic secretions (EPS)** can be examined microscopically for white blood cells (WBCs) and sent for culture.

1. In **chronic bacterial prostatitis,** urinary and EPS cultures are often recurrently positive, with at least 10 WBCs per high-power field in the EPS. Pyuria may also be present.

2. In **inflammatory CPPS,** WBCs are seen in urine, semen, and EPS, but cultures are negative.

3. WBCs are absent in secretions in **noninflammatory CPPS.**

D. An older man with typical LUTS and a digital rectal examination consistent with BPH can generally be diagnosed on clinical grounds alone. All such patients should have a UA to screen for other contributing urinary abnormalities. (SOR ◉)

1. **Prostate-specific antigen (PSA)** testing should be performed in symptomatic men expected to live at least 10 years longer if the test results would influence clinical management. PSA will typically remain elevated for up to several months after an episode of acute prostatitis.

2. No evidence supports evaluating **blood urea nitrogen (BUN)** or **creatinine** in the absence of clinical suspicion of kidney injury or disease.

3. **Renal ultrasound** can detect asymptomatic obstructive hydronephrosis. However, as ≤2% of otherwise healthy men with BPH have this condition, renal ultrasound is not recommended as a screening test.

4. **Postvoid residual (PVR)** urine volume can be measured by ultrasound or catheterization. A normal PVR is usually less than 100 mL. However, there is no clear correlation between PVR volume and symptom severity, urodynamic test results, or outcomes. In men with acute urinary retention, a Foley catheter should be left in place because retention typically recurs in hours to days, even if precipitants such as medications are removed.

5. Referral to urology is necessary for patients with atypical or complex symptoms, when surgical therapy is contemplated, or whenever cancer of the urinary tract is suspected. The urologist may perform **urodynamic tests (uroflowmetry, cystometrography,** and **pressure flow studies)**. The urologist may also perform **cystoscopy** to visualize the urothelium and obtain tissue biopsy. **Prostate biopsy** is used to evaluate for prostate cancer.

E. **An elderly man with a significant smoking history and painless hematuria should be considered to have bladder cancer** until proven otherwise, as this is the classic presentation.

1. Evaluation of an otherwise asymptomatic, low-risk patient with microscopic hematuria includes UA and culture, urine cytology, and imaging of the urinary tract with ultrasound or CT urogram (see Chapter 35).

2. Patients with gross hematuria or persistent microscopic hematuria, with or without irritative voiding symptoms, require further investigation. This includes cytology on a spontaneously voided urine specimen, and a **CT urogram** to assess for upper tract cancers, stones, or obstruction. A urologist performs **cystoscopy** to assess the bladder and **biopsy** to definitively diagnose bladder cancer. High-risk patients with a negative initial evaluation need ongoing surveillance for malignancy.

F. **When a man requests PSA screening for prostate cancer,** he needs thorough counseling on the pros and cons of testing, as recommendations have been changing. The **United States Preventive Services Task Force** (USPSTF) recommends against PSA screening for prostate cancer at any age. The **American Urological Association** (AUA) recommends against routine PSA screening in men under age 55 years who are at average risk, recommends informed decision-making for men aged 55–69 years, and suggests a screening interval of every 2 years to reduce over-diagnosis. The **American Cancer Society** (ACS) recommends that annual PSA screening be discussed with men aged 50 years and older who have a life expectancy of at least 10 years. Both these groups recommend that screening for African-Americans and those with an affected relative be individualized. A useful shared-decision-making tool can be obtained at http://www.uspreventiveservicestaskforce.org/prostatecancerscreening/prostatecancerinfo.pdf. The following points should be kept in mind when counseling men about screening PSAs:

1. **Normal PSA levels ($\leq$4 ng/mL)** are present in about 15% of men with prostate cancer.

2. **Mild elevations of PSA (4–10 ng/mL)** are frequently found, and 75% of cases are due to benign conditions, usually BPH.

3. Urologic evaluation including **transrectal ultrasound (TRUS)** and **prostate biopsy** is used to assess for prostate cancer in men with an elevated PSA.

4. PSA screening can result in detection and treatment of indolent cancer that otherwise may never have caused any health problems during the patient's lifetime, but can cause considerable anxiety and lifestyle changes from knowledge of test results and decision-making relating to treatment. Treatment for prostate cancer can also cause significant morbidity including urinary incontinence and sexual dysfunction (see Chapters 59 and 101).

5. A patient should be referred to a urologist when the PSA is greater than expected, using standardized laboratory norms. Some advocate evaluation for a PSA velocity (rise over time) of more than 0.75 ng/mL/year.

G. **Advanced prostate cancer.** A minority of men with prostate cancer present with symptoms of advanced disease, such as **advanced urinary symptoms, a markedly abnormal prostate examination, gross hematuria, bone pain, elevated alkaline phosphatase (highly suggestive of bony metastases), and generally markedly elevated PSA.** All such patients should see a urologist. When the PSA is $\geq$10 ng/mL, there is at least a 50% chance of prostate cancer, and the risk rises exponentially as PSA values do. In advanced cancer, the PSA may be $\geq$100 ng/mL. PSA is monitored to assess response to treatment.

H. If a prostate nodule is detected in the course of a screening examination or when evaluating a patient with LUTS, a diagnostic PSA should be ordered. Regardless of the results, urologic referral is indicated for further evaluation.

V. Treatment

    A. Urethritis (see Chapter 102.)

    B. Acute prostatitis

        1. Men younger than 35 years are treated with a single intramuscular dose of **ceftriaxone** 250 mg followed by oral **doxycycline** 100 mg twice daily for 10 days. (SOR ⊙)

        2. In older men, prostatitis caused by coliform bacteria is treated with a 10- to 14-day course of oral antibiotics, either with a fluoroquinolone such as **levofloxacin** 750 mg daily or **ciprofloxacin** 500 mg twice daily or with **trimethoprim-sulfamethoxazole (TMP-SMX DS)** twice daily. Some authorities recommend 4 weeks of therapy for acute prostatitis.

        3. Oral **nonsteroidal anti-inflammatory drugs (NSAIDs),** such as **ibuprofen,** 400 to 800 mg every 6–8 hours, can be used for analgesia. Oral **acetaminophen,** 500–1000 mg every 4–6 hours up to 4 g per day may also be used. **Opiates** may be needed for severe pain. However, acute urinary retention can be precipitated by opiate use, and opiate side effects such as constipation can make urinary symptoms worse.

        4. Hospitalization and **intravenous antibiotics** may be necessary for severely ill patients.

    C. Optimal treatments for **chronic bacterial prostatitis and CPPS** are being investigated in numerous ongoing clinical trials.

        1. Chronic bacterial prostatitis is treated with the antibiotics listed for acute bacterial prostatitis, in prolonged courses lasting 4 to 6 weeks for quinolones, and up to 12 weeks for TMP-SMX, repeated as necessary. (SOR ⑧)

            a. If recurrences are frequent, data support symptomatic use of oral **alpha-blockers** such as **tamsulosin** 0.4 mg once daily. (SOR ⑧)

            b. Older treatments include repetitive **prostatic massage** and **frequent ejaculation**.

            c. For severe symptoms (Table 60–1) that persist despite medical therapy, urologic consultation for possible surgery may be beneficial.

        2. CPPS. Because WBCs are seen in prostatic secretions in **inflammatory CPPS, antibiotics** as above are tried for 4 weeks. No specific therapy has emerged as clearly beneficial for CPPS. (SOR ⑧) In a usual patient, several are tried in succession, using individual response as a guide.

            a. For the obstructive symptoms of either type of CPPS, at least a 12-week trial of **alpha-blockers** is recommended (Table 60–2).

            b. Pain symptoms are treated with an oral **NSAID** such as **ibuprofen** 400 to 800 mg every 6–8 hours for at least a 6-week trial. If symptoms persist, patients are reevaluated for further therapy.

            c. Dietary modifications are often recommended, including avoidance of caffeine and other bladder irritants such as alcohol, but there is no clear evidence of benefit.

            d. Men older than 40 years with inflammatory CPPS can be offered a long-term trial of oral **finasteride** 5 mg daily or **dutasteride** 0.5 mg daily. These drugs are **5-alpha-reductase inhibitors**, blocking testosterone conversion in the prostate. These medications are used primarily in BPH to shrink enlarged tissue and can be continued long-term if the patient gets symptomatic relief (Table 60–2). They cause an artificial reduction of about 50% in PSA levels after about 6 months.

            e. Supportive counseling and psychological treatment may be necessary for patients severely affected by lifestyle limitations of their condition. (SOR ⊙) It is especially important that any fears patients have about contagion or cancer be addressed and allayed.

            f. Patients with CPPS and refractory voiding symptoms may benefit from a trial of **pentosan polysulfate sodium** 100 mg orally three times a day for a limited course of 3 to 6 months, usually under urologic supervision. This drug should be taken 1 hour before or 2 hours after food.

            g. As in chronic prostatitis, urologists may offer various **surgical interventions**. Unfortunately, there are limited data on the benefits of surgical options. Case

TABLE 60–2. MEDICATIONS FOR SYMPTOMATIC PROSTATIC HYPERPLASIA

Generic Name	Brand Name	Strength	Usual Dose	Comments	Side Effects[a]	Safety/Drug Interactions
Selective Alpha-Blockers (in general, less orthostatic hypotension than the non-selective alpha-blockers)						
Tamsulosin	Flomax	0.4 mg	0.4–0.8 mg daily	May need to titrate dose	Headache, dizziness, abnormal ejaculation, rhinitis, asthenia, backache, infectious disease Most likely to cause floppy iris syndrome	Tadalafil (orthostatic hypotension)
Alfuzosin extended release	Uroxatral	10 mg ER	10 mg daily	Reduce dosing for hepatic disease	Dizziness, fatigue, dry mouth	**Multiple Interactions** Tadalafil (orthostatic hypotension); salmeterol, azithromycin, antibiotics, amitriptyline, quinolones, fluoxetine, trazodone (QT prolongation) Contraindicated with CYP3A4 inhibitors such as ketoconazole and ritonavir
Silodosin	Rapaflo	4, 8 mg	4–8 mg daily	Renal and hepatic precautions	Nasal congestion. Most likely to cause ejaculatory problems.	Sildenafil, vardenafil (orthostatic hypotension); Not recommended with CYP3A4 inhibitors (as above) or cyclosporine Contraindicated if CrCl <30 mL/min or if liver disease at Child-Pugh Class C
Non-Selective Alpha-Blockers						
Terazosin	Hytrin	1, 2, 5, 10 mg	1–10 mg daily	Titrate dose; max dose 20 mg daily	Dizziness, headache, fatigue, edema, orthostatic hypotension	Sildenafil, vardenafil, Tadalafil, beta-blockers, verapamil (orthostatic hypotension)
Doxazosin Doxazosin extended release	Cardura Cardura XL	1, 2, 4, 8 mg 4, 8 mg ER	1–8 mg daily	Titrate dose; max dose 8 mg daily Hepatic precautions	See terazosin	See terazosin
Prazosin	Minipress	1, 2, 5 mg	0.5–5 mg twice daily	Titrate dose Hepatic precautions Rarely used for BPH; FDA-approved for hypertension, not BPH	Palpitations, nausea, dizziness, headache, fatigue, asthenia	See terazosin

(continued)

TABLE 60–2. MEDICATIONS FOR SYMPTOMATIC PROSTATIC HYPERPLASIA (*Continued*)

Generic Name	Brand Name	Strength	Usual Dose	Comments	Side Effects[a]	Safety/Drug Interactions
5-Alpha-Reductase Inhibitors (5-ARIs)[b]						
Finasteride	Proscar	1, 5 mg	5 mg daily	Decreases PSA level by about 50% at 6 months	Decreased libido, abnormal ejaculation,[c] breast tenderness	Nevirapine, St. John's wort (decreased efficacy of finasteride; can increase PSA)
Dutasteride	Avodart	0.5 mg	0.5 mg daily	As above	Reduced libido, impotence	Ciprofloxacin, ritonavir, ketoconazole, verapamil, cimetidine (increased dutasteride toxicity)
Combination 5-ARI/Alpha-Blocker[c]						
Dutasteride/tamsulosin	Jalyn	0.5/0.4 mg	0.5/0.4 mg daily	As above	See above	See above
Phosphodiesterase-5 (PDE-5) Inhibitor						
Tadalafil	Cialis	2.5, 5, 10, 20 mg	5 mg daily	Titrate dose Renal and hepatic precautions Also used for erectile dysfunction	Headache, nausea, flushing, myalgia, backache, nasopharyngitis, respiratory infection	May affect QT interval alpha₁-blockers (hypotension); protease inhibitors, itraconazole, macrolide antibiotics, rifampin (adverse effects of tadalafil); simvastatin (myopathy) Contraindicated with nitrates

[a]Alpha-blockers may cause hypotension if used with PDE-5 inhibitors, such as sildenafil, vardenafil, and tadalafil. Current or prior alpha-blocker use can lead to intraoperative floppy iris syndrome during cataract surgery.
[b]5-ARIs may reduce the overall risk of prostate cancer, but may increase the risk of high-grade prostate cancer.
[c]Sexual side effects caused by 5-ARIs are usually reversible but can be long-term.
BPH, benign prostatic hyperplasia; CrCl, creatinine clearance; ER, extended release; FDA, Food and Drug Administration; PSA, prostate-specific antigen.

series of bladder neck surgery have reported benefits in some patients with CPPS and obstructive voiding symptoms due to bladder neck obstruction. A small randomized trial demonstrated that transurethral microwave thermotherapy provided more long-term benefit than sham control in patients with Category IIIA chronic prostatitis/CPPS. Transurethral needle ablation has also been suggested, but a small sham-controlled study did not support efficacy.

  h. The most commonly tried **phytotherapy** consists of **quercetin**, a **bioflavonoid**. There is no recommended standard dose and no clear evidence of benefit. **Pollen extracts** have also been used.

  i. **Biofeedback, acupuncture,** and **neurostimulation** of the pelvic floor muscles are therapeutic adjuncts without proven benefit.

D. BPH

  1. **Watchful waiting** is the recommendation of choice for patients with mild symptom scores, which should be reassessed annually (Table 60–1). (SOR ❸) **Lifestyle changes** should include **restriction of caffeine and bedtime fluids and limitation of any sympathomimetic (e.g., decongestants) and anticholinergic medications. Frequent, regular voiding** may improve quality of life.

  2. **Drug therapy.** In patients with moderate or severe symptoms, medication should also be considered. (See Table 60–2.)

      a. Patients wishing to begin medication should initially be offered **alpha-blockers** such as **tamsulosin**. These drugs block the reversible component of obstructive symptoms (prostatic smooth muscle contraction), providing fairly prompt relief. (SOR ❹) The specific **alpha₁-blockers** (such as **tamsulosin**) cause less hypotension than the non-specific alpha₁-blockers (such as terazosin).

      b. Oral **5-alpha-reductase** inhibitors such as **finasteride** and **dutasteride** slowly reduce prostate gland volume by about 25%. PSA values in patients taking these medications are artificially lowered and should be doubled for accurate interpretation. (SOR ❹) Long-term use may decrease the total risk of prostate cancer, but may increase the risk of high-grade prostate cancer.

      c. The long-acting oral **phosphodiesterase-5 inhibitor, tadalafil 5 mg daily,** can be used for symptomatic BPH in men who also have erectile dysfunction, or in men who have incomplete relief with alpha-blockers and 5-alpha-reductase inhibitors. Hypotension may occur when phosphodiesterase-5 inhibitors are used in conjunction with alpha-blockers.

      d. **Saw palmetto**, alone or with other herbs, has been a popular choice for men with voiding symptoms, although recent trials show **no objective benefit**. (SOR ❹)

  3. **Urologic referral** is indicated for men with BPH and marked urinary retention, recurrent UTIs, gross hematuria, bladder calculi, or chronic kidney disease caused by obstruction. A variety of laser and surgical interventions are used to relieve symptoms long-term. Retrograde ejaculation may be a side effect. Less frequently seen are erectile dysfunction, UTIs, and incontinence.

E. Prostate cancer management is based on histologic tumor grading (glandular disorganization based on the Gleason system) and clinical staging is based on tumor size; local extension; spread to pelvic lymphatics; and metastases to bone, lungs, or liver. The patient's overall expected longevity should be considered based on age and medical conditions. The course of prostate cancer is quite variable, from a slow, indolent disease lasting years or decades (most common) to a rapid, invasive illness causing mortality in a few years or less. The 5-year survival rate for all stages combined is 99%, and for those with distant metastases is 28%. Survival for several years is not uncommon in metastatic disease.

  1. For **localized prostate cancer,** options may include **active surveillance, radical prostatectomy,** several forms of **radiation** therapy, or other treatments, selected in consultation with specialists in urology and radiation oncology. Risks of treatment include erectile dysfunction, urinary incontinence, and radiation injury to the bowel or bladder.

  2. In more **advanced prostate cancer, surgery** can relieve obstruction, whereas radiation can improve urinary and metastatic symptoms, such as bone pain.

  3. **Widespread prostate cancer** is often treated **palliatively**. **Orchiectomy** and various hormonal therapies are often used to cause tumor regression by inducing androgen deprivation. **Chemotherapy** may also be used. **Sipuleucel-T** is a type of **immunotherapy,** often termed a "prostate cancer vaccine," that can be used to treat some patients.

F. As with prostate cancer, **bladder cancer** management should be coordinated by a urologist knowledgeable in oncology.

1. **Superficial bladder cancer** can be treated by **local resection** during **cystoscopy. Bacille Calmette-Guérin (BCG) instillations** into the bladder are used for patients at high risk for recurrence, and **intravesical chemotherapy** may be used to prevent or treat recurrences. The average 5-year survival rate for all stages of bladder cancer at diagnosis is 78%, but rates vary widely, depending on the extent of disease.

2. For **locally invasive bladder cancer, radical cystectomy** offers a 40% to 60% 5-year survival rate. **Radiation** is an acceptable alternative.

3. **Chemotherapy** is the treatment for metastatic bladder cancer; however, there is only about a 10% 5-year survival.

SELECTED REFERENCES

American Cancer Society. Cancer facts & figures 2013. http://www.cancer.org/acs/groups/content/@epidemiologysurveilance/documents/document/acspc-036845.pdf. Accessed September 2013.

American Cancer Society. Cancer facts & figures for African-Americans, 2013–14. http://www.cancer.org/acs/groups/content/@epidemiologysurveilance/documents/document/acspc-036921.pdf. Accessed September 2013.

American Cancer Society. Prostate cancer. http://www.cancer.org/acs/groups/cid/documents/webcontent/003134-pdf.pdf. Accessed September 2013.

American Urological Association. Early detection of prostate cancer: AUA guideline. http://www.auanet.org/education/guidelines/prostate-cancer-detection.cfm. Accessed September 2013.

Anothaisintawee T, Attia J, Nickel JC, et al. Management of chronic prostatitis/chronic pelvic pain syndrome: a systematic review and network meta-analysis. JAMA. 2011;305:78–86.

Bent S, Kane C, Shinohara K, et al. Saw palmetto for benign prostatic hyperplasia. N Engl J Med. 2006;354(6):557–566.

Chowdhury S, Robinson D, Cahill D, et al. Causes of death in men with prostate cancer: an analysis of 50000 men from the Thames Cancer Registry. BJU Int. 2013;112(2):182–189.

Epstein MM, Edgren G, Rider JR, et al. Temporal trends in cause of death among Swedish and US men with prostate cancer. J Natl Cancer Inst. 2012;104(17):1335–1342.

Gore JL, Litwin MS, Yano EM, et al. Use of radical cystectomy for patients with invasive bladder cancer. J Natl Cancer Inst. 2010;102:802–811.

Kantoff PW, Higano CS, Shore ND, et al. Sipuleucel-T immunotherapy for castration-resistant prostate cancer. N Engl J Med. 2010;363:411–422.

Krieger JN, Lee SW, Jeon J, et al. Epidemiology of prostatitis. Int J Antimicrob Agents. 2008;31(Suppl 1): S85–S90.

Lipsky BA, Byren I, Hoey CT. Treatment of bacterial prostatitis. Clin Infect Dis. 2010;50:1641–1652.

McVary KT, Roehrborn CG, Avins AL, et al. Update on AUA guideline on the management of benign prostatic hyperplasia. J Urol. 2011;185:1793–1803.

National Institutes of Health, National Kidney and Urologic Diseases Information Clearinghouse. Prostatitis: Disorders of the Prostate. NIH Publication No. 08–4553. http://kidney.niddk.nih.gov/kudiseases/pubs/prostatitis/. Updated June 29, 2012. Accessed June 22, 2013.

Nickel JC. Treatment of chronic prostatitis/chronic pelvic pain syndrome. Int J Antimicrob Agents. 2008;31(Suppl 1):112–116.

Nickel JC, Forrest JB, Tomera K, et al. Pentosan polysulfate sodium therapy for men with chronic pelvic pain syndrome. J Urol. 2005;173(4):1252–1255.

Nickel JC, Gilling P, Tammela TL, et al. Comparison of dutasteride and finasteride for treating benign prostatic hyperplasia: the Enlarged Prostate International Comparator Study (EPICS). BJU Int. 2011; 108:388–394.

Potts JM. Nonpharmacological approaches for the treatment of urological chronic pelvic pain syndromes in men. Curr Prostate Rep. 2009;7:79–84.

Shariat SF, Sfakianos JP, Droller MJ, et al. The effect of age and gender on bladder cancer: a critical review of the literature. BJU Int. 2010;105:300–308.

Thompson IM Jr, Goodman PJ, Tangen CM, et al. Long-term survival of participants in the Prostate Cancer Prevention Trial. N Engl J Med. 2013;369:603–610.

U.S. Preventive Services Task Force. Screening for Prostate Cancer (published May 2012). http://www.uspreventiveservicestaskforce.org/prostatecancerscreening.htm. Accessed September 2013.

von der Maase H, Sengelov L, Roberts JT, et al. Long-term survival results of a randomized trial comparing gemcitabine plus cisplatin, with methotrexate, vinblastine, doxorubicin, plus cisplatin in patients with bladder cancer. J Clin Oncol. 2005;23:4602–4608.

Wei JT, Calhoun E, Jacobsen SJ. Urologic diseases in America project: benign prostatic hyperplasia. J Urol. 2005;173:1256–1261.

Zeegers MP, Jellema A, Ostrer H. Empiric risk of prostate carcinoma for relatives of patients with prostate carcinoma: a meta-analysis. Cancer. 2003;97:1894–1903.

61   Urticaria

Robert Ellis, MD, Montiel Rosenthal, MD, & Laura Counsell, MD

KEY POINTS

- Urticaria or "hives" is a common disorder that causes a raised erythematous intensely pruritic rash or "wheal." (SOR ❸)
- Natural course is most often self-limited and treatment is aimed at relieving symptoms and avoiding triggers. (SOR ❸)
- Unless indicated by the history or physical examination, laboratory evaluation and additional tests are usually unnecessary. (SOR ❸)
- The etiology of urticaria is often not apparent even after careful history, physical examination, and additional tests. (SOR ❸)

I. **Definition.** Urticaria are **transient,** circumscribed, raised erythematous, sometimes burning, and intensely pruritic skin lesions or wheals of varying size. In the acute form, individual lesions can last 24 hours. The evanescent nature of the wheals, or hives with their dermal edema, may lead to diagnostic confusion with other erythematous rashes. These lesions can occur in conjunction with angioedema, a nonpruritic, sometimes painful swelling of subcutaneous, dermal, and often mucosal tissue which can last up to 72 hours. In 30% of cases of urticaria where IgE is implicated, environmental, drug, dietary, and unknown factors serve as triggers to mast cells in the dermis, leading to degranulation of these cells and release of histamine. Other immune-modulating substances such as prostaglandins, kinins, and leukotrienes also lead to increased vascular permeability, vasodilation, and transudation of fluid from capillaries and small blood vessels into the surrounding tissue, resulting in dermal edema and hyperemia. Chronic urticaria lasts more than 6 weeks and has a more complex differential diagnosis.

II. **Common Diagnoses.** Urticaria is one of the most common skin conditions encountered by family physicians. The lifetime incidence is 10% to 24%. Acute urticaria is more common than chronic urticaria and females and young adults have a higher incidence. In 60% to 70% of cases of urticaria, there is no identifiable cause. This increases to 80% to 90% in chronic urticaria. The following are specific causes of urticaria:

   A. **Physical factors** (5%–10% of cases).

      1. **Dermographism** (skin writing) (Figure 61–1) is the most common physical urticaria with a lifetime prevalence of 5%; dermatographism tends to affect young adults. It presents as the formation of wheals in response to shearing forces on the skin, and forms within minutes. Common sites affected include the waist and neck where clothing tends to cause friction.

      2. **Delayed pressure urticaria** is deep and painful swelling that develops over 4 to 8 hours in response to a prolonged static pressure. It lasts 8 to 48 hours, can be associated with fever and malaise, and is typically seen on the soles, palms, buttocks, and posterior thighs. Males are more often affected.

      3. **Cold urticaria** is a reaction to cold stimuli and can also present on rewarming after cold exposure. Women are more likely to be affected. Cold urticaria can be associated with infections, autoimmune disease, and possibly neoplasia.

      4. **Heat urticaria** is a rare form occurring after exposure to temperatures greater than 38°C.

      5. **Solar urticaria** is a rare reaction to either visible or ultraviolet (UV) wavelengths between 280 and 760 nm.

      6. **Cholinergic urticaria,** induced by heat, emotional stress, or exercise, results in 2- to 3-mm scattered wheals surrounded by large erythematous macules.

   B. **Infections** (10%–15% of cases) are a significant cause of both acute and chronic urticaria. They may account for more than 80% of pediatric cases. Nonspecific viral infections are considered the most common causative agent. Other infections include hepatitis A and B, bacterial infections of the nasopharynx, HIV infection, *Helicobacter pylori infection*, infectious mononucleosis, tuberculosis, syphilis, and parasites.

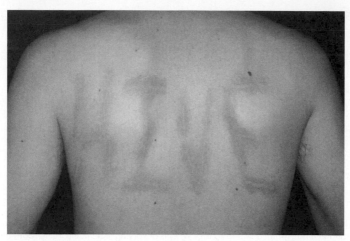

FIGURE 61-1. Dermatographism in a 21-year-old man with chronic urticarial (see color insert). (Used with permission of Richard P. Usatine, MD.)

   C. Medications (5%–10% of cases). The most common causes include penicillins, cephalosporins, and sulfa drugs. Aspirin and nonsteroidal anti-inflammatory drugs may potentiate urticaria caused by other factors. Codeine and contrast dye may cause direct degranulation of mast cells. Exogenous progesterone and preservatives, such as methylparaben used in local anesthetics and medroxyprogesterone, can also cause urticaria.

   D. Foods and **food additives** used for color, preservation, and taste may also cause urticaria. Nuts, seafood, eggs, soy, and wheat are among the foods implicated. Food as a true cause of urticaria is much less common than that perceived by patients and general physicians and accounts for 1% to 15% of cases of acute and chronic urticaria. Additives are an even rarer cause of urticaria.

   E. Other. Insect bites or stings and caterpillar toxins may cause urticaria. Collagen vascular disease, autoimmune disease, antithyroid receptor antibodies, and hereditary conditions predispose to urticaria.

   F. Emotional and psychogenic factors are implicated in urticaria, although there is insufficient research to support these in isolation from other factors.

III. Symptoms. Pruritus is most commonly present with urticaria and varies in severity. The intensity of the pruritus, like urticaria itself, is affected by extremes of heat and cold, the consumption of alcohol, and emotional distress. Angioedema (Figure 61-2) manifests as tense swelling of the lips and oral or respiratory mucosa and can lead to respiratory arrest if not addressed in sufficient time.

IV. Signs. The characteristic skin lesions of urticaria are evanescent, erythematous, well demarcated, and raised (Figure 61-3). There may be blanching of edematous central areas. Where the skin has been scratched or exposed to extremes of heat, lesions tend to be more prominent. While examining the patient, the physician should test for dermographism by firmly stroking the patient's skin (Figure 61-1) and should test for other causes of physical urticaria (pressure, cold, heat, contact irritant, aquagenic, solar, and delayed pressure) when the patient's history indicates that further testing would be appropriate.

V. Laboratory Tests (Figure 61-4).

   A. Acute urticaria

      1. Does not require laboratory evaluation unless suggested by the patient's history and physical examination or in cases of urticarial vasculitis.

      2. Urticarial vasculitis should be suspected in patients with individual lesions that persist for more than 48 hours, are painful, and are accompanied by ecchymosis or petechiae. Tests include skin biopsy, complete blood count (CBC) with differential,

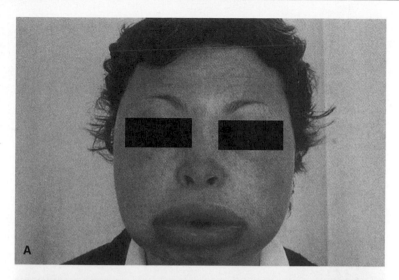

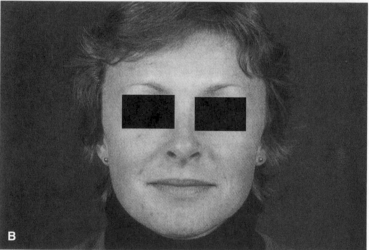

FIGURE 61–2. Hereditary angioedema. **A.** Severe edema of the face during an episode leading to grotesque disfigurement. **B.** Angioedema will subside within hours. The patient had a positive family history and had multiple similar episodes including colicky abdominal pain (see color insert). (Used with permission from Fitzpatrick's Color Atlas and Synopsis of Clinical Dermatology, 5th ed. New York, NY: McGraw-Hill; 2005.)

      erythrocyte sedimentation rate (ESR), antinuclear antibody, and serum complement assays.

    3. Consider checking for streptococcal infection in pediatric patients.

B. Chronic or persistent urticaria

    1. Tests are not required for mild disease that responds to antihistamines.

    2. For more severe symptoms and nonresponders, workup includes CBC with differential, ESR, and thyroid-stimulating hormone with antithyroid antibodies.

VI. Treatment (Table 61–1). Removal of the offending agent and management of the underlying cause are the treatments of choice when possible. If the patient has not had life-threatening

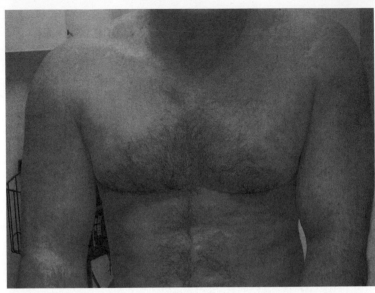

FIGURE 61–3. A 26-year-old man with acute urticaria due to trimethoprim-sulfamethoxazole (see color insert). (Used with permission of Richard P. Usatine, MD.)

angioedema as part of their symptom complex, they may benefit from a trial of provocative testing to establish a cause for urticaria if the cause was not apparent at the first visit. Patients with life-threatening angioedema or anaphylaxis should be referred for allergy testing, if no definitive cause has been identified. Referral is also indicated for patients with severe or persistent symptoms.

A. Patient education. If the cause of urticaria cannot be established during the office visit, the patient should be educated about possible offending agents, ideally with the help of a printed handout. Patients are often their own best detective in sifting through exacerbating factors they encounter between physician visits.

B. General measures

  1. The patient should avoid vasodilating influences such as heat, emotional stress, exertion, and alcohol.

  2. Cool compresses, oatmeal baths, and antipruritic lotions may provide some relief.

  3. Consider discontinuing aspirin use.

  4. Urticaria and angioedema, like other skin conditions, are highly visible to the patient and may contribute to the patient's anxiety which can aggravate the condition. **Reassuring the patient** that the condition is usually self-limited can be beneficial.

  5. Follow-up care is required when the condition is prolonged for 6 weeks or more, when the condition worsens, or when new symptoms present.

C. Medications (Tables 61–2 to 61–4).

  1. Oral **antihistamines,** including ones likely to cause sedation such as **hydroxyzine, diphenhydramine, chlorpheniramine,** and relatively nonsedating ones such as **loratadine, fexofenadine, and cetirizine,** are commonly used. There is some individual variation in response.

  a. Hydroxyzine and cetirizine are sometimes more effective than other antihistamines. Cetirizine may cause sedation but less so than hydroxyzine; higher doses of these may be used to control symptoms if tolerated.

  b. Loratadine and fexofenadine can be especially useful because they are generally nonsedating. In some patients, the combination of a nonsedating antihistamine in the morning and a sedating one in the evening will be beneficial.

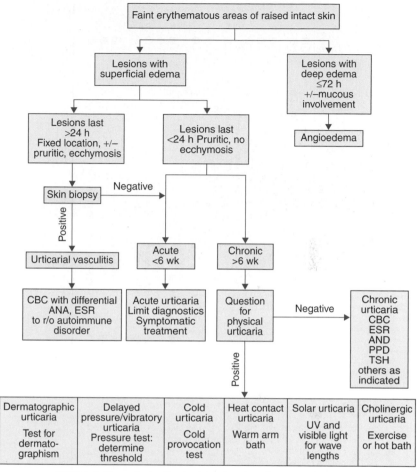

FIGURE 61-4. Diagnostic algorithm for the workup of a rash suspicious for urticaria.

    c. Diphenhydramine, chlorpheniramine, cetirizine, fexofenadine, and loratadine are available without a prescription, which may represent an advantage for some patients.

  2. Other medications that are occasionally used include the following:

    a. Systemic corticosteroids are useful in severe and poorly responsive cases of urticaria. **Prednisone** can be used in various doses for adults (see Table 61–2) and should be added to antihistamine therapy after weighing benefits and risks. Topical corticosteroids have little value in the treatment of urticaria.

    b. Leukotriene inhibitors (montelukast) may be useful in some cases of urticaria. They have been shown to provide benefit in placebo-controlled trials.

    c. The subcutaneous injection of **epinephrine** may be used to confirm the transient nature of the lesions, to provide temporary relief to the acutely symptomatic patient, and in cases of anaphylaxis.

    d. H_2 antihistamines, such as ranitidine, sometimes provide benefit when added to H_1 antihistamine treatment but are of little value when used alone. The use of **ephedrine, terbutaline, doxepin, nifedipine, colchicine,** and **dapsone** has been reported to benefit some patients.

TABLE 61–1. TYPES OF URTICARIA WITH TREATMENT OPTIONS

Types of Urticaria	Initial Treatment	SOR	Other Treatment Options	SOR
Acute	H_1 antihistamines	A	H_2 antihistamine combined with H_1	B
			Desensitization protocol for aspirin in patients with acute coronary syndrome and cardiovascular disease	B
			Epinephrine 0.3 mL SQ of 1:1000	C
Chronic	H_1 antihistamines (as above)	A	H_2 antihistamine combined with H_1	B
	Loratadine or Cetirizine, and possibly Mizolastine, appear to be treatment of choice for chronic idiopathic urticaria		Doxepin, montelukast, prednisone, nifedipine, or sulfasalazine (the latter requires intensive monitoring	C
			Cyclosporine can be effective for severe autoimmune-related urticaria but use limited by side effects and monitoring issues	A
			Dapsone 100–200 mg qd (requires intensive monitoring)	A
Physical	Avoidance of triggers	C	PUVA	C
Dermatographic	H_1 antihistamines	A	Corticosteroid burst	C
Delayed pressure	High-dose H_1 antihistamine	A	Corticosteroids, prolonged treatment	C
Cold	H_1 antihistamines	A	Inducing tolerance, montelukast	C
Heat contact	Inducing tolerance	C		
Solar	Inducing tolerance with UV light or PUVA	C	H_1 antihistamines (as above)	A
Cholinergic	H_1 antihistamines	A	Danazol	C
Urticarial vasculitis	Find and treat underlying cause of vasculitis, often autoimmune	C	Corticosteroids prolonged treatment	C

TABLE 61-2. MEDICATIONS FOR ACUTE URTICARIA (ABOVE)

Drug	Dose	Major Side Effects	Contraindications	Major Drug Interactions
Second Generation H₁ Antihistamines (nonsedating)				
Cetirizine	**Adults:** 5 or 10 mg once daily **Children:** 6–23 mo: 2.5 mg once daily; 12–23 mo: may increase to twice daily; 2–5 yr: 2.5 mg —one to two times daily or 5 mg daily; ≥6 yr: 5–10 mg daily	**Adult:** drowsiness, somnolence, fatigue, dry mouth, pharyngitis **Children:** headache, GI upset/pain, cough, diarrhea, bronchospasm, epistaxis, irritability, insomnia **Elderly:** somnolence, drowsiness, delirium	Antihistamine sensitivity Pregnancy Category B	
Desloratadine	**Adults and children 12 yr of age and older:** 5 mg once daily Renal or hepatic impairment: start at 5 mg every other day **Children:** 6–11 mo: 1 mg daily; 1–5 yr: 1.25 mg daily; 6–11 yr: 2.5 mg daily	Pharyngitis, xerostomia, somnolence, headache, fatigue, myalgia, dyspepsia	Pregnancy Category C Avoid in nursing mothers	
Fexofenadine (off label use)	**Adults and children 12 yr and older:** 60 mg twice daily or 180 mg once daily; renal impairment: start at 60 mg once daily **Children:** 6–24 mo: 15 mg twice daily; 2–11 yr: 30 mg twice daily	Headache, back pain, viral infection, GI upset, sinusitis, dizziness, drowsiness	Pregnancy Category C	Antacids (decreased fexofenadine efficacy)
Levocetirizine	**Adults and children 12 yr and older:** 2.5–5 mg daily; renal dysfunction: CrCl 50–80 mL/min: 2.5 mg daily; CrCl 30–50 mL/min: 2.5 mg every other day; CrCl 10–30 mL/min: 2.5 mg twice weekly **Children:** 6 mo to 5 yr: 1.25 mg at night; 6–11 yr: 2.5 mg at night	**Adults:** somnolence, pharyngitis, fatigue, dry mouth **Children:** pyrexia, somnolence, cough, epistaxis, diarrhea, vomiting, otitis media	Renal failure (CrCl <10 mL/min) or hemodialysis Impaired renal function in <12 y Pregnancy Category B Avoid in nursing mothers	Alcohol, CNS depressants (decreased metal alertness)
Loratadine	**Adults and children 5 yr and older:** 10 mg daily **Children:** 2–5 yr: 5 mg daily	**Adults:** headache, fatigue, dry mouth **Children:** nervousness, wheezing, hyperkinesia, abdominal pain, conjunctivitis, dysphonia, malaise, URI	Pregnancy Category B	
First-Generation H₁ Antihistamines—recommended as adjunct with second-generation for nocturnal symptoms				
Diphenhydramine	**Adults:** 25–50 mg every 4–6 h, max 300 mg/d **Children:** <6 yr and >9 kg: 5 mg/kg/d divided every 6–8 h (max 300 mg/d); 6–11 yr: 12.5–25 mg every 4–6 h (max 300 mg/d)	**Adults:** drowsiness, dizziness, anticholinergic effects **Children:** drowsiness or excitability **Elderly:** anticholinergic effects, delirium	Neonates, preterm infants, acute asthma Caution: asthma or lower respiratory disorders, CV disease, glaucoma, hyperthyroidism, hypertension, GI or urinary obstruction Pregnancy Category B Avoid in nursing mothers	Alcohol, sedatives, or other CNS depressants (additive CNS effects) Linezolid (anticholinergic toxicity)

(continued)

TABLE 61–2. MEDICATIONS FOR ACUTE URTICARIA (ABOVE) (Continued)

Drug	Dose	Major Side Effects	Contraindications	Major Drug Interactions
Chlorpheniramine (off-label use)	**Adults:** 4 mg every 4–6 h or 8–12 mg of extended-release formulation every 8–12 h **Children:** 6–11 yr: 2 mg every 4–6 h, max 12 mg/d. Not recommended in children less than 6 yr of age	**Adults:** drowsiness, dry mouth, nausea, vomiting, loss of appetite, constipation, headache, chest congestion, vision problems, difficulty urinating **Elderly:** increased risk of sedation, dizziness, hypotension	Avoid in the elderly Pregnancy Category C	Alcohol, sedatives, or other CNS depressants (additive CNS effects), amitriptyline, fentanyl, desvenlafaxine, trazodone (serotonin S)
Cyproheptadine	**Adults:** 4–20 mg daily, divided three times daily (max 0.5 mg/kg/d) **Children:** 2–6 yr: 2 mg two to three times daily (max 12 mg daily); 7–14 yr: 4 mg two to three times daily (max 16 mg daily)	Drowsiness, dizziness, paradoxical excitement, anticholinergic effects, gastritis, hypotension	Glaucoma, bladder neck, pyloric or duodenal obstruction, elderly or debilitated, prostatic hypertrophy, nursing mother, newborn or premature infant Caution: hyperthyroidism, CV disease, hypertension, asthma, increased intraocular pressure Pregnancy Category B	MAOIs (prolonged anticholinergic effect)
Hydroxyzine (off-label use)	**Adults:** 25 mg, three to four times daily **Children:** <6 yr: 50 mg daily in divided doses—three to four times daily; 6–11 yr: 50–100 mg daily in divided doses	Drowsiness, dry mouth, tremor, convulsions	Caution in the elderly and early pregnancy Pregnancy Category C Avoid in nursing mothers	Alcohol, sedatives, or other CNS depressants (additive CNS effects)
H_2 antihistamine—adjunct treatment to H_1 antihistamines				
Ranitidine[a]	**Adults:** 150 mg daily; reduce dose in renal impairment[a]	Headache, GI upset, hepatitis, rash	Pregnancy Category B Caution in renal and hepatic impairment	Amiodarone (increased amiodarone)
Steroid Burst				
Prednisone (off-label use)	**Adults:** up to 40 mg daily for short-course, up to 7 d	Weight gain, fluid retention, increased blood pressure, elevated blood sugar	Systemic fungal infection Caution: diabetes, CHF, recent MI, hypertension, immunosuppressed Pregnancy Category D	Quetiapine (decreased quetiapine levels), fluoroquinolones (tendon rupture), bupropion (reduced seizure threshold), warfarin (bleeding risk), aspirin (GI ulceration)
Prednisolone (off-label use)	**Adults:** up to 40 mg daily for short-course, up to 7 d **Children:** 1 mg/kg/d, divided in two doses (max 60 mg/d), for short-course, up to 7 d	See prednisone	See prednisone	See prednisone

[a]Off-label use for urticaria is not recommended; studies have used 150 mg twice daily for 7–9 days in adults.
CrCl, creatinine clearance; CV, cardiovascular; GI, gastrointestinal; CNS, central nervous system; MAOIs, monoamine oxidase inhibitors; MI, myocardial infarction; S, syndrome.

TABLE 61-3. MEDICATIONS FOR CHRONIC URTICARIA

Drug	Dose	Major Side Effects	Contraindications	Major Drug Interactions
Chronic Urticaria				
Second-generation H₁ antihistamines	Use as directed in Table 61–2 **Cetirizine:** use up to 40 mg daily **Loratadine:** use up to 40 mg daily	See individual agents in Table 61–2	See individual agents in Table 61–2	See individual agents in Table 61–2
First-generation H₁ antihistamines	Use as adjunct as directed in Table 61–2	See individual agents in Table 61–2	See individual agents in Table 61–2	See individual agents in Table 61–2
H₂ antihistamines	Use as adjunct as directed in Table 61–2	See individual agents in Table 61–2	See individual agents in Table 61–2	See individual agents in Table 61–2
Cyclosporine (off label use)	As adjunct to H1 antihistamine **Adults:** 3–5 mg/kg/d	Renal dysfunction/nephropathy, hypertension, headache, GI upset, hirsutism, leg cramps, tremor, paresthesia, edema, dizziness, gum hyperplasia, liver dysfunction	Concomitant PUVA or UVB therapy, concomitant radiation therapy Caution in patients with hypertension and abnormal renal function, the elderly Requires close monitoring Pregnancy Category C Do not use in nursing mothers	**Many Drug Interactions** NSAIDs (nephrotoxicity risk), statins (increased statin levels, myopathy) dronedarone (increased dronedarone), mifepristone, azoles, amphotericin B (cyclosporine increase or toxicity), St. John's wort (reduced cyclosporine levels), Fenofibrate (decline in renal function)
Doxepin	**Adults:** 10–30 mg daily (off-label use) **Children:** 1–3 mg/kg/d in single dose or divided doses (depression or anxiety dose)	Drowsiness, anticholinergic effects (e.g., dry mouth, constipation, blurred vision), nausea, vomiting, diarrhea, QT interval prolongation	Concomitant use of MAOIs (or within 2 wk), glaucoma, urinary retention Caution in patients with comorbid psychiatric disorders (suicidal ideation, cognitive abnormalities) and the elderly (increased confusion, oversedation) Pregnancy Category C	**Many Drug Interactions** linezolid (serotonin S); MAOI, phenothiazines, SSRIs, cisapride, quinolone, macrolides, trimethoprim/sulfamethoxazole and others (QT prolongation); metoclopramide (extrapyramidal reactions, neuroleptic malignant S)
Montelukast (off label use)	**Adults:** 10 mg daily for up to 6 wk; as adjunct with H₁ antihistamines (may not have value as monotherapy) **Children:** 2–12 yr: 5 mg daily; >12 yr: 10 mg daily (off-label use)	Upper respiratory infection, fever, pharyngitis, cough, abdominal pain, diarrhea, otitis media, influenza, rhinorrhea, sinusitis	Caution when withdrawing for oral steroids, do not abruptly substitute montelukast for oral corticosteroids Caution for patients with PKU (chewable form contains phenylalanine) Pregnancy Category B	Clozapine (reduced clozapine levels), gemfibrozil (increased montelukast levels), prednisone (severe peripheral edema)
Omalizumab	**Adults:** for H₁ antihistamine refractory urticarial: 300 mg single dose or 600 mg subcutaneously added to a stable dose of H₁ antihistamine	Injection site reactions, viral infections, upper respiratory infections, headache, hypersensitivity reactions and anaphylaxis	Pregnancy Category B	
Prednisone	**Adults:** 30–40 mg daily; taper slowly to lowest dose that controls symptoms	See prednisone in Table 61–2	See prednisone in Table 61–2	See prednisone in Table 61–2

GI, gastrointestinal; MAOIs, monoamine oxidase inhibitors; SSRI, selective serotonin reuptake inhibitor; PKU, phenylketonuria.

TABLE 61–4. MEDICATIONS FOR PHYSICAL AND OTHER FORMS OF URTICARIA

Drug	Dose	Major Side Effects	Contraindications	Major Drug Interactions
Physical Urticaria (Dermatographic)				
H₁ antihistamines	Use as directed in Table 61–2	See individual agents in Table 61–2	See individual agents in Table 61–2	See individual agents in Table 61–2
Physical Urticaria (Delayed Pressure)				
H₁ antihistamines	Use as directed in Chronic Urticaria	See individual agents in Table 61–2	See individual agents in Table 61–2	See individual agents in Table 61–2
Corticosteroids	Use as directed in Chronic Urticaria, can extend tapering over 3–4 wk reserved for severe cases (limited data)	See individual agents in Table 61–2	See individual agents in Table 61–2	See individual agents in Table 61–2
Montelukast	Use as directed in Table 61–3	See montelukast in Table 61–3	See montelukast in Table 61–3	See montelukast in Table 61–2
Sulfasalazine (off label use)	**Adults:** 2–3 g daily (data are limited)	Nausea, vomiting, dyspepsia, anorexia and headache. Uncommon hematologic abnormalities, proteinuria and hepatotoxicity	Intestinal or urinary tract obstruction, porphyria, Pregnancy Category B	Methenamine (crystalluria), Cyclosporine (reduced cyclosporine efficacy), digoxin (decreased digoxin levels), warfarin (bleeding risk or reduced warfarin efficacy), methotrexate (hepatotoxicity risk)
Cold Urticaria				
Second-generation antihistamines:	Use as directed in Table 61–2. **Desloratadine:** Adults can use 5 mg/d for 2 wk, 10 mg/d for 2 wk, 30 mg for 3 wk	See individual agents in Table 61–2	See individual agents in Table 61–2	See individual agents in Table 61–2
First-generation H₁ antihistamines	Use as directed	See individual agents in Table 61–2	See individual agents in Table 61–2	See individual agents in Table 61–2
Doxepin	Use as directed in Table 61–3	See doxepin in Table 61–3	See doxepin in Table 61–3	See doxepin in Table 61–3
Omalizumab	Use as directed in Table 61–3	See omalizumab in Table 61–3	See omalizumab in Table 61–3	See omalizumab in Table 61–3

Heat Urticaria

H₁ antihistamines	Use as directed in Table 61-2	See individual agents in Table 61-2	See individual agents in Table 61-2	See individual agents in Table 61-2
Omalizumab	Use as directed in Table 61-3	See omalizumab in Table 61-3	See omalizumab in Table 61-3	See omalizumab in Table 61-3

Solar Urticaria

H₁ antihistamines	Use as directed in Table 61-2	See individual agents in Table 61-2	See individual agents in Table 61-2	See individual agents in Table 61-2
ultraviolet light or psoralen and ultraviolet A for tolerance induction		Skin cancer, burns, skin aging	Avoid in pregnancy	

Cholinergic Urticaria

H₁ antihistamines	Use as directed in Table 61-2	See individual agents in Table 61-2	See individual agents in Table 61-2	See individual agents in Table 61-2
H₂ antihistamines	Use as adjunct as directed in Table 61-2	See individual agents in Table 61-2	See individual agents in Table 61-2	See individual agents in Table 61-2

Urticarial Vasculitis

Treat underlying vasculitis cause				
Corticosteroids	Prolonged treatment of 3-4 wk	See individual agents in Table 61-2	See individual agents in Table 61-2	See individual agents in Table 61-2

SELECTED REFERENCES

American Academy of Allergy, Asthma and Immunology. Consultation and referral guidelines citing the evidence: how the allergist/immunologist can help. Milwaukee,WI: American Academy of Allergy, Asthma, and Immunology; 2011.

Charlesworth E. Urticaria and angioedema. *Allergy Asthma Proc.* 2002;23(5):341–345.

Fedorowicz Z, van Zuuren EJ, Hu N. Histamine H$_2$-receptor antagonists for urticaria. *Cochrane Database Syst Rev.* 2012;(3):CD008596.

Grattan C, Powell S, Humphreys F; British Association of Dermatologists. Management and diagnostic guidelines for urticaria and angioedema. *Br J Dermatol.* 2001;144(4):708–714.

Joint Task Force on Practice Parameters. The diagnosis and management of urticaria: a practice parameter Part I: Acute urticaria/angioedema. Part II: chronic urticaria/angioedema. *Ann Allergy Asthma Immunol.* 2000;85(6 Pt 2):521–544.

Prodigy Guidance. Urticaria and angioedema. http://www.prodigy.nhs.uk, http://www.cks.library.nhs.uk/urticaria/about_this_topic.

---

62   Abnormal Vaginal Bleeding

Heather L. Paladine, MD, FAAFP & Pooja A. Shah, MD

KEY POINTS

- Anovulation and pelvic structural abnormalities are the most common causes of abnormal vaginal bleeding in reproductive-aged women. (SOR **C**)
- Premenopausal women with abnormal uterine bleeding (AUB) should have a pregnancy test and thyroid-stimulating hormone level measured. (SOR **B**)
- Adolescents with heavy menstrual bleeding and women with a history that suggests a possible bleeding disorder should have a complete blood count (CBC) with platelets, prothrombin time, partial thromboplastin time, and testing for von Willebrand disease. (SOR **C**)
- An endometrial stripe thickness of less than 4 mm on transvaginal ultrasound rules out the diagnosis of endometrial carcinoma in a postmenopausal woman with vaginal bleeding. (SOR **A**)
- Estrogen and progestin are first-line medications for AUB. (SOR **C**)

I. **Definition.** Normal vaginal bleeding follows a cyclic pattern. It starts at puberty and ends at menopause.

   A. **Phases of reproductive cycle** (Figure 62–1).

   1. The **follicular phase** begins with the onset of menses and ends on the day of the luteinizing hormone (LH) surge; it is of variable length, usually 14 to 21 days. This time is also called the proliferative phase of the endometrium, with estrogen predominance.

   2. **Ovulation** occurs 30 to 36 hours after the LH surge.

   3. The **luteal phase** begins with the LH surge and ends at the onset of menses; this phase lasts exactly 14 days. During this time, progesterone predominates often causing physical symptoms such as abdominal bloating, fluid retention, changes in mood, and appetite. This time is also called the secretory phase of the endometrium.

   4. **Menses.** On day 1 of the follicular phase, involution of the corpus luteum causes rapid decline of progesterone and estrogen, leading to the expulsion of the uterine lining (blood and endometrial tissue.)

   B. **Normal menses. The menstrual cycle** begins with the first day of bleeding of one period and ends with the first day of the next cycle. Onset of menses, called menarche, occurs normally between the ages of 9 and 16 years. It is common to have irregular periods for the first few years after menses starts, so regular period cycles usually begin about 2 years after menstruation commences. **Menopause is the permanent end of menstruation and fertility,** defined as 12 months after the last menstrual period. As menopause approaches (average age 51 years), cycle length may change, and it is

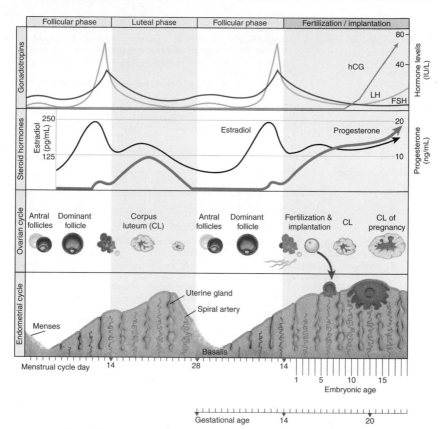

FIGURE 62-1. Phases of the reproductive cycle. FSH, follicle-stimulating hormone; hCG, human chorionic gonadotropin; LH, luteinizing hormone. (*Source:* Reproduced with permission from Gary Cunningham F, Leveno KJ, Bloom SL, Hauth JC, Rouse DJ, Spong CY, eds. *Williams Obstetrics.* 23rd ed. McGraw-Hill, Inc., 2010. Figure 3-1.)

common for the length between periods to get longer or shorter, or for the bleeding to get lighter or heavier. Table 62–1 describes normal bleeding patterns.

   C. Abnormal uterine bleeding (AUB).

      1. AUB is defined as an abnormal bleeding pattern with regards to frequency, duration, amount, etiology (nonmenstrual bleeding), or the lack of menstruation for >3 months in the absence of pregnancy. Examples of AUB include bleeding between periods, bleeding after sex, spotting anytime in the menstrual cycle, bleeding more heavily or for more days than normal, and bleeding after menopause. (Table 62–2 summarizes terms frequently used to describe AUB.)

      2. Up to 30% of women will have some type of abnormal vaginal bleeding during their reproductive years.

      3. In a cohort study of Danish women, 10.7% (95% confidence interval, 7.3%–15.0%) recorded spontaneous postmenopausal bleeding in their diaries. The incidence

TABLE 62–1. NORMAL BLEEDING PATTERNS

- Normal blood loss is between 25 and 60 cc/cycle (average 35–50 cc)
- Normal cycle length is 21 to 35 days (28 days ± 7 days)
- Normal menses lasts 2 to 7 days (average 4 days)

TABLE 62-2. TERMS TO DESCRIBE ABNORMAL BLEEDING

Menorrhagia (hypermenorrhea)	Prolonged bleeding >7 d or >80 cc menstrual fluid occurring at regular intervals. This definition is used for research purposes and, in practice, excessive blood loss should be based on the patient's perception
Metrorrhagia	Uterine bleeding between periods
Menometrorrhagia	Prolonged or excessive uterine bleeding occurring at irregular intervals and/or between periods
Polymenorrhea	Bleeding that occurs more often than every 21 d
Oligomenorrhea	Bleeding that occurs less frequently than every 35 d
Intermenstrual bleeding	Uterine bleeding of variable amounts occurring between regular menstrual periods
Midcycle spotting	Spotting occurring just before ovulation, typically from declining estrogen levels
Postmenopausal bleeding	Recurrence of bleeding in a menopausal woman at least 6 mo after cessation of cycles
Amenorrhea	The cessation of menses for a time equal to three menstrual cycles or 6 mo total in the absence of pregnancy

decreased with time since menopause, from an estimated 409/1000 person-years in the year following menopause to 42/1000 more than 3 years after menopause.

4. Abnormal bleeding is listed as an indication in 25% of all gynecologic surgeries performed each year.

II. **Causes of AUB** (Tables 62–3 and 62–4). Abnormal bleeding alone does not necessarily indicate a serious condition. Anovulation and pelvic structural abnormalities are the most common causes of AUB in premenopausal women.

A. **Pregnancy,** especially first trimester bleeding; miscarriage; ectopic pregnancy.

B. **Hormonal contraceptive methods** including oral contraceptive (OC) pills, depot medroxyprogesterone acetate (Depo-Provera), birth control implant (Implanon, Nexplanon), and hormonal and nonhormonal intrauterine devices (IUDs) (Mirena, Skyla, Paragard).

C. Other **medications** such as warfarin, heparin, nonsteroidal anti-inflammatory drugs (NSAIDs), corticosteroids, antipsychotics, selective serotonin reuptake inhibitors, thyroid replacement, and herbal and other supplements such as soy, gingko, ginseng, and motherwort. Postmenopausal bleeding may also be caused by postmenopausal hormone therapy (HT) or tamoxifen therapy.

D. **Infection of pelvic organs** (vagina, cervix, uterus, fallopian tubes, or ovaries). Sexually transmitted infections such as gonorrhea and chlamydia are often the cause of these infections (see Chapter 102). Pelvic inflammatory disease (PID) is also a cause.

E. **Structural disorders of the uterus.** Fibroids (uterine fibromyomas, leiomyomas, myomas), adenomyosis (endometriosis interna), and uterine or cervical polyps.

F. **Malignancy** of the endometrium, uterus, cervix, or vagina.

G. **Chronic disease** such as blood dyscrasias (e.g., von Willebrand disease), thyroid disorders, and diabetes.

H. Trauma, foreign bodies, nonuterine bleeding from lacerations, or abrasions as seen in sexual abuse.

I. Extreme emotional stress, anorexia nervosa, or excessive exercise can cause changes in the character of the menstrual cycle, including amenorrhea.

J. **Hypogonadism** (ovarian hypofunction), either primary ovarian insufficiency (premature ovarian failure) or secondary (deficient secretion of the pituitary gonadotropins FSH and LH), results in decreased estradiol production, resulting in irregular periods or amenorrhea.

TABLE 62-3. ACOG CLASSIFICATION OF CAUSES OF ABNORMAL VAGINAL BLEEDING

Structural (PALM)	Nonstructural (COEIN)
Polyps	**C**oagulopathy
Adenomyosis	**O**vulatory dysfunction
Leiomyoma	**E**ndometrial
Malignancy and hyperplasia	**I**atrogenic
	Not yet classified

TABLE 62–4. CAUSES OF ANOVULATORY CYCLES

Hypothalamic
- Weight loss
- Eating disorders
- Female athlete triad
- Chronic illness
- Stress
- Excessive exercise

Polycystic ovarian syndrome
Thyroid disorders
Hyperprolactinemia
Idiopathic chronic anovulation
Medication-induced (i.e., after discontinuation of hormonal contraceptives)

    K. Ovulation, causing midcycle spotting.

    L. Endometrial hyperplasia may occur during perimenopause when ovulation may not occur regularly, during menopause when ovulation stops and progesterone is no longer produced, and at other times when high levels of estrogen predominate and not enough progesterone is present. Hyperplasia can also occur with use of medications that mimic estrogen, long-term use of high-dose estrogen after menopause (in patients who have not had a hysterectomy), obesity, and ovulatory dysfunction.

    M. Ovulatory dysfunction (also known as dysfunctional uterine bleeding) is typically a result of an endocrinopathy such as polycystic ovarian syndrome (PCOS) (Tables 62–3 and 62–4).

        1. The terms **ovulatory dysfunction** and **dysfunctional uterine bleeding** are used to describe abnormal bleeding from the uterus that is not caused by pathology or systemic disease and is due to changes in hormone levels. It is a diagnosis of exclusion.

        2. Ovulatory dysfunction most commonly occurs when the ovaries do not release an egg.

        3. Changes in hormone levels may cause the patient's menses to be later or earlier and sometimes heavier than normal. It may be ovulatory or anovulatory bleeding. Dysfunctional uterine bleeding is diagnosed after pregnancy and other causes (e.g., medications, genital tract pathology, malignancy, and systemic disease) have been ruled out by appropriate investigations.

III. Signs and Symptoms

    A. Amenorrhea can be caused by pregnancy, hormonal contraceptive use, or anovulatory cycles, particularly in adolescent or perimenopausal women. An underweight appearance in the setting of amenorrhea or menstrual change can indicate excessive stress, an eating disorder such as anorexia nervosa, or excessive exercise.

    B. Fever, leukocytosis, pelvic tenderness, and cervical tenderness suggest PID, septic abortion, or other pelvic organ infection.

    C. Pelvic masses may signify pregnancy, uterine or ovarian neoplasia, fibroids, pelvic abscesses, or hematomas.

    D. A bleeding disorder may be suspected with heavy menstrual bleeding since menarche, epistaxis, frequent gum bleeding, family history of bleeding symptoms, bleeding associated with dental work, excessive bleeding associated with surgery, postpartum hemorrhage, petechiae, ecchymoses, skin pallor, and/or swollen joints. The absence of these signs does not exclude the possibility of an underlying bleeding disorder.

    E. Signs of **thyroid dysfunction** or thyroid disease include weight changes, hair/skin/nail changes, mood changes, heat/cold intolerance, thyroid nodule, or enlargement on examination.

    F. Predictable midcycle spotting is likely due to a dip in estrogen levels at ovulation.

    G. Hypogonadism and resultant estradiol deficiency may cause irregular periods or amenorrhea, anovulatory infertility, vaginal atrophy, and hot flashes.

    H. Bleeding patterns in ovulatory dysfunction and dysfunctional uterine bleeding include bleeding or spotting between periods, metrorrhagia, oligomenorrhea, irregularly spaced periods, and heavier or prolonged bleeding.

    I. Obesity and signs of insulin resistance (such as acanthosis nigricans on the neck; see Chapter 75) can indicate irregular bleeding due to endometrial hyperplasia or PCOS.

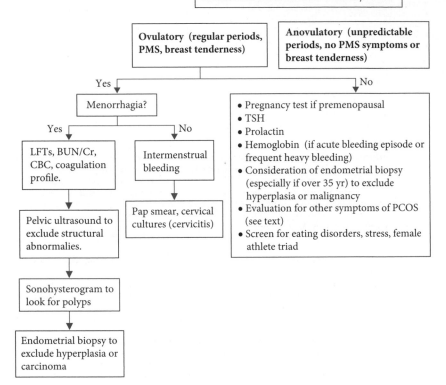

FIGURE 62–2. Evaluation of abnormal bleeding. BUN, blood urea nitrogen; CBC, complete blood count; Cr, creatinine; LFT, liver function test; PCOS, polycystic ovary syndrome; PMS, premenstrual syndrome; TSH, thyroid stimulating hormone.

Hormone level changes in women with obesity or PCOS can cause excessive growth of body hair in a male pattern (hirsutism), hot flashes, mood swings, tenderness, or vaginal dryness.

J. Perimenopause and menopausal hormonal changes can lead to symptoms such as hot flashes, mood swings, sleep disturbance, urinary incontinence, vaginal dryness, uncomfortable or painful intercourse, or atrophic vaginitis.

IV. **Laboratory Tests.** Testing should be directed by the history and physical examination (Figure 62–2).

   A. All women of reproductive age who have been or may have been sexually active should have a **pregnancy test**.

   B. **Thyroid-stimulating hormone** is helpful, as abnormal bleeding can be caused by both hypothyroidism and hyperthyroidism, and thyroid problems are relatively common. A **prolactin level** for a pituitary adenoma can also be obtained, particularly if galactorrhea is present. If bleeding has been prolonged or heavy, a **hemoglobin** can be obtained to identify anemia.

   C. **PCOS** is a clinical diagnosis; however, testing for hyperandrogenism (free and total testosterone, dehydroepiandrosterone [DHEA], follicle-stimulating hormone [FSH], and LH) can be helpful if the diagnosis is suspected but the patient does not have clinical signs of androgen excess.

D. Adolescents with heavy menstrual bleeding and women with a history that suggests a possible bleeding disorder should have a complete blood count (CBC) with platelets, prothrombin time, partial thromboplastin time, and testing for von Willebrand disease.

E. Women who are at risk should be evaluated for possible cervicitis (chlamydia and gonorrhea testing) and cervical neoplasm (including speculum exam and Papanicolau test).

F. Women who are older than 40 years or have a history of unopposed estrogen exposure (prolonged amenorrhea, obesity) are at an increased risk for endometrial carcinoma and should be evaluated to rule out malignancy if they have prolonged menstrual bleeding.

    1. In premenopausal women, the first-line test is endometrial biopsy, although ultrasound or sonohysterography can be used if other pathology (such as fibroids) is thought to be more likely. Sonohysterography is more useful than transvaginal ultrasound for evaluation of the uterine cavity (polyps, adenomyosis).

    2. Endometrial biopsy is a relatively simple procedure that can be performed in the office (http://www.nejm.org/doi/full/10.1056/NEJMvcm0803922). This procedure obtains a sample of endometrial tissue to assess for abnormalities.

G. Postmenopausal women with vaginal bleeding should also be evaluated to rule out endometrial carcinoma; in this case, either an endometrial biopsy or a transvaginal ultrasound is acceptable as an initial test. An endometrial stripe thickness of ≤ 4 mm on a transvaginal ultrasound in a postmenopausal patient rules out malignancy. Laboratory evaluation is not helpful in this age group.

V. Treatment strategies differ depending on the cause of bleeding. In bleeding with a known cause (such as pregnancy and infection), the treatment should address the underlying problem.

A. Nonpharmacologic treatments

    1. Women with ovulatory dysfunction due to PCOS may benefit from healthier diets, increased exercise, and weight loss.

    2. Complementary and alternative treatments for abnormal vaginal bleeding have not been well-researched.

B. Pharmacologic treatments. In women with nonspecific AUB, treatment depends on the amount of bleeding and interference with lifestyle. Medical treatment is the standard for initial management of AUB.

    1. For **heavy bleeding** that leads to hemodynamic instability, inpatient treatment with intravenous estrogen or surgical intervention is necessary.

    2. Combined estrogen/progesterone or progestin-only medications are standard treatments for anovulatory bleeding in women without organic pathology.

        a. While many OCs show benefit for menorrhagia, only estradiol/dienogest (Natazia) is FDA-approved. Tablets that contain varying amounts of estradiol and dienogest are color coded and given as one tablet orally daily in the order of package: one dark yellow tablet daily for 2 consecutive days, then one medium red tablet daily for 5 days, then one light yellow tablet daily for 17 days, then one dark red tablet daily for 2 days, and then one white inert tablet daily for 2 days over a total of 28 days. If a generic combined OC is chosen (e.g., 35 µg estrogen product), and spotting or irregular bleeding continues, a pill with a higher potency progestin, newer progestin, or stepped estrogen product can be tried.

        b. When using progestin-only drugs, norethindrone (5 mg three times daily) or medroxyprogesterone acetate (10 mg daily) can be given on cycle days 5 to 26 to produce optimum secretory transformation of the primed endometrium.

    3. Traxenamic acid, an antifibrinolytic drug, is a standard medication in Europe for menorrhagia. The oral form is FDA-approved in the United States and dosed as 1300 mg orally three times daily for a maximum of 5 days during menstruation. It is more effective than placebo, NSAIDs, and luteal-phase progestins and does not have an increased rate of side effects.

    4. NSAIDs (e.g., ibuprofen at 200–400 mg every 6 hours or naproxen 500 mg every 12 hours) at onset of menses are modestly effective in reducing menstrual bleeding, but less so than tranexamic acid or the levonorgestrel IUD.

    5. The **levonorgestrel IUD** and surgery are both superior to usual medical therapy in both reduction of bleeding in women with menorrhagia and patient satisfaction. Studies show the levonorgestrel IUD is not as effective as balloon ablation or endometrial resection in reducing heavy menstrual bleeding; however, no differences were seen in quality of life. Another study comparing the levonorgestrel IUD and hysterectomy showed no difference in quality of life but hysterectomy had a higher cost.

   C. Surgical options include dilation and curettage, various procedures for endometrial ablation, uterine artery embolization, and hysterectomy.

     1. Dilation and curettage can be used as a diagnostic test and for temporary relief of bleeding, but in general the abnormal bleeding will recur.

     2. Compared with hysterectomy, endometrial ablation has good patient satisfaction and fewer complications, but it is less effective at controlling bleeding and may need to be repeated.

     3. Hysterectomy is the most definitive treatment for abnormal vaginal bleeding but has a higher cost and higher complication rate than other surgical interventions.

   D. Follow-up is based on the etiology of the bleeding, the acuity, and the chronicity. Many women have recurrence of abnormal bleeding.

VI. Patient Education. Women should be educated about the cause and expected course of their vaginal bleeding.

   A. Women who have abnormal bleeding due to contraceptive medications may choose to continue these medications if the bleeding does not cause anemia or switch to a different OC.

   B. Women who are at a higher risk for endometrial carcinoma should be aware of their risk and the importance of evaluation of any abnormal bleeding.

   C. Women with PCOS are at an increased cardiovascular risk; they should be educated about lifestyle modification to decrease their risk and should be screened for other cardiovascular risk factors.

   D. Women with abnormal vaginal bleeding may have questions about fertility. Women with anovulation do have decreased fertility and may need treatment to achieve pregnancy.

SELECTED REFERENCES

American Congress of Obstetricians and Gynecologists. Diagnosis of abnormal uterine bleeding in reproductive-aged women. ACOG Committee Opinion No. 128. *Obstet Gynecol.* 2012;120:197–206.

American Congress of Obstetricians and Gynecologists. Management of acute abnormal uterine bleeding in nonpregnant reproductive-aged women. Committee Opinion No. 557. *Obstet Gynecol.* 2013;121:891–896.

Gordon P. Endometrial biopsy (video). *N Engl J Med.* 2009;361:e61.

Null DB, Weiland CM, Camlibel AR. Postmenopausal bleeding: first steps in the workup. *J Fam Pract.* 2012;61(10):597–604.

Sweet MG, Schmidt-Dalton TA, Weiss PM, Madsen KP. Evaluation and management of abnormal uterine bleeding in premenopausal women. *Am Fam Physician.* 2012;1(85):35–43.

Additional references are available online at http://langetextbooks.com/fm6e

---

63   Vaginal Discharge

L. Peter Schwiebert, MD

KEY POINTS

- A careful history, physical examination, and office laboratory studies allow arrival at an appropriate diagnosis for common causes of vaginal discharge. (SOR ⒸＣ)
- Sexually transmitted diseases (STDs) often coexist; the presence of risk factors for one should prompt screening for others. (SOR ⒸＣ)
- It is important to base treatment of vaginal discharge on solid clinical documentation to avoid inappropriate treatment and resulting drug resistance, excessive cost, and iatrogenic vaginitis. (SOR ⒸＣ)

I. Definition. From menarche to menopause, estrogen stimulates proliferation and glycogen production by vaginal squamous epithelial cells on which lactobacilli depend; these lactobacilli produce hydrogen peroxide (toxic to most vaginal pathogens) and lactic acid, resulting in a vaginal pH of 3.5 to 4.5. Normal (physiologic) discharge varies among women and with the stage of a woman's menstrual cycle, pregnancy, and sexual arousal; normal vaginal discharge is clear to slightly opaque.

This chapter focuses on vaginal discharge that is unusual in amount or odor or causes symptoms such as itching or burning. Changes in vaginal discharge and vaginal symptoms are often caused by alterations in the physiologic vaginal environment. Such unusual or symptomatic discharge may be related to

A. **Hypoestrogenic states** (in prepubertal or postmenopausal women) that thin the vaginal epithelium, decrease glycogen levels, raise pH to ≥ 5.0, and create a mixed vaginal flora.

B. **Sexually transmitted pathogens** (e.g., Neisseria gonorrhoeae, Chlamydia trachomatis, and Trichomonas vaginalis) that stimulate inflammatory response, raise vaginal pH, or both.

C. **Irritants** (e.g., douching, spermicides) that can alter physiologic vaginal pH and create a favorable environment for pathogens.

D. **Immunocompromise or suppression of normal flora by antibiotics that** permits alteration of normal vaginal flora (e.g., bacterial vaginosis [BV]) or overgrowth of opportunistic organisms (e.g., Candida species). (Candida also grows well in the glycogen-rich vaginas of reproductive-age women, but has no such substrate in premenarchal girls or postmenopausal women and is therefore rare in these groups.)

II. **Common Diagnoses.** In the ambulatory primary care setting, vaginal discharge is the most common gynecologic complaint and the 10th to 15th most common presenting complaint, resulting in more than 10 million physician office visits annually. These figures underestimate the true prevalence of the problem, since many women with discharge or odor do not seek medical attention. **Up to 90% of all cases of vaginitis are due to BV, vulvovaginal candidiasis (VVC), or trichomoniasis.**

A. **BV** accounts for up to 40% to 50% of cases of vaginitis, with prevalence varying depending on the population studied (e.g., 15%–19% of ambulatory gynecology patients and 24%–40% of patients attending sexually transmitted disease [STD] clinics). Risk factors for BV include having more than one sexual partner over the previous 3 months, use of an intrauterine device (IUD), douching, tobacco use, unprotected intercourse, receptive oral sex, and pregnancy.

B. **VVC** (approximately 20%–25% of cases) is the second most common cause of vaginitis in the United States and the most common cause in Europe. Up to 75% of women have an episode of VVC at some point and up to 5% have recurrent episodes. Risk factors for VVC include recent antibiotic use (especially penicillins, tetracycline, or cephalosporins), oral contraceptives (OCs), systemic glucocorticoid use, pregnancy, poorly controlled diabetes mellitus, obesity, immunocompromised state, or diaphragm or spermicide use. Candida albicans is the pathogen in 80% to 90% of VVC cases, with increased likelihood of non-albicans infection (e.g., Candida glabrata or Candida tropicalis) with immunocompromise, long-term anti-candidal treatment, or ≥ 4 documented episodes of VVC in 1 year (recurrent VVC).

C. **Trichomonas vaginitis** (15%–20% of cases), a true sexually transmitted infection (STI), is the third most common cause of vaginitis. Risk factors include IUD or tobacco use, multiple sex partners, history of STIs, illicit drug use, low socioeconomic status, or lack of barrier contraceptive use. Twenty to fifty percent of women with T. vaginalis are asymptomatic, and 23% of patients with this infection are also infected with N. gonorrhoeae.

D. **Cervicitis,** caused by C. trachomatis, herpes simplex virus, or N. gonorrhoeae, accounts for up to 20% to 25% of cases of vaginal discharge. Risk factors include recent new sex partners, lack of contraceptive use (including barrier contraceptives), and age less than 24 years.

E. **Physiologic discharge** (10% of cases) is a result of normal variations in cervical or vaginal secretions.

F. **Atrophic vaginitis** (10%–40% of postmenopausal women) is caused by natural or induced (e.g., radiation/chemotherapy, oophorectomy, and antiestrogenic medications) hypoestrogenic states.

G. **Group A streptococcal (GAS) vaginitis** has been isolated in up to 48% of women with chronic or recurrent vaginal discharge. Risk factors include household or personal history of GAS dermal or respiratory infection, sexual contact, or lactational or menopausal vaginal atrophy.

H. **Allergic vaginitis** (frequency unknown) is caused by topical sensitizers or irritants such as tampons, spermicides, hygienic sprays, soaps, perfumes, povidone-iodine solution, condoms (latex or lubricant/spermicide containing), lubricants, and douches. It is more common in women with an atopic history.

TABLE 63–1. SYMPTOMS AND SIGNS OF VAGINAL DISCHARGE

Condition	Symptoms and Signs	Appearance of Discharge and Mucosa
Bacterial vaginosis	Approximately 50% asymptomatic; fishy-smelling discharge	Thin, white homogeneous discharge; minimal mucosal erythema
Candida vaginitis	10%–20% asymptomatic; vulvar itching or soreness, external dysuria, superficial dyspareunia	Possibly curdy discharge; vulvar edema/erythema
Cervicitis	Mucoid discharge, intermenstrual spotting, dyspareunia	Yellow, mucoid endocervical discharge; inflamed cervix with focal hemorrhage
Trichomonas vaginitis	10%–50% asymptomatic; offensive discharge, vulvar itching, dysuria, occasionally lower abdominal discomfort	Up to 70% have vaginal discharge, frothy and yellow in 10%–30%, no signs in 5%–15%
Physiologic discharge	Discharge without itching or odor	Clear to slightly opaque cervical discharge
Atrophic vaginitis	Discharge, burning, dyspareunia, or all three	Thin and inflamed with loss of rugal folds; discharge, if present, is watery and may be foul-smelling
Group A streptococcal (GAS) vaginitis	Vaginal/perineal pain, pruritus, profuse discharge	Genital erythema/edema/tenderness, copious watery or yellow discharge

III. Symptoms and Signs (Table 63–1)
IV. Laboratory Tests (Table 63–2). A careful history and examination, coupled with office laboratory studies, allows confident assessment of common causes of vaginal discharge.
  A. A wet preparation is made by adding a drop of normal saline to a drop of vaginal discharge on a glass slide and then examining the slide with a microscope.
  B. A potassium hydroxide (KOH) preparation is made similarly using a drop of 10% KOH solution instead of saline.
  C. Nitrazine paper changes color in response to changes in the pH of vaginal discharge. A 1- to 2-inch strip of Nitrazine paper is applied to secretions on the vaginal walls or pooled in the posterior fornix.
  D. Cultures. If KOH/wet prep testing is nondiagnostic, particularly in high-risk individuals (see II.A–D), the least expensive approach is to initially perform yeast cultures, gonorrhea/chlamydia probes with gram stain, and *Trichomonas* cultures if vaginal pH is >4.9. In addition, all pregnant women should be screened for *C. trachomatis* and

TABLE 63–2. OFFICE LABORATORY FINDINGS IN VAGINAL DISCHARGE

Condition	pH (From Vaginal Walls, Not Cervix)/Color of Nitrazine Paper	Wet and Potassium Hydroxide (KOH) Preparations
Bacterial vaginosis	≥4.5/green to purple	Clue cells (bacteria obscuring epithelial cell border) 95%, few white blood cells (WBCs) on wet preparation, amine "fishy" odor on addition of KOH (≥90% sensitive)—"whiff test"
Candida vaginitis	3.5–4.5/yellow to green	Spores and pseudohyphae on KOH preparation (65% of symptomatic cases)
Cervicitis	≥4.0/yellow to purple	Mature squamous cells, ≥10 WBCs (50%–70% sensitive) on wet preparation
Trichomonas vaginitis	≥4.5/green to purple	Mature squamous cells with many WBCs on wet preparation, motile protozoa can be seen in 40%–80% of cases; usually positive whiff test
Physiologic discharge	≤4.0/yellow	Normal superficial epithelial cells, lactobacilli, no WBCs or spores on wet preparation
Atrophic vaginitis	≥5.0/green to purple	Wet preparation shows many WBCs, small round epithelial cells (parabasal cells) which are immature squamous unexposed to sufficient estrogen
Group A strep (GAS) vaginitis	≥4.5	Abundant polymorphonuclear white cells, gram-positive cocci, absent lactobacilli

N. gonorrhoeae. Confirmation of suspected GAS depends on culture showing GAS overgrowth.

1. **Nucleic acid amplification tests** (e.g., strand displacement amplification ligase chain reaction, or polymerase chain reaction testing) for *C. trachomatis* and *N. gonorrhoeae* are sensitive (90%–98% and 88.9%–95.2%, respectively), specific (98%–100% and 99.1%–100%, respectively), and cost-effective for documenting presence of these organisms.

2. **Culture for cure** following treatment of cervicitis with a recommended regimen (see Section V.E.1) is not necessary. However, cultures should be repeated 1 to 2 months after finishing treatment to detect reinfection.

E. Serologic **syphilis test (e.g., venereal disease research laboratory [VDRL]), human immunodeficiency virus (HIV) testing (e.g., enzyme-linked immunosorbent assay [ELISA])**, and counseling should be offered to patients with documented *N. gonorrhoeae* infection.

F. **Other tests**

1. The **Hansel stain** is a modified Wright–Giemsa stain that enhances eosinophils. This test should be considered in women with persistent discharge in whom the usual tests are normal and no other diagnosis is obvious. In one unpublished study of 50 patients with vaginal discharge, 12% had no evidence of infection but more than 25% eosinophils in their discharge using the Hansel stain.

2. A **PCR** test offers improved sensitivity and specificity compared with wet mount in diagnosis of trichomonas (84% and 94%, respectively, for PCR versus 52% and 78%, respectively, for wet mount).

3. New **self-administered tests for BV** (e.g., QuickVue Advance pH and Amines test and QuickVue Advance G. vaginalis test) offer rapidity and reasonably high sensitivity and specificity. A rapid yeast detection test (Savyon Diagnostics), available for home use, costs less than $10, compared with approximately $65 cost for yeast culture.

V. **Treatment**

A. **General measures.** The patient should be instructed to do the following:

1. Discontinue irritating agents (e.g., feminine hygiene products or bubble baths).

2. Wear nonocclusive, absorbent clothing (cotton rather than nylon underclothing) in cases of recurrent VVC.

3. Use barrier contraceptives (e.g., condom or diaphragm) until treatment is completed and symptoms are gone. (Oil-based intravaginal creams and suppositories can weaken latex condoms and diaphragms and risk unintended pregnancy.)

4. Restore a normal vaginal environment (i.e., pH and flora). Some clinicians recommend use of lactobacillus suppositories or oral yogurt, but efficacy is unproven.

B. **BV** is diagnosed (90% sensitivity) if three of the following four criteria are met: (1) homogeneous gray discharge adherent to vaginal walls, (2) vaginal pH of ≥4.5, (3) positive "whiff test" (fishy odor on addition of KOH to wet prep), or (4) clue cells are present (Amsel criteria). Other scoring systems (Nugent, Spiegel) focus on the mix of bacterial morphotypes, with the likelihood of BV increasing with decreasing prevalence of lactobacilli (long gram-positive rods).

1. Metronidazole (e.g., Flagyl or Protostat), 500 mg orally twice a day for 7 days, is the standard therapy. (SOR Ⓐ) Other effective regimens are metronidazole vaginal gel 0.75% (e.g., Metrogel-vaginal), 5 g vaginally twice daily for 5 days, or clindamycin (e.g., Cleocin), 300 mg twice a day orally or applied vaginally as a 2% cream for 7 days. Single-dose metronidazole (2 g) is the least expensive treatment but is not as effective for BV.

2. Although BV is associated with sexual activity, there is currently no evidence that treatment of sex partners prevents recurrences.

3. BV is associated with adverse pregnancy outcomes (preterm labor, premature ruptured membranes, chorioamnionitis, preterm birth [PTB], postpartum endometritis, and postcesarean section wound infection) in some women, especially those who have a high risk of preterm delivery.

   a. Although antibiotics are effective for treating BV in pregnancy, treatment does not prevent PTB before 37 weeks regardless of previous PTB history, even when given before 20 weeks of gestation. The United States Preventive Services Task Force (USPSTF) recommends against screening asymptomatic pregnant women for BV in the absence of a history of preterm delivery (Grade D recommendation).

   b. There is no evidence of teratogenic or mutagenic effects of metronidazole on the fetus, so it appears safe to use during pregnancy and lactation for symptomatic

TABLE 63–3. TREATMENT OF VULVOVAGINAL CANDIDIASIS[a]

Medication	Formulation	Dosage[c]
Clotrimazole	1% vaginal cream[b]	1 applicatorful (5 g) daily for 7–14 d
	2% vaginal cream[b]	1 applicatorful (5 g) daily for 3 d
Miconazole	2% vaginal cream[b]	1 applicatorful for 7 d
	4% vaginal cream[b]	1 applicatorful for 3 d
	100 mg suppository[b]	1 daily for 7 d
	200 mg suppository[b]	1 daily for 3 d
	1200 mg suppository[b]	Single dose
Butoconazole	2% cream[b]	1 applicatorful daily for 3 d
	2% cream	1 applicatorful once
Tioconazole	6.5% ointment[b]	1 applicatorful—single dose
Terconazole	0.4% cream	1 applicatorful daily for 7 d
	0.8% cream	1 applicatorful daily for 3 d
	80 mg suppository	1 daily for 3 d
Nystatin	100,000 unit vaginal tablet	1 daily for 14 d
Fluconazole	150 mg tablet	1 orally for 1 d

[a]Possible side effects from vaginal antifungals are nausea, headache, and vaginal discomfort.
[b]Available nonprescription.
[c]Unless otherwise indicated, the route of administration is intravaginal; for daily doses, the preferred administration time is at bedtime.

women. The USPSTF recommends against using intravaginal agents, especially clindamycin, during pregnancy.

4. BV has an overall recurrence rate of 30%; recurrent BV is treated with twice weekly metronidazole gel for 4 to 6 months (70% cure rate during treatment versus 39% for control group). (SOR **B**) There is a high relapse rate if treatment is discontinued. Recent controlled trials document the efficacy of vaginal probiotics and acidifying gels in reducing BV recurrence rates. (SOR **B**)

C. **VVC** (Table 63–3). A growing issue in the management of VVC is the availability and common use of nonprescription medications (VVC preparations are the 10th best-selling nonprescription products in the United States). In one study, only 28% of women who thought they had VVC actually did and only 11% of women responding to another survey recognized the classic symptoms of VVC. This results in inappropriate treatment, increasing incidence of resistant *Candida* strains and, in some situations, induction of irritant vaginitis. Use of home testing for candida vaginitis (see IV.F) may decrease inappropriate self-treatment of suspected candidal vaginitis.

1. **Uncomplicated infection** (healthy host, infrequent occurrences, mild to moderate symptoms).
   a. Imidazole creams, ointments, suppositories, or oral medications share similar efficacy (≥80%) in curing uncomplicated VVC. (SOR **A**)
   b. Tioconazole and terconazole are effective against a broader spectrum of *Candida* species than butoconazole, clotrimazole, or miconazole.
   c. Single-dose fluconazole (i.e., Diflucan) is less expensive, better tolerated, and at least as effective as standard 3- to 7-day intravaginal regimens; however, relief of itching is slower than with topical azole antifungals. Treatment with fluconazole is contraindicated during pregnancy; topical agents should be used.

2. For **complicated VVC** (moderate or severe symptoms or risk factors—see Section II.B), extending standard vaginal therapy to 10 to 14 days for acute symptoms may be effective. If using oral therapy, a second 150 mg fluconazole dose for 3 days after the initial dose improves response.

3. For **recurrent VVC** (≥4 microscopically or culture-documented episodes in a year), the following may be effective:
   a. Because of the increased likelihood of non-*albicans* infection in recurrent VVC, culture is advisable.
   b. Vaginal azole antifungals should be prescribed for 10 to 14 days, with efficacy confirmed by negative post-treatment fungal culture.
   c. This should be followed by a 6-month maintenance regimen; options include fluconazole, 100 or 200 mg per week. ***Note:*** Chronic daily use of oral medications

can interact with other medications (e.g., theophylline, anticonvulsants, anticoagulants, and OCs), can be hepatotoxic, and may be teratogenic. Approximately a 50% relapse rate occurs after cessation of maintenance therapy. One study found tapering fluconazole from 200 mg thrice weekly to once monthly achieved 90% disease-free state after 6 months and 77% after 1 year of therapy cessation.

   d. Repopulating vaginal *Lactobacillus* using intravaginal lactobacillus capsules has some efficacy in reducing recurrences and malodorous vaginal discharge.

   e. If non-*albicans* infection is documented, intravaginal terconazole or oral itraconazole may be more effective than standard regimens.

D. Trichomonas vaginitis

   1. Standard regimen. Metronidazole in a single 2 g dose for both the patient and her sex partner(s) shows a ≥90% cure rate. (SOR **Ⓐ**) To reduce recurrences, patients should be advised to avoid sexual relations until completing therapy and becoming asymptomatic.

   2. Treatment of pregnant women. The Centers for Disease Control (CDC) recommends a 2 g single dose of metronidazole, preferably after 37 weeks' gestation.

   3. Recurrent Trichomonas vaginitis. Metronidazole-resistant *T. vaginalis* has been documented. As of yet, there is no proven effective treatment for it; however, metronidazole, 2 to 4 g orally for 7 to 14 days, may be effective. (SOR **Ⓒ**)

E. Cervicitis. Empiric therapy for *C. trachomatis* or *N. gonorrhoeae* can be instituted in high-risk individuals while awaiting culture results.

   1. Because of the coprevalence of *N. gonorrhoeae* and *C. trachomatis* infection, patients should be treated with ceftriaxone (e.g., Rocephin), 250 mg intramuscularly (one dose) and azithromycin 1 g (single dose) or doxycycline, 100 mg orally twice daily for 7 days. If ceftriaxone is not available, cefixime (e.g., Suprax), 400 mg in a single dose, or ciprofloxacin (e.g., Cipro), 250 mg, or ofloxacin (e.g., Floxin), 400 mg orally for one dose are acceptable. **Pregnant or breastfeeding women should receive ceftriaxone plus azithromycin.**

   2. Acyclovir, or a similar nucleoside analog, should be given in standard doses for herpes simplex virus (see Chapter 30).

F. No treatment other than reassurance is necessary for **physiologic discharge**.

G. Although there are not yet clinical trials of treatment, GAS has been successfully treated with penicillins (penicillin V, amoxicillin, amoxicillin–clavulanate), clindamycin, or moxifloxacin. Sobel recommends penicillin V 500 mg orally four times daily for 10 to 14 days OR clindamycin 2% vaginal cream daily for 7 to 10 days.

H. First-line treatment for women with **atrophic vaginitis** is vaginal estrogen. Transvaginal estrogen creams, pessaries, or a hormone-releasing ring (e.g., Estring) are all effective. The latter offers advantages of only needing replacement every 3 months, not being messy, and allowing consistent estrogen release at levels low enough to avoid endometrial stimulation. Standard oral estrogen replacement, with added benefits of relief of vasomotor symptoms and osteoporosis prevention is also effective. (However, such benefits must be weighed against potential risks of combined estrogen/progestogen therapy.) Topical vaginal lubricants (e.g., Vagisil, Replens) can provide some relief for symptoms of atrophic vaginitis.

I. **Treatment** for **allergic vaginitis** is elimination of likely sensitizers.

SELECTED REFERENCES

Armstrong C. CDC Updates Guidelines on Diagnosis and Treatment of Sexually Transmitted Diseases. *Am Fam Physician.* 2011;84(1):123–125.

Brocklehurst P, Gordon A, Heatley E, Milan SJ. Antibiotics for treating bacterial vaginosis in pregnancy. *Cochrane Database Syst Rev.* 2013;(1):CD000262.

CDC 2010. STD Treatment Guidelines. www.cdc.gov. Accessed May 3, 2013.

Hainer GL, Gibson MV. Vaginitis: diagnosis and treatment. *Am Fam Physician.* 2011;83(7):807–815.

Mendling W, Brasch J. Guideline vulvovaginal candidosis (2010) of the German society for gynecology and obstetrics, the working group for infections and infectimmunology in gynecology and obstetrics, the German society of dermatology, the board of German dermatologists and the German speaking mycological society. *Mycoses.* 2012;55(Suppl 3):1–13.

Sherrard J, Donders G, White D, Jensen JS. European (IUSTI/WHO) guideline on the management of vaginal discharge, 2011. *Int J STD AIDs.* 2011;22(8):421–429.

Verstraelen H, Verhelst R, Vaneechoutte M, Temmerman M. Group A streptococcal vaginitis: an unrecognized cause of vaginal symptoms in adult women. *Arch Gynecol Obstet.* 2011;284(1):95–98.

64   Venous Thromboembolism

Stefani A. Hudson, MD, & Jeffrey M. Tingen, PharmD, MBA, BCPS, BCACP, CDE

KEY POINTS

- Risk factors for venous thromboembolism (VTE) include increasing age, major surgery, trauma, malignancy, previous VTE, prolonged immobility, and hypercoagulable states. (SOR ⊙)
- The diagnosis of VTE should be confirmed by objective testing. (SOR ⊙)
- Antithrombotic therapy requires frequent monitoring to minimize risk for bleeding/hemorrhage. (SOR ⊙)
- Patients should be educated about bleeding risk and possible drug and food interactions with anticoagulation drug therapy. (SOR ⊙)

I. **Definition.** The term venous thromboembolism (VTE) refers to a blood clot (thrombus) that forms within a vein. A deep venous thrombosis (DVT) is a blood clot that forms within the deep veins (tibial, popliteal, femoral, or ileac). In some instances, a DVT may detach and travel to the lungs causing a pulmonary embolism (PE). VTE manifests as both DVT and PE.

II. **Epidemiology.** VTE is a frequent cause of hospitalization. In the United States, initial VTE occurs in roughly 100 per 100,000 persons per year. However, the true incidence in the general population is unknown as an estimated 50% of patients have clinically silent disease. The incidence of VTE increases significantly with age, almost doubling for every decade of life after 50 years of age. The incidence is slightly higher in men and African-Americans. PE constitutes nearly one-third of symptomatic VTE, whereas DVT alone constitutes two-thirds. Approximately half of patients with a proximal DVT will develop a PE if untreated.

    A. **Risk factors for VTE.** Three broad categories of factors predispose patients to VTE (called Virchow triad). These are stasis of blood flow, hypercoagulability, and endothelial injury. Stasis of blood flow can occur with prolonged immobilization (including long airplane flights), recent surgery, or spinal cord injury. Conditions of hypercoagulability include genetic causes (deficiency of antithrombin III, protein C or S deficiency, Leiden V factor), polycythemia vera, autoimmune disorders, postmenopausal hormone therapy and oral contraceptive use, malignancy, changes after trauma such as lower extremity fracture or burns, and pregnancy/postpartum state. Endothelial injury is seen following implants, mechanical devices, surgery, or other circumstances that can injure blood vessels.

III. **Signs and Symptoms**

    A. Patients with **DVT** commonly present with extremity edema (swelling), pain, and warmth. Clinical signs can include erythema or discoloration of the extremity, distention of superficial veins, or tenderness to palpation. However, clinical findings do not confirm or exclude the diagnosis, as DVT can occur asymptomatically, and other disease entities may mimic the signs and symptoms of DVT.

    B. Patients with **PE** commonly present with shortness of breath and chest pain. Clinical signs include tachypnea, tachycardia, cyanosis, low-grade fever, pleural friction rub, and increased pulmonary component of the second heart sound. As with DVT, the diagnosis of PE is not made clinically, as patients with other conditions present similarly.

IV. **Diagnostic Tests**

    A. **DVT.** According to the American College of Chest Physicians' evidence-based clinical practice guidelines, the diagnostic workup for DVT begins with the risk stratification for the likelihood of DVT.

        1. **A validated tool** such as the Wells criteria (Table 64–1) should be used to assign patients with low, intermediate, or high risk. An online calculator is available for calculating the Wells score (http://www.mdcalc.com/wells-criteria-for-dvt/).

        2. Patients with a low pretest probability of first lower extremity DVT should have initial testing with a **highly sensitive D-dimer**. This test is highly sensitive but not highly specific; therefore, if the D-dimer is negative (<500 ng/mL), no further workup is needed.

        3. **If the D-dimer is positive or the pretest probability is intermediate or high, venous color duplex Doppler ultrasound imaging is recommended.** If the Doppler studies are positive, treatment for DVT should be started.

TABLE 64–1. MODEL FOR CLINICAL PREDICTION OF DVT*

Clinical Feature	Score
History	
Active cancer	1
Paralysis, recent plaster cast	1
Recent immobilization or major surgery	1
Physical examination	
Tenderness along deep veins	1
Swelling of entire leg	1
≥3 cm difference in calf circumference	1
Pitting edema	1
Collateral superficial veins	1
Clinical assessment	
Alternative diagnosis likely	−2

Source: Reproduced with permission from Wells PS, Anderson DR, Bormanis J, et al. Value of assessment of pretest probability of deep vein thrombosis in clinical management. *Lancet.* 1997;350(9094):1795–1798.
*Pretest probability of deep vein thrombosis: high if score of 3 points or greater; intermediate if score of 1–2 points; and low if score of 0 or less.

   4. If **upper extremity DVT** is suspected, Doppler ultrasound imaging should be performed. A negative Doppler ultrasound should be followed by a highly sensitive D-dimer, serial ultrasound or venographic-based imaging such as computed tomography (CT) or magnetic resonance imaging (MRI) if there is high clinical suspicion for an upper extremity DVT.
   5. **If hypercoagulability is suspected**, initial laboratory tests should be obtained including antithrombin, protein C, and protein S activity level.
      a. **Additional tests** include activated protein C resistance, prothrombin G20210A mutation testing by PCR, factor VIII level, screening tests for lupus anticoagulants (e.g., sensitive aPTT [activated partial thromboplastin time], aPTT mixing studies, dilute Russell viper venom time), and anticardiolipin antibody testing by ELISA.
      b. Testing should be considered in patients with idiopathic VTE, age under 45 years, recurrent VTE, recurrent pregnancy loss, or a family history of VTE.
      c. In the acute setting, testing should be deferred until at least 2 weeks after completing the initial course of anticoagulant therapy.
   B. **PE.** As is the case with DVT, patients are selected for testing for PE based on pretest probability. The Wells criteria (Table 64–2) can be used to risk stratify patients in whom

TABLE 64–2. WELLS CRITERIA FOR PREDICTING PULMONARY EMBOLISM*

Clinical Feature	Score
History	
Cancer (patients with cancer who were receiving treatment, those in whom treatment had been stopped within the past 6 mo, or those who were receiving palliative care)	1
Immobilization (bed rest, except to access the bathroom, for 3 consecutive days) or surgery in the previous 4 wk	1.5
Previous objectively diagnosed deep venous thrombosis or pulmonary embolism	1.5
Physical examination	
Clinical signs and symptoms of deep venous thrombosis (objectively measured leg swelling and pain with palpation in the deep vein region)	3
Heart rate higher than 100 beats/min	1.5
Hemoptysis	1.0
Clinical assessment	
Pulmonary embolism as likely as or more likely than an alternative diagnosis	3.0

Source: Wells PS, Anderson DR, Rodger M, et al. Excluding pulmonary embolism at the bedside without diagnostic imaging: management of patients with suspected pulmonary embolism presenting to the emergency department by using a simple clinical model and D-dimer. *Ann Intern Med.* 2001;135(2):98–107.
*The pretest probability of pulmonary embolism was considered low in patients with a score of less than 2.0, moderate in patients with scores 2–6, and high in patients with score greater than 6.0.

a diagnosis of PE is suspected. An online calculator is available for calculating the Wells score (http://www.mdcalc.com/wells-criteria-for-pulmonary-embolism-pe/).

1. **D-dimer testing** can be used as initial testing in patients with a low pretest probability of PE. If the D-dimer is negative, no further workup is needed.

2. **If the D-dimer is positive,** imaging should be performed. Multidetector helical CT angiography (CTA) is recommended if available. In patients with an intermediate or high pretest probability of PE, a positive CTA establishes the diagnosis of PE. If discordance occurs between imaging results and pretest probability, consider a second read of the CTA images, a ventilation/perfusion (V/Q) scan, and expert consultation from a pulmonologist or cardiologist. A normal V/Q scan eliminates a diagnosis of PE. V/Q scanning may be preferred in patients in whom CTA is contraindicated, including severe contrast allergy, renal disease, and pregnancy.

3. **Pulmonary angiography** is the standard for a diagnosis of PE; however, it is typically used when less-invasive studies are negative. A positive Doppler ultrasound may be used to diagnose PE in patients with signs and symptoms of PE who cannot tolerate other forms of testing. A negative Doppler ultrasound does not eliminate a diagnosis of PE.

V. Treatment (Table 64–3)

A. Acute management. Options include unfractionated heparin (UFH), low–molecular-weight heparins (LMWHs), fondaparinux, or rivaroxaban. UFH or LMWHs are used in the initial treatment of VTE until the patient achieves a therapeutic INR on warfarin therapy with a minimum overlap of 5 days of LMWH therapy. Therapy with rivaroxaban can be also used as monotherapy, and overlap with LMWH therapy is not needed. **Protamine sulfate** is used as a reversal agent for UFH and LMWH if needed.

1. **UFH** is used for the acute treatment of VTE. The anticoagulation effect of UFH is achieved through its binding to antithrombin which increases its anticoagulant effect through inhibition of several clotting factors. Direct inhibition of thrombin by UFH prolongs the thrombin time, allowing for monitoring of its effects by aPTT. The UFH dose and rate are adjusted based upon the results of the aPTT.

2. **LMWHs,** including dalteparin, enoxaparin, and tinzaparin, are used more commonly now than UFH because of their better pharmacokinetic profile, fewer adverse effects compared with UFH, and absence of need for routine monitoring. LMWHs bind to antithrombin and therefore inhibit several clotting factors, including factor Xa. Enoxaparin and tinzaparin are currently FDA-approved for acute VTE. Dosing and side effects are shown in Table 64–4.

   a. Plasma concentration of LMWH is most easily measured by its ability to inhibit exogenous factor Xa in an anti-Xa activity assay. **Although routine therapeutic monitoring is not required,** some patient characteristics warrant anti-Xa monitoring such as obesity, pregnancy, and renal insufficiency. Other situations requiring monitoring include the need for assessing for subtherapeutic or supratherapeutic levels when thromboembolic or hemorrhagic events occur, identifying minimal drug effects prior to major surgery or thrombolytic therapy, or determining the efficacy of reversal agents in a patient who is bleeding.

3. **Anti-Xa Inhibitors,** including fondaparinux and rivaroxaban, are another option for VTE treatment and prophylaxis. Fondaparinux is a subcutaneous injection that is dosed based upon weight (Table 64–4). Rivaroxaban received FDA approval for these indications in 2013 and is the **only oral agent** that can be used for treatment precluding the need for an injectable medication. **Routine monitoring for efficacy of rivaroxaban is not necessary**. Dosing is shown in Table 64–4, and side effects and potential drug interactions are displayed in Table 64–3. Rivaroxaban should be taken with food.

B. Subsequent management

1. **Warfarin** is the only FDA-approved **vitamin K antagonist** for the treatment of VTE. Warfarin has been the primary VTE treatment for several decades but newer agents with a more favorable drug profile (e.g., rivaroxaban) are now being used more often. Dosing can be initiated with 5 or 10 mg for the first 2 days and then 5 mg daily with subsequent dosing based on the INR. Using a lower starting dose of ≤5 mg may be appropriate in the elderly; in patients with impaired nutrition, hepatic disease, and congestive heart failure; or those at high risk for bleeding.

   a. Monitoring. INR monitoring must be conducted in patients on warfarin therapy. Drug and food interactions sometimes make it difficult for patients to maintain a therapeutic INR level (Table 64–3). The target INR for the management of VTE is 2–3.

TABLE 64–3. TREATMENT OPTIONS FOR PATIENTS WITH VENOUS THROMBOEMBOLISM

Drug[a]	Prophylaxis Dosing	Treatment Dosing	Major Side Effects	Contraindications	Drug Interactions
Unfractionated Heparin (UFH)					
Heparin[a]	Adult: 5000 units SC every 8–12 h	Adult loading: 80 units/kg Maintenance: 18 units/kg/h adjusted to aPTT	Bleeding, heparin-induced thrombocytopenia (HIT), hypersensitivity	Major or active bleeding, severe thrombocytopenia, unable to monitor levels	Aspirin, SSRIs, venlafaxine, ginkgo, garlic, St. John's wort (bleeding)
Low-Molecular-Weight Heparin (LMWH)					
Dalteparin (Fragmin) Enoxaparin (Lovenox)[a] Tinzaparin (Innohep)	See Table 64–4 for dosing	See Table 64–4 for dosing	Bleeding, HIT (much lower incidence than UFH)	Major bleeding, history of thrombocytopenia due to LMWH Caution with epidural or spinal anesthesia	SSRIs, NSAIDs (bleeding)
Anti-Xa Inhibitor					
Fondaparinux (Arixtra)	See Table 64–4 for dosing		Bleeding	Active bleeding, CrCl <30 mL/min Weight <50 kg (prophylaxis use), thrombocytopenia Caution with epidural or spinal anesthesia	SSRIs, venlafaxine, NSAIDs, garlic, ginkgo, St. John's wort (bleeding)
Rivaroxaban (Xarelto)			Bleeding	Active bleeding, hepatic impairment (Child Pugh B or C) CrCl <30 mL/min	Oral antifungals, aspirin, NSAIDs (bleeding)
Vitamin K Antagonist					
Warfarin (Coumadin)[a]	Start 5–10 mg daily and adjust dose based upon INR		Bleeding, skin necrosis, purple toe syndrome	Active bleeding, pregnancy	Multiple drug interactions Tamoxifen, aspirin, amiodarone, many antibiotics, SSRIs, methotrexate, ginkgo, St. John's wort, fish oil, oral antifungals, torsemide (bleeding)

[a]denotes medications that are available as generic products.

aPTT, activated partial thromboplastin time; CrCl, creatinine clearance; NSAIDs, nonsteroidal anti-inflammatory drugs; SSRIs, selective serotonin reuptake inhibitors.

TABLE 64–4. LOW-MOLECULAR-WEIGHT HEPARIN AND ANTI-XA INHIBITOR DOSING AND INDICATIONS

Indication	Low-Molecular-Weight Heparin			Anti-Xa Inhibitor	
	Dalteparin	Enoxaparin	Tinzaparin	Fondaparinux	Rivaroxaban
VTE Treatment					
Venous thromboembolism (deep vein thrombosis or pulmonary embolism)	No FDA-approved indication	1 mg/kg SC every 12 h **OR** 1.5 mg/kg SC every 24 h	175 units/kg SC every 24 h	Weight Based Dosing: **<50 kg:** 5 mg SC every 24 h **50–100 kg:** 7.5 mg SC every 24 h **>100 kg:** 10 mg SC every 24 h	15 mg orally twice daily for 21 days and then 20 mg once daily *Recurrent DVT/PE:* 20 mg orally once daily
Venous thromboembolism in patients with cancer	Month 1: 200 units/kg SC every 24 h Months 2–6: 150 units/kg SC every 24 h	No FDA-approved indication	No FDA-approved indication	No FDA-approved indication	No FDA-approved indication
VTE Prophylaxis					
Abdominal surgery	2500 units SC once daily **OR** 5000 units SC once daily **OR** 2500 units SC followed by 2500 units SC 12 h later and then 5000 units SC once daily	40 mg SC every 24 h initiated 2 h prior to surgery	No FDA-approved indication	2.5 mg SC every 24 h initiated 6 to 8 h after surgery	No FDA-approved indication
Hip replacement surgery	Postoperative start: 2500 units SC 4–8 h after surgery then 5000 units SC once daily Preoperative start: 2500 units SC 2 h before surgery then as above Preoperative start evening before surgery: 5000 units SC followed by 5000 units SC 4–8 h after surgery then 5000 units SC once daily	30 mg SC every 12 h initiated 12–24 h after surgery **OR** 40 mg SC every 24 h initiated 12 h prior to surgery	No FDA-approved indication	2.5 mg SC every 24 h initiated 6–8 h after surgery	10 mg orally daily for 35 days initiated 6–10 h after surgery
Knee replacement surgery	No FDA-approved indication	30 mg SC every 12 h initiated 12–24 h after surgery	No FDA-approved indication	2.5 mg SC every 24 h initiated 6–8 h after surgery	10 mg orally once daily for 12 days initiated 6–10 h after surgery
Acute medical illness	5000 units SC every 24 h	40 mg SC every 24 h	No FDA-approved indication	No FDA-approved indication	No FDA-approved indication

SC, subcutaneously.

   b. Intake of foods high in vitamin K should be limited or consumed in about the same amounts each day. These foods include kale, spinach, collards, Swiss chard, broccoli, and Brussels sprouts (http://www.cc.nih.gov/ccc/patient_education/drug_nutrient/coumadin1.pdf).

2. **Rivaroxaban** is also FDA approved for the prevention and treatment of VTE. Before deciding to prescribe rivaroxaban, assess the patient for possible drug interactions and renal and hepatic impairment and consider the financial cost to the patient. **No set reversal agent for rivaroxaban exists** although evidence supports the use of clotting factor supplement such as prothrombin complex concentrate (PCC) in the event of major bleeding.

3. The optimal **duration of anticoagulant therapy** after VTE varies depending on the clinical setting. Patients typically receive between 3 and 6 months of therapy for the first episode of VTE. If more than one episode occurs, therapy is generally warranted lifelong or until risk outweighs benefit. The American College of Chest Physicians provides recommendations for duration of treatment for VTE (http://journal.publications.chestnet.org/ss/guidelines.aspx).

   a. Patients with PE without previous VTE or with a reversible or time-limited risk factor should be treated for 3 to 6 months. Patients with metastatic cancer or recurrent VTE are generally treated for at least 6 months to 1 year followed by long-term anticoagulant therapy.

4. In the event that anticoagulation drug therapy causes complications, fails, or is contraindicated, **inferior vena cava (IVC) filters** can be used. IVC filters are surgically placed for a designated period of time to provide protection against VTE. Complications of IVC filters include thrombosis of the filter, perforation of the inferior vena cava, DVT at the insertion site, filter migration, and damage to surrounding structures.

C. **Complications**
   1. **VTE complications.** DVT may cause incompetence of the venous valves and lead to the development of postthrombotic syndrome which is characterized by pain, swelling, and ulcerations. PE complications can include cardiac arrest, pleural effusion, and pulmonary hypertension.

      a. The use of graduated compression stockings starting within 2 weeks of onset of DVT and continuing for a minimum of 2 years after DVT should be considered for most patients.

      b. VTE prophylaxis. Recommended dosing using LMWHs or anti-Xa inhibitors following abdominal, hip, or knee surgery, or during acute medical illness are shown in Table 64–4.

   2. **Complications of heparin therapy.** Heparin-induced thrombocytopenia (HIT) is an antibody-mediated adverse drug effect that can result in thromboembolism. The most common manifestation of HIT is thrombocytopenia, which typically occurs 5 to 10 days after initiation of heparin. Management of HIT involves discontinuing heparin and using an intravenous direct thrombin inhibitor such as argatroban, lepirudin, and bivalirudin.

   3. **Complications of warfarin therapy.** The annual incidence of warfarin-associated major bleeding is about 1% to 3%. If major bleeding occurs from warfarin use, rapid reversal is often warranted with a clotting factor supplement such as four-factor PCC. PCC is preferred over fresh frozen plasma because it is associated with less risk of infection transmission and more rapid INR normalization.

      a. The addition of vitamin K, 5 to 10 mg administered by slow intravenous injection, is also recommended in combination with coagulation factors.

      b. Bleeding risk rises significantly as the INR increases above 4.5. Oral vitamin K may also be considered in asymptomatic patients with significantly elevated INR (e.g., >10) or for patients with minor bleeding.

SELECTED REFERENCES

Alpert JS, Dalen JE. Epidemiology and natural history of venous thromboembolism. *Prog Cardiovasc Dis.* 1994;36(6):417–422.

Deitcher S. Hypercoagulable states. http://www.clevelandclinicmeded.com/medicalpubs/diseasemanagement/hematology-oncology/hypercoagulable-states/#s0035. Accessed October 2013.

Holbrook A, Schulman S, Witt DM, et al. Evidence-based management of anticoagulant therapy: antithrombotic therapy and prevention of thrombosis, 9th ed: American College of Chest Physicians evidence-based clinical practice guidelines. *Chest.* 2012;141(2 Suppl):e152S–e184S.

Micromedex® Healthcare Series [Internet database]. Greenwood Village, CO: Thomson Healthcare. Updated periodically.

University of Michigan Health System. Venous Thromboembolism Guideline Update, February 2009. http://www.med.umich.edu/1info/FHP/practiceguides/vte/vte.pdf. Accessed November 2013.

White RH. The epidemiology of venous thromboembolism. *Circulation.* 2003;107(23 Suppl 1):14–18.

Wilbur J, Shian B. Diagnosis of deep venous thrombosis and pulmonary embolism. *Am Fam Physician.* 2012;86(10):913–919.

Witt DM, Nutescu EA, Haines ST. Chapter 26. Venous thromboembolism. In: Wells BG, ed. *Pharmacotherapy: A Pathophysiologic Approach.* 8th ed. New York, NY: McGraw-Hill; 2011. http://www.accesspharmacy.com/content.aspx?aID=7973333. Accessed October 31, 2013.

---

65 Wheezing

Christopher Taggart, MD, & Judith Kerber Frazier, MD

KEY POINTS

- The cause of wheezing should be identified based on the patient's age; consider diseases other than asthma. (SOR **C**)
- **Respiratory distress** (cyanosis, retractions, apnea, or stridor) should be assessed immediately. Oxygen should be provided if needed and evaluation continued in the emergency department. (SOR **C**)
- A **chest x-ray** should be obtained for patients who present with new-onset wheezing. (SOR **C**)

I. Definition. Wheezing is a symptom in which the lungs produce high-pitched musical sounds due to narrowing of the tracheobronchial air passages, similar to deep breathing with a child's party kazoo in the mouth. It is usually a sign of respiratory difficulty.

II. Screening and Prevention

   A. Bronchiolitis

      1. Hand hygiene and isolation procedures reduce respiratory syncytial virus (RSV) by protecting against direct person-to-person and fomite transmission. (SOR **B**)

      2. Palivizumab (Synagis) is a monoclonal antibody against RSV indicated for high-risk children including (a) born before 35 weeks' gestation, (b) chronic lung disease requiring medical therapy, (c) congenital airway abnormality, (d) neuromuscular disease that interferes with clearance of airway secretions, (e) congenital heart disease with heart failure on medical therapy or moderate to severe pulmonary hypertension, and (f) cyanotic heart disease. (SOR **C**)

   B. Asthma. Allergen identification through formal allergy testing and a comprehensive allergen avoidance plan have been shown to reduce the severity of asthma in patients requiring daily asthma medications. (SOR **A**) Potential elements include (a) removal of pets, (b) particulate air filtration systems, (c) vacuum cleaners, (d) smoking cessation, (e) allergen-impenetrable covers for mattresses and pillows, and (f) cockroach extermination.

   C. Screening for **lung cancer** is controversial, but the American Association of Thoracic Surgery recommends that patients aged 50 years or older with a 20 pack-year history of tobacco use be offered annual chest low-dose spiral computed tomography (CT). (SOR **B**)

II. Common Diagnoses

   A. Infants younger than 2 years

      1. Acute viral respiratory tract infections are a major cause of wheezing in infants. Risk factors include: (a) fall or winter season, (b) age less than 2 years, (c) a history of atopy (allergies or allergic skin conditions), (d) hospitalization, (e) school-aged siblings, (f) day care attendance, (g) passive smoke from parents or caregivers, and (h) bottle-feeding.

      2. Acute bronchitis and pneumonia are mostly caused by viral infections. Bacterial infections can occur especially in older children and adults. Risk factors include: (a) smoke exposure (active or passive), (b) recent viral upper respiratory infection (URI), and (c) impaired gag reflex.

3. **Bronchiolitis** is caused by viral infections of the lower respiratory system. RSV accounts for a majority of these infections (>50%). Additional pathogens include parainfluenza virus, adenovirus, *Mycoplasma*, human metapneumovirus, and human bocavirus. RSV is the most important cause of bronchiolitis and pneumonia in children younger than 2 years. It is epidemic in winter and spring in temperate climates. RSV is seen in all age groups, but preterm infants are at greater risk.

4. **Aspiration**
   a. **Gastroesophageal reflux** is physiologic passive return of gastric contents into the esophagus. It peaks at 1 to 4 months of age and usually resolves by 12 months. True gastroesophageal reflux disease (GERD) is pathologic and consists of persistent respiratory symptoms, poor weight gain, and esophagitis. Prevalence of GERD is 1 in 300 infants. Risk factors for GERD include anatomic abnormalities (e.g., esophageal atresia, hiatal hernia, bronchopulmonary dysplasia), neurologic problems or delay, asthma, and cystic fibrosis (CF).
   b. **Foreign body aspiration** is an uncommon but life-threatening cause of wheezing. It must always be considered in any infant or young child with sudden onset of wheezing or respiratory distress. It occurs most often between the ages of 8 months to 4 years and is usually characterized by unilateral wheezing.

5. **CF** has an incidence of 1 in 3500 births in whites. It is an inherited autosomal recessive trait that predisposes the patient to respiratory infections. Risk factors include white race and family history.

6. **Anaphylaxis or hypersensitivity reaction** requires that the patient have prior exposure to an offending agent. Triggers include (a) drugs (e.g., nonsteroidal anti-inflammatory drugs), (b) food (e.g., peanuts), (c) bee or other insect sting, and (d) physical conditions (e.g., exercise, heat, cold).

B. **Children** (age 2 years to teenage).
1. **Respiratory tract infections**
2. **Acute bronchitis and pneumonia**
3. **Anaphylaxis or hypersensitivity**
4. **Asthma** (see Chapter 68). Ten percent of the worldwide population will have at least one asthma attack in their life. Risk factors include (a) viral URI, (b) family history, (c) environmental exposures (e.g., tobacco), and (d) atopy. Asthma in patients younger than age 2 years can be called hyperreactive airway disease.

C. **Adult** (young- to middle-aged).
1. **Respiratory tract infections.**
2. **Acute bronchitis and pneumonia.**
3. **Asthma.**
4. **Anaphylaxis or hypersensitivity.**
5. **Chronic obstructive pulmonary disease (COPD)** (see Chapter 70) affects more than 5% of the American population and is currently the third leading cause of death. Risk factors include (a) tobacco use ($\geq$20 pack-year history), (b) environmental exposures (air pollution), (c) α_1-antitrypsin deficiency, and (d) family history.
6. **Pulmonary embolus (PE)** (see Chapter 64) is an infrequent cause of wheezing. One study found that 9.1% of patients with acute PE complained of wheezing on presentation. Major risk factors include (a) fracture (hip, leg), (b) hip or knee replacement, (c) major surgery, and (d) trauma (especially spinal cord injury).

D. **Adult** (older than 50 years).
1. **RTIs.**
2. **Acute bronchitis and pneumonia.**
3. **COPD.**
4. **Congestive heart failure (CHF)** (see Chapter 73) affects more than 5 million people in the United States. Risk factors include (a) hypertension, (b) diabetes, (c) metabolic syndrome, (d) obesity, (e) atherosclerotic disease, (f) history of cardiotoxin exposure, and (g) structural heart disease (valvular disease, left ventricular hypertrophy, low left ejection fraction, history of myocardial infarction).
5. **Aspiration** (secretions, food, foreign body).
6. **Anaphylaxis or hypersensitivity.**
7. **PE.**
8. **Lung cancer** can be a rare cause of persistent wheezing. Risk factors include tobacco use, occupational exposure to carcinogens (asbestos), and positive family history.

III. Signs and Symptoms (Table 65–1)

   A. Overview. It is important to consider each patient's entire history and examination to help determine the cause of wheezing. A systematic complete chest examination is key in establishing the diagnosis. Remember that very sick patients may not wheeze even though their lungs are in imminent failure. On the other hand, healthy patients can have very loud wheezing. Below are some examination findings that can help elucidate the underlying etiology.

   B. Inspection

      1. Respiratory rate (normal *adult:* 12–20 breaths per minute [bpm]); *child:* 40–60 bpm for newborn, up to 35 bpm until age 1 year, up to 26 bpm until age 3 years, up to 24 bpm until age 6, up to 20 bpm through teen years). A person can have normal, fast, slow, or absent respiratory rate.

        a. Tachypnea is increased respiratory rate. It is usually associated with respiratory system distress and short shallow breaths (see Chapter 20).

        b. Bradypnea is low respiratory rate. This can be normal during sleep or abnormal in severe respiratory distress.

        c. Apnea is a pause or stop in respirations. It is commonly seen in patients with obstructive sleep apnea when they are asleep.

      2. Intercostal retractions are irregular breathing motions of the intercostal muscles in which these muscles are pulled into the chest cavity instead of expanding the chest with a breath. This can appear like the abdomen is breathing because the abdomen enlarges while the chest retracts. Intercostal retractions are a sign of severe lung obstruction nearing imminent complete respiratory failure and should be treated as an emergency requiring immediate attention.

      3. Anteroposterior (AP) diameter is the length between the anterior chest wall and the back. It can be increased in chronic lung diseases such as COPD, asthma, and CF.

   C. Percussion

      1. Normal percussion is symmetrical resonance at each chest level. There can be differences between levels depending upon physiologic properties and patient position during the examination.

      2. Hyperresonance sounds hollow. It is an indication of increased air volume. This can be normal or can indicate lung diseases such as asthma, COPD, CF, and pneumothorax.

      3. Dullness sounds like a "thunk." It is an indication of increased mass behind the percussed area. Duller sounds suggest a more solid structure over the percussed area. For example, a patient with pneumonia may have a mildly dull percussion sound over the site of infection, or a patient with lung cancer could have a very dull percussion sound, similar to the sound of percussion over a bone.

   D. Auscultation should be performed over the entire chest, as wheezing can sometimes only be heard in one area. Each side should be compared to the other.

      1. Breath sounds

        a. Prolonged expiratory phase is when the duration of an exhale is longer than normal (longer than inspiration). It suggests constricted airways.

        b. Rhonchi are low-pitched sounds similar to soft snoring. They are caused by increased fluid or inflammation narrowing the upper airway. They suggest pneumonia, COPD, or aspiration.

        c. Crackles (rales) are soft sounds similar to Rice Krispies© cereal in milk. They are usually heard in the distal lung and indicate alveoli opening and closing or increased fluid in the distal airway. They are suggestive of either a volume overload condition like CHF or increased fluid production like pneumonia.

      2. Voice sounds heard with your stethoscope through the normal lungs are muted and inarticulate. However, they can become louder and clearer with consolidation because sound travels better through the consolidation than through air.

        a. Whispered pectoriloquy is the transformation of whispered speech from difficult to understand to clear and understandable as if speaking to the person.

        b. Bronchophony is the transformation of a single syllable from indistinguishable to distinguishable.

        c. Egophony is the change from "Eee" to "Ay" sound when the patient says "ee".

TABLE 65–1. SYMPTOMS WITH COMMON CAUSES OF WHEEZING

	Wheeze	Fever	Cough	Sore Throat	Rhinorrhea	Lethargy	Onset	Other
Acute viral infection	X	X	X	X	X		Rapid	Coryza
Pneumonia and bronchitis	X	X	X				Rapid	
Bronchiolitis	X	X	X	X	X		Rapid	
Gastroesophageal reflux/GERD	X		X			X	Gradual	Hoarseness
Cystic Fibrosis	X					X	Gradual	Irritability Poor feeding Meconium ileus Pancreatic insufficiency
Anaphylaxis	X		X				Rapid	Urticaria Stridor Chest discomfort Lump in throat Flushing N/V/D
Asthma	X		X				Gradual	Evening wheezing or coughing
Chronic Obstructive Pulmonary Disease	X		Chronic		X		Gradual	Recurrent bronchitis Barrel chest
Congestive Heart Failure	X		X				Gradual	Lower extremity swelling JVD
Pulmonary Embolism	X		X				Rapid	Acute shortness of breath Increased respiratory rate

GERD, gastroesophageal reflux disease; JVD, jugular venous distention; N/V/D, nausea/vomiting/diarrhea.

E. Nonpulmonary
  1. **Dennie pleats** are creases under the eyes from repeated rubbing. They can be a sign of an associated allergic condition, like allergic rhinitis.
  2. **Allergic shiners** are dark circles under the eyes that can be a sign of an associated allergic condition, like allergic rhinitis.
  3. **Jugular venous distention** (see Chapter 73) is associated with CHF.
  4. **Bilateral dependent edema** (see Chapter 73) is associated with CHF.
  5. **Fever** can be a sign of pneumonia, bronchitis, or cancer.

IV. Diagnostic Tests
  A. Chest x-ray (CXR), with two images (AP and lateral), is strongly considered for patients who present with their first episode of wheezing.
    1. Patients with known asthma do not require a CXR with every episode of wheezing. If the patient's signs or symptoms (e.g., fever, rhonchi, or purulent sputum) suggest another etiology, a CXR should be considered to look for pneumonia.
    2. Potential findings to help determine etiology include
      a. Consolidations are areas with increased fluid in the air space. They are suggestive of pneumonia or atelectasis. A CXR may not show an infiltrate until 3 days into the disease.
      b. Cardiomegaly is an enlarged heart silhouette and can indicate CHF.
      c. Lung hyperexpansion is suggested when 10 or more ribs are seen in the image or the diaphragms are flat. Hyperexpansion indicates diseases like COPD which can have increased nonfunctional lung volume.
      d. A **diffuse hazy pattern** is seen in most viral illnesses.
      e. Foreign bodies, especially metallic radiopaque objects, may be apparent on CXR.
  B. Lung function tests
    1. **Peak flow** is a simple and quick test to measure a patient's current forced expiratory lung volume in 1 second (FEV_1). This can be done in the office or at home. Results vary by height, sex, and age. Peak flow is not a diagnostic test but a good method to monitor chronic lung diseases and can be an early indicator of worsening or improving obstruction.
    2. **Pulmonary function tests (PFTs)** are diagnostic lung tests that measure many different physiologic lung processes including total lung capacity, tidal volume, residual volume, forced vital capacity, forced expiratory volume at 1, 2, and 3 seconds (FEV_1, FEV_2, and FEV_3, respectively), forced expiratory flow 25% to 75%, peak expiratory flow, and others. Simple PFTs can be performed in the office, but comprehensive PFTs require a pulmonary laboratory to measure diffusing capacity. These tests differentiate obstructive from restrictive lung disease, rate the severity of lung disease in patients with chronic lung diseases like COPD, and can indicate nonrestrictive diseases. PFTs provide more information than peak flow alone.
  C. A **complete blood count (CBC)** provides information including white blood cell (WBC) count, red blood cell (RBC) count, platelets, hemoglobin, and hematocrit. A CBC with differential includes additional information such as band count and percentage of neutrophils, lymphocytes, monocytes, and eosinophils; the differential must be ordered specifically.
    1. **Elevated WBC** count can indicate infection; however, the WBC count can be **falsely elevated** in patients using intravenous or oral steroids due to demargination of cells (movement of WBCs from tissue into the blood stream).
    2. **Elevated lymphocytes** indicate viral infection.
    3. **Elevated band count** or elevated total polymorphonuclear cells (PMNs) (segs + bands) indicates a bacterial infection and is known as a "left shift."
    4. **Low hemoglobin or hematocrit** is often seen in patients with chronic diseases (anemia of chronic disease).
  D. Nasopharyngeal (NP) wash identifies five viruses causing bronchiolitis in infants and children (RSV, adenovirus, influenza A, influenza B, and parainfluenza). It can take 24 hours to process.
    1. **Rapid RSV** test is an NP wash that is primarily used in emergency departments to quickly identify RSV infection in children. It takes approximately 1 to 1.5 hours for results. Routine testing is not recommended to diagnose bronchiolitis. (SOR **C**)

E. CF testing. Sweat sodium and chloride testing is usually performed in a hospital setting. It is elevated in 90% of patients with CF. **Genetic testing** is indicated to identify CF carriers.

F. Gastroesophageal reflux disease (GERD) testing.
   1. A **24-hour pH probe** is the gold standard for diagnosing GERD testing in children. It measures the pH of the distal esophagus. An acidic result indicates reflux.
   2. Upper gastrointestinal barium swallow study can reveal structural defects.
   3. Endoscopy is usually reserved for patients unresponsive to medical management of GERD symptoms.

G. B-type natriuretic peptide (BNP) (see Chapter 73) is a blood test that measures basic natriuretic peptide, a substance secreted by stretched heart ventricles. If elevated, it can indicate CHF exacerbation as a reason for wheezing.

V. Treatment of wheezing is largely based on treating the underlying etiology.
   A. General Treatments
      1. Nonpharmacologic
         a. Oxygen is indicated in patients with an SpO2 <90% or clinical respiratory distress (increased work of breathing, cyanosis, retractions, apnea, or stridor) (see Chapter 20).
         b. IV fluids are used in patients who show signs of dehydration or shock.
      2. Pharmacologic
         a. Bronchodilators.
            (1) Albuterol/Levo albuterol are short-acting beta-agonists that relax bronchial smooth muscle and relieve obstruction and can improve wheezing. These medications are temporary ways to improve lung function, but do not address the underlying etiology.
            (2) Ipratropium is an anticholinergic agent that blocks acetylcholine and results in bronchodilation.
         b. Corticosteroids are indicated for treatment of acute asthma or COPD exacerbations.
         c. Antibiotics are indicated for suspected infectious causes of wheezing. Treatment should be based on the suspected or known pathogen.
      3. Follow-up. Frequent reassessment of respiratory status should be done after treatment is initiated.
   B. Disease-specific treatment
      1. Acute viral respiratory infection (see Chapters 54 and 56).
      2. Acute bronchitis and pneumonia (see Chapter 13 for cough).
      3. Bronchiolitis is best treated with **prevention** (see Section II). Most care is **supportive** through observation, oxygen (if indicated), hydration, and possible hospitalization (if SpO$_2$ <90%). Bronchodilators (unless initially beneficial), steroids, antiviral medications (ribavirin), or antibiotics are not routinely recommended in the treatment of bronchiolitis as they do not appear to influence morbidity or mortality or improve disease course. (SOR Ⓑ)
      4. Aspiration
         a. Gastroesophageal reflux (GERD).
            (1) Reflux precautions should be the initial treatment, especially in children. These include thickening feeds (1 tbsp rice cereal to 1 oz formula), placing the infant upright and prone, and giving small feeds (feed 1 oz, burp, repeat after every ounce consumed).
            (2) Diet changes by avoiding caffeine, alcohol, or other foods that appear to trigger symptoms.
            (3) Quit smoking.
            (4) H$_2$ blockers are useful for mild GERD and include medications like ranitidine (150 mg twice daily for adults and older adolescents; 5–10 mg/kg/d divided every 12 hours for children [1 month to 16 years]). Maintenance doses are the same as above for adults but have not been established for children; for children, therapy is continued for 6–8 weeks if improvement in symptoms is noted.
            (5) Proton pump inhibitors are indicated in moderate-to-severe GERD or if the patient fails H$_2$ blocker treatment.

(6) Metoclopramide is a prokinetic agent that works through dopamine antagonism, which results in increased gastric emptying and increased esophageal sphincter spasm. It may help control GERD that is resistant to other treatments.

b. Foreign body aspiration is a medical emergency that may require removal through bronchoscopy or surgery.

5. CF requires a team-based approach to management, and patient should be referred to a CF clinic.

6. Anaphylaxis requires immediate treatment with epinephrine injections (Epi-Pen). Patient should then be monitored in the hospital or emergency department afterward. Post-acute treatment should include corticosteroids, liberal bronchodilator use, and antihistamine medications (e.g., diphenhydramine). Prevention of recurrences includes behavior modification before another episode occurs.

7. Asthma (see Chapter 68).

8. COPD (see Chapter 70).

9. CHF (see Chapter 73).

10. Pulmonary embolus (see Chapter 64).

VI. Patient Education

A. There is no specific patient education for wheezing. Instead, see patient education for each disease or condition. An example would be an Asthma Action Plan for asthma patient education.

B. The AAFP website (www.aafp.org) and FamilyDoctor.Org (www.familydoctor.org) are excellent resources to find patient education material on many topics.

SELECTED REFERENCES

American Academy of Pediatrics: Policy statements—modified recommendations for use of palivizumab for prevention of respiratory syncytial virus infections. *Pediatrics.* 2009;124(6):1694–1701.

Calvo-Romero JM, Perez-Miranda M, Bureo-Dacal P. Wheezing in patients with acute pulmonary embolism with and without previous cardiopulmonary disease. *Eur J Emerg Med.* 2003;10(4): 288–289.

Dawson-Caswell M, Muncie HL Jr. Respiratory syncytial virus infection in children. *Am Fam Physician.* 2011;83(2):141–146.

Fitzgerald J, Dennis R, Solarte I. Clinical evidence concise: asthma. *Am Fam Physician.* 2004;70(1): 143–146.

Jaklitsch MT, Jacobson FL, Austin JH, et al. The American Association for Thoracic Surgery guidelines for lung cancer screening using low-dose computed tomography scans for lung cancer survivors and other high-risk groups. *J Thorac Cardiovasc Surg.* 2012;144(1):33–38.

Jessup M, Abraham WT, Casey DE, et al. 2009 focused update: ACCF/AHA Guidelines for the Diagnosis and Management of Heart Failure in Adults: a report of the American College of Cardiology Foundation/American Heart Association Task Force on Practice Guidelines: developed in collaboration with the International Society for Heart and Lung Transplantation. *Circulation.* 2009;119(14): 1977–2016.

Jung AD. Gastroesophageal reflux in infants and children. *Am Fam Physician.* 2001;64(11): 1853–1860.

Platts-Mills T, Leung DY, Schatz M. The role of allergens in asthma. *Am Fam Physician.* 2007;76(5): 675–680.

Qaseem A, Wilt TJ, Weinberger SE, et al. Diagnosis and management of stable chronic obstructive pulmonary disease: a clinical practice guideline update from the American College of Physicians, American College of Chest Physicians, American Thoracic Society, and European Respiratory Society. *Ann Intern Med.* 2011;155(3):179–191.

Watts K, Goodman D: Wheezing, Bronchiolitis, and Bronchitis. In *Nelson Textbook of Pediatrics.* 19th ed. Philadelphia, PA: Elsevier Saunders; 2011:1456–1460.

Weiss LN. The diagnosis of wheezing in children. *Am Fam Physician.* 2008;77(8):1109–1114.

SECTION II. **Chronic Illness**

66   Acne Vulgaris and Acne Rosacea

Paul C. Walker, PharmD, FASHP, Mindy A. Smith, MD, MS,
Brooke E. Farley, PharmD, BCPS, & Julie A. Murphy, PharmD, BCPS

KEY POINTS

- Accurate diagnosis of a patient's severity level of acne will ensure optimal medication regimen selection. (SOR **C**)
- Topical agents are often sufficient for mild-to-moderate acne vulgaris (SOR **A**) and mild forms of acne rosacea. (SOR **B**)
- For more extensive involvement in patients with acne rosacea, oral doxycycline, tetracycline, and metronidazole are effective. (SOR **A**) Systemic antibiotics are effective in patients with moderate acne, but it is not clear that they are more effective than topical agents. (SOR **C**)
- Oral isotretinoin (Accutane) is used for severe acne vulgaris or acne rosacea, (SOR **A**) but requires registration with the iPledge program to ensure safe use.
- Education of patients about the disease and the importance of compliance will improve outcomes. (SOR **C**)
- Assessment of patient progress at regular intervals will enhance the success rate of medication regimens. (SOR **C**)

ACNE VULGARIS

I. **Introduction**
   A. **Definitions**
      1. **Acne vulgaris** is a common, chronic, polymorphic skin disease of pilosebaceous units, consisting of a hair follicle and sebaceous gland, located on the face, chest, and back. It is generally a self-limited condition that begins during adolescence; however, acne can persist into adulthood. In general, acne is not a high mortality disease state; however, morbidity can be high as the disease can adversely affect self-esteem and can cause scarring and disfigurement.
      2. **Noninflammatory (obstructive) lesions** (Figure 66–1).
         a. **Open comedones,** or **"blackheads",** are wide openings on the skin surface capped with a melanin-containing blackened mass of epithelial debris.
         b. **Closed comedones,** or **"whiteheads",** have a narrow or obstructed opening on the skin surface; these may rupture, producing a low-grade dermal inflammatory reaction.

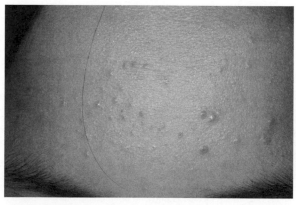

FIGURE 66–1. Comedonal acne in a 15-year-old girl. Open comedones (blackheads) and closed comedones (whiteheads) are visible on her forehead (see color insert). (Used with permission of Richard P. Usatine, MD.)

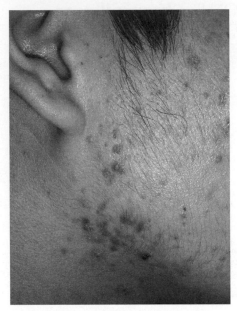

FIGURE 66–2. Inflammatory acne showing pustules and nodules in a 17-year-old boy who uses a helmet while playing football in high school (see color insert). (Used with permission of Richard P. Usatine, MD.)

3. Inflammatory lesions (Figure 66–2).
   a. Papule is a well-defined, elevated, palpable distinct area of skin generally up to 0.5 cm in diameter.
   b. Pustule is a superficial elevation of the skin, filled with purulent fluid, typically surrounding a hair follicle and up to 0.5 cm in diameter.
   c. Nodule is an elevated, firm distinct, palpable, round or oval lesion greater than 0.5 cm in diameter.
4. Severe acne variants
   a. Acne conglobata is severe cystic acne, characterized by cystic lesions, abscesses, communicating sinuses, and thickened, nodular scars, found on the upper trunk and posterior neck; this condition usually does not affect the face (Figure 66–3).
   b. Acne fulminans is severe scarring acne associated with fever, polyarthralgia, crusted ulcerative lesions, weight loss, and anemia.
B. Epidemiology. Acne vulgaris is the most common skin disorder in the United States, affecting 80% of the population between ages 12 and 25 years; however, acne can occur at any age. Prevalence does not appear to differ by gender, race, or ethnicity. Severity of disease may be influenced by race as severity of acne vulgaris appears to be lower in Asians and African-Americans than in the Caucasian population.
C. Pathophysiology. There are four primary pathologic factors, and therefore potential pharmacologic targets, identified as playing a role in the formation of characteristic acne vulgaris lesions.
   1. Excessive sebum production is caused by androgenic stimulation of the sebaceous glands. Severity of acne may be associated with the amount of sebum produced.
   2. Hyperkeratinization of the hair follicle. The normal process of dead cells being forced out of the follicle by growing hair is interrupted and instead cells do not leave the follicle as a result of keratin. This results in obstruction of the hair follicle and microcomedone formation. Continued production of sebum and keratin gives rise to visible lesions, which include closed and open comedones, as defined above.
   3. Microbial colonization of the follicle with *Propionibacterium acnes*. The microcomedone environment is a perfect place for *P. acnes*, an anaerobe, to thrive and ultimately cause inflammatory lesions.

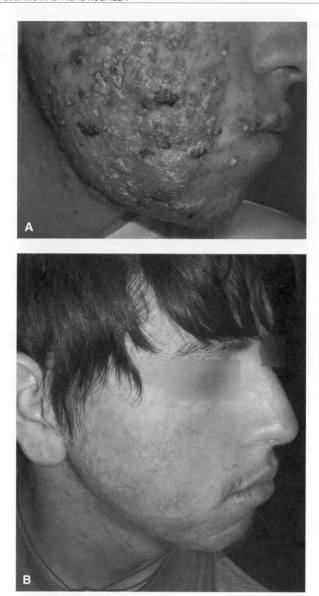

FIGURE 66–3. A. Acne conglobata in a 16-year-old boy. He has severe cysts on his face with sinus tracks between them. He required many weeks of oral prednisone before isotretinoin was started. His acne cleared completely with his treatment. **B.** Acne conglobata cleared with minimal scarring after oral prednisone and 5 months of isotretinoin therapy (see color insert). (Used with permission of Richard P. Usatine, MD.)

   4. Release of inflammatory mediators is largely related to the proliferation of
   P. acnes and free fatty acid formation within the follicle. Leakage or rupture of the
   contents of closed comedones into the dermis results in inflammatory acne lesions
   including papules, pustules, nodules, and cysts.
 II. Diagnosis is based on patient history, clinical signs, and physical examination. Severity is
   assessed by the number, type, and distribution of lesions.

TABLE 66–1. MANAGEMENT OF ACNE

	First Line	Alternatives	Alternatives for Females	Maintenance
Mild acne	TR or BPO	AA +/– BPO		TR
Comedonal	TR + BPO	AA + BPO; TD		TR +/– BP; AA
Inflammatory	TR +/– TA +/– BP			
Moderate acne	SA + TR +/– BPO; TA + TR +/– BPO	AA +/– BPO; OI	OC + TR +/– BPO	TR +/– BPO; AA
Severe acne	OI	SA + TR + BPO	OC + SA + TR +/– BPO	TR +/– BPO

AA, azelaic acid; BPO, benzoyl peroxide; OC, oral contraceptive; OI, oral isotretinoin; SA, systemic antibiotic; TA, topical antibiotic; TD, topical dapsone (single therapy or in place of TA); TR, topical retinoid.
Fixed-dose combination products are available containing BPO/TR, BPO/TA, and TA/TR.

A. **Mild acne**
   1. **Comedones** (open and closed) are the main lesions (≤20).
   2. **Papules** and **pustules** may be present but are few in number (≤10).
B. **Moderate acne**
   1. **Papules** and **pustules** (10–40) and **comedones** (20–40) are present.
   2. Few **nodules** (≤5) may also be present.
C. **Severe acne**
   1. Numerous **papules** and **pustules** are present (40–100 lesions), with many **comedones** (40–100 lesions) and occasional larger, deeper **nodules** (up to 5).
   2. **Nodulocystic acne** and **acne conglobata** may be present.
   3. Affected areas usually involve the face, chest, and back.
III. **Treatment.** A summary of treatment recommendations can be found in Table 66–1. The goals of acne management include controlling acne lesions and preventing scarring. Because multiple factors are involved in the pathogenesis of acne, combination therapy with agents that work by different mechanisms is standard. Improvement in appearance may not happen for 3 to 6 weeks, with maximum effects not being seen until after approximately 8 to 12 weeks of therapy.
   A. **Topical agents** are available as gels, solutions, creams, or lotions. Gels and solutions are best for patients with oily skin. Creams are better for patients with sensitive or dry skin. Lotions would be appropriate for any skin type. These agents should be applied after the affected area has been washed and patted dry, being sure to avoid the eyes and mucous membranes of the nose and mouth.
      1. **Benzoyl peroxide (BPO)** treats acne by its antibacterial and comedolytic properties. (SOR **Ⓐ**) A thin film of BPO is used once to twice daily and is available in various concentrations (2.5%–10%) and formulations (lotion, cream, gel, and body washes); some require a prescription. Concentrations of 2.5% to 5% are as effective as higher concentrations and are associated with fewer adverse effects. **BPO can be used as monotherapy** for comedonal acne **or in combination** with a topical retinoid or topical antibiotic for mild-to-moderate inflammatory acne.
         a. **Adverse reactions** that develop in the first few weeks of therapy include contact dermatitis (1%–2%), erythema, peeling, and dryness; these diminish with continued use. To reduce these reactions, but still maximize the benefits of the medication, the frequency of administration or the concentration of the formulation should be altered. BPO may also cause bleaching of clothing and bed linens.
      2. **Retinoids** work as effective comedolytics and also have anti-inflammatory effects. (SOR **Ⓐ**) These agents are indicated for comedonal acne and mild-to-moderate inflammatory acne.
         a. **Common adverse reactions** include erythema, scaling, dryness, pruritus, and burning. Patients should be warned of the potential exacerbation of acne within the first few weeks of therapy. Patients should be counseled to avoid prolonged exposure to the sun (this may accentuate skin irritation), wear effective sunscreen daily (sun protection factor ≥15), and start with no more than a pea-sized amount per application.
         b. The following retinoids are available:
            (1) **Tretinoin** (SOR **Ⓐ**) is to be applied nightly. It is commercially available as Retin-A cream (0.025%, 0.05%, or 0.1%), Retin-A gel (0.01% or 0.025%), and Retin-A Micro gel (0.04% or 0.1%). Although the gel is more potent than the cream, it is also more likely to be irritating to the skin, particularly at

higher concentrations. For patients with sensitive or fair skin, therapy should be initiated with 0.025% cream every other day, and then titrated up as needed. The newer delivery system (Retin-A Micro) is less irritating to the skin than the older formulations. This delivery system entraps the drug in microspheres that bring the medication directly to the follicle and serve as reservoirs for the medication. Tretinoin is a **pregnancy category C** medication.

    (2) Adapalene (SOR **A**) is available as Differin gel or cream (0.1%) and although it causes less skin irritation than the other topical retinoids, patients still need to be counseled on these adverse reactions. It is applied as a thin film to the face and other affected areas every evening. Adapalene is a **pregnancy category C** medication.

    (3) Tazarotene (SOR **B**) should be considered as a second-line topical retinoid, after tretinoin and adapalene; tazarotene is more irritating than other retinoids and may be difficult for patients to tolerate when used daily. It is available as a 0.1% gel (Tazorac) or cream (Avage or Tazorac). A thin film should be applied every evening to the affected areas. Tazarotene is a **pregnancy category X** medication.

3. Combined BPO and tretinoin therapy can be tried in patients who continue to form comedones despite monotherapy with either agent alone. (SOR **C**) BPO is generally applied in the morning and tretinoin in the evening. It is best to initiate therapy by using each medication on alternating days and advancing to day and night applications if the patient tolerates the therapy.

4. Azelaic acid (SOR **B**) treats acne through its bacteriostatic and keratolytic properties. It is available as a 20% cream (Azelex) and should be massaged into the skin twice daily. Azelaic acid is indicated for mild-to-moderate acne.

    a. Adverse reactions. Patients report transient cutaneous irritation and erythema (1%–5%). Azelaic acid can be beneficial for postinflammatory hyperpigmentation. Because of its potential to cause hypopigmentation, it should be used with caution in patients with darker complexions. It is often used when patients are unable to tolerate topical retinoids.

5. Exfoliating agents, such as salicylic acid and elemental sulfur, are less effective than BPO or retinoids and should only be used when patients are unable to tolerate the latter agents.

6. Topical antibiotics work by inhibiting the growth and activity of *P. acnes* and by impairing complement pathways and inhibiting neutrophil chemotaxis to suppress inflammation. They are to be applied once to twice daily. These agents are indicated for mild-and-moderate inflammatory acne; they have limited activity against noninflammatory lesions.

    a. Common adverse reactions include skin irritation and staining of clothes. Topical antibiotics should not be used as monotherapy due to concerns about the development of antibiotic resistance in *P. acnes.* (SOR **C**) When used in combination with BPO, there is synergistic antimicrobial action as well as a decreased risk of antibiotic resistance. (SOR **B**)

    b. Commonly used preparations include the following:

        (1) Clindamycin (SOR **A**) is available as a solution, lotion, or gel (Cleocin T 1%). Combination products include the gel formulation Duac, BenzaClin, or Clindoxyl (1% clindamycin and 5% BPO).

        (2) Erythromycin (SOR **A**) is available as a 2% gel (A/T/S or Emgel), solution (A/T/S or Eryderm), and ointment (Akne-mycin). Combination products include the gel formulation Benzamycin (3% erythromycin and 5% BPO).

7. Topical fixed-dose combination products (SOR **A**) containing adapalene with BPO, tretinoin with clindamycin, and BPO with antibiotics (clindamycin or erythromycin) may be useful in the management of inflammatory acne of all severities in patients aged 12 years and older. They may, in fact, be more effective than monotherapy with their individual components. All are **pregnancy category C** medications.

8. Topical Dapsone (SOR **B**) has both antimicrobial and anti-inflammatory actions; however, its effectiveness in acne is likely related mainly to its anti-inflammatory properties. It is available as a 5% gel (Aczone) that is applied to the affected area as a thin layer twice daily for up to 12 weeks. Common adverse effects include erythema, dryness, and peeling of the skin.

B. Systemic agents
  1. Systemic antibiotics are commonly prescribed agents for the treatment of inflammatory acne. Although commonly thought to be more effective that topical treatments, evidence supporting the superiority of systemic antibiotics is conflicting. When selecting a systemic antibiotic, preference should be given to antibiotics that have anaerobic coverage and anti-inflammatory properties. Typical duration of treatment is 3 to 4 months. After 4 months of continuous treatment, antimicrobial resistance is more likely to develop in *P. acnes*. This organism is developing increasing resistance to erythromycin, therefore making it a second-line agent after tetracycline or doxycycline. As shown in Table 66–1, systemic antibiotics can be used with topical retinoids and BPO. BPO, when used with antibiotics, reduces the risk for antimicrobial resistance. It has been suggested that if antibiotics must be used for longer than 2 months, BPO should be used for at least 5 to 7 days between antibiotic courses. (Williams HC, 2012) There is no indication for use of systemic antibiotics with topical antibiotics.
    a. Adverse effects for the systemic antibiotics consist primarily of gastrointestinal upset and vaginal candidiasis. Gram-negative folliculitis may occur as a superinfection in 1% to 4% of patients on long-term antibiotic therapy.
    b. The antibiotics most commonly prescribed for acne are **tetracycline, doxycycline,** and **erythromycin,** although others can be used.
      (1) Tetracycline (SOR Ⓐ) is administered as 250 to 500 mg twice daily. Tetracycline is **contraindicated** in pregnant women **(pregnancy category D)** and in children younger than 9 years because it may stain developing teeth. Tetracycline should be taken on an empty stomach and at least 1 to 2 hours before or 4 hours after antacids or dairy products to avoid chelation of tetracycline.
      (2) Doxycycline (SOR Ⓑ) is administered as 100 mg twice daily. Doxycycline has greater lipid solubility and better penetration into sebaceous follicles than tetracycline. The major limitation of doxycycline is increased photosensitivity. Doxycycline should not be used in children younger than 9 years and, because it is a **pregnancy category D** agent, it should not be used during pregnancy.
      (3) Erythromycin (SOR Ⓑ) is to be administered as 1 to 2 g divided two to four times daily. This is usually used for patients who cannot tolerate tetracyclines. Adherence to the regimen can be an issue for patients taking oral erythromycin because of gastrointestinal adverse effects.
      (4) Other antibiotics to consider include azithromycin, trimethoprim-sulfamethoxazole, and minocycline. The use of minocycline is controversial, because it is not superior to other therapies and poses significant risk for adverse effects including vestibular toxicity, pneumonitis, dose-related hepatotoxicity, autoimmune hepatitis, a lupus-like autoimmune syndrome, serum sickness reactions, and irreversible hyperpigmentation of the skin.
  2. Oral contraceptives (OCs) can effectively block or reduce androgens in women leading to significant reduction in lesion development. OCs that combine ethinyl estradiol with a progestin of low androgenicity (norgestimate or desogestrel) are the best choices. (SOR Ⓐ) OCs containing drospirenone (Yaz, Yasmin), which is structurally similar to spironolactone, can also be used. (SOR Ⓒ) Three OCs are FDA-approved for the treatment of acne: Ortho Tri-Cyclen (norgestimate), Estrostep (norethindrone with variable doses of ethinyl estradiol), and Yaz (drospirenone). Many other OCs have been studied and shown to be useful for treating acne; these include Alesse®, Yasmin®, Nordette®, Levlen®, and Ortho-Cept®. OCs work best to treat acne when used in combination with other agents, either topically or systemically.
  3. Oral isotretinoin (Accutane) is used for severe acne. (SOR Ⓐ) Mechanistically, it targets all pathophysiologic aspects of the disease. The prescribing of this medication is **highly regulated** by the FDA-managed iPledge Program (see below for program description). Only physicians, usually dermatologists, registered with the program may prescribe isotretinoin. The iPledge program also requires that individual pharmacies are registered in order to dispense the medication. The daily recommended weight-based dose of 0.5 to 1 mg/kg divided twice daily should be administered with food and a full glass of water. Doses of 2 mg/kg may be used in adult patients with severe disease. Initial treatment duration is usually 4 to 5 months.
    a. Adverse reactions to isotretinoin are frequent. Mucocutaneous side effects, which include cheilitis, conjunctivitis, dry mucous membranes of the nose and

mouth, xerosis, and photosensitivity, are the most common and can generally be managed by the use of topical emollients, artificial tears, or dose reduction. Other side effects include arthralgias and myalgias as well as central nervous system side effects such as headache, nyctalopia (also called night blindness— difficulty seeing in low light), and pseudotumor cerebri. Laboratory changes associated with isotretinoin include hypertriglyceridemia, elevated total cholesterol, and reduced high-density lipoprotein levels, as well as abnormalities in liver function tests and hematologic parameters. Causative associations between isotretinoin and inflammatory bowel disease and between isotretinoin and depressive symptoms have been suggested, but have not been supported by available evidence.

  (1) Isotretinoin is a teratogen, resulting in a 25-fold increase in major fetal malformations including hydrocephalus, microcephalus, external ear abnormalities, facial dysmorphia, and cardiovascular abnormalities. All female patients must be educated about risk. The iPledge program requires that female patients use two different forms of contraception while taking isotretinoin.

b. Management and monitoring. Side effects often necessitate dose reduction. Repeat courses may be necessary and can be initiated after a period of at least 2 months off therapy. If a second course of therapy is needed, it should not be initiated until at least 8 weeks after completion of the first course, because experience has shown that patients may continue to improve while off Accutane. **Laboratory tests** include a monthly lipid panel, liver function tests (all patients), and pregnancy test (female patients).

c. iPledge program (www.ipledgeprogram.com) was mandated by the FDA in 2006 for the safe prescribing, dispensing, and consumption of the medication, in particular to prevent pregnancies among females taking the medication. All parties involved, including physician, pharmacist, and patient, have monthly responsibilities in an effort to minimize adverse events. Key iPledge points include the following items:

  (1) In order to prescribe the medication, physicians must be registered with the program.

  (2) All patients, females and males, must also be registered and must sign an informed consent.

  (3) Isotretinoin cannot be prescribed for greater than a 30-day supply at any one time.

  (4) Females who can become pregnant must use two forms of acceptable, effective contraception for at least 1 month before, during, and 1 month after stopping treatment. Not all forms of contraception are acceptable for the iPledge program, and not all forms of contraception can be used together.

  (5) Urine or blood pregnancy tests are required 1 month before, during, and 1 month after treatment.

  (6) Prior to an isotretinoin prescription being dispensed by a pharmacy, patients must log onto the iPledge website monthly to answer comprehension questions and physicians must document, on same website, contraception methods being used and negative pregnancy test. Only when those responsibilities are fulfilled, can a pharmacist dispense the medication.

  (7) The patient has only a 7-day window, from the time of negative pregnancy test, to have prescription filled. If prescription is not filled in that amount of time, another pregnancy test must be done.

4. Spironolactone is an antiandrogen agent whose role in acne is generally limited to selected females with treatment-resistant acne. It is less commonly used in male patients because of potential feminization with long-term therapy. It is administered at a dose of 50 to 100 mg a day in two or three divided doses.

  a. Adverse effects. Menstrual irregularities are the most common side effects associated with its use. Less common adverse effects include breast tenderness, breast enlargement, reduced libido, and hyperkalemia.

C. Intralesional corticosteroid injection is considered adjunctive therapy in the treatment of nodulocystic acne lesions. Its use will produce a rapid reduction in inflammation and reduces the likelihood of scarring. Diluted **triamcinolone acetonide** (0.63–2.5 mg/mL) is most commonly used and may be repeated in 3 weeks if necessary. The use of a dilute solution reduces the risk of steroid-induced skin changes such as atrophy, telangiectasia, and pigment changes.

    D. Comedo extraction. Both open and closed comedones can be extracted manually by applying gentle pressure with a comedo extractor or with the opening of an eyedropper. Prior to extraction, the pore may be enlarged with a 25-gauge needle.

IV. Patient Education. The key to successful management of acne is patient education and compliance. Follow-up visits should be routinely scheduled at regular intervals. Important patient education points include the following items:

    A. Acne is not a disease of **hygiene**.

    B. Patients should **wash** their face twice daily with mild soap and water, **avoiding harsh scrubbing**. Patients should not use alcohol-based astringents that can dry and irritate the skin. Picking at lesions may cause more inflammation.

    C. Patients should be instructed to use **oil-free, noncomedogenic cosmetics and lotions**. Oil from hair products and suntan lotions can also exacerbate acne.

    D. Acne has no relationship to **diet**.

    E. It is thought that acne causes **stress,** not vice versa.

    F. Female patients should be told that acne usually worsens during the week before menses.

    G. Improvement in appearance may not happen for 3 to 6 weeks; maximum effects may require at least 8 to 12 weeks of therapy.

ACNE ROSACEA

  I. Definition. Acne rosacea is an inflammatory condition that affects the face and eyes occurring primarily in adults.

  II. Common Diagnoses. Acne rosacea is common, especially in fair-skinned people of Celtic and northern European heritage. In a general practice database study from the United Kingdom, 60,042 rosacea cases were identified for an overall incidence rate for diagnosed rosacea of 1.65 per 1000 person-years. Prevalence rates in Europe and the United States vary greatly from less than 1% to more than 20% of the adult population. In a study of 1000 randomly selected Irish individuals, the prevalence of papulopustular rosacea was 2.7%. Women are more often affected than men, although men are more prone to the extreme forms of hyperplasia, which causes rhinophymatous rosacea.

    A. Pathophysiology of rosacea involves nonspecific inflammation followed by dilation around follicles and hyper-reactive capillaries which develop into telangiectasias. Diffuse hypertrophy of the connective tissue and sebaceous glands can follow, leading to significant disfigurement, especially of the nose.

    B. There are four stages or subtypes:

        1. Erythematotelangiectatic rosacea, the mildest form, is characterized by persistent central facial erythema with frequent flushing (Figure 66–4).

        2. Papulopustular rosacea is a highly vascular stage (Figure 66–5). There are longer periods of flushing, lasting from days to weeks, and telangiectasias, papules, and pustules form.

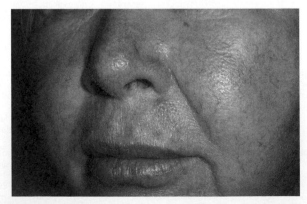

FIGURE 66–4. Erythematotelangiectatic subtype of rosacea in a middle-aged Hispanic woman (see color insert). (Used with permission of Richard P. Usatine, MD.)

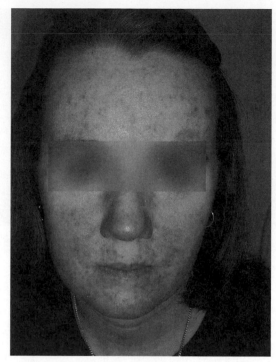

FIGURE 66–5. Rosacea in a 34-year-old woman showing erythema, papules, and pustules covering much of the face. Note her fair skin from her northern European heritage; the patient also has blue eyes (see color insert). (Used with permission of Richard P. Usatine, MD.)

    3. Phymatous or rhinophymatous rosacea is characterized by hyperplasia of the sebaceous glands. Thickened confluent plaques occur that can cause disfigurement of the nose (rhinophyma; Figure 66–6), forehead, eyelids, and chin.

    4. Ocular rosacea is the most advanced subtype characterized by severe flushing and persistent telangiectasias, papules, and pustules. Eye complaints are prominent. Corneal involvement leads to punctate erosions, infiltrates, and neovascularization that can cause blindness.

  C. Risk factors include genetic predisposition, the hair follicle mite *Demodex* infestation, and sun exposure. Alcohol can accentuate the erythema, but does not cause rosacea. Other precipitating factors are listed in Section VI.

III. Symptoms and Signs. Patients with **acne rosacea typically have** erythema, telangiectasias, papules, and pustules on the face, especially on the cheeks and nose. Erythema may also be seen on the eyelids or around the eyes. Flushing of varying severity occurs. Patients with ocular involvement may complain of watery eyes, a foreign-body sensation, burning, or dryness. Visual changes can occur including blindness. Some patients develop recurrent hordeola (stye—infection of the glands of the eyelid) and chalazia (blocked meibomian glands with lipogranulomatous reaction if ruptured).

IV. Diagnosis. The diagnosis of acne rosacea is clinical. If the diagnosis is uncertain, a punch biopsy can be obtained to differentiate acne rosacea from facial involvement of systemic lupus erythematosus, discoid lupus, or sarcoidosis.

V. Treatment

  A. For mild forms of acne rosacea, topical metronidazole (0.75% or 1% cream, gel, or lotion once daily) or topical azelaic acid (15% or 20% once or twice daily) are equally effective, but metronidazole is better tolerated. (SOR **B**) Permethrin 5% cream, active against the *Demodex* mite, was as effective as metronidazole 0.75% gel and superior to placebo in one study. (SOR **B**) Topical sodium sulfacetamide with sulfur and benzoyl peroxide were

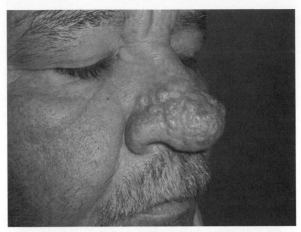

FIGURE 66–6. Rhinophymatous rosacea with hypertrophy of the skin of the nose of a 51-year-old Hispanic man. The patient acknowledges previous heavy alcohol intake. (see color insert) (Used with permission of Richard P. Usatine, MD.)

effective in single small trials. (SOR **B**) Topical brimonidine tartrate, a selective alpha-2 adrenergic receptor agonist, applied as a once-daily 0.5% gel, was significantly more efficacious than vehicle gel in treating severe facial erythema of rosacea in two trials.

   B. For more extensive involvement, oral doxycycline (40 mg daily), tetracycline, and metronidazole are effective. (SOR **A**) There is insufficient evidence about which preparation is best or whether these are more effective than topical agents. Doxycycline appears to be the most often used agent, and there does not appear to be additional benefit from higher doses (100 mg). Severe papulopustular disease refractory to antibiotics and topical treatments can be treated with oral isotretinoin (0.3 mg/kg/d). (SOR **B**)

      1. Electrosurgery, pulsed-light, and laser therapy can be used to treat the erythema and telangiectasias associated with rosacea. (SOR **C**)

      2. Rhinophyma can be treated with isotretinoin, electrosurgery, or laser. (SOR **B**)

   C. For patients with ocular involvement, cyclosporine ophthalmic emulsion is significantly more effective than artificial tears. (SOR **A**) In mild cases, oral tetracycline, lid hygiene, and warm compresses may be sufficient. (SOR **C**) **Referral to an ophthalmologist** should occur if ocular rosacea involves the cornea.

VI. Patient Education. Patients with acne rosacea should use sun protection, including use of a hat and daily sunscreen against UVA and UVB rays. (SOR **C**) Identification and avoidance of precipitating factors such as skin irritants, hot and humid weather, alcohol, hot beverages, spicy foods, and large hot meals may also be helpful. The National Rosacea Society also has excellent materials for physicians and patients (http://www.rosacea.org/).

SELECTED REFERENCES

Archer CB, Cohen SN, Baron SE. Guidance on the diagnosis and clinical management of acne. *Clin Dermatol.* 2012;37(Suppl 1):1–6.

Cunliffe WJ, Meynadier J, Alirezai M, et al. Is combined oral and topical therapy better than oral therapy alone in patients with moderate to moderately severe acne vulgaris? A comparison of the efficacy and safety of lymecycline plus adapalene gel 0.1%, versus lymecycline plus gel vehicle. *J Am Acad Dermatol.* 2003;49(Suppl):S218–S226.

Eichenfield LF, Krakowski AC, Piggott C, et al. Evidence-based recommendations for the diagnosis and treatment of pediatric acne. *Pediatrics.* 2013;131:S163–S186.

Feldman A, Careccia RE, Barham KL, et al. Diagnosis and treatment of acne. *Am Fam Physician.* 2004;69:2123–2130.

Fowler J Jr, Jackson M, Moore A, et al. Efficacy and safety of once-daily topical brimonidine tartrate gel 0.5% for the treatment of moderate to severe facial erythema of rosacea: results of two randomized, double-blind, and vehicle-controlled pivotal studies. *J Drugs Dermatol.* 2013;12(6):650–656.

Gamble R, Dunn J, Dawson A, et al. Topical antimicrobial treatment of acne vulgaris: an evidence-based review. *Am J Clin Dermatol.* 2012;13(3):141–152.

Gollnick H, Blume-Peytavi U, Szabo EL, et al. Systemic isotretinoin in the treatment of rosacea—doxycycline- and placebo-controlled, randomized clinical study. *J Dtsch Dermatol Ges*. 2010;8:505–515.

James WD. Acne. *N Engl J Med*. 2005;352:1463–1472.

Liao DC. Management of acne. *J Fam Pract*. 2003;52:43–51.

May D, Kelsberg G, Safranek S. Clinical inquiries: what is the most effective treatment for acne rosacea? *J Fam Pract*. 2011;60(2):108a–108c.

McAleer MA, Fitzpatrick P, Powell FC. Papulopustular rosacea: prevalence and relationship to photo-damage. *J Am Acad Dermatol*. 2010;63(1):33–39.

Nast A, Bettoli V, Degitz K, et al. European evidence-based (S3) guidelines for treatment of acne. *J Eur Acad Dermatol Venereol*. 2012;26(Suppl 1):1–29.

Purdy A, de Berker D. Acne vulgaris. Clinical evidence. *Clin Evid (Online)*. 2011;pii:1714.

Russell JJ. Topical therapy for acne. *Am Fam Physician*. 2000;61:357–366.

Spoendlin J, Voegel JJ, Jick SS, Meier CR. A study on the epidemiology of rosacea in the U.K. *Br J Dermatol*. 2012;167(3):598–605.

Usatine RP. Rosacea. In: *Color Atlas of Family Medicine*. 2nd ed. New York, NY: McGraw-Hill Companies, Inc.; 2013;113:659–664.

van Zuuren EJ, Kramer S, Carter B, et al. Interventions for rosacea. *Cochrane Database Syst Rev*. 2011;(3):CD003262.

Williams HC, Dellavalle RP. Acne vulgaris. *Lancet*. 2012;379:361–372.

---

67   Human Immunodeficiency Virus and Acquired Immunodeficiency Syndrome

Parya Saberi, PharmD, MAS, Megan Mahoney, MD, & Ronald H. Goldschmidt, MD

KEY POINTS

- Assess risk for human immunodeficiency virus (HIV) and sexually transmitted infections in all patients and perform HIV screening in all patients using the "opt-out" method. The U.S. Preventive Services Task Force (USPSTF) has recommended that routine HIV testing be provided to all adolescents and adults between the ages of 15 and 65 years. (SOR **A**)
- Acute HIV syndrome can be difficult to identify because of its nonspecific nature. Quantitative plasma HIV RNA testing should be considered in patients with viral syndromes, especially those presenting with fever, maculopapular rash, sore throat, lymphadenopathy, oral and genital ulcers, arthralgias, or myalgias. (SOR **C**)
- Antiretroviral therapy (ART) is recommended for all HIV-infected individuals to decrease the risk of disease progression and to decrease or prevent transmission of HIV. (SOR **A**) Individuals starting ART should be willing and able to commit to treatment, understand the benefits versus risks of therapy, and recognize the importance of treatment adherence.
- Optimize adherence by assessing patient's readiness and understanding of their regimen, identifying barriers to adherence, reducing overall pill burden by using fixed dose combination products, offering once-daily regimens that have low potential for adverse effects, incorporating the regimen into patient's daily schedule, and using a multidisciplinary HIV team approach. (SOR **B**)
- Antiretroviral failure can be the result of nonadherence to treatment or virologic resistance. Resistance testing should be conducted to guide treatment. (SOR **A**)
- Biomedical interventions, such as post-exposure prophylaxis, pre-exposure prophylaxis, and HIV treatment as prevention, can be used to minimize the risk of HIV transmission. (SOR **A**)

I. Introduction

A. Definition. HIV disease is a chronic, progressive disease caused by a retrovirus, the human immunodeficiency virus.

    1. Acute syndrome. This syndrome, which usually occurs approximately 2 to 4 weeks following HIV infection, is difficult to identify because of its nonspecific nature. The symptoms and signs are similar to those of many viral syndromes and can include fever, maculopapular rash, sore throat, lymphadenopathy, oral and genital ulcers, headache, malaise, arthralgias, and myalgias. Oral ulcers in the setting of acute viral symptoms and compatible risk factors for HIV infection are considered pathognomonic pending laboratory confirmation. Abdominal cramps, diarrhea, aseptic meningitis, encephalopathy, and neuropathies can occur rarely. The acute HIV syndrome usually resolves spontaneously within 1 to 2 weeks.

2. **Asymptomatic HIV infection.** After acquisition of HIV, an asymptomatic phase lasting 10 years or longer in some cases can occur. Although infection persists and the virus continues to proliferate, the immunologic system remains relatively intact.

3. **Symptomatic HIV infection.** Conditions such as oral candidiasis (thrush), oral hairy leukoplakia, generalized lymphadenopathy, and thrombocytopenia generally precede the development of clinical acquired immunodeficiency syndrome (AIDS). These conditions can also occur in persons who are not infected with HIV; however, laboratory confirmation is necessary for diagnosis.

4. **Clinical AIDS.** AIDS is the advanced stage of HIV disease and is defined in persons infected with HIV by characteristic opportunistic infections (OIs) (e.g., pneumocystis pneumonia [PCP]), specific cancers (e.g., Kaposi sarcoma [KS]), HIV-related encephalopathy, HIV-related wasting syndrome, or a CD4+ cell count less than 200 cells/mm^3 or less than 14% of all lymphocytes.

5. **HIV/AIDS in children.** Additional illnesses that are AIDS-defining in children but not in adults include multiple, recurrent bacterial infections and lymphoid interstitial pneumonia/pulmonary lymphoid hyperplasia. Consultation with pediatric AIDS specialists is generally necessary to guide therapy. (SOR **❸**)

B. **Epidemiology**

1. **Prevalence.** At the end of 2009, approximately 1,148,200 persons in the United States were living with HIV, including 207,600 persons whose infections had not been diagnosed. Children account for 7% of the people in the United States living with HIV. Because of extensive testing and treatment, fewer than 200 new vertical transmissions have occurred annually since 2000.

2. **Transmission.** Transmission of HIV requires the exchange of infectious body fluids including blood, semen, and vaginal secretions. HIV is not spread by casual contact.

3. The average period between initial infection and development of clinical AIDS has been estimated to be approximately 8 to 11 years.

4. Prior to the use of effective combined antiretroviral therapy (ART), the average length of survival was 15 years or less. In the era of effective ART, OIs and other complications of AIDS have declined and the average length of survival has increased dramatically.

5. **Risk factors.** The seven risk factors, defined by the Centers for Disease Control and Prevention (CDC), are male-to-male sexual contact, injection drug use, male-to-male sexual contact and injection drug use, heterosexual (male-to-female) contact, mother-to-child (perinatal) transmission, occupational exposures, and blood transfusions.

II. **Screening and Prevention**

A. **Risk-based screening.** Inquire about sexual practices and injection drug use at initial patient evaluation and periodically afterward.

B. **Routine screening.** Because a substantial number of patients do not admit to or do not appreciate their risk factors, the United States Public Health Service recommends routine testing of all persons between the ages of 15 and 64 years at least one time, regardless of risk factors. The U.S. Preventive Services Task Force (USPSTF) recommends that routine HIV testing be provided to all adolescents and adults between the ages of 15 and 65 years. (SOR **❹**) The preferred method for routine screening is by the "opt-out" method. This testing modality informs the patient that an HIV test will be ordered as part of routine care unless the patient specifically indicates he/she does not want to be tested for HIV (i.e., "opts out"). It is recommended that all pregnant women be screened for HIV along with their routine panel of prenatal screening tests unless they opt-out.

C. **Primary prevention education.** Risk assessment of sexual and drug use activities should be explored. General sexually transmitted infection and HIV prevention messages are important for both diagnosis and prevention of HIV and other sexually transmitted infections. Condom use and other prevention measures should be discussed (see Chapter 102).

D. **Prevention with HIV-positive individuals** should be provided with education on ways of preventing transmission; these patients should be screened annually for behaviors associated with HIV transmission. Some educational points include consistent condom use and attaining a viral load below the limit of assay detection (i.e., undetectable) using ART.

E. Biomedical Prevention

1. **Post-exposure prophylaxis (PEP)** should be given as soon as possible after high-risk exposure. Combination antiretroviral drugs are given for 28 days. HIV testing before and after exposure is essential. For advice, call the PEPline at 888-448-4911 or go to www.nccc.ucsf.edu.

2. **Pre-exposure prophylaxis (PrEP)** is treating HIV-uninfected persons with antiretroviral medications to prevent them from becoming infected from their HIV-positive partners. The target for this intervention is HIV-uninfected persons who continue to engage in high-risk sexual activities. Daily PrEP medications, tenofovir/emtricitabine (Truvada®) must be taken continuously. PrEP should be given in concert with risk reduction counseling and careful follow-up and monitoring for adverse effects, such as nephrotoxicity. For patients taking PrEP, adherence needs to be reassessed continuously as poor PrEP adherence can lead to HIV transmission and possible development of drug resistance. The most important decision point for the primary care clinician is patient selection. Reversion to unsafe sexual practices because of reliance on PrEP (risk compensation) has not been noted to a substantial degree. The cost of PrEP is estimated from $11,740 to $17,939 annually, including drug, laboratory and clinician visit time. Draft MMWR guidelines summarize current PrEP recommendations.

3. **Treatment as prevention** is the term used to describe the prevention benefit of ART. When ART effectively decreases viral load to undetectable or very low levels, the chances that those persons transmit HIV to their partners becomes quite low. (SOR **Ⓐ**) Therefore, effective ART not only decreases progression of HIV but also results in fewer transmissions to others.

III. Diagnosis

A. **Signs and symptoms.** Early stages of HIV can be similar to diseases of specific organ systems or nonspecific illnesses such as influenza. AIDS, with the combination of wasting syndrome, OIs, and cancers, is rarely confused with other diseases. However, many complications of HIV have presentations that are similar to other disorders; so risk assessment, counseling, and confirmation with HIV testing should be considered.

1. **Signs and symptoms.** Nonspecific symptoms such as weakness, anorexia, fever, and weight loss can be caused by HIV infection itself or OIs and cancers. Such symptoms can also be caused by bacterial or fungal sepsis, *Mycobacterium avium*–intracellulare complex (MAC) disease, or tuberculosis. Cultures can help determine the cause of significant fevers and weight loss.

2. **Common OIs and cancers.**

   a. **Skin conditions.**

      (1) KS of the skin or oral mucosa appears as red to purple lesions, usually ≥0.5 cm in diameter (Figure 67–1).

      (2) Maculopapular rashes are exceedingly common and are often associated with acute HIV infection or with drug allergy to either prescription or nonprescription drugs.

   b. **Eye diseases.** Yellow-white or hemorrhagic patches on the retina can indicate sight-threatening cytomegalovirus (CMV) retinitis.

   c. **Oral cavity.**

      (1) White plaques or erosive (erythematous) areas in the oropharynx suggest oral candidiasis (Figure 67–2). Thrush is common in acute HIV and symptomatic HIV infection and is seen almost universally in clinical AIDS.

      (2) Painless, white, somewhat hair-like lesions on the lateral borders of the tongue indicate hairy leukoplakia (Figure 67–3). This painless condition, which is caused by the Epstein–Barr virus, will disappear and can recur. Treatment is not required.

   d. **Lymph nodes** are frequently enlarged, usually reflecting a generalized response to HIV infection. Hard, asymmetric, or extremely prominent nodes require biopsy to exclude fungal infection or cancer.

   e. **Pulmonary** involvement is the most common condition in patients with AIDS.

      (1) PCP is the most common pulmonary disease in patients with AIDS. *Pneumocystis carinii* now refers only to the pneumocystis that infects rodents, and *Pneumocystis jiroveci* refers to the distinct species that infects humans. The abbreviation PCP is still used to indicate Pneumocystis pneumonia. Acute PCP is most commonly characterized by shortness of breath, dry cough, and fever. Chest x-ray (CXR) usually shows patchy infiltrates or diffused interstitial

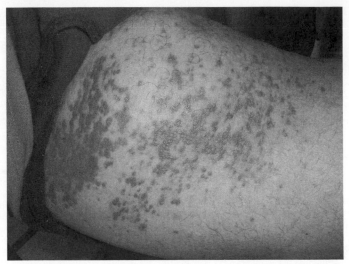

FIGURE 67–1. Kaposi sarcoma in a 43-year-old man with HIV/AIDS already on antiretroviral therapy. He presented with a diffuse rash and lymphedema in the right leg. The initial biopsy was negative, but a second biopsy demonstrated Kaposi sarcoma. The right leg is significantly larger than the left leg due to the lymphedema (see color insert). (Used with permission of Richard P. Usatine, MD.)

disease, although 5% of CXRs of patients with pulmonary disease can be normal. Thin-section, helical computerized tomography (CT) scan typically demonstrates patchy ground-glass attenuation in patients with PCP and might be useful as an adjunctive study in patients with a normal CXR.

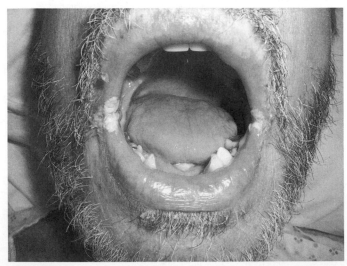

FIGURE 67–2. Thrush and perlèche in a man with AIDS. The candida infection in the corners of the mouth is called perlèche or angular cheilitis (see color insert). (Used with permission of Richard P. Usatine, MD.)

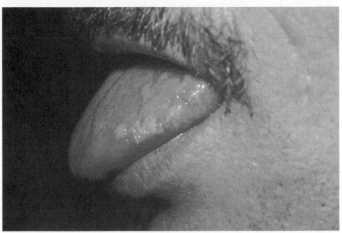

FIGURE 67–3. Oral hairy leukoplakia caused by Epstein–Barr virus on the tongue of a man with AIDS (see color insert). (Used with permission of Richard P. Usatine, MD.)

(2) Bacterial pneumonias, fungal mycobacterial infections, and KS are also important causes of pulmonary diseases.

(3) Evaluation of pulmonary disease generally requires examination of induced sputum, bronchial washings, and/or biopsies. Careful microscopic examination and cultures for *P. jiroveci, Mycobacterium tuberculosis*, bacteria, and fungi are essential.

f. Gastrointestinal conditions

(1) Esophagitis. Dysphagia, odynophagia, and substernal burning pain are symptomatic of esophagitis. Esophagitis can be caused by *Candida albicans*, CMV, or herpes simplex virus. When an empiric trial of antifungal medications for candidiasis fails, endoscopy with biopsies and cultures is essential to establish a diagnosis and direct treatment.

(2) Diarrhea is the most common gastrointestinal symptom in patients with HIV and can be caused by *Microsporidium, Cryptosporidium*, MAC, *Salmonella, Shigella*, CMV colitis, and other enteric pathogens. Diarrhea from HIV infection alone can occur and requires symptomatic treatment. Diarrhea can also be a complication of HIV medications. Among persons with profuse diarrheal illness, a single-stool specimen is usually adequate for diagnosis. Among persons with less severe disease, repeat stool sampling is recommended. Referral for a sigmoidoscopy or colonoscopy might be necessary in severe cases when stool cultures are repeatedly negative.

(3) Liver disease. Hepatomegaly, jaundice, and abnormal liver function tests indicate hepatobiliary disease. Increased alkaline phosphatase levels commonly indicate liver infection by MAC or *M. tuberculosis*. Other causes of liver disease include Bartonella, fungal infection, KS, or lymphoma. Acute and chronic viral hepatitis, drug-induced hepatitis, and HIV cholangiopathy can also occur. Ultrasound examination and CT scan are generally helpful. Biopsy, although rarely helpful, can be considered in cases in which *M. tuberculosis* infections or other treatable conditions might be present.

g. Genitourinary disease. Although vaginal candidiasis occurs more commonly and more extensively in HIV-infected women, these finding do not constitute an AIDS diagnosis. Cervical dysplasia and malignancy are more frequent and more rapidly progressive, leading to recommendations for more frequent Pap testing.

h. Neurologic problems

(1) Peripheral neuropathies can result in painful dysesthesias of the feet and legs. Presumably, HIV involvement of neural tissue causes this condition.

(2) AIDS dementia complex is characterized by behavioral changes, deficits in cognitive function, and lack of coordination. Although HIV appears to be the principal cause, other pathogenic conditions (e.g., CMV encephalitis or encephalitic toxoplasmosis) must be excluded.

(3) Meningoencephalitis, most often caused by *Cryptococcus neoformans* infection, is characterized by headache (usually slight, although at times severe), fever, and decreased mental functioning. Neck pain and nuchal rigidity can be present. Examination of cryptococcal antigen determination in serum and cerebrospinal fluid (with a baseline measurement of the opening pressure) is useful for the diagnosis of *Cryptococcus neoformans* infection.

(4) Mass lesions in the central nervous system can result in encephalopathic symptoms, seizures, or focal neurologic deficits. These lesions can be caused by *Toxoplasma gondii* infection, lymphomas, and, rarely, other OIs.

C. Laboratory tests

1. Testing for HIV. A reactive antibody test plus a positive confirmatory test is indicative of HIV infection. Generally, these tests become positive within 1 month of infection; almost all infected persons display positive HIV tests within 3 to 6 months of infection. Quantitative plasma HIV RNA testing is recommended to diagnose acute HIV syndrome.

2. Indicators of progression of HIV disease

   a. A person with AIDS usually has a CD4+ cell count of $\leq$200 cells/mm^3.

   b. Quantitative plasma HIV RNA (viral load) testing is used for staging and monitoring response to therapy. Current tests can now detect viral particles down to 20 to 50 copies per mm^3.

3. Initial laboratory evaluation of the newly diagnosed patient includes, in addition to confirmation of the HIV antibody test and baseline CD4+ cell count and HIV viral load, a complete blood count, chemistry profile, transaminase levels, BUN and creatinine, urinalysis, syphilis testing, tuberculosis screening, *Toxoplasma gondii* IgG, hepatitis A, B, and C serologies, Pap smear in women, fasting blood glucose and lipid panel, and genotype resistance test. Screening for glucose-6-phosphate dehydrogenase deficiency in persons of African, Mediterranean, Indian, or Southeast Asian descent is recommended. (SOR **A**)

4. Drug resistance testing is recommended in the patient with acute HIV and before initiating therapy for guiding therapy. (SOR **A**) Expert consultation is generally recommended to help interpret the results.

5. Follow-up testing. Generally, patients should follow-up with their primary care provider every 3 to 6 months for monitoring of disease progression and drug toxicity. (SOR **C**)

IV. Treatment. ART for treatment of HIV is complex and rapidly changing. The U.S. Department of Health and Human Services (DHHS) guidelines (http://aidsinfo.nih.gov/guidelines) and the International Antiviral Society-USA (IAS-USA) guidelines (https://www.iasusa.org) are updated regularly and serve as important sources of comprehensive guidance for HIV treatment. Starting or changing ART regimens can have personal and public health implications that affect the efficacy of future therapy; therefore, before prescribing ART, consultation with an HIV expert is recommended.

A. ART strategies

1. Initiating ART. ART is recommended for all HIV-infected individuals to decrease the risk of disease progression (pretreatment CD4+ cell count <350 cells/mm^3 [SOR **A**]; for CD4+ cell count = 350–500 cells/mm^3 [SOR **A**]; for CD4+ cell count>500 cells/mm^3 [SOR **B**]). ART is recommended for all patients to decrease or prevent transmission of HIV. (SOR **A**)

   a. Individuals starting ART should be willing and able to commit to treatment, understand the benefits versus risks of therapy, and recognize the importance of treatment adherence. Therapy may be postponed on a case-by-case basis depending on clinical and/or psychosocial factors.

   b. Initiating ART can induce an **immune reconstitution inflammatory syndrome** (IRIS). The manifestations of this syndrome are generally the activation of quiescent OIs. For some OIs, where immediate ART may increase risk of IRIS (e.g., cryptococcal meningitis or nontuberculous mycobacterial infection), a short delay before ART initiation may be warranted (SOR **C**); however, for other OIs (e.g., PCP), early ART initiation is associated with increased survival. (SOR **A**)

TABLE 67–1. ANTIRETROVIRAL MEDICATIONS

Drug[a,b]	Adult Dose (Oral)	Major Adverse Effects	Contraindications	Drug Interactions
Nucleoside/nucleotide Reverse Transcriptase Inhibitors (NRTIs/NtRTIs)				
Abacavir[a,b] (ABC, Ziagen)	300 mg twice daily **or** 600 mg daily	Hypersensitivity reaction (fever, rash, GI adverse effects, respiratory symptoms)[c]	HLA-b5701 positive	No major drug–drug interactions
Didanosine[a,b] (ddI, Videx, Videx EC)	<60 kg: 250 mg daily ≥60 kg: 400 mg daily	Nausea, vomiting, lactic acidosis, pancreatitis, steatosis, lipodystrophy, peripheral neuropathy	Coadministration with ribavirin and allopurinol	No major drug–drug interactions
Emtricitabine[b,d] (FTC, Emtriva)	200 mg daily	Headache, nausea, skin discoloration, diarrhea, rash	—	No major drug–drug interactions
Lamivudine[a,b,e] (3TC, Epivir)	150 mg twice daily **or** 300 mg daily	Headache, nausea	—	No major drug–drug interactions
Stavudine[a,b] (d4 T, Zerit)	<60 kg: 30 mg twice daily ≥60 kg: 40 mg twice daily	Steatosis, lactic acidosis, lipodystrophy, peripheral neuropathy	—	Should not be combined with AZT
Tenofovir[b,e] (TDF, Viread)	300 mg daily	Nephrotoxicity, loss of BMD	—	No major drug–drug interactions
Zidovudine[a,b] (AZT/ZDV, Retrovir)	300 mg twice daily	Anemia, neutropenia, nausea, vomiting, steatosis, myopathy, lipodystrophy, lactic acidosis	—	No major drug–drug interactions
Non-nucleoside Reverse Transcriptase Inhibitors (NNRTIs)				
Efavirenz[b] (EFV, Sustiva)	600 mg daily (on empty stomach, preferably at night)	Somnolence, vivid dreams, dizziness, depression, psychosis, hyperlipidemia, lipohypertrophy, rash	Coadministration with voriconazole, pregnancy category D	**Many drug–drug interactions**
Etravirine[b] (ETR, Intelence)	200 mg twice daily with meal	Rash	—	**Many drug–drug interactions**
Nevirapine[a,b] (NVP, Viramune)	200 mg daily × 2 wk; then 200 mg twice daily	Hepatotoxicity (black box warning), hypersensitivity, rash (dose escalation can reduce rash incidence)	Moderate to severe hepatic insufficiency	**Many drug–drug interactions**
Rilpivirine[d] (RPV, Edurant)	25 mg daily with meal of 500 calories or more	Rash, insomnia, depression, hepatotoxicity	Coadministration with proton pump inhibitors, carbamazepine, phenobarbital, phenytoin, rifabutin, and rifampin	**Many drug–drug interactions;** interaction with antacids and H₂ receptor antagonists

(continued)

TABLE 67–1. ANTIRETROVIRAL MEDICATIONS (Continued)

Drug[a,b]	Adult Dose (Oral)	Major Adverse Effects	Contraindications	Drug Interactions
Protease Inhibitors (PIs)				
Atazanavir[b] (ATV, Reyataz)	400 mg daily **or** 300 mg daily (+RTV 100 mg daily)	Indirect hyperbilirubinemia, rash, metabolic syndrome	Coadministration with lovastatin and simvastatin	**Many drug–drug interactions;** interaction with antacids, H_2 receptor antagonists, and proton pump inhibitors
Darunavir[b] (DRV, Prezista) (contains sulfonamide moiety)	800 mg daily (+RTV 100 mg daily) **or** 600 mg twice daily (+RTV 100 mg twice daily)	Metabolic syndrome, rash, hepatotoxicity, GI intolerance	Coadministration with lovastatin and simvastatin	**Many drug–drug interactions**
Fos-amprenavir[b] (Fos-APV, Lexiva) (contains sulfonamide moiety)	700 mg twice daily (+RTV 100 mg daily) **or** 1400 mg daily (+RTV 200 mg daily)	Metabolic syndrome, rash, GI intolerance, fat maldistribution	Coadministration with lovastatin and simvastatin	**Many drug–drug interactions**
Indinavir[f] (IDV, Crixivan)	800 mg every 8 h on empty stomach **or** 800 mg twice daily (+RTV 100–200 mg twice daily)	Metabolic syndrome, nephrolithiasis, GI intolerance, fat maldistribution	Coadministration with lovastatin and simvastatin	**Many drug–drug interactions**
Lopinavir/ritonavir[b] (LPV/RTV, Kaletra) (fixed dose combination)	Two tablets twice daily **or** four tablets daily	Metabolic syndrome, GI intolerance, transaminitis, fat maldistribution	Coadministration with lovastatin and simvastatin	**Many drug–drug interactions**
Nelfinavir[b] (NFV, Viracept)	1250 mg twice daily	Metabolic syndrome, GI intolerance, fat maldistribution	Coadministration with lovastatin and simvastatin	**Many drug–drug interactions**
Ritonavir[b] (RTV, Norvir)	100–200 mg, used only to boost other PIs	Metabolic syndrome, GI intolerance, fat maldistribution	Coadministration with lovastatin and simvastatin	**Many drug–drug interactions**
Saquinavir[b] (SQV, Invirase)	1000 mg twice daily (+RTV 100 mg twice daily)	Metabolic syndrome, GI intolerance, fat maldistribution	Severe hepatic insufficiency and coadministration with trazodone, lovastatin, and simvastatin	**Many drug–drug interactions**
Tipranavir[b] (TPV, Aptivus) (contains sulfonamide moiety)	500 mg twice daily (+RTV 200 mg twice daily)	Metabolic syndrome, GI intolerance, transaminitis, fat maldistribution, rash	Moderate to severe hepatic insufficiency and coadministration with lovastatin and simvastatin	**Many drug–drug interactions**

Drug	Dosing	Adverse Effects	Drug Interactions
Integrase Strand Transfer Inhibitors (INSTIs)			
Elvitegravir (ELV) (only available as Stribild)	150 mg twice daily (+cobicistat 150 mg twice daily)	—	—
Raltegravir[b] (RAL, Isentress)	400 mg twice daily	Increased CPK, myositis, rhabdomyolysis	No major drug–drug interactions; increase RAL dose to 800 mg PO BID with coadministered with rifampin
Fusion Inhibitors (FIs)			
Enfuvirtide[b] (ENF, Fuzeon)	90 mg **SQ** twice daily (Reconstituted doses are stable for 24 h)	Injection site reactions, rash	No major drug–drug interactions
CCR5 Coreceptor Antagonist			
Maraviroc (MVC, Selzentry) (requires CCR5 tropism test)	300 mg twice daily (150 mg twice daily when taken with potent CYP 3 A inhibitors)	Rash, hepatotoxicity	—	**Many drug–drug interactions**
Fixed Dose Combinations			
Atripla (TDF/FTC/EFV)	One tablet daily	—	**Many drug–drug interactions**
Combivir[a] (AZT/3TC)	One tablet twice daily	—	No major drug–drug interactions
Complera (TDF/FTC/RPV)	One tablet daily	—	**Many drug–drug interactions**
Epzicom (ABC/3TC)	One tablet daily	—	No major drug–drug interactions
Stribild (TDF/FTC/ELV/COBI)	One tablet daily with food	Decreased CrCl (not recommended if CrCl <70 mL/min), nausea, diarrhea	Coadministration with lovastatin and simvastatin	**Many drug–drug interactions**
Trizivir (AZT/3TC/ABC)	One tablet twice daily	—	No major drug–drug interactions
Truvada (TDF/FTC)	One tablet daily	—	No major drug–drug interactions

[a]Available as generic.
[b]Pediatric dose available.
[c]Hypersensitivity usually occurs during first 6 weeks of therapy; ABC should be discontinued and never rechallenged.
[d]Also used to treat hepatitis B.
[e]Use if viral load <100,000 copies/mL.
[f]Drink six or more glasses of water per day.
ARV, antiretroviral; BID, twice-daily; BMD, bone mineral density; CPK, creatine phosphokinase; CYP, cytochrome; GI, gastrointestinal; PO, orally; QD, once-daily; SQ, subcutaneous.

2. **Classes of antiretroviral agents.** Commonly used antiretroviral agents are summarized in Table 67–1.

    a. **Nucleoside and nucleotide reverse transcriptase inhibitors (NRTIs/ NtRTIs)** work by inhibiting HIV viral DNA synthesis. The combination of two NRTIs forms the backbone of most ART regimens. Emtricitabine is the fluorinated analog of lamivudine and can be used interchangeably with lamivudine. The fixed dose combination of tenofovir and emtricitabine is the preferred NRTI backbone. Tenofovir is associated with renal impairment. Other common adverse effects of most nucleoside agents include nausea, vomiting, lipoatrophy, lactic acidosis, and hepatic steatosis.

    b. **Non-nucleoside reverse transcriptase inhibitors (NNRTIs)** inhibit HIV viral DNA synthesis. A single NNRTI can be combined with two NRTIs to form an ART regimen. As a class, NNRTIs have long half-lives, high risk of resistance at time of treatment failure, and numerous drug–drug interactions and may result in liver function test abnormalities, hepatitis, and rash.

    c. **Protease inhibitors (PIs)** inhibit formation of HIV viral proteins. PI serum levels are often boosted by the addition of a small dose of ritonavir. A boosted PI can be combined with two NRTIs to form an ART regimen. PIs are associated with many drug–drug interactions and may cause nausea, vomiting, diarrhea, dyslipidemia, insulin resistance, hepatotoxicity, and fat accumulation.

    d. **Integrase strand transfer inhibitors (INSTIs)** inhibit the integration of viral DNA with human DNA. Raltegravir has few drug–drug interactions and can result in increased creatine kinase, myopathy, and rhabdomyolysis. Elvitegravir is boosted with cobicistat which has many drug–drug interactions.

    e. **Fusion inhibitors and entry inhibitors** are typically reserved for patients who have ART treatment failure.

3. **Constructing an ART regimen**

    a. Therapy should be initiated in consultation with an HIV clinical expert. The U.S. DHHS recently published guidelines containing four preferred (SOR **Ⓐ**) and nine alternative (SOR **Ⓑ**) regimens for ART naïve patients. Information regarding the dose of each ART agent is given in Table 67–1.

    b. Before selecting an initial regimen, the following factors should be considered: patient's comorbid conditions (e.g., renal or liver disease), potential adverse drug effects and drug–drug interactions, pregnancy, genotypic test results, HIV viral load, HLA-b*5701 results if considering ABC, coreceptor tropism result if considering MVC, patient preference and adherence potential, and convenience (pill burden, dosing frequency, fixed dose combinations, and food requirements).

    c. Preferred first-line ART regimens generally consist of two nucleoside reverse transcriptase inhibitors (NRTIs) combined with either a ritonavir-"boosted" PI, an NNRTI, or an integrase strand transfer inhibitor (INSTI). (SOR **Ⓐ**) These regimens consist of

       • PI-based regimens: [tenofovir + lamivudine/emtricitabine] + [atazanavir boosted with ritonavir or once-daily darunavir boosted with ritonavir]

       • NNRTI-based regimen: [tenofovir + lamivudine/emtricitabine] + [efavirenz]

       • INSTI-based regimen: [tenofovir + lamivudine/emtricitabine] + [raltegravir]

    d. Other alternative regimens include the use of abacavir, rilpivirine, fosamprenavir boosted with, lopinavir boosted with ritonavir, and elvitegravir boosted with cobicistat. Patients initiating abacavir-containing regimens should be screened for HLA-B5701 to assess for hypersensitivity reaction.

    e. Certain ART combinations (e.g., all NRTI mono-, dual-, triple-, or quadruple-regimens) should be avoided as initial therapy because of inferior virologic outcomes, inconvenient dosing, overlapping toxicities, or limited clinical trial experience.

4. **Preferred initial regimens**

    a. NNRTI-based regimen. The combination of efavirenz + tenofovir + emtricitabine, available in the fixed-dose combination Atripla®, is a preferred regimen. Potential side effects include rash, renal impairment, neuropsychiatric symptoms, dyslipidemia, and hepatotoxicity. Efavirenz is pregnancy category D.

    b. PI-based regimens. Atazanavir/ritonavir + tenofovir + emtricitabine OR darunavir/ritonavir (once-daily dosed) + tenofovir + emtricitabine are two PI-based preferred options. The combination of tenofovir + emtricitabine is available as Truvada®. Potential side effects from these regimens include but are not limited to renal impairment, gastrointestinal adverse effects, hepatotoxicity, and metabolic complications. Atazanavir is association with indirect hyperbilirubinemia and nephrolithiasis.

    c. INSTI-based regimen. The combination of raltegravir + tenofovir + emtricitabine is the only INSTI-based preferred option. The combination of tenofovir + emtricitabine is available as Truvada®. Raltegravir has been associated with increased creatine kinase and myopathy.

  5. Adherence. Optimal adherence to ART is necessary to achieve and maintain durable viral suppression, reduce drug resistance, increase survival, and improve quality of life. It is important to optimize adherence by assessing patient's readiness and understanding of their regimen, identifying barriers to adherence, reducing overall pill burden by using fixed-dose combination products, offering once-daily regimens that have low potential for adverse effects, incorporating the regimen into patient's daily schedule, and using a multidisciplinary HIV team approach. Tools such as pill boxes or alarms can be useful in enhancing adherence. Patients should be counseled on the importance of adherence.

  6. Discontinuation or interruption of therapy. ART discontinuation can result in increased viral load, decreased CD4+ cell count, and clinical progression. In general, planned long-term therapy interruptions are not recommended.

B. OIs and other manifestations

  1. Prophylaxis to prevent OIs is indicated when CD4+ cell count decreases to specific threshold values, as described in Table 67–2.

  2. Cryptococcal meningitis and other cryptococcal infections should be treated acutely with amphotericin B 0.7 mg/kg intravenously (IV) daily + flucytosine (5-FC) 25 mg/kg orally four times daily for at least 2 weeks for those with normal renal function. (SOR **Ⓐ**) Lipid formulation of amphotericin B 4 to 6 mg/kg IV daily + flucytosine can be considered for those with renal dysfunction. After at least 2 weeks of induction, defined as significant clinical improvement and negative cerebrospinal fluid cultures, therapy can be consolidated to fluconazole at 400 mg orally daily for 8 weeks. (SOR **Ⓐ**) Preferred maintenance therapy with fluconazole 200 mg orally daily can be continued lifelong (SOR **Ⓐ**) or discontinued if patient has completed a course of initial therapy, remains asymptomatic, and CD4+ cell count has increased to ≥200 cells/mm^3 for >6 months in response to ART. (SOR **Ⓑ**)

  3. CMV retinitis. Ganciclovir, foscarnet, cidofovir, and valganciclovir administered for an induction period of 14 to 21 days followed by lifelong maintenance therapy are effective in slowing the progression of CMV retinitis. (SOR **Ⓐ**) It is possible to discontinue maintenance therapy with inactive disease, sustained CD4+ cell count >100 cell/mm^3 for 3 to 6 months or more, and consultation with ophthalmologist. (SOR **Ⓑ**)

    a. After discontinuing maintenance therapy, patients should undergo eye examinations every 3 months. (SOR **Ⓑ**) Selection of initial therapy depends on location and severity of lesion(s), level of immunosuppression, adverse effects, and adherence.

    b. For immediate sight-threatening lesions, ganciclovir intraocular implants are used with valganciclovir 900 mg orally twice daily for induction and then once daily for maintenance. (SOR **Ⓐ**) **For small peripheral lesions,** valganciclovir is dosed at 900 mg orally twice daily during induction, followed by 900 mg orally once daily for maintenance. (SOR **Ⓑ**) Alternatively, ganciclovir can be used at a dose of 5 mg/kg IV every 12 hours during induction and 5 mg/kg IV once daily for maintenance. (SOR **Ⓐ**) Other alternatives include foscarnet 90 mg/kg IV every 12 hours for induction followed by 90 to 120 mg/kg IV every 24 hours for maintenance (SOR **Ⓐ**) and cidofovir 5 mg/kg IV once weekly for induction, followed by 5 mg/kg IV once every other week for maintenance. (SOR **Ⓐ**) All four medications must be dose-adjusted for renal impairment.

  4. Diarrhea caused by specific bacterial or parasitic organisms may respond to standard therapy. Symptomatic treatment should be offered when antibiotics are not effective or when no causative organisms can be identified. Early initiation of ART

TABLE 67–2. PRIMARY PROPHYLAXIS FOR OPPORTUNISTIC INFECTIONS^a

CD4 Cell Count (cells/mL)	Provide Prophylaxis Against
<200	*Pneumocystis jiroveci* pneumonia (PCP)
<100	Toxoplasmosis
<50	*Mycobacterium avium-intracellulare* complex (MAC)

^{a}If ART results in a CD4 cell count increase to >200 for >3 months, primary prophylaxis can be discontinued.

should prevent diseases such as cryptosporidiosis and microsporidiosis. (SOR ❶) Patients should be advised to wash hands thoroughly with soap and water after handling pets, avoid contact with pets' feces (SOR ❸), avoid drinking water from lakes or rivers (SOR ❶), and avoid eating raw oysters (SOR ❸).

5. **Esophageal candidiasis** can be treated with oral fluconazole 100 mg (up to 400 mg) orally daily or itraconazole oral solution 200 mg orally daily for 14 to 21 days. (SOR ❶) Alternative therapies include voriconazole 200 mg orally twice daily, posaconazole 400 mg orally twice daily, caspofungin 50 mg IV daily, or micafungin 150 mg IV daily. (SOR ❸) Suppressive therapy is generally not recommended (SOR ❸) as chronic or prolonged use of azoles may promote development of drug resistance. For suppressive therapy, consider fluconazole 100 to 200 mg orally daily or posaconazole 400 mg orally twice daily. (SOR ❸) Failure to respond to therapy necessitates endoscopic evaluation for herpes esophagitis or CMV esophagitis.

6. **KS** of the skin and oral mucosa does not require treatment unless the lesions are uncomfortable or cosmetically disturbing. ART should be initiated in all patients with KS. (SOR ❸) Widespread disease can be treated with chemotherapeutic agents. (SOR ❸)

7. **MAC** can cause a wide range of localized or systemic problems, including fevers, weight loss, night sweats, diarrhea, anemia, and hepatic or other gastrointestinal disease. Preferred treatment includes clarithromycin 500 mg orally twice daily + ethambutol 15 mg/kg orally daily. (SOR ❶) Addition of rifabutin 300 mg orally daily may be considered for advanced immunosuppression (CD4+ cell count <50 cells/mm^3), high mycobacterial load (>2 log CFU/mL), or absence of effective ART. (SOR ❸) Alternative therapy includes azithromycin 500 to 600 mg orally daily + ethambutol 15 mg/kg orally daily. (SOR ❶)

   a. **Chronic maintenance therapy can be discontinued** when patients have completed 12 or more months of MAC treatment, have remained asymptomatic, and have a CD4+ cell count >100 cells/mm^3 for >6 months in the presence of ART. (SOR ❸) Primary prophylaxis against MAC should be initiated when CD4+ cell count is <50 cells/mm^3 with azithromycin 1200 mg orally once weekly or clarithromycin 500 mg orally twice daily. (SOR ❶) Primary prophylaxis can be discontinued when CD4+ cell count increases to >100 cells/mm^3 for 3 or more months in the presence of ART. (SOR ❶)

8. **Oropharyngeal candidiasis** can be treated with fluconazole 100 mg orally daily (SOR ❶), clotrimazole troches 10 mg orally five times daily (SOR ❸), nystatin suspension 4 to 6 mL swish-and-swallow four times daily (SOR ❸), nystatin pastilles one to two pastilles —four to five times daily (SOR ❸), or miconazole mucoadhesive tablet orally daily (SOR ❸).

9. **PCP.**

   a. **Acute PCP.** Clinical evidence of response to therapy usually takes 3 to 5 days. Acute PCP can be treated on an inpatient or outpatient basis. Outpatient therapy is preferred for mild-to-moderate PCP when adequate home support is available. Secondary prophylaxis can be discontinued when CD4+ cell count increases to >200 cells/mm^3 for >3 months as a result of ART. (SOR ❸)

      (1) **Trimethoprim-sulfamethoxazole (TMP-SMX)** administered IV for moderate-to-severe PCP (15–20 mg/kg TMP and 75–100 mg/kg SMX per day divided into—three to four doses to be given every 6–8 hours) or orally for mild-to-moderate PCP (two double-strength tablets orally three times a day), is the drug of choice. (SOR ❶) TMP-SMX has the advantage of providing additional treatment against other bacterial pulmonary pathogens. The duration of therapy is 21 days. Skin rashes are common. Nephrotoxicity and hepatotoxicity can also occur.

      (2) **Corticosteroids** such as prednisone starting at 40 mg daily and tapered over 21 days are indicated for patients with a PaO2 <70 mmHg.

      (3) **Other agents** for moderate-to-severe PCP include Pentamidine at 4 mg/kg IV daily over ≥60 minutes, primaquine 15 to 30 mg orally daily + clindamycin 600 to 900 mg IV every 6 to 8 hours (or 300–450 mg orally every 6–8 hours). Alternative therapy for mild-to-moderate PCP include dapsone 100 mg orally daily + TMP 5 mg/kg orally three times daily, atovaquone 750 mg orally twice daily with food, or primaquine 15 to 30 mg orally daily + clindamycin 300 to 450 mg orally every 6 to 8 hours.

b. PCP prophylaxis. Patients with a CD4+ cell count <200 cells/mm³ or history of oropharyngeal candidiasis should receive primary PCP prophylaxis. (SOR **A**) Primary prophylaxis can be discontinued when CD4+ cell count increases to >200 cells/mm³ for >3 months as a result of ART. (SOR **A**)

    (1) TMP-SMX is the drug of choice. The dosage is one double-strength tablet orally daily (SOR **A**), one single-strength tablet orally daily (SOR **A**), or one double-strength tablet orally three times per week. (SOR **B**)

    (2) Dapsone 100 mg orally daily is a suitable alternative. (SOR **B**)

    (3) Other options include aerosolized pentamidine or atovaquone. (SOR **B**)

10. Toxoplasmosis of the central nervous system can be treated with pyrimethamine 200 mg once, then 50 mg (<60 kg) to 75 mg (≥60 kg) orally daily, plus sulfadiazine 1000 mg (<60 kg) to 1500 mg (≥60 kg) orally every 6 hours, plus leucovorin 10 to 25 mg orally daily (SOR **A**) for at least 6 weeks. (SOR **B**)

a. Chronic maintenance therapy includes pyrimethamine 25 to 50 mg orally daily, plus sulfadiazine 2000 to 4000 mg orally daily (in two to four divided doses), plus leucovorin 10 to 25 mg orally daily. (SOR **A**) Clindamycin (600 mg IV or orally every 6 hours) can be substituted for sulfadiazine in patients with sulfa allergy. (SOR **A**) Anticonvulsants should be administered to those with a history of seizures. Chronic maintenance therapy can be discontinued after successful completion of therapy and an increase in CD4+ cell count to >200 cells/mm³ for >6 months on ART. (SOR **B**)

b. For primary prophylaxis, the TMP-SMX double-strength daily dose for PCP prophylaxis is also effective against toxoplasmosis. (SOR **A**) However, for those with CD4+ cell count <100 cells/mm³, who are unable to tolerate TMP-SMX, dapsone plus pyrimethamine plus leucovorin is the recommended alternative. (SOR **B**)

V. Management Strategies. Patients with HIV infection require comprehensive primary care. Ideally, one primary care provider who is responsible for health care maintenance, early intervention, and treatment of common OIs or an HIV specialist who also manages primary care issues should be identified. Consultation with specialists for specific problems can augment primary care. A team of medical staff, social workers, pharmacists, nurses, and family members that are organized around the care of the patient is essential for the treatment of patients with HIV disease.

A. Patient education. Special attention to the psychosocial impact of HIV disease is essential to the development of therapeutic strategies. Especially, important interventions include discussions about natural history of HIV, infectiousness and transmission, treatment strategies, and consideration of the quality of life. Aftercare for the family of a patient who has died of HIV is also very helpful.

B. Follow-up testing: Generally, patients should follow-up with their provider every 3 to 6 months for monitoring of disease progression with viral load and CD4+ cell count testing, as well as monitoring for potential adverse effects of ART.

C. HIV and pregnancy. Given the recommendations for universal prenatal HIV counseling and testing, ART prophylaxis, scheduled cesarean delivery, and avoidance of breastfeeding, the rate of perinatal HIV transmission has dramatically diminished to less than 2% in the United States and in Europe. ART during antepartum and intrapartum periods as well as prophylaxis to the infant is recommended to prevent perinatal HIV transmission. (SOR **A**)

1. All pregnant HIV-infected women should receive ART regardless of their viral load or CD4+ cell count (SOR **A**) for their own health (SOR **A**) and for prevention of perinatal transmission in those who do not yet require therapy. (SOR **A**) It is important to coordinate services among prenatal care providers, primary care and HIV specialty care providers, mental health and drug abuse treatment services, and public assistance programs to ensure high levels of ART adherence. (SOR **A**)

2. The National Perinatal HIV Hotline (1-888-448-8765) provides free clinical consultation on perinatal HIV care.

VI. Prognosis. Because of the effectiveness of combination ART, the prognosis for persons living with HIV infection continues to improve dramatically.

A. The mean survival of HIV-infected persons in the United States before the advent of effective ART was approximately 11 years from time of infection. The CD4+ cell count and viral load at the time of diagnosis were closely correlated with the prognosis, with persons with high viral load and CD4+ cell counts ≤200 cells/mm³ having an 80% likelihood of developing AIDS within 3 years, whereas persons with high viral load but

CD4+ cell counts ≥ 350 cells/mm^3 having a 40% chance of developing AIDS within 3 years. In contrast, the patient with a CD4+ cell count ≥ 500 cells/mm^3 and viral load $\leq 20,000$ has less than a 20% chance of developing AIDS within 3 years. These data continue to apply to persons with HIV disease who are not receiving effective ART, including the nearly 300,000 persons in the United States infected with HIV disease but unaware of their HIV diagnosis.

B. The life expectancy of most HIV-infected persons who receive effective ART has increased by many years and, as a result, HIV-infected individuals can have near-normal life expectancy. Deaths from AIDS have decreased dramatically, and clinical manifestations of HIV infection and AIDS have partially or completely resolved in many patients. The quality of life for persons receiving effective ART can improve dramatically. However, the pill burden and side effects from ART can be considerable, so quality of life is not invariably improved. The clinician, therefore, needs to help each patient make the best possible decisions about their use of ART.

SELECTED REFERENCES

Because advances in HIV/AIDS occur frequently, the principal federal guidelines that represent current standards in treatment are continually updated. The following guidelines were used for the treatment data in this chapter:

Cohen MS, Chen YQ, McCauley M, et al. Prevention of HIV-1 infection with early antiretroviral therapy. *N Engl J Med.* 2011;365(6):493–505.

Kaplan JE, Benson C, Holmes KH, et al; Centers for Disease Control and Prevention. Guidelines for prevention and treatment of opportunistic infections in HIV-infected adults and adolescents. *MMWR.* 2009;58(RR-4):1–207.

Panel on Antiretroviral Guidelines for Adults and Adolescents. Guidelines for the use of antiretroviral agents in HIV-1-infected adults and adolescents. Department of Health and Human Services. http://aidsinfo.nih.gov/ContentFiles/AdultandAdolescentGL.pdf. Accessed April 2013.

Panel on Treatment of HIV-Infected Pregnant Women and Prevention of Perinatal Transmission. Recommendations for Use of Antiretroviral Drugs in Pregnant HIV-1-Infected Women for Maternal Health and Interventions to Reduce Perinatal HIV Transmission in the United States. http://aidsinfo.nih.gov/contentfiles/lvguidelines/PerinatalGL.pdf.

More information and other guidelines can be viewed on sites such as:
www.aidsinfo.nih.gov
http://www.cdc.gov/hiv (http://www.cdc.gov/hiv/prevention/research/prep/index.html)
www.iasusa.org
www.hivinsite.com
www.nccc.ucsf.edu

---

68   Asthma

Jonathan MacClements, MD, FAAFP

KEY POINTS

- Current guidelines emphasize the importance of asthma control and focus on current impairment and future risk to assess asthma severity (for initiating therapy) and asthma control (for ongoing monitoring). (SOR **A**)
- Effective control of asthma is necessary to prevent fibrosis of the basement membrane and remodeling of the airways, which can lead to irreversible obstructive lung disease. This control is accomplished by using anti-inflammatory agents, most commonly inhaled corticosteroids. (SOR **A**)
- Successful control of asthma requires high-quality ongoing patient education in which the patients understand their medications and how to avoid factors that aggravate asthma including controlling environmental exposures. (SOR **B**)

- Patients with asthma are at a significant risk for high morbidity and death and should be monitored in a systematic and careful manner by their primary care provider. Spirometry and patient-monitored peak flow meters play an important role in the management. (SOR **A**)
- The principal goals for treating asthma exacerbations are correction of significant hypoxemia, rapid reversal of airflow obstruction, and reduction of the likelihood of relapse of the exacerbation or future recurrence of severe airflow obstruction by intensifying therapy. (SOR **A**)

I. Introduction

A. Definition. Asthma is a disease of the airways, manifested by recurrent or persistent inflammatory and obstructive processes, or both. Asthma is due to multifactorial causes and frequently results in irreversible loss of lung function and major disability. It is important to assess asthma severity before therapy is initiated; the degree of control after treatment; and understand the effect of these symptoms on the daily activities of the patient. **The terms describing asthma severity are intermittent, mild persistent, moderate persistent, and severe persistent,** defined by frequency and severity of symptoms (Table 68–1). The control of asthma is classified as well controlled, not well controlled, and poorly controlled (Table 68–2).

B. Epidemiology

1. **Onset** is before age 5 years in 75% to 90% of cases, with peak prevalence between 5 and 17 years of age.

2. **Risk factors** include a family history of asthma or atopy, parental smoking, ambient air pollution, obesity, poor nutrition, and viral respiratory infections, especially bronchiolitis from respiratory syncytial virus. Females and blacks are at greater risk. There is an association with exposure to cats, cockroaches, and house dust mites.

3. The **prevalence** of asthma in the United States has increased during the last two decades; in 2011, it was estimated that 25.9 million Americans currently have asthma, including 7.1 million children under age 18 years. Asthma is one of the leading causes of school absenteeism, with 5% to 10% of all children experiencing the disease during childhood. Asthma is the third leading cause of hospitalization among children under age 15 years. The annual healthcare cost of asthma is approximately $56.0 billion dollars (direct and indirect costs).

C. Pathophysiology

1. **Expiratory airflow obstruction** is initiated by bronchial wall inflammation, resulting in bronchospasm, bronchial gland mucus exudates, airway edema, and airway remodeling.

2. **Resultant pathophysiologic changes** include increased airway resistance and hyperinflation.

3. The **etiology** is not completely understood, but encompasses a wide variety of genetic, immunologic, infectious, and environmental factors.

II. Diagnosis.
Although patients with asthma typically present with recurrent episodes of wheezing, not all asthma episodes are characterized by wheezing and not all wheezing indicates asthma. Undiagnosed asthma is a common reason for referral to pediatric and adult pulmonary outpatient departments.

A. Symptoms and signs

1. **Symptoms** usually include wheezing, coughing, dyspnea, chest tightness, and sometimes sputum production. Most patients report symptom-free intervals, but a rapidly changing and variable clinical picture is common.

    a. **Coughing** may be the initial symptom of asthma and is essentially the only symptom in cough-variant asthma. This form of asthma presents with nonproductive cough occurring both day and night. Pulmonary function studies can be normal. Therapy is similar to standard asthma treatment.

    b. **Atelectasis,** often misdiagnosed on chest x-ray as pneumonia, is a common clue to undiagnosed asthma.

    c. A **patient or family history of atopy or asthma** supports the diagnosis.

2. **Signs** may be absent in the patients with asthma, especially early in the disease and during asymptomatic intervals. Forceful expiration occasionally uncovers otherwise unnoticed end-expiratory wheezing.

TABLE 68–1. INITIAL VISIT: CLASSIFICATION OF SEVERITY AND INITIATING THERAPY (NOT CURRENTLY ON LONG TERM CONTROL)

Components of SEVERITY		Age (yr)	Classification of Asthma			
				Persistent		
			Intermittent	Mild	Moderate	Severe
Impairment	Symptoms	All	≤2 d/wk	>2 d/wk but not daily	Daily	Throughout the day
	Nighttime awakenings	0–4	0	1–2×/mo	3–4×/mo	>1×/wk
		≥5	≤2×/month	3–4×/mo	>1×/wk but not nightly	Often 7×/wk
	SABA used for symptom control	All	≤2d/wk	>2 d/wk but not daily	Daily	Several times a day
	Interference with normal activity	All	None	Minor limitation	Some limitation	Extremely limited
	Lung function:					
	FEV_1 (predicated) or PEF (personal best)	≥5	Normal FEV_1 between exacerbations >80%	>80%	60%–80%	<60%
	FEV_1/FVC	5–11	≥85%	>80%	75%–80%	<60%
		≥12	Normal	Normal	Reduced 5%	Reduced >5%
Risk	**Exacerbations requiring oral corticosteroids**	0–4	≤1/yr	≥2 × 6mo or ≥4 wheezing episodes/ yr lasting >1 d AND risk factors for persistent asthma		
		5–11		≥2×/yr		
		≥12		Consider severity and interval since last exacerbation. Frequency and severity may fluctuate over time for patients in any severity category. Relative annual risk of exacerbations may be related to FEV_1		
Recommended step for starting treatment		0–4	Step 1	Step 2	Step 3	Step 3
		5–11				Step 3 or 4
		≥12				Step 4 or 5
		All			Consider short course of oral corticosteroids	
		All	In 2–6 wk, evaluate level of asthma control that is achieved and adjust therapy accordingly. For 0–4-year-old children, if no clear benefit is observed in 4–6 wk, consider alternative diagnosis or adjusting therapy			

FEV_1, forced expiratory volume in 1 second; FVC, forced vital capacity; PEF, peak expiratory flow; SABA, short-acting β_2-agonist

Source: Data from National Heart, Lung, and Blood Institute, National Asthma Education and Prevention Program. Expert panel report 3: guidelines for the diagnosis and management of asthma. Bethesda, MD: National Heart, Lung, and Blood Institute; Revised August 2007. NIH publication no. 07-4051. http://www.nhlbi.nih.gov/ guidelines/asthma/asthgdln.pdf. Accessed May 23, 2013.

    a. Severe asthma may be characterized by both expiratory and inspiratory wheezing, prolongation of the expiratory phase, thoracic cage retractions, tachypnea, cyanosis, accessory muscle recruitment, and apprehension.

    b. Pulsus paradoxus (a pulse pressure that markedly decreases in size during inspiration), a silent chest, or chest wall crepitus caused by subcutaneous emphysema may signify severe airway obstruction requiring urgent care.

TABLE 68–2. FOLLOW-UP VISIT: CLASSIFICATION OF ASTHMA CONTROL AND ADJUSTING THERAPY

Components of Control		Age (yr)	Levels of Asthma Control		
			Well Controlled	**Not Well Controlled**	**Very Poorly Controlled**
Impairment	Symptoms	0–4	≤2 d/wk but ≤ 1 d	>2 d/wk or multiple times on ≤ 2 d/wk	Throughout the day
		5–11			
		≥12	≤2 d/wk	>2 d/wk	
	Nighttime awakenings	0–4	<1×/mo	>1×/mo	>1×/wk
		5–11		≥2×/mo	>2×/wk
		≥12	<2×/mo	1–3×/wk	>4×/wk
	SABA used for symptom control	All	≤2×/wk	>2×/wk	Several times a day
	Interference with normal activity	All	Minor limitation	Some limitation	Extremely limited
	Lung function:				
	FEV1 or PEF	≥5	>80%	60%–80%	<60%
	FEV1/FVC	5–11	>80%	75%–80%	<75%
		≥12	Not applicable	Not applicable	Not applicable
	Validated Questionnaires				
	ATAQ	≥12	0	1–2	3–4
	ACQ	≥12	≤0.75	≥1.5	Not applicable
	ACT	≥12	≥20	16–19	≤15
Risk	Exacerbations requiring oral corticosteroids	0–4	≤1×/yr	2–3×/yr	>3×/yr
		5–11		≥2×/yr	
		≥12		Consider severity and interval since last exacerbation	
	Reduction in lung volume	5–11	Evaluation requires long-term follow-up care		
	Loss of lung function	≥12	Evaluation requires long-term follow-up care		
	Treatment-related adverse effects	All	Medication side effects can vary in intensity from none to concerning		
Recommended treatment actions		All	**Maintain current step:** regular follow-up at every 1–6 mon; consider stepping down if well controlled for ≥3 mo	**Step up 1 step** Before stepping up, review adherence to medication, inhaler technique, environmental control, and comorbid conditions. If an alternative treatment option was used in a step, discontinue and use the preferred treatment for that step Reevaluate the level of asthma control in 2–6 wk and adjust therapy accordingly. For side effects, consider alternative treatment options	**Step up 1–2 steps** and consider short course of oral corticosteroids

ACQ, Asthma Control Questionnaire; ACT, Asthma Control Test; ATAQ, Asthma Therapy Assessment Questionnaire; FEV$_1$, forced expiratory volume in 1 second; FVC, forced vital capacity; PEF, peak expiratory flow; SABA, short-acting β$_2$-agonist.

Source: Data from National Heart, Lung, and Blood Institute, National Asthma Education and Prevention Program. Expert panel report 3: guidelines for the diagnosis and management of asthma. Bethesda, MD: National Heart, Lung, and Blood Institute; Revised August 2007. NIH publication no. 07–4051. http://www.nhlbi.nih.gov/guidelines/asthma/asthgdln.pdf. Accessed May 23, 2013.

    c. Chronic changes may include such chest wall deformities as pectus carinatum or an increased anteroposterior diameter. Clubbing is rarely associated with asthma and suggests a diagnosis of cystic fibrosis or cancer.

B. Diagnostic tests

    1. Peripheral blood smear and a **sputum examination** showing eosinophilia may suggest allergic asthma.

    2. Allergy skin tests, allergen-specific IgE, and the **radioallergosorbent test** can be used to test specific allergens. These tests may identify specific allergens that can be avoided or treated with immunotherapy desensitization. Skin tests are the least costly of the three tests. Radioallergosorbent test and IgE blood tests are usually reserved for patients who cannot undergo skin testing because of a history of severe reaction or other intolerance. Positive tests should correlate with the patient's history of allergies before acting on them. Total IgE levels are usually elevated in atopic asthma.

    3. The chest x-ray is useful for selected patients in ruling out other diseases. It may show hyperinflation, atelectasis, pneumonia, or, rarely, pneumomediastinum. Criteria for ordering chest films include tachypnea, tachycardia, localized rales, localized decreased breath sounds, or cyanosis. Portable chest x-rays may be appropriately ordered for critically ill patients, but two-view posteroanterior and lateral chest films are helpful when the view requires clarification, such as when the physician suspects that a posteroinferior lung infiltrate that could be concealed behind the cardiac silhouette.

    4. Pulmonary function tests

        a. Indications for pulmonary function tests include confirmation of the diagnosis of asthma, objective measurement of the response to therapy, and measurement of pulmonary dysfunction.

        b. Forced expiratory volume in 1 second (FEV$_1$) is very useful in assessing acute asthma, but the **peak expiratory flow rate (PEFR)** parallels the FEV$_1$ and is usually easier to obtain. Devices that measure PEFR are inexpensive and can be prescribed to allow patients with asthma to monitor their progress at home. Patients with a PEFR below 70% of their baseline value should be evaluated. An FEV$_1$ or PEFR below 40% after aggressive therapy indicates severe obstruction, and the patient should be hospitalized. The accuracy of peak flow meters varies, however, and can deteriorate over time.

        c. The **peak flow–zone system** allows patients to monitor the PEFR and make clinical decisions about their asthma, under the physician's supervision, using an asthma action plan designed for each patient (http://www.nyc.gov/html/doh/downloads/pdf/asthma/aamap.pdf).

           (1) The **green zone** (PEFR = 80%–100% of the patient's best score) indicates that the patient can continue the usual course of medicine.

           (2) The **yellow zone** (PEFR = 50%–80%) is a warning to the patient to take additional medicine or call the physician.

           (3) The **red zone** (PEFR ≤ 50%) indicates that the patient should both use their inhaler, take additional medication, and call the physician or go to the emergency room immediately.

    5. Provocative testing with either methacholine or histamine is indicated for the rare patient for whom a definitive diagnosis is sought when the clinical picture is unclear. These tests carry a minimal risk of producing life-threatening bronchospasm. They must be performed under experienced supervision with resuscitative support immediately available.

    6. Arterial blood gases are indicated for patients who have poor respiratory status or a poor response to therapy. Impending respiratory failure should be suspected, even when the PCO$_2$ is normal or slightly elevated (≥40 mm Hg), in the presence of hypoxia (PO$_2$ ≤ 70 mm Hg). Pulse oximetry monitoring is noninvasive and very useful in monitoring the oxygenation of patients with asthma.

    7. Nitric oxide test system monitors exhaled nitric oxide levels, which are elevated in the lungs in a variety of inflammatory diseases including asthma. This test has proven beneficial in diagnosing and monitoring the response of lung inflammation to asthma therapy.

C. Differential diagnosis

    1. Common diseases to be excluded are bronchiolitis, cystic fibrosis, and foreign bodies (see Chapter 65), chronic bronchitis (see Chapter 70), and congestive heart failure (see Chapter 73).

2. Less common diseases to be considered are vocal cord dysfunction, bronchopulmonary dysplasia, allergic bronchopulmonary mycoses, and bronchiolitis obliterans.

III. **Treatment** goals include maintenance of normal activities (including exercise) and optimal pulmonary function values while minimizing symptoms, exacerbations, and adverse drug effects. Long-term therapy directed at suppressing inflammation early in the course of illness is now felt necessary to modify the disease process and prevent irreversible lung dysfunction. (SOR **Ⓐ**)

A. **Environmental control** can provide significant relief by avoiding triggers identified in the clinical history and known to produce deleterious effects.

   1. **Inhaled allergens** cannot be totally avoided, but much of the exposure can be eliminated.

      a. **Tobacco smoke** should be banned from the home and automobile. The use of nonsmoking hotel rooms, rental cars, and restaurants is beneficial.

      b. **House dust mites** are difficult to eradicate. Frequent household cleaning can help reduce their numbers.

         (1) **Rooms**, when practical, should be free of carpets, stuffed toys, and other dust-collecting items.

         (2) **Central air-conditioning systems** should have frequently cleaned mechanical or electrostatic air filters. Portable, high-efficiency, particulate air filters can be used in patients' bedrooms. Attempt to reduce the humidity level to between 30% and 50% relative humidity.

         (3) **Nonallergenic mattress covers** should be used, down fillings avoided, and bed linens should be washed weekly.

      c. **Other irritants** to be avoided include pets, flowering plants, molds, perfumes, hair sprays, paints, and aerosolized chemicals.

   2. **Emotional factors** can play a significant role in triggering asthma in some patients and must be minimized.

      a. **Parents** should avoid overcompensating behavior that can create opportunities for manipulation by the child with asthma. They should also avoid the other extreme of ignoring the child's plight.

      b. The **family** should offer the child support, consistency, and loving parental guidance.

   3. **Exercise** and exposure to cold air frequently aggravate asthma. Acute exacerbations resulting from exercise can be lessened by appropriate premedication and by restricting activities to participation in such sports as water sports, which typically cause less bronchial irritation than do other athletic activities. Weight loss in patients with obesity is beneficial.

B. **Drug therapy** involves two groups of drugs: long-term-control and quick-relief medications. (Table 68–3).

   1. **Long-term-control medications** are usually given daily over the long term to control persistent asthma. They include corticosteroids, cromolyn, long-acting bronchodilators, leukotriene modifiers, and theophylline.

      a. **Corticosteroids** are very effective anti-inflammatory drugs for treating acute and chronic asthma, (SOR **Ⓐ**) but can cause many serious adverse effects. In children, suppression of linear growth and adverse effects on the hypothalamic–pituitary–adrenal axis are a major concern of systemic steroids. In adults, bone demineralization, cataract formation, gastrointestinal hemorrhage, and psychiatric problems sometimes occur with systemic usage. Corticosteroids should be initiated early in the course of treatment and in adequate doses for patients with severe asthma. The mode of action of corticosteroids is unclear, but current consensus suggests they improve airflow by decreasing inflammatory activity in the arachidonic acid, leukotriene, prostaglandin, and inflammatory cell systems and by increasing smooth muscle responsiveness to β-agonists.

         (1) **Inhaled corticosteroids (ICS)** are first-line drugs and are often prescribed with inhaled β-agonists. (SOR **Ⓐ**) Inhaled corticosteroids available in metered dose inhalers (MDIs) include budesonide (Pulmicort), fluticasone (Flovent), beclomethasone (Vanceril or Beclovent), flunisolide (AeroBid), mometasone (Asmanex), and triamcinolone (Azmacort).

            (a) Administration is by MDI with dosages listed in Table 68–3. Budesonide and fluticasone are also available in powder MDI preparations and budesonide is available in solution for updraft inhalation. Withdrawal of ICS should be done slowly to avoid worsening of asthma.

TABLE 68–3. MEDICATIONS FOR ASTHMA

Drug[a]	Dose Per Age (yr)	Major Side Effects	Drug Interactions
β₂-Agonists			
Albuterol	≥4: 2 puffs every 4–6 h prn	Anxiety, paradoxical bron-	
MDI 90 µg/puff	>12: 2.5–5 mg four times daily	chospasm, tachycardia,	
Nebulizer soln.[a]	prn	upper respiratory infection,	
0.63–5 mg/3 mL	2–12: 2.5 mg four times daily prn	rhinitis, throat irritation	
Levalbuterol	≥4: 2 puffs every 4–6 h prn		
MDI 45 mcg/puff,	≥12: 0.63–1.25 mg three times		
Nebulizer soln.	daily prn		
0.31–1.25 mg/3	5–11: 0.31–0.63 mg three times		
mL	daily prn		
	≤5: 0.31–1.25 mg every 3–4 h prn		
Formoterol[b]	>5: 12 µg every 12 h	Paradoxical bronchospasm,	
Dry-powder inhaler		asthma exacerbation, chest	
12 µg/capsule		pain, palpitations, tremor,	
		headache	
Salmeterol[b]	≥4: 50 µg every 12 h	Paradoxical bronchospasm,	
Dry-powder inhaler		asthma exacerbation, mus-	
50 µg/puff		culoskeletal pain	
Pirbuterol	≥12: 2 puffs every 4–6 h	Tremor, anxiety, paradoxical	
MDI 200 mcg/puff	≤12: 4 to 8 puffs every 1–4 h	bronchospasm	
Mast Cell Stabilizers			
Cromolyn sodium[a]	>2: 20 mg (nebulizer) or 800 µg	Throat irritation, nasal irrita-	
MDI or nebulizer	(MDI) four times daily	tion, cough, bronchospasm	
soln. 800 µg/puff			
Inhaled Corticosteroids			
Beclomethasone	≥12: 40–160 µg twice daily	Headache, pharyngitis, oral	Systemic effects and
MDI 40/80 µg/puff	Max: 640 µg/d	Candidiasis	drug interactions
	5–11: 40 µg twice daily		are minimal
	Max: 160 µg/d		
Budesonide	≥6: 180–360 mg twice daily	Diarrhea, nausea, respiratory	
DPI 90, 180 µg/puff	Max: Adults 1440 µg/d	tract infection, headache,	
Nebulizer soln.[a]	Children 720 µg/d	arthralgia, syncope	
0.25, 0.5 mg/	1–8: 0.25- 1 mg/day in one or		
2 mL	two divided doses		
Ciclesonide	≥12: 80–320 µg twice daily	Bronchospasm, arthralgias,	
MDI 80, 160 µg/	Max: 640 µg/d	headache, upper respira-	
puff		tory infection, nasal	
		congestion, increased	
		intraocular pressure	
Fluticasone	>12: 88–880 µg twice daily	Oral candidiasis, headache,	
MDI 44/110/220	Max: 1760 µg/d	upper respiratory infection,	
µg/puff	4–11: 88 µg twice daily	pneumonia, throat irritation	
Dry-powder inhaler	Max: 176 µg/d		
100/250 µg/puff			
Mometasone	>12: 220 to 440 µg twice daily	Nausea, headache, muscu-	
Dry-powder inhaler	Max: 880 µg/d	loskeletal pain, dysmenor-	
110, 220 µg/puff	4–11: 110 µg each evening	rhea, allergic rhinitis, upper	
	Max: 110 µg/d	respiratory tract infection	
Systemic Corticosteroids			
Prednisone[a]	≥12: 7.5–60 mg as single dose	Impaired glucose control,	Live vaccines,
Methyl-prednis-	daily or every other day as	hypertension, weight gain,	fluoroquino-
olone[a]	needed for control	osteoporosis, mood distur-	lones, lopinavir,
Prednisolone[a]	*Short-course:* 40–60 mg in single	bance, impaired wound	ritonavir, telaprevir,
	or two divided doses for 5–10 d	healing, edema, Cushing	bupropion, que-
	≤12: 0.25–2 mg/kg as single	syndrome, increased infec-	tiapine, clozapine
	dose daily or every other day	tion risk[c]	
	as needed		
	Short-course: 1–2 mg/kg/d, max-		
	imum 60 mg/d for 3–10 d		

TABLE 68-3. MEDICATIONS FOR ASTHMA (*Continued*)

Drug[a]	Dose Per Age (yr)	Major Side Effects	Drug Interactions
Combination Medications			
Budesonide /formoterol[b] MDI 80/4.5, 160/4.5 μg/puff	≥12: 80/4.5–160/4.5 μg twice daily Max: 640 μg/18 μg/d	See individual drugs	
Fluticasone/ salmeterol[b] MDI 45/21, 115/21, 230/21 μg/puff Dry-powder inhaler 100/50, 250/50, 500/50 μg/dose	≥12: 1–2 puffs twice daily Max: 920 μg/84 μg/d	See individual drugs	
Mometasone /formoterol[b] MDI 100/5, 200/5 μg/spray	≥12: 2 puffs twice daily Max: 400 μg/20 μg/d	See individual drugs	
Methylxanthines			
Theophylline[a] (Extended-release tablets or capsules)	≥15: 300–600 mg/d in three to four divided doses 1–15 (≤45 kg): 12–14 mg/kg/d in four to six divided doses; max. 600 mg/d Therapeutic range: 10–20 mg/L	Headache, insomnia, tremor, restlessness, irritability, atrial fibrillation, tachy-cardia, seizures, Stevens–Johnson syndrome	Can increase toxic effects of mifepristone, azole antifungals, boceprevir, caffeine, bupropion, fluoroqui-nolones, imipenem, macrolides, halo-thane, vemurafenib, peginterferon α-2A, zileuton, oral contra-ceptives, deferasirox
Leukotriene Modifiers			
Montelukast[a] Tablets 10 mg Chewable tablets 4 or 5 mg Granule packet 4 mg	≥15: 10 mg each evening 6–14: 5 mg each evening 1–5: 4 mg each evening	Headache, Stevens–Johnson syndrome, altered or aggressive behavior, suicidal ideation; contraindicated in patients with hepatic impair-ment including cirrhosis	Dabrafenib, clozap-ine, gemfibrozil
Zafirlukast[a] Tablets 10, 20 mg	≥12: 20 mg twice daily 5–11: 10 mg twice daily	Headache, hepatitis, abnor-mal LFTs, aggressive behavior, agitation, hal-lucinations, dream disorder, Stevens–Johnson syndrome	
Zileuton Tablets 600 mg IR or 1200 mg CR	≥12: 600 mg IR four times daily or 1200 mg CR twice daily after meals	Headache, sinusitis, upper abdominal pain, hepato-toxicity, behavioral distur-bance, dream disorder; contraindicated in patients with hepatic disease	
Humanized Monoclonal Antibody			
Omalizumab Only used for IgE-mediated asthma	≥12: 150–375 mg SQ every 2 or 4 wk; do not administer more than 150 mg per injection site	Headache, upper respiratory infection, viral disease, serum sickness, malignancy, thrombocytopenia (severe), injection site reaction (severe)	

[a]Available as generic.
[b]LABA increases the risk of asthma-related death; LABA should only be used in patients with long-term asthma.
control treatment such as ICS. Do not use LABA if asthma is adequately controlled on low/medium dose ICS.
[c]Most adverse effects are associated with duration of therapy; with short course, adverse drug reactions are transient.
LFTs, liver function tests; LABAs, long-acting β₂-agonists; PRN, as needed; SQ subcutaneously; SABA, short-acting β₂-agonist.

(b) **Significant adverse effects** of inhaled corticosteroids are much less than those of systemic corticosteroids. Studies are conflicting regarding the long-term effect of inhaled corticosteroids on children's growth; the 1-year studies show a small, dose-dependent effect although the influence on final adult height is uncertain. Recent studies show that a high-dose regimen may be as effective as a daily low-dose regimen of budesonide in reducing asthma exacerbations and reduces long-term exposure to the drug. (SOR **A**) Budesonide and fluticasone are considered to be more potent and have less gastric absorption and fewer active metabolites than the older drugs. Minor adverse effects include oropharyngeal candidiasis, cough, and, rarely, dysphonia, but they are seldom severe enough to warrant discontinuation. The use of spacer devices and oral rinses after inhalation can lessen these side effects.

(2) Systemic steroids are indicated when other modes of therapy fail to control severe asthma.

(a) **Oral tablets** of prednisone, methylprednisolone, and prednisolone are given in doses of 1 to 2 mg/kg/d (usually, 20–80 mg/d) and gradually reduced over 1 to 3 weeks, depending on disease severity.

(b) **Liquid preparations** of prednisolone include Prelone (15 mg/5 mL) and Pediapred (5 mg/5 mL). Liquid preparations of prednisone include Liquid Pred Syrup (5 mg/5 mL) and Prednisone Intensol (5 mg/1 mL). See Table 68–3 for dosing.

(c) **Drug interactions with** fluoroquinolones, lopinavir, ritonavir, telaprevir, bupropion, quetiapine, and clozapine. Should not administer live vaccines while on systemic steroids.

b. Cromolyn sodium, an anti-inflammatory medication used prophylactically to control chronic asthma and exercise-induced asthma, (SOR **C**) inhibits both early- and late-response allergic reactions. Although cromolyn's mechanism of action is not fully understood, it probably stabilizes mast cells by preventing their degranulation and release of inflammatory mediators.

(1) Adverse effects are few, but cromolyn requires dedicated patient compliance, since an adequate therapeutic response may not occur until after 4 to 6 weeks of therapy. Children appear to respond to cromolyn better than do adults.

(2) Preparations of cromolyn (Intal) include an MDI, an aerosolized solution that can be combined in an aerosol with a β_2 drug, and an inhaled powder capsule. The recommended dose is two inhaled metered sprays (800 µg per spray) four times daily at regular intervals. It seems more effective in children with asthma.

c. Long-acting β_2-agonists (LABAs). LABAs increase the risk of asthma-related death when used as monotherapy. These drugs are **contraindicated without concurrent use of long-term asthma control treatment** such as ICS. They should not be used if asthma is adequately controlled on low/medium dose ICS alone.

(1) Salmeterol (Serevent), available as an MDI and inhaled powder, is a long-acting (every 12 hours) β-agonist indicated for maintenance therapy and contraindicated for acute treatment. (SOR **A**) It is approved for children 6 years and older. Salmeterol acts as a bronchodilator, relaxing smooth muscle by adenylate cyclase activation and increased cyclic AMP production. Its onset of action is 15 to 30 minutes and the duration of action is greater than 12 hours. It is especially useful for controlling nocturnal symptoms.

(2) Formoterol (Foradil Aerolizer) is a dry powder inhaler (DPI), which is similar to salmeterol and is dosed at 12 µg every 12 hours. Both salmeterol and formoterol have an FDA warning that long-acting β_2-adrenergic agonists may increase the risk of asthma-related death. It is recommended for use only as an additional treatment if symptoms are not controlled on low-to-medium dose inhaled corticosteroids, or if disease severity warrants initial treatment with two maintenance drugs.

(3) Albuterol sustained-release (Vospire ER) is an oral sustained-release form of albuterol that tends to have more side effects than the inhaled LABAs.

d. The combination of inhaled fluticasone and salmeterol (Advair Diskus, DPI, and Advair HFA) offers the advantage of improved compliance and may also enhance efficacy through drug synergy. Dosages are listed in Table 68–3.

e. Theophylline is a methylxanthine bronchodilator that is usually well absorbed from the gastrointestinal tract. Theophyllines are considered second-line agents and are used as adjuncts with anti-inflammatory and other bronchodilator drugs. (SOR **Ⓐ**) Monitoring theophylline levels may be useful to reduce toxicity.

(1) Dosage requirements of theophylline vary considerably with age and the individual patient. Blood levels should be monitored and maintained between 5 and 15 µg/mL. When possible, therapy should be initiated slowly to minimize side effects. Children tend to clear the drug significantly more rapidly than do adults.

(2) Adverse effects are similar to those of caffeine and include nervousness, anorexia, irritability, nausea, vomiting, enuresis, insomnia, poor school performance, and behavioral problems. Factors that can increase serum levels of theophylline and give rise to toxicity include impaired liver function, age older than 55 years, chronic heart and lung disease, sustained high fever, viral illnesses, and drug interactions, including those with cimetidine, allopurinol, ciprofloxacin, erythromycin, rifampin, propranolol, oral contraceptives, phenytoin, clarithromycin, and lithium carbonate.

(3) Overdose usually manifests as nausea and vomiting but can cause arrhythmias, seizures, and, very rarely, death. Patients and their family members should be taught to recognize signs of theophylline toxicity.

(4) Oral preparations of theophylline include liquid, tablets, and capsules. Capsules (Theo-24, TheoCap, and others) can be given to young children by sprinkling the medication on food to facilitate administration and accurate dosing.

f. Leukotriene modifiers are indicated for the treatment of mild-to-moderate non-acute asthma by modifying the inflammatory effects of leukotrienes. (SOR **Ⓒ**)

(1) Preparations include orally administered zileuton (Zyflo), a 5-lipoxygenase inhibitor; zafirlukast (Accolate) and montelukast (Singulair), leukotriene receptor antagonists. These drugs offer better compliance because of their oral administration, especially with montelukast's once-daily dosing. However, they are less effective than inhaled corticosteroids, being indicated for mild intermittent and mild persistent asthma, and are less well supported in their ability to block lung inflammation and sequelae.

(2) Drug interactions with dabrafenib, clozapine, and gemfibrozil for montelukast and clozapine, theophylline, dabrafenib, amiodarone, warfarin, primidone, and tizanidine for zileuton.

g. Recombinant humanized monoclonal antibody omalizumab (Xolair), that blocks IgE, has shown promise in reducing corticosteroid dosage in patients with persistent and severe allergic asthma who aged 12 years and older. It is administered subcutaneously every 2 to 4 weeks, but its use may be limited by its cost.

h. Other drugs used to treat asthma:

(1) Antihistamines, which formerly were believed to have adverse effects on asthma, are now considered safe. These agents act as weak bronchodilators.

(2) Antiviral agents, such as ribavirin for treatment of respiratory syncytial virus, and oseltamivir for influenza not prevented by vaccination, may be helpful.

(3) Antibacterial drugs are useful for the treatment of patients with pneumonia, bacterial sinusitis, and other specific bacterial infections. Antibiotics are frequently overused in the treatment of patients with asthma, especially when atelectasis is confused with pneumonia.

(4) Expectorants and **mucolytics** (e.g., guaifenesin and iodides) have not been proven effective. Aerosolized acetylcysteine (Mucomyst) is contraindicated in asthma, since it may cause severe bronchospasm.

(5) Sedatives and anxiolytic agents are also contraindicated. (SOR **Ⓒ**)

(6) Immunosuppressive drugs such as methotrexate, cyclosporine, and hydroxychloroquine have been considered as therapy, but are not well accepted because of their potential toxicity, low efficacy, or both. **Tumor**

necrosis factor-α inhibitor infliximab may be effective in reducing the rate of exacerbations in patients with moderate asthma; (SOR ❸) however, trials are inconclusive.

i. **Immunotherapy,** also called desensitization, allergy injection therapy, or allergen immunotherapy, remains controversial, inconvenient, and expensive, but may benefit a few selected patients with allergic asthma. (SOR ❸) Immunotherapy also involves a small but significant risk of anaphylaxis and even death.

j. **Complementary alternative medicine** includes relaxation techniques, herbal medicines, vitamin supplements, dietary changes, acupuncture, homeopathy, and chiropractic spinal manipulation. Although these alternative healing processes are not recommended as substitutes for conventional pharmacologic therapy, they are used by up to 40% of patients with asthma in the United States and continue to grow in popularity.

  (1) Herbal remedies used to treat asthma have a worldwide origin involving hundreds of plants as well as minerals, animals, and mixtures of all three.

  (a) The **herb ma huang (ephedra)** contains ephedrine (a bronchodilator) and is perhaps the most commonly used agent. This drug was formerly included in several asthma prescriptions and nonprescription drugs, but the FDA has banned its sale in the United States. Ephedrine is no longer recommended to treat asthma because of its adverse effects including sudden death, high blood pressure, nephrolithiasis, and hyperglycemia.

  (b) Traditional Chinese medicine is widely used in the United States and involves the use of many unfamiliar herbs, some having been used for hundreds of years. The typical Chinese remedy may contain 10 or more herbs, including ma huang, gingko extracts, Cordyceps, reishi mushroom, flavescent sophora root, licorice, magnolia, and others. While some of these have some efficacy, their clinical value remains unproven. (SOR ❸)

  (2) Hydrotherapy (cold baths) is commonly used in Japan to open constricted airways.

  (3) Acupuncture is very popular, especially in Europe, and has been investigated in a number of controlled studies. It has not been shown to be as effective as conventional therapy. (SOR ❸) Deaths have been reported in patients with asthma who relied only on acupuncture and avoided conventional therapy. Furthermore, acupuncture carries some risks including organ puncture and infection from contaminated needles.

  (4) Relaxation techniques are designed to relieve stress, which is believed to aggravate asthma. These include yoga and biofeedback training, especially emphasizing breathing techniques. (SOR ❸)

  (5) Dietary supplementation to maintain normal levels of vitamin antioxidants, vitamin D, selenium, and zinc may improve asthma outcomes. (SOR ❸)

2. **Quick-relief medications**

  a. **Short-acting inhaled β_2-agonists** are most frequently delivered as aerosols through MDIs and, less commonly, as solutions via compressed-air nebulizers (Pulmo-Aide, among others). The MDI delivery system should be enhanced by the use of a reservoir spacer device (e.g., AeroChamber, Inhal-Aid, InspirEase, or Brethancer). Some spacers have masks that allow for infant and toddler use. Heliox-driven albuterol nebulization may be useful for life-threatening exacerbations. (SOR ❹) Inhaled β_2-agonists are most commonly prescribed as needed, rather than with firm dosage times, because of concerns about tachyphylaxis and adverse effects.

  (1) Preparations include albuterol (AccuNeb, Proair, Proventil, Ventolin), levalbuterol (Xopenex), metaproterenol (Alupent, Metaprel), pirbuterol (Maxair), and terbutaline (Brethine).

  (a) Albuterol (Ventolin, Proair HFA, or Proventil) is available in syrup, tablets, MDI, and nebulizer solutions for inhalation. The cost of albuterol inhalers has increased with the recent introduction of the HFA delivery system as generics are presently not readily available.

  (b) Terbutaline (Brethaire, Brethine, or Bricanyl) is available in tablets, MDI, nebulizer solution, and an aqueous solution for subcutaneous injection. It is classified as an FDA-category B drug in pregnancy.

      (c) Levalbuterol (Xopenex), the *R*-enantiomer of racemic albuterol, is available for nebulization (0.63 mg and 1.25 mg per 3 mL unit-dose vials). Levalbuterol may cause fewer adrenergic effects than albuterol while providing excellent bronchodilation.

    (2) Indications include the rapid relief of acute bronchospasm and prevention of exercise-induced bronchospasm. (SOR **Ⓐ**) These drugs are generally administered on a need basis rather than regularly scheduled. The inhaled route is preferred because of faster onset of action, fewer adverse effects, and greater effectiveness.

    (3) Adverse effects include tachycardia, nervousness, irritability, tremor, headache, hypokalemia, and hyperglycemia. The less selective β_2-agonists (epinephrine, metaproterenol, isoproterenol, isoetharine) are no longer recommended for therapy. Patients should be warned against overuse of these drugs (e.g., ≥ 200 puffs of albuterol per month) and encouraged to use more of their anti-inflammatory medications.

  b. Ipratropium bromide (Atrovent), an anticholinergic quaternary derivative of atropine, is indicated for the relief of acute cholinergically mediated bronchospasm. (SOR **Ⓐ**) This drug is frequently used with a β_2-agonist, but has a slightly slower onset of action. Tiotropium (Spiriva) may also improve bronchodilation in poorly controlled asthmatics.

  c. Systemic corticosteroids (methylprednisolone, prednisolone, prednisone) are indicated in doses of 1 to 2 mg/kg for patients with acute exacerbations of moderate or severe asthma. (SOR **Ⓐ**) They are usually given for 3 to 10 days and continued until the patients' PEFR is 80% of their personal best value. Prolonged therapy, ≥ 1 to 2 weeks, requires tapering of the dosage to prevent pituitary–adrenal–cortical dysfunction, but tapering per se does not prevent relapse of symptoms of asthma.

  d. Intravenous magnesium sulfate relaxes bronchial smooth muscle, may reduce inflammation, and appears to be beneficial for people with severe asthma attacks for whom bronchodilators and steroids are not working.

C. Bronchial thermoplasty is an experimental outpatient procedure performed through a standard flexible bronchoscope and uses catheter-delivered radiofrequency energy to thermally ablate airway smooth muscle. Ongoing trials show significant decrease in asthma exacerbations in moderate or severe asthma.

IV. Management Strategies. The 2007 National Asthma Education and Prevention Program expert committee applied evidence-based methods to review the scientific literature. The consensus panel's asthma management guidelines include recommendations to move away from a rigid categorization of asthma, and to identify separate but related concepts of severity, control, and treatment responsiveness. The guidelines recommended asthma care that includes assessment and monitoring, patient education, control of factors contributing to asthma severity, and pharmacologic treatment.

  A. Education is a critical tool in the care of the patient with asthma. Family members, teachers, and athletic coaches should understand the disease process. (SOR **Ⓑ**) Asthma support groups and camps for children with asthma can also be very helpful. All patients should have a written asthma action plan based on signs and symptoms and/or PEF. (SOR **Ⓑ**)

    1. Patient compliance is much better when patients are given the opportunity to acquire an adequate understanding of both the disease process and the prescribed medications.

    2. Office counseling should be provided to patients and their families, especially to patients with special educational or behavioral problems.

    3. Referral to an outside counselor may occasionally be necessary to provide parents with additional help in the management of the children with difficult-to-control asthma.

  B. Treatment guidelines. Classifying severity is emphasized for initiating therapy; assessing control is emphasized for monitoring and adjusting therapy. Asthma control is now as important as asthma severity in determining appropriate therapy, since asthma severity can change over time, and the emphasis is on the continuum of care of the asthmatic.

    1. Definitions. Severity is the intrinsic intensity of the disease process. Severity is most easily and directly measured in a patient who is not receiving long-term control therapy. Severity can also be measured, once asthma control is achieved, by the amount of medication required to maintain control. **Control** is the degree to which the manifestations of asthma are minimized by therapeutic intervention and the goals of therapy are met. A "rule of twos" may be used to describe control: in children under the age of 12 years, asthma is not well-controlled if they have had symptoms or used a β-agonist for symptom relief more than twice per week, had two or more nocturnal awakenings due to asthma symptoms in the past month, or had two or more exacerbations requiring systemic corticosteroids in the past year. For patients over 12 years of age, there must be more than two nocturnal awakenings per month to classify their asthma as not well controlled. **Responsiveness** is the ease with which asthma control is achieved by therapy.

2. A "six-step" stepwise approach to managing control is used to prescribe medications for increasing severity from **intermittent asthma** (step 1) to **persistent asthma** (**mild**, step 2; **moderate**, step 3 or 4; **severe**, step 5 or 6) (Table 68–4).

   a. **Stepping therapy up or down** is based on how well asthma is controlled or not controlled. The goal of asthma therapy is to maintain long-term control of asthma with the least amount of medication and hence minimal risk for adverse

TABLE 68–4. STEPWISE TREATMENT OF ASTHMA

	Step	0–4 Years of Age	5–11 Years of Age	>12 Years of Age & Adults
Assess control (Step up if needed; OR Step down if possible, and asthma is well controlled at least 3 mo)	1	*Preferred:* SABA as needed (use as rescue for all stages)	*Preferred:* SABA as needed (use as rescue for all stages)	*Preferred:* SABA as needed (use as rescue for all stages)
	2	*Preferred:* Low-dose ICS *Alternative:* Montelukast or Cromolyn	*Preferred:* Low-dose ICS *Alternative:* LTRA, Cromolyn, Nedocromil, or Theophylline	*Preferred:* Low-dose ICS *Alternative:* Cromolyn, LTRA, Nedocromil, or Theophylline
	3	*Preferred:* Medium-dose ICS	*Preferred:* Either Low-dose ICS + LABA, LTRA, or Theophylline OR Medium-dose ICS	*Preferred:* Either Low-dose ICS + LABA OR Medium-dose ICS *Alternative:* Low-dose ICS + either LTRA, Theophylline, or Zileuton
	4	*Preferred:* Medium-dose ICS AND Either: Montelukast or LABA	*Preferred:* Medium-dose ICS + LABA *Alternative:* Medium-dose ICS + either LTRA or Theophylline	*Preferred:* Medium-dose ICS + LABA *Alternative:* Medium-dose ICS + either LTRA, Theophylline, or Zileuton
	5	*Preferred:* High-dose ICS AND Either: Montelukast or LABA	*Preferred:* High-dose ICS + LABA *Alternative:* High-dose ICS + either LTRA, or Theophylline	*Preferred:* High-dose ICS + LABA AND Consider Omalizumab for patients who have allergies
	6	*Preferred:* High-dose ICS AND Either: Montelukast or LABA AND Oral corticosteroid	*Preferred:* High-dose ICS + LABA + oral corticosteroid *Alternative:* High-dose ICS + either LTRA, or Theophylline + oral corticosteroid	*Preferred:* High-dose ICS + LABA + oral corticosteroid AND Consider Omalizumab for patients who have allergies

SABA, short-acting β_2-agonist; LABA, long-acting β_2-agonist; ICS, inhaled corticosteroid; LTRA, leukotriene receptor antagonist.
Source: Data from National Heart, Lung, and Blood Institute, National Asthma Education and Prevention Program. Expert panel report 3: guidelines for the diagnosis and management of asthma. Bethesda, MD: National Heart, Lung, and Blood Institute; Revised August 2007. NIH publication no. 07–4051. http://www.nhlbi.nih.gov/guidelines/asthma/asthgdln.pdf. Accessed May 23, 2013.

effects. If very poorly controlled, consider an increase by two steps, or add oral corticosteroids or both.

   b. Before increasing medication therapy, evaluate exposure to environmental triggers, adherence to therapy, proper device technique, and comorbidities.

   c. Encouraging the **earlier use of inhaled steroids** is one of the preferred methods of management for mild persistent and more severe asthma. (SOR **Ⓐ**)

   d. Consider consulting an asthma specialist for moderate persistent asthma or for patients who are not well controlled (consider earlier consultation for children less than 4 years of age). In patients with nocturnal symptoms who respond poorly to therapy, diagnosis and therapy for gastroesophageal reflux should be considered.

  3. The **severity of an asthma exacerbation** in the urgent care or emergency room setting is classified as mild, moderate, severe, or life threatening, and the clinical course can be managed as per protocols given in Table 68–5.

  4. In **pregnancy,** asthma control should be checked at all prenatal visits and medications adjusted as needed. Taking medication is safer for the mother and fetus than having poorly controlled asthma. Inhaled corticosteroids are the preferred long-term control medication.

  5. Inactivated flu vaccine is safe in patients with asthma more than 6 months of age. Vaccination prevents substantial morbidity from influenza infection and its associated hospitalization costs because of complications. (SOR **Ⓐ**)

V. Prognosis

  A. Total remission of symptoms occurs in as few as 24% of patients with asthma by late adolescence or early adulthood. Most patients retain airway hyper-reactivity (as demonstrated by provocative testing).

  B. Onset of disease is not a reliable factor in predicting either the length or the severity of symptoms.

  C. Initial severity of the illness, especially the length of the episode and the need for hospitalization, is a more reliable indicator than the age of onset in predicting whether the child's asthma will persist into adulthood.

  D. Persistence of reduced pulmonary function and the presence of atopy (eczema, allergic rhinitis, and skin test reactivity to antigens) are associated with continued and more severe disease.

TABLE 68–5. CLASSIFYING SEVERITY OF ASTHMA EXACERBATIONS IN THE URGENT CARE OR EMERGENCY ROOM SETTING

Severity	Symptoms and Signs	Initial PEF (or FEV_1)	Clinical Course
Mild	Dyspnea only with activity (assess tachypnea in young children)	PEF ≥70% predicted or personal best	• Usually cared for at home • Prompt relief with inhaled SABA • Possible short course of oral systemic corticosteroids
Moderate	Dyspnea interferes with or limits usual activity	PEF 40%–69% predicted or personal best	• Usually requires office or ED visit • Relief from frequent inhaled SABA • Oral systemic corticosteroids; some symptoms last 1–2 d after treatment is begun
Severe	Dyspnea at rest; interferes with conversation	PEF <40% predicted or personal best	• Usually requires ED visit and likely hospitalization • Partial relief from frequent inhaled SABA • PO systemic corticosteroids; some symptoms last >3 d after treatment is begun • Adjunctive therapies are helpful
Subset: Life threatening	Too dyspneic to speak; perspiring	PEF <25% percent predicted or personal best	• Requires ED/hospitalization; possible ICU • Minimal or no relief from frequent inhaled SABA • Intravenous corticosteroids • Adjunctive therapies are helpful

ED, emergency department; ICU, intensive care unit; PEF, peak expiratory flow; SABA, short-acting β_2-agonist.
Source: Data from National Heart, Lung, and Blood Institute, National Asthma Education and Prevention Program. Expert panel report 3: guidelines for the diagnosis and management of asthma. Bethesda, MD: National Heart, Lung, and Blood Institute; Revised August 2007. NIH publication no. 07–4051. http://www.nhlbi.nih.gov/guidelines/asthma/asthgdln.pdf. Accessed May 23, 2013.

E. Control of the disease process through good pharmacotherapy is a known predictor of future disease. Patients with very poorly controlled asthma are more likely to have a negative outcome, and recent severe exacerbations are a strong independent risk factor for predicting severe exacerbations. In addition, early introduction of inhaled corticosteroids in high-risk children will control but not prevent asthma and may not prevent the natural course of asthma. Most children do not follow-up with a primary care doctor after an emergency room visit for asthma, and even those who do have not been shown to have a reduction of emergency room revisits and hospitalizations in the following year.

F. Mortality of patients with asthma in the United States continues to decline, with less than 3400 deaths reported in 2009. Mortality rates are higher in blacks, females, the elderly, and patients with coexistent chronic obstructive pulmonary disease. Historical events of concern for exacerbation with a potentially fatal outcome include previous history of respiratory acidosis with or without intubation, history of episodes of cyanosis, frequent hospitalizations, multiple emergency department visits during a short period, episodes of loss of consciousness, minimal response to a major therapeutic regimen, and presence of severe anxiety and depression.

SELECTED REFERENCES

American Lung Association, Epidemiology and Statistic Unit, Research and Program Service, November 2012. Trends in asthma morbidity and mortality. http://www.lung.org/finding-cures/our-research/trend-reports/asthma-trend-report.pdf. Accessed May18, 2013.

Bartholow AK, Deshaies DM, Skoner JM, Skoner DP. A critical review of the effects of inhaled corticosteroids on growth. *Allergy Asthma Proc.* 2013;34(5):391–407.

Chipps BE, Zeiger RS, Borish L, et al. Key findings and clinical implications from The Epidemiology and Natural History of Asthma: Outcomes and Treatment Regimens (TENOR) study. *J Allergy Clin Immunol.* 2012;130(2):332–342.

Doeing DC, Mahajan AK, White SR, et al. Safety and feasibility of bronchial thermoplasty in asthma patients with very severe fixed airflow obstruction: a case series. *J Asthma.* 2013;50(2):215–218.

Li P, To T, Guttmann A. Follow-up care after an emergency department visit for asthma and subsequent healthcare utilization in a universal-access healthcare system. *J Pediatr.* 2012;161(2):208–213.

National Heart, Lung, and Blood Institute, National Asthma Education and Prevention Program. Expert panel report 3: guidelines for the diagnosis and management of asthma. Bethesda, MD.: National Heart, Lung, and Blood Institute; Revised August 2007. NIH publication no. 07–4051. http://www.nhlbi.nih.gov/guidelines/asthma/asthgdln.pdf. Accessed May 23, 2013.

O'Byrne PM, Pedersen S, Schatz M, et al. The poorly explored impact of uncontrolled asthma. *Chest.* 2013;143(2):511–523.

Szefler SJ. Advances in pediatric asthma 2006. *J Allergy Clin Immunol.* 2006;119:558–562.

Wechsler ME, Kelley JM, Boyd IO, et al. Active albuterol or placebo, sham acupuncture, or no intervention in asthma. *N Engl J Med.* 2011;365(2):119–126.

Zeiger RS, Mauger D, Bacharier LB, et al. Daily or intermittent budesonide in preschool children with recurrent wheezing. *N Engl J Med.* 2011;365(21):1990–2001.

---

69   Cancers of the Breast, Lung, and Colon

Elizabeth R. Menzel, MD, & Kathryn Jacobe, MD

KEY POINTS

- Breast, lung, and colon cancers are common and are believed to follow the accepted two-hit hypothesis of genetic and environmental factors combining to create susceptibility and/or disease. (SOR **C**)
- Diagnosis of breast, lung, and colon cancers is based on pathology and treated based on TNM (tumor, node, and metastasis) stage. (SOR **C**)
- Breast cancer screening guidelines are established, but somewhat controversial. Mammograms have demonstrated a 15% to 20% relative reduction in breast cancer mortality in women aged 40 to 74 years. (SOR **B**)

- With the majority of lung cancer caused by smoke exposure and radon exposure, it is one of the most preventable common cancers. (SOR **C**)
- Screening for colon cancer by colonoscopy is recommended for all adults starting at age 50 years (earlier if high risk) and has a 95% sensitivity for cancer detection. (SOR **A**)

I. Introduction

Breast, lung, and colon cancers are three of the most common cancers in the United States. The annual US incidence of breast cancer is 135/100,000 women, lung cancer is 60/100,000 people, and colorectal is about 50/100,000 people. Most cancers are thought to result from a combination of factors, including genetic predisposition and environmental exposures (e.g., viruses, sunlight, tobacco, ionizing radiation, hormones).

A new diagnosis of cancer is always a sensitive topic and should be approached with great care by any healthcare provider who might be involved in delivering such a diagnosis. Generally, this news is best delivered face-to-face in a situation where the patient has appropriate support (e.g., family member(s) or other support person(s)) and is able to have the undivided attention of the healthcare provider discussing the news. Generally, patients need help determining their "next step" in diagnosis and treatment, and they often remember very little of the initial conversation of their diagnosis. Some patients describe being unable to process any information presented to them after the word "cancer." Appropriate follow-up is important to ensure the patient's medical and psychosocial needs are addressed.

II. Epidemiology

A. Breast cancer primarily affects women (99% of cases) with an estimated 232,340 new cases of invasive breast cancer and 39,620 associated deaths in US women in 2013. Excluding skin cancers, breast cancer is the leading cancer diagnosis in women, and the second leading cause of cancer death in women.

B. Lung cancer. Of the common cancers, lung cancer is one of the most fatal. More people in the United States die from lung cancer than any other type of cancer and it accounts for more deaths than colon, breast, and prostate cancers combined. It is the second most commonly diagnosed cancer in both men and women. The median age at diagnosis is 70 years and the median age of death is 72 years. Lifetime risk of lung cancer for men is 1 in 13, for women, 1 in 16 (when smokers and non-smokers are considered together). Race and gender account for some variation in incidence, with black men being about 20% more likely than white men and black women about 10% less likely than white women to develop lung cancer. The past two decades have shown a continued decline in lung cancer incidence among men, but women's rates have just begun to decline. In 2013, an estimated 228,190 new diagnoses and 159,480 lung-cancer deaths will occur in the United States, accounting for 27% of all cancer-related deaths.

C. Colon cancer is the third most common cancer for both men and women in the United States and globally. In 2009, 136,717 people in the United States were diagnosed with colorectal cancer (CRC) (70,223 men, 66,494 women). Estimates for 2013 suggest that there will be 142,820 new diagnoses and 50,830 deaths. According to Centers for Disease Control and Prevention (CDC) data, the incidence decreased by 1.6% to 3.2% from 2000 to 2009 and mortality also decreased by the same amount during that period, except among American Indians/Alaskan natives. Incidence and mortality remained stable in women. Five percent of Americans are expected to develop the disease within their lifetime. Risk begins to increase around age 40 years and increases more rapidly starting around age 52 years, doubling with every subsequent decade. Median age at diagnosis is 69 years and median age of death is 74 years.

III. Risk Factors

A. Breast cancer

1. Non-modifiable risk factors include the following:

   a. Increasing age is associated with higher risk of diagnosis. For example, a 30-year-old woman has a 1 in 250 risk of diagnosis over the next 10 years, whereas a 50-year-old woman's risk is 1 in 42 and a 60-year-old woman's risk is 1 in 29.

   b. Personal history of invasive breast cancer, ductal carcinoma in situ (DCIS) or lobular carcinoma in situ is associated with a higher risk of a new diagnosis of breast cancer and/or contralateral breast cancer diagnosis.

    c. Family or genetic history. The presence of one first-degree relative with breast cancer (independent of BRCA gene mutation) increases breast cancer risk almost twofold, whereas two first-degree relatives with breast cancer pose a threefold increased risk. Women with BRCA1 and BRCA2 mutations have an increased risk of breast, ovarian, and possibly colon cancers. Breast cancer tends to occur earlier in these women. BRCA2 is also associated with male breast cancer, prostate and pancreatic cancers, and lymphomas.

    d. Endogenous estrogen is a common link to many of the risk factors for development of breast cancer including nulliparity, older age at first birth, early menarche, late menopause, and possibly obesity. Estrogen and progestin cause growth of breast cells, and women with breast cancer have been shown to have higher endogenous estrogen and androgen levels.

    e. Dense breast tissue (noted on mammogram) carries a threefold risk of breast cancer compared to nonradiologically dense breast tissue.

2. Potentially modifiable risk factors include the following:

    a. Combination (estrogen plus progesterone) hormone therapy (HT) has been associated with increased breast cancer risk based on multiple randomized trials, including the Women's Health Initiative (WHI). A portion of the WHI trial was terminated early due to observed breast cancer rates; women who received combined HT had higher rates of abnormal mammograms, breast cancer and breast-cancer-related mortality than the women who received placebo. The increased risk was later noted to decrease significantly after stopping HT.

    b. Ionizing radiation exposure increases the risk of breast cancer. This risk has been observed in women with exposures such as fluoroscopy for tuberculosis and radiation treatments for Hodgkin lymphoma, acne, or postpartum mastitis. The risk increases with younger age at the time of radiation exposure.

    c. Obesity is associated with increased breast cancer risk, especially in postmenopausal women not taking HT. This risk factor was observed in the WHI trial.

    d. Alcohol consumption increases breast cancer risk by about 7% for each extra drink per day.

3. Factors associated with decreased breast cancer risk.

    a. Postmenopausal use of estrogen (without progestin) by women following hysterectomy is associated with decreased risk of breast cancer and breast-cancer mortality. Unopposed estrogen in women with a uterus is contraindicated as it increases uterine cancer risk

    b. Exercise is associated with decreased breast cancer risk based on observational studies. One large study found that heavy manual labor or exercising >4 hours per week decreased risk, particularly among premenopausal women with normal- or low-body mass index (BMI).

    c. Early pregnancy, particularly full-term pregnancy prior to age 20 years, is associated with decreased breast cancer risk.

    d. Breastfeeding. Every year of breastfeeding decreases the relative risk of breast cancer by 4.3%, plus 7% for each birth.

B. Lung cancer. For most factors below, the risk of lung cancer is even greater when the factor is combined with cigarette smoking.

    1. Cigarette smoking is the leading cause of lung cancer. In the United States, smoking causes 90% of lung cancers. At least 70 of the chemicals contained in cigarettes are known carcinogens. Smoking is associated with a 15- to 30-fold increase in incidence of and mortality from lung cancer. The risk is dose-related and smoking cessation decreases this risk.

    2. Radon exposure is the second leading cause of lung cancer. Radon is a naturally occurring gas that comes from rocks and dirt, specifically from the breakdown of uranium. Radon outdoors is not considered dangerous, but the gas can be trapped in buildings (basements) and become more concentrated. High levels are found in 1 of 15 US homes. Radon cannot be seen, smelled, or tasted. Radon causes 20,000 cases of lung cancer annually.

    3. Use of other types of tobacco including cigar and pipe smoke increases risk nearly as much as cigarettes.

    4. Secondhand smoke exposure. Annually about 3000 people in the United States who never smoked die from lung cancer caused by secondhand smoke.

5. Asbestos exposure. Most commonly used in mines, mills, shipyards, places with insulation, and textile plants. Smoking plus asbestos exposure often leads to mesothelioma (cancer of the pleura). It is not considered lung cancer.

6. Family history of lung cancer, specifically in first-degree relatives, increases lung cancer risk, likely through a combination of behavior, environment, and genetics.

7. Personal history of radiation therapy to the chest, with a higher risk if the individual was treated for Hodgkin disease or if a women was treated with radiation after mastectomy.

8. Other carcinogens. Risk factors include arsenic (found in drinking water from private wells), diesel exhaust, some forms of silica, and chromium.

C. Colon cancer. About 75% of CRCs occur in people with no known risk factors.

1. Inflammatory bowel disease. Crohn disease or ulcerative colitis increases risk likely from abnormal cell growth due to chronic inflammation.

2. Personal or family history of CRC or colorectal polyps. Greater risk comes with closer relationship, younger age of the related person at diagnosis, and larger number of affected family members.

3. Genetic syndromes—only 5% of CRCs are attributable to these which include familial adenomatous polyposis and hereditary non-polyposis CRC (Lynch Syndrome).

4. Health habits including lack of regular physical activity, low fruit and vegetable intake, and low fiber or high fat intake.

5. Obesity and overweight. The Nurses' Health Study found that a BMI of 29 compared to BMI <21 increased the relative risk for incidence of CRC to 1.45 (95% CI, 1.02–2.07).

6. Alcohol consumption. Many studies have shown links between alcohol intake and CRC, some of which indicate a dose–response relationship with increased consumption leading to increased mortality from CRC when compared with non-drinkers.

7. Tobacco use leads to increased risk of adenomas in general and increased risk of recurrent adenoma after polypectomy; risk increases after 20+ years of smoking. Based on the Cancer Prevention Study II, 12% of US CRC deaths in 1997 were attributed to smoking.

IV. Prevention

A. Breast cancer. In addition to avoiding modifiable risk factors and increasing factors associated with decreased risk, there are multiple interventions associated with decreased risk of breast cancer.

1. Selective estrogen receptor modulators (SERMs). Both tamoxifen and raloxifene reduce the incidence of breast cancer in postmenopausal women; tamoxifen may be slightly more effective, but there are no head-to-head trials for primary prevention. Tamoxifen also decreases breast cancer risk in high-risk premenopausal women. Both of these effects have been demonstrated to continue for several years after cessation of therapy. However, tamoxifen and raloxifene also increase the risk of cataracts and vascular events, such as pulmonary embolus and deep vein thrombosis. Tamoxifen also increases the risk of endometrial cancer.

a. The United States Preventive Services Task Force (USPSTF) and American Academy of Family Physicians (AAFP) recommend that clinicians discuss chemoprevention with women at a high risk for breast cancer and a low risk for adverse effects of chemoprevention. (SOR **B**) This guideline is currently under revision. The USPSTF and AAFP recommend against tamoxifen or raloxifene for primary prevention of breast cancer in low- or average-risk women. (SOR **B**) This guideline is also currently under revision.

2. Aromatase inhibitors/inactivators (AIs). These agents decrease risk of invasive breast cancer in postmenopausal women with at least one risk factor. AIs are associated with adverse effects including hot flashes and fatigue.

3. Prophylactic mastectomy reduces risk of breast cancer by up to 90% according to studies, but is associated with operative and postoperative complications including psychological effects such as anxiety, depression, impaired body image, and regret.

4. Prophylactic oophorectomies in women with BRCA mutations and prophylactic oophorectomies or ovarian ablations in women with a history of thoracic radiation reduce the risk of breast cancer by up to 50%. However, oophorectomies are also associated with operative and postoperative complications as well as menopausal effects (e.g., hot-flashes, sleep and mood disturbance, decreased bone mineral density).

5. Genetic testing for BRCA mutations can be used to identify persons at risk for development of breast cancer to aid in determination of need or desire for prophylactic therapies. BRCA mutations are associated with an increased risk of breast and ovarian cancer. By the age of 70 years, a woman with a relevant BRCA mutation is estimated to have 35% to 84% risk for breast cancer and a 10% to 50% risk for ovarian cancer. Based on this risk, the USPSTF recommends referral for genetic counseling (and possible BRCA testing) for women whose family history is associated with an increased risk for BRCA1 or BRCA2 mutations. (SOR **B**) However, they recommend against routine referral for women whose family history is not associated with an increased risk for these mutations. (SOR **B**) These recommendations are currently under revision.

B. Lung cancer
   1. Quit smoking/never start smoking.
   2. Avoid secondhand smoke. Do not allow smoking in the home or car.
   3. Radon testing in the home or workplace using qualified testers or radon detectors.
   4. Avoid carcinogens in the work place.
   5. Choose a healthy diet. Fruits and foods rich in carotenoids probably protect against lung cancer.

C. Colon cancer
   1. Daily aspirin (ASA) for at least 5 years reduces the incidence of CRC. In an American Cancer Society study, investigators found that regular users of ASA had 40% lower mortality rate for colon and rectal cancers. There is ongoing research into whether non-aspirin NSAIDs can reduce the risk of colon (but not rectal) cancer.
   2. Decreased dietary fat intake. Ongoing research, some of which is contradictory, suggests that lower dietary fat intake may be associated with less risk of colon cancer. Right now there is inadequate evidence to clearly indicate if this is protective.

V. Screening
A. Breast Cancer. Screening is a much-studied and discussed topic of scientific and media focus. Guidelines are varied and controversial.
   1. Mammogram screening has demonstrated a 15% to 20% relative reduction in breast cancer mortality in women age 40 to 74 years. However, the risks of mammogram include over diagnosis associated with treating cancers that otherwise would not cause symptoms or death. The risks associated with treatment of those cancers include surgical deformity, lymphedema, new cancers, and cardiac toxicity. Up to 54% of breast cancers are estimated to be a result of over diagnosis. Additional risk is associated with false-positive mammograms, which occur at an estimated rate of 50% of women screened annually for 10 years. Of those with false positives, 7% to 17% will have biopsies, which can complicate evaluation of future mammograms.
      a. The USPSTF notes a false-positive rate nearly double for women under 50 years compared with women older than 50 years. They also note a much higher number needed to screen to prevent one cancer death in women aged 39 to 49 years compared with women aged 50 years and older. False negatives (estimated rate of 6%–46%) are an additional risk, potentially delaying necessary diagnosis.
      b. Mammogram accuracy is affected by factors such as patient age, breast density, availability of comparison, tumor characteristics (mucinous, lobular, and rapidly growing cancers are less likely to be detected), and radiologist experience. Based on this evidence, national organizations have published guidelines that vary in recommended mammogram frequency, starting age, and duration of screening. These guidelines are outlined in Table 69–1.
   2. Clinical breast examination (CBE) has not been well studied. Evidence suggests that it may be associated with equivalent mortality rate compared with CBE plus mammogram. One study showed a sensitivity of 54% and a specificity of 94%. Risks of CBE include false positives (and associated risk of additional evaluation and anxiety) and false negatives, which can lead to delayed diagnosis.
   3. Breast self-examination (BSE) does not decrease mortality from breast cancer when compared to no screening. Research has also failed to find benefit from BSE in the rate of diagnosis of breast cancer or the tumor size or stage. Studies support that formal instruction and encouragement to perform BSE increases breast biopsies and diagnosis of benign breast lesions. Based on this evidence, some organizations are recommending "breast self-awareness" the recognition of the normal appearance and feel of one's breasts without systematic approach. Others recommend against this practice (Table 69–1).

TABLE 69–1. BREAST CANCER SCREENING GUIDELINES

Screening Modality	AAFP	ACS	ACOG	USPSTF
Breast self-examination	Recommends against	Counsel benefits and limitations	Breast self-awareness	Recommends against
Clinical breast examination	Insufficient evidence	Every 3 yr aged 20–39 yr, annually age 40 yr and older	Every 1–3 yr age 20–39 yr, annually age 40 yr and older	Insufficient evidence
MRI	Insufficient evidence	Offer annually with mammogram to women at high risk	Offer annually with mammogram to women at high risk	Insufficient evidence
Mammography				
Frequency interval	2 yr	1 yr	1 yr	2 yr
Screening age	50–74 yr	40 yr or older	40 yr or older	50–74 yr

AAFP, American Academy of Family Physicians; ACS, American Cancer Society; ACOG, American College of Obstetricians and Gynecologists; USPSTF, United States Preventive Services Task Force.

4. **Magnetic resonance imaging (MRI)** has a higher sensitivity than mammogram in detecting breast cancer; however, due to non-standardized approach, it has been associated with poor reliability. Some organizations are recommending use of mammogram in certain high-risk women, such as those with BRCA mutation in themselves or a first-degree relative, or women with a lifetime risk of at least 20% (Table 69–1). MRI is very sensitive but not very specific so women have an increased risk of biopsy.

5. **The Breast Cancer Risk Assessment Tool** from the National Cancer Institute is available online (http://www.cancer.gov/bcrisktool/) and estimates a woman's 5-year and lifetime risks of developing breast cancer based on the following risk factors: age, age at first menstrual period, age at first live delivery, race/ethnicity, number of first-degree relatives with breast cancer, history of breast biopsy, number and outcome (positive/negative) of breast biopsies, or history of at least one biopsy with atypical hyperplasia.

B. **Lung cancer.** Chest x-rays (CXRs) are not recommended for screening. The American Lung Association recommends low-dose CT scan for screening in some high-risk people. Risks include current or former smoker (has quit in last 15 years), AND age 55 to 74 years, AND at least a 30 pack-year history, AND no history of lung cancer. People with different risk levels should not be screened due to the lack of evidence of benefit. This may reduce lung cancer mortality by 20% and new guidelines are currently under development.

C. **Colon cancer** (Table 69–2)

1. People with known genetically based colon cancer syndromes (familial adenomatous polyposis or hereditary nonpolyposis colon cancer) and those with inflammatory bowel diseases should have their screening recommendations made by a specialist. They typically are screened earlier and more frequently.

2. According to the CDC, 6 of 10 deaths from CRC could be prevented if all men and women were screened appropriately. The screening rate in the United States is between 54.1% and 75.2%.

3. **Screening tests are shown in Table 69–2.** (SOR Ⓐ) High-sensitivity fecal occult blood testing (FOBT) uses antibodies to detect blood in the stool and is recommended every 5 years or yearly with Guaiac testing. Flexible sigmoidoscopy is used to check for polyps or cancer inside the rectum and lower third of the colon. Colonoscopy is used to check for polyps or cancer inside the rectum and entire colon. Colonoscopy is considered to be the "gold standard" for screening. It is 90% specific and 95% sensitive for detection of cancer. Other tests used by some to assist in CRC screening are digital rectal examinations and virtual colonoscopy.

VI. **Signs and Symptoms**

A. **Breast cancer**

1. Early, small tumors, which are the most treatable, are generally asymptomatic, which is why screening guidelines to enhance early detection have been developed.

TABLE 69–2. COLON CANCER SCREENING GUIDELINES

Who to Screen	When to Screen	How to Screen	Frequency
Adults from age 50 to 75 yr with average risk	Starting at age 50 yr	Fecal occult blood testing (FOBT) Sigmoidoscopy Colonoscopy	Annually or every 5 yr with high-sensitivity FOBT Every 3 yr Every 10 yr if normal
One first-degree relative with CRC or adenomatous polyps before age 60 yr	Age 40 or 10 yr before earliest diagnosis in family	Colonoscopy	Every 5 yr if normal
Two or more second-degree relatives diagnosed at any age	Age 40 or 10 yr before earliest diagnosis in family	Colonoscopy	Every 5 yr if normal
One first-degree relative with CRC or adenoma-tous polyps at age 60 yr or later	Age 50 yr (manage as those with average risk)	FOBT Sigmoidoscopy Colonoscopy	Annually or every 5 yr with high-sensitivity FOBT Every 3 yr Every 10 yr if normal
One or more third-degree relatives with CRC	Age 50 yr (manage as those with average risk)	FOBT Sigmoidoscopy Colonoscopy	As above
Familial adenomatous polyposis	Age 10–12 yr	Refer for genetic testing or annual screening by sigmoidoscopy	
Hereditary nonpolyposis colorectal cancer	Age 20–25 yr OR 10 yr younger than youngest age of colorectal cancer diagnosis in family	Refer for genetic testing OR colonoscopy every 1–2 yr	

Sources: Information from Zauber AG, Lansdorp-Vogelaar I, Knudsen AB, et al. Evaluating test strategies for colorectal cancer screening: a decision analysis for the U.S. Preventive Services Task Force. *Ann Intern Med.* 2008;149:659–669; Levin B, Lieberman, DA, McFarland B, et al. Screening and surveillance for the early detection of colorectal cancer and adenomatous polyps, 2008: a joint guideline from the American Cancer Society, the US Multi-Society Task Force on Colorectal Cancer, and the American College of Radiology. *CA Cancer J Clin.* 2008;58(3):130–160.

    2. Clinically evident breast cancer usually presents as a palpable mass, classically a hard, immobile, painless mass with irregular borders. Symptoms can also include breast thickening or swelling, asymmetry, ulceration, or retraction of the nipple.

    3. Additional skin findings suggestive of inflammatory breast cancer include erythema, thickening, or dimpling of the overlying skin (peau d'orange).

    4. Locally advanced disease can present as axillary lymphadenopathy. Metastatic disease can present with signs and symptoms associated with the location of the metastases such as liver (abdominal pain, nausea, jaundice), bone (pain), or lung (dyspnea, cough).

    5. Breast pain is usually associated with benign conditions rather than with cancer.

  B. Lung cancer. Often, people with lung cancer do not have symptoms until the cancer is advanced. Coughing that persists longer than 8 weeks should be evaluated with a CXR; worsening cough is also concerning. Other symptoms include chest pain, shortness of breath, wheezing, fatigue, unintentional weight loss, bloody sputum, recurrent pneumonia, and hilar lymphadenopathy.

  C. Colon cancer. Potential symptoms include bright red or dark blood in or on stool; change in stool caliber; diarrhea or constipation; persistent stomach pain; feeling of incomplete emptying; frequent gas pain, cramps, fullness, or bloating; unintentional/unexplained weight loss; feeling tired all the time; and nausea or vomiting.

VII. Differential Diagnosis

  A. Breast cancer. The differential diagnosis of breast cancer is based on the presentation:

    1. Breast mass. The differential of breast masses is broad (see Chapter 8). While it includes breast cancer, it also includes many benign conditions, including fibrocystic breast, simple cyst, fibroadenoma, fat necrosis, intraductal papilloma, and abscess.

    2. Abnormal mammogram. The description of abnormal findings on mammogram is determined by the Breast Imaging Reporting and Data System (BI-RADS), which classifies the likelihood an abnormality is benign or malignant. BI-RADS categories are numbered 0 through 6 and include incomplete, normal, benign, probably benign, suspicious abnormality, highly suggestive of malignancy, and biopsy-proven carcinoma.

3. Pathology. While pathology is considered the gold standard for the diagnosis of breast cancer, other diagnoses must still be considered. The differential includes DCIS (with or without microinvasion), benign breast lesions, and other cancers (e.g., Paget disease, lymphoma, breast sarcoma, Phyllodes tumor).

B. Lung cancer. The differential diagnosis for lung cancer is broad and depends upon presentation. It includes diagnoses such as infection (e.g., tuberculosis, pneumonia), chronic obstructive pulmonary disease, chronic bronchitis, asthma, congestive heart failure, and other cancers.

C. Colon cancer. Differential diagnosis for colon cancer includes other conditions that can cause bleeding or abdominal pain such as arteriovenous malformation, inflammatory bowel disease, irritable bowel syndrome, ileus, diverticulitis, ischemic bowel, infectious colitis, hemorrhoids, and anal fissure.

VIII. Diagnosis of breast, lung and colon cancer is based on malignant epithelial cells identified on pathology.

A. Breast cancer

1. Specimens are usually obtained by fine-needle aspiration (FNA), core-needle biopsy, or excision of a mass or lymph node. Cellular types include carcinoma NOS, ductal (intraductal/in situ, invasive, comedo, inflammatory, medullary with lymphocytic infiltrate, mucinous/colloid, papillary, scirrhous, tubular), lobular (in situ, invasive with predominant in situ component, or invasive), and nipple/Paget disease (NOS, with intraductal carcinoma or with invasive ductal carcinoma).

2. Receptor status is also an important part of diagnosis as it affects treatment and prognosis. Immunohistochemical assays are used to determine the presence of estrogen and progestin receptors. Additionally, some breast cancers overexpress or amplify the gene for human epidermal growth factor receptor (HER2), and it is recommended that an assay for HER2 be performed in all cases at the time of diagnosis. The preferred assay is controversial.

B. Lung cancer. Diagnosis of lung cancer is made using history and physical examination, CXR, contrast computed tomography (CT) scan, sputum cytology, FNA biopsy of lung, bronchoscopy, thoracoscopy, or thoracentesis to obtain fluid to send for evaluation by pathology, light and electron microscopy, and immunohistochemistry. Lung cancer is typically described as non-small cell or small cell.

1. Non–small-cell lung cancer is most common and comprises 85% to 90% of lung cancers. Treatments typically do not cure this type of cancer. Non–small-cell lung cancer may arise from the following types of cells:

a. Adenocarcinoma begins in the cells that line the alveoli and make mucous. Comprises 40% of all lung cancers. Occurs in smokers, but is the most common type found in nonsmokers. Adenocarcinoma tends to occur in the outer parts of the lung and is more slow-growing. **Adenocarcinoma in situ** (previously called bronchoalveolar carcinoma) has best prognosis of all lung cancer.

b. Squamous cell carcinoma, also called epidermoid carcinoma, makes up 21% of all lung cancers. Typically, this cancer is found in the middle of the lung, near a bronchus.

c. Large cell carcinoma comprises less than 5% of all lung cancers and can occur anywhere in the lung. It grows and spreads quickly and tends to be more difficult to treat.

2. Small-cell lung cancer comprises 10% to 15% of all lung cancers and occurs almost exclusively in smokers. It tends to start near a bronchus and spread widely throughout the body early in its course; consequently, treatments typically do not cure the cancer. There are two main types: small-cell carcinoma (also called oat cell cancer) and combined small-cell carcinoma.

3. Other uncommon lung cancers include pleomorphic, carcinoid tumor (rare, cured by surgery, better prognosis than non–small-cell or small-cell cancers), salivary gland carcinoma, unclassified carcinoma, and metastatic cancer from other sites (e.g., skin, breast, pancreas, or kidney).

C. Colon cancer. Colorectal cancer is a cancer that occurs in the colon or rectum. Typically, these cancers arise from adenomatous polyps, which are areas of overgrowth of the cells of glandular structures (parts of the colon that make mucus and fluid) that line the colon.

TABLE 69-3. COLON CANCER POLYP TYPES

Polyp Type	Features	Risk	Follow-Up
Hyperplastic	Occur in the descending colon and rectum, less than 0.25 inches in diameter BUT can be larger if they grow on the right side	Noncancerous	If <10 mm needs repeat colonoscopy in 10 yr
Adenomatous	Three types: villous, tubular, and tubulovillous Adenomas are the most common type (70%)	Potential to become cancerous	One to two tubular adenomas <10 mm: needs 5–10-yr follow-up 3–10 tubular adenomas <10 mm: 3-yr follow-up >10 tubular adenomas <10 mm: <3-yr interval One or more tubular adenomas ≥10 mm: 3 yr One or more adenomas with villous features of any size: 3 yr One or more adenomas with high-grade dysplasia: 3 yr
Inflammatory	Usually due to inflammatory bowel disease	Noncancerous	

Sources: Information from Ahnen DJ, Macrae FA, Bendell J. Clinical presentation, diagnosis, and staging of colorectal cancer. In *UpToDate.* Savarese DM, Grover S, eds.; National Cancer Institute. *Breast Cancer Treatment (PDQ®).* Bethesda, MD: National Cancer Institute. Updated May 9, 2013. http://www.cancer.gov/cancertopics/pdq/treatment/breast/Patient. Accessed August 2013.

1. **Diagnostic tests.** Colonoscopy can be both a screening test and diagnostic test. Diagnosis requires pathologic assessment of tissue, which can be accomplished if the patient has a polypectomy or biopsy. If the patient had an alternate initial screening test, they will likely need to undergo colonoscopy for diagnosis.
2. **The main types of polyps** are hyperplastic, adenomatous, and inflammatory. These are further classified by shape (pedunculated or sessile) and degree of dysplasia. High-grade dysplasia is associated with higher risk of cancer. The type of the polyp determines what further treatment and follow-up the patient will need (Table 69–3).

IX. **Staging**

A. **Breast cancer.** Staging of breast cancer is based on tumor, node, metastases (TNM) classification designated by the American Joint Committee on Cancer (http://www.cancer-staging.org/staging/). The goal of this staging is to group patients based on prognosis.

B. **Lung cancer.** Staging tests for lung cancer include MRI, CT, positron emission tomography (PET), radionuclide bone scan, pulmonary function tests, endoscopic ultrasound, mediastinoscopy, lymph node biopsy, and bone marrow aspiration and biopsy.

1. For details on staging of non–small-cell lung cancer, see http://www.cancer.org/cancer/lungcancer-non-smallcell/detailedguide/non-small-cell-lung-cancer-staging.
2. Small-cell lung cancer has two stages:

   a. Limited-stage small-cell lung cancer in which cancer is localized to the lung but may have spread to the area between the lungs or to supraclavicular lymph nodes.

   b. Extensive-stage small-cell lung cancer in which cancer has spread beyond the lung and mediastinum and supraclavicular nodes to other places in the body. The most common sites of metastasis are the adrenal gland, bone, brain, liver, and lung.

C. **Colon cancer.** Staging involves a clinical stage (physician estimate of extent of disease from physical exam, biopsy, and imaging) and a pathologic stage (combines factors used in clinical staging AND pathology results from surgery).

1. **Tests** used to perform staging include CT scan or MRI, PET, CXR, lymph node biopsy, complete blood count, and carcinoembryonic antigen (CEA) assay. CEA is a tumor marker, but can also be found with other types of cancer, with other diseases, and in people who smoke. Surgery is performed to remove the cancer and determine the spread through the colon and deep into the colon wall (often this includes samples sent to pathology).

2. **The staging system** can be found at http://www.cancer.org/cancer/colonandrectumcancer/detailedguide/colorectal-cancer-staged.

3. The most likely sites of colon cancer metastases are the liver, lung, and peritoneum.

X. Treatment

A. Breast cancer. Treatment is determined by taking into account the stage, tumor size, lymph node status, receptor status (estrogen, progesterone, and HER2), menopausal status, and patient's overall health.

1. **Breast-conserving therapy (BCT),** which includes breast-conserving surgery (lumpectomy) and radiation therapy, is an option for women with early stage breast cancer (clinical stage I, IIA, or IIB and some IIIA). Depending on other factors (e.g., receptor status, lymph node involvement, and tumor grade), adjuvant systemic therapy may be offered. The goal of BCT is to provide a mastectomy-equivalent survival rate with low recurrence risk and improved cosmetic outcome.

   a. BCT for early disease (no spread to skin, chest wall, or distant organs) results in survival rates equivalent to those of mastectomy.

   b. Women with the following factors are not candidates for BCT: multicentric disease, large tumor to breast ratio, diffuse imaging findings consistent with malignancy, prior chest radiation, pregnancy, and re-excision attempts with positive margins. Some women are candidates to undergo neoadjuvant systemic therapy and subsequently become candidates for BCT.

2. **Mastectomy** is recommended for women who are not candidates for BCT (or who are candidates for BCT but prefer mastectomy). Women who undergo mastectomy may choose breast reconstruction, which can be done at the time of surgery or at a later time.

3. **Lymph node evaluation** is performed by FNA, sentinel lymph node biopsy at time of surgery, or complete axillary dissection. This evaluation is based on risk of lymphatic invasion, which is related to tumor size, tumor location, histologic grade, and presence of lymphatic invasion of primary tumor. Breast cancer classically spreads initially to the axillary nodes, with rare involvement of internal mammary or supraclavicular nodes first. A sentinel node is considered any node that receives direct drainage from the primary tumor. **Sentinel lymph node biopsy is as effective as complete axillary dissection.**

4. **Radiation therapy** is performed in women with BCT as well as women with mastectomy who have a high risk of recurrence.

5. **Adjuvant therapy** includes medical interventions such as HT, HER2-targeted therapy, and chemotherapies.

   a. **HT** (SERMs, AIs, ovarian ablation) is recommended for hormone (estrogen or progestin) receptor-positive breast cancer. Some populations are targeted with specific agents. For example, AIs are the first-line adjuvant for postmenopausal women.

   b. **HER2/neu-targeted adjuvant therapy** (e.g., trastuzumab) is recommended for HER2-positive breast cancers (usually in addition to chemotherapy), usually for 1 year. Cardiac toxicity is a known adverse effect.

   c. **Chemotherapy** includes agents such as cyclophosphamide, doxorubicin, taxol, docetaxel, paclitaxel, and fluorouracil. They are used in varied combinations, although no combination has been proven superior to others. **Chemotherapeutic agents have been shown to decrease the risk of relapse and death from breast cancer in younger women.** However, they are also associated with multiple and often intolerable side effects.

      (1) Chemotherapy is used in multiple circumstances, including for HER2-postive breast cancers and as the recommended adjuvant for women with "triple-negative disease" (ER/PR and HER2-negative) as they are not candidates for endocrine or biologic therapies.

      (2) Women with triple negative breast cancer and small primary tumors should not undergo chemotherapy.

   d. **Neoadjuvant** systemic therapy is recommended for women with locally advanced breast cancer, with the goal of inducing tumor response prior to surgery and potentially allowing for BCT.

B. Lung cancer. Treatment options are determined based on staging (Table 69–4). Non–small-cell cancer is often treated with a combination of treatment modalities. Small-cell lung cancer is often treated with (only) radiation therapy and chemotherapy.

TABLE 69–4. LUNG CANCER TREATMENT OPTIONS BASED ON CANCER TYPE AND STAGE

Type of Cancer	Stage	Type of Surgery	Chemotherapy	Radiation Therapy	Other Adjuvant Treatment Options
Nonsmall cell	Stage 0	Wedge resection or segmental resection	No	No	Photodynamic therapy, electrocautery, cryosurgery, or laser surgery
Nonsmall cell	Stage I	Wedge OR segmental OR sleeve OR lobectomy	Yes, after surgery	Yes, primary treatment if can't or won't have surgery and can join a trial after surgery	Could do a clinical trial of surgery followed by chemoprevention OR photodynamic therapy through an endoscope
Nonsmall cell	Stage II	Wedge OR segmental OR sleeve OR lobectomy OR pneumonectomy	Yes, can try before surgery or after	Yes, primary treatment if opt not for surgery and can trial after	Could participate in trials
Nonsmall cell	Stage IIIA	Yes, if cancer may be removed, any of the typical surgeries OR if cancer is nonoperable, no surgery	Yes, before or after surgery OR for nonoperable cancer, chemo plus radiation concurrently	Yes, may combine with surgery alone or with surgery and chemotherapy OR for nonoperable cancer, chemo plus radiation concurrently OR radiation alone (if can't tolerate chemo) for palliation	Could participate in trials OR laser surgery to relieve symptoms and improve quality of life
Nonsmall cell	Pancoast tumor	May have surgery alone or after trial of combined chemo plus radiation or after radiation	May try combined chemo and radiation prior to surgery No chemo alone	May have radiation alone or radiation followed by surgery	Could participate in trials
Nonsmall cell	Stage IIIB	Yes, any of the types after chemo	Chemo followed by or concurrently with radiation or chemo followed by surgery	Radiation alone if not a chemo candidate OR radiation for palliation	Could participate in trials
Nonsmall cell	Stage IV	No	Combination chemo	Radiation as palliation	Maintenance with anticancer drug after combination chemo OR combination chemo + targeted therapy with monoclonal antibody OR targeted therapy with tyrosine kinase inhibitor OR laser therapy OR trial participation
Small cell	Limited stage	Any of the surgeries	Combination chemo and radiation OR if not a radiation candidate just chemo, either before or after surgery	Yes, in combination with chemotherapy OR radiation to the brain may be given if the lung cancer is gone to prevent spread to the brain	Could participate in trials

TABLE 69–4. LUNG CANCER TREATMENT OPTIONS BASED ON CANCER TYPE AND STAGE (Coninued)

Type of Cancer	Stage	Type of Surgery	Chemotherapy	Radiation Therapy	Other Adjuvant Treatment Options
Small cell	Extensive stage	No	Combination chemo alone	Palliative radiation to sites of metastasis OR radiation to brain to prevent spread	May participate in clinical trials

Sources: Information from National Cancer Institute. *Non-Small Cell Lung Cancer Treatment (PDQ®).* Bethesda, MD: National Cancer Institute. Date last modified May 30, 2013. http://www.cancer.gov/cancertopics/pdq/treatment/non-small-cell-lung/healthprofessional. Accessed July 31, 2013; National Cancer Institute. *Small Cell Lung Cancer Treatment (PDQ®).* Bethesda, MD: National Cancer Institute. Date last modified June 25, 2013. http://www.cancer.gov/cancertopics/pdq/treatment/small-cell-lung/healthprofessional. Accessed July 31, 2013.

1. **Surgery.** Surgical options include wedge resection (removes tumor and some normal surrounding tissue), lobectomy (removes entire lung lobe containing the tumor), pneumonectomy (removes one entire lung), and sleeve resection (removes part of the bronchus).
2. **Chemotherapy.** Multiple agents are used in both small-cell and non–small-cell lung cancer, sometimes as adjuvant therapy. In non–small-cell lung cancer, chemotherapy is generally used as an adjuvant to surgical intervention, although in patients with advanced disease, systemic treatments like chemotherapy may be the only option. Small-cell lung cancer, however, usually presents in late stage, so chemotherapy is a primary component of the treatment of these patients. For those who present at an earlier stage, radiation is used in conjunction with chemotherapy.
3. **Radiation therapy.** The type used depends on the location and stage of the cancer. For tumors in the airway, radiation can be given directly through an endoscope.
4. **Targeted therapy.** Medicines that prevent growth and spread of cancer cells.
5. **Laser therapy.** Uses a laser to kill cancer cells.
6. **Photodynamic therapy.** Uses a drug and special laser where the drug travels to the cancer cells and is then activated when laser light is delivered to the cancer cells. This treatment preserves healthy tissues and is good for tumors on or under the skin, in lining of internal organs, or in the airways.
7. **Cryosurgery** can be used to freeze and destroy abnormal tissue. The procedure can be done through an endoscope for airway tumors.
8. **Electrocautery** is the use of a heated probe or needle to destroy abnormal tissue. This procedures can also be done through an endoscope for airway tumors.
C. **Colon cancer.** The treatment goals are to decrease cancer burden, minimize side effects, extend life, and relieve symptoms. Treatment options vary based on the stage of disease. Options include
   1. **Surgical resection only.**
      a. **Stage 0.** Tumors at this stage can often be completely removed during colonoscopy, larger tumors may require colectomy.
      b. **Stages 1 through 3.** Usually requires partial colectomy or diverting colostomy.
      c. **Stage 4.** Surgery is unlikely to be curative. Partial colectomy plus, if possible, surgery to remove metastatic disease, if only small number of areas are found.
   2. **Adjuvant chemotherapy**
      • **Stage 1** requires no chemotherapy.
      • **Stage 2.** Chemotherapy is considered.
      • **Stage 3.** Six months of chemotherapy is recommended after initial surgical management.
      • **Stage 4.** Individualized approach, often involving chemotherapy.
      a. Research is ongoing using "targeted therapies," drugs that work on specific portions of the pathology of colon cancer. These therapies often have different and less severe side effects. They can be used with traditional chemotherapy or alone if typical chemotherapy is no longer effective. Examples include bevacizumab, cetuximab, and panitumumab.

TABLE 69–5. RECOMMENDATIONS FOR INTENSIVE FOLLOW-UP AFTER COLON CANCER

Stage	Colonoscopy Recommendations	History and Physical Examination	CEA Test	Chest/ Abdomen/ Pelvis CT
Stage 1	Colonoscopy at 1 yr, repeat at 3 yr, then every 5 yr If villous polyp, >1 cm polyp or high-grade dysplasia, annual colo-noscopy			
Stage 2 with no known residual disease	As above May recommend more frequently if colon cancer diagnosed at <50 yr of age	Every 3–6 mo for 2 yr, then every 6 mo for 5 yr	If the patient is a potential candidate for aggressive curative surgery, obtain at baseline and every 3–6 mo for 2 yr, then every 6 mo for a total of 5 yr	Annually up to 5 yr ONLY if high risk for recurrence
Stage 3 with no known residual disease		As above	As above	Annually for up to 5 yr
Stage 4 after curative-intent surgery and chemotherapy				Every 3–6 mo for the first 2 yr, then every 6–12 mo for a total of 5 yr

CEA, carcinoembryonic antigen.
Source: Information from Haggstrom DA, Cheung WY. Approach to the long-term survivor of colorectal cancer. In *UpToDate.* Savarese DM, ed. www.uptodate.com. Accessed July 2013.

3. **Adjuvant chemoradiation.** Usually targeted radiation plus 5-FU chemotherapy. This is only for patients with T4 tumors penetrating to a fixed structure or patients with recurrent disease. Health providers also use radiation to the tumor bed and any remaining surgical clips.

4. **Complementary therapies** can be added to treat symptoms: these include meditation, acupuncture, and peppermint tea for nausea.

5. After initial treatment, **intensive follow-up** is recommended because early identification of recurrence can limit severity (Table 69–5). Patients with a history CRC are at an increased risk for developing a second cancer, particularly in the first 2 years. There are no recommendations for monitoring with PET/CT. Patients should follow-up with their primary care provider for routine immunizations, cancer screening, medical care aimed at reducing risk factors for cancer and other chronic conditions, monitoring for late sequelae of treatment, and management of any treatment side effects such as chronic diarrhea or stool incontinence.

XI. Prognosis

A. **Breast cancer.** The prognosis is widely variable and depends on many factors including age, menopausal status, stage, histologic grade of the primary tumor, receptor status, and recurrence.

1. Overall 5-, 10-, and 15-year survival rates of breast cancer are 89%, 83%, and 73%, respectively. When broken down by stage at diagnosis, 5-year survival rates for local, regional, and distant stages are 98%, 84%, and 24%, respectively. However, these numbers do not necessarily reflect the effectiveness of current treatments (e.g., 15-year survival rates are reflective of patients diagnosed as early as 1991).

B. **Lung cancer.** Based on the data from 2006 to 2010, the age-adjusted death rate in the United States was 49.5 per 100,000 men and women per year. There are about 380,000 lung cancer survivors alive today. The overall 5-year survival rate of lung cancer based on SEER data from 2001 to 2007 was 15.6%. Estimates for 5-year survival for non–small-cell lung cancer by stage are Stage IA 73%, Stage IB 65%, Stage IIA 46%, Stage IIB 36%, Stage IIIA 24%, Stage IIIB 9%, and Stage IV 13%. For small-cell lung cancer, median survival for those with limited disease is about 15 to 20 months and for those with more advanced disease, median survival is about 8 to 13 months.

C. **Colon cancer.** From 2006 to 2010 in the United States, the age-adjusted death rate was 16.4 per 100,000 per year. Five-year survival rates vary based on the stage of disease as follows: stage I, 74%; stage IIA, 67%; stage IIB, 59%; stage IIC, 37%; stage IIIA, 73%; stage IIIB, 46%; stage IIIC, 28%; stage IV, 6%.

XII. Special Populations

A. **Male breast cancer** represents less than 1% of all breast cancer cases. Risk factors include radiation exposure, exogenous estrogen, hyperestrogenic states (e.g., Klinefelter syndrome or cirrhosis), and family history (e.g., BRCA2 mutation).

  1. Pathology most commonly reveals infiltrating ductal carcinoma. Overall, pathology is similar in men and women, but lobular carcinoma-in-situ has not been observed in men. Approximately 85% of the tumors are estrogen-receptor-positive and 70% are progesterone-receptor-positive.

  2. Staging is the same for men and women.

  3. **Treatment** for men includes modified radical mastectomy with axillary dissection. Lumpectomy with radiation has also been used with men. Surgical outcomes are similar in men and women. Adjuvant therapy is recommended in men under the same guidelines as women. Hormonal therapy is recommended in all cases with receptor-positive diagnoses. Tamoxifen side effects (e.g., hot flashes and impotence) are significant treatment limitations, but response to treatment is similar for men and women.

  4. **Prognosis** is similar for men and women, although on average, men are diagnosed at a later stage than women.

SELECTED REFERENCES

Ahnen, DJ, Macrae FA, Bendell J. Clinical presentation, diagnosis, and staging of colorectal cancer. In UpToDate. Savarese DM, Grover S, eds. http://uptodate.com. Accessed July 1, 2013.

American Academy of Family Physicians. Summary of Recommendations for Clinical Preventive Services. Updated October 2012. www.aafp.org. Accessed August 2013.

American Cancer Society. Cancer Facts & Figures 2013. Atlanta: American Cancer Society; 2013.

American Lung Association. Providing Guidance on Lung Cancer Screening to Patients and Physicians. Report on Lung Cancer Screening. April 23, 2012.

Centers for Disease Control and Prevention. Colorectal (Colon) Cancer. Basic Information About Colorectal Cancer. http://www.cdc.gov/cancer/colorectal/basic_info/index.htm. Last updated 2/26/13.

Centers for Disease Control and Prevention. Lung Cancer. Basic Information. Symptoms. Last updated July 15, 2013. http://www.cdc.gov/cancer/lung/basic_info/symptoms.htm.

Centers for Disease Control and Prevention. U.S. Cancer Statistics: An Interactive Atlas. http://apps.nccd.cdc.gov/DCPC_INCA/DCPC_INCA.aspx. Accessed August, 2013.

Haggstrom DA, Cheung WY. Approach to the Long-Term Survivor of Colorectal Cancer. In UpToDate. Savarese DM, ed. http://uptodate.com. Accessed July 2013.

Howlader N, Noone AM, Krapcho M, et al. SEER Cancer Statistics Review, 1975–2010. Bethesda, MD: National Cancer Institute, Updated June 14, 2013. http://seer.cancer.gov/csr/1975_2010/. Accessed August 21, 2013.

Levin B, Lieberman, DA, McFarland B, et al. Screening and surveillance for the early detection of colorectal cancer and adenomatous polyps, 2008: a joint guideline from the American Cancer Society, the US Multi-Society Task Force on Colorectal Cancer, and the American College of Radiology. CA Cancer J Clin. 2008;58(3):130–160.

Mandel J, Stark P. Differential Diagnosis and Evaluation of Multiple Pulmonary Nodules. In: UpToDate. Muller NL, Kin TE, eds. http://uptodate.com. Accessed July 1, 2013.

Morice AH, McGarvey, LM, Pavord I. Recommendations for the management of cough in adults. Thorax. 2006;61(Suppl 1):i1–i24.

National Cancer Institute. Breast Cancer Treatment (PDQ®). Bethesda, MD: National Cancer Institute. Updated May 9, 2013. http://www.cancer.gov/cancertopics/pdq/treatment/breast/Patient. Accessed August, 2013.

Tria Tirona M. Breast cancer screening update. Am Fam Physician. 2013;87(4):274–278.

US Preventive Services Task Force. Chemoprevention of Breast Cancer. http://www.uspreventiveservicestaskforce.org/uspstf/uspsbrpv.htm. Accessed August, 2013.

US Preventive Services Task Force. Genetic risk assessment and BRCA mutation testing for breast and ovarian cancer susceptibility: recommendation statement. Ann Intern Med. 2005;143:355–361.

Zauber A, Lansdorp-Vogelaar I, Knudsen AB, et al. Evaluating test strategies for colorectal cancer screening: a decision analysis for the U.S. Preventive Services Task Force. Ann Intern Med. 2008;149:659–669.

70   Chronic Obstructive Pulmonary Disease

H. Bruce Vogt, MD, FAAFP

KEY POINTS

- Chronic obstructive pulmonary disease is a preventable and treatable disease characterized by airflow obstruction that is generally progressive and associated with an amplified chronic inflammatory response to noxious gases or particles. (SOR **A**)
- Primary differential diagnoses include asthma, bronchiectasis, and congestive heart failure. (SOR **C**)
- The single most important factor to prevent COPD is avoidance of cigarette smoking. (SOR **A**)
- Spirometry is required to make the diagnosis ($FEV_1/FVC < 0.70$), but a combined assessment of a patient's symptoms along with spirometric classification and/or risk of exacerbations is important for appropriate management. (SOR **C**)
- Bronchodilators are the mainstay of chronic treatment, although inhaled corticosteroids are important in patients with more advanced airflow obstruction and/or higher risk of exacerbations. (SOR **A**)
- Surgery, including lung volume reduction surgery and lung transplantation, is only considered in carefully selected patients. (SOR **C**)

I. Introduction

A. Definition. Chronic obstructive pulmonary disease (COPD) is a preventable and treatable disease characterized by airflow limitation that is generally progressive. It is associated with an amplified chronic inflammatory response of the lung to noxious particles or gases. It also causes significant extrapulmonary effects, and these along with acute exacerbations and other comorbidities can contribute to the severity of the disease in individual patients.

The terms emphysema and chronic bronchitis are no longer used in the definition of COPD, although emphysema is one element of the pathologic changes of COPD and chronic bronchitis is a useful clinical designation. The latter is defined as the presence of a chronic productive cough for three consecutive months in two successive years.

B. Epidemiology. Over 13 million adults older than 18 years were estimated to have COPD in 2008; however, nearly twice that many have evidence of decreased pulmonary function, indicating underdiagnosis. The number of women with COPD has increased dramatically to the point that prevalence in men and women is almost equal. Preliminary 2011 data from the Division of Vital Statistics of the Centers for Disease Control and Prevention (CDC) indicates that unlike the other top three causes of death in the United States (heart disease, cancer, cerebrovascular diseases), the age-adjusted mortality rate for chronic respiratory diseases continues to rise. COPD is a leading cause of morbidity and mortality worldwide with an increasing social and economic impact. The prevalence of the disease is significantly higher in those older than 40 years, in smokers, and in ex-smokers.

C. Risk factors

1. Cigarette smoking is the major cause of COPD, accounting for greater than 80% of cases. Not all smokers develop clinically significant COPD and non-smokers can develop COPD. Cigarette smokers, however, have a higher prevalence of abnormalities in pulmonary function including a greater annual decline in forced expiratory volume in 1 second (FEV_1). Pack-years of cigarette smoking is the best but only one predictor of FEV_1. Environmental tobacco smoke (secondhand smoke) also contributes to the disease process.

2. Occupational exposure to hazardous airborne substances (e.g., dusts, gases, fumes), when intense or prolonged, is an independent risk factor for COPD and, when associated with smoking, increases the risk of disease. Indoor pollution from biomass cooking and heating in poorly ventilated dwellings is also a risk factor. Urban air pollution is harmful to persons with lung disease, but its role in the etiology of COPD is uncertain.

3. Alpha-1 antitrypsin deficiency is a well-established genetic abnormality that accounts for a relatively small percent of cases of COPD, but studies of the human genome

have demonstrated other genetic associations. An interaction between genetic and environmental factors influences disease susceptibility.

4. Factors that negatively affect lung growth in utero and during childhood may increase the risk of an individual developing COPD. Impairment of pulmonary function has been associated with maternal smoking during pregnancy, low birth weight, and early childhood lung infections. Although the pathologic process is different in asthma, bronchial hyper-reactivity appears to be a risk factor for COPD. Younger patients with chronic bronchitis who smoke have an increased incidence of COPD.

5. The specific and likely multiple reasons for the increased risk posed by poverty have not been determined, but this relationship has been established.

D. **Pathology and pathophysiology.** The pathologic changes in COPD are characterized by chronic inflammation and this inflammatory response to respiratory irritants is modified and exaggerated in patients with COPD. Oxidative stress may also play a role and is known to be increased during exacerbations. An imbalance between destructive proteases and protective antiproteases has been identified.

Chronic inflammation causes parenchymal (alveolar) destruction. This includes the protease-mediated destruction of elastin resulting in loss of elastic recoil. This chronic inflammation, along with fibrosis and luminal exudates, causes chronic narrowing of small airways and resultant airflow obstruction and air trapping during expiration. These pathologic changes lead to progressive decline in FEV_1. Hypoxemia and hypercapnia typically worsen with disease progression, and pulmonary hypertension can develop from loss of capillary beds due to scarring and hypoxia-related vasoconstriction of small pulmonary arteries.

II. Screening and Prevention

A. Generalized screening for COPD has not been found to be effective and is not advised. Assessment for the disease, however, including performance of spirometry should be considered in patients older than 40 years with dyspnea that is persistent, progressive, or worse with exercise; chronic cough or chronic production of sputum; exposure to tobacco, biomass smoke or occupational dusts and chemicals; or a family history of COPD.

B. Screening for patients with alpha-1 antitrypsin deficiency should be considered in patients who present with COPD prior to age 45 years, in patients who have no history of smoking or environmental exposure to other known risk factors, in patients with unremitting asthma or unexplained hepatic cirrhosis, and when there is a family history of the disorder.

C. The single most important factor in the prevention of COPD is avoidance of cigarette smoking. (See Section V below.) Attention should also be given to limiting exposure to all forms of tobacco, including secondhand smoke, as well as to other environmental and occupational risk factors such as organic and inorganic dusts, chemical agents, and fumes.

III. Diagnosis

A. **Differential diagnosis.** The primary differential diagnoses for COPD are asthma (Chapter 68), bronchiectasis, and congestive heart failure (Chapter 73). Bronchiectasis is a disease in which destruction of the structural components of the bronchial walls leads to permanent dilation of bronchi. Infection is the primary cause. Clinical features include persistent cough productive of purulent sputum and episodic exacerbations of increased sputum production and fever. Tuberculosis (Chapter 13), obliterative bronchiolitis, and diffuse panbronchiolitis are other diagnostic considerations in certain clinical situations.

B. **Symptoms and signs**

1. Chronic and progressive dyspnea is the cardinal symptom of patients with COPD, although chronic cough is often the first symptom.

2. Cough may initially be intermittent. Sputum production is variable and usually mucoid except during exacerbations, when it may become purulent.

3. Other cardiopulmonary symptoms of COPD include wheezing, chest tightness, and recurrent respiratory infections, which are often prolonged.

4. Anorexia, weight loss, and fatigue are common in advanced disease.

5. Anxiety, commonly due to dyspnea, and depression are also frequent problems in severe COPD.

6. COPD is characterized by acute exacerbations, and there may be shorter intervals between episodes as the disease progresses.

7. The physical examination is characteristically normal or reveals only prolonged expiration or wheezing on forced expiration with early or mild disease.

    a. With later-stage disease, hyperinflation is manifested by a barrel-shaped chest, hyper-resonance to percussion, decreased breath sounds, and distant heart sounds. Crackles may be heard, particularly in chronic bronchitis, and wheezing is common. In advanced disease, there is dyspnea at rest and may be cyanosis. The patient often uses pursed lip breathing during expiration and use of the accessory muscles of respiration. The latter may be exhibited by a patient sitting, leaning forward, and resting (supporting) their arms on their thighs or another surface (tripod position).

   8. Physical findings unrelated to heart failure can include a palpable but normal-sized liver due to chest hyperexpansion and neck vein distention as a result of increased intrathoracic pressure. When right heart failure is present, increased jugular venous distention, tender hepatomegaly, and peripheral edema are typical.

 C. Clinical assessment/diagnostic tests. Spirometry is required to establish a diagnosis of COPD; however, the diagnosis is made in the clinical context of assessing a symptomatic patient with risk factors. The extent and severity of the patient's symptoms, risk for exacerbations, and presence of comorbidities must be determined as well as the severity of the spirometric abnormalities as part of the assessment of the disease burden. FEV_1, however, correlates poorly with a patient's symptoms and quality of life and is a poor indicator of disease status. Staging, which previously was based upon spirometric classification alone, has been replaced with a combined assessment of symptomatology along with the patient's spirometric classification and/or risk of exacerbations.

   1. Symptomatic assessment can be aided through use of one of several validated and reliable instruments. The Modified British Medical Research Council (mMRC) Questionnaire measures the severity of breathlessness specifically, whereas the COPD Assessment Test (CAT) is a broader measure of impairment, which correlates well with the St. George Respiratory Questionnaire. The Clinical COPD Questionnaire is designed to detect exacerbations, but requires further validation. In addition, use of the COPD Questionnaire can be of value to the physician in providing individualized patient education. Symptomatic assessment along with a knowledge of previous exacerbations and spirometry are used to classify patients (GOLD categories A–D). (See Section III.C.3.)

   2. Office spirometry is necessary not only to establish the diagnosis of COPD but also to assess disease severity and monitor response to treatment.

     a. Measurements of airflow include forced vital capacity (FVC), FEV_1, forced expiratory flow rate over the interval from 25% to 75% of the total FVC ($FEF_{25\%-75\%}$), and the calculated FEV_1/FVC ratio.

     b. Active lung infection, hemoptysis, or an acute coronary syndrome are among the contraindications to spirometry.

     c. The Global Initiative for Chronic Obstructive Lung Disease (GOLD) uses $FEV_1/FVC < 0.70$ (postbronchodilator) as the diagnostic criterion for airflow limitation and hence COPD. Results should be compared to reference values based on race, gender, age, and height.

     d. The spirometric grading classification for COPD in patients with an $FEV_1/FVC < 0.70$ is determined by the FEV_1 as established by the GOLD criteria (GOLD levels 1–4) (Table 70–1). For standardization, testing is to be accomplished following administration of an appropriate dose of a short-acting bronchodilator.

   3. Combined assessment involves determination of a patient's current symptomatology, GOLD spirometric classification (FEV_1), and/or exacerbation history. Based on

---

TABLE 70–1. CLASSIFICATION OF SEVERITY OF AIRFLOW LIMITATION IN COPD (BASED ON POSTBRONCHODILATOR FEV_1)

In patients with $FEV_1/FVC < 0.70$:

GOLD 1	Mild	$FEV_1 \geq 80\%$ predicted
GOLD 2	Moderate	$50\% \leq FEV_1 < 80\%$ predicted
GOLD 3	Severe	$30\% \leq FEV_1 < 50\%$ predicted
GOLD 4	Very severe	$FEV_1 < 30\%$ predicted

FEV_1, forced expiratory volume in one second; FVC, forced vital capacity.
Source: Reproduced with permission from the Global Initiative for Chronic Obstructive Lung Disease (GOLD) 2013. *Pocket guide to COPD Diagnosis, Management and Prevention.* A Guide for Health Care Professionals. Updated 2013.

this system, patients are classified into four groups: A, B, C, and D (Figure 70–1). Patients in groups A and B (typically, GOLD 1 or GOLD 2 and/or having 0–1 exacerbations per year) are at a lower risk for future exacerbations, with group A patients being less symptomatic. Patients in groups C and D (typically, GOLD 3 or GOLD 4 and/or having >2 exacerbations per year) are at a higher risk for future exacerbations, with group D patients being more symptomatic.

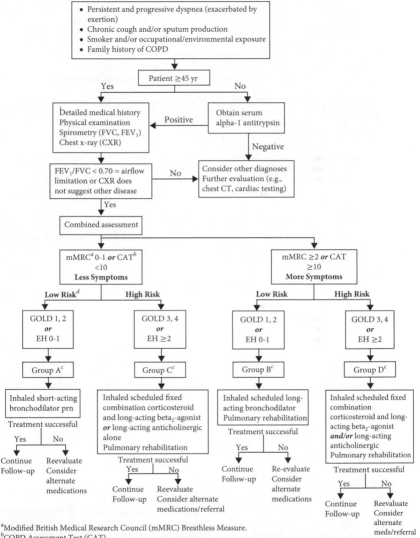

[a]Modified British Medical Research Council (mMRC) Breathless Measure.
[b]COPD Assessment Test (CAT).
[c]If there is a discrepancy in risk category (Groups A–D) as determined by the combined assessment-spirometric classification (GOLD 1–4) and the history of previous exacerbations (0-1, ≥2), the category denoting the highest risk should be used.
[d]Risk of future events as determined by yearly exacerbations, hospitalizations and 3-year mortality risk.

FIGURE 70–1. Approach to the patient with suspected COPD. COPD, chronic obstructive pulmonary disease; GOLD, Global Initiative for Chronic Obstructive Lung Disease; EH, exacerbation history; prn, as needed.

In classifying patients, symptoms are first assessed using either the mMRC or the CAT scale. Then, the risk of exacerbations is determined by either spirometry to grade the severity of airflow obstruction or by the number of exacerbations suffered over the previous 12 months. When there is a discrepancy between the patient's spirometric classification (GOLD 1–4) and the patient's history of previous exacerbations, the assessment denoting the higher risk should be used.

4. **Arterial blood gas measurements** are usually normal in early or mild COPD. They should be obtained in patients with an FEV_1 <35% of predicted; oxygen saturation of <92% via peripheral oximetry; or findings suggestive of respiratory or right heart failure, polycythemia, dysrhythmias, or an altered mental state. A PaO_2 ≤60 mm Hg (hypoxemia) with or without a $PaCO_2$ of ≥50 mm Hg (hypoventilation, respiratory acidosis) on room air is diagnostic of respiratory failure. An O_2 saturation of ≤90% generally indicates hypoxemia. Arterial blood gases should also be obtained if oxygen therapy is initiated and periodically thereafter. Finger or ear pulse oximetry can be used for follow-up of patients in both the hospital and outpatient settings, but is less reliable.

5. **Complete blood counts** are indicated to screen for polycythemia and when the patient is febrile and/or a superimposed infection is suspected. Eosinophilia suggests atopy and possibly an element of reversible bronchospasm (i.e., allergic asthma).

6. **Chest x-rays (CXRs)** are unremarkable in early disease, but abnormalities are apparent with advanced disease.
   a. CXR findings include hyperexpansion characterized by a low and flat diaphragm; increased anteroposterior diameter of the thorax; hyperlucency; increased retrosternal airspace; and a vertically positioned, narrow heart shadow. Bullae may or may not be seen and, if present, only indicate focal severe disease, not necessarily diffuse disease.
   b. CXRs are of value in ruling out other diagnoses, helping determine associated comorbidities, and at the time of clinical exacerbations. High-resolution computerized tomographic scans of the chest have a much greater sensitivity and specificity than CXRs, but are not part of routine care unless the diagnosis is in doubt or if a surgical procedure is considered.

7. Electrocardiograms are not routinely indicated, although in patients with long-standing COPD can show low voltage, right axis deviation, poor R wave progression, and, if cor pulmonale is present, may demonstrate right atrial enlargement (P pulmonale) and right ventricular hypertrophy with strain.

IV. **Treatment**
A. **Goals.** COPD is preventable and it is critical to address factors known to cause the disease and influence its progression. Although mentioned earlier, generalized screening is ineffective, early identification of patients with the disease is advised. Treatment of patients with established disease should be individualized and is directed at reducing symptoms of stable COPD to improve health quality of life and limiting the frequency and severity of exacerbations, the latter being associated with a more rapid decline in pulmonary function (FEV_1) and worsening health status. Treatment includes both pharmacologic and nonpharmacologic therapy. Although drug therapy does not reduce COPD-related deaths or slow disease progression, it can decrease symptoms (improve quality of life) and reduce the likelihood of acute exacerbation. Attention should also be given to comorbidities as concomitant diseases can markedly affect health status and mortality.

B. **Nonpharmacologic treatment.** Attention to smoking cessation, environmental control, surgery, home oxygen therapy, and pulmonary rehabilitation are among nonpharmacologic modalities discussed in section V.

C. **Pharmacologic treatment**
   1. **Bronchodilators** are the principal medications to treat COPD.
      a. Classes include both short- and long-acting beta₂-agonists and anticholinergic agents. Beta₂-agonists produce sympathetic-mediated bronchodilation, whereas anticholinergic agents reduce parasympathetic-mediated bronchoconstriction. Both reduce symptoms and improve exercise capacity (SOR **Ⓐ**). (See Table 70–2 for a listing of agents.)
      b. Long-acting agents are more convenient and effective (i.e., reducing dyspnea, improved exercise capacity, and improved health-related quality of life) compared with short-acting agents (SOR **Ⓐ**). Their duration of action provides more sustained effects, although consideration should be given to cost as they are more expensive.

TABLE 70–2. INHALED BRONCHODILATORS AND CORTICOSTEROIDS FOR COPD

Drug[a]	Dose	Major Side Effects	Contraindications	Drug Interactions
Anticholinergics				
Ipratropium Bromide[a] (Atrovent) *Short-Acting*	MDI: two puffs four times daily (max 12/d) Nebulized: 0.5 mg —three to four times daily (separate doses by 6–8 h)	Paradoxical bronchospasm, acute angle-closure glaucoma, cough, xerostomia, taste perversion, bronchitis		No known interactions where it is recommended to avoid concomitant use
Aclidinium Bromide (Tudorza Pressair) *Long-Acting*	DPI: one puff twice daily	Paradoxical bronchospasm, acute angle-closure glaucoma, diarrhea, urinary retention, xerostomia, nasopharyngitis	Caution in patients with hypersensitivity to milk proteins	Avoid coadministration with other anticholinergic agents
Tiotropium Bromide (Spiriva) *Long-Acting*	DPI: one inhalation capsule daily via two oral inhalations	Paradoxical bronchospasm, acute angle-closure glaucoma, xerostomia, urinary retention, upper respiratory tract infection, sinusitis	Hypersensitivity to ipratropium or lactose	No known interactions where it is recommended to avoid concomitant use
Beta₂-Agonists				
Albuterol[a] *Short-Acting*	MDI: two puffs every 4–6 h as needed for bronchospasm (max. 12 inhalations/24 h) Nebulized: 2.5 mg over 5–15 min three to four times daily (max. 10 mg/24 h)	Paradoxical bronchospasm, throat irritation, cough, tremor, ECG changes (arrhythmias, tachycardia), angina, hypokalemia	History of hypersensitivity to albuterol (cross-reactivity within class cannot be ruled out)	**Multiple Drug Interactions** Cisapride, amiodarone, dronedarone, phenothiazines, TCAs (QT prolongation), linezolid, MAOIs, TCAs (may potentiate albuterol effect on vascular system), beta-blockers (block pulmonary effect), terbutaline (risk of CV effects), theophylline (may augment bronchodilation response), diuretics (may acutely worsen ECG changes, hypokalemia)

(continued)

TABLE 70–2. INHALED BRONCHODILATORS AND CORTICOSTEROIDS FOR COPD (*Continued*)

Drug[a]	Dose	Major Side Effects	Contraindications	Drug Interactions
Levalbuterol[a] (Xopenex) *Short-Acting*	MDI: two puffs every 4–6 h Nebulized: 0.63–1.25 mg three times daily (every 6–8 h) as needed for bronchospasm	Paradoxical bronchospasm, tremor, nervousness, tachycardia	History of hypersensitivity to albuterol	**Multiple Drug Interactions** Cisapride, amiodarone, dronedarone, phenothiazines, TCAs (QT prolongation), other short-acting sympathomimetic bronchodilators, epinephrine (CV effects), beta-blockers (block pulmonary effect), diuretics (may acutely worsen ECG changes, hypokalemia), MAOIs or TCAs (increased levalbuterol action in vascular system), lobenguane
Formoterol (Foradil) *Long-Acting*	DPI: one puff twice daily (inhale contents of 1–12 mcg capsule every 12 h via Aerolizer inhaler) Nebulized: 20 mcg twice daily	Paradoxical bronchospasm, arrhythmias, diarrhea, nausea, chest pain, tremor, palpitations, dizziness		**Multiple Drug Interactions** Cisapride, amiodarone, dronedarone, phenothiazines, TCAs (QT prolongation), adrenergic agents, beta-blockers (block pulmonary effect), diuretics (hypokalemia), linezolid, MAOIs or TCAs (increased formoterol action in vascular system), methylxanthines (hypokalemia), steroids (hypokalemia and hyperglycemia), lobenguane
Arformoterol (Brovana) *Long-Acting*	Nebulizer: 15 mcg twice daily (max. 30 mcg/d)	Paradoxical bronchospasm, QT prolongation, arrhythmias, chest pain, diarrhea	History of hypersensitivity to formoterol (cross-reactivity within class cannot be ruled out)	**Multiple Drug Interactions** Cisapride, amiodarone, dronedarone, phenothiazines, TCAs (QT prolongation), linezolid or MAOIs (increased arformoterol action in vascular system), methylxanthines (may potentiate hypokalemia), beta-blockers (block pulmonary effect), steroids (may potentiate hypokalemia and hyperglycemia), diuretics (may worsen ECG changes or hypokalemia)

Drug	Dosage	Adverse Effects	Contraindications	Multiple Drug Interactions
Indacaterol (Arcapta) *Long-Acting*	DPI: one capsule/inhalation daily	Paradoxical bronchospasm, angina, atrial fibrillation, cough, nasopharyngitis; headache	Phenothiazines, history of hypersensitivity to other long-acting beta-agonists (cross-reactivity within class cannot be ruled out)	**Multiple Drug Interactions** Cisapride, amiodarone, dronedarone, phenothiazines, TCAs (QT prolongation), beta-blockers (block pulmonary effect), beta-agonists (risk of overdose), adrenergic agents (may potentiate sympathetic effects), steroids, xanthine derivatives (may potentiate hypokalemia), diuretics (may potentiate ECG changes, hypokalemia), MAOIs, TCAs (risk of CV effects)
Salmeterol (Serevent) *Long-Acting*	DPI: 1 (50 mcg) puff twice daily	Paradoxical bronchospasm, arrhythmias, throat irritation, headache	As for indacaterol	**Multiple Drug Interactions** Cisapride, amiodarone, dronedarone, phenothiazines, TCAs (QT prolongation), beta-blockers (blocks pulmonary effect), erythromycin (increases salmeterol concentrations, CV risks), linezolid, TCAs, MAOIs (may potentiate action on vascular system), other long-acting beta-agonists (additive effects, overdose risk), diuretics (may potentiate ECG change, hypokalemia), lobenguane
Corticosteroids				
Beclomethasone (Qvar) [40 mcg, 80 mcg]	DPI: one to four puffs twice daily (max. 640 mcg/d)	Bronchospasm, headache, hoarseness, oral candidiasis, HPA suppression		Amphotericin B, leflunomide, diuretics, natalizumab (beclomethasone may increase drug levels/effects), trastuzumab (may increase beclomethasone effects)
Budesonide (Pulmicort) (90 mcg, 180 mcg)	DPI: two puffs twice daily (max 1440 mcg/d)	Bronchospasm, hoarseness, oral candidiasis, syncope	Hypersensitivity to milk proteins	Potent CYP3A4 inhibitors (e.g., clarithromycin, indinavir, itraconazole, ketoconazole, nefazodone), warfarin (may increase anticoagulation), barbiturates, carbamazepine (may decrease budesonide effects), phenytoin (may decrease effects of each drug)

(continued)

TABLE 70–2. INHALED BRONCHODILATORS AND CORTICOSTEROIDS FOR COPD (*Continued*)

Drug[a]	Dose	Major Side Effects	Contraindications	Drug Interactions
Fluticasone (Flovent HFA: 44 mcg, 110 mcg, 220 mcg) (Flovent Diskus: 50 mcg, 100 mcg, 250 mcg)	MDI: two to four puffs twice daily (max. 1760 mcg/d) DPI: one to four puffs twice daily (max. 200 mcg/d)	Bronchospasm, headache, throat irritation, hoarseness, oral candidiasis, HPA suppression	Hypersensitivity to milk proteins	Potent CYP3A4 inhibitors (e.g., ketoconazole)
Combination Inhalers				
Albuterol/Ipratropium[a] (Combivent: 90 mcg/18 mcg per actuation) (Combivent Respimat: 100 mcg/20 mcg per actuation) (DuoNeb: 3 mg/0.5 mg per 3 mL)	MDI (Combivent): two puffs four times daily (max. 12/d) MDI (Combivent Respimat): one puff four times daily (max. 6/d) Nebulizer (DuoNeb): 3 mL four times daily (max. six doses/24 h)	See Individual Agents	See Individual Agents	See Individual Agents
Fluticasone/Salmeterol (Advair Diskus 250/50 mcg and Advair HFA 45/21, 115/21, 230/21 mcg)	DPI: one puff twice daily MDI: two puffs twice daily	See Individual Agents	See Individual Agents	See Individual Agents
Mometasone/Formoterol (Dulera) (100/5, 200/5 mcg)	MDI: two puffs twice daily	See Individual Agents	See Individual Agents	See Individual Agents
Budesonide/Formoterol (160 mcg/4.5 mcg) (Symbicort)	MDI: two puffs twice daily, 160 mcg/4.5 mcg per inhalation	See Individual Agents	See Individual Agents	See Individual Agents

[a]Available as generic.

MDI, metered-dose inhaler; DPI, dry-powder inhaler; ECG, electrocardiogram; TCAs, tricyclic antidepressants; MAOIs, monoamine oxidase inhibitors; CV, cardiovascular; HPA, hypothalamic–pituitary axis.

    c. Bronchodilators are either given on a routine basis to prevent or decrease symptoms or as needed for relief of acute or persistent symptoms. Short-acting beta$_2$-agonists are preferred for "rescue" over ipratropium as the latter has a slower onset of action. Long-acting preparations of bronchodilators are not suited for "rescue" as maximal effect is seen only after several hours.

    d. Inhaled preparations are preferred based on efficacy and side effects which are less common and resolve more quickly than with oral medications. (SOR **A**)

    e. Short-acting beta$_2$ agonists improve FEV$_1$ and reduce symptoms. (SOR **B**)

    f. Long-acting beta$_2$-agonists improve FEV$_1$, reduce symptoms, reduce the rate of exacerbations, improve quality of life (SOR **A**), and decrease the rate of hospitalizations. (SOR **B**)

    g. Long-acting anticholinergics improve symptoms, reduce exacerbations, and decrease the rate of hospitalizations (SOR **A**). They do not cause tachyphylaxis whereas this can occur with beta$_2$-agonists. Inhaled anticholinergics (short-acting and long-acting) have been associated with an increased risk of all-cause mortality possibly due to the risk of cardiac arrhythmias. Cardiovascular risk should be assessed prior to initiation of anticholinergic therapy.

    h. Combinations of short-acting beta$_2$-agonists and anticholinergics improve FEV$_1$ and symptoms to a greater extent than either alone. (SOR **B**) This may also prevent or reduce side effects that could result from increasing the dose of a single agent. This usually, however, increases cost.

    i. Combining a long-acting beta$_2$-agonist with tiotropium (long-acting anticholinergic) may improve health-related quality of life compared to tiotropium alone. (SOR **B**)

    j. Formoterol (long-acting beta$_2$-agonist) in combination with tiotropium appears to have a greater effect on FEV$_1$ than either alone. (SOR **C**)

    k. Proper technique for use of inhalers must be assured. Routine use of a spacer is preferred, particularly for patients less facile with their use and in the setting of an acute exacerbation.

    l. Theophylline, a non-selective phosphodiesterase, is reported to have effects in addition to causing bronchodilation. Given its narrow therapeutic range and the potential for serious toxicity, it is not recommended for routine use.

2. Corticosteroids

    a. Regular use of inhaled corticosteroids improves symptoms, pulmonary function, quality of life, and decreases exacerbations in patients with FEV$_1$ <60% of predicted. (SOR **A**) Corticosteroids are not recommended as monotherapy for COPD and do not alter the natural history of COPD, FEV$_1$, or mortality rates. (SOR **A**)

    b. Corticosteroids used along with long-acting beta$_2$-agonist bronchodilators produce a greater improvement in pulmonary function, improve health status, and decrease the frequency of exacerbations in patients with moderate (SOR **B**) to very severe COPD. (SOR **A**) An association between corticosteroids and increased risk of pneumonia has been reported. (SOR **A**)

    c. Long-term use of oral corticosteroids is not recommended due to serious side effects including osteoporosis, steroid myopathy, cataracts, glaucoma, and adrenal suppression. Inhaled corticosteroids may increase the risk for pneumonia and osteoporosis/bone fracture and their long-term use is associated with increase in the risk for cataracts and glaucoma.

    d. Table 70–2 lists bronchodilator/corticosteroid combination agents.

3. Phosphodiesterase-4 (PDE4) inhibitors

    a. PDE4 inhibitors improve lung function and decrease the likelihood of exacerbations, however, have little impact on symptoms or quality of life. They may reduce exacerbations in patients with severe COPD, chronic bronchitis, and a history of frequent exacerbations, (SOR **B**) and also decrease hospitalizations.

    b. PDE4 inhibitors should only be used in combination with a long-acting bronchodilator.

4. Antibiotics. There is no benefit to chemoprophylaxis with antibiotics in patients with COPD, (SOR **B**) although they are indicated in acute exacerbations (see IV.E.10.d).

5. Immunizations

    a. Annual influenza vaccination is important and has been shown to be effective in decreasing serious lower respiratory illnesses and death. (SOR **A**)

    b. In addition to its recommended use in all patients aged 65 years or older, pneumococcal polysaccharide vaccine is indicated in younger patients with COPD who have serious concomitant illnesses.

TABLE 70–3. COMMON ORAL ANTIBIOTICS FOR CHRONIC COPD EXACERBATIONS

Drug[a]	Dose	Major Side Effects	Contraindications	Drug Interactions
First-Line Agents				
Sulfamethoxazole/ Trimethoprim[a,b] (Bactrim, Septra, Sulfatrim)	160 mg/800 mg twice daily for 14 days	Anorexia, nausea, vomiting, rash, Stevens–Johnson syndrome, toxic epidermal necrolysis, fulminant hepatic necrosis, agranulocytosis	History of sulfonamide or trimethoprim-induced immune thrombocytopenia or hypersensitivity, marked hepatic damage, folate-deficient megaloblastic anemia, nursing or pregnancy, severe renal insufficiency	**Multiple Drug Interactions** Dofetilide, methenamine bepridil, thioridazine, levomethadyl, mesoridazine, cisapride, terfenadine, pimozide, gemifloxacin, TCAs (QT prolongation), warfarin (increased bleeding), ACE inhibitors (hyperkalemia, cardiac effects), diuretics (primarily thiazides; thrombocytopenia), phenytoin (increased phenytoin levels), MTX (MTX toxicity)
Tetracycline[c] (Sumycin)	500 mg four times daily	Nausea/Vomiting, diarrhea, anaphylaxis, angioedema, photosensitivity	Pregnancy, concomitant use of acitretin and other retinoic acid derivatives (increased intracranial pressure), methoxyflurane (nephrotoxicity)	Digoxin (digoxin toxicity), aluminum, calcium, magnesium-containing antacids (drug binding, decreased efficacy), anticoagulants (bleeding)
Doxycycline[c] (Vibramycin, Doryx, Monodox)	100 mg twice daily	Anaphylaxis, angioedema, photosensitivity	Hypersensitivity to tetracycline, concomitant use of Acitretin and other retinoic acid derivatives (increased intracranial pressure), pregnancy	See tetracycline MTX (MTX toxicity), methoxyflurane (nephrotoxicity)
Erythromycin (Eryc, E-Mycin, EES)[c]	250 mg every 6 h, **or** 500 mg every 12 h, **or** 333 mg every 8 h	QT prolongation, ventricular arrhythmias, hepatitis, nausea/ vomiting, diarrhea		**Multiple Drug Interactions** Amiodarone, dronedarone, dofetilide, cisapride, ergot alkaloids, pimozide, terfenadine, TCAs (QT prolongation), simvastatin, lovastatin, atorvastatin (myopathy), sertraline (serotonin syndrome), everolimus (everolimus toxicity), ranolazine (increased ranolazine levels)
Second-Line Agents				
Amoxicillin[d] (Amoxil, Polymox, Trimox)	250–500 mg three times daily	Diarrhea, anaphylaxis, urticaria, Stevens–Johnson Syndrome, erythema multiforme, serum sickness, toxic epidermal necrolysis	Hypersensitivity to other beta-lactam antibiotic	Probenecid (increased or prolonged amoxicillin levels), OCs (reduced OC effectiveness), MTX (risk of MTX toxicity), venlafaxine (risk of serotonin syndrome), warfarin (risk of bleeding)

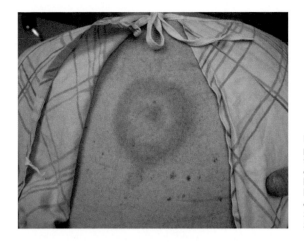

FIGURE 7–1. A 32-year-old woman presents having 5 days of low-grade fevers and the typical eruption of erythema migrans on her upper back. Note the expanding annular lesion with a target-like morphology. (Used with permission from Gil Shlamovitz, MD.) (www.VisualDx-Series.com)

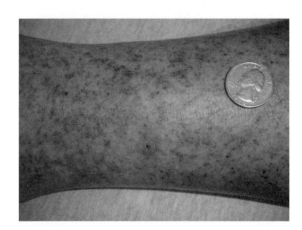

FIGURE 7–2. Rocky Mountain spotted fever with many petechiae visible around the original tick bite. This rickettsial disease looks similar to vasculitis (Used with permission of Tom Moore, MD.)

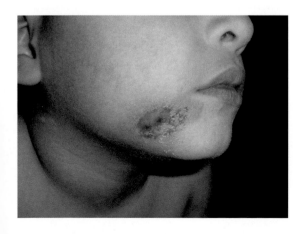

FIGURE 9–1. Impetigo. (Used with permission of Dr. Richard Usatine.)

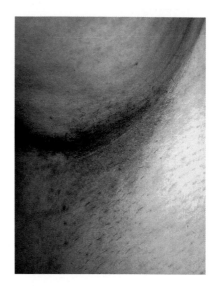

FIGURE 9–2. Erythrasma. (Used with permission of Dr. Richard Usatine.)

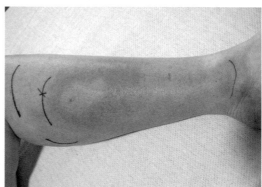

FIGURE 9–3. **Cellulitis.**

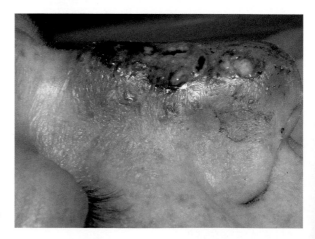

FIGURE 9–4. Carbuncle of the nose.

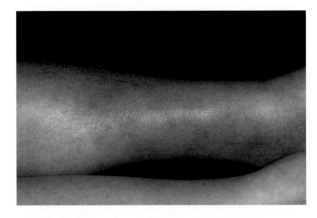

FIGURE 9–5. Erysipelas. (Used with permission of Dr. Richard Usatine.)

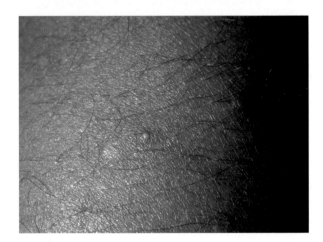

FIGURE 9–6. Folliculitis. (Used with permission of Dr. Richard Usatine.)

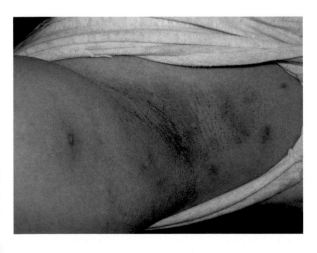

FIGURE 9–7. Hidradenitis suppurativa. (Used with permission of Dr. Richard Usatine.)

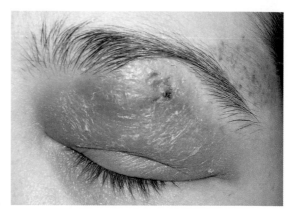

FIGURE 9–9. **Periorbital cellulitis.**

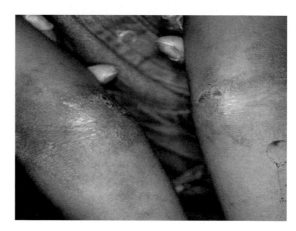

FIGURE 14–1. Atopic dermatitis. (This photograph has been taken by and is the property of Dick Anstett, MD, MPH. Faculty, Family Medicine Residency of Idaho, Boise, Idaho.)

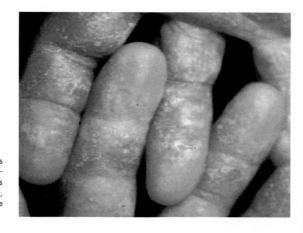

FIGURE 14–2. Contact dermatitis from dishwasher water. (This photograph has been taken by and is the property of Dick Anstett, MD, MPH. Faculty, Family Medicine Residency of Idaho, Boise, Idaho.)

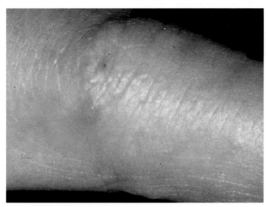

FIGURE 14–3. Scabies. (This photograph has been taken by and is the property of Dick Anstett, MD, MPH. Faculty, Family Medicine Residency of Idaho, Boise, Idaho.)

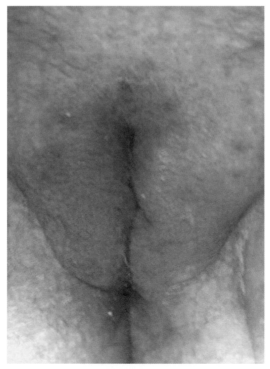

FIGURE 14–4. Lichen simplex chronicus. (This photograph has been taken by and is the property of Dick Anstett, MD, MPH. Faculty, Family Medicine Residency of Idaho, Boise, Idaho.)

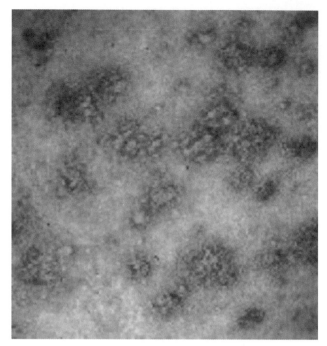

FIGURE 14–5. Lichen planus. (This photograph has been taken by and is the property of Dick Anstett, MD, MPH. Faculty, Family Medicine Residency of Idaho, Boise, Idaho.)

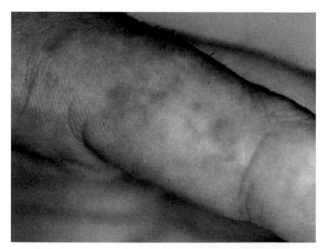

FIGURE 14–6. Dyshidrotic eczema. (This photograph has been taken by and is the property of Dick Anstett, MD, MPH. Faculty, Family Medicine Residency of Idaho, Boise, Idaho.)

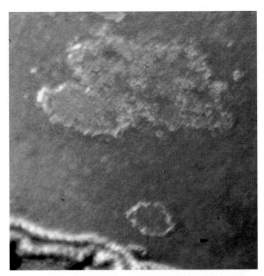

FIGURE 14–7. Herald patch, pityriasis rosea. (This photograph has been taken by and is the property of Dick Anstett, MD, MPH. Faculty, Family Medicine Residency of Idaho, Boise, Idaho.)

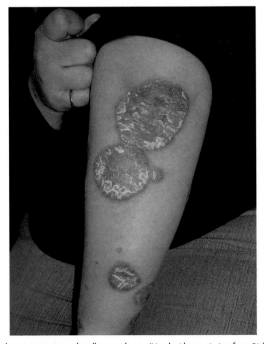

FIGURE 14–8. Typical plaque psoriasis on the elbow and arm. (Used with permission from Richard P. Usatine, MD.)

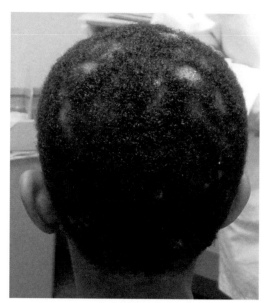

FIGURE 14–9. Tinea capitis in a young black boy. (Used with permission from Richard P. Usatine, MD.)

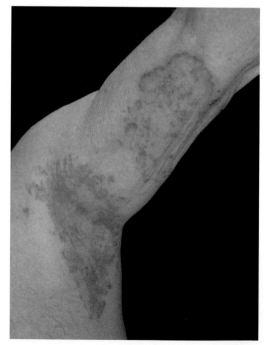

FIGURE 14–10. Extensive tinea corporis in the axilla and arm of this older adult. (Used with permission from Richard P. Usatine, MD.)

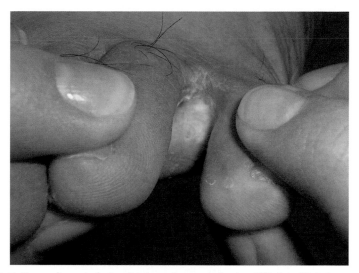

FIGURE 14–11. Tinea pedis seen in the interdigital space between the fourth and fifth digits. This is the most common area to see tinea pedis. (Used with permission from Richard P. Usatine, MD.)

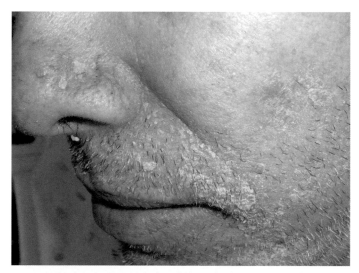

FIGURE 14–12. Severe seborrheic dermatitis on the face of a hospitalized man. The stress of his illness has worsened the otherwise mild seborrhea. (Used with permission from Richard P. Usatine, MD.)

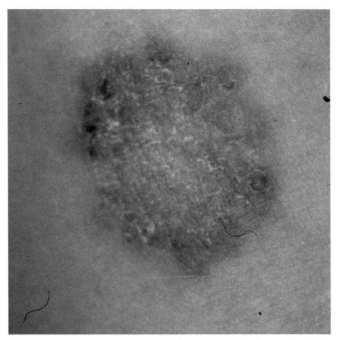

FIGURE 14–13. Nummular eczema. (This photograph has been taken by and is the property of Dick Anstett, MD, MPH. Faculty, Family Medicine Residency of Idaho, Boise, Idaho.)

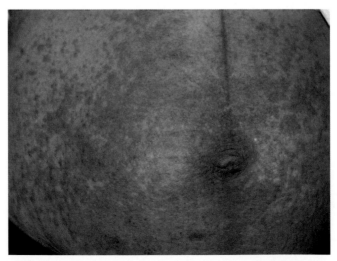

FIGURE 14–14. PUPP. (This photograph has been taken by and is the property of Dick Anstett, MD, MPH. Faculty, Family Medicine Residency of Idaho, Boise, Idaho.)

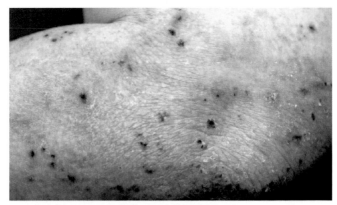

FIGURE 14–15. Delusion of parasitosis. (This photograph has been taken by and is the property of Dick Anstett, MD, MPH. Faculty, Family Medicine Residency of Idaho, Boise, Idaho.)

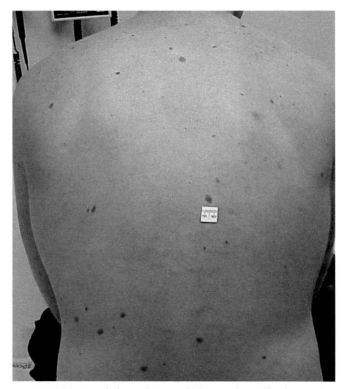

FIGURE 15–1. AMS; note multiple macular to papular lesions with variable coloring and size.

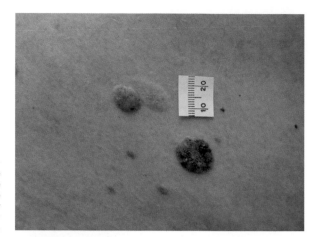

FIGURE 15–2. Multiple macular cherry angiomas. More advanced lesions may be raised or even polypoid. Note several verrucous irregularly pigmented seborrheic keratoses which are also age related.

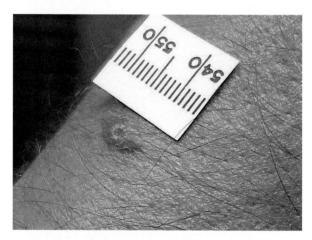

FIGURE 15–3. Keratoacanthoma with raised borders and central keratin plug.

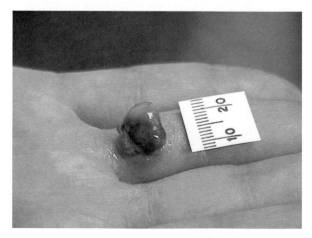

FIGURE 15–4. Pyogenic granuloma with glistening fragile overgrowth of capillaries and epithelium.

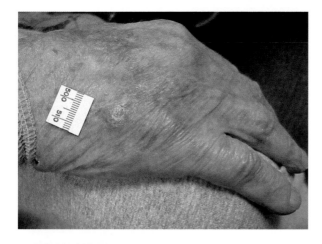

FIGURE 15–5. Actinic keratosis which has reached the raised actinic horn stage and also note the diffuse raised erythematous base of progression to squamous cell cancer.

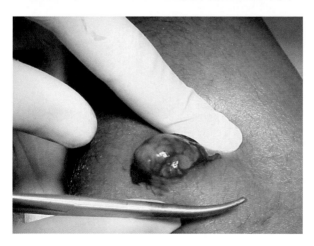

FIGURE 15–6. Basal cell cancer. Note similar appearance to keratoacanthoma with raised borders, but has telangiectasias and central ulceration.

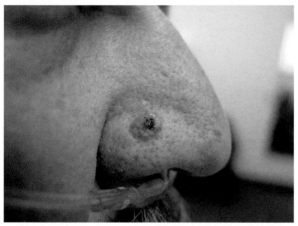

FIGURE 15–7. Lipoma with capsule being expressed after blunt dissection from a relatively small incision.

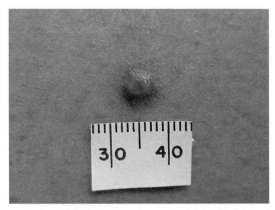

FIGURE 15–8. Dermatofibroma typically pigmented and sometimes raised.

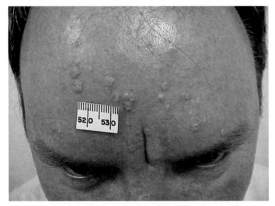

FIGURE 15–9. Sebaceous hyperplasia, common on the forehead and face looks similar to early BCCs, but is often seen as multiple lesions.

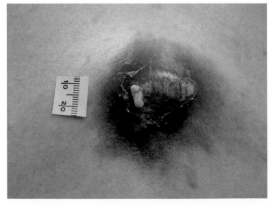

FIGURE 15–10. Epidermal cyst which has become infected, inflamed, and painful which requires incision and drainage.

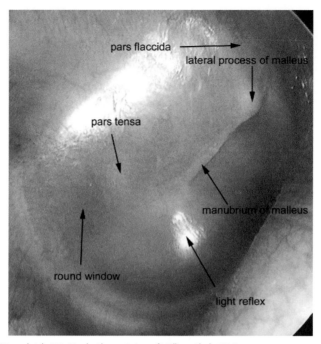

FIGURE 22–1. Normal right TM. (Used with permission of William Clark, MD.)

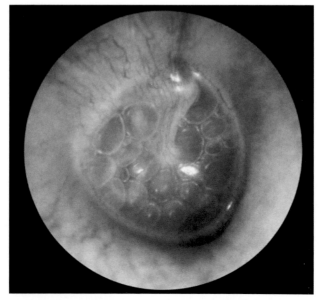

FIGURE 22–2. OME (otitis media with effusion) in the right ear. Note multiple air-fluid levels in this slightly retracted, translucent, nonerythematous TM. (Used with permission of Frank Miller, MD.)

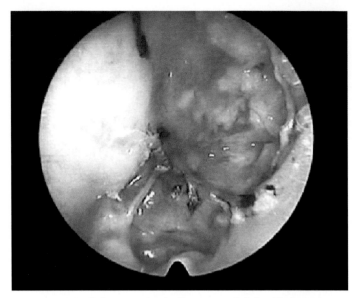

FIGURE 22–3. Cholesteatoma. (Used with permission of Vladimir Zlinsky, MD.)

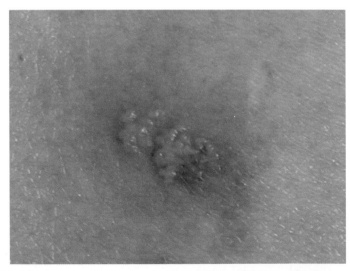

FIGURE 30–1. Tightly grouped vesicles 1 to 3 mm in diameter forming a lobulated irregular plaque over a larger erythematous base represent a herpetic lesion about 2-day-old. (Reproduced with permission from Tomás P. Owens, Jr., MD.)

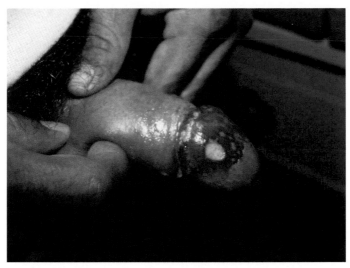

FIGURE 30–2. Primary syphilis with a large chancre on the glands of the penis. The multiple small surrounding ulcers are part of the syphilis and not a second disease. (Used with permission from Richard P. Usatine, MD.)

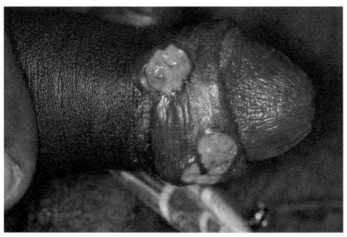

FIGURE 30–3. Culture-proven indurated beefy chancroid lesions in an HIV-positive man. (Used with permission from Richard P. Usatine, MD.)

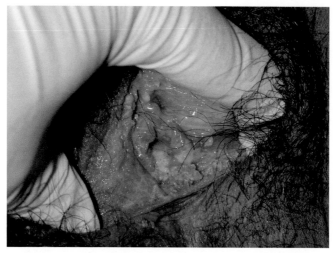

FIGURE 30–4. A peach-colored cauliflower-like lesion is noted on the comisure of the labia majora immediately caudal to the fourchette. Single coniform lighter pink lesions are also present at the R periurethral area, R superior labia majora, and L labia minora. (Used with permission from Tomás P. Owens, Jr., MD.)

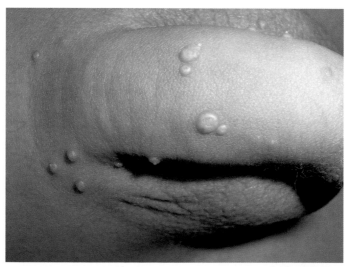

FIGURE 30–5. Molluscum contagiosum on and around the penis of a young boy. There was no evidence for sexual abuse. (Used with permission from Richard P. Usatine, MD.)

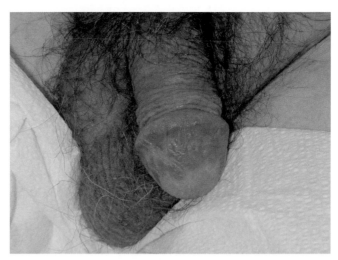

FIGURE 30–6. Irregular erythematous plaques following cleansing of smegma and debris. These lesions completely disappeared after topical antifungals, confirming the absence of Bowenoid disease. (Used with permission from Tomás P. Owens, Jr., MD.)

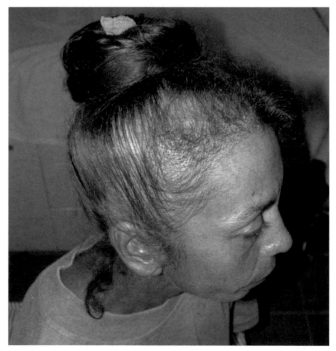

FIGURE 31–1. Traction alopecia from pulling the hair up in a tight bun. (Used with permission from Richard P. Usatine, MD.)

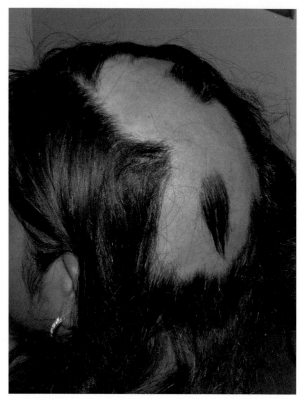

FIGURE 31-2. Extensive alopecia areata for over 6 months in an adult woman. (Used with permission from Richard P. Usatine, MD.)

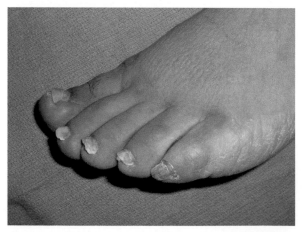

FIGURE 31-3. Onychomycosis in all toenails of a 29-year-old woman. Note the nail plate thickening and discoloration along with the subungual keratosis. She also has tinea pedis in a moccasin distribution. (Used with permission of Richard P. Usatine, MD.)

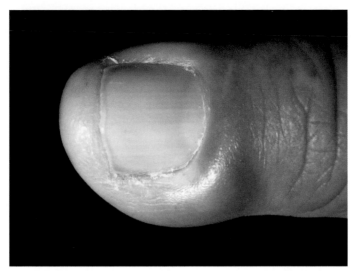

FIGURE 31–4. Painful acute paronychia around the fingernail of a 41-year-old woman. Note the swelling and erythema with a small white-yellow area suggesting purulence. (Used with permission from Richard P. Usatine, MD.)

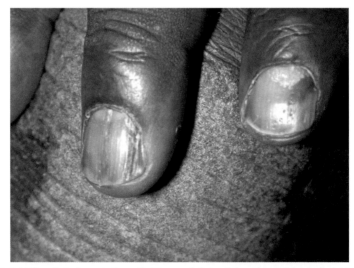

FIGURE 31–5. Nail psoriasis demonstrating nail pitting, onycholysis, oil-drop sign, and longitudinal ridging. Nails held over the silvery plaque on the knee. (Used with permission from Richard P. Usatine, MD.)

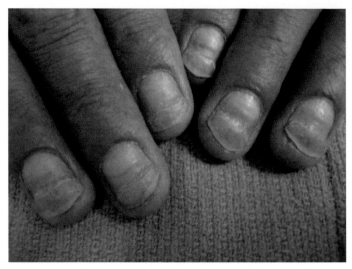

FIGURE 31–6. Beaulines most likely due to an acute cholecystitis episode before a couple of months. (Used with permission from Richard P. Usatine, MD.)

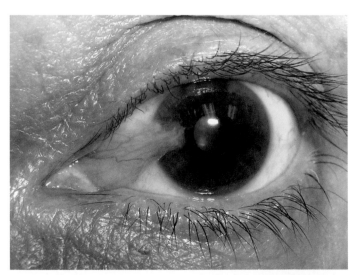

FIGURE 53–1. Pterygium that has grown into the cornea but not covering the visual axis. This fibrovascular tissue has the shape of a bird's wing (literal definition of pterygium). The small vessels are prominent in this view. (Used with permission from Richard P. Usatine, MD.)

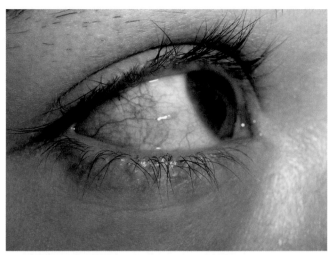

FIGURE 53–2. Episcleritis showing inflammation of only the conjunctival and episcleral tissues. Note the absence of violaceous color that is seen in scleritis. (Used with permission from Richard P. Usatine, MD.)

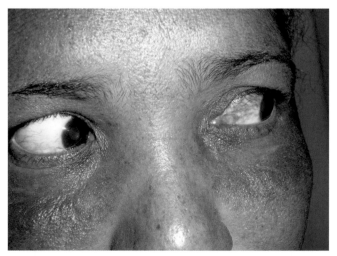

FIGURE 53–3. Scleritis in a young woman with systematic lupus erythematosus. Note the malar rash that is also present. (Used with permission from Richard P. Usatine, MD.)

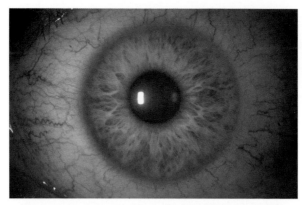

FIGURE 53–4. Iritis (anterior uveitis) with a limbal flush, red to purple perilimbal ring. This patient has eye pain and vision loss, which are absent in conjunctivitis. (Used with permission from Paul D. Comeau.)

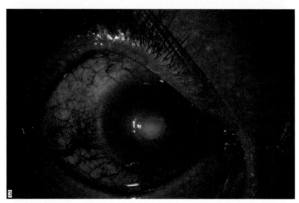

FIGURE 53–5. Diffuse ciliary injection and cloudy cornea demonstrating keratitis with corneal ulcer formation and a leukocyte infiltration. (Used with permission from Paul D. Comeau.)

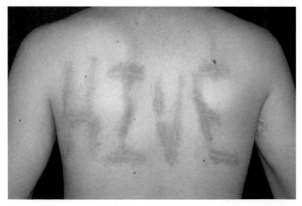

FIGURE 61–1. Dermatographism in a 21-year-old man with chronic urticarial. (Used with permission of Richard P. Usatine, MD.)

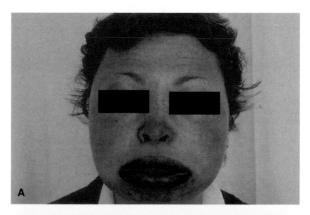

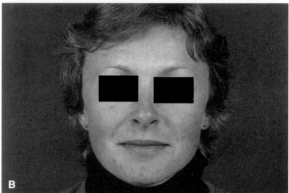

FIGURE 61–2. Hereditary angioedema. **A.** Severe edema of the face during an episode leading to grotesque disfigurement. **B.** Angioedema will subside within hours. The patient had a positive family history and had multiple similar episodes including colicky abdominal pain. (With permission from Fitzpatrick's Color Atlas and Synopsis of Clinical Dermatology, 5th ed. New York, NY: McGraw-Hill; 2005.)

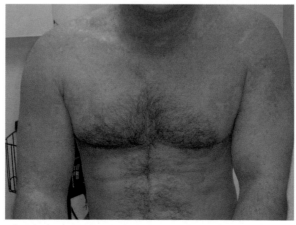

FIGURE 61–3. A 26-year-old man with acute urticaria due to trimethoprim-sulfamethoxazole. (Used with permission of Richard P. Usatine, MD.)

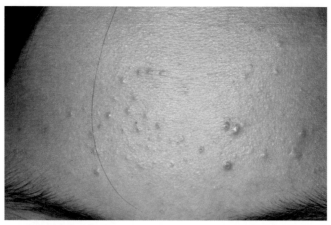

FIGURE 66–1. Comedonal acne in a 15-year-old girl. Open comedones (blackheads) and closed comedones (white-heads) are visible on her forehead. (Used with permission of Richard P. Usatine, MD.)

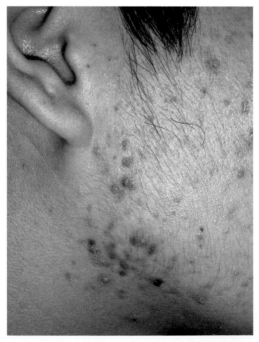

FIGURE 66–2. Inflammatory acne showing pustules and nodules in a 17-year-old boy who uses a helmet while playing football in high school. (Used with permission of Richard P. Usatine, MD.)

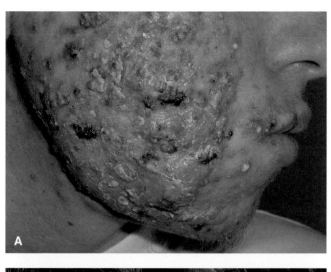

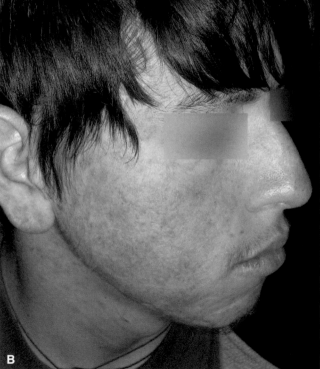

FIGURE 66–3. **A.** Acne conglobata in a 16-year-old boy. He has severe cysts on his face with sinus tracks between them. He required many weeks of oral prednisone before isotretinoin was started. His acne cleared completely with his treatment. **B.** Acne conglobata cleared with minimal scarring after oral prednisone and 5 months of isotretinoin therapy. (Used with permission of Richard P. Usatine, MD.)

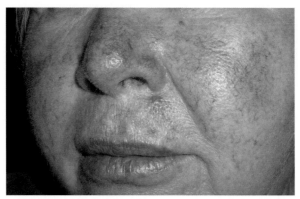

FIGURE 66–4. Erythematotelangiectatic subtype of rosacea in a middle-aged Hispanic woman. (Used with permission of Richard P. Usatine, MD.)

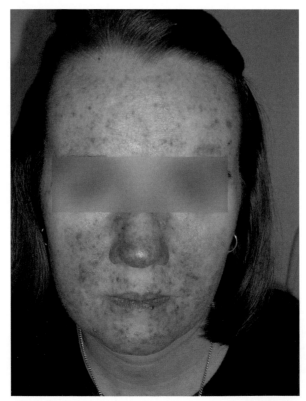

FIGURE 66–5. Rosacea in a 34-year-old woman showing erythema, papules, and pustules covering much of the face. Note her fair skin from her northern European heritage; the patient also has blue eyes. (Used with permission of Richard P. Usatine, MD.)

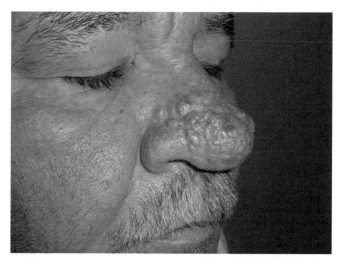

FIGURE 66–6. Rhinophymatous rosacea with hypertrophy of the skin of the nose of a 51-year-old Hispanic man. The patient acknowledges previous heavy alcohol intake. (Used with permission of Richard P. Usatine, MD.)

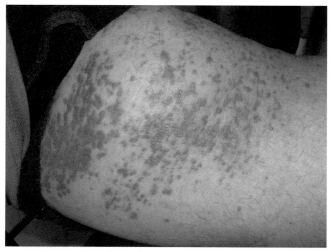

FIGURE 67–1. Kaposi sarcoma in a 43-year-old man with HIV/AIDS already on antiretroviral therapy. He presented with a diffuse rash and lymphedema in the right leg. The initial biopsy was negative, but a second biopsy demonstrated Kaposi sarcoma. The right leg is significantly larger than the left leg due to the lymphedema. (Used with permission of Richard P. Usatine, MD.)

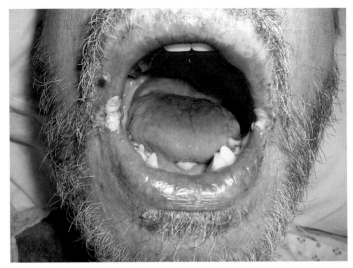

FIGURE 67–2. Thrush and perlèche in a man with AIDS. The candida infection in the corners of the mouth is called perlèche or angular cheilitis. (Used with permission of Richard P. Usatine, MD.)

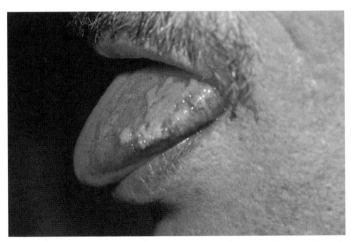

FIGURE 67–3. Oral hairy leukoplakia caused by Epstein–Barr virus on the tongue of a man with AIDS. (Used with permission of Richard P. Usatine, MD.)

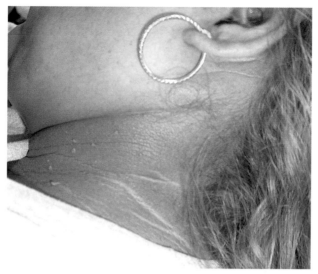

FIGURE 75–1. Acanthosis nigricans on the neck of an obese Hispanic woman with type 2 diabetes. (Used with permission Richard P. Usatine, MD.)

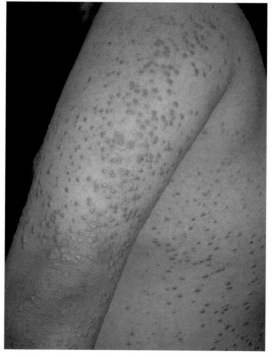

FIGURE 76–1. Eruptive xanthomas on the extremities and trunk of a young man with untreated type 2 diabetes and hyperlipidemia. (Used with permission of Richard P. Usatine, MD.)

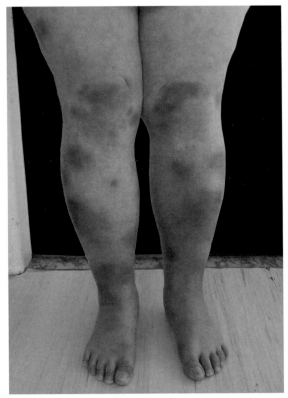

FIGURE 78–1. Erythema nodosum in a middle-aged woman with no known cause. These lesions are bright red, warm, and painful.(Used with permission from Richard P. Usatine.)

Drug	Dosage	Adverse Reactions	Contraindications	Drug Interactions
Amoxicillin/Clavulanate Potassium[c] (Augmentin)	875 mg/125 mg twice daily or 500 mg/125 mg three times daily	See Amoxicillin	History of cholestatic jaundice or hepatic dysfunction associated with amoxicillin/clavulanate, extended-release formulation, patients with severe renal impairment (CrCl < 30 mL/min) or on hemodialysis	See Amoxicillin; Allopurinol (increased incidence of rash)
Cefuroxime (Ceftin)[c]	250–500 mg twice daily	Diarrhea, nausea/vomiting, eosinophilia, transient increase in liver function tests, anaphylaxis, angioedema, Stevens–Johnson syndrome, toxic epidermal necrolysis, interstitial nephritis	Hypersensitivity to any cephalosporin	Drugs that increase gastric pH (e.g., antacids, H_2 antagonists) (may reduce bioavailability), probenecid (increased cefuroxime concentrations)
Cefprozil (Cefzil)[c]	500 mg twice daily	Nausea/vomiting, anaphylaxis, Stevens–Johnson Syndrome, elevated BUN, serum creatinine, seizures	See cefuroxime	Probenecid (increased serum cefprozil)
Cefixime (Suprax)	400 mg once daily or 200 mg every 12 h	Diarrhea, abdominal pain, anaphylaxis, erythema multiforme, Stevens–Johnson Syndrome, toxic epidermal necrolysis, acute renal failure	See cefuroxime	Warfarin (bleeding)
Cefpodoxime (Vantin)[c]	100–400 mg twice daily	Anaphylaxis, diarrhea, nausea, Stevens–Johnson syndrome, toxic epidermal necrolysis, Clostridium difficile colitis	See cefuroxime	Warfarin (bleeding), antacids, H_2 antagonists (reduced absorption), probenecid (increased serum cefpodoxime)
Cefdinir (Omnicef)[c]	14 mg/kg/d up to 600 mg divided daily or twice daily	Diarrhea, vaginitis, anaphylaxis, Stevens–Johnson syndrome, toxic epidermal necrolysis, erythema multiforme	See cefuroxime	Warfarin (bleeding), iron products (reduced drug levels), aluminum, calcium, magnesium-containing antacids (drug binding, decreased cefdinir levels), probenecid (increased serum cefdinir)

(continued)

TABLE 70–3. COMMON ORAL ANTIBIOTICS FOR CHRONIC COPD EXACERBATIONS (*Continued*)

Drug[a]	Dose	Major Side Effects	Contraindications	Drug Interactions
Azithromycin[e] (Zithromax)	500 mg on day 1 then 250 mg days 2–5, **OR** 500 mg daily for 3 d	Nausea/vomiting, headache, angioedema, anaphylaxis, hepatotoxicity, prolonged QT interval	Hypersensitivity to any other macrolide or ketolide antibiotic, hepatic dysfunction, or cholestatic jaundice with prior azithromycin therapy	**Multiple Drug Interactions** Aluminum, calcium, magnesium-containing antacids (drug binding, decreased azithromycin levels), ergot derivatives (ergotism risk), cisapride, dronedarone, amiodarone, phenothiazines, TCAs (QT prolongation), warfarin (bleeding risk), simvastatin (myopathy risk), rifabutin (neutropenia risk)
Clarithromycin (Biaxin)	250–500 mg twice daily for 7–14 d	*Clostridium difficile*, diarrhea, hepatotoxicity, QT prolongation, headache, diarrhea	Hypersensitivity to any other macrolide or ketolide antibiotics, history of QT prolongation or ventricular cardiac arrhythmias, concomitant use with colchicine in patients with renal or hepatic impairment	**Multiple Drug Interactions** Dutasteride, tamsulosin, colchicine, ergot derivatives, lurasidone, simvastatin, lovastatin (myopathy), cisapride, amiodarone, dronedarone, phenothiazines, TCAs (QT prolongation), benzodiazepines, maraviroc, lurasidone, silodosin, conivaptan, tolvaptan
Levofloxacin[c] (Levaquin)	500 mg daily	Dizziness, headache, insomnia, nausea, constipation, anaphylaxis, phototoxicity, *Clostridium difficile*, diarrhea	Hypersensitivity to other quinolones	**Multiple Drug Interactions** Cisapride, amiodarone, dronedarone, phenothiazines, TCAs (QT prolongation), aluminum, calcium, magnesium-containing antacids (drug binding, decreased levofloxacin levels), NSAIDs, tramadol (CNS stimulation, seizure risk), antidiabetic agents (blood glucose changes), warfarin (bleeding risk)

[a]Available as generic.
[b]Available in single-strength (80 mg/400 mg) or double-strength (160 mg/800 mg) tablets.
[c]Not FDA-labeled for acute infective exacerbation of COPD.
[d]Amoxicillin, although recommended by GOLD as a first-line agent, may not be as effective because it is inactive against most nontypeable *H. influenza* and *M. catarrhalis*.
[e]Five-day course.
TCA, tricyclic antidepressants; ACE, angiotensin converting enzyme; MTX, methotrexate; OC, oral contraceptive; CrCl, creatinine clearance.

6. Neither **mucolytics** nor **antitussives** are recommended for routine use in COPD. Although N-acetylcysteine has antioxidant effects, no significant effect on quality of life has been found. (SOR **B**) Most antitussives contain narcotics that may cause sedation, respiratory depression, and resultant hypercapnia. (SOR **B**)

7. **Opiates.** Oral and parenteral opiates may benefit some patients with severe dyspnea, although care is required, given the potential for serious adverse effects. There is insufficient evidence to support the use of nebulized opioids.

8. **Respiratory stimulants and immunoregulators** require further study and are not currently recommended.

9. **Alpha-1 antitrypsin therapy** should only be considered in young patients with severe deficiency of this protease inhibitor. (SOR **C**) It is very expensive and not readily available.

D. Management of stable COPD

1. A **combined baseline assessment** of current symptomatology, review of exacerbation frequency, and spirometric classification (GOLD 1–4) is important in determining a rational approach to individualized management of patients with COPD. This combined assessment, which classifies patients into GOLD categories A to D, forms the basis for treatment guidelines.

2. As mentioned earlier, the mMRC Questionnaire, the CAT, the St. George Respiratory Questionnaire, and the Clinical COPD Questionnaire are validated instruments for **assessing symptomatology or control.**

4. **Pharmacotherapy.** The initial pharmacologic management of patients with stable COPD is based upon the combined baseline assessment described earlier. A **proposed management strategy** for patients classified by GOLD as groups A to D (section II.IC.3) is depicted in the algorithm illustrated in Figure 70–1.

   a. **Inhaled bronchodilators** (short-acting in group A; long-acting in groups B–D) **are the principal medications used in all groups**. Bronchodilators alone are recommended for the initial management of patients in groups A and B (Figure 70–1).

   b. In Group A patients who are not responding adequately to "as needed" use of a short-acting bronchodilator or a combination of short-acting agents from different classes, the introduction of a long-acting agent (beta$_2$-agonist or anticholinergic) is an alternative.

   c. In Group B patients who are not responding optimally to a single long-acting bronchodilator, the addition of a long-acting agent from the other class of agents is an alternative.

   d. For Group C patients who are not adequately responding to their current drug regimen (a long-acting anticholinergic or a fixed combination of a long-acting beta$_2$-bronchodilator/corticosteroid preparation), a corticosteroid (in the case of the former), or a second long-acting bronchodilator (in the case of the latter) is an alternative. Inhalers that combine a long-acting beta$_2$-agonist with a corticosteroid are available. Use of a PDE4 and a long-acting bronchodilator is another option.

   e. In Group D patients, use of an inhaled steroid along with agents of both classes of long-acting bronchodilators is an alternative for initial management. For those failing to respond to the initially prescribed regimen, the addition of theophylline, a selective phosphodiesterase-4 inhibitor (e.g., roflumilast) or carbocysteine are options. Further diagnostic evaluation and/or referral to a pulmonologist should also be considered.

   f. As mentioned earlier, antibiotics are not indicated in patients with stable COPD. Their use in acute exacerbations is discussed below.

5. **Nutrition** should be addressed as a component of the comprehensive approach to patients with COPD.

   a. Patients with COPD are prone to nutritional deficiencies and have below-normal muscle mass, including respiratory muscles. Weight loss can be due to reduced caloric intake and hypermetabolism.

   b. Low body weight is associated with impaired lung function, exercise capacity, and a higher mortality rate. A recent Cochrane review showed that in malnourished patients receiving at least 2 weeks of supplemental nutritional support, there were significant improvements in respiratory muscle strength and health quality status. (SOR **B**)

   c. Scheduling inhaled bronchodilators as well as chest physiotherapy, if part of a patient's treatment plan, 1 hour before or after meals may prevent or reduce nausea.
   d. For the patient with advanced disease, frequent small meals may help avoid loss of appetite and the adverse metabolic and ventilatory effects of a high caloric load.
   e. Adequate protein intake (approximately 20% of calories or 1.2–1.5 g of protein per kilogram) is important to maintaining muscle mass. Liquid high-calorie protein supplements can enhance caloric intake.
   f. Sodium restriction is appropriate in patients with cor pulmonale or congestive heart failure.
   g. Fluid intake should be adequate to maintain good hydration and help thin secretions, thereby promoting expectoration.
   h. Consultation with a nutritionist can be helpful in developing a plan tailored to the individual patient.
  6. Exercise
   a. Exercise has both physiologic and psychological benefits and is recommended for all patients with COPD (GOLD groups A–D).
   b. A combination of muscle strength (weightlifting) and endurance (aerobic) training is recommended. Programs should relate to daily activities such as walking and use of the arms.
   c. A more prescriptive plan for exercise training is one facet of a pulmonary rehabilitation program.
E. Treatment of acute exacerbations. Periodic acute exacerbations are the rule throughout the natural course of COPD and increase in frequency with worsening disease. A history of exacerbations is the best predictor for future episodes. GOLD defines exacerbations as "an acute event characterized by a worsening of the patient's respiratory symptoms that is beyond normal day-to-day variations and leads to a change in medication."
   1. Patients suffering two or more episodes per year are considered "frequent exacerbators."
   2. Presenting complaints include a worsening of dyspnea, cough, sputum production, or a combination.
   3. Exacerbations reduce the patient's quality of life, accelerate disease progression (decline of pulmonary function), and can be the immediate cause of the patient's death.
   4. The most common etiology for an acute COPD exacerbation is an acute respiratory infection (viral or bacterial). Up to 15% to 25% are caused by viruses including rhinovirus, influenza, parainfluenza, and adenovirus. Air pollution and interruption of maintenance therapy can also precipitate episodes. In up to one-third of cases, the cause cannot be determined.
   5. Upon patient presentation, the **first step is to assess the severity and potential causes**. The evaluation should typically entail:
   a. Pulse oximetry or, particularly in the hospital setting, an initial measurement of arterial blood gases.
   b. Complete blood cell count.
   c. Additional laboratory evaluation depending upon the patient's condition, other comorbidities, and medications (e.g., electrolytes in a patient on diuretics).
   d. A CXR is important to assess a patient for possible pneumonia or to rule out other causes of acute respiratory distress (i.e., pleural effusion, congestive heart failure).
   8. Most acute exacerbations can be treated in the outpatient setting. Risk of death increases with respiratory acidosis, the need for ventilatory support, and when the patient has significant comorbidities. **Hospitalization should be considered under the following circumstances:**
   a. Marked increase in the intensity of symptoms (e.g., development of dyspnea at rest).
   b. Acute exacerbations failing to respond to outpatient treatment.
   c. Onset of new physical findings (e.g., cyanosis, peripheral edema).
   d. Impaired level of consciousness or acute confusion.
   e. Severe COPD or a history of frequent exacerbations.
   f. Significant comorbidities, both pulmonary (e.g., pneumothorax, pleural effusion, pneumonia, pulmonary contusion) and nonpulmonary (e.g., rib or vertebral body fracture, severe steroid myopathy).

  g. New-onset cardiac dysrhythmias.
  h. Lack of sufficient home support by either family or supplementary home health-care services.
 9. Hospital-at-home management is an alternative option for patients with acute exacerbations who are at a low risk of dying (i.e., absence of severe hypoxemia or respiratory acidosis); do not require ventilator support; lack serious comorbidities; and arrangements can be made for nurse-administered home care.
 10. Regardless of setting, a modification in the patient's usual pharmacologic regimen is required.
  a. An increased dosage and/or addition of a second short-acting bronchodilator (beta$_2$-agonist, anticholinergic) is indicated. Beta$_2$-agonists have a quicker onset of action and are preferred for "rescue."
  b. Spacers should be used with inhalers. An alternative is delivery of the short-acting bronchodilators by nebulization, which can deliver a high concentration of medication and be easier to use for sicker patients.
  c. Failure to respond to an increase in the dose or frequency of short-acting agents or a combination of bronchodilators is an indication for corticosteroids. Authors of a Cochrane review determined that systemic corticosteroids (oral or parenteral) administered to hospitalized patients with acute exacerbations of COPD improved dyspnea and blood gases; reduced the need for additional medication and treatment failure; and shortened duration of hospitalization. They also reduce early relapse. The optimal dosage has not been established. Parenteral steroids are commonly used in the hospitalized patient. In patients treated with oral medication, prednisolone in doses of 30 to 40 mg daily for 10 to 14 days is one recommended regimen.
  d. A Cochrane review supports the **use of antibiotics in acute exacerbations of COPD**. GOLD recommends their use in patients who have the three cardinal symptoms of increased dyspnea, sputum volume, and sputum purulence or in patients with increased sputum purulence (suggests a bacterial infection) and one other cardinal symptom. Antibiotics are also indicated for patients requiring mechanical ventilation. Antibiotics reduce the risk of treatment failure and death for patients with exacerbations. (SOR **Ⓐ**)
   (1) Empiric antibiotic therapy is appropriate, as obtaining sputum for culture and sensitivity (C&S) is not always practical and results are not typically available for 48 hours. In patients who are not responding to antibiotic therapy, however, or in those who are hospitalized, obtaining a C&S should be attempted.
   (2) Agents selected should cover the most common offending bacteria, namely *Streptococcus pneumoniae*, *Haemophilus influenza*, and *Moraxella catarrhalis*, and are dictated by local patterns of sensitivity/resistance. The severity of underlying COPD influences the likely etiology, with *Pseudomonas aeruginosa* more important in patients categorized as GOLD 3 or 4. Table 70–3 lists common oral antibiotics used for acute COPD exacerbations.
 11. Oxygen
  a. As mentioned earlier, oximetry or arterial blood gases should be obtained at the time of an acute exacerbation to determine the level of the patient's oxygenation and assess whether there is evidence of carbon dioxide retention and respiratory acidosis.
  b. Oxygen should be administered to maintain an oxygen saturation level of at least 92%. High flow Venturi masks deliver more reliable oxygen concentrations, but are often not tolerated by patients as well as nasal prongs. Arterial blood gases should be checked 30 to 60 minutes after administration to ensure satisfactory oxygenation and recheck the acid–base status. Reversal of hypoxemia supersedes concern about CO_2 retention, which is rare. Prior to hospital discharge, the possible need for long-term home oxygen therapy should be determined.
  c. Use of home oxygen therapy is discussed in section V.E.
 12. Ventilatory support is required in the setting of acute respiratory failure. Options include noninvasive mechanical ventilation (NIV) and invasive mechanical ventilation (IMV).
  a. NIV has become increasingly popular in appropriate patients. Randomized controlled trials have proven its success by decreasing respiratory rate, severity of breathlessness, work of breathing, ventilator associated pneumonia, rates of

intubation, length of hospitalization, and mortality. (SOR **Ⓐ**) Indications for NIV include at least one of the following: (1) respiratory acidosis (pH ≤ 7.35 and/ or $PaCO_2$ ≥ 45 mm Hg or (2) severe dyspnea as judged by clinical signs of respiratory muscle fatigue and increased work of breathing (e.g., use of accessory muscles of respiration, intercostal retractions).

b. IMV is indicated in the patient in respiratory failure who cannot tolerate or fails NIV, or with further deterioration such as respiratory or cardiac arrest, obtundation or psychomotor agitation unresponsive to medication, difficulty in managing secretions, massive aspiration, life-threatening ventricular dysthymias, and hemodynamic instability unresponsive to fluid and drug management. Risks associated with the use of IMV include ventilator-acquired pneumonia, barotrauma, and failure to wean in some cases. It should be noted, however, that acute mortality for patients with COPD requiring intervention with IMV is lower than patients on ventilators for other reasons. A variety of factors influence the likelihood of successful weaning and the decision to employ IMV can be made easier if the patient has an advance directive.

13. Attention to hydration is always important, and for patients ill for several days, parenteral nutrition should be considered. Oral and/or parenteral fluid intake and urine output must be followed closely and insensible water loss from tachypnea considered. Serum creatinine, BUN, and electrolytes must be monitored.

14. In those patients who require hospitalization, **discharge criteria** include: the patient has been clinically stable (including a PaO_2 >60 mm Hg for at least 12 hours); the patient and/or family or home health caregiver understands the drug regimen and how to properly administer bronchodilators; the patient is not requiring short-acting bronchodilators more often than every 4 hours; eating and sleeping are not interrupted frequently by dyspnea; and, if previously ambulatory, the patient can tolerate walking across the room without significant dyspnea.

15. Pulmonary rehabilitation is beneficial after acute exacerbations and is described in Section V.F.

16. Follow-up office visits are important to monitor the patient's progress and to allow early modification of the patient's regimen if there has been deterioration since discharge. The timing of the first follow-up visit and frequency of ongoing visits will depend on the physician's judgment based upon the severity of the exacerbation and patient's hospital course, the severity of the patient's underlying COPD, comorbidities, and the patient's home setting (e.g., lives alone, others in the house, family caregiver, home health aid).

V. Management Strategies. The primary care physician should develop an individualized plan for the patient and coordinate the care given by others.

A. Smoking cessation. For patients who smoke, **smoking cessation is the most crucial intervention**. (SOR **Ⓐ**) This is often the most difficult challenge for the patient. Smoking cessation slows disease progression by decreasing the otherwise rapid decline in FEV_1 and mortality rates. Smoking cessation also decreases cough and sputum production, reduces the risk of respiratory failure, and lowers the patient's risk of contracting other smoking-related illnesses.

1. The physician should be persistent in educating patients about the benefits of and methods for discontinuing smoking; success in cessation often involves combined approaches. Practical individualized counseling, behavior modification, self-help materials, group cessation programs, social support, and pharmacotherapies (nicotine replacement, bupropion, varenicline) all have a place in assisting the patient. For a comprehensive discussion on this topic, see Chapter 104.

a. Nicotine replacement includes nonprescription oral forms (2 mg or 4 mg tablet or lozenge) and patch (7 mg, 14 mg, and 21 mg [24-hour release]) and prescription spray (0.5 mg) and inhaler (10 mg cartridge delivering 4 mg of nicotine vapor). For oral forms, dosing begins with one piece every 1 to 2 hours for the first 6 weeks decreasing the frequency in weeks 7–9 (every 2–4 hours) and weeks 10–12 (every 4–8 hours). The spray (one spray in each nostril) and inhaler cartridges (continuous puffing for 20 minutes) are also dosed initially every 1 to 2 hours and tapered over 3 to 6 months. Cautions include recent myocardial infarction or serious underlying arrhythmias or angina, peripheral vascular disease, uncontrolled hypertension, active peptic ulcer disease, pregnancy or breast-feeding (pregnancy category D), and those younger than 18 years.

    b. Bupropion (Zyban) is started 1 to 2 weeks before the quit date with dosing at 150 mg orally once each morning for 3 days, then twice daily for 7 to 12 weeks with maintenance up to 6 months if needed. There is a black-box warning for neuropsychiatric symptoms, and bupropion is contraindicated in patients with seizure disorder, current or previous anorexia nervosa or bulimia, simultaneous use of bupropion for depression, simultaneous abrupt discontinuation of alcohol, sedatives or benzodiazepine, and monoamine oxidase inhibitor use in the previous 14 days. There are multiple drug interactions, and concurrent use is contraindicated with metoclopramide, theophylline, and cyclobenzaprine. Use with caution in patients on medications is known to lower the seizure threshold (e.g., systemic corticosteroids, methylphenidate), severe hepatic cirrhosis, pregnancy or breastfeeding (pregnancy category C), and those younger than 18 years.

    c. Varenicline (Chantix®) is prescribed as 0.5 mg orally each morning on days 1 to 3, twice daily on days 4 to 7, and then as 1 mg twice daily for weeks 2 to 12. An additional 12-week course can be used in selected patients. There is a black-box warning for neuropsychiatric symptoms and cardiovascular adverse events with existing cardiovascular disease and is used with caution in patients with renal impairment, pregnancy or breastfeeding (pregnancy category C), and those younger than 18 years. There are no known drug interactions.

B. Environmental control

    1. Patients should avoid exposure to secondhand tobacco smoke and remain indoors when air quality is poor.

    2. Patients who are sensitive to extremes of humidity and temperature may find that use of a humidifier in the winter and a dehumidifier or air conditioner in the summer improves symptoms.

    3. Air cleaners, whether directed against indoor or outdoor generated air contaminants, are ineffective.

    4. Commercial aircraft are usually pressurized between 5000 and 10,000 feet. Most patients with COPD do not require supplemental oxygen to fly. A general guideline is that a patient able to walk 50 m without stopping is able to fly. Patients who normally use oxygen should increase their flow rate by 2 L. Patients should contact their travel airline a few days prior to flights to learn specifics for making the necessary arrangements. Patients should avoid flying in unpressurized aircraft, and patients with large bullae should probably not fly at all because of the potential for pneumothorax.

C. Surgery

    1. Surgery can be considered in carefully selected patients.

    2. Lung volume reduction surgery typically involves stapled resection of 20% to 30% of the apices bilaterally. Success is variable with the best results in those who primarily have upper lobe disease and poor exercise tolerance despite rehabilitation. These patients have improved functional status and quality of life. In a large multicenter trial of lung volume reduction surgery, patients with upper lobe emphysema and low exercise capacity had a greater survival rate at 4.3 years and improved maximal work capacity and health-related quality of life compared with similar patients who received medical therapy. This palliative operation, however, is expensive and associated with a risk of serious postoperative pulmonary and cardiac complications.

    3. Bronchoscopic lung volume reduction requires further study.

    4. Lung transplantation is an alternative for patients meeting specific criteria. It is a consideration in patients <60 years with FEV_1 <25%, severe hypercapnia, or severe pulmonary hypertension.

D. Home oxygen therapy. Treatment of resting daytime hypoxemia with oxygen therapy prolongs survival. The administration of oxygen for at least 15 hours per day in patients with a PaO_2 less than 55 mm Hg or an O_2 saturation less than 88% increases survival. (SOR **B**) It positively impacts hemodynamics, hematologic characteristics, exercise capacity, lung mechanics, and mental state. It also improves sleep and cognitive performance. Reversal of hypoxemia supersedes concerns about CO_2 retention, which is rare. Oxygen is the most potent treatment for cor pulmonale and mitigates right heart failure secondary to it.

    1. Guidelines

        a. $PaO_2 \leq 55$ mm Hg or $SaO_2 \leq 88\%$ (waking values), with or without hypercapnia; **or** PaO_2 between 55 mm Hg and 60 mm Hg; **or** SaO_2 of 88% with pulmonary hypertension, congestive heart failure, or polycythemia.

b. The goal is to increase baseline SaO_2 to, at least, 90% at rest. The usual starting point is 2 L/minute by nasal cannula. The flow rate should be adjusted upward over baseline for exercise and sleep if required to prevent desaturation.

c. Oxygen is indicated for those who desaturate with ambulation. It will decrease dyspnea, improve exercise tolerance, and may allow greater exercise intensity training in pulmonary rehabilitation during aerobic exercise.

2. Oxygen delivery systems include:

    a. Low-flow systems—transtracheal catheter, nasal cannula, simple mask, and reservoir mask (partial rebreather, non-rebreather).

    b. High-flow systems—Venturi masks and reservoir nebulized blenders (blenders— generally with artificial airways).

3. Oxygen source

    a. Liquid gas (in canisters) is the only practical system for active individuals, but is more expensive and may be of limited availability in small communities.

    b. Compressed gas (in high-pressure cylinders) is widely available and inexpensive. However, multiple tanks are needed and the tanks are heavy and unsightly.

    c. Concentrators are convenient for home use and cost less. Disadvantages include the lack of portability, noise, and need for electricity. A back-up system (e.g., small, compressed oxygen cylinders, liquid O_2 reservoirs) must be readily accessible in the event of power failure.

4. Oxygen-conserving devices allow more efficient oxygen delivery. They either collect O_2 flowing during expiration or only permit O_2 flow during inspiration (demand system).

5. Monitoring. A patient should initially be assessed via arterial blood gases. Monitoring may then be accomplished by either arterial blood gases or pulse oximetry done periodically. This is particularly important in the patient with worsening symptoms. Pulse oximetry should also be checked with typical exertion (e.g., walking in the hallway) and during sleep, as a patient's resting oxygen saturation may be normal.

E. Pulmonary rehabilitation is a multidisciplinary, multidimensional approach to care of patients with chronic respiratory diseases and is recommended for patients with COPD and an FEV_1 <50% (GOLD B–D). (SOR **B**)

1. Small studies have shown pulmonary rehabilitation to be highly effective and safe; it reduces hospital admissions, improves mortality, and improves health-related quality of life in patients who have had recent exacerbations. Some gain over pre-rehabilitation levels can be sustained with continued exercise training. (SOR **B**)

2. Goals include reducing symptoms, preventing complications, improving quality of life, and achieving the individual's maximum level of function and independence. Major components include education, nutrition counseling, exercise training, breathing retraining, and inspiratory muscle training.

3. Baseline assessment prior to a patient's participation in a rehabilitation program includes a history and physical examination, spirometry, evaluation of exercise capacity, a measurement of health status and impact of breathlessness, and an assessment of inspiratory and expiratory muscle strength and quadriceps strength in patients with muscle wasting. Outcomes assessment includes retesting exercise capacity and muscle strength.

4. Patient benefits from exercise training include decreased breathlessness, less fatigue, and improved exercise capacity all improving their quality of life. (SOR **A**) Recommendations for frequency, intensity, and duration vary based on baseline functional status, needs, and goals.

5. Regular lower extremity exercise improves exercise tolerance, particularly endurance, enhances performance of daily activities, and reduces dyspnea. Walking, jogging, bicycling, stair climbing, and swimming are examples of aerobic (endurance) exercise. Treadmills, Exercycle, and stair steppers are also effective devices as well as cross-country ski and rowing machines, which provide the added benefit of upper extremity exercise.

6. Upper extremity exercise is associated with a higher ventilatory and metabolic demand than lower extremity exercise. Upper extremity training, endurance and strength, improves arm muscle endurance and sense of well-being.

7. Breathing retraining should be part of a rehabilitation program with the aim of helping the patient relieve and control dyspnea and of counteracting physiologic abnormalities such as hyperinflation. Pursed-lip and diaphragmatic breathing assist in slowing the respiratory rate and increasing tidal volume, while inhibiting airspace collapse and enhancing gas exchange. Both help alleviate dyspnea. Leaning forward and resting the arms on one's thighs or on a table (*tripoding*) may also help relieve dyspnea. Breathing exercises may be useful to improve exercise tolerance in selected individuals unable to participate in exercise training.

    9. Inspiratory muscle training likely increases respiratory muscle strength, but its effect on quality of life improvement is not clearly established. (SOR **B**)

F. Immunizations, which have been addressed earlier, are an important component of the management of COPD.

G. Personalized patient education should address the disease process and provide information about medications (e.g., rationale, side effects, inhaler technique, and home oxygen, if prescribed). Use of the Chronic Obstructive Pulmonary Disease Questionnaire can be of value in providing individualized patient education. Patient education and patient–physician agreement on short- and long-term goals improve adherence to the therapeutic regimen. This should include helping identify a way for the patient to monitor progress toward goals. Persistence in supportively stressing the importance of smoking cessation regardless of disease stage is imperative. Sensitive issues such as sexual activity should be addressed. Patients should be counseled about the importance of early attention to worsening symptomatology with the goal of preventing or reducing the severity of exacerbations. Education of family members, particularly those involved in the patient's care, is also important and, given the considerable adaptation they must make in their own lives; caregivers may need supportive therapy themselves.

H. Comorbidities are common in patients with COPD and can impact the patient's quality of life and prognosis. Cardiac disease (e.g., ischemic heart disease, congestive heart failure, atrial fibrillation), hypertension, osteoporosis, anxiety, and depression are examples. Treatment of these comorbidities should follow the usual management guidelines for these problems and, similarly, the treatment of a patient's COPD is not modified because of their presence. Lung cancer is the most common cause of death in patients with mild COPD.

VI. Prognosis

A. Death rate. COPD is the fourth leading cause of death in the United States (CDC) and mortality rates continue to rise. There has been a dramatic increase in mortality in women over the past 25 years. This reflects an increased smoking rate for women. The year 2007 marked the eighth consecutive year in which women exceeded men in the number of deaths from COPD.

B. FEV_1 declines with normal aging, but COPD is characterized by a much greater progressive decline in pulmonary function. Although variable, FEV_1 decreases by an average of 45 mL/year in smokers and by 50 to 75 mL/year in patients with COPD, compared to 25 to 30 mL/year (beginning at around age 35 years) in nonsmokers without pulmonary disease. Age, lifetime smoking, and the number of cigarettes currently smoked are all risk factors for more rapid decline in pulmonary function.

    1. The multidimensional BODE index (body mass index, obstructive ventilator defect, severity, dyspnea severity, and exercise capacity) is an excellent prognostic tool. Besides age, FEV_1 is the best predictor of mortality. The mortality rate for patients with COPD and an FEV_1 <35% is about 10% per year. Other predictors of poor prognosis include severe dyspnea, severe hypoxemia, resting tachycardia, cor pulmonale, poor nutrition, and frequent exacerbations.

    2. In severe COPD, death is related to recurrent episodes of hypoxia, leading to the development of pulmonary vascular hypertension and cor pulmonale. Acute respiratory failure, severe pneumonia, pneumothorax, pulmonary embolism, and cardiac dysrhythmias are medical complications often responsible for death. The mortality rate 10 years after diagnosis is ≥50%.

C. Regular follow-up is important to the successful management. The purpose of such visits includes supporting the patient in smoking cessation, monitoring and modifying as necessary the therapeutic regimen, monitoring changes in pulmonary function, early identification of complications, ongoing education, and emotional support. Attention to the pulmonary illness must not entirely supplant addressing other health promotion/disease prevention issues. Advance directives should also be reviewed periodically.

SELECTED REFERENCES

American Lung Association. Chronic Obstructive Pulmonary Disease fact sheet. http://www.lung.org/lung-disease/COPD/resources/facts-figures/COPD-fact-sheet.html. Accessed April 2013.

Decramer M, Janssens W, Miravitlles M. Chronic obstructive pulmonary disease. *Lancet.* 2012;379: 1341–1351.

Evensen A. Management of COPD exacerbations. *Am Fam Physician.* 2010;81(5):607–613, 616.

Global Strategy for the Diagnosis, Management and Prevention of COPD, Global Initiative for Chronic Obstructive Lung Disease (GOLD) 2013. http://www.goldcopd.org./. Accessed May 2013.

Gross N, Levin D. Primary care of the patient with chronic obstructive pulmonary disease-part 2: pharmacologic treatment across all stages of disease. *Am J Med.* 2008;121(Suppl 7a):S13–S24.

Nannini LJ, Lasserson TJ, Poole P. Combined corticosteroid and long-acting beta 2-agonist in one inhaler versus long-acting beta 2-agonists for chronic obstructive pulmonary disease. *Cochrane Database Syst Rev.* 2012;(9):CD006829.

Qaseem A, Wilt TJ, Weinberger SE, et al. Diagnosis and management of stable chronic obstructive pulmonary disease: a clinical practice guideline update from the American College of Physicians, American College of Chest Physicians, American Thoracic Society, and European Respiratory Society. *Ann Intern Med.* 2011;155:179–191.

Ram FSF, Rodriguez-Roisen R, Granados-Navarrete A, et al. Antibiotics for exacerbations of chronic obstructive pulmonary disease. *Cochrane Database Syst Rev.* 2011;(1):CD004403.

Ray SM, Helmer RS, Stevens AB, et al. Clinical utility of the chronic obstructive pulmonary disease knowledge questionnaire. *Fam Med.* 2013;45(3):197–200.

Reilly JJ Jr, Silverman EK, Shapiro SD. Chronic obstructive pulmonary disease. In: *Harrison's Principles of Internal Medicine.* 18th ed. New York, NY: McGraw-Hill; 2012:2151.

Spencer S, Karner C, Cates CJ, et al. Inhaled corticosteroids versus long-acting beta 2-agonists for chronic obstructive pulmonary disease. *Cochrane Database Syst Rev.* 2011;(12):CD007033.

Walters JAE, Gibson PG, Wood-Baker R, et al. Systemic corticosteroids for acute exacerbations of chronic obstructive pulmonary disease. *Cochrane Database Syst Rev.* 2009;(1):CD001288.

Additional references are available online at http://langetextbooks.com/fm6e

---

71   Chronic (Persistent) Pain

Michael P. Temporal, MD

KEY POINTS

- The biopsychosocial context is important in the assessment and management of chronic pain conditions to understand both the perception of severity and the effect of treatment. (SOR **C**)
- Pain scales and pain medication contracts can help decrease the risk of inappropriate pain medication prescribing. (SOR **C**)
- A multidisciplinary approach using multiple modalities is usually needed to manage chronic pain. (SOR **C**)
- Routine, rather than as-needed, dosing of medications results in better pain control. (SOR **A**)
- Acetaminophen and nonsteroidal anti-inflammatory drugs (NSAIDs) are used as first-line pain medications (SOR **A**); among NSAIDs all appear to have equivalent efficacy. (SOR **A**)
- Narcotic pain medications should be used when patients have failed NSAID therapy alone. They should not be used as a sole agent and should be titrated to the most effective dose and then changed to long-acting preparations when available. (SOR **C**)
- Adjuvant medications can be particularly helpful for chronic, relapsing pain. (SOR **C**) Antidepressants are also useful for both the emotional component of pain and analgesia. (SOR **B**)

I. Introduction
   A. Pain is the most common reason for which people seek medical care. **Pain** is an unpleasant sensory and emotional experience associated with actual or potential tissue damage. **Persistent pain** is defined as recurrent or chronic pain lasting more than 3 months, which may or may not be directly related to the inciting disease process. Persistent pain

affects 30% of the population and accounts for over $60 billion annually in lost productivity in the United States.

B. The transition from acute pain to a chronic pain state involves neuroplastic changes in the dorsal horn of the spinal cord. These changes cause allodynia, defined as a lower pain threshold resulting from a loss of inhibition of dorsal horn neurons. The neuropathic upregulation of pain fibers results in multiple abnormal pain pathways that also connect different pelvic organs through common spinal cord innervation. As an example, pain in one pelvic organ can cause pain in a neighboring organ, which underlies the multifactorial cause of most pelvic pain syndromes.

C. Persistent pain may be classified as nociceptive or neuropathic. Although acute pain can be a protective reflexive response to limit further tissue destruction, persistent pain does not have a similar useful purpose.

   1. Nociceptive pain stems from ongoing tissue damage such as arthritis or tumor. Pain signals are transmitted through nonmyelinated C-fiber nerves mediated by calcium and sodium. Persistent nociceptive pain is related to N-methyl-D-aspartate (NMDA) receptors that are both more easily stimulated and require higher antinociceptive activity to quiet. Released endorphin and enkephalin binding to mu- and gamma-opioid receptors reduce nociceptive pain.

   2. Neuropathic pain results from the sustained transmission of pain signals in the absence of ongoing tissue damage. Injury or damage to the sensory nerves, central ganglia, or spinal cord has occurred. Common descriptions of this chronic pain include numbness (hypoesthesia), pins-and-needles sensation (paresthesia), or severe pain from usually innocuous stimuli (allodynia). It is more difficult to treat and usually does not respond to treatment with nonsteroidal anti-inflammatory drugs (NSAIDs) or acetaminophen alone.

II. Diagnosis

A. The **assessment of pain** must include the type, severity, onset, location, duration, and previous history. Persistent pain may have variable duration (less than once per week, multiple times per week, daily, or constant). Within a psychosocial context, more intense pain may be associated with certain activities, emotions, or events (work, mood, menstrual cycle).

B. An important **measure of persistent pain** is the associated impairment or loss of function. Associated symptoms such as nausea, dizziness, diaphoresis, and weakness; comorbid conditions such as diabetes mellitus, connective tissue disease, and psychiatric illness (which may affect treatment response); as well as hepatic disease, renal disease, history of gastrointestinal (GI) bleeding, and medication sensitivity (which may limit treatment choices) should be sought. Previous treatment strategies (including complementary and alternative therapies) and response to those strategies provide important historical information and can guide the current management.

C. Pain rating scales allow quantification of baseline and relative response to pain therapies (http://onlinelibrary.wiley.com/doi/10.1002/art.11440/pdf). The simplest range from 0 (no pain) to 10 (worst pain possible). Mild pain ranges from 1 to 4, moderate pain ranges from 5 to 6, and severe pain ranges from 7 to 10. Multidimensional pain assessments include the McGill Pain Questionnaire (https://www.google.ca/#q = McGill+Pain+questionnaire) and the Edmonton Symptom Assessment Scale (http://meds.queensu.ca/assets/palliative-care/ppcip_esas.pdf). These tools rate pain and other symptom domains, including tiredness, nausea, depression, anxiety, drowsiness, appetite, well-being, shortness of breath, and other problems, that can be queried over time to assess response to treatment.

D. Physical assessment can give more objective data to the necessarily subjective sensation of pain. However, instability of vital signs or alterations of consciousness seen in acute pain situations may be blunted in persistent pain. Important functional information of endurance, range of motion, and palpable inflammation, point tenderness, or spasm should be identified.

III. Treatment. The management of persistent pain requires the use of multiple modalities. Framed within the biopsychosocial context, the goal of treatment is not elimination of pain, but alleviation to allow maximal function and quality of life with tolerable side effects.

A. Physical therapy has been used in the management of acute pain to help with stretching, strengthening, and improving endurance. The primary impairments, directly caused by the injury, may or may not be responsive to physical therapy. The secondary impairments—lack of exercise, poor body alignment, shortening and weakening of the joint structures, and over guarding of the injured area—which can limit function and exacerbate the perception of pain, are often responsive in the motivated patient.

Physical reconditioning in a gradual, directed program will help the patient who has been immobile. With the goal of increasing function, decreasing disability, and establishing effective pain coping and management skills, exercise programs can include the following: aerobic exercise to 65% to 80% of predicted maximal heart rate; stretching exercises for shortened muscles; endurance exercise for major postural muscles; and coordination and stabilization exercises. (SOR **Ⓒ**)

1. **Transcutaneous electrical nerve stimulation (TENS)** has been helpful in mild-to-moderate pain. (SOR **Ⓑ**) It works through counter-stimulation of the pain-transmitting nerves.

2. Scheduled use of **ice or heat** may provide a similar benefit. (SOR **Ⓑ**) Typically, most heat can be applied from 10 to 20 minutes at a time, three to four times per day. Ice can be tolerated for 10 to 15 minutes at a time.

B. **Occupational therapy** can be used to help moderate total activity and develop compensatory techniques for activities of daily living. The provision of adaptive equipment can enhance the effectiveness of other treatment modalities.

C. **Acupuncture** has demonstrated effectiveness in the chronic pain of fibromyalgia, knee osteoarthritis, and low back pain. (SOR **Ⓑ**)

D. **Biofeedback, self-hypnosis,** and **relaxation** can also be taught to help manage the sensation of pain and the response to painful stimuli. (SOR **Ⓒ**)

E. **Cognitive therapy.** Understanding the pain cycle and how the individual is affected can be a step toward moving the focus away from the pain and more toward adaptive behaviors. (SOR **Ⓒ**) Cognitive therapies seek to bring an awareness of the triggers and responses the body has to pain in the context of daily life activities. Educating the patient and the family regarding pain, tension, and the physiologic response is a therapeutic intervention. Reframing the language and associations of pain may bring control for a person who has not had control of pain for a long time. Relaxation techniques, stress management, and pain diary records help to respond productively to pain.

F. **Pharmacologic therapy.** The World Health Organization (WHO) organizes pain medication management into three tiers. Step 1 medications are used for mild-to-moderate pain and include acetaminophen, aspirin, and NSAIDs. Step 2 medications are commonly used for moderate pain and include tramadol, codeine, and opioid medications coformulated with a step 1 medication. Step 3 medications are used for severe pain and typically are narcotics. Within each of these tiers, adjuvant medications can be used to treat pain through other pathways. Table 71–1 displays medications used for persistent pain.

1. **Non-opioid Analgesics**
   a. **Acetaminophen** is an excellent analgesic for mild-to-moderate nociceptive pain. The maximum total daily dose for acetaminophen for adults is 4 g/24 hours. However, because of the risk for hepatotoxicity, emerging guidance is to limit total daily dose of all sources of acetaminophen to 3 g/24 hours and to 2 g/24 hours in the elderly, consumers of three or more servings daily of alcohol, or known liver disease. Although it has no anti-inflammatory properties, acetaminophen is thought to work through NMDA receptors and substance P.
   b. **Salicylates** (aspirin) have good efficacy in mild-to-moderate pain for short-term use and can be administered in oral, rectal, or parenteral forms. Regularly scheduled chronic aspirin use is usually not tolerated due to nausea and vomiting, and gastric bleeding risk. Non-acetylated forms, choline magnesium salicylate (Trilisate), diflunisal (Dolobid), or salsalate (Disalcid) may be better tolerated with less GI irritation/bleeding and platelet inhibition.
   c. **NSAIDs** are effective agents for mild-to-moderate pain with an inflammatory component. They work at the peripheral site of action and are effective in the chronic management of arthritis and myalgias. They also can be effectively combined with centrally acting opioid medications for other persistent pain. No one NSAID is superior to others for chronic pain, but periodic substitution between classes may afford an improved response. (SOR **Ⓑ**) The risks of NSAIDs are related to prostaglandin inhibition and include gastric irritation, bleeding, and renal dysfunction. Allergic reactions including angioneurotic edema, asthma, and hypotension have been reported. Because of sodium retention, caution is advised in the setting of congestive heart failure. A topical NSAID, diclofenac (Voltaren Gel), offers a direct effect with less risk for systemic side effects. (SOR **Ⓑ**) For information on dosing, see Table 71–2; additional information on NSAID selection, preventing side effects, and potential drug interactions can be found in Chapter 82.

TABLE 71–1. TREATMENT OPTIONS FOR PATIENTS WITH PERSISTENT PAIN

Drug	Dose	Major Side Effects/ Contraindications	Drug Interactions
Acetaminophen	2000–4000 mg/d in divided doses	Nausea, vomiting, constipation, agitation, insomnia, headache, itching, rash/ blisters/other skin reaction[b]/alcohol use	Sodium nitrite, prilocaine (↑ risk methemoglobin-emia)
Salicylates			
Aspirin[a]	325–650 mg up to six times daily	GI upset, bleeding, easy bruising, tinnitus/ triad of asthma, rhinitis and nasal polyp	**Multiple Interactions** Anticoagulants/antiplatelet agents, SSRIs/SNRIs, ginkgo (bleeding); methotrexate (methotrexate toxicity); antihypertensives (↓ antihypertensive efficacy); sulfonylureas (hypoglycemia)
Choline-Mg-salicylate[a] (Trilisate)	1500 mg twice daily	See Aspirin	See Aspirin
Diflunisal[a] (Dolobid)	250–500 mg twice daily	Nausea, diarrhea, headache, rash/asthma, urticaria, or allergic reaction to aspirin; CABG surgery perioperative pain	See Aspirin
Salsalate[a] (Disalcid)	1500 mg twice daily	Nausea, tinnitus/As above	
Nonsteroidal Anti-inflammatory Drugs (NSAIDs)			
Propionic acids Ibuprofen[a]	200–800 mg three times daily	Nausea, heartburn, GI bleed, dizziness, nephrotoxicity, exacerbation of heart failure and hypertension, rebound headache/as above	**Multiple Interactions** ACE inhibitors, cyclosporine (↑ nephrotoxicity); anticoagulants, antiplatelet agents, SSRI/SNRI, ginkgo, corticosteroids (↑ bleeding risk); lithium (lithium toxicity); methotrexate (methotrexate toxicity); antihypertensives (↓ antihypertensive efficacy); sulfonylureas (hypoglycemia)
Cox-2 selective Celecoxib[a] (Celebrex)	100–200 mg daily		
Fenamates Meclofenamate[a] (Meclomen)	50–100 mg three to four times daily		
Heteroaryl acetic acids Diclofenac[a] (Voltaren)	50–75 mg two to three times daily (ER) 100 mg one to two times daily		
Diclofenac topical (Voltaren Gel)	LE or UE joints 2–4 g joints 2–4 g four times daily		
Tolmetin[a] (Tolectin)	200–600 mg three times daily		
Indole acetic acid Indomethacin[a] (Indocin)	25–50 mg two to three times daily (ER) 100 mg one to two times daily		
Sulindac[a] (Clinoril)	150 mg twice daily		
Naphthylokanone Nabumetone[a] (Relafen)	1000 mg one to two times daily		
Enolic Acids Piroxicam[a] (Feldene)	10–20 mg once daily		

(continued)

TABLE 71–1. TREATMENT OPTIONS FOR PATIENTS WITH PERSISTENT PAIN

Drug	Dose	Major Side Effects/ Contraindications	Drug Interactions
Meloxicam[a] (Mobic)	7.5–15 mg daily		
Naproxen[a]	250–500 mg twice daily		
Flurbiprofen[a] (Ansaid)	100 mg two to three times daily		
Ketoprofen[a] (Orudis, Oruvail SR)	50–75 mg three times daily (ER) 200 mg once daily		
Oxaprozin[a] (Daypro)	1200–1800 mg once daily		
Pyranocarboxylic acid Etodolac[a] (Lodine)	200–1000 mg two to three times daily (ER) 400–1000 mg daily		
Opioid Like Agents			
Tramadol[a] (Ultram, Ultram ER)	50–100 mg four times daily ER 100–300 mg once daily	Nausea, constipation, somnolence, dizziness, headache, insomnia, pruritis/severe asthma or respiratory depression	**Multiple Interactions** Carbamazepine, fluoxetine, haloperidol, clarithromycin (seizures); venlafaxine, mirtazapine, trazodone (serotonin syndrome); warfarin (bleeding); digoxin (digoxin toxicity)
Tapentadol (Nucynta ER)	50–250 mg twice daily	Nausea, constipation, somnolence, dizziness, headache/asthma or respiratory depression, GI obstruction	**Multiple Interactions** MAOI, venlafaxine, SSRI, TCAs, triptans (serotonin syndrome)
Antidepressants			
Tricyclic Antidepressants			
Amitriptyline[a] (Elavil)	25–150 mg at bedtime (0.1 mg/kg/d titrated over a few weeks)	Sedation, constipation, dry mouth, blurred vision, weight gain, dizziness, headache, urinary retention/cardiac arrhythmia, hypotension, depression, hepatotoxicity, agranulocytosis, thrombocytopenia	**Multiple Interactions** MAOI, tramadol (seizures, serotonin syndrome); metoclopramide (extrapyramidal reactions); fluconazole, SSRI, phenothiazines, sulfamethoxazole/trimethoprim, buspirone, methadone, solifenacin, macrolide and quinolone antibiotics, (QT prolongation); warfarin (bleeding); cimetidine (TCA toxicity)
Imipramine[a] (Tofranil)	0.2–3 mg/kg to 300 mg at bedtime (100 mg max. in the elderly)		
Nortriptyline[a] (Pamelor)	5–10 mg three times daily		
Serotonin Norepinephrine Reuptake Inhibitor			
Duloxetine (Cymbalta)	30–60 mg once daily	Nausea, dry mouth, constipation, diarrhea, decreased appetite, headache, dizziness, fatigue, insomnia, sweating/abnormal bleeding, liver toxicity, suicidal thoughts	**Multiple Interactions** MAOI, SSRI, triptans, methadone, venlafaxine, tramadol, dextromethorphan, trazodone (serotonin syndrome); metoclopramide (extrapyramidal reactions); NSAIDs, anticoagulants, anti-platelet agents (bleeding); Class 1C antiarrhythmics (QT prolongation)

Drug	Dosage	Adverse Effects	Drug Interactions/Cautions
Milnacipran (Savella)	12.5–50 mg twice daily	Nausea, constipation, sweating, headache, increased blood pressure and heart rate, palpitations/abnormal bleeding, depression, suicidal thoughts	MAOI, SSRI, triptans, methadone, venlafaxine, tramadol, dextromethorphan, trazodone, antipsychotics (serotonin syndrome); NSAIDs, anticoagulants, antiplatelet agents (bleeding)
Anticonvulsants (see Chapter 87 for drug information) Gabapentin [a,c] (Neurontin) Pregabalin (Lyrica) Carbamazepine[a] (Tegretol) Valproate[a] (Depakene) Clonazepam[a] (Klonopin)			
Local Anesthetics			
Lidocaine patch 5% (Lidoderm)	One to three patches up to 12 h/d	Hypotension	Dihydroergotamine (severe hypertension); beta-blockers, cimetidine (lidocaine toxicity); Class 1 and Class 3 antiarrhythmics, phenytoin, antiretroviral therapy (cardiac toxicity)
Mexiletine[a]	150–1200 mg/d (start at 150 mg at bedtime, ↑ weekly to 150 mg three times daily, then up to a max. dose of 10 mg/kg/d or 1200 mg/d)	Dizziness, tremor, hypotension, ataxia, dyspepsia, rash second or third degree AV block	Clozapine (clozapine toxicity); fluvoxamine (mexiletine toxicity); ritonavir, quinidine (cardiotoxicity)
Antispasmodics			
Baclofen[a]	5–20 mg three to four times daily	Nausea, dizziness, asthenia, headache, somnolence hypotension, urinary problems, GI bleeding	Fentanyl (CNS depression); loxapine (impaired cognitive and motor function, respiratory depression)
Cyclobenzaprine[a] (Flexeril)	5–10 mg three times daily	Somnolence, dizziness, dry mouth, cholestasis, cardiac arrhythmia, abnormal liver function, thrombocytopenia/CHF, arrhythmia	**Multiple Interactions** MAOI, SSRIs, SNRIs, TCAs, verapamil, trazodone, bupropion, fentanyl (serotonin syndrome); fluoxetine (QT prolongation, serotonin syndrome); tramadol (seizures, serotonin syndrome)
Tizanidine[a] (Zanaflex)	2–8 mg three to four times daily	Somnolence, dry mouth, asthenia, dizziness, hypotension, hepatotoxicity	Ciprofloxacin, oral contraceptives, fluvoxamine, ticlopidine, cimetidine, (hypotension, sedation); phenytoin (phenytoin toxicity)

[a]Generic available.

[b]Rare but serious skin reactions (rash, blisters, other skin reaction) may occur in users of acetaminophen which may be indicative of Stevens-Johnson Syndrome or toxic epidermal necrolysis (TEN). Problems usually begin with flu-like symptoms followed by skin symptoms. If this occurs patients should be advised to seek medical care immediately.

[c]Adjust dose in renal insufficiency

ACE, angiotensin-converting enzyme; CABG, coronary artery bypass graft; CHF, congestive heart failure; CNS, central nervous system; ER, extended release; GI, gastrointestinal; LE, lower extremity; MAOIs, monoamine oxidase inhibitors; NSAIDs, nonsteroidal anti-inflammatory drugs; SNRI, serotonin norepinephrine reuptake inhibitors; SSRIs, selective serotonin reuptake inhibitors; TCAs, tricyclic antidepressants; UE, upper extremity; URI, upper respiratory infection.

TABLE 71-2. OPIOID THERAPY

Drug	Equianalgesic Dose (mg)	Starting Oral Dose and Frequency	Duration of Action (h)
Morphine	10 IM, 30 oral	15–30 mg every 2–4 h	3–4
Codeine	75 IM, 130 oral	60 mg every 4–6 h	3–4
Hydrocodone	30 oral	5 mg every 4–6 hours	3–4
Oxycodone	15 IM, 30 oral	15–30 mg every 4–6 h	2–4
Hydromorphone	1.5 IM, 7.5 oral	2–4 mg every 4–6 h	2–4
Levorphanol	2 IM, 4 oral	4–8 mg every 6–8 h	4–8
Methadone	10 IM, 20 oral	5–10 mg every 8–12 h	4–8
Fentanyl patch	25 µg/h = 1 mg/h	25 µg every 72 h	72

2. **Opioid analgesics.** Although opioid medications are readily accepted in the management of cancer pain, their use in persistent, nonmalignant pain is characterized by provider fear of regulatory scrutiny, fostering addiction, and overuse. However, the use of opioids is appropriate when other modalities have failed to provide adequate analgesia. In cancer pain, opioid dose is titrated to patient response and limited by side effects such as respiratory depression. In persistent nonmalignant pain, there is evidence that continued escalation of dose results in worsened analgesic response. (SOR **B**) This is because NMDA receptors are upregulated leading to tolerance, while pain receptors become more sensitive to similar stimuli. Low-to-moderate total dosage of opioid agents may provide the best response in persistent pain. (SOR **C**) Short-acting agents can be used initially to titrate quickly to effect, and then converted to long-acting agents for chronic use. In situations of tolerance to medication with a desire to change receptor response, it is appropriate to switch from one opioid agent to another, usually starting at half the equivalent dose of the alternate medication. (SOR **C**)

   a. **Tramadol** (Ultram) is a centrally acting, synthetic opioid agonist oral analgesic useful in moderate-to-severe pain. It has been used for chronic osteoarthritis, low back pain, and other chronic pain. (SOR **B**) In some regions, it is a nonscheduled medication. It binds to mu-opioid receptors and inhibits serotonin and norepinephrine reuptake. An extended release preparation is also available and may be a better choice for persistent pain. (SOR **A**)

   b. **Coformulated hydrocodone or oxycodone** with acetaminophen, aspirin, or ibuprofen is commonly used for acute pain and may be necessary for persistent pain. They are considered **Step 2 medications within the WHO paradigm**. The combination is believed to provide better pain relief with lower doses of either agent. Prescription coformulated acetaminophen products are now limited to no more than 325 mg of acetaminophen per tablet (becomes FDA rule January 14, 2014).

   c. **Single formulation opioid analgesics are considered Step 3 medications by WHO.** Equal analgesic doses (Table 71-2) can be used as a general guide, but when switching between medications, a lower total dose is prudent. (SOR **C**) Options of medication delivery include pill and oral concentrates, as well as transdermal formulation fentanyl. **Transdermal fentanyl** may be an attractive option to convert patients on stable multiple oral doses of narcotic.

   d. The FDA has approved a **Risk Evaluation and Mitigation Strategy (REMS)** for extended release and long-acting opioids, including the fentanyl patch (http://www.fda.gov/Drugs/DrugSafety/InformationbyDrugClass/ucm163647.htm). REMS is part of a multiagency Federal effort to address prescription drug abuse and misuse. Safety measures, including education programs and training for prescribers, an updated medication guide and patient counseling document, and monitoring should help reduce risks and improve safe use of extended release/long-acting (ER/LA) opioids while continuing to provide access to these medications for patients with persistent pain.

   e. **Tapentadol** (Nucynta ER) is a Schedule II agent that also binds to mu-opioid receptors as well as inhibiting norepinephrine reuptake. It is indicated for persistent pain but has efficacy and risk similar to any opioid agent. (SOR **B**)

   f. **Chronic use of opioid medications for persistent pain requires safeguards** for both the prescriber and the patient. A **pain management contract** should be signed (Table 71-3). Periodic monitoring including pill counts

TABLE 71-3. COMPONENTS OF A NARCOTIC MEDICATION PAIN CONTRACT

The risks, side effects, and benefits have been discussed in detail.

Only one physician will be responsible for prescribing narcotic pain medications.

Other providers caring for the patient must be aware of the pain medication plan.

Patient must make regular scheduled visits to receive prescriptions.

Narcotic prescriptions will not be mailed.

Patient agrees to random urine or blood tests to assess compliance.

Lost, misplaced, destroyed, or stolen medications will not be replaced. Refills will not be given early for any reason.

If there is no observed improvement in quality of life or function for the patient, narcotic pain medication will be tapered.

and the use of random urine drug tests can be useful to identify overuse or diversion of medication. **Prescription monitoring programs** should be accessed to identify other controlled medications or prescribers.

3. **Antidepressants.** Whether considered independent pain management choices or adjuvant therapies, psychopharmacologic agents are used for persistent pain. (SOR ●) Randomized control trials have shown efficacy in painful diabetic peripheral neuropathy (DPN), postherpetic neuralgia (PN), trigeminal neuralgia, and peripheral neuropathy. (SOR ❶) Although it is true that mood affects both perception and response to pain, these agents have been shown to have independent effect on pain.

   a. **Tricyclic antidepressants** have analgesic properties in low doses, but maximal analgesic effect is achieved at increased doses. Dosing then should be titrated over weeks and increased to the maximum efficacy that dose-related side effects will allow. Commonly used agents include amitriptyline (Elavil), tertiary amines imipramine (Tofranil), clomipramine (Anafranil), and doxepin (Sinequan). The quaternary amines may be better tolerated in older patients and tend to have less central activity and hypotension. (SOR ❸) These include desipramine (Norpramin), nortriptyline (Pamelor), protriptyline (Vivactil), and amoxapine (Asendin).

   b. **Serotonin-norepinephrine reuptake inhibitors** (SNRIs) work through signal inhibition mediated by these neurotransmitters at the level of the brainstem and the spinal cord. Norepinephrine modulates signal transmission in damaged nerves (neuroplasticity) and augments endogenous opioid receptors. Duloxetine (Cymbalta) is a balanced SNRI that is indicated in PN, DPN, and fibromyalgia. Milnacipran (Savella) is indicated for fibromyalgia. Venlafaxine (Effexor, Effexor XR) and desvenlafaxine (Pristiq) have also been used, but do not have FDA indications for pain and may be dose limited due to potential hypertension.

   c. **Selective serotonin reuptake inhibitors** (SSRIs) were introduced in the late 1980s as a novel antidepressant. They were soon found to be useful in a variety of conditions including panic disorder, generalized anxiety, chronic fatigue, premenstrual syndrome, and chronic pain. (SOR ❸) Their use to treat persistent pain seems best explained as their amelioration of the distressing effects of pain rather than through direct pain pathways. (SOR ●) Common side effects include headache, stimulation or sedation, cardiac effects (bradycardia or tachycardia), GI effects (increased or decreased appetite, nausea, vomiting, bloating, diarrhea), sedation, fine tremor, and tinnitus. They variably affect libido. Agents include fluoxetine (Prozac), fluvoxamine (Luvox), paroxetine (Paxil), sertraline (Zoloft), citalopram (Celexa), and escitalopram (Lexapro). See Chapter 94 on depression for further dosing information.

4. **Anticonvulsants.** Stabilizing neuronal membranes; alteration of sodium, calcium, and potassium ion channels; and effects on other neurotransmitters (e.g., norepinephrine, gamma-aminobutyric acid, serotonin) are the proposed mechanisms for anticonvulsants. Efficacy is usually seen at therapeutic drug levels. For information on doses, side effects, and drug interactions, see Chapter 87, Table 87-4.

   a. **Gabapentin** (Neurontin) has been used for a variety of neuropathic pain conditions. It is indicated in the management of PN. (SOR ❸) Gabapentin has relatively few side effects and its absorption is not affected by food.

   b. **Pregabalin** (Lyrica) works through calcium channels to mediate neurotransmitter pain response. It can be helpful for diabetic, postherpetic, and other neuropathic pain. (SOR ❸) Doses of 75 mg twice daily have been efficacious for fibromyalgia. (SOR ❸)

    c. Carbamazepine (Tegretol) is dosed as shown in Table 87–4; slower titration may minimize side effects. Monitoring of the drug includes a complete blood count and liver function studies.

    d. Valproic acid also requires monitoring with baseline and periodic liver function tests. GI side effects will often improve over time. An extended release preparation (Depakote ER) can be used for once daily dosing.

    e. Clonazepam (Klonopin) is a benzodiazepine with anticonvulsant activity. Abrupt cessation of this medication can result in a withdrawal syndrome.

  5. Local anesthetics have been used as blocking agents subcutaneously, along nerve roots, and at the spinal cord for acute conditions and procedures. In persistent pain, they may be helpful for continuous and lancinating pain, neuropathic pain of herpes zoster, phantom limb pain, and diabetic neuropathy. The mechanism of action is direct stabilization of nerve membranes and decreased ion flux in sodium channels.

  6. Antispasmodics are often used to treat spasticity associated with chronic conditions, but they are also believed to have analgesic properties that may augment opioid-induced analgesia. Baclofen has been useful for painful spasticity, trigeminal neuralgia, and lancinating neuropathic pain. Cyclobenzaprine (Flexeril) relieves muscle spasm without interfering with muscle function. It should not be used for more than 2 to 3 weeks, so it may not be a good choice for chronic conditions. Tizanidine (Zanaflex) is an α2-agonist that decreases sympathetic transmission at the level of the dorsal horn and is indicated for sympathetic maintained pain as well as pain described as lancinating, electrical, or burning.

G. Topical agents. The use of topically applied gels and ointments can help in painful arthritic conditions and work locally, whereas other agents have effect at the level of the peripheral nerve. Topical analgesics include methyl salicylate/menthol (Ben-Gay), trolamine salicylate (Aspercreme), and camphor/phenol (Campho-Phenique). They are best for localized pain in muscles and joints. (SOR **C**) Capsaicin cream (Capsin 0.025%, Zostrix HP 0.075%) depletes substance P at the local area and can provide relief in PN. (SOR **B**). An 8% capsaicin patch (Qutenza) is available but must be placed under medical supervision for no more than 60 minutes, no more frequently than every 3 months. Users of capsaicin should be cautioned to avoid inadvertently having capsaicin make contact with mucus membranes. Finally, the lidocaine patch (Lidoderm 5%) can be used for PN, applied up to 12 hours per day. (SOR **B**)

H. Complementary and alternative therapies. Patients in persistent pain are usually willing to try anything to help relieve their pain. Complementary approaches including homeopathy, naturopathy, and spiritual healing may have a therapeutic effect on the patient, although randomized controlled trials have not been conducted. The provider must help the patient find a balance between maintaining hope while limiting potential harm.

I. Surgical therapies include implanted nerve stimulators (TENS), injected anesthetics (intrathecal or continuous infusion), epidural steroids, nerve blocks, and nerve ablation. (SOR **A**) Specialized anesthesiologists can assist in these techniques.

IV. Management Strategies

  A. Effective care of persistent pain is best delivered using multiple disciplines and modalities. Biochemical pain may respond better to usual or adjuvant pharmacotherapies. Physical pain may respond to massage, cold/heat, and medication. Emotional pain response may depend on effective communication with the provider as much as any other treatment. Caregivers must be included in discussions and may be a critical component to implementing care plans.

  B. The patient and care provider must negotiate and agree on the goals of treatment—the reduction rather than elimination of pain; the improvement or restoration of function; the ability to resume social activities; or the improvement of mood. They must also discuss possible limitations including medication side effects (e.g., sedation, confusion) or tolerance and risk of addiction. Both patient and provider must be willing to acknowledge when a particular treatment is not working and should be abandoned.

SELECTED REFERENCES

American Geriatric Society Panel on Persistent Pain in Older Adults. The management of persistent pain in older persons. *J Am Geriatr Soc.* 2002;50(6 Suppl):S205–S224.

American Pain Society. *Pain Control in the Primary Care Setting.* Glenview, IL: American Pain Society; 2005.

Ballantyne J, ed. *The Massachusetts General Hospital Handbook of Pain Management.* 3rd ed. Philadelphia, PA: Lippincott, Williams & Wilkins; 2005.

Caritas Health Group. Guidelines for using the 2010 revised Edmonton Symptom Assessment System (ESAS-r). http://www.palliative.org/newpc/_pdfs/tools/ESAS-r%20guidelines.pdf. Accessed October 29, 2013.

Melzack R. The McGill Pain Questionnaire: major properties and scoring methods. *Pain.* 1975;1:277–299.

VA/DoD Clinical Practice Guideline: Management of Opioid Therapy for Chronic Pain (2010). http://www.healthquality.va.gov/COT_312_Full-er.pdf. Accessed October 29, 2013.

72   Cirrhosis

Mark C. Potter, MD, & Mari Egan, MD, MHPE

KEY POINTS

- Cirrhosis is the 10th leading cause of death in the United States. Alcohol abuse is the most common cause of cirrhosis, followed by hepatitis C. (SOR **C**)
- Treatment for alcoholic cirrhosis is total alcohol abstinence. (SOR **A**) Prednisolone and pentoxifylline have been shown to reduce complications from alcoholic hepatitis. (SOR **B**)
- Treatment for hepatitis C is currently indicated for patients with biopsy-proven active hepatitis and detectable serum levels of hepatitis C RNA. (SOR **A**)
- The primary care physician should monitor patients with cirrhosis for signs of ascites, spontaneous bacterial peritonitis (SBP), encephalopathy, coagulopathy, varices, and hepatocellular carcinoma (HCC). (SOR **B**)
- Vaccinations should be administered (hepatitis A and B, influenza, and pneumococcus). (SOR **C**) Education should be given on avoiding medical toxicity (e.g., acetaminophen), (SOR **C**) eating a low-salt diet with 1 to 1.5 g protein/kg/day, (SOR **B**) and being aware of increased risks for infection. (SOR **C**)
- Patients with cirrhosis are at an increased risk for HCC. Patients should be screened for cancer with a serum α-fetoprotein test and liver ultrasound every 6 to 12 months. (SOR **A**)

I. Introduction

A. Liver cirrhosis is characterized by diffuse hepatocellular injury that progresses with nodular regeneration to eventual irreversible fibrosis. Because of loss of normal hepatocytes and distorted hepatic architecture, the liver is unable to perform its synthetic or metabolic functions normally. As the normal portal architecture is destroyed, blood flow is diverted around the liver rather than through it (portosystemic shunting). This process has major effects on many other organ systems, which manifest as the important complications of cirrhosis.

B. Cirrhosis ranks as the 10th leading cause of death in the United States and is most prevalent in the 36- to 54-year-old age group with a slight male predominance. Chronic liver disease often takes 20 to 40 years to progress from hepatitis to cirrhosis. Once cirrhosis is advanced, liver transplantation is often required to extend life. In the United States, there are four times as many patients who are candidates for liver transplants as the number that will eventually receive one.

C. When a physician first evaluates a patient with signs or symptoms of liver disease, it is important to search for potential contributing factors. History should be elicited for risk factors for viral infection (prior blood transfusions, hemodialysis, hemophilia, organ transplant, sexual practices, multiple sexual partners, travel), toxic insults (alcohol intake, hepatotoxic drugs, vitamins, and herbal remedies), occupational exposures, family history, diabetes mellitus, and autoimmune diseases.

D. The physician must manage complications of liver damage if they occur. However, not all patients with cirrhosis will develop life-threatening complications. Forty percent of patients with cirrhosis are asymptomatic, and the diagnosis is commonly made at autopsy. Mortality rates are higher in patients with alcoholic cirrhosis.

E. Among patients infected with hepatitis C virus (HCV), 20% to 30% will develop cirrhosis in 20 to 40 years.

II. Diagnosis

A. Symptoms and signs. The clinical presentation of patients with cirrhosis varies widely. It ranges from asymptomatic disease found incidentally to liver disease to multiple end-stage disease with complications. The symptoms and signs of cirrhosis can be separated into three major groups:

1. **Symptoms and signs of hepatocellular dysfunction.** These include fatigue, weight loss, jaundice, nausea and vomiting, coagulopathy, palmar erythema, gynecomastia, testicular atrophy, menstrual dysfunction, loss of pubic hair, muscle wasting, spider angiomas, peripheral edema, ascites, gastrointestinal bleeding and confusion, or sleep disturbances which could indicate encephalopathy.

2. **Symptoms and signs of portal hypertension.** These are caused by increased intrahepatic vascular resistance, which causes ascites, lower extremity edema, splenomegaly, esophageal and gastric varices, and dilated abdominal wall veins (caput medusa).

3. **Symptoms and signs caused by another disease which has also caused cirrhosis.** This includes withdrawal symptoms in chronic alcoholics or cardiomyopathy in patients with hemochromatosis.

B. Identifying the underlying cause. The gold standard for diagnosis of cirrhosis is examination of the whole liver at autopsy, but in clinical practice **liver biopsy** is used. Since cirrhosis is a syndrome caused by many diseases, a diagnostic work-up should be undertaken in all patients with cirrhosis to identify all contributing underlying causes (see Table 72–1). (SOR ⊙) Treatment can slow the progression of liver injury, morbidity, or mortality in most cases of cirrhosis.

1. **Viral hepatitis. Chronic hepatitis C, chronic hepatitis B, and coinfection with hepatitis D** are major viral causes of cirrhosis. Since most patients with chronic viral hepatitis are asymptomatic or have nonspecific symptoms, complications of cirrhosis may be their earliest sign of infection.

   a. Patients presenting with cirrhosis should be **tested for hepatitis B surface antigen** (HBsAg), **surface antibody, core antibody, and hepatitis C antibody**. Patients with chronic hepatitis C infection will have a positive test for anti-HCV antibody (anti-HCV enzyme-linked immunoassay (EIA)-2 or EIA-3). Patients with a positive anti-HCV antibody test should have the presence of HCV RNA determined with either a quantitative (preferred if antiviral treatment is likely) or a qualitative polymerase chain reaction (PCR) test. Patients with a positive anti-HCV antibody test, who also have a high-risk history for hepatitis C infection (e.g., injection drug users), can be assumed to have hepatitis C infection and can proceed to quantitative HCV antibody testing. Such patients can also be offered HCV genotyping and liver biopsy if they are candidates for treatment.

   b. **Elevated alanine aminotransferase** (ALT) may also be found in viral hepatitis, but because ALT levels often fluctuate and may even have periods in the normal range, ALT levels are not a reliable guide as to the severity of liver injury.

   c. Patients with chronic hepatitis B infection will have persistently positive HBsAg for longer than 6 months.

   d. **Additional testing for Hepatitis B e antigen** (HBeAg) and **serum HBV DNA** should be ordered in patients with positive tests for hepatitis B to make treatment decisions.

   e. A positive test for hepatitis D virus indicates coinfection by hepatitis D.

2. **Alcoholic cirrhosis** usually occurs 10 or more years after a period of excessive alcohol ingestion. Between 8% and 20% of chronic alcoholics develop cirrhosis. Liver failure is common in patients with alcoholic cirrhosis, with 25% developing decompensation within 1 year and 50% within 5 years following diagnosis.

   a. **The first step in diagnosis** is to obtain a history of alcohol use. Laboratory evidence in patients who are currently drinking can include a ratio of aspartate aminotransferase (AST) to ALT of greater than two to one. **An AST-to-ALT ratio greater than 2 is rarely seen in other causes of cirrhosis**. In alcoholic liver disease, the **gamma-glutamyl transpeptidase** (GGT) is often elevated to 8 or more times the upper limit of normal.

   b. Malnourished alcoholics may have hyponatremia, hypomagnesemia, hypophosphatemia, low blood urea nitrogen levels, and an elevated mean corpuscular volume.

   c. **Hepatic steatosis or fatty liver** can be an early sign of alcoholic liver disease. Alcohol overuse should be considered if steatosis is found on imaging or

TABLE 72–1. COMMON CAUSES OF CIRRHOSIS

Etiology of Cirrhosis	Diagnosis (Biopsy May be Required for Definitive Diagnosis)	Management (Transplant May Be Required If Severe, Immunizations and Screening as in Text)
Alcohol	Alcohol abuse history AST-to-ALT ratio >2 GGT >8 times normal limits	Abstinence from alcohol (SOR Ⓐ) Nutritional support (SOR Ⓑ) Prednisolone and pentoxifylline (SOR Ⓑ)
Hepatitis C	Hepatitis C antibodies (anti-HCV EIA-2 or EIA 3) HCV RNA and HCV genotyping	HCV 1-triple therapy of peginterferon, ribavirin, and a protease inhibitor (SOR Ⓐ) HCV 2, 3, and 4 treated with peginterferon and ribavirin (SOR Ⓐ)
Hepatitis B	HBsAg, HBsAB, HB core AB, HBeAg, and HBV DNA	Several treatment options (see text) (SOR Ⓐ)
Nonalcoholic steatohepatitis (NASH)	Hepatic steatosis No alcohol history Metabolic syndrome: hyperlipidemia, hypertension, obesity, and diabetes	Gradual weight loss and exercise (SOR Ⓒ)
Primary biliary cirrhosis	Elevated alkaline phosphatase, antimitochondrial antibodies	UDCA 13–15 mg/kg/d (SOR Ⓐ)
Autoimmune hepatitis (adults)	Antinuclear antibodies and antismooth muscle antibody	Corticosteroids with azathioprine (SOR Ⓐ)
Wilson disease	Kayser–Fleischer rings, low ceruloplasmin, high urinary copper excretion	Penicillamine 750 to 1000 mg/day for maintenance treatment (SOR Ⓐ)
Alpha-1 antitrypsin (AAT) deficiency	No alpha-1 globulin peak on protein electrophoresis, AAT levels <120 mg/dL	IV infusion of pooled human AAT (SOR Ⓒ)
Hemochromatosis	Elevated transferrin saturation, iron and ferritin	Phlebotomy 500 mg weekly for 18 months (SOR Ⓐ)

ALT, alanine aminotransferase; AST, aspartate aminotransferase; DNA, deoxyribonucleic acid; EIA, enzyme-linked immunoassay; GGT, gamma-glutamyl transpeptidase; HBeAg, hepatitis B e antigen; HBsAg, hepatitis B surface antigen; HBsAB, hepatitis B surface antibody; HCV, hepatitis C virus; RNA, ribonucleic acid; UDCA, ursodeoxycholic acid.

biopsy. Patients with suspected alcohol-related liver disease should, however, have other causes ruled out before a diagnosis of alcoholic liver disease is accepted.

3. **Primary biliary cirrhosis** is a chronic, progressive disease of the liver characterized by destruction of the intrahepatic bile ducts. The cause probably has an autoimmune basis. Genetic variants of HLA class II, IL12A, and IL12RB2 loci may be risk factors for developing the disease. Ninety-five percent of those diagnosed with primary biliary cirrhosis are women aged 30 to 65 years. The prevalence of this disease in recent years has been increasing.

   a. **More than half of patients are asymptomatic when diagnosed,** although fatigue is a common presenting symptom, along with pruritus and right upper quadrant pain. Hepatomegaly is seen in 50% of patients, and 10% to 50% will have splenomegaly. A quarter to a half of patients will present with hyperpigmentation of the skin. This pigmentation change is not due to jaundice but due to melanin deposition.

   b. **Laboratory tests** may show an isolated elevation of serum alkaline phosphatase often more than twice the upper limit of normal. All patients with significant suspicion for primary biliary cirrhosis should be tested for antimitochondrial antibodies for which over 90% of those with primary biliary cirrhosis will test positive. Serum lipids, antinuclear antibodies (ANAs), and eosinophils have also been shown to be elevated in this disease.

4. **Hemochromatosis** is an autosomal recessive disorder that can lead to cirrhosis. It is associated with increased absorption of iron and deposition of iron in the liver and other organs. Clinical symptoms are not usually seen until after age 40 years when body iron stores reach 4 to 10 times normal. The disease affects men more often than women, and at an earlier age. C2827 mutations of the HFE gene cause the majority of cases but only around one percent of homozygotes appear to develop clinical manifestations.

   a. **Most patients are asymptomatic when diagnosed,** but may present with one or more of diabetes mellitus, hyperpigmentation, fatigue, arthralgias, or impotence.

   b. **Laboratory tests** reveal serum transferrin saturation elevated to greater than 50%, an elevated ferritin concentration of >400 ng/mL, and serum iron >180 mcg/dL. In such patients, genotypic analysis for HFY C282Y mutation should be done.

5. **Other hereditary diseases** can be the cause of cirrhosis.

   a. **Wilson disease** is a rare autosomal recessive disorder of copper metabolism which leads to copper deposition that affects the liver, brain, and eyes. The mean age of diagnosis is 12 to 24 years. Kayser–Fleischer rings, a deposition of copper in the cornea, can be detected by slit-lamp examination. Patients are found to have reduced serum levels of ceruloplasmin, increased 24-hour urine copper excretion, and increased hepatic copper concentrations. Many patients will also have Coombs negative hemolytic anemia. Untreated Wilson disease is usually fatal, but patients who adhere to treatment have an excellent prognosis.

   b. **Alpha-1-antitrypsin (AAT) deficiency** is an autosomal recessive (or codominant) disorder of the Pi gene. Patients present with symptoms of early onset emphysema and cirrhosis. Serum protein electrophoresis will show no alpha-1-globulin peak and ATT levels <120 mg/dL. Genetic testing is confirmatory.

6. **Nonalcoholic steatohepatitis (NASH).** This entity is diagnosed when a liver biopsy reveals hepatic steatosis, but the patient's history is repeatedly confirmed to exclude significant alcohol consumption. Patients with NASH often have components of the metabolic syndrome, which include hyperlipidemia, hypertension, obesity, and diabetes. The pathogenesis of NASH is not clear, but the strongest theory implicates insulin resistance as the key mechanism leading to hepatic steatosis.

   a. **Most patients with NASH are asymptomatic** and come to medical attention with elevated liver enzymes or when hepatic steatosis is found incidentally on imaging.

   b. **Diagnosis** requires evidence of hepatic steatosis by imaging or biopsy, exclusion of significant alcohol consumption, and exclusion of other causes of hepatic steatosis. NASH carries a better prognosis than alcoholic liver disease, but still increases the likelihood of eventual cirrhosis.

7. **Autoimmune hepatitis** is progressive inflammation of the liver without other identifiable cause in the presence of circulating autoantibodies and hypergammaglobulinemia. Type 1 that accounts for 80% of the cases mainly occurs in women and

is characterized by the presence of antinuclear antibodies and antismooth muscle antibody. Type 2 occurs mostly in children and is correlated with antibody to liver/kidney microsome type 1 (anti-LKM1), antibody to liver cytosol type 1 (anti-LC1), and antibody to liver/kidney microsome type 3 (anti-LKM3).

8. **Other causes of cirrhosis** include secondary biliary obstruction, **primary sclerosing cholangitis,** cardiac cirrhosis, schistosomiasis, and systemic mastocytosis. Toxins (e.g., industrial cleaning solvents) and drugs (e.g., methotrexate, isoniazid, acetaminophen, methyldopa, and estrogen) can cause cirrhosis. In 10% to 15% of patients, there is no identifiable cause of the liver damage, and this is called **cryptogenic cirrhosis**.

C. **Diagnostic tests.** First signs of cirrhosis in patients may be found in laboratory tests that evaluate liver enzymes and synthetic function of the liver. Laboratory tests that can be helpful in diagnosis include serum aminotransferase, bilirubin, albumin, prothrombin time, and a complete blood count.

1. **Liver enzymes** (ALT and AST) assess acute liver injury. They are usually moderately increased in cirrhosis, although they may be minimally elevated or normal in as many as 10% of patients. Paradoxically, the enzymes may be virtually normal in severe liver disease, since many of the normal liver cells have been replaced by fibrous tissue. ALT is found predominantly in the liver and is a more specific indicator of liver damage.

2. **Lactate dehydrogenase** is a marker of hepatocyte injury, although less specific than AST or ALT. It is elevated disproportionally after ischemic injury to the liver.

3. **Alkaline phosphatase** originates mostly from the liver and bones. Elevated levels are seen when there is a blockage of the bile ducts or impaired bile formation. It is also elevated when there is injury to the bile ducts. It is elevated disproportionately to AST or ALT in primary and secondary biliary cirrhosis as well as primary sclerosing cholangitis.

4. **Serum bilirubin levels, albumin levels, and prothrombin time** represent hepatocyte function rather than acute hepatocellular injury. Hepatocyte injury or destruction inhibits the secretion and conjugation of bilirubin. The conjugated **bilirubin** level will not become elevated until the liver has lost more than 50% of its excretory capacity. **Serum albumin** is often depressed in cirrhosis and can serve as a gauge of the liver's synthetic function. Because the liver manufactures the blood-clotting factors, **prothrombin time** can be prolonged in cirrhosis. A prolonged prothrombin time that does not correct after parenteral vitamin K (10 mg subcutaneously every day for 3 days) suggests severe liver damage.

5. **Serum ammonia** is often measured in patients with hepatic encephalopathy. Although elevated serum ammonia levels suggest a hepatic cause for encephalopathy, the ammonium concentration does not correlate tightly with the level of stupor or coma.

6. **Imaging**
   a. **Ultrasonography of the biliary tree and liver** is the initial diagnostic imaging modality of choice in evaluating patients with liver dysfunction. (SOR ❸) Beyond evaluating for obstructive causes of liver dysfunction, the echotexture or nodularity of the liver parenchyma and dimensions of the portal vessels often provide useful information. Ultrasonography is very sensitive at detecting ascites and can detect as little as 100 mL of peritoneal fluid.
   b. **Computerized tomography** usually does not add much to ultrasound information. **MRI** has been used in the evaluation of cirrhosis, but a clear role has not yet been established.
   c. A **radionucleotide scan of the liver and spleen** in patients with cirrhosis will show decreased, patchy uptake in the liver and increased uptake in the spleen and bone marrow. This test does not often add to information gained by other testing.

7. **Liver biopsy.** A liver biopsy provides information on the grade (inflammatory severity) and stage (degree of fibrosis) of liver disease. A liver biopsy is usually indicated if a treatable cause of cirrhosis, such as Wilson disease or hepatitis C is suspected. This procedure may also be used to help establish a prognosis and to determine whether a patient with antibody evidence of hepatitis B or C infection would benefit from antiviral therapy.

8. **Factors that best predict cirrhosis** in patients with liver disease include
   - Presence of ascites (likelihood ratio [LR] 7.2)
   - Platelet count $<160 \times 10^3$ (LR 6.3)
   - Spider nevi (LR 4.3)
   - Bonacini cirrhosis discriminant score >7 (LR 9.4)

    a. The **Bonacini Cirrhosis Discriminant Score** can be used to predict the likelihood of cirrhosis. Patients with a score of 8 or more out of 11 total points are highly likely to have cirrhosis. Calculation of the score is computed by giving points for the following factors:
- Platelets (x1000/mm^3): >340, zero points; 280 to 399, one point; 220 to 279, two points; 160 to 219, three points; 100 to 159, four points; 40 to 99, five points; and <40, six points.
- ALT/AST ratio: >1.7, zero points; 1.2 to 1.7, one point; 0.6 to 1.19, two points; <0.6, three points.
- International normalized ratio (INR): <1.1, zero points; 1.1 to 1.4, one point; >1.4, two points.

III. Treatment. The treatment of cirrhosis consists of preventing further liver damage, managing the potential complications of cirrhosis, treating the underlying cause of cirrhosis when possible, and considering liver transplantation (see Table 72–1).

  A. Preventing further liver damage

    1. Avoidance of alcohol and drug toxicity. Safe levels of alcohol consumption in cirrhosis have not been established, so complete abstinence is the most prudent recommendation. Alcohol also acts synergistically with hepatitis C, so abstinence from alcohol should also be strongly recommended to those with chronic hepatitis C, even without established cirrhosis. The liver is also vulnerable to injury from medications, vitamins, and herbs.

      a. Common hepatotoxic medications include tricyclic antidepressants, muscle relaxants, lipid-lowering drugs, antidiabetic agents, isoniazid, nitrofurantoin, antifungal agents, and anticonvulsant agents. **Nonsteroidal anti-inflammatory drugs** are especially important to avoid in cirrhosis. Because they inhibit platelet function, they may exacerbate coagulopathy. In addition, as a prostaglandin inhibitor, they may decrease renal blood flow and precipitate renal failure. **Acetaminophen should be used with caution** if at all, and should be restricted to a dose of 500 mg four times a day in well-nourished patients who are not actively consuming alcohol. Patients and physicians should attempt to assess all vitamins and herbal therapies for hepatotoxicity.

    2. Vaccinations against hepatitis A and B viruses should be performed in patients with cirrhosis if they are not already immune. (SOR **©**) Superinfection with these viruses can worsen liver disease. In addition, the pneumococcal and influenza vaccines should be given.

    3. Diet. A nutritious low-salt diet is desirable because cirrhotic patients have increased sodium retention. In early cirrhosis with muscle-wasting malnutrition, a diet containing 1 to 1.5 g of protein/kg/day with vitamin supplementation is optimal. (SOR **®**) Dietary treatment in severely malnourished alcoholics has demonstrated shorter- and longer-term survival benefit. (SOR **®**) With worsening cirrhosis and increased risk of encephalopathy, protein should be restricted to no more than 1 g/kg/day. (SOR **®**)

  B. Managing complications of cirrhosis

    1. Ascites is the most common complication of cirrhosis.

      a. Restriction of sodium intake is the cornerstone of therapy. Sodium intake should be limited to less than 2 g per day. One of the goals of treatment is to increase urinary excretion of sodium so that it exceeds 78 mmol per day. Restriction of fluid intake to 1500 mL per day may be necessary for treating ascites in patients with sodium levels less than 125 mEq/L.

      b. Diuresis is frequently needed and the usual regimen is a morning dose of **spironolactone,** 100 mg, and **furosemide,** 40 mg, daily. This combination treatment shortens time to mobilization of the ascites. The medication doses can be increased every 3 to 5 days to maintain weight loss and natriuresis with a maximum of 400 mg per day of spironolactone and 160 mg per day of furosemide. (SOR **©**)

      c. For tense ascites, a single large-volume paracentesis (5 L) followed by diet and diuretic therapy is appropriate treatment. (SOR **©**)

      d. Angiotensin-converting enzyme inhibitors, angiotensin receptor blockers, and nonsteroidal anti-inflammatory medications should be avoided in patients with ascites. (SOR **©**)

      e. Evaluation for liver transplant should be undertaken when ascites develops. (SOR **®**)

2. **Spontaneous bacterial peritonitis (SBP)** is one of the major potential complications of cirrhosis. **Paracentesis** to exclude SBP should be considered for patients with ascites that is new in onset or who have fever, hypotension, abdominal pain, decreased bowel sounds, and an abrupt onset of hepatic encephalopathy.

   a. Patients with an ascitic fluid neutrophil count ≥ 250 cells/mm^3 in a community-acquired setting should receive **empiric antibiotics** preferably intravenous cefotaxime 2 g every 8 hours or another third-generation cephalosporin. (SOR **Ⓐ**) Oral ofloxacin (400 mg twice daily) may be used for stable patients. (SOR **Ⓑ**).

   b. Certain at-risk patients (as above) with a clinical suspicion of SBP should receive albumin 1.5 g/kg body weight within 6 hours of detection and 1.0 g/kg on day 3. (SOR **Ⓑ**)

   c. **Recurrence of SBP is high in certain patients.** Patients who have survived one episode of SBP should be placed on daily norfloxacin (400 mg daily) for long-term prevention. (SOR **Ⓐ**) Patients with SBP should also avoid the use of proton-pump inhibitors.

3. **Hepatic encephalopathy** should be considered when the patient with cirrhosis exhibits a change in mental status. The pathogenesis of this condition is still unclear, but an increase in ammonia concentration is the leading hypothesis.

   a. **Common symptoms** are forgetfulness, impaired arousability, and asterixis (flapping tremor).

   b. Hepatic encephalopathy is reversible and often has a **precipitating factor** that increases ammonia levels such as infection, gastrointestinal bleeding, increased protein intake, and constipation. Other causes are linked to hypoxia or medications. The first step in treatment is to identify and treat precipitating factors. Most patients will improve when the precipitating cause has been treated.

   c. In patients who do not improve, the second step is to **reduce the serum ammonia concentration. Lactulose,** 45 to 90 g per day, can be given initially with subsequent adjustment (usually to 30–45 mL or 20–30 g per day orally three to four times daily) to allow for two or three soft stools a day. Most patients will improve with lactulose. (SOR **Ⓒ**) For patients who do not improve in 48 hours, antibiotics are added and **neomycin** is used at a dose of 4 to 12 g per day orally in divided doses for 5 to 6 days (maximum 2 weeks). An alternative medication is **rifaximin** 550 mg twice daily.

   d. There have not been good clinical studies supporting protein restriction in patients with acute hepatic encephalopathy.

4. **Coagulopathy** can be improved by administration of vitamin K, 10 mg subcutaneously every day for 3 days. Replacement therapy for coagulopathy is recommended only in the setting of hemorrhage or prior to invasive procedures. (SOR **Ⓒ**)

5. **Varices** occur due to chronic high pressure in the portal veins. Bleeding from varices is the most common lethal complication in the patient with cirrhosis. Fifty percent of patients with cirrhosis will have varices on endoscopic examination and their presence correlates with the severity of cirrhosis.

   a. **Patients with cirrhosis should be endoscopically screened for varices** at the time of their diagnosis. (SOR **Ⓒ**) Patients with compensated cirrhosis with no varices on initial screening should be rescreened in 2 to 3 years. Patients who are diagnosed with small varices should be rescreened in 1 to 2 years and patients with decompensated cirrhosis should be screened annually.

   b. **Prevention of hemorrhage.** Variceal wall diameter and tension determine the **likelihood of rupture**. In patients with medium to large varices, the use of nonselective beta-blockers or endoscopic variceal ligation is recommended for the prevention of hemorrhage. (SOR **Ⓐ**) The usual dose is propranolol, 20 mg two times daily, or nadolol, 40 mg once daily. Nitrates, sclerotherapy, or shunt therapy should not be used for the prevention of variceal bleeding. (SOR **Ⓐ**)

C. **Specific treatment for underlying causes of cirrhosis**

1. **Treatment for alcoholic cirrhosis** includes arranging all necessary support for total alcohol abstinence. Prevention and treatment of alcohol withdrawal must be part of treatment. (SOR **Ⓑ**) Nutritional support interventions have also been shown to decrease infections and reduce liver disease mortality. (SOR **Ⓑ**) Both prednisolone and pentoxifylline individually have been shown to reduce complications, but may not reduce mortality in patients with severe alcoholic hepatitis. (SOR **Ⓑ**)

2. Treatment for chronic hepatitis C
  a. Antiviral therapy is indicated when HCV RNA is positive or there is evidence of inflammation, fibrosis or cirrhosis on liver biopsy; compensated cirrhosis; acceptable hematologic markers; and no major contraindications exist (e.g., uncontrolled depression or substance use). Regimens for treatment of viral hepatitis have been evolving rapidly. Treating physicians should consider referring to frequently updated sources of treatment recommendations (see References) or consider specialist consultation for treatment initiation.
    (1) The current regimen of first choice for patients with hepatitis C genotypes 2, 3, and 4 is pegylated interferon alpha-2b (PEG-Intron), 1.5 IU/kg subcutaneously weekly **or** pegylated interferon alpha-2a (Pegasys), 180 µg subcutaneously weekly, with ribavirin (Rebetol), 0.8 to 1.2 g/kg/day divided for twice daily. (SOR Ⓐ) Dosing of ribavirin depends on whether you are using peginterferon alpha-2a or peginterferon alpha-2b. Therapy should be administered for 24 weeks for patients infected by genotype 2 or 3 and 48 weeks to patients infected by genotype 4. (SOR Ⓑ)
    (2) Patients with chronic hepatitis C genotype 1 should have a protease inhibitor added to the regimen, either boceprevir or telaprevir. (SOR Ⓐ) Treatment should be continued for 48 weeks. The addition of a protease inhibitor to these two medications significantly increases the sustained viral response in patients. Telaprevir and boceprevir appear to be similar in efficacy. Telaprevir is given as 750 mg three times a day and boceprevir is given as 800 mg three times daily.
    (3) Patients should have a HCV viral load checked at 4, 12, and 24 weeks of therapy to assess treatment response.
3. Treatment for chronic hepatitis B should be considered in patients when they have HBV DNA levels greater than 20,000 IU/mL, serum ALT levels two times normal, and evidence of severe hepatitis on liver biopsy. Deciding when and with what medications is complicated for patients with hepatitis B infections and one should consider the patient's age, severity of liver disease, likelihood of response, and potential adverse events associated with the treatment.
  a. The American Association for the Study of Liver Disease (AASLD) **treatment guidelines** can be found at www.aasld.org.
    (1) For patients who are HBeAg positive, start treatment with any of approved antiviral medications, but peginterferon alpha, tenofovir, or entecavir are preferred.(SOR Ⓐ)
    (2) Patients with compensated cirrhosis who either have ALT more than two times normal or patients with normal or minimally elevated ALT, but high serum HBV DNA levels should also be considered for treatment. Patients with compensated cirrhosis are best treated with nucleoside analogs because there is a risk of hepatic decompensation associated with interferon; tenofovir and entecavir are preferred. (SOR Ⓑ)
    (3) For patients with compensated cirrhosis due to hepatitis B, peginterferon should be avoided as there is a risk of hepatic decompensation with this medication. (SOR Ⓑ)
4. Treatment for primary biliary cirrhosis is ursodeoxycholic acid (UDCA), 13 to 15 mg/kg/d. (SOR Ⓐ) Treatment should be continued indefinitely. For patients who worsen while on UDCA, either colchicine or methotrexate can be added to their regimen. The **pruritus of primary biliary cirrhosis** may be improved by cholestyramine, 4 to 16 g per day divided and mixed with food or juice with each meal. (SOR Ⓑ)
5. Hemochromatosis is treated when there is an evidence of iron overload. Removing 500 mL of blood weekly by phlebotomy to maintain ferritin at 50 to 100 mcg/L in the first 18 months of the disease increases life expectancy. (SOR Ⓑ) A diet that avoids iron and vitamin C supplements is also advised. (SOR Ⓒ) For patients unable to undergo phlebotomy, oral chelation with deferoxamine may be considered.
6. Treatment for Wilson disease is d-penicillamine, initially 1000 to 2000 g per day in four divided doses beginning with 250 mg daily and increasing by 250 to 500 mg daily. After 4 to 6 months of initiation treatment, the dose can be reduced to 750 to 1000 mg daily in two divided doses for lifelong maintenance. (SOR Ⓑ) Children are usually dosed 20 mg/kg/day divided twice daily.

    a. For patients who do not tolerate penicillamine, trientine can be used, 750 to 1500 mg orally divided two to three times daily (maximum daily dose of 2 g). (SOR **B**) Dosing for children can be 20 mg/kg/day divided two to three times daily.

    b. Zinc can be used as a third-line agent to block copper absorption.

    c. Copper excretion, complete blood count, urinalysis, and serum creatinine should be monitored for patients on treatment.

  7. Treatment for alpha-1 antitrypsin (AAT) deficiency is intravenous infusion of pooled human AAT (alpha-1 antiprotease), which elevates AAT levels. (SOR **C**) There are limited data suggesting that this treatment may slow lung decline, but it does little to treat the liver disease. Cessation of cigarette smoking is crucial for these patients.

  8. Treatment for NASH is weight loss and regular exercise. (SOR **C**) Management should also include blood glucose control and treatment of hyperlipidemia.

  9. Treatment for autoimmune hepatitis in adults should begin with combination treatment prednisone (30 mg per day, tapering down to 10 mg per day within 4 weeks) plus azathioprine (50 mg per day or 1–2 mg/kg body weight). (SOR **A**) In children, treatment should include prednisone (1–2 mg/kg/day up to maximum dose of 60 mg per day) plus azathioprine (1–2 mg/kg/day) or 6-mercaptopurine (1.5 mg/kg/day). (SOR **B**) Maintenance therapy usually consists of prednisone alone and should continue until transaminase levels are normal.

IV. Management Strategies. Management of cirrhosis consists not only of treatment but also of monitoring for complications, deciding when hospitalization is required, providing education for the patient, and, if needed, referring the patient for liver transplantation.

A. Monitoring

  1. Laboratory parameters to be followed, on an interval based on severity, include serum transaminases (AST, ALT), prothrombin times, serum albumin, electrolytes, bilirubin, and complete blood counts. The patient should be checked clinically for ascites, signs of volume depletion, bleeding, and encephalopathy. Surveillance for hepatocellular carcinoma (HCC) should be performed every 6 to 12 months with ultrasound and serum alpha-fetoprotein (AFP). (SOR **A**)

  2. Hospitalization is indicated for gastrointestinal bleeding, worsening encephalopathy, increasing azotemia, or intractable ascites.

  3. Diagnostic paracentesis should be considered for new-onset or worsening ascites, or when SBP is suspected.

  4. Hepatocellular carcinoma should be suspected in patients with an unexplained clinical deterioration of chronic cirrhosis or watery diarrhea.

B. Patient support for adherence to diet is essential. Abstinence from alcohol is also essential; most patients will require considerable skill and support from the primary care physician, the family, and rehabilitation programs in order to abstain (see Chapter 90).

C. Liver transplantation

  1. A physician should consider referring a patient for transplantation when they develop evidence of hepatic dysfunction (Child-Turcotte–Pugh score >7; http://www.hepatitis.va.gov/provider/tools/child-pugh-calculator.asp) or when they experience their first cirrhotic complication (ascites, hepatic encephalopathy, or variceal bleeding.

    a. Absolute contraindications to liver transplantation include portal vein thrombosis, severe medical illness, malignancy, hepatobiliary sepsis, or lack of patient understanding. Among the **relative contraindications** are active alcoholism, human immunodeficiency virus (HIV) positivity, hepatitis B surface antigen positivity, extensive previous abdominal surgery, and lack of a family or personal support system.

V. Prognosis. The prognosis for cirrhosis is determined by the cause and the presence of complications. Complications of cirrhosis include portal hypertension, variceal bleeding, splenomegaly, ascites, edema, and hepatic encephalopathy.

A. Prognosis related to complications of cirrhosis

  1. Portal hypertension contributes to the development of splenomegaly, varices, and ascites and carries a significant negative prognosis.

  2. Hepatic encephalopathy is a complex, neuropsychiatric disorder most likely caused by one or more substances of intestinal origin that are not metabolized because of hepatocellular dysfunction and portal systemic shunting. As a late-stage finding in cirrhosis, unless an acute reversible liver insult is identified and removed, hepatic encephalopathy tends to recur.

B. Patients without gastrointestinal bleeding, encephalopathy, low albumin, and ascites have a better prognosis than those with such complications.

C. The prognosis of alcoholic cirrhosis is dependent on abstinence. The 5-year survival rate is 60% or greater for patients who abstain compared to 40% for patients who continue to drink alcohol.

D. In a 20-year prospective study of individuals with cirrhosis, liver failure, HCC, and gastrointestinal hemorrhage accounted for three-quarters of the deaths. The 5-year survival rates were 14% for cryptogenic cirrhosis and 60% for chronic active hepatitis.

SELECTED REFERENCES

Bacon BR, Adams PC, Kowdley KV, Powell LW, Tavill AS; American Association for the Study of Liver Diseases. Diagnosis and management of hemochromatosis: 2011 practice guideline by the American Association for the Study of Liver Diseases. *Hepatology.* 2011;54(1):328–343.

Bonacini M, Hadi G, Govindarajan S, Landsay KL. Utility of a discriminant score for diagnosing advanced fibrosis or cirrhosis in patients with chronic hepatitis C virus infection. *Am J Gastroenterol.* 1997;92(8):1302–1304.

European Association for the Study of the Liver. EASL Clinical Practice Guidelines: Wilson's disease. *Hepatology.* 2012;56:671–685.

Farrell GC, Larter CZ. Nonalcoholic fatty liver disease: from steatosis to cirrhosis. *Hepatology.* 2006; 43(2 Suppl 1):S99–S112.

Ferenci P, Runyon B. Hepatic encephalopathy in adults: treatment. www.uptodate.com. Accessed July 18, 2013.

Gilbert D, Moellering RC, Eliopoulos GM, et al., eds. *The Sanford Guide to Antimicrobial Therapy.* 37th ed. Sperryville, VA: Antimicrobial Association; 2008.

Goldberg E, Chopra S. Overview of complications, prognosis and management of cirrhosis. www.uptodate.com. Accessed July 17, 2013.

Goldberg E, Chopra S. Diagnostic approach to patients with cirrhosis. www.uptodate.com. Accessed July 17, 2013.

Lindor KD, Gershwin ME, Poupon R, et al. Primary biliary cirrhosis. *Hepatology.* 2009;50(1):291–308.

Manns MP, Czaja AJ, Gorham JD, et al. Diagnosis and management of autoimmune hepatitis. *Hepatology.* 2010;51:2193–2213.

Pawlotski J. Therapy of hepatitis C: from empiricism to eradication. *Hepatology.* 2006;43:S207–S220.

Runyon BA. Introduction to the revised American Association for the Study of Liver Diseases Practice Guideline management of adult patients with ascites due to cirrhosis 2012. *Hepatology.* 2013; 57(4):1651–1653.

---

73 Congestive Heart Failure

Philip M. Diller, MD, PhD, & Christopher R. Bernheisel, MD

KEY POINTS

- Heart failure (HF) is a common progressive terminal condition with a poor prognosis. The prevalence of HF is increasing with the aging of the population. (SOR **C**)
- Optimal management of HF begins with identifying the stage (A–D) and type of HF (systolic versus diastolic). (SOR **B**) Therapies include those that prevent HF (BP control, lipid lowering [SOR **A**]), slow the progression of cardiac remodeling (angiotensin-converting enzymes and beta-blockers [SOR **A**]), achieve euvolemia (diet and diuretics [SOR **C**]), and digitalis (SOR **A**).
- Angiotensin-converting enzymes, beta-blockers, aldosterone, and angiotensin II receptor blockers have been shown to reduce mortality rates in clinical trials of patients with HF and left ventricular systolic dysfunction. (SOR **A**)
- Diastolic HF therapies are directed to the underlying cause—typically, ischemia, hypertension, and rate control if a tachycardia is present. (SOR **C**)

I. Introduction

A. Definition. HF is a clinical syndrome of symptoms and signs that may include fatigue, exercise intolerance, dyspnea, peripheral edema, and pulmonary congestion. HF signs and symptoms result when the heart is unable to fill with or eject blood sufficient to perfuse body tissues and meet metabolic demands. "Heart failure" is preferred over the term "congestive heart failure" because up to one-third of ambulatory patients with HF do not manifest pulmonary or systemic congestion.

B. Classification. In clinical practice, HF is commonly classified in two ways. First, according to left ventricular ejection fraction (LVEF): systolic if LVEF <40% or diastolic if LVEF >45% to 50% and documented diastolic dysfunction. Second, HF is classified according to the stage of progression in recognition of the early, often asymptomatic onset of HF. The stages are

1. Stage A. At risk for developing HF, but no structural disorders of the heart (in the United States, 50–60 million individuals).

2. Stage B. No experience of HF symptoms, but with a structural disorder of the heart (in the United States, 8–10 million individuals).

3. Stage C. Structural heart disease and is experiencing or has experienced the HF symptoms (in the United States, 5 million individuals).

4. Stage D. Advanced heart disease with severe HF symptoms and specialized treatment approaches (in the United States, 50,000–200,000 individuals).

This staging system emphasizes the important role of preventing HF for the primary care physician.

C. Epidemiology

1. Prevalence. Close to 5 million people in the United States have HF, with nearly 500,000 new cases diagnosed each year. HF is the primary reason for more than 1 million hospital admissions each year and is the most common reason for hospital admission among persons older than 65 years (one in five admissions). Approximately 300,000 HF-related deaths occur each year in the United States and the number increases despite treatment advances. Approximately 6% to 10% of people older than 65 years have HF.

In primary care practice, approximately 40% of patients present with signs and symptoms of HF and have normal systolic function; the other 60% have left ventricular systolic dysfunction. HF causes with a normal LVEF are shown in Table 73–1.

TABLE 73–1. COMMON CAUSES OF HEART FAILURE WITH NORMAL LVEF

Inaccurate diagnosis of HF (e.g., COPD)
Inaccurate measurement of LVEF
LV systolic function overestimated by LVEF (e.g., mitral regurgitation)
Episodic LV systolic dysfunction, normal at the time of evaluation (severe hypertension, ischemia, tachycardia, infection, volume overload, spontaneous variability of EF)
Obstruction of LV inflow (mitral stenosis)
Diastolic dysfunction because of:
  Abnormal LV relaxation
  Ischemia
  Hypertrophy
  Cardiomyopathies
  High-output states
  Volume overload
  Aging
  Diabetes mellitus
  Amyloidosis
  Pericardial disease

COPD, chronic obstructive pulmonary disease; EF, ejection fraction; HF, heart failure; LV, left ventricular; LVEF, left ventricular ejection fraction.
Source: Adapted with permission from Dauterman KW, Massie BM, Gheorghiade M. Heart failure associated with preserved systolic function: a common and costly clinical entity. *Am Heart J.* 1998;135:S310–S319.

2. Etiology. Underlying the signs and symptoms of HF are diverse causes that lead to an inability of the heart to perfuse tissues and meet the metabolic demands of the body. Some of the most important predisposing factors include the following:

a. Hypertension. In the Framingham study, 5143 adults without HF at baseline were followed for an average of 14 years. Of the 392 persons who developed HF, 357 (91%) had hypertension that antedated initial HF diagnosis. Hypertension accounted for 39% of new HF cases in men and 59% of new cases in women. Chronic hypertension leading to left ventricular hypertrophy (LVH) is a common pathway in the development of HF.

b. Coronary artery disease is the cause of HF in two-thirds of patients with left ventricular (LV) systolic dysfunction. Measurable decreases in systolic function may be present for months or years before overt HF symptoms develop. Acute myocardial ischemia and myocardial infarction can result in sudden changes in systolic and diastolic ventricular function and acute HF with systemic congestion.

c. Other causes of cardiomyopathy. Viral infections, diabetes mellitus, and excessive alcohol intake have direct effects on the myocardium and can lead to cardiomyopathy and ventricular dysfunction. Diabetes is emerging as a significant causative factor for the development of HF.

d. Valvular disease. Significant valvular stenosis, regurgitation, or both, particularly in the mitral or aortic valves, are well-documented factors that contribute to ventricular dysfunction, and are commonly seen in the elderly as a contributing factor for HF.

e. Cardiovascular changes that occur with normal aging help explain why HF incidence and prevalence increase with age. Arterial stiffening with increased afterload and peripheral vascular resistance occurs with advancing age even in normotensive individuals. An increase in LV mass that often occurs with aging may lead to impaired ventricular diastolic filling.

D. Pathophysiology

1. The HF syndrome is a heterogeneous, progressive condition caused by various combinations of central and peripheral pathophysiologic mechanisms. These mechanisms are often dynamic, leading to wide fluctuations in measured ventricular function and physical impairment that can be observed over time in individual patients.

2. Central/cardiac factors. HF begins with some injury to or stress on the myocardium that leads to impaired ventricular function during systole, diastole, or both. Initially, the effects of inadequate cardiac output may only be experienced with physical exertion, but eventually in advanced HF dyspnea at rest occurs. This progression of symptoms correlates with changes in the geometry of the left ventricle: dilatation, hypertrophy, and assumption of a more spherical shape. Such cardiac remodeling leads to inefficient hemodynamic performance that is sustained and progressive.

3. Peripheral factors. Peripheral compensatory responses to diastolic or systolic LV dysfunction or both may initially help maintain cardiac function and organ perfusion, but eventually they lead to worsening HF signs and symptoms.

a. Renin–angiotensin–aldosterone system (RAAS). In response to LV dysfunction, the RAAS is activated, resulting in increased levels of angiotensin II, aldosterone, increased preload and afterload, and sodium and water retention. Initially, RAAS activation may help maintain or even improve LV function, but continued increases in intravascular volume and peripheral resistance become detrimental to LV function and lead to volume overload.

b. The **sympathetic nervous system** is also activated in response to LV dysfunction to maintain blood pressure and organ perfusion through increased catecholamine levels that augment cardiac contractility and increased heart rate. Prolonged sympathetic activation causes chronic elevations in afterload (peripheral vasoconstriction) and eventual worsening of LV function. Elevated resting plasma norepinephrine levels are independent predictors of clinical outcomes and mortality among patients with severe HF.

c. Natriuretic peptides and other parahormones. Atrial natriuretic peptide and brain natriuretic peptide (BNP) are produced from cardiac myocytes in response to increased pressures in the cardiac chambers. These peptides initially promote natriuresis and diuresis, but resistance occurs to these effects over time in chronic HF. Endothelins are endogenous peptides with strong vasoconstrictor and vasopressor activities and are found at high levels in patients with HF. Elevated levels of the natriuretic and endothelin peptides correlate with worsening HF and higher mortality rates among patients with HF. N-terminal-proBNP is also available for measurement and this or measurement of BNP is helpful in the diagnosis of HF (see Section II.C.1).

II. Prevention. The common etiologic factors leading to HF suggest potentially useful strategies to HF prevention. Preventive measures include adequate blood pressure control using medications known to limit or reverse LVH, (SOR **A**) smoking cessation, (SOR **A**) aggressive lipid lowering, (SOR **A**) achieving target blood sugar control in patients with diabetes, (SOR **A**) alcohol abstention, (SOR **C**) surgical valve replacement when indicated, improvement of coronary blood flow with appropriate revascularization strategies, (SOR **A**) and use of angiotensin-converting enzyme inhibitors (ACEIs) for patients with asymptomatic LV systolic dysfunction. (SOR **A**)

III. Diagnosis. HF diagnosis requires, first, the recognition of the clinical syndrome based on the characteristic constellation of clinical signs and symptoms and, second, the determination of the underlying structural abnormality of the heart that produced those symptoms. Clinical criteria used to aid in the diagnosis of HF include the Framingham Criteria and the Boston Criteria (Table 73–2). These criteria may not identify individuals with LV dysfunction who have mild or intermittent symptoms. Determination of plasma BNP levels can assist in the differentiation between cardiac and noncardiac causes of dyspnea. (SOR **B**)

A. Clinical symptoms and signs
   1. Symptoms
      a. Shortness of breath can range from mild to severe. Exertional dyspnea may occur with any level of activity, depending on the severity of the HF syndrome. The absence of dyspnea on exertion makes the diagnosis of HF unlikely. (SOR **B**) With

TABLE 73–2. CRITERIA USED FOR DIAGNOSIS OF CONGESTIVE HEART FAILURE IN CLINICAL STUDIES

The Framingham Heart Study Criteria	The Boston Scale Criteria
Major criteria • Paroxysmal nocturnal dyspnea • Neck vein distension • Rales • Cardiomegaly • Acute pulmonary edema • S_3 gallop • Increased venous pressure (>16 cm) • Circulation time ≥25 s • Hepatojugular reflux positive	*Category I: History* • Rest dyspnea (4 points) • Orthopnea (4 points) • Paroxysmal nocturnal dyspnea (3 points) • Dyspnea climbing (1 point)
Minor criteria • Ankle edema • Night cough • Hepatomegaly • Pleural effusion • Vital capacity reduced by one-third from predicted • Tachycardia (≥120) • Major or minor criterion • Weight loss of more than 4.5 kg over 5 days in response to treatment	*Category II: Physical examination* • Heart rate: 91–110 (1 point): >110 (2 points) • Jugular venous pressure elevation: >6 cm H_2O plus hepatomegaly or leg edema (3 points) • Lung rales: Basilar (1 point); more than basilar (2 points) • Wheezing (3 points) • Third heart sound (3 points)
	Category III: Chest radiography • Alveolar pulmonary edema (4 points) • Interstitial pulmonary edema (3 points) • Bilateral pleural effusion (3 points) • Cardiothoracic ratio ≥0.50 (3 points) • Upper zone flow redistribution (2 points)
Definite congestive heart failure • Two major criteria or one major and two minor criteria	*Determine score* • Point value within parentheses and no more than 4 points from each category allowed. The maximum possible is 12 points. *Definite congestive heart failure* • 8–12 points *Possible congestive heart failure* • 5–7 points

Source: Data from McKee PA, Castelli WP, McNamarra PM, et al. The natural history of congestive heart failure: the Framingham study. *N Engl J Med.* 1971;285:1441–1446; Remes J, Miettenen H, Rennanen A, et al. Validity of clinical diagnosis of heart failure in primary health care. *Eur Heart J.* 1991;12:315–321; and Young JB. The heart failure syndrome. In: Mills RM, Young JB, eds. *Practical Approaches to the Treatment of Heart Failure.* Philadelphia, PA: Lippincott Williams & Wilkins; 1998.

orthopnea, patients will report feeling short of breath while lying flat, may be using pillows to prop themselves up at night, or may need to sleep sitting up if HF is severe. **Paroxysmal nocturnal dyspnea or nighttime cough** are suggestive of HF. **Dyspnea at rest** occurs in advanced HF or during acute exacerbations and volume overload.

    b. Fatigue and weakness. These symptoms are nonspecific and are in part caused by abnormal autoregulation of blood flow to the extremities and muscle deconditioning.

2. Clinical signs. Physical examination findings for HF include the following:

    a. Tachycardia is present in many patients with HF and reflects increased adrenergic activity. Other symptoms related to increased adrenergic activity are pallor and coldness of the extremities and cyanosis of the digits (peripheral vasoconstriction).

    b. Moist crackles, usually heard in both lung bases, are a consequence of transudation of fluid into the alveoli. Pleural effusion collecting in the bases may lead to dullness on percussion. If the bronchial mucosa is congested, then bronchospasm and associated high-pitched wheezes may also be present.

    c. Systemic venous hypertension is suggested by a jugular venous pressure level higher than 4 cm above the sternal angle when the patient is examined sitting at a 45-degree angle. In advanced cases, venous pressure is so high that peripheral veins on the dorsum of the hand are dilated and fail to collapse when elevated above the shoulder.

    d. Hepatojugular reflux is helpful in differentiating hepatomegaly resulting from HF from other conditions. The neck veins are observed, and then the right upper quadrant of the abdomen is compressed continuously for 1 minute. The patient is instructed to breathe normally. This maneuver increases venous return to the heart. In patients with HF, the jugular veins expand during and immediately after compression because of the inability of the heart to respond to the increased venous supply.

    e. Hepatomegaly is due to liver congestion. If this occurs acutely, the liver may be tender to palpation. With advanced HF, the liver is still enlarged, but is typically nontender.

    f. Peripheral edema is a nonspecific yet a very common sign in HF. A corresponding symptom of weight gain is often elicited from patients. The edema is typically bilateral and symmetrical in the dependent portions of the body. For ambulatory patients, the edema worsens as the day progresses and resolves after a night's rest.

    g. Cardiomegaly is also a nonspecific yet very common sign in HF. A normal apical impulse is located in the fourth or fifth intercostal space and is a brief tap. It is only palpable in approximately 50% of patients with HF. If the apical impulse involves more than one intercostal space, cardiomegaly is present. Precordial percussion is more sensitive than the apical impulse for detecting abnormal LV size. A percussion dullness distance greater than 10.5 cm in the fifth intercostal space has a sensitivity of 91% and a specificity of 30% for increased LV size.

    h. The presence of an S_3 gallop occurs from ventricular vibration with rapid diastolic filling. It is a low-pitched sound best heard with the bell of the stethoscope over the apical impulse. Having the patient in the 45-degree left lateral decubitus position doubles the yield.

B. Chest x-ray (CXR). Findings in patients with HF may include the following:

    1. Cardiomegaly. A cardiothoracic ratio of 50% or more on anteroposterior CXR.

    2. Pulmonary edema marked by equalization of the caliber of blood vessels in the apex and the lung bases (cephalization), interstitial edema (development of Kerley B lines, sharp linear densities of interlobular interstitial edema), and alveolar edema (central butterfly or cloud-like appearance of fluid around the hila).

C. Laboratory testing in a patient with a new HF diagnosis should include an electrocardiogram (for arrhythmia, ischemia, LVH); a complete blood count (anemia); a urinalysis and tests of levels of serum creatinine, potassium (renal function), and albumin; and thyroid studies (T4, thyroid-stimulating hormone, hypothyroidism). Screening evaluation for arrhythmias using Holter monitoring is not routinely warranted.

    1. Measuring BNP in patients with suspected HF. BNP is elevated in both systolic and diastolic HFs. BNP can be helpful when the physician is unclear if the patient has dyspnea caused by HF or noncardiac causes. Using a cutoff level of 100 pg/mL, BNP has a sensitivity of 90%, a specificity of 76%, and a positive predictive value of 83% in identifying patients with LV dysfunction. This can be compared to the Framingham clinical criteria which have a sensitivity of 83%, a specificity of 67%, and a positive predictive value of 73%. Obesity (BMI 30 and higher) lowers BNP levels decreasing the sensitivity of BNP in this patient population. Elevated pulmonary hypertension and pulmonary embolus can cause elevations of BNP in the intermediate range between 100 and 400 pg/mL. So, if these conditions are suspected based on clinical presentation, then appropriate tests should be obtained to diagnose these disorders.

D. **Diagnosing the heart's structural abnormality (the type of HF)** helps establish the physiologic goals of treatment and individualize pharmaceutical therapy.

1. Two-dimensional echocardiography coupled with Doppler flow (SOR **B**) studies allows the physician to determine whether the structural abnormality is myocardial, valvular, or pericardial, and if myocardial, whether the dysfunction is systolic or diastolic. Measurement of LVEF is determined with this study; patients with LVEF <40% have systolic dysfunction. Physiologic goals and the evidence base for specific therapeutic decisions differ between patients with LV systolic dysfunction and those who have normal LVEF and isolated diastolic dysfunction. Doppler flow measures of diastolic filling need to be interpreted in the context of the individual patient, since they are often abnormal in healthy elderly patients without HF and may be deceivingly normal in patients with progressively restrictive filling patterns or difficult to assess in obese patients.

2. Coronary angiography should be performed in patients with HF who have angina or evidence of ischemia and are considered prior to revascularization if indicated.

E. **Assessing the level of HF severity. The level of functional impairment** from HF is a strong prognostic marker, allows the physician to monitor the effects of treatment, and determines whether patients will benefit from certain therapies (see Section V). **The New York Heart Association (NYHA) Functional Classification** is the simplest and most widely used tool for assessing physical functioning (Table 73–3). Other objective tests of functional capacity include the six-minute walk test (distance covered in 6 minutes), formal exercise testing, and maximal oxygen uptake (VO_{2max}).

IV. **Treatment.** The heterogeneous nature of HF mandates an individualized approach to treatment with attention to etiology, type of HF, noncardiac comorbid conditions, and, if systolic HF, the stage. Most of the large clinical trials on treatment of HF have only included patients with systolic dysfunction. The treatment of diastolic HF continues to be based on the underlying pathophysiologic mechanism(s).

A. **Treatment of specific underlying cardiac factors** may significantly improve ventricular function and HF symptoms. Special attention should be given to surgical correction of significant valvular disease when appropriate and reversal of myocardial ischemia with stent placement or surgical bypass when indicated. Ventricular rate control and/or conversion to sinus rhythm may improve ventricular function for patients with atrial fibrillation and HF.

B. **Using BNP level to guide therapy** has been shown to reduce all-cause mortality and hospital readmission rates. (SOR **A**)

C. A number of **noncardiac comorbid conditions** may affect the proper diagnosis and clinical course of HF and should be carefully assessed and treated:

1. **Chronic obstructive pulmonary disease.** Dyspnea, exercise intolerance, nighttime cough, and other symptoms of chronic pulmonary disease may be misinterpreted

TABLE 73–3. NEW YORK HEART ASSOCIATION FUNCTIONAL CLASSIFICATION

Class I	No limitation of activity. Ordinary activity does not cause undue fatigue, palpitation, dyspnea, or anginal pain.
Class II	Slight limitations of physical activity. Patient is comfortable at rest. Ordinary activity results in fatigue, palpitation, dyspnea, or anginal pain.
Class III	Marked limitation of physical activity. Patient is comfortable at rest, but less than ordinary activity causes fatigue, palpitation, dyspnea, or anginal pain.
Class IV	Inability to carry out physical activity without symptoms. Symptoms of heart failure often present at rest. Increased symptoms or discomfort with even minor physical activity.

Source: Data from Criteria Committee, New York Heart Association. *Nomenclature and Criteria for Diagnosis of Diseases of the Heart and Great Vessels.* 9th ed. Boston, MA: Little, Brown; 1994:253–256.

as HF symptoms. Treatment of chronic obstructive pulmonary disease should be optimized (see Chapter 70).

2. **Diabetes mellitus** may predispose patients to silent myocardial ischemia that worsens LV function, "stiff" ventricles, and diastolic dysfunction. For both types of HF, diabetes control is an important goal (see Chapter 75). The thiazolidinediones class of medications can cause fluid retention and acute volume overload episodes, and, therefore, must be used cautiously in patients with HF.

3. **Renal insufficiency** will influence fluid and electrolyte problems in HF and may limit usefulness or lead to changes in dosing for HF medications, particularly ACEIs and diuretics.

4. **Significant arthritis** may further limit physical activity and worsen the skeletal muscle changes that occur in patients with HF. Nonsteroidal anti-inflammatory drugs and COX-II inhibitors can cause sodium retention and peripheral vasoconstriction leading to reduced efficacy and can potentially enhance the toxicity of diuretics and ACEIs. Such anti-inflammatory drugs should be used cautiously in patients with HF.

5. **Depression and poor social support** have been shown to be important predictors of clinical outcomes, hospitalizations, and deaths among patients with ischemic heart disease. Depression is common is patients with HF.

6. **Substance abuse.** Smoking cessation should be encouraged. Patients with a component of LV dysfunction resulting from alcohol abuse may show significant functional improvement with abstention from alcohol.

7. Hypothyroidism or hyperthyroidism may aggravate HF symptoms.

8. **Nephrotic syndrome, hypoalbuminemia, or both** may worsen volume overload in HF.

D. **Treatment of systolic dysfunction HF.** The treatment of systolic HF is guided by stage (see Section I.B) as shown in Table 73–4. The centerpiece of these recommendations is the use of ACEIs and beta-blockers **to reduce mortality in all patients with**

TABLE 73–4. TREATMENT RECOMMENDATIONS ACCORDING TO HEART FAILURE STAGE

Stage A. At risk for heart failure but without structural heart disease or symptoms of HF
Treat hypertension
Encourage smoking cessation
Treat lipid disorders
Encourage regular exercise
Discourage alcohol intake, illicit drug use
ACE inhibition in appropriate patients

Stage B. Structural heart disease but without symptoms of HF
All measures under Stage A
ACE inhibitors in appropriate patients
Beta-blockers in appropriate patients

Stage C. Structural heart disease without prior or current symptoms of HF
All measures under Stage A
Drugs for routine use:
  Diuretics
  ACE inhibitors
  Beta-blockers
  Digitalis
  Dietary salt restriction

Stage D. Refractory HF requiring specialized interventions
All measures under Stages A, B, and C
Mechanical assist devices
Heart transplantation
Continuous (not intermittent) intravenous inotropic infusions for palliation
Hospice care

ACE, angiotensin-converting enzyme.
Source: Data from Hunt SA, Abraham WT, Chin MH, et al. ACC/AHA 2005 Guideline Update for the Diagnosis and Management of Chronic Heart Failure in the Adult: a report of the American College of Cardiology/American Heart Association Task Force on Practice Guidelines. *Circulation.* 2005;112:e154–e235.

systolic HF. (SOR **Ⓐ**) Additional mortality reductions are possible with the addition of aldosterone antagonists in patients with severe HF. (SOR **Ⓐ**) In addition to the mortality prevention goal, there are physiologic treatment goals for stage C patients. The following discussion reviews the necessary management steps to achieve those goals.

1. **Achieving and maintaining optimal volume status.** Although ACEIs should be considered first-line therapy for chronic HF resulting from systolic dysfunction, an initial presentation of a patient with HF and pulmonary and systemic congestion dictates acute treatment with diuretics to lessen fluid overload and rapidly improve symptoms. Intravenous administration of diuretics may be necessary to relieve acute pulmonary congestion. (SOR **Ⓐ**) The discussion that follows is geared more toward management of the patient with chronic HF.

   a. **The loop diuretic furosemide** is the most frequently prescribed diuretic for treatment of volume overload in HF. (SOR **Ⓐ**) Initial oral doses of 10 to 40 mg once a day should be administered to patients with dyspnea on exertion and signs of volume overload who do not have indications for acute hospitalization. Severe overload and pulmonary edema are indications for hospitalization and intravenous furosemide. Other considerations for prescribing diuretics in HF include the following:

      (1) Some patients with mild HF can be treated effectively with thiazide diuretics. Those who have persistent volume overload on 50 mg of hydrochlorothiazide per day should be switched to an oral loop diuretic.

      (2) Oral absorption of furosemide is diminished by physiologic changes in HF, particularly if the oral dose is taken on a full stomach. Torsemide is an alternative loop diuretic that is extremely well absorbed from the gastrointestinal tract in patients with HF.

      (3) Patients with poor oral absorption, renal insufficiency, or both may require much higher doses of a loop diuretic to reach a threshold level for diuresis, up to a maximum of 300 mg twice a day of furosemide.

      (4) Important adverse effects of diuretics that require periodic monitoring include orthostatic hypotension, prerenal azotemia, hyponatremia, hypomagnesemia, and hypokalemia. Most patients taking 40 mg or more of furosemide daily should supplement their oral potassium intake through dietary changes, prescribed potassium supplements, or both. ACEIs, however, can cause hyperkalemia, so periodic monitoring is helpful.

      (5) Once volume overload is corrected and an ACEI is initiated, the diuretic dose can often be carefully decreased or even eliminated. Some patients may only need intermittent diuretic therapy when symptoms and increases in daily weights signal a return of excess fluid volume.

   b. **Adding a second diuretic** is sometimes necessary to maintain optimal fluid balance. (SOR **Ⓒ**) Adding **metolazone,** 2.5 to 10 mg per day, to a daily furosemide dose can significantly increase diuresis for outpatient treatment of moderate volume overload. Prolonged combined therapy with metolazone should be avoided because of the increased risk of electrolyte depletion.

   c. **Spironolactone or eplerenone,** aldosterone-blocking agents, should also be added to standard regimens (diuretics, ACEI, digoxin, and a beta-blocker) to increase diuresis and reduce all-cause mortality in patients with NYHA Classes II–IV and left ventricular ejection fraction under 30%. Spironolactone should be started at 12.5 to 25 mg daily and eplerenone at 25 mg daily. Patients should have careful monitoring of their potassium and creatinine, checking 3 days and 7 days after initiation, monthly for 3 months followed by every 3months. The medications should be discontinued in patients with serum potassium level >5.0 mmol/L, creatinine >2.5 mg/dL, or creatinine clearance <30 mL/min.

   d. **Sodium restriction.** Patients should limit sodium intake to 2 to 3 g per day or less by avoiding salty tasting foods, not adding salt at the table, and reading nutritional labels to choose lower-sodium food options. (SOR **Ⓒ**) A sudden increase in dietary sodium intake is a frequent cause of acute fluid overload, pulmonary congestion, and hospitalization.

   e. Patients should **weigh themselves daily,** record their weight, and report any gain or loss of more than 3 lbs from their baseline weight. Baseline weight is determined when the patient is in optimal fluid balance on a stable medical regimen. Reliable patients may be instructed to increase daily diuretic dose for 2 to 4 days when they see an increase in daily weights.

2. **Decreasing preload and afterload by blunting the exaggerated peripheral compensatory response** using ACEIs.
   a. **ACEIs.** Many clinical trials have provided consistent evidence that ACEIs result in decreased symptoms, improved quality of life, fewer hospitalizations, and reductions in mortality for patients with NYHA class II–IV HF. (SOR **A**) In addition, ACEIs slow the progression to HF among patients with asymptomatic LV systolic dysfunction. (SOR **A**) **All patients with HF and LV systolic dysfunction should be prescribed ACEIs unless they have a contraindication to these drugs.**
   (1) Contraindications to ACEI use include pregnancy, bilateral renal artery stenosis, angioedema or other allergic responses, or documented persistent intolerance to ACEI (symptomatic hypotension, severe renal dysfunction, hyperkalemia, or cough).
   (2) The positive effects of ACEI probably apply to all available drugs in this class, but preference should be given to drugs with the most evidence for improved clinical outcomes. Enalapril, captopril, lisinopril, and ramipril have the strongest evidence for mortality reductions. (SOR **A**)
   (3) To minimize the risk of symptomatic hypotension, one-half the normal starting dose should be given to patients with hyponatremia (<135 mEq/L), recent increase in diuretic dose, serum creatinine levels >1.7 mg/dL, and patients older than 75 years. Patients at a high risk for symptomatic hypotension should be given a test dose of a short-acting ACEI (captopril, 6.25 mg) and be observed in the physician's office for 2 hours before starting daily ACEI therapy.
   (4) Laboratory tests (blood urea nitrogen, serum creatinine, and potassium) and blood pressure should be obtained before starting ACEI therapy, 1 to 2 weeks after initiating therapy, after changes in dose, and every 3 to 4 months thereafter. The average increase in creatinine is 0.4 mg/dL, with most of the change observed in the first 6 weeks. The reversible renal impairment caused by ACEIs may resolve with a careful decrease in diuretic dose. As long as creatinine stabilizes at approximately 3.5 mg/dL or less, and hyperkalemia or symptomatic hypotension is not persistent, ACEIs should be continued and titrated up to target doses (Table 73–5). If target doses are not tolerated, lower doses should be used because they also appear to confer some benefit. (SOR **C**) Systolic blood pressure of 90 to 100 mm Hg should not deter the physician from titrating to target doses unless hypotension becomes symptomatic.
   (5) Nonproductive cough is a common adverse effect of ACEIs, secondary to increased bradykinin levels. Cough is not necessarily attributable to ACEIs since it is a common HF symptom. Only 1% to 2.5% of patients in clinical trials discontinued ACEI because of cough. For patients with cough on an ACEI, switching to an alternative ACEI may diminish cough symptoms.
   (6) Concomitant use of aspirin may attenuate the hemodynamic actions of ACEIs and their effects on survival, whereas clopidogrel does not. However, there is insufficient evidence to avoid concurrent use of aspirin and ACEIs in appropriate patients.
   b. For patients unable to use ACEIs, a trial of **hydralazine and isosorbide dinitrate (HYD-ISDN)** should be initiated to decrease preload and afterload (SOR **A**) (Table 73–5). Patients at a high risk for symptomatic hypotension should receive lower initial doses and be monitored for adverse effects. The HYD-ISDN combination has resulted in decreased mortality in African-American men in HF clinical trials, but compliance with this combination is poor owing to the high number of tablets needed and the high incidence of adverse effects (headache and gastrointestinal complaints).
   c. **Angiotensin II receptor blockers (ARBs)** are an alternative therapy for patients who cannot use ACEIs. (SOR **A**) ARBs do not affect bradykinin levels, and thus, do not induce angioedema and cough to the same extent as ACEIs. Evidence is mounting that these medications alone confer mortality reductions equivalent to ACEIs, and that addition of ARBs to standard regimens of ACEIs and beta-blockers reduces hospitalizations for HF. (SOR **A**) A recent study suggests that addition of ARBs to patients taking ACEIs and a beta-blocker may also lead to further mortality reductions. However, the addition of an ARB to the drug regimen for patients with HF already on an ACEI and a beta-blocker is not recommended pending further supporting evidence.

TABLE 73–5. TARGET DOSES FOR ACEIs AND HYD-ISDN COMBINATION

	Starting Dose/ Maximum Daily Dose (mg)	Target Dose (mg)	Side Effects and Notes
Preferred ACEIs (see text)		Monitor Renal function with ACEIs	
Captopril[a,b]	12.5–25 three times daily/450 mg/d	50–100 three times daily	**Common:** rash, angioedema, hyperkalemia, hypotension, loss of taste, cough, neutropenia, increased serum creatinine **Black Box Warning:** d/c captopril if pregnancy is detected **Serious:** angioedema, Steven–Johnson syndrome, agranulocytosis, neutropenia
Enalapril[b]	2.5 twice daily/ 20 twice daily	10 twice daily	**Serious:** in addition to above—acute renal failure, renal impairment
Lisinopril[b]	5 daily/40 daily	5–20 daily	**Common:** For lisinopril and ramipril in addition to above, headache and dizziness **Serious:** in addition to above—cholestatic jaundice (rare)
Ramipril[b]	1.25–2.5 twice daily/ 10 daily	5 twice daily	Same as other ACEIs **Serious:** in additional to above—hepatic necrosis
Fosinopril[b]	5–10 daily/40 daily	20–40 daily	Same as other ACEIs **Serious:** same as other ACEIs and acute renal failure, azotemia, oliguria
Quinapril[b]	5 twice daily/ 20 twice daily	10–20 twice daily	Same as other ACEIs **Serious:** same as Fosinopril
Hydralazine-Isosorbide dinitrate (HYD-ISDN) Combination (BiDil)			
HYD[b]	25–37 three times daily/ 150 four times daily	75 four times daily	**Common:** headache, dizziness, and GI complaints, chest pain, tachycardia, hypotension, fluid-sodium retention **Serious:** agranulocytosis, leucopenia, hepatotoxicity, lupus pneumonia (acute), systematic lupus erythematosus **Caution:** renal failure
ISDN[b]	20 three times daily/ 120 mg/d	40 three times daily	**Common:** hypotension, headache, lightheadedness **Serious:** syncope, methemoglobinemia **Caution:** sildenafil (risk of severe hypotension)

[a]Give a single dose of captopril 6.25 mg with observation of the patient for 2 hours for patients at high risk for symptomatic hypotension.
[b]Available as generic.
ACEIs, angiotensin-converting enzyme inhibitors; GI, gastrointestinal.

   d. The first- and second-generation **calcium channel blockers** such as nifedipine, diltiazem, and nicardipine may worsen systolic dysfunction symptoms because of their negative inotropic effects. Amlodipine is better tolerated, with evidence of a neutral if not beneficial effect on HF survival. Amlodipine can be considered for patients with continued hypertension who take ACEI and diuretics, or those with symptomatic ischemia not controlled by nitrates, beta-blockers, or both.

    e. Exercise training is an effective intervention that reverses some of the exaggerated peripheral compensatory changes in patients with stable mild-to-moderate (classes I–III) systolic dysfunction HF. A series of randomized trials has shown improvements in a number of peripheral hemodynamic parameters, with diminished symptoms and improved physical functioning. Most trials have used supervised aerobic exercise on treadmills or stationary cycles. A single study evaluating the long-term effect of exercise training showed a reduction in hospitalization and deaths. Exercise training should be considered for all patients with stable HF, even though there is limited clinical trial evidence using mortality as an endpoint.

3. Delaying the clinical progression of systolic dysfunction HF and further improving symptoms may be accomplished with two other pharmaceutical interventions. One has gained acceptance in recent years (beta-blockers) and the other has been a part of HF treatment for some 200 years (cardiac glycosides/digoxin).

    a. Beta-blockers inhibit the adverse effects of sympathetic nervous system activation (e.g., cardiac hypertrophy and apoptosis, provoked arrhythmias, increased ventricular volumes). Three drugs have been studied in clinical trials involving >10,000 patients: β_1-adrenergic receptor selective blockers (bisoprolol and metoprolol) and α_1, β_1, and β_2-adrenergic receptor blockers (carvedilol). The collective experience indicates that treatment with beta-blockers in patients with HF and systolic dysfunction reduces HF symptoms, improves quality of life, reduces the risk of death by 35%, and prevents hospitalizations. (SOR **A**) The patients in these trials were also taking ACEIs, diuretics, and digoxin; thus, the benefits of beta-blockers were in addition to those already seen with the ACEIs. Beta-blockers should be prescribed in all patients with stable HF caused by LV systolic dysfunction unless they have a contraindication (symptomatic bradycardia, allergy) or are unable to tolerate them (patients with asthma).

      (1) Starting beta-blockers should be delayed in patients who are not euvolemic. Volume overload should be treated before starting a beta-blocker.

      (2) Starting at very low doses followed by a gradual up-titration once the lower dose is well tolerated (approximately every 2–4 weeks). If fluid retention occurs, then the diuretic can be increased until the weight returns to its pretreatment levels. The goal is to get the patient to the target doses achieved in the clinical trials. Table 73–6 shows the starting and target doses for beta-blockers in patients with HF. Some patients require a longer up-titration period to achieve the target dosing goal.

      (3) Patients should be monitored for the most common complications of beta-blockade: hypotension/poor perfusion, bradycardia or atrioventricular block, and bronchospasm.

      (4) Patients should be informed that achieving benefit and desired clinical response might take 2 to 3 months. Fatigue is a common side effect and usually resolves spontaneously after several weeks except in a small percentage of patients.

    b. Digoxin is considered the preferred agent among a number of available cardiac glycoside preparations. Digoxin neither improves nor worsens HF survival, but does decrease symptoms, increase exercise capacity, and decrease the need for hospitalization in systolic dysfunction HF. (SOR **A**) Digoxin is particularly appropriate for patients who remain symptomatic on ACEI, beta-blockers, and diuretics, and for patients with atrial fibrillation and rapid ventricular response.

      (1) Loading doses are generally unnecessary. A daily oral dose of 0.125 to 0.25 mg will lead to steady-state serum levels in 1 to 2 weeks.

      (2) Once a steady state is reached, a serum digoxin level, an electrocardiogram, blood urea nitrogen/creatinine levels, and serum electrolytes should be obtained.

      (3) Results of the Digitalis Investigation Group (DIG) trial suggest that a serum concentration in the lower therapeutic range (0.7–1.2 ng/mL) retains the clinical benefit of digoxin while avoiding toxicity. Levels should be checked yearly and at the time of significant changes in HF symptoms or renal function.

E. Isolated diastolic dysfunction. In comparison to the large evidence base for treating systolic dysfunction, there are minimal data available to guide the treatment of HF resulting from diastolic dysfunction. The only evidence for any treatment effects comes

TABLE 73-6. STARTING AND TARGET DOSES FOR BETA-BLOCKERS

Drug	Starting Dose/ Maximum Daily Dose (mg)	Target Dose (mg)	Side Effects and Notes (Should Be Euvolemic When Starting
Bisoprolol[a]	1.25 daily/10 daily	10 daily	**Common:** GI, headache, rhinitis, upper respiratory infection, Drowsiness, insomnia, decreased libido, bradycardia, depression **Serious:** bronchospasm **Contraindication:** AV block—second or third degree, cardiac failure, cardiogenic shock, sinus bradycardia (severe)
Carvedilol[a]	3.125 twice daily/ 50 twice daily	25 twice daily	**Common:** hypotension, dizziness, fatigue/weakness, hyperglycemia, weight gain, diarrhea, bradycardia, edema, headache, erectile dysfunction **Serious:** AV block, Stevens–Johnson syndrome, TEN, aplastic anemia, intraoperative floppy iris syndrome, asthma with status asthmaticus (rare)
Metoprolol[a] Immediate release	6.25 twice daily/ 225 twice daily[b]	50 twice daily	**Common:** bradycardia, hypotension, dizziness, fatigue, depression, rash, pruritus, dyspnea, wheezing **Serious:** bronchospasm **Contraindication:** systolic BP <100 mm Hg, HR <45 beats/min, peripheral arterial circulatory disorder (hypertension and angina)
Extended release NYHA classes II–IV EF <40% NYHA classes II–IV EF <25%	12.5–25 daily/ 400 daily[b] 12.5–25 daily 12.5 daily	200 daily 150–200 daily 100–200 daily	**Caution:** abrupt withdrawal may exacerbate angina pectoris or MI, bronchospastic disease, mask symptoms of hypoglycemia (tachycardia) in diabetic patient

[a]Available as generic
[b]There is no well-established maximum dose.
AV, atrioventricular; GI, gastrointestinal; NYHA, New York Heart Association Classification; TEN, toxic epidermal necrolysis.

from small studies where patients with diastolic HF taking verapamil increased exercise performance and improved HF symptom score. Treatment is largely empiric and directed toward reversing presumed underlying pathophysiology. (SOR **C**) There are a number of ongoing trials of ACEIs, beta-blockers, and ARBs in patients with HF and preserved systolic function.

1. Reduce the congestive state. The methods for achieving and maintaining optimal fluid balance are similar to those described for systolic dysfunction. Rapid or overdiuresis should be avoided since small changes in intravascular volume may cause significant decreases in diastolic filling and cardiac output.
2. Treatment of cardiac ischemia may improve diastolic function. Nitrates, beta-blockers, and calcium channel blockers may all be useful, but there is little direct evidence for their effectiveness in treating diastolic dysfunction. Coronary revascularization should also be considered for appropriate patients with ischemia.
3. Effective treatment of hypertension is indicated with drugs that may limit or even reverse LVH (ACEI, ARBs, CCB > beta-blockers) and thus improve the compliance of the ventricle. Beta-blockers are attractive in this regard in addition to their anti-ischemic and rate-limiting properties, all of which may improve diastolic filling. ACEIs are often appropriate, but compared with systolic dysfunction there is no evidence for specific indications for diastolic dysfunction HF. Candesartan has demonstrated decreased hospitalizations in patients with preserved systolic function, but not a mortality benefit (CHARM preserved trial).
4. Conversion of atrial fibrillation to sinus rhythm will restore the atrial component of diastolic filling and may improve cardiac output. If conversion to sinus rhythm is not feasible, then ventricular rate control with a rate-limiting calcium channel blocker or digoxin may allow more complete ventricular filling in diastole.

TABLE 73-7. SPECIFIC INSTRUCTIONS FOR PATIENTS ABOUT WHEN TO CONTACT A PHYSICIAN'S OFFICE

Weight gain 3 lbs or more, not responding to predesignated diuretic change
Uncertainty about how to increase diuretics
New swelling of the feet or abdomen
Worsening shortness of breath with mild exercise
Onset of inability to sleep flat in bed or awakening from sleep because of shortness of breath
Worsening cough
Persistent nausea/vomiting or inability to eat
Worsening dizziness or new spells of sudden dizziness not related to sudden changes in body position
Prolonged palpitations

If you, the patient, experience any sudden severe symptoms, you may need to call 911 or the equivalent emergency phone number to arrange a trip to the emergency department. (These sudden severe symptoms may include **but are not limited** to chest pain, severe shortness of breath, loss of consciousness not because of sudden standing, new cold or painful arm or foot, sudden new visual changes, or impairment of speech or strength in an extremity.) Note: This is only a sample list and is not intended to include all potential problems for which a patient with heart failure should seek urgent medical advice.
Source: Reprinted with permission from Goldman L, Braunwald E. *Primary Cardiology.* 2nd ed. Philadelphia, PA: Saunders; 2003.

   5. Attention to controlling the heart rate is important in managing patients with diastolic dysfunction. Slowing the heart rate will improve cardiac output in patients with HF and diastolic dysfunction who have tachycardia. Overdiuresis often leads to tachycardia in these patients, compounding the problem of dyspnea in the acute setting.

   6. Theoretically, digoxin would not be indicated for patients with diastolic dysfunction; however, a subgroup analysis of the recent DIG clinical trial showed surprising improvement in clinical outcomes for the small number of patients in the study who had normal LVEF. Until more evidence is available, however, digoxin should be reserved for patients with diastolic dysfunction who have a separate indication such as atrial fibrillation.

V. Management Strategies

   A. Patient education and self-care are important components of maintaining clinical stability. (SOR **B**) Topics include explanation of symptoms, causes, and prognosis; activity recommendations including exercise prescription when appropriate; proper use of medications; sodium restriction; daily weights; and instructions for monitoring symptoms and when to contact the physician (Table 73-7).

   B. Case management strategies have been shown to improve quality of life and decrease the need for hospitalization. (SOR **A**) Nurse case managers work with patients to improve patient education; promote adherence to medication and dietary regimens; improve home-based self-monitoring; and coordinate medical, community, and social support resources.

   C. Consultation or referral to a cardiologist or HF specialty clinic should be considered for patients who remain symptomatic on standard HF therapy, have underlying valvular or pericardial infiltrative disease, or have potentially reversible ischemic heart disease. Patients may also benefit from comanagement with a cardiologist to ensure reaching target doses of an ACEI or to initiate beta-blocker therapy. Those with symptomatic atrial or ventricular tachyarrhythmias should also be assessed by a cardiologist. Evaluation for possible cardiac transplantation includes exercise evaluation with measurement of VO_{2max}. Patients with VO_{2max} <14 mL/kg/min and no severe comorbid conditions may be candidates for transplantation.

VI. Prognosis

   A. Exacerbations and hospitalization frequently occur in HF. More than 40% of hospitalized patients with HF require readmission to the hospital within 6 months of discharge. Patients often experience a fluctuating clinical course marked by periods of fluid overload and diminished exercise tolerance. Common preventable reasons leading to hospitalization include poor adherence to sodium restriction or medication regimens, inadequate social support systems, or failure to seek medical attention when symptoms worsen or daily weights increase. Hospitalization rates are similar for patients with systolic and diastolic dysfunction HF.

   B. Mortality risk for patients with HF is substantial, with annual rates as high as 50% mortality for patients with advanced disease (NYHA class IV). LVEF is one of the most consistent predictors of mortality, with a marked increase in mortality risk for patients with LVEF less than 20%. Hyponatremia, elevated plasma norepinephrine levels, BNP levels, and significant ventricular arrhythmias are also independent markers for increased mortality risk. Mortality rates are lowest for patients with HF and normal LVEF.

SELECTED REFERENCES

Adorisio R, De Luca L, Rossi J, Gheorghiade M. Pharmacological treatment of chronic heart failure. *Heart Fail Rev.* 2006;11:109–123.
Aurigemma GP, Gaasch WH. Clinical practice, diastolic heart failure. *N Engl J Med.* 2004;351:1097–1105.
Fonarow GC, Adams KF, Abraham WT, et al. Risk stratification for in-hospital mortality in acutely decompensated heart failure: classification and regression tree analysis. *JAMA.* 2005;293:572–580.
McMurray JJ. Clinical Practice. Systolic heart failure. *N Engl J Med.* 2010;362(3):228–238.
Porapakkham P, Porapakkham PB, Zimmet H, et al. B-type natriuretic peptide-guided heart failure therapy: a meta-analysis. *Arch Intern Med.* 2010;170(6):507–514.
Redfield MM, Jacobsen SJ, Burnett JC, et al. Burden of systolic and diastolic ventricular dysfunction in the community: appreciating the scope of the heart failure epidemic. *JAMA.* 2003;289:194–202.
Takeda A, Taylor SJ, Taylor RS, et al. Clinical service organization for heart failure. *Cochrane Database Syst Rev.* 2012;(9):CD002752.
Yancy CW, Jessup M, Bozkurt B, et al., 2013 ACCF/AHA Guidelines for the Management of Heart Failure. *J Am Coll Card.* 2013;S0735-1097(13):02114-1.

74   Dementia

Radha Ramana Murthy Gokula, MD, CMD, & Leelasri Vanguru, MD

KEY POINTS

- A complete history and cognitive assessment should be followed by a thorough neurologic examination. Consider neuropsychological testing in patients with borderline cognitive impairment or those at risk for dementia. (SOR **C**)
- Screen for reversible causes of dementia such as B_{12} deficiency, hypothyroidism, and depression (pseudo-dementia), as these conditions are easily treatable. (SOR **C**)
- Address advance directives and end-of-life issues early in the disease process. (SOR **B**)
- Consider nonpharmacologic approaches for prevention and behaviors in dementia. (SOR **B**)
- Encourage social interaction, physical fitness, cognitive stimulation exercises, and a vegetarian diet rich in antioxidants. (SOR **B**)

I. Introduction

A. Dementia is a progressive neurodegenerative disorder characterized by impairment and diminished capacity in at least one cognitive domain (recent memory, language, spatial ability, and executive function). As the disease progresses, there is a decline in function and quality of life leading to increased frailty, dependence, and death.

B. Definition of dementia. The Diagnostic and Statistical Manual of Mental Disorders defines dementia as evidence from the history and mental status examination that indicates major impairment in learning and memory as well as at least one of the following abilities:

- Impairment in handling complex tasks
- Impaired reasoning ability
- Impaired spatial ability and orientation
- Impaired language

1. Cognitive symptoms must significantly interfere with the individual's work performance, usual social activities, or relationships with other people.
2. The condition must represent a significant decline from the previous level of functioning.

     3. Disturbances are of insidious onset and progressive, based on evidence from the history or serial Mini-Mental Status Examinations.

     4. Disturbances do not occur exclusively during the course of delirium and are not explained by a major psychiatric diagnosis or by a systemic disease or another brain disease.

  C. Causes for dementia are multifactorial and comorbidities exacerbate the condition in the elderly population. Risk factors for dementia are shown in Table 74–1. Despite recent advances in medicine, thorough in-person evaluation combined with historical information from a reliable informant provides most information needed to ascertain the cause of dementia.

TABLE 74–1. RISK FACTORS FOR DEMENTIA

Risk Factor	Discussion	Level of Evidence
Age	Strongest risk factor	A
Genetic Factors	Autosomal dominant mutations of the amyloid precursor protein gene on chromosome 21 and genes encoding presenilin 1 on chromosome 14 and presenilin 2 on chromosome 1. ApoE epsilon 4 gene has strongest evidence as a risk factor in late life nonfamilial AD	A
Smoking	Compared with never smokers, current smokers have 1.79 times the risk of incident AD, 1.78 times the risk of incident vascular dementia, and 1.27 times the risk of any dementia. Current smokers also show a significantly larger yearly decline in Mini-Mental State Examination scores vs. never smokers	A
Infection	AIDS dementia complex and Creutzfeldt–Jacob disease are viral and prion infections, respectively, and place the patient at an increased risk for dementia (SOR **Ⓐ**) as do meningitis, encephalitis, untreated syphilis, Lyme disease	B
Trauma	Traumatic brain injury	A
Medical Conditions	Parkinson disease and Down syndrome (SOR **Ⓐ**) and other conditions including chronic kidney disease, high and low blood pressure, vitamin B_{12} and folate deficiency, gait impairment, hearing loss, dehydration, hydrocephalus, immunosuppression (e.g., leukemia, multiple sclerosis [MS]), thyroid problems, hypoglycemia, high or low sodium or calcium, and chronic hypoxia	B
Gender	Women are at a higher risk than men	B
Family History	Early onset familial AD places a 50% risk of inheriting the same mutation for siblings and children	B
Mild Cognitive Impairment (MCI)	Patients with either amnesic or nonamnesic MCI	B
Vascular Pathology	Vascular diseases (e.g., hypertension, diabetes, cerebral infarction)	B
Depression	Depression increases the risk for dementia	B
Toxins	Organophosphates, excessive alcohol, recreational drugs, heavy metals like aluminum and lead, organic solvents like benzene, and carbon monoxide poisoning are associated with increased dementia	B
Hemoglobin	Anemic participants and participants with high hemoglobin levels have a 60% increased risk for developing AD and decline in global cognitive function	B
Education level	Lower education increases risk (less cognitive reserve)	B
Medication-induced	Medications associated with dementia include diphenhydramine, tolterodine, metoclopramide, zolpidem, eszopiclone, drugs with anticholinergic effects, NSAIDs, digoxin, beta-blockers, corticosteroids, anticonvulsants, and long-acting benzodiazepines	B

AD, Alzheimer disease; AIDS, acquired immunodeficiency syndrome; NSAIDs, nonsteroidal anti-inflammatory drugs.

1. Alzheimer disease (AD) is the most common cause of dementia accounting for 60% to 80% of dementia cases. AD is estimated to affect more than 5 million Americans including up to 10% of the population aged 65 years and over and 40% of the population above age 85 years.

    a. Incidence. About 15 per 1000 person-years, with rates for men and women at 13.0 and 16.9 per 1000 person-years, respectively.

    b. Costs. These high rates indicate that there are 2.4 to 3.1 million caretakers (spouses, relatives, and friends) for patients with AD. The cost of caring for one person with AD at home or in a nursing home is more than $47,000 per year. In 2011, the cost of health care, long-term care, and hospice services for people aged 65 years and older with dementias in the United States was estimated to be $183 billion, which does not include services provided by unpaid caregivers.

D. Various **dementia syndromes** have been recognized including:
- Mild cognitive impairment (MCI)—preclinical
- AD (60%–80% of all dementia cases)
- Dementia with Lewy bodies (DLB)
- Frontotemporal dementia (FTD)
- Vascular (multi-infarct) dementia (10%–20% of all dementia cases)—more common in blacks and in patients with hypertension or diabetes
- Parkinson disease (PD) with dementia (5% of all dementia cases)
- Alcohol-related dementia
- Reversible dementia (i.e., vitamin B_{12} deficiency, hypothyroidism, neurosyphilis, depression, medication-induced cognitive dysfunction)
- Medical conditions causing cognitive deficits such as human immunodeficiency virus/acquired immunodeficiency syndrome, head trauma, PD, Huntington chorea, Pick disease, Creutzfeld–Jacob corticobasal syndrome, progressive supranuclear palsy, normal-pressure hydrocephalus, limbic encephalitis, some toxins, and some metabolic disorders.

E. Pathophysiology

    1. The majority of cases of **AD** are sporadic and likely caused by the interaction of genetic and environmental factors. Genetic mutations (Table 74–1) account for about 3% of cases and are characterized by early onset (as early as the third or fourth decade of life).

        a. Pathologic characteristics for AD include extracellular amyloid beta (Aβ) plaques and intracellular neurofibrillary tangles. Recent advances in diagnosis such as cerebrospinal fluid (CSF) biomarkers (i.e., Aβ, tau, and phosphorylated tau) as well as structural and functional imaging aid in early diagnosis and treatment.

    2. Levels of acetylcholine (Ach), a neurotransmitter linked to the interpretation of sensory and cognitive stimuli, memory retention and awareness, are linked to dementia. Plaque deposition on Ach-containing nerve cells causes abnormal levels of Ach and resultant altered memory and awareness.

    3. Deficits in a number of neurotransmitters, especially Ach and glutamate, are the basis of most approved medical treatments (see below).

II. Screening and Prevention

    A. In 2003, the United States Preventive Services Task Force concluded that evidence is insufficient to recommend for or against routine screening for dementia in older adults.

    B. Recent studies indicate that dementia can be prevented or delayed. Lifestyle modifications such as regular exercise, healthy diet rich in antioxidants and omega-3 polyunsaturated fatty acids, vitamin B supplementation, quality sleep, stress reduction, smoking cessation, control of high blood pressure and elevated blood glucose, consistent involvement in "brain activities" that involve learning, thinking, analyzing, and practicing and being socially active play an important role in prevention of dementia. Participating in favorite hobbies, listening to music, remembering and thinking of favorite vacations, or game playing can be helpful in delaying dementia or as secondary prevention of dementia.

III. Diagnosis and Evaluation. Early diagnosis is very important for dementia, particularly for AD. Early diagnosis allows for potentially more treatment benefits; appropriate medical, financial, and legal planning; and more benefit from support services. Early diagnosis allows families to prepare and develop a person-centered care plan including interventions for decreased cognitive ability, abnormal behaviors, and overall function. Preparation to adapt to changing patient condition results in improving patient outcomes as well as reduced costs, care giver burden, and stress.

TABLE 74–2. EARLY SYMPTOMS AND SIGNS OF ALZHEIMER DISEASE

Symptoms	Signs During Office Evaluation
Worsening memory loss	Cannot remember recent information
Losing things	Defers to caregiver
Repetitive questions	Dresses inappropriately
"Slowing down"	Poor hygiene or grooming
Driving problems	Trouble expressing thoughts
Financial mistakes	Persistently a "no show" or comes at wrong day/time
Aggressive or inappropriate behavior	Nonadherent
(e.g., shoplifting, sexuality, explosive outbursts)	Procrastinates excessively
"Depressed"	Weight loss and/or "failure to thrive"
Weight loss	
Poor hygiene	
Irritability	
Suspiciousness	

Unfortunately, primary care physicians miss the diagnosis of dementia approximately half of the time. Providers should be alert to any changes in cognitive function and the activities of daily living performance as indicators of mild cognitive impairment. It is clinically useful to describe the manifestations of dementias in three domains: cognitive, functional, and behavioral while recognizing that the early symptoms may be in only one or two domains. For both diagnosis and management, it is useful to record characteristic symptoms from these three domains, asking direct questions if necessary. Early detection of dementia risk factors (Table 74–1) and subsequent medical intervention is important for dementia prevention. Thorough assessment of vascular risk factors is particularly critical. Table 74–2 lists some "hints" based on symptoms or observations that early dementia may be present.

A. History (Step 1; Table 74–3). The initial and crucial step in the evaluation of a patient with suspected dementia should focus on the history. Family members or other informants who know the patient well are invaluable resources for providing an adequate history of cognitive and behavioral changes. Dementia often presents insidiously making the diagnosis difficult for caregivers and health care providers. Often, patient and family do not like to bring it to the physician's attention due to misconception about loss of independence or fear of being labeled with a diagnosis. Most times, it is the spouse who brings it to the attention of the health care provider.

    1. Onset of dementia can be dated based on when the patient lost use of instrumental activities of daily living (IADL) such as driving and financial management. Ask questions like "When did you first notice the memory loss?" and "How has the memory loss progressed since then?" History must include onset, duration, progression, frequency, and any precipitating factors (Table 74–3).

    2. Symptoms. Clues to dementia include frequent falls, functional decline in activities of daily living (ADLs) and instrumental (I) ADLs, and urinary incontinence. Patients with dementia may also have difficulty with one or more of the following:

        a. Learning
        b. Retaining new information
        c. Handling complex tasks (i.e., balancing a checkbook)
        d. Reasoning and abstract thinking
        e. Inability to cope with unexpected events
        f. Spatial ability and orientation (i.e., getting lost in familiar places)
        g. Language (i.e., word retrieval)
        h. Behavior or personality changes
        i. Mood changes
        j. Performing previously routine tasks
        k. Judgment

    3. A comprehensive **medication history** must be obtained including all the current and past prescribed, nonprescription, homeopathic/herbal medications, and nutritional supplementations.

        Occasionally, medications alone will be the cause of apparent dementia, and often medication adjustment can reduce AD symptoms.

TABLE 74–3. STEPWISE APPROACH TO DIAGNOSING AND ASSESSING ALZHEIMER DISEASE IN PRIMARY CARE

Stage	Purpose	Tools to Use/Information to Obtain
Step 1: Prediagnostic tests	Differential diagnosis and determination of coexisting disorders	Risk factors: including age, female sex, apolipoprotein E4 gene, prior head injury, low education, and family history of AD; stroke, obesity, hypertension, hyperlipidemia, hyperhomocystein-emia, diabetes, hyperinsulinemia, and smoking
		Medical history:
		• Other ailments that mimic dementia include normal age-associated memory changes, depression, delirium, drug reactions, vision and hearing problems
		Key questions to ask:
		• Has the patient had any recent illnesses?
		• Has the patient used any new prescription or nonprescription medications that could cause memory loss, such as benzodiazepines, anticholinergic drugs for urinary incontinence
		• Has the patient used or been exposed to illicit drugs?
		• Has there been any exposure to environmental toxins, e.g., fuels or solvents?
		• Has the patient had any head injuries recently?
		• Is there any personal or family history of epilepsy?
		Laboratory/medical tests:
		• Complete blood cell count (to ascertain presence of anemia/infection), glucose and thyroid function tests, serum electrolytes, serum B_{12} levels (to identify vitamin deficiency), liver function tests, renal function tests, and urinalysis, if appropriate
		• Patients with AD frequently have comorbid medical conditions, e.g., cardiovascular disease, infection, pulmonary, renal insufficiency, and arthritis.
		Early warning signs of preclinical dementia:
		• Increased frequency of patient visits to the PCP prior to diagnosis, over a period up to 5 years prior to the diagnosis
		• Accelerated weight loss, late-life depression, gait disturbances, and physical frailty
Step 2: Assess performance	Cognitive assessments that help screen for/diagnose AD	Cognitive tests:
		• MMSE
		• Mini-Cog
		• MoCA
		Informant-rated tool:
		• AD8
Step 3: Assess daily functioning	Determine level of independence and degree of disability	Daily function assessment tool:
		• IADL
Step 4: Assess behavioral symptoms	Determine presence and degree of behavioral symptoms	Behavioral assessment tool:
		• NPI-Q
		Assess the patient for drug toxicity and medical psychiatric, psychosocial, or environmental problems that may underlie behavioral changes.
Step 5: Identify caregiver and assess needs	Identify the primary caregiver and assess adequacy of family and other support systems	Identify primary caregivers and establish collaboration:
		• Family caregivers are central to the PCP's assessment and care of the patient.
		• Establish and maintain collaboration with caregivers.
		• Routinely incorporate caregivers' reports of patients' changes in daily routine, mood, behavior, and sleeping patterns.
		Assess health of primary caregiver:
		• Regularly monitor the physical and emotional health of the primary caregiver as well as that of the patient.
		• The PCP should assess the caregiver or refer them to a psychologist, social worker, or other member of the health care delivery team.

(continued)

TABLE 74–3. STEPWISE APPROACH TO DIAGNOSING AND ASSESSING ALZHEIMER DISEASE IN PRIMARY CARE (Continued)

Stage	Purpose	Tools to Use/Information to Obtain
Special considerations	Identify culture, language, and literacy of patient and caregiver	Culture: • Recognize the caregiving patterns of ethnic minority groups, e.g., African-American and Hispanic families often distribute care among several family members, rather than one primary career. • Ethnic minority groups may place different interpretations on memory and behavioral problems. Language: • Be aware of the preferred language of the patient and family. Literacy: • Recognize that paper-and-pencil tests and forms may not work well with diverse patient populations if basic literacy is not present, even when such forms are in the person's native language. • Some experts suggest that patients be tested only on what they reasonably may be expected to know, e.g., a person with little schooling may not know how to do the serial sevens on the MMSE, but may be competent at applying simple math, such as subtraction, when handling monetary transactions.

AD, Alzheimer disease; AD8, 8-item Ascertain Dementia tool; IADL, instrumental (or intermediate) activities of daily living; MMSE, Mini-Mental State Examination; Mini-Cog, Mini Cognitive Assessment Instrument; MoCA, Montreal Cognitive Assessment; NPI-Q, Neuropsychiatric Inventory Questionnaire; PCP, primary care physician. *Source:* Reproduced with permission from Galvin JE, Sadowsky CH, Nincds Adrda. Practical guidelines for the recognition and diagnosis of dementia. *Journal of the American Board of Family Medicine: JABFM* . 2012;25(3):367–382.

    a. The anticholinergic side effects of many nonprescription allergy (e.g., diphenhydramine), cold, and even sleep or pain medications are a frequent cause of abrupt worsening of cognition in old people, and especially in those with dementia. The anticholinergic effects of different concurrent drugs can be additive. Consider a trial of discontinuing such medications in all patients with cognitive problems, and avoid using them in general with elders unless the benefits truly outweigh this huge disadvantage.

  4. Past medical history should include queries for cardiovascular diseases, brain injuries, mental illnesses, neurologic problems, HIV/AIDS infection, recent sudden environmental or emotional changes, drug abuse, and chronic medical conditions. Family history should include queries regarding any family member, particularly first-degree relatives who had or has dementia.

  5. Comprehensive review of systems is important to rule out reversible causes and multisystem disease. Assess for cardiovascular and neurologic problems, injuries, diabetes or other metabolic disorders, infections, sarcoidosis, immunodeficiency conditions, Behcet disease, or multiple sclerosis.

B. Physical assessment. The next important step in the assessment in any patient with possible cognitive impairment for dementia is the neurologic examination. Neurologic status is often normal in the early stages of most dementias. Any specific signs in early stages may be due to reversible or very rare causes.

  Look for the following signs/symptoms in the neurologic examination (Table 74–4):

- Any involuntary movements at rest such as chorea, tremor, dystonia, myoclonus, fasciculations, visual acuity, or hearing problems
- Ocular signs—abnormal pupillary reflexes, eye movements, optic disc, and visual field
- Speech and swallowing difficulties
- Pyramidal or extrapyramidal signs
- Motor apraxia (loss of the ability to execute or carry out learned purposeful movements)
- Increased muscle tone
- Peripheral neuropathy
- Gait abnormalities
- Primitive reflexes

C. Diagnostic tests

  1. Laboratory tests should be aimed at assessments that could affect cognitive functioning or become the primary cause of dementia. These include complete blood count, biochemical profile (electrolytes, blood glucose, calcium, renal function, and hepatic function), thyroid function, and serum vitamin B_{12} and folate levels. (SOR **Ⓐ**) Additional

TABLE 74–4. ABNORMAL NEUROLOGIC SIGNS AND IMPORTANCE IN DEMENTIA

Physical Sign	Seen in
Eyes and Nose	
Abnormal eye movements	Progressive supranuclear palsy (PSP), Wernicke–Korsakoff syndrome, Whipple disease, corticobasal degeneration (CBD), mitochondrial cytopathies, cerebellar tumors, causes of raised intracranial pressure, Creutzfeldt–Jakob disease (CJD), mitochondrial disorders, Huntington disease (HD), Niemann–Pick type C
Cortical blindness	Vascular disease, Alzheimer disease (AD), CJD
Optic disc pallor	MS, vitamin B_{12} deficiency
Papilledema	Tumor, subdural hematoma, hydrocephalus
Pupillary abnormalities	Neurosyphilis (Argyll Robertson pupil)
Visual field defect	Tumor, vascular disease, CJD
Anosmia	Subfrontal meningioma, head injury, AD, Parkinson disease (PD), HD
Neurologic Examination	
Ataxia	Paraneoplastic disease, cerebellar tumor, Whipple disease, CJD, AIDS dementia complex, spinocerebellar ataxia (SCA), Wernicke–Korsakoff syndrome, Hallervorden–Spatz disease, ornithine transcarbamylase deficiency, Niemann–Pick disease, mitochondrial disorders, adrenoleukodystrophy, neurodegeneration with brain iron accumulation (NBIA), lead poisoning
Extrapyramidal signs	Dementia with Lewy bodies, PD, PSP, vascular dementia, frontotemporal dementia (FTD), CJD, Wilson disease, HD, dentatorubropallidoluysian atrophy (DRPLA), neuroacanthocytosis, cerebral autosomal dominant arteriopathy with subcortical infarcts and leukoencephalopathy (CADASIL), Niemann–Pick disease, mitochondrial disorders, NBIA
Fasciculations	Frontal dementia (motor neuron disease), rarely CJD
Involuntary movements	HD, inherited metabolic disorders including Wilson disease, CJD, CBD, systemic lupus erythematosus (SLE), Whipple disease, Hallervorden–Spatz disease, Lesch–Nyhan syndrome
Myoclonus	Postanoxia, CJD, AD, subacute sclerosing panencephalitis (SSPE), myoclonic epilepsies, Hashimoto encephalopathy, dementia with Lewy bodies, CBD
Other cranial nerve signs	Sarcoidosis, tumors, neoplasia, tuberculous meningitis, frontal dementia (motor neuron disease; bulbar features)
Peripheral neuropathy	Vitamin B_{12} deficiency, paraneoplastic disorders, neuroacanthocytosis, SCA, Hallervorden Spatz, adrenoleukodystrophy, NBIA, lead poisoning, SLE
Pyramidal signs	Motor neuron disease, CJD, LCBD, vitamin B_{12} deficiency, MS, SCA, multisystem atrophy, hydrocephalus, AD, Hallervorden–Spatz disease, CADASIL, mitochondrial disorders, adrenoleukodystrophy, frontal lobe dementia
Seizures	Vasculitis, neoplasia, primary angiitis of the nervous system, limbic encephalitis, AIDS dementia complex, neurosyphilis, SSPE, Hashimoto encephalopathy
Other Findings	
Alien hand[a]	Corticobasal degeneration
Early onset incontinence	Tumor, hydrocephalus, PSP
Grimacing facial expression	Wilson disease

[a]Hand does not seem to belong to the person.

tests for the patient with dementia include blood sedimentation rate, syphilis, HIV, RPR/VDRL, serum toxin levels, serum antinuclear antibodies, and urinalysis. (SOR Ⓑ)

2. Routine CSF test or genetic testing not recommended

   a. CSF analysis should be performed in patients when there is clinical suspicion of certain diseases and in patients with atypical clinical presentations. (SOR Ⓑ) Examination of CSF (with routine cell count, protein, glucose, and protein electrophoresis) is mandatory if inflammatory disease, vasculitis, or demyelination is suspected as a cause of dementia. CSF testing for total tau, phospho tau, and β-amyloid (Aβ42) should be used as an adjunct in cases of diagnostic doubt. For the identification of Creutzfeldt–Jakob disease in cases with rapidly progressive dementia, assessment of the 14-3-3 protein should be performed.

   b. Genetic testing must only be undertaken with consent from the patient and caregivers. Appropriate scenarios for genetic testing include the presence of an appropriate phenotype with a family history of autosomal dominant dementia or an asymptomatic adult individual with a clear family history of dementia with a known mutation in an affected family member. Routine Apo E genotyping is not recommended. (SOR Ⓑ)

3. Brain biopsy should only be undertaken in carefully selected cases for diagnosis of rare dementias.

4. **Brain imaging.** Structural imaging should be used in the evaluation of every patient suspected of dementia. (SOR **Ⓐ**)

   a. **Computed tomography (CT)** can be used to identify surgically treatable lesions and vascular disease.

   b. **Magnetic resonance imaging** (including T1, T2, and fluid-attenuated inversion recovery [FLAIR] sequences) can be used to increase specificity for diagnosis.

   c. **Functional imaging** (i.e., SPECT and PET) may be useful in those cases where diagnostic uncertainty remains after clinical and structural imaging. They should not be used as the only imaging measure.

5. **EEG** is routine only when Creutzfeldt–Jakob disease is suspected.

D. **Cognitive assessment** (Step 2; Table 74–3) is essential for the diagnosis and evaluation of dementia and should be performed on all patients with dementia or suspected of dementia. Evaluation of cognitive function and mental state should be conducted using standardized neuropsychological examination(s).

   1. Standardized assessments should include those targeting memory, language, attention and concentration, judgment, calculation, executive function, and visuospatial abilities. (SOR **Ⓐ**) Screening tools for AD are shown in Table 74–5. More detailed

TABLE 74–5. SCREENING TOOLS FOR ALZHEIMER DISEASE IN PRIMARY CARE

Screening Tools	Key Features Relevant to Clinical Practice	Number of Items	Maximum Score
MMSE (Mini-Mental State Examination)	• Assesses orientation, registration, attention and calculation, recall, language, and ability to copy a figure • Disadvantages of the MMSE is that it is copyrighted and does not pick up mild cognitive impairment	30 items	30 (cutoff score 23–26)
SLUMS[a] (Saint Louis University Mental Status)	• Adopted by the Veterans Administration	11 items	30 (cutoff score 20 or 19 if <high school education)
Mini-Cog	Combines an uncued three-item recall test with a Clock Drawing Test (CDT) that serves as a recall distracter	2 items	5[b]
MoCA (Montreal Cognitive Assessment Tool)	Addresses frontal/executive functioning	12 items	30 (cutoff score 26)
AD8 interview	• Informant-rated change • Screening interview: brief, sensitive measure of memory, orientation, judgment, and function	8 Yes/No	Scores of 0 to 1 are normal Scores of 2 or more probable cognitive impairment
Clock Drawing Test	To differentiate between normal aging and early stage dementia May be used as an adjunct to MMSE	4 (0–3)	3 is normal 0–2 represents memory deficit.
IADL	Evaluates patient's ability to perform more complex activities that are necessary for optimal independent functioning	7	Three answer choices per question: I—Completely independent A—Assistance required D—Dependent on help for each activity
Behavioral assessment NPI-Q (neuropsychiatric inventory questionnaire)	Rates frequency and severity of behavioral symptoms commonly seen in dementia, and caregiver distress	12 symptoms/ questions	Each question is scored as either present or absent

[a]Download copy from http://www.elderguru.com/download-the-slums-dementia-alzheimers-test-exam/.
[b]0, cognitive impairment; 1 to 2+ with an abnormal CDT, cognitive impairment; 1 to 2+ with a normal CDT, no cognitive impairment; 3, negative for dementia and no need to score the CDT.

psychological batteries are aimed at differentiating questionable or mild dementia from normal cognitive decline, differentiating among subtypes of dementia, and providing information for treatment.

   2. Comprehensive neuropsychological testing should be considered in all patients with nonsevere dementia including prodromal dementia. (SOR **Ⓒ**)

E. Activities of daily living (Step 3; Table 74–3). Patient-based assessment tools and/or caregiver interviews should be used for an objective "ADL" assessment. (SOR **Ⓐ**)

F. Behavioral and psychological symptoms often have somatic comorbidity or complications (Step 4; Table 74–3). Assessment for possible causative comorbidity or complication should be included in evaluation. Visual or auditory hallucinations and paranoia may also be reported.

   1. For depression screening, a geriatric depression scale (http://www.stanford.edu/~yesavage/GDS.english.short.score.html) is one option for assessing depression in older people. This scale, however, does not work well in individuals with dementia.

   2. In patients with dementia, screening for depression can be accomplished with either the Cornell scale (http://www.scalesandmeasures.net/files/files/The%20Cornell%20Scale%20for%20Depression%20in%20Dementia.pdf) or the Patient Health Questionnaire (PHQ)-9 (http://www.cqaimh.org/pdf/tool_phq9.pdf). The former involves interviews with the caregiver (19 items) and a brief interview with the patient. The latter consists of nine items representing symptoms of depression that are completed by the patient. An advantage of the PHQ-9 is that CMS mandates its use for nursing home residents as part of data gathering for the Minimum Data Set-3.0. A positive screen requires further evaluation and depression management.

G. Staging and Typing for Dementia. Staging of dementia is commonly accomplished using the Global Deterioration Scale (http://www.alzheimer.ca/en/About-dementia/Alzheimer-s-disease/What-is-Alzheimer-s-disease/Global-Deterioration-Scale), Brief Cognitive Rating Scale (http://www.iowahealthcare.org/userdocs/Documents/BCRS_GDS_assessments02262010.pdf), and Functional Assessment Staging (http://www.mciscreen.com/pdf/fast_overview.pdf) measures. Following initial diagnosis, it is important to differentiate the type of dementia to optimize disease management. Table 74–6 shows the characteristics of different types of dementia.

   1. In the oldest dementia patients, it can be extremely difficult to determine the contribution of cognitive loss to the loss of functional abilities because of comorbid conditions, sensory loss, physical disability, fragility, and fatigue. Determination of the dementia etiology is therefore challenging.

   a. With advancing age, the correlation between neuropathology and clinical dementia decreases. Approximately one-half of clinically demented very elderly individuals have sufficient neuropathology to account for dementia and half of such individuals without dementia meet the neuropathologic criteria for AD. In another study, 22% did not have sufficient neuropathology to explain their cognitive loss. Other reports do not substantiate a relationship between clinical dementia and neuropathologic observations in the oldest-old.

   2. Delirium is another important differential diagnosis that can result in poor cognitive performance which may or may not be related to a person's actual level of cognition when not acutely ill. Delirium in the elderly can be related to a number of medical illnesses and medications. Lewy body dementia can also cause delirium along with fluctuating levels of attention and cognitive performance.

IV. Treatment of Dementia

A. The management of people with dementia requires a **multidisciplinary team** approach. The most effective management can be achieved by extensive and frequent communication among team members. Team members should include physicians, nurses, clinical psychologists, social workers, and occupational therapists. Roles include evaluation of concurrent illnesses, treatment prescription, facilitation of hospital and community services, general care of inpatients and nursing home residents, initiation and conduct of behavior modification regimes, education, support and counseling of the patient, caregiver and family members, and ensuring provision of local services such as residential care, respite care, home care, and environmental design.

B. Advance directives. The need for and importance of advance directives to the patient newly diagnosed with dementia or AD must be clearly explained. These should be completed with the help of a psychiatrist, geriatrist, and law attorney. It is always useful to

TABLE 74-6. DIFFERENT TYPES OF DEMENTIA

Type	Features
Alzheimer disease	**Symptoms:** • Difficulty remembering names and recent events • Apathy and depression • Later symptoms include impaired judgment, disorientation, confusion, behavior changes, and difficulty speaking, swallowing, and walking **Brain changes:** Deposits of the beta-amyloid (plaques) and twisted tau strands (tangles), nerve cell damage
Vascular dementia	**Symptoms:** • Impaired judgment and ability to organize and plan are initial symptoms. **Brain changes:** Blood vessel occlusion
Dementia with Lewy bodies (DLB)	**Symptoms:** • Memory loss and thinking problems • Early sleep disturbances, well-formed visual hallucinations when compared to AD. • Muscle rigidity or other movement problems like Parkinson disease. **Brain changes:** Lewy bodies are abnormal aggregations (or clumps) of the protein alpha-synuclein in the cortex[a]
Mixed dementia	**Brain changes:** Abnormalities of more than one type of dementia—mostly AD, vascular dementia, and DLB
Parkinson disease	**Symptoms:** • Initial symptoms are movement-related • Dementia develops later and will be mostly similar to DLB **Brain changes:** Alpha-synuclein aggregates in the substantia nigra
Frontotemporal dementia	**Symptoms:** • Personality and behavior changes and difficulty with language • Younger person (age about 60 years) and survival is much less than AD **Brain changes:** No specific microscopic features can be seen in all cases
Creutzfeldt–Jakob disease	**Symptoms:** • Rapidly progressive disease and fatal • Memory and coordination impairment • Behavior changes **Brain changes:** Misfolded prion protein throughout the brain
Normal pressure hydrocephalus	**Symptoms:** • Difficulty walking • Memory deficit • Urinary incontinence **Brain changes:** Fluid in the ventricles
Huntington disease	**Symptoms:** • Abnormal involuntary movements • Severe thinking and reasoning deficit • Mood changes such as irritability, depression, and anxiety **Brain changes:** Abnormalities in Huntington brain protein due to gene deficit
Wernicke–Korsakoff syndrome	**Symptoms:** • Severe memory deficit • Reasoning, thinking, and social skills are relatively less affected **Brain changes:** Nerve cell damage

[a]Alpha-synuclein aggregates are seen if the patient also has Parkinson disease, but their appearance and pattern are different from Lewy body aggregations.

have an advance directive. The patient should be counseled about the concept of allowing natural death and the benefits of hospice care.

C. **Pharmacologic treatment for AD.** Despite decades of research, there is currently no cure for AD. Instead, therapy is directed at treating symptoms. The mainstays of therapy are still pharmacologic although nonpharmacologic interventions can be excellent adjuncts.

1. **Donepezil** inaugurated the second generation of cholinesterase inhibitors. With fewer side effects and once-daily dosing, it remains a popular choice for patients with

AD. Authors of a Cochrane review found benefits of donepezil up to 1 year in cognitive function, activities of daily living, and behavior, but not in quality of life. (SOR **Ⓐ**) The recommended dose is 5 mg orally once daily for 4 weeks and 10 mg orally once daily thereafter, although the Cochrane authors found little added benefit and more side effects with the 10-mg dose. Since the cholinomimetic side effects of donepezil are usually well tolerated, it is a viable option for long-term therapy. In fact, studies have shown the adverse effects to be mild and transient (20% of patients).

2. **Rivastigmine.** Like donepezil, rivastigmine is a second-generation cholinesterase inhibitor with similar efficacy, but with a more troubling adverse effect profile (nausea, vomiting, anorexia, and headaches). The FDA warning includes increased risk of GI symptoms. In addition, the manufacturer advises slow titration of the drug (initiating therapy at 1.5 mg twice daily with titration every 2 weeks up to 6 mg twice daily); if treatment is interrupted for more than a few days, it should be restarted at the lowest daily dose and then titrated again. Fortunately, rivastigmine is now available as a transdermal patch that has been shown to have fewer GI symptoms but similar efficacy at the highest dose (6 mg twice daily). It shows similar small benefits in cognition, activities of daily living, and behavior as donepezil for patients with AD. (SOR **Ⓐ**)

3. **Galantamine.** This drug is an alkaloid manufactured synthetically or derived from the bulbs and flowers of *Galanthus caucasicus* (Caucasian snowdrop, Voronov's snowdrop). Galantamine has a long history of usage in Eastern Europe and Russia for myasthenia and motor and sensory dysfunction of the central nervous system. In the United States, it is FDA, approved for the treatment of mild-to-moderate AD. Like rivastigmine it seems to be as efficacious as donepezil but with more intense GI symptoms, and the dose needs to be titrated. (SOR **Ⓐ**) Galantamine has the advantage of once daily dosing.

4. **Memantine** has fewer side effects compared to cholinesterase inhibitors, mostly dizziness and rarely confusion and hallucination. Thus, it is a useful adjunct especially in moderate-to-severe AD when options are few. Authors of a Cochrane review found small beneficial effects at 6 months on cognition, activities of daily living, and behavior that were clinically notable. (SOR **Ⓐ**) Some physicians advocate memantine alone in advanced disease since it may have a disease modifying effect. Memantine can be added to the existing regimen in patients progressing to moderate AD and can be continued, even if only to alleviate caretaker burden.

5. In addition to decreased acetylcholine synthesis in the cerebral cortex, the pathophysiology of AD also involves both oxidative stress and excessive glutamate activity. These two mechanisms are of relevance in as much as they are amenable to pharmacologic manipulation. Drug development is under way to target these pathways.

D. **Pharmacologic treatment for non-Alzheimer dementia.** Despite advances in identifying non-Alzheimer dementias, there are no effective treatments except for symptomatic relief for individual behaviors. However as our understanding improves with the proteinopathies of each dementia type, we can hope for targeted therapies attacking the pathologic protein responsible for particular dementias. Table 74–7 provides more information about the drugs used for these conditions. Rivastigmine was shown in one large 24-week trial to improve cognition in patients with vascular dementia, but not global impression of change or noncognitive measures. (SOR **Ⓑ**)

E. **Nonpharmacologic and alternative treatments for dementia.** Table 74–8 lists the nonpharmacologic approaches to treat dementia symptoms. Research is also ongoing to determine whether phototherapy and aromatherapy can help patients with dementia.

F. **Nutrition** should be addressed throughout the course of the illness. Early in the disease, patients will not eat if overwhelmed by choices. Later, they may need to be spoon-fed, as self-feeding becomes difficult. Later still, the issue comes up about maintenance with tube feeding. In most authorities' opinions, long-term tube feeding in the later stages of a dementing illness is inappropriate. However, individuals (or their families as surrogates) must make their own decisions; sometimes it may be reasonable to maintain an individual who has relatively early loss of appetite or dysphagia out of proportion to the degree of dementia.

G. **Management of the behavioral and psychological symptoms of dementia (BPSD)** is a challenge. The behaviors manifest as repetitive speech, aggression, wandering, delusions, agitation, hallucinations along with depression, and insomnia. Other commonly seen behaviors in severe dementia are repetitive vocalizations, shadowing, resistance to care, wandering, and argumentativeness. One or more of these symptoms are seen in 61% to 92% of patients and the prevalence increases with disease progression. If untreated, these symptoms lead to functional decline and increased caregiver burden,

TABLE 74–7. PHARMACOLOGIC TREATMENT FOR NON-ALZHEIMER DISEASE DEMENTIA

Dementia Type	Pharmacologic Treatment	Level of Evidence
Frontotemporal lobe degeneration (FTLD)	Cholinesterase inhibitors (ChEIs)	C
	Memantine	
• Frontotemporal dementia	Antidepressants(SSRIs and Trazodone)	A
• Semantic dementia	Dopaminergic agents for motor symptoms	C
• Progressive nonfluent aphasia		
Dementia of Lewy body type	Rivastigmine	B
	Memantine	B
	Antipsychotics	None
Dementia of Parkinson disease	Rivastigmine	B
	Memantine	B
	Antipsychotics	None
Progressive supranuclear palsy	ChEIs	None
Corticobasal syndrome	ChEIs	None
Limbic encephalitis	Intravenous immunoglobulin, plasma exchange, corticosteroids, cyclophosphamide, rituximab	None
Huntington disease	ChEIs, vitamin E, idebenone, baclofen, lamotrigine, coenzyme Q, ethyl-eicosapentanoic acid, creatine	None
Prion disease	Quinacrine (ChEIs), memantine, antidepressants	None
Vascular dementia	ChEIs and memantine	B
Reversible dementias	Vitamin B_{12}	A
	Hypothyroidism (levothyroxine)	A
	Depression (antidepressants)	A

frequently resulting in nursing home placement. The mainstay of treatment is nonpharmacologic. The effectiveness of pharmacologic agents is modest and there is an increased risk of coronary and cerebrovascular events with antipsychotics, the most commonly used drugs to treat these specific symptoms. We often see specific behaviors associated with a particular type of dementia such as depression with vascular dementia; hallucinations with DLB; and disinhibition, wandering, social inappropriateness, and apathy with FTD.

1. **Hallucinations and delusions** occur spontaneously, sometimes precipitated by intercurrent physical illness. Benign hallucinations are very frequent in the earliest stages of AD. They often involve children, and even if the patient realizes they are not quite "real," they are not particularly frightening. These therefore do not require treatment. However, if hallucinations become vivid and frightening, directive, or fostering a delusional system, efforts should be made to ensure that the environment is not contributing to delusional activity (e.g., the patient may be misinterpreting noises they hear in the night, or shadows on the drapes). Treatment with an antipsychotic in these cases is justified. Much lower doses than are usually recommended for patients with schizophrenia should be used.

2. Always use a **standardized screening tool** (e.g., Neuropsychiatric Inventory Questionnaire [NPI-Q], http://www.medafile.com/cln/NPI-Qa.htm) to identify these

TABLE 74–8. NONPHARMACOLOGIC AND ALTERNATIVE TREATMENTS IN DEMENTIA

Non-pharmacologic Treatments	Complementary/Alternative Treatments
• Structured group cognitive stimulation program	• Multisensory stimulation
• Treatment for depression	• Therapeutic music or dancing
• Treat pain or discomfort	• Animal assisted therapy
• Life history and person-centered activities	• Massage
• Active social engagement	
• Correct environmental factors	
• Educate—behavioral and functional evaluation with direct care providers	

Source: Information from National Institute for Health and Clinical Excellence and Social Care Institute for Excellence, London, UK, 2006.

behaviors. If the patient screens positive, identify the behavior's onset, safety to self, others and caregiver burden due behaviors. It is important to rule out underlying medical illness, review medications, and make sure that patient does not have pain, constipation, dehydration, under-nutrition, and sleep–wake cycle dysfunction. A care plan that addresses safety strategies and education of the caregiver is a very important step. Screen caregivers for depression.

3. **Treatment of BPSD.** The first step is to screen for and identify specific problem behaviors that are occurring and discuss them with the patient and caregiver. Identifying and addressing underlying causes and modifying potential triggers is the next step. Once these are addressed, a treatment plan is developed. Periodic assessment of treatment effectiveness and monitoring for new behaviors follows with continued support provided to the patient and family by the care team. Table 74–9 presents nonpharmacologic approaches and strategies for addressing BPSD.

4. **Patient and family support.** A major advantage of early diagnosis is early training of the caregiving family in how to work with and support the patient with AD, in order to improve the quality of life for both caregiver and patient and to minimize (or at least manage) the behavioral problems that will arise. The agency perhaps best equipped to teach the family is the Alzheimer's Association, many of whose chapters operate local instructional and support groups. Table 74–10 lists potential resources.

One randomized, controlled trial of a counseling and support intervention for caregivers of patients with AD found that the intervention was associated with a 28% reduction in the rate of nursing home placement or a 557-day delay to placement, compared to control patients. In addition, two-thirds of caregivers in the intervention group were satisfied with the social support, response to behaviors, and improvement

TABLE 74–9. NONPHARMACOLOGIC APPROACHES FOR BEHAVIORAL AND PSYCHOLOGICAL SYMPTOMS OF DEMENTIA (BPSD)

Domain	Intervention
Activities	• Obtain the patient's life history to develop cognitively stimulating activities that are person-centered • Involve the patient in repetitive activities such as folding towels, block building, cleaning doors and windows, stuffing envelopes
Caregiver education and support	• Help caregivers understand that behaviors do not represent the person • As disease progresses there is a decline in cognitive abilities, so do not start activities at the previous level of function; use frequent cueing and reminders • Keep the environment safe • Do not argue with the patient during aggression • Ensure breaks during caregiving to reduce caregiver burden and stress • Create a network with Alzheimer's Association and support groups
Communication	• Follow routine communication rules • Frequently introduce the individual involved in care • Face the patient directly • Sit at eye level • Speak slowly and use a calm and reassuring voice • Ask open-ended questions: "What would you like me to do for you?" • Keep commands and choices simple (1–2 at a time) • If the patient has hearing deficits, raise voice volume accordingly • Consider writing requests or questions in large print • Allow ample time for the patient to answer queries • Assist the patient in word retrieval during conversation • Place your hand on the patient while talking to create a sense of comfort
Environment modification	• Clear clutter to reduce falls • Use labels to identify objects • Reduce noise to a minimum to prevent distractions during interactions • Avoid bright colors to prevent distraction • Develop visual clues to perform activities of daily living like bathing, dressing, and toileting
Direction for tasks	• Simplify complex tasks to a few steps • Provide prompts for each step • Create a structured routine for all activities

TABLE 74–10. RESOURCES FOR CAREGIVERS

Alzheimer's Association	www.alz.org
National Association of Home Care	www.nahc.org
Administration on Aging (Department of Health and Human Services)	www.aoa.gov
Alzheimer's Disease Education and Referral (ADEAR) Center (National Institute on Aging)	www.nia.nih.gov/alzheimers
ABA Commission of Legal problems in Elderly	www.abanet.org
National Institute of Neurological Disorders and Stroke	www.ninds.nih.gov
Family Caregiver Alliance	www.caregiver.org
The American Geriatrics Society	www.americangeriatrics.org
The Associate of Frontotemporal Dementias	www.ftd-picks.org
Eldercare Locator (Administration on Aging)	www.eldercare.gov

in their own depression. A recent meta-analysis of 13 studies found that care support and education decreased the odds of institutionalization.

V. Patient Care
  A. Mild dementia. Understanding the disease and respecting the patient are key. Patients with mild dementia may not need much care, but caregivers can benefit from social and emotional support.
    1. Caregivers should try to maintain a positive attitude and be truthful in expressing their emotions. They should also be encouraged to express the need for time for themselves and socializing.
      a. Caregivers should consider counseling to help them with the following: (1) managing daily activities and behavioral changes; (2) understanding and being patient and kind; (3) encouraging the patient's favorite activities and cognitive stimulation activities; (4) preventing burn out; (5) preventing influenza (immunization) in the patient and caregiver; (6) caring for their own health; (7) discussing issues with family and friends; (8) facilitating good communication with the health care team regarding the patient; (9) identifying behavioral changes in the patient and themselves; and (10) planning for long-term care, considering both financial and legal issues.
      b. Both the patient and the caregiver should be given information about available support from the local Alzheimer's Association such as patient and caregiver education, patient support groups, adult day programs, home nursing care, meals on wheels, and caregiver support groups.
    2. Safety. People with dementia need safe surroundings. Caregivers and professionals must survey the home regularly and ensure safe conditions at each inspection; an orderly environment can be achieved by modifications in the kitchen and bathroom to prevent patient wandering in search of basic needs and to prevent falls. Emergency calling options should be available in all places from the foyer to the bathroom.
  B. Moderate dementia. As dementia progresses, the patient and the caregiver will likely need additional support. Suggestions should be offered to seek help at home or to consider an assisted living center. Patient and caregiver needs must be considered.
  C. Severe dementia. In severe dementia, patients depend on others for all care and daily activities and may need to be moved to a nursing home. This can be quite distressing to the caregivers and family, and additional support and guidance are needed from both support groups and the healthcare team. It is important to talk to patients, even when they do not respond or understand. An occupational therapist, a physiotherapist, and a community nurse can play crucial roles in the management of the loss of mobility and its consequences. Proper nutrition and hydration are important to fight infections. Care must be taken to prevent choking due to impaired swallowing reflexes. Referral to a nutritionist and speech therapist may help at this stage. Incontinence needs to be addressed properly to prevent bedsores and infections. Support will be needed to manage behavioral changes, minimize discomfort, and prevent polypharmacy (specifically the administration of more medications than are clinically indicated).
VI. Patient Safety. Safety issues are important in the care of patients with dementia because of the decreased ability of affected individuals to make rational decisions. Safety planning must involve proactive planning and execution. Important issues for recognition, management of safety, and societal issues related to dementia are outlined in Table 74–11.

TABLE 74–11. SAFETY MEASURES FOR DEMENTIA PATIENTS

Safety Concern	Recognition	Assessment	Management
Driving	• Recent (1–5 yr) history of motor vehicle accident or citation • Self-restricted driving • Aggressive or impulsive behaviors • Caregiver's assessment of marginal or unsafe driving • Mini-Mental State Examination (MMSE) score of 24 or less	Clinical Dementia Rating (CDR) Scale (http://alzheimer.wustl.edu/cdr/aboutcdr.htm) CDR = 2 = high risk for unsafe driving CDR = 0.5 or 1 = intermediate risk for unsafe driving; consider other risk factors	The individual with dementia should stop driving; ensure that state guidelines are followed Consider voluntary surrender of driving privileges, limiting driving to daylight hours, and/or referral for a professional driving evaluation
Finances	Look for signs of financial mismanagement, vulnerability to scams and exploitation	Financial Capacity Instrument (http://archneur.jama-network.com/article.aspx?articleid=776646)	• Execute Financial Durable Power of Attorney • Court-appointed guardian if needed • Create online banking, direct deposit, automatic bill-pay, joint bank accounts, over-draft protections, and use of living trusts • Educate patients and families on advance financial planning • Refer to appropriate medical and legal sources
Wandering and getting lost	• Taking more time for a regular walk or drive than usual • Has difficulty locating familiar places • Appears lost in a new or changed place	Taking thorough history	• Maintain a daily plan • Monitor at times when wandering usually occurs • Help set up identifiable aids for basic needs • Avoid confusing places
Falls	• History of falls, rigidity • Difficulty with gait and balance • New medications • Fear of falling • Lower extremity weakness, older age, female gender, arthritis, psychotropic drug use, history of stroke, orthostatic hypotension, dizziness, and anemia	Check for orthostatic hypotension; Timed 'Get up & Go' Test 'Functional reach' Test 'Short Performance Physical Battery', visual acuity and hearing testing, complete blood count, basic metabolic panel **Special Tests:** Holter monitor, X-ray, echocardiogram	• Remove offending medications • Treat underlying cause or disease • Physical and occupational therapy
End of Life	• Dependence for all ADLs, wheel chair dependent, speaking less than five intelligible words in 24-h period • Poor nutritional status or oral intake with continued involuntary weight loss • Recurrent aspiration pneumonia, UTIs, pyelonephritis, sepsis • Stage 3–4 decubitus ulcers • Recurrent fever after antibiotics	Functional Assessment of Staging Dementia (www.mciscreen.com/pdf/fast_overview.pdf)	• Refer for hospice consultation • Engage in advance care planning (see below) • Avoid percutaneous endoscopic gastrostomy tubes in patients with severe dementia

(continued)

TABLE 74–11. SAFETY MEASURES FOR DEMENTIA PATIENTS (*Continued*)

Safety Concern	Recognition	Assessment	Management
Advance Care Planning	Bring up advance care planning during initial visits	Establish decision-making capacity[a]	• Educate patient and family on the course of the disease and available resources • Explore patient and family preferences and values regarding end of life issues • Foster ongoing discussion regarding end of life issues
Living Alone	• Assess for signs of self-neglect, poor judgment and disorientation • Presence of COPD, stroke • Functional history (ADLs/IADLs)	Conduct cognitive testing (see text); lower scores indicate increased risk of living alone Total dependence on more than three ADLs	• Educate and improve knowledge and acceptance of available resources and support • Help patient and family transition to supported living
Cooking	Easy distractibility, need frequent reminders and consistently misplaces things	Katz Activities of Daily Living (http://consultgerirn.org/uploads/File/tryhis/try_this_2.pdf)	• Disable stoves • Suggest microwave oven • Meals on wheels • Group meals
Suicide Risk	Identify risk factors: Lower SES Suicidal ideation Use of alcohol, illicit drug use, prescription drug abuse Screen for depression	Depression screen, Patient Health Questionnaire-9, query regarding suicide ideation	• Antidepressants (best evidence for citalopram and sertraline in the elderly • Cognitive behavioral therapy

[a]Can the patient communicate, does the patient understand implications of proposed care and the impact of his/her decisions, can the patient express or decide plan of care, is there a rationale for making decisions.

ADLs, activities of daily living; COPD, chronic obstructive pulmonary disease; IADL, instrumental ADL; SES, socioeconomic status.

A. Driving. This is one of the most difficult issues for patients and their families as it represents patient independence. The following characteristics can be useful for identifying patients at an increased risk for unsafe driving (in addition to the information given in Table 74–11): a caregiver's rating of a patient's driving ability as marginal or unsafe (SOR **B**), a history of crashes or traffic citations (SOR **C**), reduced driving mileage or self-reported situational avoidance (SOR **C**), Mini-Mental State Examination scores of 24 or less (SOR **C**), and aggressive or impulsive personality characteristics (SOR **C**). On the other hand, the following characteristics are not useful for identifying patients at an increased risk for unsafe driving: a patient's self-rating of safe driving ability (SOR **A**) and lack of situational avoidance. (SOR **C**) There is insufficient evidence to support or refute the benefit of neuropsychological testing, after controlling for the presence and severity of dementia, or interventional strategies for drivers with dementia. Patients and families should be encouraged to develop alternative sources of transportation early on.

SELECTED REFERENCES

Alzheimer's Association. 2010 Alzheimer's disease facts and figures. *Alzheimer's Dement.* 2010;6(2): 158–194.
Alzheimer's Association. Know the 10 signs. Early detection matters. http://www.alz.org/national/documents/checklist_10signs.pdf. Accessed July 2013.
Birks J. Cholinesterase inhibitors for Alzheimer's disease. *Cochrane Database Syst Rev.* 2006;(1): CD005593.
Birks J, Harvey RJ. Donepezil for dementia due to Alzheimer's disease. *Cochrane Database Syst Rev.* 2006;(1):CD001190.
Craig D, Birks J. Rivastigmine for vascular cognitive impairment. *Cochrane Database Syst Rev.* 2013;(5):CD004744.
Galvin JE, Sadowsky CH, NINCDS-ADRDA. Practical guidelines for the recognition and diagnosis of dementia. *J Am Board Fam Med.* 2012;25:367–382.
Gitlin LN, Kales HC, Lyketsos CG. Nonpharmacologic management of behavioral symptoms in dementia. *JAMA.* 2012;308:2020–2029.
Knopman D, Boeve BF, Petersen RC. Essentials of the proper diagnoses of mild cognitive impairment, dementia, and major subtypes of dementia. *Mayo Clin Proc.* 2003;78:1290–1308.
McShane R, Areosa Sastre A, Minakaran N. Memantine for dementia. *Cochrane Database Syst Rev.* 2006;(2):CD003154.
Rikkert MG, Tona KD, Janssen L, et al. Validity, reliability, and feasibility of clinical staging scales in dementia: a systematic review. *Am J Alzheimers Dis Other Demen.* 2011;26:357–365.
Rolinski M, Fox C, Maidment I, McShane R. Cholinesterase inhibitors for dementia with Lewy bodies, Parkinson's disease dementia and cognitive impairment in Parkinson's disease. *Cochrane Database Syst Rev.* 2012;(3):CD006504.

Additional references are available online at http://langetextbooks.com/fm6e

---

75   Diabetes Mellitus

Stuart D. Rockafellow, PharmD, BCACP, Caroline R. Richardson, MD, & Mark B. Mengel, MD, MPH

KEY POINTS

- The prevalence of type 2 diabetes mellitus (DM) is increasing, mirroring the increase in the prevalence of obesity. (SOR **C**)
- Type 2 DM is the most common type of diabetes, representing approximately 95% of diabetes cases in the United States. (SOR **C**)
- Type 2 DM is a largely a preventable disease. Intensive lifestyle intervention resulting in a 7% weight loss and increased physical activity decreases incident type 2 diabetes by 58% in people with prediabetes. (SOR **B**)
- Because type 2 DM can be asymptomatic for many years, screening may improve outcomes, but evidence supporting screening is limited. The U.S. Preventive Services Task

Force recommends screening for type 2 DM in patients with an elevated blood pressure regardless of age, body mass index, or other risk factors. (SOR **B**) Tests used to screen for diabetes also detect prediabetes.
- Patients with type 1 DM require insulin. (SOR **A**)
- For patients with type 2 DM, instituting a healthy diet with just enough calories to maintain ideal body weight and engaging in regular exercise is the cornerstone of treatment. (SOR **B**) Patients with type 2 DM are usually started on metformin 500 mg daily to twice daily increased to 1000 mg twice daily, or other oral agents or insulin added as needed. (SOR **A**)
- Hemoglobin A1c is the best measure of diabetic control; it should be checked every 3 to 6 months, (SOR **C**) in order to ensure that patients are meeting their individualized glycemic goals to minimize diabetic complications. (SOR **B**)
- Control of blood pressure, lipids, and smoking cessation are also important to reduce the chance of macrovascular complications. (SOR **A**)
- Clinicians should also assess and reduce common barriers to care which prevent achievement of control goals such as depression, family dysfunction, lack of financial resources, and low health literacy. (SOR **B**)

I. Introduction
A. Diabetes mellitus (DM) is a metabolic disorder in which the body does not properly process food resulting in a state of hyperglycemia. Hyperglycemia results from either an absolute deficiency in insulin or cellular resistance to insulin. It can also result from a combination of both.

1. **Prevalence.** According to the Centers for Disease Control and Prevention (CDC), in 2011, approximately 21 million Americans had been diagnosed with diabetes and an additional 7 million had undiagnosed diabetes. In addition, another 80 million patients are prediabetic and at an increased risk for developing diabetes. Gestational diabetes complicates about 7% of pregnancies in the United States.

2. **Associated complications.** Potential complications of diabetes, especially when poorly controlled, include macrovascular complications (those due to damage of large blood vessels such as coronary artery disease, stroke, and peripheral vascular disease) and microvascular complications (those due to damage of small vessels such as diabetic nephropathy, neuropathy, and retinopathy).

3. **Defining control.** Diabetes control is usually evaluated with a hemoglobin A1c test. Glucose glycates with molecules of hemoglobin inside red blood cells. The more glucose in the blood, the more hemoglobin becomes glycated. Measuring the percentage of A1c in the blood provides a reasonable surrogate for average blood glucose control for the past few months.

a. **Targets.** The American Diabetes Association (ADA) recently issued updated consensus guidelines for A1c targets. The new recommendations emphasize **individualizing A1c targets** for patients and stratifies patients into three broad groups.

(1) The first group has an A1c target of <7%. Patients in this group could benefit from the reduction in microvascular complications seen in patients achieving this level of control. Achieving tight glycemic control at this level early in disease is associated with a long-term (20 years) modest reduction in cardiovascular disease (absolute risk reduction, 2.8 myocardial infarctions/1000 patient-years) and all-cause mortality (absolute risk reduction, 3.5 deaths/1000 patient-years). Very long-term (>20 years) outcomes have not been studied.

(2) A second group of patients could target an A1c of <6.5% in order to minimize the long-term risk of diabetic complications. This may be appropriate in patients who are young, have a long life expectancy despite their diagnosis of diabetes, have had diabetes a short time, and can achieve this level of control without undue burden or incidence of hypoglycemia.

(3) The final group of patients has a recommended A1c goal of <8%. Patients for whom this represents a rational A1c goal include patients with a limited life expectancy who may not be anticipated to survive to see any benefit of tight control, those who have already developed the microvascular or

macrovascular complications of diabetes, patients who have a history of severe hypoglycemia, and patients for whom a tighter goal has not been able to be achieved despite optimized medication and lifestyle efforts.

(4) The current guideline from the American Association of Clinical Endocrinologists is for a target A1c level of 6.5% or less for most nonpregnant women if it can be achieved safely.

b. Although tighter glycemic control has been shown to reduce the risk of some microvascular complications in patients with type 1 and type 2 DM, the picture is less clear for macrovascular complications. Long-term studies have shown a reduced risk of cardiovascular complications in patients who achieved tighter glycemic control early. However, a number of recent studies failed to show this benefit in patients with type 2 DM, although there were concerns expressed about many of these studies. Intensive treatment of diabetes is also associated with a greater risk for hypoglycemia. The 2012 ADA guidelines appear to strike a balance between achieving improved glycemic control to minimize future diabetic complications and minimizing the risk of hypoglycemia. The evolving work in this area could mean that A1c targets may shift in one direction or the other in the future. The reader is encouraged to maintain a current knowledge of ongoing diabetic research in order to apply the best clinical judgment when caring for their patients with diabetes.

c. In order to optimize treatment, health systems may need to track quality metrics that assess overtreatment and associated adverse outcomes. This would require improved documentation of medication side effects, frequency of hypoglycemic events, comorbidities, life expectancy, functional status, and patient preferences. Until such algorithms are developed, it will remain the job of the physician to negotiate appropriate glycemic targets with each patient individually taking into consideration all of these factors.

B. Prediabetes is a state in which patients have blood sugar levels above normal, but do not meet criteria for diabetes. These patients are at an increased risk for developing type 2 diabetes.

C. Type 1 DM represents approximately 5% of cases of diabetes. In these patients, autoimmune-mediated destruction of pancreatic beta-cells results in an absolute insulin deficiency. These patients require all insulin to be provided exogenously in order to maintain euglycemia. Patients most commonly present with type 1 DM before the age of 15 years, but can present at any age.

1. The 65-kD isoform of glutamic acid decarboxylase (GAD65) is a major autoantigen in type 1 DM, among other pancreatic islet antigens. Type 1 DM in children and particularly in teenagers and adults is strongly associated with autoreactivity to GAD65. Autoantibodies to GAD65 are common at the time of clinical diagnosis and may be present for years prior to the onset of hyperglycemia.

D. Type 2 DM represents 95% of cases of diabetes. In these patients, increasing resistance to the body's own insulin places an increasing demand on the pancreas to produce higher levels of insulin in order to maintain euglycemia. Insulin resistance is associated with being overweight or obese.

1. Although previously rarely seen in patients younger than 40 years, the increasing rate of obesity in younger individuals has also led to increased prevalence of DM in this population.

2. Known risk factors for type 2 DM include age, a family history of type 2 diabetes, obesity and overweight status, sedentary lifestyle, a previous diagnosis of prediabetes or gestational diabetes, or a history of polycystic ovary syndrome (PCOS). Type 2 diabetes is more common in African-Americans, Latinos, Native Americans, and Asian Americans/Pacific Islanders.

E. Latent autoimmune diabetes in adults (LADA), sometimes known as diabetes type 1.5, is currently classified as a slowly progressive form of type 1 diabetes that occurs after age 30 years. Patients are initially controlled through diet and exercise alone, but generally progress to needing insulin in 3 to 10 years. These patients generally exhibit a positive response to antibody testing that indicates that the patient's own immune system has played a role in their diabetes. Current estimates indicate that this population represents somewhere between 10% and 20% of patients initially diagnosed with type 2 diabetes. This means the population likely equals or is larger than the population of people with type 1 diabetes.

      1. GAD65 autoantibodies predict conversion to insulin dependence when present in patients classified with type 2 DM.

      2. Early treatment with insulin has been associated with improved outcomes in some initial studies in this population. Glucagon-like peptide 1 (GLP-1) agents also have shown some initially positive results.

  F. Gestational diabetes is an insulin resistance dominant form of diabetes that occurs in pregnancy. Clinical detection is important to prevent perinatal morbidity. Diabetes usually resolves postpartum, but these women remain at a higher risk for developing type 2 DM later in life.

II. Screening and Prevention

  A. No routine screening for type 1 diabetes is currently recommended.

  B. Screening criteria for type 2 DM in adults are currently evolving. The **U.S. Preventive Services Task Force** recommends screening for type 2 DM in patients with an elevated blood pressure regardless of age, BMI, or other risk factors. (SOR **B**) The **ADA** recommends screening all adults for diabetes beginning at age 45 years. Additionally, the ADA recommends that adults who are overweight and have risk factors should be considered for testing regardless of age. (SOR **C**)

      1. Additional risk factors include a previous history of abnormal blood sugar including an A1c >5.7%, impaired glucose tolerance, or impaired fasting glucose; sedentary lifestyle; a first-degree relative with diabetes, high-risk race (African-American, Latino, Native American, Asian American, Pacific Islander); previous history of gestational diabetes or who delivered a bay weighting more than 9 pounds; hypertension; high-density lipoprotein <35 mg/dL; a history of polycystic ovary syndrome; a history of cardiovascular disease; a history of other conditions that are associated with insulin resistance such as severe obesity or acanthosis nigricans (Figure 75–1).

      2. Repeat testing should be performed every 3 years in the absence of abnormal results. More frequent testing should be considered in patients at a high risk for developing diabetes such as patients meeting criteria for prediabetes, for whom testing should recur annually based on the ADA. (SOR **C**)

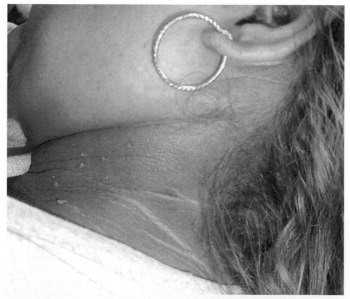

FIGURE 75–1. Acanthosis nigricans on the neck of an obese Hispanic woman with type 2 diabetes. (see color insert) (Used with permission Richard P. Usatine, MD.)

3. **Screening criteria for type 2 DM in children** should be considered for children at age 10 years if they have at least two of the following risk factors and are overweight.
   a. **Overweight is defined** as a BMI greater than the 85th percentile for age and sex, weight for height greater than the 85th percentile, or weight is >120% of ideal for height.
   b. **Risk factors** include a family history of type 2 DM in a first-degree or second-degree relative, high-risk racial background, signs of insulin resistance such acanthosis nigricans, hypertension, dyslipidemia, PCOS, or small-for-gestational-age birth weight; maternal history of diabetes or mother with gestational diabetes during the child's gestation.
4. **Screening for diabetes in pregnancy.**
   a. **Screening for undiagnosed type 2 DM** should occur at the first prenatal visit in women with risk factors.
   b. **Screening for gestational diabetes** should occur between 24 and 28 weeks' gestation. Screening should be by 75-g 2-hour oral glucose tolerance test (OGTT) administered after an overnight fast or fasting for at least 8 hours. The test is considered positive if any of the following values are exceeded: fasting blood glucose >92 mg/dL; 1-hour glucose level ≥180 mg/dL; or 2-hour glucose level >153 mg/dL. The American Congress of Obstetrics and Gynecology recommends screening all pregnant women based on patient history, clinical risk factors, or a 50-g, 1-hour glucose challenge test at 24 to 28 weeks' gestation with confirmation made based on the result of the 100-g, 3-hour OGTT.
5. **Screening for LADA.** No specific screening guidelines for LADA currently exist. Checking GAD65 in a lean young patient with type 2 DM may be reasonable. This is particularly true if the patient has increasing A1c or deteriorating diabetes control inconsistent with current lifestyle efforts.
6. **Screening for prediabetes.** There are no current recommendations for screening for prediabetes. However, testing used in diabetes screening is the same as that used for prediabetes screening. Individuals who are screened for diabetes but whose test results fall in the prediabetes range should be informed of their prediabetes status and referred to a lifestyle modification diabetes prevention program.

III. Diagnosis
   A. **Fasting plasma glucose, hemoglobin A1c, and 2-hour glucose tolerance tests** are the three tests used routinely in clinical medicine to diagnose diabetes. Meeting any one of the criteria shown in Table 75–1 establishes the diagnosis in nonpregnant women. Criteria for prediabetes are shown in Table 75–2.
   1. **Antibody testing.**
      a. **C-peptide** measures residual B-cell function. It is high in type 2 DM, low in type 1 DM, and low to moderate in LADA.
      b. **A positive GAD** is indicative of type 1 DM or LADA. A negative result is expected in type 2 DM.
      c. **Islet cell antibodies** can be helpful in differentiating type 2 DM from LADA. It is negative in in patients with type 2 DM and positive in patients with LADA.

TABLE 75–1. CRITERIA FOR THE DIAGNOSIS OF DIABETES

- A1c ≥6.5%. The test should be performed in a laboratory rather than point-of-care testing.
- Fasting plasma glucose >126 mg/dL. Fasting is defined as no caloric intake for 8 h or more.
- Two-hour plasma glucose ≥200 mg/dL during an oral glucose tolerance test. The test should be performed as described by World Health Organization, using a glucose load containing the equivalent of 75 g anhydrous glucose dissolved in water.
- A random plasma glucose ≥200 mg/dL in a patient with classic symptoms of hyperglycemia or hyperglycemic crisis.

TABLE 75–2. CRITERIA FOR THE DIAGNOSIS OF PREDIABETES

- A1c 5.7%–6.5%.
- Impaired fasting glucoses as defined by a fasting plasma glucose level of 100–125 mg/dL.
- Impaired glucose tolerance as defined by a 2-hour plasma glucose level between 140 and 199 mg/dL in the 75-g oral glucose tolerance test.

TABLE 75–3. COMPONENTS OF PERIODIC EVALUATION IN PATIENTS WITH DIABETES

I. Height, weight, BMI
II. Blood pressure determination
III. Fundoscopic examination
IV. Thyroid palpation
V. Skin examination (for acanthosis nigricans and insulin injection sites)
VI. Comprehensive foot examination, performed annually
    a. Visual inspection
    b. Palpation of dorsalis pedis and posterior tibial pulses
    c. Presence/absence of patellar and Achilles reflexes
    d. Determination of proprioception, vibration, and monofilament sensation
VII. Laboratory evaluation
    a. A1c, if results are not available within past 2–3 mo. Retest every 6 months if controlled and quarterly until control is achieved
    b. If results are not available within past year
        i. Fasting lipid profile, including total, LDL, and HDL cholesterol, and triglycerides
        ii. Microalbumin
        iii. Test for urine albumin excretion with spot urine albumin-to-creatinine ratio
        iv. Serum creatinine and calculated GFR
        v. TSH, dyslipidemia, or women older than 50 years
VIII. Referrals
    a. Annual dilated eye examination by eye care professional
    b. Family planning for women of reproductive age
    c. Registered dietitian for Medical Nutrition Therapy
    d. Diabetes self-management education
    e. Dentist for comprehensive periodontal examination
    f. Mental health professional, if needed

BMI, body mass index; GFR, glomerular filtration rate; HDL, high-density lipoprotein; LDL, low-density lipoprotein; TSH, thyroid-stimulating hormone.

      d. Insulin antibody tests can be helpful in distinguishing types of diabetes. The test would be negative for patients with type 2 DM or gestational diabetes and positive in patients with type 1 DM. Patients with LADA can test positive or negative for this antibody.

   B. Symptoms and signs
      1. Type 1 DM. Polyuria, polydipsia, polyphagia (the 3 Polys), weight loss, malaise, fatigue, abdominal pain, and irritability are typical presenting complaints of patients with type 1 diabetes. Many patients are in diabetic ketoacidosis at the time of diagnosis.
      2. Type 2 DM. Many patients with type 2 DM are asymptomatic. Physicians should suspect type 2 DM in patients with symptoms of polyuria, polydipsia, polyphagia, recurrent infections, visual difficulties, unexplained peripheral neuropathy, and signs of other insulin resistance states such as polycystic ovarian syndrome, acanthosis nigricans (Figure 75–1), or the metabolic syndrome. (SOR **©**) The presence of risk factors for type 2 DM should lower the threshold for both screening and diagnostic testing.
      3. Physical examination. Table 75–3 summarizes the components of a physical examination for a patient with diabetes. Note that the emphasis of the examination is on the evaluation of relevant comorbidities and consequences of uncontrolled hyperglycemia.

  IV. Treatment
   A. The goals of treatment are (1) reduction in incident diabetes among individuals with prediabetes, (2) reduction of diabetic symptoms, (3) prevention of acute complications (e.g., diabetic ketoacidosis, hyperosmolar nonketotic coma, hypoglycemia), (4) encouragement of normal growth and development in children with DM, and (5) prevention of chronic complications.
   B. Treatment for prediabetes
      1. Patients meeting criteria for prediabetes should be referred to an effective ongoing **support program**. Targets of the program should include dietary strategies to reduce caloric intake and the percent of fat in the diet; weight loss of 7% of body weight and increasing physical activity with a goal of at least 150 min/week of

moderate activity such as walking. Additional dietary strategies include meeting the USDA-recommended fiber intake of 14 g daily and reducing and limiting the intake of sugar-sweetened drinks. (SOR **Ⓐ**) Recommendations for fiber vary by age and gender, but some authors suggest a higher daily intake of between 25 and 35 g. The CDC's National Diabetes Prevention Program provides support, intervention materials and health coach training for institutions and providers interested in implementing diabetes prevention group classes.

2. **The Mediterranean diet** has been shown to reduce incidence of diabetes even in the absence of weight loss. (SOR **Ⓑ**)

3. **Metformin therapy** for prevention of progression from prediabetes to overt diabetes can be considered in high-risk patients such as those with a BMI >35 kg/m^2, age >60 years, or women with a previous history of gestational diabetes who are unwilling or unable to participate in lifestyle interventions. Metformin therapy is less effective than lifestyle interventions for preventing incident diabetes. While the evidence is limited, adding metformin to lifestyle interventions does not appear to further reduce incident diabetes.

C. **Nonpharmacologic treatment for diabetes.** Figure 75–2 outlines an approach to the patient suspected of having type 2 DM.

1. A **healthy diet** is recommended for any individual with DM to achieve patient goals for energy balance and weight loss. Registered dieticians with expertise in

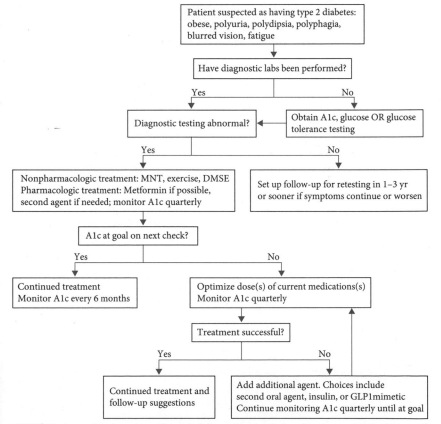

FIGURE 75–2. Approach to the patient with type 2 diabetes. MNT, medical nutrition therapy; DSME, diabetes self-management education; SMBG, self-monitoring of blood glucose.

diabetes management can help individuals with diabetes adopt a healthy diabetic diet. The mix of carbohydrate, protein, and fat can be adjusted to meet individual patient goals and preferences, but monitoring and limiting carbohydrate intake remains essential. Some patients perform carbohydrate counting, particularly those with type 1 DM. Saturated fat should be limited or reduced to <7% of calories. Likewise, limiting trans fats such as those found in many prepared foods and baked goods can help improve cholesterol.

2. **Exercise.** Patients with diabetes should target a total of 150 minutes per week of moderate-intensity aerobic exercise such as walking. This should optimally occur on five out of seven days of the week for 30 minutes or more daily. Most patients with diabetes can also benefit from resistance training with a goal of at least two times each week. Exercise goals should be modified based on patient comorbidities and contraindications to exercise. Patients may moderate postprandial glucose excursions by exercising.

3. **Weight management.** Patients with diabetes should work to maintain a normal weight, as indicated by a BMI <25. Most patients with type 2 DM meet criteria for overweight status or obesity. The positive effects of moderate weight loss in type 2 DM, defined as a loss of 5% of body weight, have been well established for improving insulin resistance, glycemic control, blood pressure control, and lipid control. The long-term benefit on cardiovascular risk of these improvements, however, remains unclear. One study, Look Ahead, demonstrated little cardiovascular benefit from weight loss.

   a. **Bariatric surgery** may be considered for patients with diabetes and a BMI >35; however, the high cost and high rate of postsurgical complications have limited adoption of this intervention. Surgery may be a good option in patients with significant comorbidities and difficulty controlling their diabetes through lifestyle and pharmacologic therapy. There are insufficient current data supporting bariatric surgery in overweight patients with DM whose BMI is <35.

D. **Pharmacologic treatment for diabetes**

1. All patients with **type 1 DM** are managed with insulin therapy. (SOR **Ⓐ**) For the vast majority of patients with type 1 DM, intensive insulin therapy is used consisting of multiple injections of prandial insulin daily using rapid or fast-acting insulin and one or more injections with a basal insulin, either intermediate or long-acting insulin. Many patients with type 1 diabetes utilize an insulin pump for their intensive therapy. Although conventional therapy with twice-daily prandial insulin and twice-daily neutral protamine hagedorn (NPH) was previously considered the standard of care, regimens structured in this way have been demonstrated to be inferior to intensive therapy. Table 75–4 provides additional information about individual insulin preparations. There are currently no available oral antidiabetic medications for patients with type 1 DM.

2. For patients with **type 2 DM,** oral antidiabetic medications form the most common treatment regimens, but insulin may be an appropriate therapy from some patients.

TABLE 75–4. INSULIN TYPES

Type	Onset of Action (h)	Peak Action (h)	Duration of Action (h)
Rapid-acting			
Lispro (Humalog)	<0.25	1–2	3–6
Glulisine (Apidra)	<0.25	1–2	3–6
Aspart (Novolog)	<0.25	1–2	3–6
Short-acting			
Regular	0.5–1	2–3	4–12
Intermediate-acting			
Neutral protamine hagedorn (NPH)	1–2	4–8	10–20
Long-acting			
Glargine (Lantus)	1–2	No peak	24
Detemir (Levemir)	1–2	Usually none	12–20
Regular U500	0.5–1	2–4	Up to 24 h

For instance, insulin therapy may be the best choice in newly diagnosed patients who have significant symptoms or highly elevated A1c at diagnosis.

a. Currently, there is **strong evidence for starting metformin** first in all patients with type 2 DM for whom it is not contraindicated. (SOR **A**) If control is not achieved and maintained within 3 to 6 months, therapy should be intensified by dose optimization, addition of another oral agent, or addition of an injectable antidiabetic agent including GLP-1 agonist or insulin.

b. When insulin therapy is instituted for patients with type 2 DM, it is often initiated as a once-daily dose of basal insulin. As disease progresses, patients with type 2 DM may need to move to an intensive insulin regimen similar to patients with type 1 DM in order to achieve glycemic goals. Conventional insulin therapy is an option in patients with type 2 DM, although it is associated with a higher incidence of hypoglycemia and weight gain.

c. Over the last decade, as the medical community has gotten more aggressive in efforts to control blood glucose in patients with type 2 diabetes, concerns have been raised about harms caused by overtreatment, particularly in older and sicker patients. For example, in a recent study of patients with diabetes in the Veterans Affairs healthcare system, 44% of those on insulin and/or sulfonylureas were not appropriate candidates for tight-control therapy based on age and comorbidities, and of those 48% had HbA1c <7%. Hypoglycemia, a well-documented outcome of tight control that is more common in older and sicker patients, is associated with morbidity, mortality, and increased healthcare costs as well as with depression and reduced quality of life.

   (1) The American Geriatrics Society recommends that medications other than metformin should not be routinely used to lower hemoglobin A1c below 7.5% in patients older than 65 years. The group further recommends an HbA1c target of 8% to 9% for those with serious comorbid conditions.

d. **Classes of oral antidiabetic agents** (Table 75–5).

   (1) Biguanides. Metformin, the only available biguanide in the United States, is currently available in both branded and generic formulations that are immediate release and long acting. It is also available in several combination products with sulfonylureas, DDP4 inhibitors, and thiazolidinediones (TZDs).

   (a) Mechanism of action. Metformin is generally considered to be the first-line antidiabetic agent in type 2 diabetes. It acts by restoring insulin sensitivity, largely in the liver, but also in peripheral tissues. Metformin does not affect insulin secretion, and in fact, insulin secretion may be decreased due to improved glycemic control.

   (b) Efficacy. A1c reductions of 1.5% to 2% can be expected, and coupled with increased exercise and improved diet, some patients experience greater reductions.

   (c) Safety. Patient must have adequate renal function, and metformin is contraindicated in women with a creatinine level of 1.4 or greater and men with a creatinine level of 1.5 or greater. Caution should be used in patients with heart failure, renal insufficiency, or other conditions that affect perfusion and increase the risk of lactic acidosis. Although a recommendation exists against using metformin in patients older than 80 years, consensus agreement and general practice show that it is safely used in patients who do not meet one of the other criteria.

   (d) Notes on dosing. A large number of patients have difficulty tolerating metformin due to gastrointestinal side effects. The extended release formulation may be better tolerated in these patients. Also, starting at the lowest dose, 500 mg daily, and slowly titrating as needed helps with tolerance. Taking metformin with food can also help.

   (2) Sulfonylureas. Generic glipizide, glyburide, and glimepiride are currently available.

   (a) Mechanism of action. Sulfonylureas act by enhancing insulin secretion.

   (b) Efficacy. Second-generation agents lower hemoglobin A1c levels by 1% to 2% on average.

   (c) Safety. Sulfonylureas can cause hypoglycemia and weight gain. All the sulfonylureas undergo hepatic metabolism and should be used with

TABLE 75–5. ORAL HYPOGLYCEMIC AGENTS

Drug	Starting Dose/Maximum Daily Dose	Side Effects and Notes
Biguanides		
Metformin (Glucophage and Glucophage XR)	500 mg daily or twice daily/ 2550 mg/d (2000 mg/d for XR)	Nausea, vomiting, diarrhea, lactic acidosis/contraindicated if ethanol abuse, CHF, or renal insufficiency[a]
Sulfonylureas		
Glimepiride (Amaryl)	1–2 mg daily/8 mg	Hypoglycemia, weight gain, rash, increased LFTs
Glipizide (Glucotrol and Glucotrol XL)	5 mg daily/40 mg (20 mg for XL)	As above
Glyburide (Diabeta, Micronase)	1.25–2.5 mg daily/20 mg	As above
Glyburide-micronized (Glynase PresTab)	1.5–3 mg daily/12 mg	As above
Alpha-Glucosidase Inhibitor		
Acarbose (Precose)	25 mg three times daily before meals/300 mg	Bloating, flatulence, diarrhea; contraindicated in IBD
Miglitol (Glyset)	25 mg three times daily with meals/300 mg	As above
Nonsulfonylureas Secretagogues		
Nateglinide (Starlix)	60 mg three times daily before meals/360 mg	Hypoglycemia, weight gain, increased LFTs
Repaglinide (Prandin)	0.5 mg three times daily before meals/16 mg	As above
Thiazolidinediones		
Pioglitzone (Actos)	15 mg daily/45 mg	Hepatitis, edema
Rosiglitazone (Avandia)[b]	4 mg daily to twice daily/8 mg	MI, Hepatitis, edema
DPP-4 Inhibitors ("gliptins")		
Sitagliptin (Januvia)	100 mg daily/100 mg[c]	URIs, headaches/lower dose in those with renal disease[d]
Saxagliptin (Onglyza)	5 mg daily/5 mg[c]	URIs, UTIs, headache[d]
Linagliptin (Tradjenta)	5 mg daily/5 mg daily	URI, diarrhea, cough[d]
SLGT2 Inhibitors		
Canagliflozin (Invokarna)	100 mg daily/100 mg[c]	Hypotension, UTI

[a]Contraindicated in women with a creatinine of 1.4 mg/dL or greater and men with a creatinine of 1.5 mg/dL or greater.
[b]Restricted availability.
[c]Adjustment of dose required or recommended in renal insufficiency.
[d]Emerging data indicate that there may be an increased risk of pancreatitis with agents in this class.
CHF, congestive heart failure; IBD, irritable bowel disease; LFTs, liver function tests; MI, myocardial infarction; URI, upper respiratory infection; UTI, urinary tract infection.

caution in patients with liver abnormalities. Glyburide also has a significant portion of renal elimination and should be used with caution in patients with renal compromise and in the elderly. Glipizide is preferred in patients with renal abnormalities including the elderly.

  (d) **Notes on dosing.** These medications need to be dosed prior to eating a meal for optimal effect. This can also help minimize the risk of hypoglycemia.

(3) **Dipeptidyl peptidase 4 (DPP-4) inhibitors.** Sitagliptin (Januvia), saxagliptin (Onglyza), and linagliptin (Tradjenta) are currently available. No generic formulation is available for these agents.

  (a) **Mechanism of action.** DPP-4 inhibitors (gliptins) slow the inactivation of incretin hormones by blocking the effect of DPP-4, the enzyme that breaks down GLP-1 in the body. The net physiologic effects are related to increased levels of GLP-1, which increases insulin release and decreases glucagon release.

(b) Efficacy. Gliptins lower hemoglobin A1c by 0.5% to 1%, over 6 months, either as monotherapy or in combination with metformin or a TZD.

(c) Safety. Although there is little risk of hypoglycemia when used as monotherapy, these agents can increase the risk for and severity of hypoglycemia when used with other agents that can cause hypoglycemia.

(d) Notes on dosing. The dosage of sitagliptin must be reduced in patients with renal disease. Saxagliptin and linagliptin are metabolized through the cytochrome P450 system and can interact with other agents that undergo hepatic metabolism.

(4) TZD. Pioglitazone (Actos) is available for both new starts and maintenance. At the time of this writing, rosiglitazone (Avandia) is currently subject to a Risk Evaluation and Mitigation Strategy (REMS) program that restricts its use only to prescribers who acknowledge the potential increased risk of myocardial infarction associated with its use and patients who have been advised of this increased risk AND are either already taking rosiglitazone or, if not already taking rosiglitazone, are unable to achieve glycemic control on other medications, including pioglitazone.

(a) Mechanism of action. TZD agents are insulin sensitizers. They increase insulin sensitivity by direct stimulation of nuclear receptors in hepatic and skeletal muscle cells.

(b) Efficacy. TZDs can be expected to lower A1c by 1% to 1.5%. Full effect may take 6 months to achieve. These agents can be used as monotherapy or in combination with other oral hypoglycemic agents.

(c) Safety. Liver function tests, though indicated, are not likely necessary on a routine basis. Weight gain can be significant. Fluid retention is also a problem, and these medications have been associated with exacerbation of heart failure and new onset heart failure. TZDs are contraindicated in patients with class III or IV heart failure. Rosiglitazone is associated with an increased risk of myocardial infarction.

(5) Non-sulfonylureas secretagogues. Nateglinide (Starlix) and repaglinide (Prandin) are currently available. No generic is currently available.

(a) Mechanism of action. Meglitinides are rapid-acting agents that stimulate insulin release postprandially, and thus must be taken before each meal. If a meal is missed, the drug should not be taken.

(b) Efficacy. Meglitinides lower hemoglobin A1c by 0.5% to 1% on average.

(c) Safety. Although less likely than with sulfonylureas, these agents can cause hypoglycemia and weight gain. They have a short duration of action that may make hypoglycemia easier to treat. Because they are metabolized in the liver, these agents should be used cautiously in patients with liver abnormalities.

(d) Notes on dosing. These drugs are more expensive than oral sulfonylureas, but may prove useful in patients with renal impairment or patients who do not eat on a regular schedule. They also may be helpful for patients who experience nocturnal hypoglycemia on sulfonylurea therapy.

(6) Alpha-glucosidase inhibitors. Acarbose (Precose) and miglitol (Glyset) are currently available; acarbose is available as a generic.

(a) Mechanism of action. These agents inhibit the alpha-glucosidase enzyme that lines the brush border of the small intestine delaying absorption of simple sugars.

(b) Efficacy. On an average, these agents lower hemoglobin A1c by 0.5% to 1.0%.

(c) Safety. Patients taking these agents will have trouble treating hypoglycemic attacks with complex carbohydrates and so should have oral glucose tablets readily available. These agents are contraindicated in patients with bowel disease.

(d) Notes on dosing. These drugs must be taken with each meal in order to lower postprandial glucose levels. These agents can be used in combination with other oral hypoglycemic agents.

(7) SLGT2 inhibitors. Canagliflozin (Invokana) is the only current medication in this class. It is relatively new to the market and not available as a generic.

TABLE 75–6. NONINSULIN INJECTIBLE MEDICATIONS

Drug	Starting Dose/Maximum Daily Dose	Side Effects and Notes
GLP-1 Mimetics		
Exenatide (Byetta)	5 mcg twice daily/10 mcg twice daily	Nausea, diarrhea, vomiting[a]
Liraglutide (Victoza)	0.8 mg daily	As above
Exenatide LA (Bydureon)	2 mg weekly[b]	As above
Amylin Mimetic		
Pramlintide (Symlin)	Type 1 DM	Hypoglycemia
	15 mg three times daily/60 mg three times daily[c]	
	Type 2 DM	
	60 mg three times daily/120 mg three times daily[c]	

[a]Emerging data indicate that there may be an increased risk of pancreatitis with agents in this class.
[b]Requires reconstitution.
[c]Recommended 30%–50% dose reduction for prandial insulin at initiation.

(a) **Mechanism of action.** Canagliflozin inhibits subtype 2 sodium-glucose transport protein, the enzyme responsible for reabsorption of glucose in the kidney.

(b) **Efficacy.** Hemoglobin A1c is reduced by 0.5% to 0.7%.

(c) **Safety.** Hypotension, hypoglycemia, an increase in mycotic urinary and genital infections, and increased low-density lipoprotein (LDL) have all been reported.

(8) **Noninsulin injectable, GLP-1 mimetics** include Byetta (exenatide), Victoza (liraglutide), and Bydureon (exenatide LA) (Table 75–6). None are currently available as a generic.

(a) **Mechanism of action.** These agents work like GLP-1, a naturally occurring gut hormone. They increase insulin release, lower glucagon, delay gastric emptying, and suppress appetite.

(b) **Efficacy.** These agents can be expected to lower A1c by 1% to 2%. Weight loss is expected and ranges upward from 2 to 4 kg. Weight loss may not be maintained beyond 1 year.

(c) **Safety.** Side effects include nausea and vomiting, which usually occur at the start of treatment or with dose escalation. In some patients, this does not improve and can be dose limiting or lead to discontinuation. These agents can cause or potentiate hypoglycemia.

(d) **Notes on dosing.** GLP-1 mimetics are indicated in patients with type 2 diabetes who have not achieved glucose control goals while taking metformin or combination therapy with metformin. They should NOT be used in patients with type 1 DM. Exenatide carries a recommended initial dose of 5 μg twice daily before meals that may be titrated to a maximum dose of 10 μg twice daily if tolerated. Liraglutide carries indicated doses of 0.6, 1.2, and 1.8 mg daily and should be titrated slowly as needed beyond the initial dose. Bydureon requires reconstitution from a powder which can be difficult for some patients. One potential advantage of this formulation is that dosing is once weekly. Of these agents, only exenatide currently carries an indication for concurrent use with basal insulin.

(9) **Noninsulin injectable, amylin mimetics.** Symlin (pramlintide) is the only agent available in this class.

(a) **Mechanism of action.** Pramlintide is an analog of amylin that slows food absorption, inhibits glucagon, and reduces appetite.

(b) **Efficacy.** Pramlintide can be expected to lower A1c by 0.5% to 0.8%.

(c) **Safety.** The main side effect is nausea. Hypoglycemia occurs more commonly in patients with type 1 DM. Delayed gastric emptying may delay the absorption of orally administered medication.

(d) **Notes on dosing.** Pramlintide is injected along with premeal insulin (separate syringes) and improves glucose control, while lowering body weight. The starting dose is 15 μg, increased by 15 μg increments to 30 or 60 μg as tolerated in patients with type 1 DM before each meal.

The starting dose for patients with type 2 DM is 60 µg, with the dose increasing to 120 µg twice a day if tolerated. Insulin doses should be reduced by 50% when pramlintide is started.

3. Insulin therapy

a. **Characteristics of insulin preparations.** Selection from available insulin preparation is based on concentration (usually, U-100, although U-500 regular insulin is available) and the pharmacokinetic/pharmacodynamic characteristics of the various insulins. Table 75–4 summarizes these characteristics for currently available insulins. All insulins currently on the market are human or modified human insulins. Animal, derived insulins are no longer marketed in the United States.

   (1) Rapid-acting insulins. Insulin lispro, insulin aspart, and insulin glulisine have been shown to be more effective than regular insulin in controlling postprandial blood sugar.

   (2) Long-acting insulins. Insulin glargine and detemir have no peak onset of action and mimicking basal insulin secretion. As monotherapy these insulins have the lowest risk of hypoglycemia, but it can still be significant. In patients with type 1 and type 2 DM, use of insulin glargine given once daily (rather than twice a day NPH), is associated with less hypoglycemia, less weight gain, and better glucose control. Insulin detemir has been found to be less potent on a unit-by-unit basis and may require higher insulin doses than insulin glargine. Insulin detemir also frequently requires twice-daily dosing to maintain control. A third long-acting insulin has been approved for human use in the European Union and is undergoing additional requested testing in the United States. If approved for the market, it is expected to carry an indication for every other day injections.

b. **Insulin dosing in type 1 DM.** Based on the Diabetes Control and Complications study, we know that the best control and lowest risk of complications comes with intensive insulin therapy composed of four or more injections of insulin designed to mimic the physiologic processes in nondiabetics. This type of regimen, also known as split-dose, closely mimics what the pancreas provides in healthy, nondiabetic patients. Under this regimen, the patient takes multiple insulin injections daily of prandial insulin at mealtimes and a basal insulin.

   Alternatively, these patients may use an insulin pump to deliver a constant infusion of insulin to cover their basal needs and then boluses of the same insulin to cover their meal time needs. These patients often count their carbohydrate intake (http://www.upmc.com/patients-visitors/education/diabetes/Pages/basic-carb-counting.aspx) and establish a ratio of units of insulin needed to cover grams of carbohydrate. They use this ratio to calculate their meal-time insulin needs. These patients will often have a modifier, sometimes called a correction factor, that works like a sliding scale to correct hyperglycemia at the start of a meal. The calculated modifier dose is added to the dose calculated with the carbohydrate/insulin ratio for the total meal time dose.

c. **Initiating insulin in type 1 DM.** Patients newly diagnosed with type 1 DM either receive education and begin their insulin regimen while hospitalized or, if not in ketoacidosis, can begin their insulin treatment as an outpatient. Patients may first be placed on preprandial and nighttime injections of either regular insulin or rapid-acting insulin based upon preprandial blood glucose.

   (1) Patients should start with a **total daily dose of 0.6 units/kg of body weight**. When intensive therapy is going to be used, two-thirds of the total amount of insulin is given in the morning and one-third in the evening. The morning and evening dosages can then be split into 75% basal and 25% preprandial insulin. If insulin glargine with rapid-acting insulin before each meal is used, then 40% to 50% of the total dose is given as insulin glargine first thing in the morning or at bedtime with the other 50% to 60% split up and given as rapid-acting insulin prior to each meal based upon preprandial glucose values. Patient's self-monitoring can then be used to adjust insulin therapy.

   (2) Intensification of insulin therapy. The ideal insulin regimen in type 1 DM includes basal insulin and prandial insulin dosed prior to meals based on carbohydrate counting. A correction factor can be used to adjust for premeal high blood glucose readings.

(3) Honeymoon period. Soon after insulin therapy is initiated, a "honeymoon period" of 12 to 18 months occurs in nearly all patients with type 1 or type 2 DM. During this time, patient's insulin requirements usually are drastically reduced. This phenomenon is thought to be due to reduced glucose toxicity. Therefore, patients should be encouraged to utilize self-blood glucose monitoring, and protocol should be designed so that they can reduce insulin therapy as their insulin requirements are reduced.

d. Initiating insulin therapy in type 2 DM. Patients with type 2 DM may reach a point where they need additional coverage to achieve adequate glycemic control despite optimal doses of oral medications. For these patients, the next step may be to add insulin.

(1) Initiating insulin therapy. Although most patients first lose the ability to maintain postprandial control, the most common insulin regimen initiated is basal insulin because of the lower risk of hypoglycemia and the ability to greatly improve control with a simple insulin regimen. Common starting regimens include using insulin glargine or detemir 10 units daily and titrating as needed.

(2) Intensification of insulin. As type 2 DM progresses, patients often need additional coverage beyond basal insulin. These patients add prandial insulin sometimes just at the largest meal and sometimes at all meals. Doses are adjusted based on home monitoring results. The ideal prandial insulin dosing regimen would be based on carbohydrate counting after establishing an insulin-to-carbohydrate ratio as discussed in Section IV.D.3.b. For patients in whom carbohydrate counting is not feasible, fixed doses that are adjusted to meet their average carbohydrate needs can be administered. Ideally a correction factor may be added to these fixed doses. In no circumstance does sliding scale dosing of prandial insulin alone give adequate glycemic control and it is considered suboptimal dosing in ambulatory settings. Sliding scale alone may be used in hospitalized patients where glycemic goals are different from those in ambulatory chronic care patients.

(3) Notes. Metformin can be continued as long as renal function permits. Metformin confers some cardioprotective effect in overweight and obese patients. Sulfonylurea medications offer little to no benefit once prandial insulin is started and should be stopped once prandial insulin is initiated.

V. Self-Monitoring of Blood Glucose (SMBG). The value of SMBG is limited for people with type 2 DM on oral agents or diet alone. For patients with type 2 DM on basal insulin only or on oral antidiabetic medications, testing is recommended only if used to guide treatment and when prescribed as part of broader educational plan in which the readings will be evaluated and acted upon.

A. SMBG is an important component of self-management for individual using insulin to achieve tight glucose control and for those using an insulin pump to manage their diabetes.

B. The ADA issued new recommendations for self-testing in January 2013. These newest recommendations suggest that patients on intensive insulin therapy test multiple times daily, at least before eating and taking insulin, and additionally sometimes after meals and before bedtime with no limit on the number of times per day that patients test. This changed the three times per day limit that was previously recommended. Payers may only reimburse to this level of testing.

VI. Reducing barriers to care. Certain nonmedical factors are associated with improved control in patients with DM.

A. Patient-centered care. A team-based approach that encourages patient involvement in decision-making regarding goal setting and management options improves glucose control. (SOR **B**) The patient centered medical home is an example of this care model.

B. Knowledge and self-management skills. Patients with DM should be enrolled in an education program that discusses a wide range of topics pertinent to their care and encourages patient decision-making and self-management. A meta-analysis showed that such an approach increases knowledge about DM; increases the frequency, accuracy, and usefulness of SMBG; improves dietary habits; and improves glucose control. (SOR **A**) Education in either individual or group settings has been found to be of benefit. More frequent contact between patients and the caregiver team improves control.

TABLE 75-7. ADDITIONAL MEDICATIONS TO CONSIDER IN PATIENTS WITH DIABETES

Medication	Target Population
Nicotine replacement or smoking cessation aid (see Chapter 70)	Patients, who are current smokers, who meet criteria for prescribing and have no contraindications
Angiotensin converting enzyme inhibitor	All patients with hypertension and diabetes Patients with nephropathy
Angiotensin receptor blocker	Patients who develop cough on ACE inhibitor
Statin	All patients older than 40 years regardless of LDL level Patients younger than 40 years with LDL >100 mg/dL
Aspirin 81 mg daily	Patients older than 40 years Patients younger than 40 years with a personal history of coronary artery disease or a strong family history of heart disease

C. **Psychosocial factors.** The following psychosocial factors have been linked with poor diabetic control: pessimistic attitudes about DM, poor social support and social isolation, low self-efficacy skills, an external locus of control, excessive stress, being in precontemplation regarding necessary behavior change, and a passive pessimistic coping style. Screening for depression and family dysfunction is recommended for all patients with DM periodically and can direct appropriate treatment.

D. Determining use of complementary and alternative therapies and discussing the efficacies of those therapies with patients have been shown to improve glucose control, as patients rely less on ineffective therapies.

E. **Health literacy.** Low health literacy is common among all patients and is associated with several negative health outcomes. These negative outcomes include decreased adherence to treatment regimens, inability to keep appointments, and not understanding instructions and patient education. All educational materials utilized by clinicians should be appropriately targeted to reading level and language. Clinicians should consider using practice aids like the Health Literacy Universal Precautions Toolkit to assess their practice and work with staff to improve communication with patients and their patient's health literacy (http://www.ahrq.gov/legacy/qual/literacy/healthliteracytoolkit.pdf).

F. **Financial.** Even with health insurance, the cost of medications and supplies for DM can be prohibitive. Clinicians should make every attempt to use the most cost-effective treatment options available. Assistance programs through the manufacturer are available for many diabetic medications, including most insulins. Referring patients to appropriate resources or to a social worker to coordinate these efforts may allow patients to obtain diabetic medications and supplies at a price that is affordable to them.

VII. **Prevention and Early Detection of Complications**

A. **Risk factor reduction.** Management of contributing comorbidities is essential to minimizing macrovascular complications. This includes smoking cessation, maintaining blood pressure control, and treating to diabetic goals for hyperlipidemia. Additional medications to consider in patients with diabetes are shown in Table 75-7. Targets and goals for patients with comorbid hypertension and hyperlipidemia are shown in Table 75-8.

1. **Smoking cessation** is critically important, and offering pharmacotherapeutic options such as nicotine replacement product, varenicline, or bupropion is effective.

2. The ADA released **new goals for blood pressure** for people with diabetes in 2013, relaxing the standard somewhat to a goal of <140/80 mm Hg in all patients, with tighter control in certain patients in whom it does not cause an undue burden.

TABLE 75-8. TARGETS AND GOALS FOR COMORBID CONDITIONS FOR PATIENTS WITH DIABETES

Condition	Target and goal
Hypertension	Blood pressure <140/80 mm Hg (ADA) OR <140/90 mm Hg (JNC 8) in all patients Blood pressure <130/80 mm Hg in selected patients such as young patients in whom this does not present undue burden (ADA)
Hyperlipidemia	LDL <100 mg/dL (with an option of targeting <70 mg/dL in high-risk patients) HDL >40 mg/dL Triglycerides <150 mg/dL

    a. The **JNC 8** evidence-based treatment goals for the general population are a blood pressure of <150/90 mm Hg for people aged 60 years and over and a diastolic goal of <90 mm Hg for all other individuals. (SOR **Ⓐ**) For patients aged 18 years and over with diabetes, pharmacologic treatment should be initiated to lower blood pressure to <140/90 mm Hg. (SOR **Ⓒ**)

  3. All patients over the age of 40 years with diabetes should be considered for a **statin medication,** even if their LDL is at goal.

  4. Aspirin 81 mg oral daily to prevent cardiovascular complications is also indicated in all patients with type 2 diabetes over the age of 40 years per most guidelines, and in all patients with a personal history of coronary artery disease or a strong family history regardless of age.

  5. Immunizations. Adult patients with DM should receive a yearly flu vaccine, a pneumococcal vaccine every 5 to 7 years, and a tetanus vaccine every 10 years. The CDC now recommends that the hepatitis B series of vaccinations be given as soon after diagnosis of diabetes as possible.

B. Achieving near, normal diabetic control. Design of an effective treatment regimen and the assessment and correction of factors associated with poor diabetic control and barriers to care help to prevent complications of DM.

C. Screening for complications. Routine diabetic eye examinations, diabetic foot examinations, and renal assessment (measurement of serum creatinine and urinary microalbumin) aid early diagnosis of diabetic complications (Table 75–3). Examining the feet of a patient with diabetes at each visit has been associated with a decreased risk of morbidity including amputation. The frequency of other examinations with the exception of annual ophthalmologic examinations and annual testing for serum creatinine and microalbuminuria has not been well studied.

D. Quarterly physician visits are recommended for individuals on insulin while visits every six months may be sufficient for patients not on insulin. More frequent visits are needed if adherence to the treatment program, including risk factor reduction, is poor.

E. Treating complications as they develop. Once complications are diagnosed, risk factor reduction and symptomatic treatment remain the mainstays of complication management.

  1. Painful peripheral neuropathies can often be treated with a low dose of a tricyclic antidepressant, such as amitriptyline, 50 mg orally at bedtime. Gabapentin (300 mg/dose up to 3600 mg per day as tolerated), duloxetine (60 mg once daily), pregabalin (50 mg three times daily up to 300 mg per day), oxycodone (initial dose 5–15 mg every 4–6 hours up to 30 mg every 4–6 hours), and tramadol (25 mg per day up to 100 mg per day in divided doses) are also effective for the symptomatic treatment of painful diabetic neuropathy. (SOR **Ⓐ**)

  2. The progression of diabetic nephropathy can be slowed with an angiotensin-converting enzyme (ACE) inhibitor (even if the patient is not hypertensive) such as lisinopril, 10 mg orally daily, or an angiotensin receptor 2 blocking agent such as losartan 50 mg daily if the ACE inhibitor is not tolerated.

VIII. Office Management. An organized evidenced-based approach to the management of patients with DM in medical offices has been shown to improve diabetic control in patients visiting those offices.

A. Use of multiple interventions has been associated with better patient management. Interventions include clinician education through materials and meetings, developing a local consensus process regarding care protocols, auditing outcomes, and providing that feedback to practitioners, using reminders for clinicians regarding when to conduct certain interventions, such as annual ophthalmologic examinations, enhancing the professional role of nurses in the office, and utilizing case management and disease management for patients who need that additional support.

B. A multidisciplinary treatment team is needed for many patients, particularly those on intensive insulin treatment regimens.

C. Group visits focused on lifestyle change for individuals with prediabetes yield reductions in incident diabetes similar to those seen in the original intensive and expensive diabetes prevention program intervention but at a much lower cost.

  1. The CDC's National Diabetes Prevention Program (http://www.cdc.gov/diabetes/prevention/) provides support, intervention materials, and health coach training for institutions and individual providers interested in implementing diabetes prevention group classes.

2. Group visits for individuals with diabetes may also be a cost-effective way to support diabetes self-management. There is currently little evidence that these visits improve glycemic control, but several studies are ongoing. During these visits, approximately 20 patients with DM receive a group educational session, discuss supportive strategies among themselves, and receive a brief visit from the clinician. Patients generally like the group sessions, appreciating the camaraderie and social interaction.

D. The National Diabetes Education Program website (http://ndep.nih.gov/) includes an extensive list of high-quality diabetes education materials for providers and patients.

IX. Prognosis. The outcome of DM in a particular patient depends on several factors. These factors include the nature and severity of the disease, the simultaneous occurrence of other diseases, the presence of risk factors for diabetic complications (disease duration is the most important), genetic susceptibility to specific complications, and how well the patient responds to treatment. The patient's ability to adapt constructively to the disease also influences the course of the illness.

A. The mean survival of patients with type 1 DM diagnosed before age 30 years is currently 10 to 15 years less than that of the general population. Death usually results from end-stage renal disease (40% to 50%) or coronary artery disease, although ketoacidosis and hypoglycemic coma continue to cause significant mortality.

B. Life expectancy in patients with type 2 DM is roughly one-third less than that of age-matched non-diabetic patients. Cardiovascular disease accounts for 75% of the deaths in patients with type 2 DM after age 60 years.

C. Complications. Except for ketoacidosis, all the complications associated with type 1 DM occur in patients with type 2 DM. However, macrovascular complications are more common in type patients with 2 DM. Hyperosmolar nonketotic coma, an acute complication, is seen almost exclusively in patients with type 2 DM.

SELECTED REFERENCES

American Diabetes Association. Summary of Revisions for the 2013 Clinical Practice Recommendations. Diabetes Care 2013;36(Suppl1):S3.

American Diabetes Association website. www.diabetes.org. Accessed March 1, 2013.

Boussageon R, Bejan-Angoulvant T, Saadatian-Elahi M, et al. Effect of intensive glucose lowering treatment on all cause mortality, cardiovascular death, and microvascular events in type 2 diabetes: meta-analysis of randomised controlled trials. BMJ. 2011;343:d4169.

Executive summary: Standards of medical care in diabetes–2013. Diabetes Care. 2013;36(Suppl 1): S4–S10.

Feil DG, Rajan M, Soroka O, et al. Risk of hypoglycemia in older veterans with dementia and cognitive impairment: implications for practice and policy. J Am Geriatr Soc. 2011;59(12):2263–2272.

Feit S. Putting evidence into practice: Outpatient management of type 2 diabetes mellitus. Clinical Evidence. A report funded by United Health Foundation. London: BMJ Publishing Group; 2006.

Funnel, MM, Brown TL, Childs BP, et al. National standards for diabetes self-management education. Diabetes Care. 2012;35(Suppl 1):S102–S108.

Handelsman Y, Mechanick JI, Blonde L, et al. American Association of Clinical Endocrinologists medical guidelines for clinical practice for developing a diabetes mellitus comprehensive care plan. Endocr Pract. 2011;17(Suppl 2):1–53.

Holman RR, Paul SK, Bethel MA, et al. 10-year follow-up of intensive glucose control in type 2 diabetes. N Engl J Med. 2008;359(15):1577–1589.

Inzucchi SE, Bergenstal RM, Buse JB, et al. Management of hyperglycemia in type 2 diabetes: a patient-centered approach. Position statement from the American Diabetes Association (ADA) and the European Association for the Study of Diabetes (EASD). Diabetologia. 2012;55(6):1577–1596.

Ismail-Beigi F, Craven T, Banerji MA, et al. Effect of intensive treatment of hyperglycaemia on microvascular outcomes in type 2 diabetes: an analysis of the ACCORD randomised trial. Lancet. 2010;376(9739): 419–430.

James PA, Oparil S, Carter BL, Cushman WC, Dennison-Himmelfarb C, Handler J, et al. 2014 evidence-based guideline for the management of high blood pressure in adults: report from the panel members appointed to the eight Joint National Committee (JNC-8). JAMA. 2014;311(5):507–520.

Peterson KA, Hughes M. Readiness to change and clinical success in a diabetes educational program. JABFP. 2002;15(4):266–271.

Additional references are available online at http://langetextbooks.com/fm6e

76   Dyslipidemias

Trisha D. Wells, PharmD, Amanda M. Cox, MD, Mindy A. Smith, MD, MS, &
Michael A. Crouch, MD, MSPH

KEY POINTS

- One-half of all American adults have unhealthy blood lipid levels. Although higher cholesterol levels pose the greatest *relative* risk, more than one-half of all myocardial infarctions occur in those with suboptimal or borderline low-density lipid (LDL) cholesterol levels. (SOR **C**)
- Lowering intake of dietary saturated fats, trans fats, and cholesterol is the cornerstone for treating hypercholesterolemia and reducing risk for coronary heart disease (CHD). (SOR **A**) Other useful dietary measures include regular intake of fiber, fish, or fish oil (omega-3 fatty acids), nuts, soy protein, and plant sterols or stanols. (SOR **B**) Weight loss and exercise raise high-density lipid (HDL) cholesterol and lower triglycerides, but do not improve LDL cholesterol. (SOR **A**)
- Patients in the four benefit groups should receive medication treatment with statins in addition to dietary modification to achieve the recommended treatment intensity (Table 76–2). (SOR **A**)
- For other patients who are not in the benefit groups, it is appropriate to consider a trial of statins if they have primary LDL ≥160 mg/dL or other evidence of genetic hyperlipidemias, a family history of or CHD-equivalent (peripheral arterial disease, carotid artery disease, abdominal aortic aneurysm), or an LDL between 70 and 189 mg/dL with an atherosclerotic CVD risk between 5% and 7.5%. (SOR **C**)
- Long-term adherence is poor for statin therapy. Many patients are apprehensive about potential adverse drug effects and do not have a clear understanding of the benefit/risk ratio. Repetitive patient education in verbal, textual, and graphic formats, focused on specific patient concerns, may foster long-term statin compliance and maximize treatment benefit. (SOR **C**)

I. Introduction

A. Dyslipidemia is a broad term that includes several lipid disorders such as elevated total cholesterol, elevated low-density lipid (LDL) cholesterol, elevated triglycerides (TGs), low high-density lipid (HDL) cholesterol, or any combination of these. Factors contributing to dyslipidemia include familial (primary disorder), metabolic (secondary disorder), lifestyle, and iatrogenic (e.g., medication-induced).

1. **Primary** lipid disorders are **familial,** being transmitted across generations by both genetic factors and learned behaviors.
2. **Secondary** causes of dyslipidemias include diabetes mellitus, hypothyroidism, pregnancy, nephrotic syndrome, chronic renal failure, obstructive liver disease, anorexia nervosa, obesity, acute intermittent porphyria, and glycogen storage disease. Diets high in saturated fats, added sugars, and alcohol, along with sedentary lifestyle, are common lifestyle contributors. Medications that can cause dyslipidemia include progestins, estrogens, raloxifene, tamoxifen, thiazide diuretics, glucocorticoids, beta-blockers, amiodarone, bile acid sequestrants, protease inhibitors, and cyclosporine.

B. Hyperlipidemia refers to elevated total blood cholesterol, LDL cholesterol, or TG levels (or both). **Familial combined (mixed) hyperlipidemia** refers to elevated LDL cholesterol and TGs.

C. Hypercholesterolemia is elevated total blood cholesterol.

1. Familial heterozygous and homozygous (more adversely affected) hypercholesterolemia display autosomal dominant inheritance, but most cases of hypercholesterolemia are polygenic.
2. The prevalence of hypercholesterolemia increases with age until the fifth decade for men and sixth decade for women at which time the levels plateau.
3. Total cholesterol <200 mg/dL is considered desirable, borderline high is 200 to 239 mg/dL, and total cholesterol ≥240 mg/dL is considered high.

4. About half (46.8%) of American adults over the age of 20 years have a total cholesterol at or above 200 mg/dL and 17% have high cholesterol. Half of patients with elevated cholesterol are unaware that they have an elevated level.

D. Hypertriglyceridemia is elevated fasting TGs. Saturated fat and cholesterol are absorbed from the gastrointestinal tract and packaged into TG-rich particles called chylomicrons. These chylomicrons are broken down into very low-density lipoprotein (VLDL) particles that are rich in TGs.

1. TGs <150 mg/dL are considered desirable, TGs of 150 to 199 mg/dL are "borderline high," high TG is ≥200 mg/dL, and very high TG is ≥500 mg/dL.

2. Elevated TGs are seen in 20% to 30% of American adults.

3. Excessive **alcohol intake,** dietary **sugars,** and rapidly digested **starches** elevate TGs. **Physical inactivity** or being **overweight** or **obese** also elevates TGs.

E. Hyperbetalipoproteinemia is elevated LDL cholesterol. Very low-density lipid particles are catalyzed by the enzyme lipoprotein lipase into cholesterol-rich LDL particles. LDL particles attach to LDL receptors on cell membranes. Cholesterol from the LDL particles passes into cells. The influx of cholesterol into the cells suppresses the activity of the rate-limiting enzyme in cholesterol synthesis, 3-hydroxy-3-methylglutaryl coenzyme A (HMG-CoA) reductase. LDL cholesterol is one of the main risk factors for atherosclerotic cardiovascular disease (ASCVD), which includes coronary heart disease (CHD), stroke, and peripheral arterial disease, and is the primary target for therapy.

1. Optimal LDL cholesterol is ≤100 mg/dL, "above optimal" LDL cholesterol is 100 to 129 mg/dL, "borderline high" LDL cholesterol level is 130 to 159 mg/dL, and high LDL cholesterol is ≥160 mg/dL. The 2013 American College of Cardiology (ACC)/ American Heart Association (AHA) Guideline on Treatment of Blood Cholesterol to Reduce Atherosclerotic Cardiovascular Risk in Adults moves away from categorizing lipid targets in favor of a benefit group approach that includes those with high LDL levels.

2. Excessive dietary intake of **saturated fat and cholesterol** raises LDL and total cholesterol.

3. Drug-associated causes of lipid elevations are common.

    a. Thiazide diuretics, especially in higher doses, can increase LDL and total cholesterol. Some studies report that this effect lasts about 1 year, after which the cholesterol returns to pretreatment levels despite continuing use of diuretics.

    b. Nonselective and beta-1 selective **beta-blockers** cause a slight decrease in HDL. Nonselective beta-blockers can also increase TGs. Beta-blockers with intrinsic sympathomimetic activity (such as acebutolol and pindolol) and labetalol do not affect cholesterol levels.

    c. Oral contraceptives with strong androgen/progestin effects lower HDL cholesterol, raise TGs, and sometimes raise LDL cholesterol.

    d. High-dose corticosteroids raise TGs.

F. Hypoalphalipoproteinemia is low HDL cholesterol. HDL particles facilitate LDL metabolism, which results in cholesterol being carried back to the liver from peripheral tissues. Patients with low HDL cholesterol and elevated TGs tend to have smaller, more dense LDL particles that are more atherogenic.

1. In men, an HDL >40 mg/dL and in women, an HDL >50 mg/dL is considered ideal. Low HDL cholesterol is ≤40 mg/dL.

2. Physical inactivity or being overweight or obese decreases HDL cholesterol as does cigarette smoking.

3. Alcohol in moderation (no more than one drink per day for women and two drinks per day for men) raises HDL cholesterol in males over the age of 45 years and females over the age of 55 years.

G. Atherogenic dyslipidemia includes TG levels ≥150 mg/dL and low HDL cholesterol <40 mg/dL.

H. Metabolic syndrome is a constellation of risk factors that occurs in about 20% to 25% of US adults. Metabolic syndrome is associated with a high risk for ASCVD. Per the National Cholesterol Education Program (NCEP)–Adult Treatment Panel (ATP) III guidelines, metabolic syndrome is present if a patient has three or more of the following characteristics:

- Waist size >40 in (102 cm) for men or >35 in (89 cm) for women (NCEP criterion), or body mass index (BMI) ≥30 (World Health Organization criterion).
- TG level at or above 150 mg/dL.

TABLE 76–1. RISK FACTORS TO BE CONSIDERED IN TREATMENT DECISIONS FOR THOSE NOT FALLING INTO THE FOUR BENEFIT GROUPS

Factors cited by the ACC/AHA 2013 Guideline
Genetic hyperlipidemia
Primary LDL cholesterol ≥160 mg/dL
Family history of premature ASCVD in a first-degree relative (onset in men <55 yr and women <65 yr)
C-reactive protein elevation ≥2 mg/L
Coronary artery calcium score ≥300 Agatston units or ≥75 percentile for age, sex, and ethnicity
Ankle-brachial index <0.9
Elevated lifetime risk of ASCVD

- Blood pressure at or above 130/85 mm Hg.
- Fasting glucose value at or above 110 mg/dL.
- HDL-C level less than 40 mg/dL for men or less than 50 mg/dL for women.

II. **Screening and Prevention.** The 2013 ACC/AHA Guideline notes the importance of a patient-centered approach. Before statins are initiated for primary prevention of ASCVD, the individual patient's potential ASCVD risk reduction, adverse effects, drug–drug interactions, and preferences should be considered. Statins for secondary prevention in patients with ASCVD (one of the four benefit groups described later) are recommended based on strong evidence. (SOR **Ⓐ**)

1. **The U.S. Preventive Services Task Force** (USPSTF) strongly recommends screening men aged 35 years and older for lipid disorders. (SOR **Ⓐ**) There is strong evidence that drug therapy reduces CHD events and mortality in middle-aged men (aged 35–70 years) with abnormal lipids and a potential risk of CHD events greater than 1% per year.

2. **The USPSTF** strongly recommends screening women aged 45 and older if they are at an increased risk for CHD. (SOR **Ⓐ**) The USPSTF also recommends screening men aged 20 to 35 years and women aged 20 to 45 years if they are at an increased risk for CHD (Table 76–1). (SOR **Ⓑ**) There is less direct evidence suggesting effectiveness of drug therapy in other adults with similar levels of risk.

3. **The USPSTF** found insufficient data to assess the efficacy of screening children and adolescents for dyslipidemia for delaying the onset and reducing the incidence of CAD-related events. However, **the Expert Panel on Integrated Guidelines for Cardiovascular Health and Risk Reduction in Children and Adolescents,** updated in 2011 by National Heart Lung Blood Institute, recommend the following:
   - 2 to 8 years: No routine lipid screening. (SOR **Ⓑ**) Measure fasting lipid profile twice if the family history is positive for elevated cardiovascular risk or the child has a high-level risk factor (e.g., hypertension requiring drug therapy, BMI ≥97th percentile, or current cigarette smoker) or condition (e.g., diabetes mellitus, chronic kidney disease/end-stage renal disease/postrenal transplant, postorthotopic heart transplant, and Kawasaki disease with current aneurysms).
   - 9 to 11 years: Universal screening with nonfasting lipid profile and calculate non-HDL (TC-HDL). (SOR **Ⓑ**) If non-HDL is ≥145 mg/dL and HDL <40 mg/dL, repeat fasting lipid profile twice as discussed earlier to obtain average level.
   - 12 to 16 years: No routine screening. (SOR **Ⓑ**) If new knowledge of positive family history, new risk factor or new high risk condition is identified in the patient, obtain fasting lipid panel (use the average of two readings).
   - 17 to 21 years: Universal screening once in this time period, obtain nonfasting lipid profile and calculate non-HDL; if non-HDL ≥145 mg/dL and HDL <40 mg/dL, obtain fasting lipid panel (use the average of two readings). (SOR **Ⓑ**)

4. **Screening** is recommended by the NCEP every 3 to 5 years for most adults starting at age 20 years. (SOR **Ⓒ**) Patients with multiple risk factors may need to be screened more frequently. Children and adolescents with a family history of severe dyslipidemia or early atherosclerotic disease should also be screened. (SOR **Ⓒ**)

III. **Diagnosis**
   A. **Symptoms and signs.** Lipid problems are usually asymptomatic for several decades prior to clinical disease.
      1. **Symptoms are related to end-organ effects.** Common symptoms of coronary artery disease include chest pain (angina pectoris), shortness of breath, palpitations, diaphoresis, difficulty with speech, anxiety, and abdominal pain (Chapter 79). Some

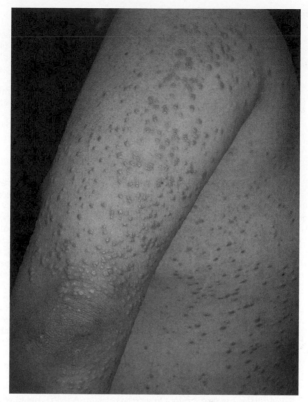

FIGURE 76–1. Eruptive xanthomas on the extremities and trunk of a young man with untreated type 2 diabetes and hyperlipidemia (see color insert). (Used with permission of Richard P. Usatine, MD.)

patients do not experience symptoms. Intermittent claudication, erectile dysfunction, and transient neurologic symptoms can herald advanced atherosclerosis.

2. Signs include eruptive xanthomas (Figure 76–1), high blood pressure, increased BMI or waist circumference, and acute pancreatitis in the setting of very high TG.

3. Myocardial infarction (MI), cerebrovascular accident (stroke), and sudden death are often the first sign of a lipid problem.

B. Laboratory tests

1. A **random or fasting lipid profile** (with total, LDL, and HDL cholesterol and TGs) should be obtained; the latter is preferred by ACC/AHA. If the profile is done nonfasting, total cholesterol and HDL are accurate, but LDL and TG levels can be different from fasting levels by 10% and 20%, respectively. If the nonfasting profile produces a total cholesterol ≥200 mg/dL or HDL <40 mg/dL, then a fasting lipid profile should be obtained. Fasting lipid profiles should be performed after a 9- to 12-hour fast.

2. Interpreting cholesterol results

a. Blood lipids change acutely in response to food intake. The TG level is lowest in the fasting state. As the TG level rises, total and LDL cholesterol each fall by an average of 5 to 15 mg/dL. Thus, total and LDL cholesterol tend to be higher when fasting. HDL cholesterol varies little between the fasting and postprandial states.

b. Blood lipids can fluctuate within minutes, days, or weeks in response to illness, emotional stress, pregnancy, or malnutrition. Blood lipid levels also may fluctuate seasonally. In colder climates, cholesterol and TG levels tend to be somewhat higher in winter, presumably because of higher fat intake and reduced activity.

3. Diagnosing lipid disorders

a. If a screening lipid profile shows elevated LDL cholesterol, low HDL cholesterol, or high TGs, a **second lipid profile** should be obtained (fasting) before starting treatment, to confirm elevation and establish an accurate baseline. (SOR **C**)

b. Excluding secondary causes. If symptoms or signs are suggestive, the clinician should consider ordering thyroid, renal, or liver function tests to rule out secondary causes of dyslipidemia.

c. Additional testing for secondary causes of hyperlipidemia. Individuals with an LDL >190 mg/dL or TG >500 mg/dL should be evaluated for secondary causes of hyperlipidemia (see Section 1A.2) (SOR **B**).

(1) Patients with markedly elevated LDL cholesterol levels (≥190 mg/dL) are at an increased risk for ASCVD even if they have HDL cholesterol levels at or above average.

(2) Patients with high fasting TG levels are at an increased risk, especially obese patients with diabetes mellitus.

d. Additional tests sometimes can be helpful to refine a patient's estimated risk and adjust the aggressiveness of treatment, especially in those with a strong family history of CHD or stroke.

(1) It is recognized that chronic inflammatory processes are involved in atherosclerosis. **C-reactive protein (CRP)** is an inflammatory marker that can predict risk for MI. Metabolic syndrome and obesity are associated with higher CRP levels. If CRP levels are obtained and are elevated, lowering LDL levels to below goal could be considered. However, NCEP does not recommend routine monitoring of CRP levels.

(2) Homocysteine elevation is correlated with an increased risk for MI and stroke. Intervention outcome study results, however, have shown no benefit from lowering homocysteine with the combination of folate, pyridoxine, and vitamin B_{12}.

(3) Apolipoprotein levels predict outcome more accurately than do LDL cholesterol or HDL cholesterol, but their clinical usefulness has not been proven. Apolipoprotein levels can sometimes help in the decision about how aggressively to treat patients with elevated LDL cholesterol levels. A low level of **apolipoprotein A-I,** the main apolipoprotein in HDL, also indicates an increased risk for CHD. Apolipoprotein A-I is usually low when HDL is low.

(4) Lipoprotein (a) is also associated with an increased CHD risk. Small LDL particles are also thought to increase risk for ASCVD, but to what extent risk is increased is unknown.

IV. Treatment. The 2013 ACC/AHA Guideline, released in November 2013, contains the following changes from the previous guideline: (1) a focus on ASCVD risk reduction and the identification of four statin-benefit groups, (2) a move away from specific LDL-C and/or non-HDL–C treatment targets that are not supported by evidence to targeting groups most likely to benefit from statin therapy, (3) a global risk assessment for primary prevention using the new Pooled Cohort Equations to estimate 10-year ASCVD risk (www.static.heart.org/ahamah/risk/Omnibus_Risk_Estimator.xls or http://cvdrisk.nhlbi.nih.gov/), (4) addresses patient safety considerations and management of statin-associated adverse effects, and (5) discusses the role of biomarkers and noninvasive tests in informing treatment decisions.

A. Treatment groups. Four benefit groups have been identified for whom the ASCVD risk reduction clearly outweighs the risk (Table 76–2). These groups are based on the patient's age, clinical status, and estimated 10-year risk for ASCVD.

1. The estimated 10-year risk for ASCVD is a key step in evaluating candidacy for statin therapy for patients not known to fall into the first three risk groups. A web-based calculator and downloadable spread sheet is available at http://my.americanheart.org/cvriskcalculator and http://www.cardiosource.org/science-andquality/practice-guidelines-and-quality-standards/2013-prevention-guideline-tools.aspx. Treatment is also considered for patients with primary LDL ≥160 mg/dL or other evidence of genetic hyperlipidemias, a family history of or CHD-equivalent (peripheral arterial disease, carotid artery disease, abdominal aortic aneurysm), and for individuals with LDL 70 to 189 mg/dL with an ASCVD risk between 5% and 7.5%. (SOR **C**)

B. Lifestyle approaches often improve lipid levels effectively. It is appropriate to encourage lifestyle changes in anyone with LDL cholesterol ≥130 mg/dL or HDL cholesterol ≤40 mg/dL. (SOR **B**) Those with HDL cholesterol levels in the 40- to 49-mg/dL range are also appropriate candidates for exercise counseling.

TABLE 76-2. BENEFIT GROUPS FOR STATIN THERAPY AND TREATMENT RECOMMENDATIONS

Benefit Groups for Statin Therapy	High-Intensity Statin Therapy (Daily Dose Lowers LDL by Approximately 50% or More)[a]	Moderate-Intensity Statin Therapy (Daily Dose Lowers LDL by 30% to 49%)
Patients with known ASCVD	Age ≤75 yr (SOR **A**)	Age >75 yr or not a candidate for high-intensity therapy (SOR **A**)
Patients with primary elevation of LDL ≥190 mg/dL	All candidates (SOR **B**)	Not a candidate for high-intensity therapy (SOR **B**)
Patients aged 40–75 yr without ASCVD who have DM, and an LDL of 70–189 mg/dL	Estimated 10-yr ASCVD risk ≥7.5%[b] (SOR **C**)	All others with DM (SOR **A**)
Other patients aged 40–75 yr without ASCVD or DM with an estimated 10-yr ASCVD risk ≥7.5%[b]	Clinical decision (SOR **A**)	Clinical decision (SOR **A**)

[a]Percent LDL reduction can be used as a measure of treatment response and adherence, but is not in itself a treatment goal.
[b]10-year risk of ASCVD, defined as nonfatal myocardial infarction, coronary heart disease death, and nonfatal and fatal stroke.
ASCVD, atherosclerotic cardiovascular disease (includes acute coronary syndromes or a history of MI, stable or unstable angina, coronary or other arterial revascularization, stroke, TIA, or peripheral arterial disease presumed to be of atherosclerotic origin); LDL, low-density lipoprotein.

1. **Dietary modification.** Depending on a patient's baseline diet, eating a diet lower in saturated fat and cholesterol can lower LDL by 20% to 30%. Following are the key dietary changes for lowering elevated cholesterol:
   a. Eat **less beef and pork** (especially fatty cuts).
   b. Eat **cold-water fish** twice a week (salmon, tuna, herring, mackerel). Fish that tend to have high mercury content (e.g., swordfish) should be limited to once a month.
   c. Eat more **chicken** and **turkey** (white "skinless" meat).
   d. Eat 40 to 50 g of **soy protein** a day (tofu, soy burger, soy dog, soy milk).
   e. Drink **nonfat,** 0.5%, **or 1% fat milk,** instead of 2% or whole milk (3.5% fat). Eat minimal amounts of other whole-milk dairy products such as cheese, butter, ice cream, and sour cream.
   f. Use **polyunsaturated oil products** (safflower, corn, soybean) or **monounsaturated oil products** (olive) for margarine and cooking oil (desired ratio of polyunsaturated to saturated fat is ≥1.5:1). **Avoid hydrogenated oils** present in **stick margarines;** instead use **tub margarines** (preferably small amounts).
   g. Minimize intake of commercial **fried foods,** which are the main source of **trans fats**.
   h. Eat **oat bran** as cereal or muffins, three to six servings per day. Oat bran can reduce total cholesterol and LDL cholesterol an average of 5% to 10% in some patients with elevated LDL cholesterol.
   i. Eat **nuts** (walnuts, pecans, almonds, peanuts, cashews) as a protein source, 1 oz a day. Nuts are high in alpha-linolenic acid, which is converted to omega-3 fatty acids in the body. Mounting evidence links nut intake with reduced risk for ASCVD events.
   j. **Fish oil** high in omega-3 fatty acids (i.e., eicosapentaenoic [EPA] and docosahexaenoic [DHA]) has been shown to be beneficial. Fish oils decrease secretion of TGs by the liver, and reduce blood TGs, but there is little or no effect on total blood cholesterol level and HDL cholesterol. LDL-cholesterol level is unchanged or may increase with fish oil consumption. If regular intake of cold-water fish is ineffective or unacceptable, three capsules a day of fish oil provides close to the 1 g per day of EPA plus DHA that is recommended for preventive intake. To lower TGs, the recommended dose is 2 to 4 g per day of EPA plus DHA daily. Lovaza is a prescription fish oil product with a dose of 4 g orally daily or 2 g orally twice daily. High doses of fish oil can increase risk of bleeding.

k. **Plant stanols** or **sterols** can be beneficial as dietary supplements. Plant stanols derived from soybeans and corn are available in nonprescription products (e.g., Benecol, Take Control). Stanols block absorption of dietary and biliary cholesterol in the intestine. Sterols work similarly, but are absorbed more readily than stanols. Benecol can be used as a food spread, like margarine. It has no significant drug interactions and no demonstrated side effects. At the recommended dose of two to three servings per day, plant stanols lower LDL-C by 6% to 15%, but there are no identified ASCVD outcomes from clinical trials for these supplements.

2. **Exercise.** Regular aerobic exercise, at least 30 minutes at a time, most days of the week raises HDL cholesterol, lowers TG and VLDL cholesterol, and sometimes lowers LDL cholesterol. Walking daily for several miles has been shown to have smaller favorable effects on lipids.

3. **Weight loss** lowers TG and VLDL cholesterol, raises HDL cholesterol, but lowers LDL cholesterol only transiently during the weight reduction period.

4. **Smoking cessation** increases HDL cholesterol but does not affect LDL cholesterol, VLDL cholesterol, or TGs. (SOR **Ⓐ**)

C. **Medications.** Both the ACC/AHA guideline and the NCEP Adult Treatment Panel III recommend treatment if LDL cholesterol remains ≥190 mg/dL despite lifestyle management, regardless of the patient's clinical status and other CHD risk factors. For patients with diabetes, coronary or carotid artery disease, statin medication is recommended regardless of LDL cholesterol level. The four benefit groups for prescribing drug therapy with statins are shown in Table 76–2.

1. **Nonprescription medications** are an option to lower cholesterol, although they may not be as effective as prescription medications and there are limited data on ASCVD outcomes.

a. **Psyllium hydrophilic mucilloid** (Metamucil and other brands). Psyllium, which lowers LDL cholesterol and total cholesterol an average of 5% to 10%, is an option to treat mildly elevated LDL cholesterol (130–159 mg/dL) when HDL cholesterol is ≥45 mg/dL. (SOR **Ⓒ**) It promotes bowel regularity but sometimes causes flatulence, although there are no serious adverse effects.

b. **Niacin** is an option for treating the healthy patient with moderately elevated LDL cholesterol who also has either low HDL cholesterol (≤35 mg/dL) or high TGs. Niacin has demonstrated value for preventing MI and CHD death. (SOR **Ⓐ**)

(1) When taken in a dose of 2 to 3 g per day, niacin lowers LDL cholesterol by 15% to 30%, lowers elevated TGs by 20% to 50%, and raises HDL cholesterol by 15% to 35%. Patients should begin with a low dose of 100 to 200 mg of the regular release form or 250 to 500 mg of the sustained-release form (Slo-Niacin); the dose should be gradually increased to a maximum of 2 to 3 g per day based on patient tolerance.

(2) Most patients experience minimal flushing and itching when taking sustained-release niacin. Patients who experience flushing and itching can block much of the adverse symptoms by taking 325 mg of aspirin daily shortly before niacin ingestion. Some patients also develop tolerance to flushing with extended use.

(3) Although it is sometimes well tolerated and usually safe, **niacin can worsen diabetic hyperglycemia, exacerbate gout, precipitate serious arrhythmias in patients with heart disease, or cause severe reversible liver toxicity**. These effects increase with increased doses of niacin, especially 2 g or more.

(4) Long-term use of niacin in some patients can be limited by drug side effects.

c. **Red yeast rice supplements** were shown in several randomized trials to reduce LDL and total cholesterol but data on patient-oriented outcomes are lacking. (SOR **Ⓒ**)

2. **Prescription drugs for modifying lipids** are the mainstay of cholesterol treatment (Table 76–3). Available drug therapies include the HMG-CoA reductase inhibitors (statins), bile acid sequestrants, nicotinic acid (niacin, as discussed earlier), fibric acid derivatives (fibrates), and cholesterol absorption inhibitors. Statins have the strongest evidence supporting benefit for cardiovascular outcomes. Second-line agents including bile acid sequestrants, nicotinic acid, and omega-3 fatty acid supplements have shown some cardiovascular benefit, but data are less robust. Data are

TABLE 76–3. MEDICATIONS USED IN THE TREATMENT OF LIPID DISORDERS

Generic Name (Brand)	Dosing	Cholesterol Lowering	Side Effects	Contraindications	Drug Interactions
HMG-CoA Reductase Inhibitors (statins)					
Atorvastatin[a] (Lipitor)	Adults: 10–80 mg once daily Peds: 10–17 yr: 10 mg daily, max. 20 mg; <10 yr: safety and efficacy not established **High intensity:**[b] 80 mg **Moderate intensity:** 10 mg	Average decrease in LDL: 10 mg: 35%–39% 20 mg: 43% 40 mg: 50% 80 mg: 55%–60%	Diarrhea, arthralgia, myalgia, UTIs, nasopharyngitis, pain in extremities, increased liver enzymes, rhabdomyolysis	Active liver disease, persistent ↑ serum transaminases, pregnancy, nursing mothers	Antiretrovirals, gemfibrozil fenofibrate, clarithromycin, cyclosporine, erythromycin, clofibrate, diltiazem, verapamil, azole antifungals, colchicine (myopathy)
Fluvastatin[a] (Lescol)	Adults: 20–40 mg daily to twice daily Peds: 10–17 yr: as for adults; <10 yr: safety and efficacy not established **Moderate intensity:**[b] 40 mg twice daily or 80 mg XL once daily	Average decrease in LDL: 20 mg: 22% 40 mg: 25% 80 mg: 35% (as XL product)	Indigestion, nausea, headache, pancreatitis, autoimmune hepatitis, liver failure, SLE, rhabdomyolysis	As above	Fibrates, gemfibrozil, colchicine, erythromycin (myopathy); phenytoin (phenytoin toxicity); warfarin (bleeding)
Lovastatin[a] (Mevacor)	Adults: immediate release, 10–80 mg with evening meal; extended release, 20–60 mg at bedtime Peds: 10–17 yr: 10–40 mg daily Elder: immediate release: no dosage adjustment; extended release: 20 mg at bedtime **Moderate intensity:**[b] 40 mg daily	Average decrease in LDL: 10 mg: 21% 20 mg: 24%–27% 40 mg: 30%–31% 80 mg: 40%–42% (as 40 mg twice daily)	Abdominal pain, constipation, arthralgia, increased liver enzymes, autoimmune disease, SLE, rhabdomyolysis	As for atorvastatin plus concomitant use with strong CYP3A4 inhibitors, immune-mediated myopathy	See atorvastatin
Pitavastatin (Livalo)	Adults: 2 mg once daily, max. 4 mg Peds: safety and efficacy not established	Average decrease in LDL: 1 mg: 31%–32% 2 mg: 36%–39% 4 mg: 41%–45%	Constipation, diarrhea, backache, myalgia, limb pain, rhabdomyolysis	As for atorvastatin plus concomitant use with cyclosporine	Antiretrovirals, gemfibrozil fenofibrate, niacin, rifampin, erythromycin, cyclosporine, (myopathy)

(continued)

TABLE 76–3. MEDICATIONS USED IN THE TREATMENT OF LIPID DISORDERS (*Continued*)

Generic Name (Brand)	Dosing	Cholesterol Lowering	Side Effects	Contraindications	Drug Interactions
Pravastatin[a] (Pravachol)	Adults: 40–80 mg once daily; Peds: 14–18 yr: 40 mg daily; 8–13 yr: 20 mg daily; **Moderate intensity:**[b] 40 mg daily	Average decrease in LDL: 10 mg: 22% 20 mg: 32% 40 mg: 34% 80 mg: 37%	Rash, diarrhea, nausea, vomiting, musculoskeletal pain, headache, cough, rhinitis, upper respiratory tract infection, pancreatitis, increased liver enzymes, rhabdomyolysis	As for atorvastatin	See atorvastatin
Rosuvastatin (Crestor)	Adults: 5–40 mg daily; Peds: 10–17 yr, 5–20 mg once daily; **High intensity:**[b] 20 mg; **Moderate intensity:**[b] 10 mg	Average decrease in LDL: 5 mg: 45% 10 mg: 46%–52% 20 mg: 47%–55% 40 mg: 55%–63%	Abdominal pain, nausea, arthralgia, myalgia, asthenia, dizziness, headache, pancreatitis, abnormal liver enzymes, rhabdomyolysis, acute renal failure	Active liver disease, pregnancy, breastfeeding	Antiretrovirals, gemfibrozil fenofibrate, niacin, clarithromycin, cyclosporine, azole antifungals, (myopathy); warfarin (bleeding); OCs (OC adverse effects); amiodarone (transaminase elevations)
Simvastatin[a] (Zocor)	Adults: 5–40 mg daily; Peds: as for adults; safety and efficacy not established in <10 yr; **Moderate intensity:**[b] 20–40 daily	Average decrease in LDL: 5 mg: 26% 10 mg: 30% 20 mg: 38% 40 mg: 29%–41%	Abdominal pain, constipation, nausea, headache, upper respiratory tract infections, cholestatic hepatitis, ↑ liver enzymes, jaundice, liver failure, rhabdomyolysis	Concomitant use with gemfibrozil, cyclosporine, danazol, strong CYP3A4 inhibitors, active liver disease, nursing mothers, pregnancy	Antiretrovirals, gemfibrozil fenofibrate, niacin, macrolide antibiotics, ciprofloxacin, cyclosporine, nefazodone, diltiazem, verapamil, diltiazem, amlodipine, azole antifungals, colchicine, tadalafil, amiodarone (myopathy); warfarin (bleeding)
Bile Acid Sequestrants					
Cholestyramine[a] (Questran, others)	Adults: 8–16 g in divided doses, max. 24 g daily; Peds: 80 mg/kg three times daily	12.6% more LDL reduction compared to placebo	Constipation, abdominal discomfort, flatulence, nausea, vomiting	Complete biliary obstruction	Should be administered several hours before or after many medications to avoid decreasing effectiveness of other agents

Drug	Dosage	Efficacy	Adverse effects	Contraindications	Drug interactions
Colestipol[a] (Colestid)	Adults: powder: 5–30 g once daily or divided; tablet: initial: 2 g once or twice daily; maintenance: 2–16 g once daily or divided Peds: safety and efficacy not established		Constipation, vomiting		See cholestyramine
Colesevelam (Welchol)	Adults: 1875 mg twice daily or 3750 mg once daily Peds: 10–17 yr; as for adults; <10 yr or children with diabetes: safety and efficacy not established	Decreased LDL 15%–20% in clinical trials	Constipation, indigestion, nausea, nasopharyngitis	History of bowel obstruction, history of pancreatitis, serum triglycerides >500 mg/dL	See cholestyramine
Fibrates					
Fenofibrate[a] (Fenoglide, Lipofen, Lofibra, Tricor, Triglide)	Triglide: 50–160 mg, Lipofen: 50–150 mg, Fenoglide: 40–120 mg, Tricor: 48–145 mg once daily Peds: safety and efficacy not established Elderly: starting dose: Tricor, 48 mg; Triglide, 50 mg	Fenoglide lowered LDL an average of 20%–30%, except in those with very high TGs; reduces TG	Abdominal pain, nausea, ↑ liver enzymes, backache, rhinitis, pancreatitis, cholestatic hepatitis, rhabdomyolysis, ↑ SCr	Gallbladder disease, active liver disease, severe renal impairment, nursing mothers	Statins, colchicine (myopathy); oral anticoagulants (bleeding); cyclosporine (impaired renal function); ezetimibe (risk of gallstones)
Gemfibrozil[a] (Lopid)	Adults: 600 mg 30 min before morning and evening meal Peds: safety and efficacy not established	Lowered LDL 5% in clinical trials, reduces TG	Abdominal pain, acute appendicitis, indigestion, ↑ liver enzymes, rhabdomyolysis	Concomitant use with repaglinide, preexisting gallbladder disease, hepatic dysfunction, hypersensitivity, severe renal impairment	Simvastatin (CI)/statins, colchicine (myopathy); repaglinide (CI), glyburide, pioglitazone (hypoglycemia); ezetimibe (risk of gallstones); montelukast (montelukast adverse effects); warfarin (bleeding)

(continued)

TABLE 76–3. MEDICATIONS USED IN THE TREATMENT OF LIPID DISORDERS (*Continued*)

Generic Name (Brand)	Dosing	Cholesterol Lowering	Side Effects	Contraindications	Drug Interactions
Other					
Ezetimibe[a] (Zetia)	Adults: 10 mg once daily Peds: >10 yr, 10 mg once daily; <10 yr, safety and efficacy not established	Lowers LDL 16%–19% and increases HDL 3%–3.5%	Diarrhea, arthralgia, myalgia, nasopharyngitis, sinusitis, URI, hepatitis, anaphylaxis, rhabdomyolysis	Liver disease, persistent ↑ in hepatic transaminases	Gemfibrozil, clofibrate, fenofibrate (gallstones); warfarin (bleeding)
Niacin[a] (various brands)	Adults: regular release, 2 g three times daily, ER: 500 mg daily up to 2 g daily Peds: safety and efficacy not established	Decreases LDL 10%–15%	Flushing, headache, nausea, vomiting, hepatic necrosis, hepatotoxicity, rhabdomyolysis	Active liver disease, active peptic ulcer, arterial bleeding	Statins (myopathy); warfarin (bleeding)
Omega-3 acid ethyl esters (Lovaza, Omacor)	Four 1 g capsules daily or in divided doses	Increases LDL, however lowers TGs up to 45%	Burping, indigestion, taste sense alteration, anaphylaxis	Hypersensitivity	Anticoagulants, antiplatelet agents (bleeding)

[a]Available as generic.

[b]High- and moderate-intensity doses are from the 2013 ACC/AHA guideline and are based on doses used in randomized clinical trials.

CI, contraindicated; ER, extended release; LDLs, low-density lipids; OCs, oral contraceptives; SCr, serum creatinine; SLE, systemic lupus erythematosus; TG, triglyceride; URI, upper respiratory infection; UTI, urinary tract infection.

inconsistent with respect to fibrates. As of yet, there are no data to show that adding a nonstatin drug(s) to high-intensity statin therapy will provide incremental ASCVD risk reduction benefit with an acceptable margin of safety.

a. Statins (HMG-CoA reductase inhibitors). This category is the gold standard therapy for patients with moderately or severely elevated LDL cholesterol and for most high-risk patients. (SOR **Ⓐ**) In addition to lowering LDL cholesterol, statins can increase HDL by 5% to 15% and decrease TG by 7% to 30%.

(1) In controlled trials, statins reduce MI, stroke, CHD death, and total mortality by 25% to 40%. Cost-effectiveness analyses of this class of agents have shown favorable cost–benefit ratios. The ACC/AHA guideline notes that there is a high-level evidence that high-intensity statin therapy with atorvastatin 40 to 80 mg reduced ASCVD risk more than moderate-intensity statin therapy with atorvastatin 10 mg, pravastatin 40 mg, or simvastatin 20 to 40 mg twice daily. Target doses for high-intensity and moderate-intensity statin therapy are provided in Table 76–3.

(2) Most statins are available as generics.

(3) Statins are usually well tolerated, and serious **adverse effects** are uncommon. Common side effects of statins and contraindications are shown in Table 76–3. Patients predisposed to statin adverse effects include those with multiple or serious comorbidities, history of previous statin intolerance or muscle disorders, unexplained threefold or greater elevations in alanine transaminase (ALT), concomitant use of drugs affecting statin metabolism, and age over 75 years.

(4) Statin use is contraindicated in patients with active **hepatic disease** or significantly elevated serum transaminase levels (≥3 times normal upper limit). Because significant (but asymptomatic) elevation of ALT occurs in 1% to 2% and mildly elevated ALT (≤3 times normal) occurs in approximately 5% to 10% of treated patients, it is prudent to obtain a baseline ALT level. Recent opinion does not require a recheck of AST or ALT after starting statins unless symptoms warrant. No cases of serious or life-threatening liver toxicity have thus far been attributed to statin therapy.

(5) **Myalgias** or muscle weakness occur in approximately 10% of patients, either early on or after prolonged treatment. Muscle symptoms caused by statins usually resolve within a few days to weeks after drug discontinuation. **Myopathy** occurs less frequently, sometimes leading to **rhabdomyolysis** and **acute renal failure**. Muscle toxicity occurs somewhat more often when statins are used concurrently with niacin, gemfibrozil, fenofibrate, and other drugs (Table 76–3).

(a) If **unexplained severe muscle symptoms** develop during statin therapy, discontinue the statin and test for rhabdomyolysis by obtaining CK, creatinine, and a urinalysis for myoglobinuria.

(b) If **mild-to-moderate muscle symptoms** occur, discontinue the statin and evaluate for other conditions that may contribute to muscle symptoms (e.g., hypothyroidism, reduced renal or hepatic function, rheumatologic disorders, steroid myopathy, vitamin D deficiency, or primary muscle diseases). If symptoms resolve, a trial back on the original or a lower statin dose can be tried. Use of fewer doses per week has also been tried with atorvastatin and rosuvastatin to reduce myalgia with some success

(c) Taking coenzyme Q-10 (suggested dose of 100 mg twice a day) with a statin appears to prevent muscle symptoms in some patients complaining of myalgias.

(6) Numerous medications may interact with statins to increase their blood level and increase the risk for serious adverse effects. The medications in Table 76–3 should be avoided if possible when taking a statin, or the statin dose should be adjusted downward. Because they are metabolized differently from other statins, pravastatin, rosuvastatin, and fluvastatin are least likely to cause drug interactions.

(7) Grapefruit juice interferes with the metabolism of simvastatin, atorvastatin, and lovastatin and raises their blood level, which can create an increased risk of adverse effects. Because this effect of grapefruit juice consumption

lasts 24 hours or more, it should be avoided or minimized by patients taking these statins.

(8) Supplemental intake of the antioxidant **vitamin E** does not appear to be advisable, since it interfered with the beneficial effects of statin therapy in the Heart Protection Study.

(9) Once started, statin therapy should be continued indefinitely, barring unacceptable side effects or allergic reactions.

(10) Perceived side effects from one statin can often be avoided by switching to a different statin. Because they are hydrophilic, pravastatin or fluvastatin may be least likely to cause side effects. Neither drug is recommended as high-intensity treatment.

(11) Pregnancy. Because of potential teratogenicity, statins should not be used in women of childbearing age unless contraception effectiveness is maximized and the potential benefits appear to exceed the risks.

(12) Children. Statins are used in children who have homozygous familial hypercholesterolemia, children over age 9 years whose LDL-C remains ≥190 mg/dL despite 6 months of lifestyle change, (SOR **Ⓐ**) and children with LDL-C between 160 to 189 mg/dL who fail a trial of lifestyle/diet management and who have a positive family history of premature CVD/events in first-degree relatives or at least one high-level risk factor or risk condition or at least two moderate-level risk factors or risk conditions (SOR **Ⓑ**). Treatment should be prescribed in conjunction with a lipid specialist. All statins except pitavastatin are approved for use in children with familial hypercholesterolemia by the US Food and Drug Administration (FDA). Treatment should begin at the lowest available dose.

(13) Statin choices along with dosing, side effects, contraindications, and drug interactions are listed in Table 76–3. The number needed to treat to prevent one additional death in patients with CHD is approximately 30 to 50. There do not appear to be important differences by type of statin in head-to-head trials.

    (a) Rosuvastatin is the most potent available statin, followed by **atorvastatin; these two drugs are recommended for high-intensity therapy**. Proteinuria occasionally occurs with rosuvastatin, so periodic spot microalbumin/creatinine ratio testing may be advisable.

    (b) It may be **harmful to initiate simvastatin at 80 mg daily** or increase the dose of simvastatin to 80 mg daily because of increased muscle damage. (SOR **Ⓑ**) Simvastatin 80 mg should be used only in patients who have been taking this dose for 12 months or more without evidence of muscle injury (myopathy). Simvastatin 80 mg should not be started in new patients, including patients already taking lower doses of the drug. In addition to these new limitations, FDA is requiring changes to the simvastatin label to add new contraindications (should not be used with certain medications such as itraconazole, ketoconazole, erythromycin, HIV protease inhibitors, nefazodone, and gemfibrozil) and dose limitations for using simvastatin with certain medicine (e.g., not to exceed 10 mg with concurrent use of verapamil or diltiazem or 20 mg with amiodarone, amlodipine, or ranolazine).

    (c) Pravastatin is associated with fewer drug interactions. It is the only statin with prominent renal excretion (approximately 50% renal), so it should be used with caution, if at all, in patients with renal insufficiency or renal failure.

b. Bile acid sequestrants decrease LDL by 15% to 30%, increase HDL by 3% to 5%, but have no effect or increase in TG. (SOR **Ⓑ**) They lower LDL by binding bile acids in the intestine leading to cholesterol conversion to bile acids in the liver and enhanced LDL receptor expression. Dosing, side effects, and drug interactions are listed in Table 76–3. These medications can decrease the absorption of other medications.

(1) Bile acid sequestrants are contraindicated for use in patients with TG >300 mg/dL or type III hyperlipoproteinemia.

(2) Cholestyramine is available as a powder to be mixed with water or food. Questran Light may be more palatable for long-term compliance. Colesevelam is the only medication in this class available via tablets.

c. **Fibric acid derivatives (fibrates).** Effects on lipids include decreasing LDL by 5% to 20% (but may be increased in patients with high TG), increasing HDL cholesterol by 10% to 35%, and decreasing TG by 20% to 50%. The mechanism of action of fibrates is to increase the activity of lipoprotein lipase and decrease the formation of VLDL particles. Major uses of fibrates are in patients with high TGs or atherogenic dyslipidemia. These drugs decrease the risk of pancreatitis, which can occur with TG levels >1000 mg/dL. In clinical trials, there is inconsistent evidence of cardiovascular benefit, with only some trials showing a decreased CHD risk. (SOR ❸) In addition, noncardiovascular mortality has been slightly but consistently elevated in most fibrate trials. Dosing, side effects, and drug interactions are listed in Table 76–4.

(1) **Gemfibrozil** (Lopid) changes the hepatic metabolism of lipoproteins. Gemfibrozil is a logical choice for the patient with low HDL cholesterol and moderately or severely elevated TGs. (SOR ❹) The drug is well tolerated and appears to be relatively safe for long-term use. It should not be used with patients on statin therapy (see Table 76–3).

(2) **Fenofibrate** (Tricor) is similar to gemfibrozil and is appropriate for the same patients. (SOR ❸) It does not interact as much with HMG-CoA reductase inhibitors and has fewer drug interactions overall when compared to gemfibrozil.

d. **Ezetimibe** (Zetia), approved in 2002, lowers cholesterol by interfering with the absorption of cholesterol in the intestines. Used alone, ezetimibe lowers LDL cholesterol and TGs only modestly (15% to 20%). Since ezetimibe is minimally absorbed, its combined use with low-dose statin may produce less adverse effects than high-dose statin therapy. It has a low risk of interaction with other medications.

e. **Statin combinations with other drugs**

(1) Vytorin (simvastatin–ezetimibe), low dose (10 mg of each), lowers LDL cholesterol as much or more than the maximal dose of simvastatin alone. Currently the use of Vytorin is questioned due to the results of the ENHANCE trial showing lack of evidence that ezetimibe has effects on atherosclerosis progression. The COURAGE trial demonstrated that ezetimibe helped patients at maximum statin dose achieve LDL targets, but data on patient-oriented outcomes are sparse.

(2) Caduet (atorvastatin–amlodipine) combines a statin with a calcium channel blocker. It is a reasonable option for patients with hyperlipidemia and hypertension.

D. **Partial ileal bypass surgery,** in conjunction with a low-fat diet, lowers LDL cholesterol by 40% to 50%. The operative and postoperative morbidity and mortality are low. This surgery is a reasonable option for patients with severely elevated LDL cholesterol that cannot be managed satisfactorily with any tolerable combination of lipid-altering medications. (SOR ❸)

V. **Management Strategies**

A. **Long-term adherence** to lifestyle measures and lipid-altering medications is quite poor. Many patients are reluctant to take preventive medications for asymptomatic conditions. Fear of potential adverse effects from chronic medications appears to be a major deterrent to adherence.

B. **Patient education** and discussions with key family members are vital in order to foster a good understanding of the importance of long-term commitment to a healthy lifestyle and adherence to medical management of lipid disorders to prevent complications. Many educational materials are available from the American Heart Association (www.heart.org), the NCEP (http://www.nhlbi.nih.gov/about/ncep/), and commercial sources.

C. **Elderly patients** are at a greatly increased risk for MI or sudden death. Randomized controlled trials have shown that treating dyslipidemia in patients aged 65 to 85 years can decrease the risk of first and recurrent coronary events. Data are limited for patients older than 85 years. Since outcome studies show similar benefits and no increase in adverse effects for elderly patients, treatment of lipid disorders in this population is reasonable. (SOR ❸)

D. **Children and adolescents** with dyslipidemias should receive ongoing family-oriented education about diet, exercise, and weight control. Extreme low-fat diets should be avoided in children younger than 6 years because of the risk of essential fatty acid malnutrition having deleterious effects on nervous system development. Medication therapy is not recommended until the age of 8 years. Bile acid sequestrants have been recommended as first-line treatment in the past, although newer evidence shows that statins are safe in children (see Section IV.C.2.a.12).

E. Secondary prevention focuses on identifying and treating persons who have already developed clinical atherosclerosis with statins. They are the **most** likely to benefit from treatment to prevent further atheroma progression, prevent atheroma rupture, and regress existing atheromas. The lowering of LDL cholesterol has clearly demonstrated benefit in secondary prevention trials, which primarily include statin therapy. (SOR **A**) Long-term adherence is improved when statin therapy is started **prior** to hospital discharge for patients admitted with acute MI or unstable angina. (SOR **C**)

1. The 2013 ACC/AHA Guideline made no recommendations for or against specific LDL or non-HDL goals for the primary or secondary prevention of ASCVD because of the absence of data on the value of titrating drug therapy to specific goals.

2. **Laboratory monitoring**

   (a) **Prior to initiation of statins,** obtain a fasting lipid panel, alanine ALT (SOR **B**), and creatine kinase (CK) (SOR **C**) and consider evaluation for secondary causes (see Section 1A.2). If the patient has a primary lipid disorder, consider screening of family members. **Following initiation of statin therapy,** therapeutic response and safety should be regularly assessed with a fasted lipid panel (within 4–12 weeks of initiation or dose adjustment then every 3–12 months). Other tests should be obtained if clinically indicated. (SOR **A**)

   (b) **Prior to initiation of niacin,** baseline hepatic transaminases, fasting blood glucose or hemoglobin A1c, and uric acid should be obtained. (SOR **B**)

   (c) **Prior to initiation of a bile acid sequestrant,** obtain a fasted lipid panel and then follow with a fasted lipid panel at 3 months and every 6 to 12 months. (SOR **C**)

   (d) **Prior to initiation of fibrate,** evaluate renal status then again within 3 months and every 6 months afterwards. Fenofibrate should not be used in patients with moderate or severe renal impairment (GFR <30 mL/min) and for those with a GFR of 30 to 59 mL/min; the dose of fenofibrate should not exceed 54 mg per day. (SOR **B**) If the GFR decreases persistently to ≤30 mL/min, fenofibrate should be discontinued.

   (e) **Prior to initiation of ezetimibe,** consider obtaining hepatic transaminases and discontinue the drug if ALT elevations of >3 times the upper limit of normal. (SOR **C**)

3. **Consideration may be given to decreasing the stain dose** when two consecutive values of LDL levels are <40 mg/dL. (SOR **C**)

4. For individuals who are ≥21 years of age with an untreated primary LDL-C ≥190 mg/dL after maximum intensity statin therapy has been achieved, addition of a non-statin drug may be considered to further lower LDL. (SOR **C**) This should be individually tailored by evaluating the potential for ASCVD risk reduction benefits, adverse effects, drug–drug interactions, and patient preferences.

G. Systematic follow-up at regular intervals is essential for effective long-term management of lipid disorders. A manual or computerized flowchart in the medical record documenting blood lipid results, dietary and exercise modifications, and medication regimens facilitates the evaluation and alteration of treatment for best results.

V. Prognosis. The clinical course of lipid disorders depends on its type and severity and on the presence of other risk factors for atherosclerosis, especially cigarette smoking, diabetes mellitus, and hypertension.

A. Acute pancreatitis can occur with severe TG elevation ≥1000 mg/dL. This serious lipid problem requires urgent treatment with fluid replacement, pain medication, and treatment for the cause of pancreatitis. Intravenous heparin, apheresis, and insulin are potential therapies for severe acute pancreatitis.

B. Other valuable measures for curtailing atherosclerosis or minimizing its damage include smoking cessation, good control of hypertension and diabetes, and daily aspirin (81 or 325 mg, enteric coated). Some studies indicate that getting a flu shot annually may lower risk for ASCVD events.

SELECTED REFERENCES

Ballantyne CM. Current and future aims of lipid-lowering therapy: changing paradigms and lessons from the Heart Protection Study on standards of efficacy and safety. *Am J Cardiol.* 2003;92(4B):3K–9K.

Eiland LS, Luttrell PK. Use of statins for dyslipidemia in the pediatric population. *J Pediatr Pharmacol Ther.* 2010;15(3):160–172.

Expert Panel on Detection, Evaluation, and Treatment of High Blood Cholesterol in Adults. Executive Summary of the Third Report of the National Cholesterol Education Program (NCEP) Expert Panel on Detection, Evaluation, and Treatment of High Blood Cholesterol in Adults (Adult Treatment Panel III). *JAMA.* 2001;285:2486–2497.

Food and Drug Administration. Mercury content of selected fish. U.S. Food and Drug Administration Center for Food Safety and Applied Nutrition, Office of Seafood. http://www.fda.gov/food/foodborneillnesscontaminants/buystoreservesafefood/ucm110591.htm. Accessed May 15, 2001.

Grundy SM, Cleeman JI, Merz NB, et al. Implications of recent clinical trials for the National Cholesterol Education Program Adult Treatment Panel III guidelines. *Circulation.* 2004;110:227–239.

Heart Protection Study Collaborative Group. MRC/BHF Heart protection study of cholesterol lowering with simvastatin in 20,536 high risk individuals: a randomized placebo-controlled trial. *Lancet.* 2002;360:7–22M.

Hu FB, Willett WC. Optimal diets for prevention of coronary heart disease. *JAMA.* 2002;288:2569–2578.

Jones PH, Davidson MH, Stein EA, et al. Comparison of the efficacy and safety of rosuvastatin versus atorvastatin, simvastatin, and pravastatin across doses (STELLAR trial). *Am J Cardiol.* 2003;92(2):152–160.

Kris-Etherton PM, Harris WS, Appel LJ; American Heart Association. Nutrition Committee. Fish consumption, fish oil, omega-3 fatty acids and cardiovascular disease. *Circulation.* 2002;106(21):2747–2757.

Maron DJ, Hartigan PM, Neff DR, et al.; COURAGE Trial Investigators. Impact of adding ezetimibe to statin to achieve low-density lipoprotein cholesterol goal (from the Clinical Outcomes Utilizing Revascularization and Aggressive Drug Evaluation [COURAGE] trial). *Am J Cardiol.* 2013;111:1557–1562.

National Heart, Lung, and Blood Institute. *Expert Panel on Integrated Guidelines for Cardiovascular Health and Risk Reduction in Children and Adolescents. Summary Report.* NIH publication No. 12-7486A. October 2012. http://www.nhlbi.nih.gov/guidelines/cvd_ped/peds_guidelines_sum.pdf. Accessed April 2013.

Preiss D, Sattar N. Lipids, lipid modifying agents and cardiovascular risk: a review of the evidence. *Clin Endocrinol.* 2009;70(6):815–828.

Sidu D, Naugler C. Fasting time and lipid levels in a community-based population: a cross-sectional study. *Arch Intern Med.* 2012;172(22):1707–1710.

Stone NJ, Robinson J, Lichtenstein AH, et al. 2013 ACC/AHA Guideline on the Treatment of Blood Cholesterol to Reduce Atherosclerotic Cardiovascular Risk in Adults. A Report of the American College of Cardiology/American Heart Association Task Force on Practice Guidelines. *J Am Coll Cardiol.* 2013;pii:S0735-1097(13)06028-2. http://content.onlinejacc.org/article.aspx?articleid=1770217. Accessed November 2013.

Talbert RL. Dyslipidemia. In: DiPiro JT, Talbert RL, Yee GC, et al. eds. *Pharmacotherapy: A Pathophysiologic Approach.* 8th ed. New York, NY: McGraw-Hill Medical; 2011. Chapter 28.

United States Preventive Services Task Force. Screening for lipid disorders in adults. 2008. http://www.uspreventiveservicestaskforce.org/uspstf/uspschol.htm. Accessed April 2013.

Verhoeven V, Lopez Hartmann M, Remmen R, et al. Red yeast rice lowers cholesterol in physicians—a double blind, placebo controlled randomized trial. *BMC Complement Altern Med.* 2013;13(1):178 [Epub ahead of print].

Zhou Z, Rahme E, Pilote L. Are statins created equal? Evidence from randomized trials of pravastatin, simvastatin, and atorvastatin for cardiovascular disease prevention. *Am Heart J.* 2006;151:273–281

77   Hypertension

Ann E. Evensen, MD, FAAFP, & Charles B. Eaton, MD, MS

KEY POINTS

- The relationship between blood pressure and risk of cardiovascular disease events is continuous, consistent, and independent of other risk factors. (SOR **C**)
- Normal blood pressure is systolic blood pressure (SBP) <120 mm Hg and diastolic blood pressure (DBP) <80 mm Hg; prehypertension is SBP 120 to 139 mm Hg or DBP of 80 to 89 mm Hg; and hypertension is SBP ≥140 mm Hg or DBP ≥90 mm Hg. These results should be based on the average of two or more readings, taken at each of two or more visits. (SOR **C**)
- Evaluation for secondary causes of hypertension should be done only when a secondary cause is suspected based on history, physical evaluation, and routine laboratory evaluation. (SOR **C**)
- Lifestyle modifications (Dietary Approaches to Stop Hypertension [DASH] diet, sodium restriction, weight loss, exercise, and moderate alcohol consumption) should be used for all patients with hypertension and prehypertension. (SOR **A**)
- Blood pressures that are not to goal should be treated with antihypertensive medication to reduce risk of cardiovascular, cerebrovascular, and renal disease. (SOR **A**) Goal blood pressure in people over age 60 years is under 150/90 mm Hg. For those under age 60 years or with diabetes, the diastolic goal is under 90 mm Hg. (SOR **A**)
- The most effective first-line treatment for preventing the occurrence of cardiovascular morbidity and mortality is an angiotensin-converting enzyme inhibitor, angiotensin receptor blocker, calcium channel blocker, or thiazide diuretic. (SOR **B**)
- The majority of patients will require two or more medications to reach their blood pressure goal. Reducing the complexity of the medication regimen improves blood pressure control. (SOR **A**)
- Patients with certain comorbid conditions including diabetes mellitus, chronic kidney disease and cardiovascular disease, have stricter blood pressure goals and may benefit from drug classes other than thiazide diuretics. (SOR **A**)

I. Introduction

A. Definitions. A patient is diagnosed with **hypertension** if his or her systolic blood pressure (SBP) is 140 mm Hg or higher or diastolic blood pressure (DBP) is 90 mm Hg or higher or if he or she is taking antihypertensive medication.

1. **Prehypertension** is defined as SBP of 120 to 139 mm Hg or DBP of 80 to 89 mm Hg.
2. **Stage 1** hypertension is defined as SBP of 140 to 159 mm Hg or DBP of 90 to 99 mm Hg. **Stage 2** hypertension is defined as SBP of 160 mm Hg or more or DBP of 100 mm Hg or more.
3. Hypertension without an identifiable cause is termed **essential or primary hypertension**.
4. **Secondary hypertension** is hypertension due to an identifiable cause. It is less common than primary hypertension and more common in patients with resistant hypertension. Causes of secondary hypertension are listed in Table 77–1.
5. **Resistant hypertension** is defined as blood pressures that remain above goal in spite of the concurrent use of three antihypertensive agents of different classes, preferably at optimal doses and including a diuretic. Causes of resistant hypertension are listed in Table 77–2.

B. Epidemiology. Hypertension affects approximately 67 million people in the United States, or 30% of adults. Another 70 million people have prehypertension. Approximately 60% of Americans with hypertension are aware of the diagnosis and 45% are treated. However, only 46% of patients with hypertension are under good control. The lifetime risk of developing hypertension in patients who are normotensive at age 55 years is 90%. The higher the BP, the greater the risk of cardiovascular disease (CVD) and kidney disease. Those with prehypertension have a risk of developing CVD similar to that of patients with hypertension.

TABLE 77-1. CAUSES OF SECONDARY HYPERTENSION

Common
- Obstructive sleep apnea
- Medications or other interfering substances
- Primary aldosteronism
- Renal parenchymal disease
- Renal artery stenosis

Uncommon
- Increased intracranial pressure
- Cushing disease
- Pheochromocytoma
- Thyroid disease
- Coarctation of the aorta
- Primary hyperparathyroidism

II. Diagnosis

A. Symptoms. Hypertension is typically asymptomatic, unless the blood pressure is extremely elevated. Symptoms of hypertension can include fatigue, headache, lightheadedness, flushing, epistaxis, chest pain, visual or speech disturbances, and dyspnea.

Other symptoms may be present that could suggest the etiology of a secondary cause of hypertension: leg claudication from lower extremity ischemia (coarctation of the aorta); hirsutism; easy bruising (Cushing syndrome); excessive perspiration, sustained or intermittent hypertension, paroxysmal headaches, palpitations, anxiety attacks, pallor, tremor, nausea, or vomiting (pheochromocytoma); hypokalemia, muscle weakness, cramps, polyuria, paralysis, or nocturia (primary hyperaldosteronism); or flank pain (renal or renovascular disease).

B. Signs. Because patients rarely feel symptoms from mildly to moderately elevated blood pressures, it is necessary to screen patients for hypertension. It is appropriate to screen adults who have normal blood pressure every 2 years and adults with prehypertension every year.

1. Measuring blood pressure accurately. Ideally, blood pressure measurement should be performed after the patient has been sitting with feet supported for at least 5 minutes (i.e., not on an examination table). The bladder of the blood pressure cuff should encircle at least 80% of the circumference of the arm and be placed at heart level. The cuff should be inflated 30 mm Hg above where the radial pulse can no longer be felt. The systolic reading is made at the onset of Korotkoff sounds (phase I), and the diastolic reading is taken when the sounds completely disappear (phase V). The blood pressure should be measured in both arms; if there is a discrepancy in reading, the higher reading should be used. In the absence of target organ damage and/or pregnancy, the diagnosis of hypertension should not be made unless blood pressures are elevated on at least two separate occasions separated by 1 week or more.

TABLE 77-2. COMMON CAUSES OF RESISTANT HYPERTENSION

- "Pseudoresistance" (improper BP measurement or medication nonadherence)
- Obesity
- Physical inactivity
- Excess dietary sodium
- Excess alcohol use
- Use of interfering medications or other substances:
  - Corticosteroids
  - Nonsteroidal anti-inflammatory drugs
  - Caffeine
  - Illicit drugs (e.g., cocaine)
  - Medications for attention deficit (e.g., methylphenidate)
  - Chemotherapy agents (e.g., cyclosporine, tacrolimus)
  - Real black licorice (not anise)
  - Weight loss agents
  - Decongestants

TABLE 77-3. RISK FACTORS FOR DEVELOPMENT OF CARDIOVASCULAR DISEASE

- Hypertension
- Tobacco use
- Obesity (BMI ≥30), especially truncal obesity
- Physical inactivity
- Dyslipidemia
- Diabetes mellitus
- Men older than 55 yr
- Women older than 65 yr
- Family history of premature cardiovascular disease (men younger than 55 yr, women younger than 65 yr)
- Microalbuminuria (or estimated GFR ≤60 mL/min)

2. **Ambulatory blood pressure monitoring.** Intermittent home blood pressure monitoring and 24-hour ambulatory blood pressure monitoring are also useful in diagnosing and monitoring hypertension. An ambulatory blood pressure goal of less than 135/85 mm Hg is appropriate for patients who have an office blood pressure goal of less than 140/90 mm Hg. Guidelines such as the National Institute for Health and Clinical Excellence (NICE; www.nice.org.uk) can be used for further interpretation of blood pressures taken outside of the clinic setting. Routine use of automated ambulatory blood pressure monitoring or home monitoring devices, however, is not currently recommended as their value has not been established.

C. **Evaluation for new diagnosis of hypertension.** Once the diagnosis of hypertension has been established, further workup is indicated. To tailor therapy, the clinician should
- Assess other cardiovascular risk factors (listed in Table 77-3).
- Assess potential comorbidities.
- Assess presence of target organ damage.

Secondary causes of hypertension should be sought only in patients whose age, history, abruptness of onset of hypertension, severity of presentation, and initial laboratory work-up suggest a secondary cause.

1. **Physical examination.** Table 77-4 lists the suggested components of a physical examination for a patient with newly diagnosed hypertension.

   a. **Evaluate for cardiovascular risks.** See Table 77-3 for potential comorbid conditions. The presence of comorbidities may affect one's choice of antihypertensive medication, blood pressure goals, and/or use of additional agents such as aspirin or smoking cessation aids.

   b. **Identify target organ damage.** Organs potentially injured or at risk for injury by hypertension include the heart (left ventricular hypertrophy, coronary artery disease, or heart failure), brain (cerebrovascular accent [CVA] or transient ischemic attack [TIA]), kidneys (chronic kidney disease), peripheral arteries (peripheral arterial disease [PAD]), and retina (retinopathy).

   Signs of target organ damage include arteriolar narrowing, arteriovenous compression, hemorrhages, exudates, or papilledema on fundoscopic examination; carotid bruits and distended jugular veins in the neck; loud aortic second sound, precordial heave, arrhythmia, or early systolic click on cardiac examination; diminished or absent peripheral arterial pulses, peripheral edema of the extremities; aneurysm of the abdominal aorta; and abnormal neurologic assessment.

   c. **Be alert for signs of secondary hypertension.** Medications that can cause elevated blood pressure include nonsteroidal anti-inflammatory agents, corticosteroids, migraine medications, serotonin norepinephrine receptor inhibitors

TABLE 77-4. SUGGESTED PHYSICAL EXAMINATION COMPONENTS FOR PATIENTS WITH NEWLY DIAGNOSED HYPERTENSION

- Calculation of BMI and measurement of waist circumference
- Complete examination of the fundi, thyroid, heart, lungs, skin, and abdomen
- Complete neurologic examination
- Vascular examination to include auscultation of carotid, femoral, renal, and aortic arteries and palpation of aorta and peripheral pulses

(e.g., venlafaxine, sibutramine), estrogens (including birth control pills) and other hormones, nonprescription cough/cold and asthma medications (particularly when the cough/cold medicine is taken with certain antidepressants like tranylcypromine or tricyclics), and nasal decongestants. Also ask about excessive alcohol use or cocaine abuse.

Signs suggestive of secondary hypertension include abdominal or flank masses (polycystic kidneys); absence of femoral pulses (aortic coarctation); tachycardia, diaphoresis, or orthostatic hypotension (pheochromocytoma); abdominal bruits (renovascular disease); truncal obesity or elevated body mass index (BMI), ecchymoses, or pigmented striae (Cushing syndrome); and an enlarged or nodular thyroid gland (hyperthyroidism).

2. **Laboratory tests.** Testing is used to assess target organ damage, to determine whether other cardiovascular risk factors exist, and, if appropriate, to evaluate for causes of secondary hypertension.

   a. **Routine tests** for all patients with newly diagnosed hypertension include hematocrit; potassium; creatinine; fasting glucose; calcium; fasting lipid profile including total cholesterol, HDL cholesterol, LDL cholesterol, and triglycerides; urinalysis; and resting electrocardiogram. Obtaining a urinary albumin excretion or albumin/creatinine ratio is optional. More extensive testing for identifiable causes is generally not indicated. (SOR **C**)

   b. **Laboratory tests to identify secondary causes.** The following laboratory tests may be helpful when specific secondary causes are suspected based on history, physical evaluation, and routine laboratory evaluation:

   (1) Chest x-ray may reveal coarctation of the aorta.

   (2) In patients with an acute worsening of renal function with use of angiotensin-converting enzyme (ACE) inhibitors or who are at a higher risk for fibromuscular dysplasia (young females) or atherosclerotic disease (older adults), consider imaging to rule out renal artery stenosis. Imaging options include magnetic resonance imaging or arteriography (MRI/MRA), computed tomography (CT) scan, and ultrasonography. The preferred method will depend on the capabilities of the institution and personnel. Use of intravenous contrast (including gadolinium) may worsen renal function, especially in patients with poor renal function at baseline.

   (3) 24-hour urine collection for metanephrines, creatinine clearance, total protein, aldosterone, sodium, and/or potassium can be done to assess for renal disease and pheochromocytoma. Testing plasma metanephrines is another reasonable screen for pheochromocytoma.

   (4) Paired, morning plasma aldosterone and plasma renin or plasma renin activity can be done to evaluate for primary aldosteronism.

   (5) Serum thyroid-stimulating hormone (TSH) can be used to screen for thyroid disease.

   (6) A sleep study could be obtained for patients with suspected obstructive sleep apnea (e.g., excessive snoring, daytime sleepiness, obesity).

III. Treatment

A. **Decision to treat.** If a patient has hypertension, therapy is indicated to lower the risk of cardiovascular, cerebrovascular, and renal morbidity and mortality. (SOR **A**) The Joint National Committee 8 (JNC 8) recommends treatment of blood pressure to a goal of 150/90 mm Hg in people older than 60 years, and to a diastolic goal of less than 90 mm Hg in all other individuals. (SOR **A**) The recommendations for all individuals, based on expert opinion, is to treat to a goal of less than 140/90 mm Hg. (SOR **C**)

1. **Patients with diabetes mellitus** have an SBP goal less than 140 mm Hg and a DBP goal less than 80 mm Hg.

2. **Patients with coronary artery disease, coronary artery disease equivalents** (carotid artery disease, peripheral arterial disease, or abdominal aortic aneurysm), **or high cardiovascular risk** (10-year Framingham risk score 10% or more) have an SBP goal less than 130 mm Hg and a DBP goal less than 80 mm Hg.

3. **Patients with chronic kidney disease** have an SBP goal less than 130 to 140 mm Hg and a DBP goal less than 80 to 90 mm Hg, depending on their urine protein excretion.

B. **Lifestyle modifications** are important for all patients with prehypertension and hypertension. Lifestyle changes reduce the number and dosage of medications needed

TABLE 77-5. LIFESTYLE MODIFICATIONS TO MANAGE HYPERTENSION[a]

Modification	Recommendation	Approximate Systolic BP Reduction, Range
Weight reduction	Maintain normal body weight (BMI, 18.5–24.9)	4–5 mm Hg/4-kg weight loss
Adopt DASH eating plan	Consume a diet rich in fruits, vegetables, and low-fat dairy products with a reduced content of saturated and total fat	8–14 mm Hg
Dietary sodium reduction	Reduce dietary sodium intake to 5–6 g/d, preferably less than 3 g/d	4–6 mm Hg
Physical activity	Engage in regular aerobic physical activity such as brisk walking (at least 30 min/d, most days of the week)	3–5 mm Hg
Moderation of alcohol consumption	Limit consumption to no more than two drinks per day in most men and no more than one drink per day in women and lighter-weight persons[b]	3 mm Hg

[a]For overall cardiovascular risk reduction, stop smoking. The effects of implementing these modifications are dose- and time-dependent and could be higher for some individuals.
[b]A standard drink is equal to 0.6 ounces of pure alcohol such as 12 ounces of beer, 5 ounces of wine, or 1.5 ounces of 80-proof distilled spirits or liquor.
BMI, body mass index calculated as weight in kilograms divided by the square of height in meters; BP, blood pressure; DASH, Dietary Approaches to Stop Hypertension.
Source: Data from Calhoun et al. (2008); Chobanian et al. (2003); Siebenhofer et al. (2011); Whelton et al. (2002); Xin et al. (2001).

to control hypertension. Evidence-based lifestyle modifications include weight reduction for those who are overweight, Dietary Approaches to Stop Hypertension (DASH) diet, dietary sodium reduction, physical activity, and moderate alcohol consumption (Table 77–5). (SOR **A**)

1. **Weight loss.** A meta-analysis of eight studies involving 2100 participants showed an average weight loss of 4 kg was associated with a decrease in SBP of 4.5 mm Hg and DBP of 3.2 mm Hg. The long-term risks of benefits of weight loss could not be assessed in this meta-analysis. Weight loss can reduce the dosage requirement of people using antihypertensive medications. (SOR **A**)

2. **DASH diet.** The DASH study found that diets high in fruits and vegetables (8–10 daily servings of fruits and vegetables for a person with moderate physical activity) significantly decreased SBP and DBP in patients with hypertension. The DASH-diet eating plan is now recommended for most patients with prehypertension and hypertension. (SOR **A**) Recipes and patient education materials are available at http://www.nhlbi.nih.gov/health/public/heart/hbp/dash/index.htm.

3. **Sodium restriction.** Reducing salt intake significantly reduces blood pressure. A meta-analysis of 34 trials involving 3400 patients showed that lowering sodium intake to 5 to 6 g per day reduced SBP by 4 to 6 mm Hg and DBP by 2 mm Hg. Further benefits were noted with a sodium intake of less than 3 g per day. (SOR **A**) The degree of blood pressure lowering by sodium restriction appears to vary, with certain "salt-sensitive" individuals experiencing a significant effect, and others receiving little apparent benefit. Therefore, if sodium restriction is burdensome for a patient, a trial of sodium restriction can be performed in order to tailor therapy.

4. **Physical activity.** A meta-analysis of trials has shown that physical activity is effective in lowering blood pressure in normal weight and overweight individuals and in those with prehypertension and hypertension. Aerobic exercise is associated with a 3 to 5 mm Hg reduction in the SBP and a 2 to 3 mm Hg reduction in the DBP. The PREMIER study showed that increasing physical activity could be successfully added to a DASH-sodium diet, with allowance for moderate alcohol consumption, to lower blood pressure. All sedentary patients with prehypertension and hypertension should be encouraged to participate in 30 minutes of moderate or vigorous physical activity between 5 and 7 days per week. (SOR **A**)

5. Moderate alcohol consumption. A meta-analysis of 15 randomized clinical trials concluded that reduction in alcohol consumption results in a modest reduction in SBP of 3 mm Hg and DBP of 2 mm Hg. Individuals with prehypertension and hypertension should be encouraged to limit alcohol intake—two drinks per day for men and one drink per day for women; neither men nor women should consume more than five drinks in any 24-hour period. (SOR **Ⓐ**)

C. Pharmacologic treatment. Treatment of prehypertension with medication is not recommended. In fact, for patients without established CVD, treatment of stage 1 hypertension does not reduce morbidity or mortality over 4 to 5 years. In contrast, pharmacologic treatment of patients with known CVD reduces the risk of a subsequent event even if blood pressures are already at goal. (SOR **Ⓐ**)

1. Setting of initial treatment. The majority of patients can be treated in the outpatient setting. If a patient is experiencing a hypertensive emergency or crisis (elevated blood pressures plus experiencing target organ damage such as mental status changes, aortic dissection, chest pain, pulmonary edema, or acute renal failure), he or she should be managed in the hospital. (SOR **Ⓒ**) Hypertension in a pregnant woman should be assumed to be preeclampsia, and prompt evaluation should be performed. (SOR **Ⓒ**)

2. Patient education. Patient (and family, if appropriate) education begins with the initial diagnosis. Patient beliefs should be elicited regarding the necessity and effectiveness of treatment, risks of inadequate treatment, and concerns about treatment side effects. Barriers to adherence such as cost should be identified. The patient should participate in determining the strategies to reach their blood pressure goals. Shared decision-making tools are available to assist in this conversation (such as http://sdm.rightcare.nhs.uk/shared-decision-making-sheets/high-blood-pressure). Instructions including lifestyle changes, medications, monitoring of blood pressure, and laboratory testing should be discussed and/or written at a level appropriate for the patient's health literacy. (SOR **Ⓒ**)

3. Initial drug therapy. The most effective first-line treatment for preventing the occurrence of cardiovascular morbidity and mortality is **an ACE inhibitor, angiotensin receptor blocker, calcium channel blocker, or thiazide diuretic**. (SOR **Ⓐ**) In the black hypertensive population, a calcium channel blocker or thiazide diuretic is recommended as initial therapy. (SOR **Ⓑ**)

a. Ethnicity. Patients with African or Caribbean ancestry may respond better to CCB and less well to ACE inhibitors or ARB as compared to Caucasian patients. African-American patients also have an increased risk of ACE inhibitor-induced angioedema. However, the use of any class of antihypertensive medication is appropriate, especially for patients with compelling indications such as diabetes mellitus.

4. Ongoing management. The three most common causes of uncontrolled hypertension are patient nonadherence (responsible for the majority of treatment failures), inadequate therapy, and inappropriate therapy.

a. Appointment frequency. Monthly check-ups can be done until blood pressures are controlled. Evaluation should include a measurement of blood pressure and weight as well as an interval history to identify medication side effects, symptoms of CVD, and common habits that affect blood pressure (e.g., physical activity, use of caffeine, tobacco, or alcohol). More frequent visits may be needed if blood pressures are extremely high or for patients at a high risk of complications.

Although elevated SBP is considered a stronger risk factor than elevated DBP, lifestyle modification and medication (if necessary) should be used in a vigorous stepped-care approach. Treating patients to less than the recommended BP targets may not reduce morbidity or mortality and may increase risk due to potential adverse medication effects/interactions, cost of medications, falls, and decreased cerebral perfusion. (SOR **Ⓐ**)

b. Drug regimen management. Drug regimens can be tailored based on many factors including severity of hypertension, age, cost, safety, side effects, effectiveness, convenience, possibility of drug interactions, consideration of pathophysiologic mechanisms, concurrent risk factors and diseases, history of response to other agents, and the potential use of the medication for other medical problems. Control of blood pressure is better with bedtime dosing when compared with dosing upon awakening, but the clinical significance of this finding is unknown. Table 77–6 lists

TABLE 77–6. COMMON ORAL ANTIHYPERTENSIVE DRUGS

Drug (Trade Name)	Starting Dose (Maximum Dose)	Common Side Effects	Drug Interactions
Thiazide Diuretics			
Chlorothiazide (Diuril)	0.5 g (2 g) once or twice daily	Phototoxicity, vertigo, electrolyte disorders (hyponatremia, hypercalcemia, hypokalemia, hypomagnesemia, hypophosphatemia), hyperuricemia	Dofetilide, sotalol (QT Prolongation); lithium (lithium toxicity); methotrexate, cyclophosphamide (antineoplastic agent toxicity); ACE inhibitors (first-dose postural hypotension)
Chlorthalidone (generic)	12.5 (25) mg once daily		
Hydrochlorothiazide (Microzide, HydroDIURIL)	12.5 (50) mg once daily		
Indapamide (Lozol)	1.25 (5) mg once daily		
Metolazone (Mykrox)	0.5 (1) mg once daily		
Metolazone (Zaroxolyn)	2.5 (5) mg once daily		
Loop Diuretics			
Bumetanide (Bumex)	0.5 (2) mg once daily	Electrolyte disorders (hypomagnesemia, hypochloremia, hypokalemia) polyuria, hyperuricemia, azotemia	Dofetilide, sotalol, droperidol (QT prolongation); lithium (lithium toxicity); aminoglycoside antibiotics (ototoxicity and nephrotoxicity); cephaloridine (cephaloridine toxicity)
Furosemide (Lasix)	20 (80) mg once daily		See bumetanide
Torsemide (Demadex)	2.5 (10) mg once daily		See bumetanide; warfarin (bleeding)
Potassium-Sparing Diuretics			
Amiloride (Midamor)	5 (10) mg once or twice daily	Electrolyte disorders, hyperuricemia,	ACE inhibitors, tacrolimus (hyperkalemia); dofetilide, sotalol, droperidol (QT prolongation); methotrexate (methotrexate toxicity)
Triamterene (Dyrenium)	50 (100) mg once or twice daily	As above plus nausea, loss of appetite, diarrhea	
Aldosterone-Receptor Blockers			
Eplerenone (Inspra)	50 (100) mg once or twice daily	Hyperkalemia, increased serum creatinine, cough	Azole antifungals, macrolide antibiotics, verapamil, nefazodone, antiretrovirals (eplerenone toxicity); ACE inhibitors (hyperkalemia)
Spironolactone (Aldactone)	25 (50) mg once or twice daily	Hyperkalemia, gynecomastia, impotence, menstruation disorder	Sulfamethoxazole–trimethoprim, ACE inhibitors, tacrolimus (hyperkalemia); sotalol, droperidol (QT prolongation); lithium (lithium toxicity)
β-Blockers			
Atenolol (Tenormin)	25 (100) mg once daily	Fatigue, cold extremities, depression, confusion, dizziness, headache, dyspnea/wheezing	Amiodarone, dronedarone, calcium channel blockers (hypotension, bradycardia); clonidine (bradycardia); beta-2 agonists (bronchospasm); antidiabetic agents (hypo- or hyperglycemia); alpha-adrenergic blockers (first dose hypotension)
Bisoprolol (Zebeta)	2.5 (10) mg once daily		
Metoprolol (Lopressor)	50 (100) mg once or twice daily		
Metoprolol extended release (Toprol XL)	50 (100) mg once daily		Propranolol only: thioridazine (QT prolongation); fluoxetine (heart block)
Nadolol (Corgard)	40 (120) mg once daily		
Propranolol (Inderal)	40 (160) mg twice daily		
Propranolol long-acting (Inderal LA)	60 (180) mg once daily		
Timolol (Biocadren)	20 (40) mg twice daily		
Nebivolol (Bystolic)	5 (40) mg once daily		

TABLE 77–6. COMMON ORAL ANTIHYPERTENSIVE DRUGS (Continued)

Drug (Trade Name)	Starting Dose (Maximum Dose)	Common Side Effects	Drug Interactions
β-Blockers with Intrinsic Sympathomimetic Activity			
Acebutolol (Sectral)	200 (800) mg twice daily	Dizziness, headache, fatigue, Pindolol only: edema, myalgias, arthralgia, anxiety, insomnia	Amiodarone, dronedarone, calcium channel blockers (hypotension, bradycardia); clonidine (bradycardia); beta-2 agonists (bronchospasm); antidiabetic agents (hypo- or hyperglycemia); alpha-adrenergic blockers (first dose hypotension)
Penbutolol (Levatol)	10 (40) mg once daily		
Pindolol (generic)	10 (40) mg twice daily		
			Pindolol only: Thioridazine (QT prolongation)
Combined Alpha- and Beta-Blockers			
Carvedilol (Coreg)	12.5 (50) mg twice daily	Dizziness, weight gain, diarrhea, fatigue, hyperglycemia, erectile dysfunction, peripheral edema	Amiodarone, dronedarone, calcium channel blockers (hypotension, bradycardia); beta-2 agonists (bronchospasm); antidiabetic agents (hypo- or hyperglycemia); alpha-adrenergic blockers (first dose hypotension)
Labetalol (Normodyne, Trandate)	200 (800) mg twice daily	Dizziness, fatigue, nausea, tingling sensation	
ACE (Angiotensin-Converting Enzyme) Inhibitors			
Benazepril (Lotensin)	10 (40) mg once or twice daily	Cough, hyperkalemia, dizziness, headache Captopril: disorder of taste Enalapril: increased BUN and creatinine	Potassium sparing diuretics, potassium (hyperkalemia); lithium (lithium toxicity); capsaicin (cough); loop and thiazide diuretics (first dose hypotension)
Captopril (Capoten)	25 (100) mg twice daily		See benazepril; azathioprine (myelosuppression); interferon alfa-2a (hematologic abnormalities); allopurinol (hypersensitivity reactions, Stevens-Johnson S), aspirin (↓captopril effect)
Enalapril (Vasotec)	2.5 (40) mg once or twice daily		See captopril; metformin (lactic acidosis)
Fosinopril (Monopril)	10 (40) mg once daily		See benazepril; azathioprine (myelosuppression)
Lisinopril (Prinivil, Zestril)	10 (40) mg once daily		See benazepril; azathioprine (myelosuppression)
Moexipril (Univasc)	7.5 (40) mg once daily		See benazepril; azathioprine (myelosuppression)
Quinapril (Accupril)	10 (40) mg once daily		See benazepril; azathioprine (myelosuppression)
Ramipril (Altace)	2.5 (20) mg once daily		See benazepril; azathioprine (myelosuppression); telmisartan (renal dysfunction)
Angiotensin-Receptor Blockers			
Candesartan (Atacand)	4 (32) mg once daily	Hyperkalemia, diarrhea, cough, dizziness, hypoglycemia, backache, myalgia, chest pain Irbesartan: upper respiratory infection Losartan: anemia	Potassium-sparing diuretics, potassium (hyperkalemia)
Irbesartan (Avapro)	75 (300) mg once daily		As above
Olmesartan (Benicar)	5 (40) mg once daily		As above
Losartan (Cozaar)	25 (100) mg once daily		As above plus lithium (lithium toxicity); fluconazole—oral, rifampin (↓ efficacy of losartan)
Telmisartan (Micardis)	40 (80) mg once daily		Potassium-sparing diuretics, potassium (hyperkalemia); ramipril (renal dysfunction); lithium (lithium toxicity); digoxin (digoxin toxicity)
Valsartan (Diovan)	40 (320) mg once daily		Potassium-sparing diuretics, potassium (hyperkalemia); lithium (lithium toxicity)

(continued)

TABLE 77–6. COMMON ORAL ANTIHYPERTENSIVE DRUGS (Continued)

Drug (Trade Name)	Starting Dose (Maximum Dose)	Common Side Effects	Drug Interactions
Direct Renin Inhibitors			
Aliskiren	150 (300) mg once daily	Diarrhea, headache, dizziness	Potassium-sparing diuretics, potassium (hyperkalemia)
Calcium Channel Blockers: Non-Dihydropyridines (non-DHP)			
Verapamil immediate release (Calan)	240 (480) mg in three divided doses	Constipation, edema, dizziness, head-	**Multiple Interactions**
Verapamil sustained release (Verelan, Calan SR)	180 (480) mg once daily	ache, pharyngitis, sinusitis, influenza-like symptoms	Dofetilide (QT prolongation); colchicine (colchicine toxicity); digoxin (digoxin toxicity); dabigatran, clopidogrel (VTE); statins (myopathy); beta blockers, amiodarone, clonidine, clarithromycin (bradycardia); phenytoin (↓ verapamil efficacy); lithium (lithium toxicity); aspirin (bleeding)
Diltiazem (Cardizem CD)	120 (480) mg once daily	Peripheral edema, headache, diz-	Cisapride, erythromycin (QT prolonga-tion); colchicine (colchicine toxicity);
Diltiazem (Diltia XT, Cardizem LA)	180 (540) mg once daily	ziness, cough, fatigue	statins (myopathy); atazanavir, cimeti-dine (cardiovascular toxicity); clopido-grel (VTE); beta blockers, amiodarone (bradycardia); phenytoin, rifampin (↓ diltiazem efficacy); aspirin (bleed-ing); digoxin (digoxin toxicity)
Calcium Channel Blockers: Dihydropyridines (DHPs)			
Nifedipine (Nifedical, Procardia)	30 (90) mg once daily	Peripheral edema, flushing, head-ache, palpitations, dizziness, nausea, fatigue	**Multiple Interactions** clopidogrel (↑ VTE); fentanyl (severe hypo-tension); amiodarone, (AV block); beta-adrenergic blockers, clarithromycin (hypotension, bradycardia); tacrolimus (tacrolimus toxicity); cimetidine, azole antifungals, ginkgo, ginseng (nifedipine toxicity)
Amlodipine (Norvasc)	5 (10) mg once daily		Clopidogrel (↑ VTE); antiretroviral agents, azole antifungals (amlodipine toxicity); simvastatin, (myopathy); amiodarone (AV block); beta-adrenergic blockers (hypotension, bradycardia); St. John's wort (↓ efficacy of amlodipine); fentanyl (severe hypotension)
Felodipine (Plendil)	5 (10) mg once daily		Itraconazole (cardiotoxicity); other azole antifungals, cyclosporine, antiretrovirals (felodipine toxicity); amiodarone (AV block); beta-adrenergic blockers, (hypotension, bradycardia)
Isradipine (Dynacirc)	2.5 (20) mg twice daily		Ziprasidone, pimozide, thioridazine, bepridil, mefloquine, gemifloxacin,
Isradipine controlled release (Dynacirc CR)	5 (20) mg once daily		fluconazole, cisapride, Class I or III anti-arrhythmic agents, tricyclic antidepres-sants (cardiotoxicity); azole antifungals, antiretrovirals (isradipine toxicity); rifampin (↓ isradipine efficacy)
Centrally Acting Agents			
Clonidine (Catapres)	0.2 to 0.6 (2.4) mg once daily 0.1 (initial)—0.6 mg transdermal patch daily	Dry mouth, drowsi-ness, dizziness, constipation Transdermal: contact dermatitis, ery-thema (in addition to above)	Doxepin, tricyclic antidepressants, mir-tazapine (↓ antihypertensive efficacy); verapamil, diltiazem, beta blockers (bradycardia); cyclosporine (cyclospo-rine toxicity)

TABLE 77-6. COMMON ORAL ANTIHYPERTENSIVE DRUGS (Continued)

Drug (Trade Name)	Starting Dose (Maximum Dose)	Common Side Effects	Drug Interactions
Reserpine	0.5 mg daily for 1 to 2 weeks; then 0.1 to 0.25 mg once daily	Depression, nasal congestion, dizziness, somnolence, headache, abdominal pain, xerostomia	Tetrabenazine, MAOIs (release of catecholamines); colchicine (colchicine toxicity); phenytoin (↓phenytoin efficacy)
Guanfacine (Intuniv)	1 (2) once daily	Constipation, xerostomia, somnolence, impotence, headache, insomnia	Tricyclic antidepressants (↓ antihypertensive efficacy)
Methyldopa	250 mg in 2–3 divided doses (max 3000 mg daily)	Asthenia, dizziness, headache, sedation, impotence, disorder of ejaculation, reduced libido, drug fever	MAOIs, pseudoephedrine (hypertensive crisis); beta-blockers, entacapone (tachycardia); haloperidol (reversible dementia or Parkinsonism); iron (↓ methyldopa efficacy)
Alpha-1 Blockers			
Terazosin (Hytrin)	1 mg at bedtime (max 40 mg in 1–2 divided doses)	Dizziness, asthenia, headache, somnolence, nasal congestion, palpitations, peripheral edema, nausea	Phosphodiesterase-5 enzyme inhibitors (hypotension); beta-blockers (first alpha-1 blocker dose hypotension)
Prazosin (Minipress)	1 mg at bedtime (max 20 mg in 1 to 2 divided doses)		
Doxazosin (Cardura)	1 (16) mg daily		
Direct Vasodilators			
Hydralazine (Apresoline)	10 (40) mg four times daily	Chest pains, palpitations, tachycardia, loss of appetite, headache	No significant interactions
Minoxidil	5 (100) mg once or twice daily	Hirsutism, hypertrichosis, edema, hypernatremia	

VTE, venous thromboembolism.

the common oral antihypertensive agents along with dosing, common side effects, and drug interactions.

(1) **Most patients with hypertension do not reach their blood pressure goal with a single medication.** If the initial agent does not control BP sufficiently, a second (or more, if needed) agent of a different class can be added. Using agents at low doses will decrease side effects, although one should not diagnose resistant hypertension until blood pressures are not controlled despite the concurrent use of three agents (including a diuretic) at optimal doses. (SOR ❸) Reducing the number of daily doses is effective in increasing adherence to blood pressure medications. (SOR ❶) It may be possible to accomplish these disparate tasks with the use of combination formulations (e.g., diuretic and ACE inhibitor in a single tablet). Many combination antihypertensives are now available to reduce cost and treatment complexity. Generic combination medications include chlorthalidone plus atenolol as well as hydrochlorothiazide plus one of the following: triamterene, bisoprolol, propranolol, irbesartan, losartan, candesartan, and most ACE inhibitors. Numerous brand name combinations are also available.

(2) **A memory-assist device,** such as an automated voice reminder system, a cellular phone alarm, weekly or monthly pill boxes, and/or pill boxes with alarms, are appropriate for patients receiving complex regimens or with a memory disturbance.

   (3) **Medication prices** for individuals without prescription insurance can be
       found at websites such as http://www.drugpriceinfo.com/. Many pharmacy
       retailers have limited formularies of deeply discounted generic medications
       that can make treating hypertension more affordable for patients.
   c. **Laboratory testing.** Electrolytes and renal function (urinalysis, albumin/cre-
      atinine ratio, serum creatinine, and/or glomerular function rate) should be mea-
      sured periodically. More frequent or complex testing may be needed based on
      the patient's comorbid conditions such as diabetes mellitus or collagen vascu-
      lar disease. **Renal function and serum potassium should be checked
      shortly after initiation of an ACE inhibitor, ARB, direct renin inhibitor
      (DRI), or diuretic.** If there is greater than 30% increase in serum creatinine after
      initiation of an ACE inhibitor, ARB, or DRI, consider evaluation for renal artery
      stenosis. Periodic screening for hyperlipidemia and diabetes screening should be
      completed. (SOR **C**)
   d. **Home monitoring.** Home blood pressure monitoring improves blood pressure
      control and accurately predicts target organ damage. (SOR **A**) Patients should use
      a blood pressure cuff assessed regularly for reliability.
5. **Medications for comorbid conditions**
   a. **Aspirin.** The use of aspirin by patients with well-controlled hypertension is recom-
      mended based on a combination of factors including age, gender, and history of
      CVD and diabetes. Individualized risk–benefit assessments are needed to balance
      the risk of bleeding against the reduced risk of cardiovascular events and possible
      reduced risk of colorectal cancers. Most patients with known CVD who do not use
      other anticoagulants would benefit from daily aspirin use. (SOR **A**)
   b. **Statins.** Use of a statin in primary prevention of CVD reduces all-cause mortality,
      even in low-risk populations (number need to treat [NNT] of 96 patients treated
      for 5 years to prevent one death) and coronary heart disease events (NNT of
      56 patients treated for 5 years). (SOR **A**) The new 2013 American College of
      Cardiology (ACC)/American Heart Association (AHA) Guideline on Treatment of
      Blood Cholesterol to Reduce Atherosclerotic Cardiovascular Risk in Adults is dis-
      cussed in Chapter 76 and can be found at http://content.onlinejacc.org/article.
      aspx?articleid=1770217.
6. **Smoking cessation.** Quitting smoking may have a small effect on SBP and DBP
   and will significantly reduce morbidity and mortality including CVD, chronic obstructive lung disease, kidney disease, CVA/TIA, and lung cancer. (SOR **A**)
7. **Benefits of treatment.** Antihypertensive drug therapy is associated with a 35% to
   40% reduction in stroke, 20% to 25% reduction in myocardial infarction, and 50%
   reduction in heart failure in subjects with hypertension. (SOR **A**) A Cochrane meta-
   analysis found **treatment of moderate-to-severe hypertension** decreased
   cardiovascular morbidity and mortality in all patients including those over 80 years of
   age. All-cause mortality was reduced by treating those patients less than 80 years of
   age. (SOR **A**)

SELECTED REFERENCES

Appel LJ, Brands MW, Daniels SR, et al. Dietary approaches to prevent and treat hypertension: a scientific statement from the American Heart Association. *Hypertension.* 2006;47(2):296–308.
Arguedas JA, Perez MI, Wright JM. Treatment blood pressure targets for hypertension. *Cochrane Database Syst Rev.* 2009;(3):CD004349.
Bliziotis IA, Destounis A, Stergiou GS. Home versus ambulatory and office blood pressure in predicting
   target organ damage in hypertension: a systematic review and meta-analysis. *J Hypertens.* 2012;(7):
   1289–1299.
Calhoun DA, Jones D, Textor S, et al. Resistant hypertension: diagnosis, evaluation, and treatment: a
   scientific statement from the American Heart Association Professional Education Committee of the
   Council for High Blood Pressure Research. *Circulation.* 2008;117(25):e510–e526.
Centers for Disease Control. Vital signs: awareness and treatment of uncontrolled hypertension among
   adults–United States, 2003-2010. *MMWR Morb Mortal Wkly Rep.* 2012;61:703–709.
Chobanian AV, Bakris GL, Black HR, et al. The Seventh Report of the Joint National Committee on
   Prevention, Detection, Evaluation, and Treatment of High Blood Pressure: the JNC 7 report. *JAMA.* 2003;
   289(19):2560–2572.
Diao D, Wright JM, Cundiff DK, Gueyffier F. Pharmacotherapy for mild hypertension. *Cochrane Database Syst Rev.* 2012;8:CD006742.

Glynn LG, Murphy AW, Smith SM, et al. Interventions used to improve control of blood pressure in patients with hypertension. *Cochrane Database Syst Rev.* 2010;(3):CD005182.

He FJ, Li J, Macgregor GA. Effect of longer-term modest salt reduction on blood pressure. *Cochrane Database Syst Rev.* 2013;4:CD004937.

James PA, Oparil S, Carter BL, et al. 2014 evidence-based guideline for the management of high blood pressure in adults: report from the panel members appointed to the eight Joint National Committee (JNC-8). *JAMA.* 2013;284427. Published online December 18th, 2013.

Krause T, Lovibond K, Caulfield M, McCormack T, Williams B, Group GD. Management of hypertension: summary of NICE guidance. *BMJ.* 2011;343:d4891.

Siebenhofer A, Jeitler K, Berghold A, et al. Long-term effects of weight-reducing diets in hypertensive patients. *Cochrane Database Syst Rev.* 2011;(9):CD008274.

Thompson AM, Hu T, Eshelbrenner CL, et al. Antihypertensive treatment and secondary prevention of cardiovascular disease events among persons without hypertension: a meta-analysis. *JAMA.* 2011;305(9): 913–922.

Taylor F, Huffman MD, Macedo AF, et al. Statins for the primary prevention of cardiovascular disease. *Cochrane Database Syst Rev.* 2013;(1):CD004816.

U.S. Preventive Services Task Force. Screening for high blood pressure: U.S. Preventive Services Task Force reaffirmation recommendation statement. *Ann Intern Med.* 2007;147(11):783–786.

Wright JM, Musini VM. First-line drugs for hypertension. *Cochrane Database Syst Rev.* 2009;(3): CD001841.

Additional references are available online at http://langetextbooks.com/fm6e

---

78   Inflammatory Bowel Disease

Russell Lemmon, DO, & David M. Lessens, MD, MPH

KEY POINTS

- Inflammatory bowel disease consists of Crohn's disease (CD) and ulcerative colitis (UC), which vary in presentation and underlying histopathology. (SOR **C**)
- Both conditions typically present with abdominal pain and diarrhea, but UC usually involves hematochezia while CD does not. (SOR **C**)
- The diagnosis is most reliably made with colonoscopy and biopsy, with CD showing intermittent, transmural lesions and UC displaying continuous, superficial mucosal inflammation starting at the rectum. (SOR **C**)
- Treatment options are similar for both types, and focus on reducing inflammation and inducing remission. (SOR **C**)
- Patients with UC, but not those with CD, require increased colon cancer surveillance depending on the extent of disease. (SOR **A**)

I. Introduction

A. Definition. Inflammatory bowel disease (IBD) is a chronic, relapsing, immune-mediated, systemic condition mainly affecting the intestines. Evidence suggests that IBD results from an inappropriate inflammatory response to intestinal microbes in a genetically susceptible host. IBD consists of two distinct types: ulcerative colitis (UC) and Crohn's disease (CD), which share common features and treatment options, but vary in presentation and underlying histopathology.

    1. UC is characterized by inflammation of the mucosal layer of the large bowel, typically starting at the rectum and extending proximally in a continuous fashion. Forty to fifty percent of patients have disease limited to the rectosigmoid region, and 20% have involvement of all segments of the colon. UC only affects the colon.

    2. CD, in contrast, is characterized by transmural inflammation that can affect any part of the gastrointestinal (GI) tract from the mouth to the anus. The inflammatory process is normally discontinuous and produces segments of uninvolved mucosa known as skip lesions. It typically affects the ileum and the colon.

B. Epidemiology. There is geographic variance in the incidence of IBD with highest rates reported in northern Europe, the United Kingdom, and North America. The incidence in countries where IBD was previously rare is increasing, however. The prevalence of IBD is approximately 1.4 million in the United States and 2.2 million in Europe.

    1. IBD can be diagnosed at any age. The **peak incidence age for IBD** is 20 to 30 years with a smaller peak later in life at approximately 50 to 60 years. The peak incidence for UC is thought to be 5 to 10 years later than CD. Pediatric IBD accounts for 7% to 20% of IBD cases with CD being more common than UC in children.

    2. Men and women are affected at an equal rate overall. Whites and those of Jewish descent are at higher risk in the United States, although geography may play a larger role than race.

C. Risk factors

    1. Genetics. Genome studies have identified many IBD-associated loci on multiple chromosomes. Approximately one-third of these mutations have shared risk factors between UC and CD, which could account for overlap of some disease characteristics. Genetics seem to play a larger role in CD as there is a 50% disease concordance found in monozygotic twins versus a 6% rate found in UC.

    2. Smoking is one of the most consistently reported modifiable risk factors for CD; however, there appears to be variance within geographic regions and ethnic groups as to how much risk smoking imparts. Smoking likely does not cause CD, but rather modulates the disease once present.

    3. Appendectomy. Having an appendectomy for confirmed appendicitis appears to confer a protective benefit for UC, but the association in CD is less clear. Those with a prior appendectomy who develop UC appear less likely to have severe disease.

    4. Diet. The incidence of IBD has been shown to increase as a country becomes "Westernized" or when groups migrate to high-incidence regions, and it is thought that diet plays a large role; it is unclear to what extent a specific food type, additive, or pollutant confers risk. Population and prospective studies from Europe have shown an increased risk of IBD with increased intake of animal protein, omega-6 fats, and foods high in sugar.

    5. Antibiotic use. Observational data have shown an association between childhood antibiotic use and the subsequent development of IBD, but no causal relationship has been established.

    6. Geography. IBD is more prevalent in areas of higher latitude and, as such, low vitamin D levels and reduced exposure to sunlight have been proposed as risk factors. Although these observational associations have been made, they do not explain the rising incidence of IBD in regions of lower latitude. No causal relationship has yet been established.

II. Diagnosis

A. Signs and symptoms. UC commonly presents with abdominal pain, diarrhea, hematochezia, tenesmus, and passage of mucus or pus. This can be a dramatic presentation with frequent stools, abdominal distension, and sometimes a toxic appearance. CD also presents with abdominal pain and diarrhea, but typically does not involve blood or mucus in stools. CD often has a more insidious onset that can lead to weight loss by the time of diagnosis. A tender mass of the right lower quadrant may be appreciated. CD can also present with stomatitis, small bowel or colonic obstruction, and anal fistulae.

    1. Extraintestinal manifestations. There are many possible extraintestinal manifestations of IBD which may be present at diagnosis.

        a. Erythema nodosum are tender, erythematous nodules most often on the extremities present in about 10% of patients (Figure 78–1).

        b. Seronegative arthritis often affects the large joints asymmetrically.

        c. Other possible manifestations include **primary sclerosing cholangitis, granulomatous hepatitis, uveitis, and hypercoagulability**.

    2. Extramural manifestations, such as fistula and abscesses, can be present with more severe disease.

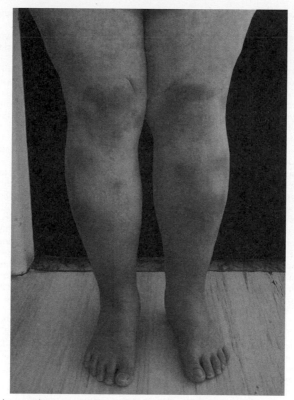

FIGURE 78–1. Erythema nodosum in a middle-aged woman with no known cause. These lesions are bright red, warm, and painful (see color insert). (Used with permission from Richard P. Usatine.)

B. Laboratory assessment. The diagnosis of IBD is based on characteristic endo-scopic and histologic findings, in the absence of other causes. Laboratory assessment cannot make the diagnosis, but is often necessary to help rule out other causes of bowel inflammation and assess for secondary problems such as anemia. Possible studies include a complete blood cell count, metabolic panel and hepatic function tests, celiac testing, and stool cultures or biopsies to evaluate for infectious causes of inflammation. Depending on the clinical picture, it may also be prudent to screen for human immunodeficiency virus, and, in the case of proctitis, to obtain herpes simplex virus serologies.

C. Imaging/diagnostics. The goals of imaging studies in IBD are to establish a diag-nosis (including differentiation between UC and CD), rule out other causes, determine disease severity, and screen for colon cancer in long-standing colonic IBD. The current diagnostic **standard is colonoscopy,** which is ideal for visualization of the bowel wall and the ability to easily obtain biopsies. The main disadvantages of colonoscopy are the invasive nature of the procedure and inability to visualize the small bowel proxi-mal to the terminal ileum. Therefore, other imaging modalities are frequently necessary during the evaluation of suspected IBD.

    1. Abdominal plain film may be indicated on initial presentation with concern for an acute abdomen. A plain film can reveal free air from a perforation, show signs of bowel obstruction, or show colonic dilation. Toxic megacolon is a dramatic presentation of severe UC, which can be detected on a plain x-ray.

2. **Small-bowel follow-through** is often necessary to indirectly visualize the small bowel, helping to differentiate CD from UC. CD may show a narrowed terminal ileum on a small bowel series, known as the string sign.

3. **Ultrasound** can be useful for ruling out other etiologies of abdominal pain and can be used to identify CD. However, the large bowel is difficult to visualize with ultrasound, so overall the diagnostic value in IBD is limited.

4. **Computed tomography (CT) imaging** relies on contrast medium to identify bowel wall thickening, the hallmark of IBD on a CT scan. CT is also useful for evaluating for extramural complications such as abscesses and fistula and excludes other etiologies of abdominal pain, such as appendicitis. CT imaging can miss superficial ulcerations or mild inflammatory changes. Sensitivity for colonic IBD is thought to be between 69% and 84%.

5. **Magnetic resonance imaging** colonography has been found to have similar specificity and possibly greater sensitivity in detecting bowel wall thickening when compared with CT imaging. This could be used in a similar diagnostic manner as a CT scan, but is limited by cost and availability.

6. **Endoscopy** is the gold standard for the diagnosis of IBD to identify characteristic ulcerations and inflammatory changes and to confirm the distinctive histology from a colonic biopsy. The ulcerations of UC will typically be superficial, starting at the rectum and extending proximally in a continuous fashion. More severe disease can show deeper ulcerations, bleeding, and pseudopolyps. CD lesions are normally characterized by transmural ulcerations, skip lesions, pseudopolyps, fissures, and rectal sparing.

III. **Treatment.** The focus of treatment is to reduce inflammation by focusing on inducing remission during a flare and by maintaining remission once acute symptoms are under control. Active patient participation in decision-making is encouraged, given that long-term treatment is required and many treatment options need to be considered. Other treatment goals include optimizing patient well-being, ensuring adequate nutrition, minimizing medication side effects, preventing complications, and avoiding emergent surgery. In addition, disease location and associated symptoms should be considered. Although CD and UC are separate entities, similar treatments are used for both conditions.

A. **Nonpharmacologic treatment**

1. **Supportive measures.** Patients diagnosed with IBD should be counseled to stop using tobacco products, avoid nonsteroidal anti-inflammatory medications and oral contraceptives (can exacerbate symptoms), receive age-appropriate vaccines (patients on immunomodulators and anti-TNF therapies should not receive any live virus vaccines), and, for women of childbearing age, avoid pregnancy while on certain medications. Improving stress management may also improve the patients' approach to care and degree of suffering.

2. **Nutrition.** No single diet has been found to be universally helpful in patients with IBD. However, a higher prevalence of food sensitivities exists in this population, and enteral nutrition is considered first-line therapy in some countries. Although not all patients respond equally well to dietary modifications, certain recommendations should be considered.

   a. Given the higher than average prevalence of food sensitivities, using a **food-symptom diary** followed by a customized elimination diet for 2 to 4 weeks (focusing on dairy, wheat, corn, certain fruits, and vegetables) can be helpful. (SOR **B**) It may also be prudent to avoid carrageenan, a food additive used to stabilize milk proteins in processed foods, which has been experimentally used to induce UC in animals.

   b. **Lactose malabsorption** occurs in about one-quarter to one-third of those with CD or UC, respectively. Thus, lactose restriction may be beneficial to relieve diarrhea or bloating symptoms.

   c. **Vitamin B, antioxidant, and iron deficiencies** may be common due to poor dietary intake, poor absorption, or interaction with medications. Treatment of documented deficiencies is indicated and it may be prudent to recommend all patients take a daily multivitamin.

   d. In cases of active colitis, total parenteral nutrition may be indicated when severe caloric protein malnutrition is present.

B. Complementary and alternative treatment

1. Omega-3 fatty acids, though known to decrease systemic inflammation, are not effective for relapse prevention in CD. (SOR **B**)

2. Probiotics. Given the possible role of altered gut immunity or existence of pathogenic colonic bacteria, probiotics may play a role in restoring healthy gut flora. These are the most common complementary therapies used by patients. Use of a combination preparation (VSL #3), which contains *Bifidobacterium*, *Lactobacillus*, and *Streptococcus* species, and a single preparation of *Saccharomyces boulardii*, may lead to fewer relapses in those with CD. (SOR **C**) The role of probiotics continues to be an area of active study and few conclusions can be made on their class efficacy. Be cautious if the patient is also on immunosuppressive medication.

3. Curcumin. When administered at doses of 2 g per day, this has been shown to be an effective therapy for the maintenance of remission in UC when given along with sulfasalazine or mesalamine. (SOR **B**)

B. Pharmacologic treatment (Table 78–1). It remains controversial which treatments should be initiated first. A "bottom-up" approach starts with 5-aminosalicylic acid (5-ASA) compounds and steroids, whereas a "top-down" approach starts with immunomodulators or biologic medications; most often, the bottom-up approach is used. Anti-inflammatory medications, such as **nonsteroidal anti-inflammatory drugs and aspirin should be AVOIDED,** as these can impair healing of the GI tract. (SOR **C**)

1. 5-ASA compounds have a variety of anti-inflammatory and immunosuppressive effects and are most effective and often used in patients with UC to induce and maintain remission. (SOR **B**) They exhibit their effects topically and are only minimally absorbed by the colon. Often, these are used in patients with mild-to-moderate disease activity. Although they can be used in the active phase of mild-to-moderate CD (with the best evidence for sulfasalazine), use in maintenance therapy after surgery is limited.

    a. Mesalamine is available in both oral and topical formulations. Oral forms have pH-sensitive resins or timed-release capsules. Topical forms include suppositories and enemas, and these can provide much higher local concentrations of medication with less systemic absorption.

    b. Azo compounds are activated by colonic bacteria, which cleave a molecule and render them active. This class of compounds interferes with folate metabolism, so supplements are recommended. They also contain sulfa, so should not be used in sulfa-allergic patients. Sulfasalazine is the oldest and least expensive in this class; because of side effects, it is used less often than other 5-ASA compounds.

2. Corticosteroids

    a. Systemic. These are a mainstay of therapy for moderate to severe disease. Steroids are often used along with 5-ASA compounds and are more effective as mono-therapy than 5-ASA compounds or placebo. (SOR **A**) Budesonide is a newer agent that exhibits extensive first-pass hepatic metabolism and so has high topical anti-inflammatory activity with minimal systemic effects; a controlled release formulation is available that targets delivery to the terminal ileum and proximal colon. Budesonide has been shown to be more beneficial than placebo or mesalamine for induction of remission in patients with ileal and right-sided colonic CD and in those with UC. Corticosteroids are often used if patients have failed first-line therapies. Corticosteroids are not efficacious in the maintenance treatment of CD or UC. For those who do not respond to 5-ASA compounds and budesonide, prednisone is often used, and if one requires hospitalization, hydrocortisone or methylprednisolone can be considered for intravenous therapy. (SOR **B**) Improvement is usually rapid over a few days, and prednisone doses are usually slowly tapered until discontinued.

    b. Topical. For those with UC located in the rectum or sigmoid colon, enemas can be effective. Foam preparations may be more effective than liquid, given that they facilitate greater contact time. Topical hydrocortisone (SOR **A**) or budesonide (SOR **B**) is effective for distal colon inflammation. Topical steroids may be slightly less effective than topical 5-ASA therapies.

3. Antibiotics. Metronidazole and ciprofloxacin are widely used and have both anti-infective and anti-inflammatory properties. However, controlled trials have not documented consistent, beneficial effects.

TABLE 78–1. COMMON TREATMENTS FOR IBD

Class/Drug	Brand Name	Site of Action	Dose Range	Adverse Effects	Selected Drug Interactions
5-ASA Mesalamine	Apriso	Colon	0.375 g extended-release capsule	Abdominal pain, belching, diarrhea, nausea, vomiting, arthralgia, headache, GI hemorrhage, agranulocytosis, renal failure	Azathioprine (increased risk of myelosuppression), antacids (decrease mesalamine)
	Asacol/Asacol HD	Colon/terminal ileum	400 and 800 mg delayed-release tablets; Asacol: 800 mg oral three times daily for 6 wk; Asacol HD: 1600 mg three times daily for 6 wk	Same as above	Same as above
	Canasa	Rectum	1000 mg rectal suppository once daily at bedtime for 3–6 wk	Same as above	Same as above
	Lialda	Colon	1.2 g delayed release tablet; 2.4 or 4.8 g daily with a meal for up to 8 wk	Same as above	Same as above
	Pentasa	Small bowel, ileum, colon	250 and 500 mg extended-release capsules; 1 g oral four times daily up to 8 wk	Same as above	Same as above
	Rowasa[a]	Descending colon	4 g per 60 mL rectal enema suspension at bedtime for 3–6 wk	Same as above; fewer systemic effects	Same as above
Balsalazide	Colazal[a]	Colon	750 mg capsule; 2250 mg three times daily for 8–12 wk	Abdominal pain, diarrhea, nausea, vomiting, arthralgia, headache, ulcerative colitis exacerbation, renal failure, hepatic failure	Azathioprine, mercaptopurine (increased risk myelosuppression), ACEI (decrease effectiveness of ACEI), valproic acid (increase valproic acid)
Olsalazine	Dipentum	Colon	250 mg capsule; 500 mg twice daily	Abdominal pain, diarrhea, indigestion, nausea, headache, blurred vision, hypertension	Varicella virus (risk of Reye syndrome), mercaptopurine (increased risk of myelosuppression)
Sulfasalazine	Azulfidine[a]	Colon	500 mg tablet and 250 mg per 50 mL oral suspension; up to 4 g daily in evenly divided doses no exceeding 8-h intervals	Pruritus, rash, abdominal pain, indigestion, loss of appetite, nausea, vomiting, headache, oligospermia (reversible), fever, agranulocytosis, hepatotoxicity	Methanamine[b] (crystalluria), riluzole (increased hepatotoxicity), cyclosporine (decrease cyclosporine efficacy), digoxin (decrease digoxin), folic acid (decrease folic acid), live vaccines
Corticosteroids Budesonide	Entocort EC[a]	Systemic	Up to 9 mg every morning for up to 8 wk	Diarrhea, arthralgia, headache, Cushing syndrome	HIV protease inhibitors, boceprevir, antifungals, clarithromycin (increase budesonide)

Prednisone[a]	Deltasone, Cortan, Delta-Dome, Fernisone, Meticorten, Orasone, Paracort, Prednicen-M, Rayos, Servisone	Systemic	10–60 mg/d	Hypertension, decreased body growth, edema, hypernatremia, osteoporosis, mood changes, hyperglycemia, Cushing's syndrome	Rotavirus vaccine[b]; quetiapine (decrease quetiapine); HIV protease inhibitors, clarithromycin, antifungals (increase prednisone); phenytoin (decrease prednisone)
Corticosteroid Enema	Cortenema[a]	Colon	One enema (100 mg/60 mL) per day rectally	As above	As above
Immunomodulators					
Azathioprine	Imuran[a]	Systemic	50 mg/d	Nausea, vomiting, pancreatitis, lymphoma, myelosuppression	Febuxostat[b], ACEI (increased risk myelosuppression), allopurinol (increase azathioprine toxicity), mycophenolate, mercaptopurine, mesalamine (increase azathioprine), live vaccines
6-Mercaptopurine	Purinethol[a]	Systemic	50–100 mg/d	Hyperuricemia, hypoglycemia, pancreatitis, hepatotoxicity, myelosuppression	Febuxostat[b], allopurinol (increase 6-mercaptopurine toxicity), azathioprine (increased toxicity), methotrexate, sulfasalazine (increase bone marrow suppression), live vaccines
Methotrexate	Methotrexate[a]	Systemic	15–25 mg/wk	Alopecia, thrombocytopenia, nausea, vomiting, stomatitis, hepatotoxicity, nephrotoxicity	Cotrimoxazole, NSAIDs, leflunomide, amoxicillin, PPI (increase methotrexate toxicity), warfarin (increase warfarin), live vaccines
Cyclosporine	Cylosporin[a]	Systemic	8–10 mg/kg/d orally	Hypertension, hirsutism, gingival hyperplasia, headache, tremor, hyperkalemia, hypomagnesemia, hepatotoxicity, nephrotoxicity	Simvastatin[b], dronedarone[b], lovastatin (increase lovastatin), antifungals (increase cyclosporine), colchicine (increase both drugs), methotrexate (increase methotrexate toxicity)

(continued)

TABLE 78–1. COMMON TREATMENTS FOR IBD (*Continued*)

Class/Drug	Brand Name	Site of Action	Dose Range	Adverse Effects	Selected Drug Interactions
Anti-Tumor Necrosis Factor (TNF)					
Adalimumab	Humira	Systemic	160 mg SQ once on day 1, then 80 mg once on day 15, then 40 mg every other week starting at week 4	Headache, injection site reaction, upper respiratory infection, heart failure, opportunistic infections, Stevens–Johnson syndrome	Cyclosporine (decrease cyclosporine), tacrolimus (decrease tacrolimus), live vaccines
Certolizumab	Cimzia	Systemic	400 mg SQ once at weeks 0, 2, 4, then 400 mg every 4 wk	As above	Live vaccines
Infliximab	Remicade	Systemic	5 mg/kg IV once at weeks 0, 2, 6, then 5 mg/kg every 8 wk; max 20 mg/kg IV every 8 wk in patients who become unresponsive	Rash, abdominal pain, nausea, headache, respiratory tract infection, fatigue, heart failure, leukemia, opportunistic infections	Sirolimus (decrease sirolimus), warfarin (decrease warfarin), phenytoin (decrease phenytoin), cyclosporine (decrease cyclosporine), tacrolimus (decrease tacrolimus)
Anti-Integrin					
Natalizumab	Tysabri	Systemic	50 mg/day	Dermatitis, rash, nausea, arthralgia, headache, infection, bowel obstruction, hepatotoxicity, depression	

*a*Available as generic.
*b*Contraindicated.
ACEI, angiotensin-converting enzyme inhibitor; GI, gastrointestinal; NSAIDs, nonsteroidal anti-inflammatory drugs; PPI, proton-pump inhibitor.

4. Immunomodulators are often used for intractable or inoperable disease. They are often better tolerated than long-term corticosteroids but also have the potential for severe side effects. Because of this potential of adverse events, including leukopenia and associated infections, regular laboratory testing is indicated. Unlike corticosteroids, they can take up to 3 months to have a clinical effect.

    a. 6-Mercaptopurine and azathioprine. These two medications are used primarily for inducing remission for intractable perianal CD, (SOR **A**) although evidence for use in UC is increasing. They are also used for the long-term maintenance of remission of CD and UC and are often combined with low doses of corticosteroids. (SOR **A**) These medications can also be used as monotherapy for those intolerant to mesalamine, sulfasalazine, and corticosteroids.

    b. Methotrexate. This is an alternative therapy for patients intolerant of other immunomodulating medications, although its clinical evidence for efficacy is not as robust. The best evidence is for inducing remission and enabling withdrawal from corticosteroids in patients with refractory CD. (SOR **B**) There is insufficient evidence to support the use of methotrexate in patients with UC. Given that it interferes with folate metabolism, supplementation should be prescribed. This medication is relatively inexpensive and it is often used when other options are not financially available.

    c. Cyclosporine is effective as a means to avoid surgery in patients with severe corticosteroid-refractory UC (SOR **A**) and is often given along with corticosteroids. It is initially effective in the majority of patients and is often used to delay surgery to a later time when the surgical risks are reduced. It is often reserved for individuals not responding to other medications, given the potential of severe side effects, including nephrotoxicity. It should not be used for maintenance therapy, and it has no demonstrated role in the treatment of CD.

5. Biologics. Given that IBD may be due to abnormal cellular immunity to luminal substances, targeting aspects of the immune system has proven beneficial. This class of agents can be helpful for those with steroid-dependent or refractory disease and may alter the disease's natural history. However, these agents are often expensive and can have life-threatening side effects that result in severe infections. Although there has been some concern about an increased risk of lymphoma while taking these medications, this has not been supported by recent data. (SOR **B**)

    a. Anti-TNF. Tumor necrosis factor (TNF) is a pro-inflammatory cytokine that works as part of the TH1 immune response. Anti-TNF medications are indicated for moderate-to-severe CD or UC and should be considered in patients who do not respond to corticosteroids or immunosuppressive therapy. The best evidence supports induction and maintenance of remission for CD. (SOR **A**) The anti-TNF medications available include Infliximab (Remicade), Adalimumab (Humira), and Certolizumab (Cimzia).

    b. Anti-integrin. Natalizumab (activity against alpha-4 integrin) has been shown to be effective for induction of remission in some patients with moderate-to-severe active CD. (SOR **A**) However, its use has been limited due to an association with progressive, multifocal leukoencephalopathy.

C. Surgery. Common indications for surgery include perforation, obstruction, abscess, refractory or fulminant disease, cancer, intractable hemorrhage, or dysplasia. Procedures most often performed include surgical resection of the involved colon or abscess drainage. Over half of all patients require surgery within 10 years of a CD diagnosis, and the postoperative recurrence of disease is 40% to 60%. About one-third of those with UC will require surgery during their lifetime.

IV. Management Strategies

    1. Patient education. Involving patients in the decision-making process is important, given the range of treatments available and potential for serious, adverse side effects. The websites shown in the below box can be recommended to patients.

Websites for Information on IBD

- Centers for Disease Control and Prevention: inflammatory bowel disease http://www.cdc.gov/ibd/

- Family Doctor.org: inflammatory bowel disease http://familydoctor.org/familydoctor/en/diseases-conditions/inflammatory-bowel-disease.html
- Medline Plus (Spanish available): Crohn's disease http://www.nlm.nih.gov/medlineplus/crohnsdisease.html
- Medline Plus (Spanish available): ulcerative colitis http://www.nlm.nih.gov/medlineplus/ulcerativecolitis.html

2. Tests for screening and follow-up
A. Cancer screening. UC is associated with an increased risk of **colon cancer,** though this risk varies based on the site(s) of disease and duration of symptoms (and not its activity). Epidemiologic data have shown that proctitis alone confers no additional risk, but pancolitis that began in childhood confers a 162 times higher risk than for those without UC.

   1. Screening for colon cancer is best performed when the disease is in remission.

   2. The frequency of screening has not been rigorously studied and should be individualized. Many guidelines recommend screening initiation 10 years after diagnosis with follow-up every 1 to 5 years. Patients with CD do not appear to have an increased risk of colon cancer, although this is still being investigated; however, they may have an increased risk of small bowel cancer, but no reliable screening exists for this.

   3. Women taking immunosuppressive therapy may be at a higher risk for **cervical cancer,** and close adherence to current screening guidelines is recommended.

B. Follow-up related to medications

   1. Long-term corticosteroid use (beyond 3 months) increases risk of osteoporosis. In these patients, vitamin D and calcium supplementation as well as bisphosphonate therapy may be appropriate. In addition, obtain a baseline dual-energy x-ray absorptiometry and perform annual ophthalmologic examinations. Secondary hypertension can also develop so blood pressure should be monitored at every visit.

   2. Immunomodulator medications (i.e., azathioprine, methotrexate). To monitor for side effects, complete blood count and kidney and liver function tests are indicated both at baseline and for routine follow-up. A chest x-ray is indicated to look for infections.

   3. Anti-TNF therapies. In addition to the tests needed to monitor treatment for the immunosuppressive medications, a purified protein derivative test is indicated, given these medications are associated with reactivation of latent tuberculosis.

V. Prognosis. IBD is a chronic and often relapsing disease that can often be managed with medical therapy. New medications have improved rates of people living with well-controlled IBD symptoms for many years.

SELECTED REFERENCES

Botoman VA, Bonner GF, Botoman DA. Management of inflammatory bowel disease. *Am Fam Physician.* 1998;57:57–68.

Lashner B. Inflammatory bowel disease. In: *Cleveland Clinic: Current Clinical Medicine.* 2nd ed. Philadelphia, PA: Saunders; 2010:463–467.

Lichtenstein GR, Abreu MT, Cohen R, Tremaine W; American Gastroenterological Association. American Gastroenterological Association Institute medical position statement on corticosteroids, immunomodulators, and infliximab in inflammatory bowel disease. *Gastroenterology.* 2006; 130(3):935–939.

Ng SC, Bernstein CN, Vatn MH, et al. Geographical variability and environmental risk factors in inflammatory bowel disease. *Gut.* 2013;62(4):630–649.

Wilkins T, Jarvis K, Patel J. Diagnosis and management of Crohn's Disease. *Am Fam Physician.* 2011; 84:1365–1375.

Additional references are available online at http://langetextbooks.com/fm6e

79   Ischemic Heart Disease and Acute Coronary Syndromes

Damon F. Lee, MD, Lovedhi Aggarwal, MD, & Allen L. Hixon, MD

KEY POINTS

- The highest priority in the evaluation of patients with chest pain is distinguishing cardiac from noncardiac causes. (SOR **C**)
- The clinical history including cardiac risk factors remains critical in the evaluation of each patient. Evidence-based primary and secondary prevention should be targeted at modifiable risk factors. (SOR **C**)
- A normal electrocardiogram result cannot be used to exclude ischemic heart disease (IHD). An exercise treadmill test remains the most valuable diagnostic tool. (SOR **B**)
- Consensus guidelines should be used to determine management of patients with chronic stable IHD and acute coronary syndromes. (SOR **C**)
- Aspirin (SOR **A**) and beta-blockers (SOR **B**) should be considered in all patients with IHD; the latter are especially important in patients with a prior myocardial infarction. (SOR **A**)

I. Introduction

A. Definition. Ischemic heart disease (IHD) is a condition in which there is an inadequate supply of blood and oxygen to a portion of the myocardium, typically occurring when there is an imbalance between myocardial oxygen supply and demand. Most commonly caused by coronary atherosclerosis, IHD may be stable and chronic or it may present as an acute coronary syndrome (ACS). See Figure 79–1.

1. ACS is a cluster of clinical symptoms that are associated with acute myocardial ischemia. These symptoms typically result from the disruption of atherosclerotic plaques, leading to obstruction of myocardial blood flow. The term ACS encompasses conditions including unstable angina, non–ST-elevation myocardial infarction (NSTEMI) and ST-elevation myocardial infarction (STEMI). Myocardial infarction (MI) is injury to the heart due to lack of blood supply.

B. Epidemiology

1. Cardiovascular disease is the leading cause of death in both men and women. Heart disease is responsible for 28% of male and 27% of female deaths in the United States. It accounts for approximately half of all deaths in the developed world and one-quarter of all deaths in the developing world. More than 1 million men and women die annually in the United States alone from coronary artery disease or stroke. Fifty percent of postmenopausal women die of coronary artery disease or its sequelae. It is estimated that by the year 2020, cardiovascular disease will surpass infectious diseases as the leading cause of death and claim 25 million lives worldwide.

2. IHD has an enormous economic impact on medical care in this country. The cost of treatment is expected to rise with the aging of the US population. In industrialized nations, economic loss, disability, and death from coronary artery disease exceeded any other cluster of illnesses.

3. Unrecognized MIs are common and as lethal as symptomatic infarcts. At least 25% of MIs are silent and another 25% present with atypical chest pain. Only 20% of MIs are preceded by angina. Many MIs occur at rest and nearly as many occur during sleep as during heavy physical activity. Distressing life events reportedly occur with increased frequency in the months preceding an MI.

C. Pathogenesis. The heart muscle functions almost exclusively as an aerobic organ, with little capacity for anaerobic metabolism. At rest, the heart extracts approximately 80% of the oxygen it receives, leaving it more susceptible to effects of decreased perfusion. ACSs arise from a mismatch of myocardial oxygen supply and demand. This mismatch is most often initiated by disruption of an atherosclerotic plaque, causing blockage of normal coronary blood flow. Partial or complete mechanical obstruction may result from thrombus or dynamic obstruction from coronary vasoconstriction. Inflammation as well as systemic hemodynamic factors also play a role in the development or severity of IHD. This process causing myocardial ischemia results in a variety of signs and symptoms. It

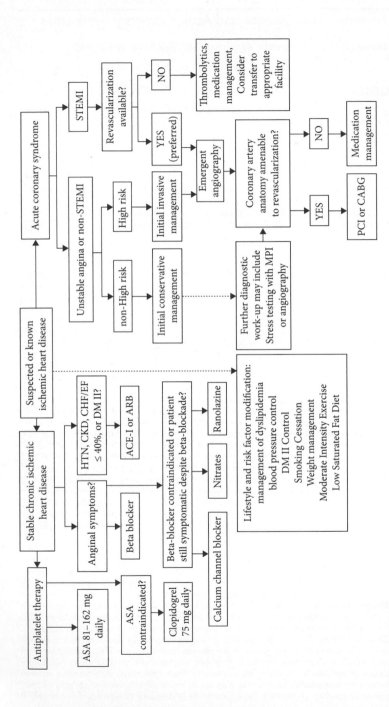

FIGURE 79-1. Approach to the patient with suspected or known ischemic heart disease. ACE-I, angiotensin-converting enzyme inhibitor; ARB, angiotensin receptor blocker; ASA, aspirin; CABG, coronary artery bypass graft; HTN, hypertension; CKD, chronic kidney disease; CHF, congestive heart failure; DM II, type 2 diabetes mellitus; EF, ejection fraction; MPI, myocardial perfusion imaging; PCIs, percutaneous coronary interventions; STEMI, ST-elevation myocardial infarction.

TABLE 79–1. USPSTF SCREENING RECOMMENDATIONS AND LEVEL OF EVIDENCE

Condition or Intervention	Demographic	Level of Evidence[a]
Aspirin chemoprevention discussion	Adults with increased coronary heart disease risk	A
Tobacco cessation	All adults	A
Hypertension (HTN)	Age 18 yr and older	A
Intensive dietary behavioral counseling	Adults with hyperlipidemia and cardiovascular/diet-related chronic disease risk factors	B
Cholesterol	Men ≥35 yr, women over age 44 yr at high risk	A
	Men 20–34 yr at high risk, women over age 20–44 yr at high risk	B
Obesity screening	Adults	B
Promotion of physical activity	Primary care settings	I
Type 2 diabetes screening	Asymptomatic adults	I
	Adults with HTN or hyperlipidemia	B
Screening EKG or ETT	Asymptomatic adults	D

[a]Key: A, strongly recommends providing the service to eligible patients; B, recommends providing the service to eligible patients; D, recommends against providing the service; I, insufficient evidence for or against routinely providing the service.
Source: Data from Agency for Healthcare Research and Quality, U.S. Preventive Services Task Force. The Guide to Clinical Preventive Services. www.uspreventiveservicestaskforce.org/. Accessed October 2013.

is important for clinicians to recognize the many manifestations of this disease process. Chest pain is the foremost manifestation of myocardial ischemia and results from a disparity between myocardial oxygen demand and coronary blood flow.

II. Prevention

A. **Primary prevention** should target smoking cessation, blood pressure and cholesterol screening, maintaining a normal BMI, and discussing aspirin therapy. See Table 79–1 for the U.S. Preventive Services Task Force screening guidelines and levels of evidence and Chapter 105 for a more complete list of recommendations.

   1. **Hormone therapy for women.** The Women's Health Initiative (WHI) trial and the Estrogen/Progestin Replacement Study helped to clarify the role of hormone therapy (HT) in relation to IHD prevention. Combination HT (estrogen plus progestin) led to an increase in IHD; **for every 10,000 women treated per year, there would be about 7 more MIs**. Based on these studies, and consistent with American College of Cardiology and the American Heart Association (ACC/AHA) recommendations, HT is not recommended for either primary or secondary prevention of IHD. (SOR **A**) The WHI trial of unopposed estrogen versus placebo in women who have undergone hysterectomy showed no increase in heart disease, but showed an increase in stroke in the treatment group.

B. **Secondary prevention** in patients diagnosed with hypertension (see Chapter 77), dyslipidemia (see Chapter 76), or diabetes mellitus (see Chapter 75) should focus on controlling blood pressure, cholesterol, and blood sugar in accordance with consensus guidelines such as the Seventh Report of the Joint National Committee on Prevention, Detection, Evaluation, and Treatment of High Blood Pressure (JNC 7); the National Cholesterol Education Program (NCEP); and the American Diabetic Association's Standards of Medical Care in Diabetes. These and other important consensus guidelines may be found at the National Guideline Clearinghouse (www.guideline.gov).

C. **Annual influenza vaccination** is recommended for all patients with IHD. (SOR **B**)

III. Diagnosis.
Chest pain is one of the common reasons for patients to visit primary care physicians. The major diagnostic considerations for chest pain are addressed in Chapter 10. The highest priority is generally given to distinguishing cardiac from noncardiac chest pain. Studies have demonstrated that 10% to 30% of patients with chest pain who undergo coronary arteriography have no arterial abnormalities. Of the many noncardiac causes of chest pain, gastrointestinal (esophageal), bronchopulmonary, and psychiatric (panic attacks

and major depression) are common. Less common causes include chest wall (herpes zoster, costochondritis), aortic dissection, and referred pain from the abdomen.

A. Risk factors. Cigarette smoking, hyperlipidemia, hypertension, diabetes, older age, and male gender are commonly recognized risk factors for IHD. In addition, elevated homocysteine levels and markers of vascular inflammation such as the highly sensitive C-reactive protein are associated with IHD. Mental stress has increasingly been recognized as related to IHD.

B. Symptoms and signs

1. **Angina** is not simply one type of pain; it is a constellation of symptoms related to cardiac ischemia. The description of angina may fit several patterns.

   a. **Typical (classic) angina** presents as an ill-defined chest pressure, heaviness (feeling like a weight), or squeezing sensation. The location of classic anginal pain is most often substernal and left-sided. It may radiate to the jaw, interscapular area, or down the arm. Angina usually begins gradually and lasts only a few minutes. Aggravating factors include exertion or stress. Typical angina is alleviated by rest or nitroglycerin (NTG). It is important to appreciate that the qualitative description of pain may be greatly influenced by socioeconomic status, education, culture, and personality.

   b. **Atypical angina.** The patient has some but not all of the features of typical angina. For example, there may be a sense of heaviness that is not consistently related to exertion or relieved by rest. Conversely, the pain may have an atypical character—sharp or stabbing—but the precipitating or alleviating factors are anginal. This is the category of chest pain that is most prone to a diagnostic error. All presentations of chest pain should be taken seriously until proven to be benign.

   c. **Nonanginal pain.** The pain has neither the quality nor precipitating or alleviating characteristics of typical angina. Chest pain quality not consistent with IHD includes the following descriptive terms: needlelike, shooting, tingling, stabbing, jabbing, knifelike, and cutting.

   d. **Anginal equivalent.** The sensation of dyspnea may be the sole or major manifestation.

   e. **Metabolic syndrome, insulin resistance, and diabetes.** IHD is the leading cause of death in adult patients with diabetes. Hypertension, obesity, and hyperlipidemia cluster in patients with diabetes who have accelerated development of atherosclerotic vascular disease. Insulin resistance promotes atherosclerosis even before the diagnostic criteria for diabetes mellitus are met. Atypical clinical presentations have been thought to occur more frequently in patients with diabetes than in the general population; however, this notion has recently been challenged.

   f. **Women** are twice as likely as men to present with angina and less likely to present with infarction or sudden death. Diabetes in women increases both the risk and mortality of MI. Women are often overlooked as having significant IHD. Women older than 65 years are as vulnerable to IHD mortality as men. There is a precipitous increase in IHD in women after either natural or surgical menopause.

2. **Probability of IHD based on history.** Despite the well-known problems experienced in determining the cause of chest pain, the clinical history remains critical in the evaluation of each patient. From the information gathered in the history, the clinician should strive to **categorize the patient's symptoms as nonanginal, atypical angina, or typical angina**. Table 79–2 provides a guideline as to the likelihood of whether a patient has significant IHD based on the history. The Framingham Global Prediction model includes age, total cholesterol, LDL-C, HDL-C, blood pressure, diabetes, and tobacco use. It may be used to calculate the 10-year coronary heart disease risk. An online version is available at http://cvdrisk.nhlbi.nih.gov/calculator.asp.

3. **Use of nitrate and response to NTG.** NTG is thought to act by reducing left ventricular preload and afterload as a result of venous (predominantly) and arterial dilation with a more efficient distribution of blood flow within the myocardium. The response of the chest pain to sublingual NTG may be used (with caution) as an adjunct for determining whether a patient's chest pain is from IHD. For example, a prompt response of ≤3 minutes increases the probability of IHD; however, esophageal spasm and biliary colic may also respond favorably to nitrate administration. **Failure to respond to NTG should not be used to exclude the possibility of IHD.**

TABLE 79-2. PRETEST PROBABILITY OF CORONARY ARTERY DISEASE BY AGE, GENDER, AND SYMPTOMS

Age (yr)	Gender	Typical/Definite Angina Pectoris	Atypical/ Probable Angina Pectoris	Nonanginal Chest Pain	Asymptomatic
30–39	Men	Intermediate	Intermediate	Low	Very low
	Women	Intermediate	Very low	Very low	Very low
40–49	Men	High	Intermediate	Intermediate	Low
	Women	Intermediate	Low	Very low	Very low
50–59	Men	High	Intermediate	Intermediate	Low
	Women	Intermediate	Intermediate	Low	Very low
60–69	Men	High	Intermediate	Intermediate	Low
	Women	High	Intermediate	Intermediate	Low

Source: Data from Gibbons RJ, Balady GJ, Bricker JT, et al. ACC/AHA 2002 guideline update for exercise testing: summary article. A report of the ACC/AHA Task Force on Practice Guidelines (Committee to Update the 1997 Exercise Testing Guidelines). *Circulation.* 2002;106:1883–1892.

4. **Signs.** There are no reliable, consistent physical signs found on examination for IHD. The main purposes of the examination are to assess the patient for evidence of complications from atherosclerotic disease (e.g., peripheral vascular disease, cerebrovascular disease, congestive heart failure) and to exclude other causes of chest pain. The clinician should pay attention to the vascular examination, including blood pressure measurement, peripheral artery bruits, retinal arteriolar changes, and the presence of an S_3 or S_4 heart sound, and for the consequences of diminished myocardial contractility, such as lower extremity edema. Signs of hyperlipidemia and therefore increased cardiovascular risk, such as xanthomas and xanthelasma may also be appreciated (see Chapter 76).

C. **Diagnostic tests**
   1. **12-Lead electrocardiogram (ECG)** and **serial cardiac enzymes** are frequently used to rule out an MI. Cardiac enzymes typically followed include cardiac troponin I or T and CK-MB. ECG changes of significance are noted below.
   2. The standard provocative test for IHD is the **exercise treadmill test (ETT)**. The ETT can be performed with or without nuclear medicine myocardial perfusion imaging (MPI) or echocardiography. For patients unable to exercise on a treadmill, a pharmacologic stress test can be performed. The ACC) and the AHA have developed consensus guidelines for exercise treadmill testing as follows:
      a. ETT is appropriate as a diagnostic test to determine the presence or absence of coronary artery disease in patients with an intermediate pretest probability (Table 79–1). (SOR ❸) This includes patients with complete right bundle branch block or less than 1 mm of resting ST depression.
      b. ETT may be useful for patients with known or suspected IHD who have experienced a change in clinical status. (SOR ❸)
      c. Low-risk patients with unstable angina 12 hours after presentation who are free of ischemic symptoms or heart failure may be appropriate for stress testing. Similarly, intermediate-risk patients with unstable angina 2 to 3 days after presentation and free of ischemic symptoms or heart failure may also be appropriate for stress testing.
      d. Many protocols exist; however, the Bruce protocol (www.youtube.com/watch?v= y3Zq4n3WSyc) has become the most widely used.
      e. **Prognostic value of an ETT.** In addition to the diagnostic value of an ETT, there are prognostic implications. The following are considered to be parameters associated with a poor prognosis or increased disease severity: failure to complete stage II of a Bruce protocol, failure to achieve a heart rate ≥120 beats per minute (off beta-blockers), onset of ST-segment depression at a heart rate of ≤120 beats per minute, ST-segment depression ≥2.0 mm, ST-segment depression lasting ≥6 minutes into recovery, ST-segment depression in multiple leads, poor systolic blood pressure response to exercise, angina with exercise, and exercise-induced ventricular tachycardia. Recently, heart rate recovery and the Duke treadmill exercise score, based on exercise time, ST deviation and angina during the test (http://www.zunis.org/Duke%20Treadmill%20Score%20-%20CAD%20Predictor.htm) have been determined to be independent predictors of mortality.

3. **Resting ECG.** A resting ECG, while important to obtain on all patients with suspected IHD (SOR **B**), must be interpreted with caution. The ECG will be normal or show nonspecific changes in more than 50% of patients with IHD. **A normal resting ECG may not be used to rule out IHD.**
  a. The ACC guidelines define an "interpretable" ECG as a normal 12-lead or one with minimal (<0.5 mm) resting ST-T changes. The classic ECG changes of acute ischemia are peaked, hyperacute T waves, T-wave flattening or inversion with or without ST-segment depression, horizontal ST-segment depression, and ST-segment elevation. ACC guidelines for further diagnostic work up are based, in part on whether or not the resting ECG is "interpretable" or "uninterpretable."
  b. To view ECG tracings, the reader is referred to one of the many online resources and teaching aids including http://www.learntheheart.com/ecg-review/ecg-quiz/, http://www.practicalclinicalskills.com/ekg.aspx, and http://highered.mcgraw-hill.com/sites/dl/free/007351098x/451682/sample_ch05.pdf.
4. **Laboratory studies**
  a. Studies to help stratify a patient's risk include a fasting lipid profile, diabetes screen (fasting blood glucose or hemoglobin A1C), and hemoglobin and hematocrit.
  b. Serum markers used to diagnose MI include troponins T or I, creatinine kinase, creatinine kinase myocardial bands, and myoglobin. Of these, the most sensitive and specific for myocardial injury is troponin. Normal troponin (troponin T <0.18 ng/mL) at 10 hours after onset of symptoms rules out MI. Serial normal troponin Ts with a normal ECG also effectively rules out MI (negative likelihood ratio of 0.003) and elevated troponin T, even with a normal ECG, is diagnostic of MI.
5. **Chest X-ray** may show cardiomegaly or signs of congestive heart failure. It is also useful in evaluating other diagnoses such as aortic dissection (widened mediastinum), pneumonia (infiltrates), or pulmonary embolus (wedge-shaped shadows).
6. **Angiography.** Cardiac catheterization is not routinely recommended for initial evaluation of patients with stable angina. Patients who warrant such an evaluation are those who exhibit evidence of severe myocardial ischemia on noninvasive testing (SOR **B**) and who have symptoms that are refractory to antianginal medications. (SOR **C**) In patients who undergo catheterization, the most important determinant of survival is left ventricular function, followed by the number of diseased vessels.
7. **Coronary CT angiography (CCTA)** may be considered in patients unable to undergo stress testing with MPI, those with ongoing symptoms despite prior normal stress testing, or those with inconclusive prior stress testing. (SOR **C**)

IV. **Treatment**
  A. **Chronic stable IHD.** Stable angina is characterized by no change in frequency, severity, duration, or precipitating factors for at least the past 2 months. The treatment of patients with stable IHD includes identification and management of specific cardiovascular risk factors, aspirin, and antianginal drug therapy (see Figure 79–1). Treatment goals include mortality reduction, prevention of MI, and symptom relief. With appropriate therapy some patients become asymptomatic.
    1. **Risk factor modification** may include smoking cessation, maintaining a BMI of 18.5 to 24.9 kg/m^2, and moderate intensity aerobic activity for 30 to 60 minutes at least 5 days a week (SOR **B**).
    2. **Treatment of associated disease.** Diabetes, hypertension, hyperlipidemia, thyroid disease, anemia, congestive heart failure, valvular disease, and arrhythmias should be aggressively identified and managed.
      a. Lipid lowering. Patients with high cholesterol should have their LDL cholesterol lowered to a target of ≤100 mg/dL with consideration of ≤70 mg/dL, according to ATP III guidelines (see Chapter 76). Blood pressure should be managed according to JNC 7 guidelines (see Chapter 77). All patients with IHD should also be screened for depression with positive screens treated appropriately.
    3. **Antiplatelet therapy.** Most experts recommend a range of 75 to 162 mg of aspirin per day to decrease platelet aggregation. (SOR **A**) Clopidogrel can be used in patients for whom aspirin is contraindicated. (SOR **B**)
    4. **Antianginal drug therapy.** The goals are to abolish or reduce anginal attacks and myocardial ischemia and to promote a more normal lifestyle. Three classes of antianginal drugs commonly used are beta-blockers, calcium channel blockers, and nitrates. No greater efficacy in relieving chest pain or decreasing exercise-induced

ischemia has been shown for one or another group of these drugs, although specific clinical indications may favor one over another (e.g., diastolic dysfunction, left ventricular hypertrophy, hypertension, asthma, depression, diabetes mellitus). See Medication Table 79–3.

a. Beta-blockers. Beta-blockade decreases heart rate, contractility, and arterial blood pressure, reducing myocardial oxygen demand and subsequently anginal symptoms. Beta-blockers reduce morbidity and mortality in patients with IHD versus placebo and are recommended as initial therapy for patients with chronic angina and prior MI (SOR **A**) as well as for those without prior MI. (SOR **B**) All beta-blockers, regardless of their selective properties, are equally effective in relieving anginal symptoms; however, the 2012 ACC Guidelines for management of stable IHD recommend carvedilol, metoprolol succinate, or bisoprolol in patients with LVEF ≤40%, because they have been shown to reduce the risk of death. (SOR **A**) The dose of the beta-blocker should be adjusted to achieve a heart rate of 50 to 60 beats per minute.

   (1) Approximately 20% of patients do not respond to beta-blockers. Those who do not are more likely to have severe IHD. **Contraindications** to beta-blockers include heart block, sick sinus syndrome, and severe bradycardia. **Caution** should be used in patients with asthma/obstructive lung disease, severe depression, or peripheral vascular disease.

b. Calcium channel blockers. These are a diverse group of compounds that have different effects on the atrioventricular node, heart rate, coronary arteries, diastolic relaxation, cardiac contractility, systemic blood pressure, and afterload. Most studies show equal effects between beta-blockers and calcium channel blockers, including effect on all-cause mortality. Calcium channel blockers may be preferred in patients who cannot tolerate beta-blockers or who have contraindications to their use. (SOR **B**)

   (1) The most troublesome **side effects** are constipation, edema, headache, and aggravation of congestive heart failure. Studies suggest that short-acting dihydropyridine calcium channel blockers such as nifedipine should be avoided because of an increased risk of adverse cardiac events. There is no evidence of a similar effect with long-acting calcium antagonists (Table 79–3).

c. Nitrates improve myocardial blood flow and oxygen demand via endothelial vasodilatation. Short-acting NTG tablets or spray are useful for the immediate relief of angina. (SOR **B**) Long-acting nitrates are used for symptom prevention in patients with contraindications to beta-blockade. (SOR **C**) There is no mortality benefit to these agents.

   (1) The most significant issue for this class of drugs is **tolerance**. Most studies show that tolerance develops rapidly to long-acting nitrates. Tolerance can develop within 24 hours. When prescribing a patch, it is important to have patch-free intervals of 10 to 12 hours to retain the antianginal effect.

   (2) Patients should be warned about the **potential for severe hypotension** when a phosphodiesterase type 5 inhibitor for the treatment of erectile dysfunction (e.g., sildenafil, tadalafil, vardenafil, avanafil) is taken within 24 hours after any nitrate preparation has been taken.

d. Ranolazine inhibits the late inward sodium current and decreases myocardial oxygen consumption by decreasing ventricular diastolic tension. It may be useful in patients for whom beta blockade is contraindicated, produces untoward side effects, or is ineffective. (SOR **B**) Ranolazine usually has no effect on heart rate and blood pressure.

   (1) Contraindications include severe hepatic dysfunction and concomitant medications that are potent inhibitors of the CYP3A4 pathway (e.g., azole antifungals, macrolides).

e. Combination therapy. Calcium channel blockers or long-acting nitrates given with beta-blockers may provide greater antianginal effects than when used independently. (SOR **B**) Combination therapy may be considered when initial therapy with beta-blockers is unsuccessful. Calcium antagonists and nitrates can be used in combination therapy and substituted for beta-blockers as initial treatment in patients who cannot tolerate beta-blockers. (SOR **C**) Calcium channel antagonists (in particular, the nondihydropyridines verapamil and diltiazem) and beta-blockers

TABLE 79–3. ANTIANGINAL MEDICATIONS

Drug	Usual Statin Dose	Max Daily Dose	Common Adverse Effects	Drug Interactionsa	Comments
Beta-Blockers—Non-Cardioselective					
Propranolol	20 mg four times daily	320 mg/d divided twice daily to four times daily	Fatigue (dose-related), dizziness, exacerbation of bronchospasm, bradycardia, AV conduction defects, left ventricular failure	Thioridazine (QT prolongation, cardiac arrest); fluoxetine, amiodarone (bradycardia, cardiac arrest, heart block); calcium channel blockers (bradycardia, AV conduction disturbances); beta-2-agonists (bronchospasm); antidiabetic agents (hypo- or hyperglycemia)	Beta-blockers are particularly useful in treating the following conditions that occur with IHD: hypertension, ventricular arrhythmia, supraventricular arrhythmias
Propranolol (Long acting)	80 mg/d	320 mg/d			
Nadolol	40 mg/d	240 mg/d	Fatigue (dose-related), dizziness, Raynaud phenomenon, impotence, nightmares, mild increase in lipids; may block symptoms of hypoglycemia	Amiodarone (bradycardia, cardiac arrest, heart block); calcium channel blockers (bradycardia, AV conduction disturbances); beta-2-agonists (bronchospasm); antidiabetic agents (hypo- or hyperglycemia)	There is no advantage in using a beta-blocker with ISA or alpha₁-sympathomimetic blockade. Cardioselectivity will be overcome as the dose is raised. Abrupt discontinuation may exacerbate angina.
Carvedilol	6.25 mg twice daily	25–50 mg twice daily	Dizziness, hypotension, erectile dysfunction, edema, weight gain, diarrhea, hyperglycemia, bradycardia, AV block	See nadolol	Consider in post-MI with LVEF ≤40%. May titrate after 3–7 d. Monitor for fluid retention, bradycardia, or hypotension
Carvedilol (extended release)	20 mg/d × 3–10 d	80 mg/d			
Beta Blockers—Cardioselective					
Atenolol	25–50 mg/d	100 mg/d	Hypotension, fatigue, dizziness, depression, cold extremities, bradycardia	See nadolol	
Metoprolol Tartrate	50 mg twice daily	400 mg/d	Hypotension, fatigue, dizziness, heart failure, bradycardia, dyspnea, depression	See nadolol	
Metoprolol Succinate	100 mg/d	400 mg/d	fatigue, dizziness, bradycardia, dyspnea, depression	See nadolol	

Calcium Channel Blockers—Short-Acting Formulations

Drug					
Diltiazem	30 mg four times daily	360 mg/d divided three to four times daily	Edema, headache, fatigue, dizziness, bradycardia	Erythromycin, cisapride (QT prolongation); colchicine (colchicine toxicity); statins (myopathy); clopidogrel (↓ antiplatelet effect); amiodarone (AV block, bradycardia)	Useful in treating IHD, hypertension, and supra-ventricular arrhythmias; may be drugs of choice in vasospastic (Prinzmetal) angina. All calcium channel blockers may induce hypotension; it is important to titrate the dose, especially in the elderly
				Use caution with combined use of beta-blockers or digitalis (exacerbation of CHF or conduction delays)	
Verapamil	80–120 mg three to four times daily	480 mg/d	Constipation, headache, dizziness, edema, sinusitis/pharyngitis, hypotension	Digoxin (dig toxicity); statins (myopathy); erythromycin (prolonged QT); amiodarone (AV block, bradycardia); clopidogrel (↓ antiplatelet effect)	

Calcium Channel Blockers—Long-Acting Formulations

Drug					
Diltiazem	120–180 mg/d	360–480 mg/d	As above	As above	Dosage may vary by brand and formulation
Nifedipine	30–60 mg/d	120 mg/d	Edema, headache, dizziness, flushing, nausea, palpitations, nervousness	Clopidogrel (↓ antiplatelet effect); fentanyl (severe hypotension); amiodarone (bradycardia, AV block); clarithromycin (hypotension, bradycardia); cimetidine (edema, tachycardia); fluconazole (dizziness, edema); NSAIDs (GI bleeding)	Caution with doses ≥90 mg when treating angina
Verapamil	180 mg/d	480 mg/d	See above	See nifedipine	See nifedipine

Second-Generation Calcium Channel Blockers (Dihydropyridines)

Drug					
Amlodipine	2.5–5 mg/d	10 mg/d	Edema, palpitations, dizziness, flushing, headache	See nifedipine	Plasma T½ 36 h, little negative inotropic effect, may be useful in treatment of angina and hypertension
					Use lowest dose in elderly and those with hepatic dysfunction
Felodipine (Off-label use)	2.5–5 mg/day	10 mg/day	Edema, headache, flushing, GI upset, URI	Itraconazole, cyclosporine (cardiotoxicity); amiodarone (bradycardia, AV block); clopidogrel (↓ anti-platelet effect); fluconazole (edema, dizziness); NSAIDs (GI bleeding)	

(continued)

TABLE 79–3. ANTIANGINAL MEDICATIONS (Continued)

Drug	Usual Statin Dose	Max Daily Dose	Common Adverse Effects	Drug Interactions[a]	Comments
Nitrates—Short-Acting Nitroglycerin					
Nitrostat	0.4 mg every 5 min ×3		Headache, dizziness, hypotension; potential for hypotension greater when used in combination with a calcium channel blocker	Phosphodiesterase-5 enzyme inhibitors (severe hypotension)	Tolerance is the most significant issue in the use of nitrates. Oral nitrates are more effective, given twice daily at a high dose than more frequently at a low dose
Nitrospray	400 µg one to two sprays every 5 min ×3				
Nitrates—Long-Acting Nitroglycerin					
Transderm NTG patch	0.2–0.4 mg/h for 12–14 h	0.8 mg/h	See above	Phosphodiesterase-5 enzyme inhibitors (severe hypotension); aspirin (additive anti-platelet effect)	Long-acting nitrates should not be used for acute anginal attacks. Nitroglycerin patches should be removed at night to prevent tolerance. Nitrates work well with either beta-blockers or calcium channel blockers
Isosorbide Dinitrate					
Immediate-release	5–20 mg two to three times daily	160 mg	Headache, dizziness, hypotension	Phosphodiesterase-5 enzyme inhibitors (severe hypotension)	Elderly start at lower dose; allow 14-h, dose-free interval
Extended-release	40 mg once or twice daily	160 mg		Caution in patients taking medications for erectile dysfunction; potential hypotension	Allow 18-h, dose-free interval. Severe hypotension may result
Isosorbide Mononitrate					
Immediate-release	20 mg twice daily		Headache, dizziness	Phosphodiesterase-5 enzyme inhibitors (severe hypotension)	First dose on awakening and then 7 h later
Extended-release	30–60 mg/d	120–240 mg/d			
Other					
Ranolazine	500 mg twice daily	1000 mg twice daily	Dizziness, headache, constipation, nausea, bradycardia, hypotension	Rifampin, carbamazepine, phenytoin (↓ ranolazine effect); oral azole antifungals, clarithromycin (QT prolongation)	Contraindicated in hepatic cirrhosis. Not to be used in acute attacks

[a]Beta-blockers, calcium channel blockers, and ranolazine have multiple drug interactions.

AV, atrioventricular; CHF, congestive heart failure; IHD, ischemic heart disease; ISA, intrinsic sympathomimetic activity; NSAIDs, nonsteroidal anti-inflammatory drugs; URI, upper respiratory infection.

in combination should be used with caution because of the increased risk of extreme bradycardia or heart block. Ranolazine may be used in combination with beta-blockers when treatment with a beta-blocker alone is insufficient to relieve symptoms. (SOR **B**)

5. **Renin–Angiotensin–Aldosterone Blocker Therapy.** Studies such as the Heart Outcomes Prevention Evaluation (HOPE) trial have suggested that use of an angiotensin-converting enzyme (ACE) inhibitor substantially lowers the risk of death, MI, stroke, coronary revascularization, and heart failure in high-risk patients with preexisting vascular disease. ACE inhibition may have vasculoprotective effects. ACE inhibitors should be considered in all patients with IHD who also have hypertension, CKD, diabetes, or LVEF ≤40%. (SOR **A**) For those who are unable to tolerate ACE inhibitors, angiotensin II receptor blockers (ARBs) may be considered. (SOR **A**).

6. **Antioxidants.** Oxidized low-density lipoprotein particles are implicated in the development and progression of atherosclerosis. Recent studies have found **no benefit** of vitamin C or E or beta-carotene supplementation with regard to mortality, MI, and cardiovascular events. (SOR **A**)

7. **Vitamins B₆ and B₁₂ and folate.** Elevated homocysteine levels are associated with IHD. Although the mechanisms are not well understood, alteration in coagulation profile or endothelial damage is postulated to play a role. Supplementation with vitamins B_6 and B_{12} and folate reduce plasma homocysteine levels; however, these reductions have not been found to decrease risk or reduce mortality in IHD. (SOR **A**)

8. **Other therapies.** Chelation therapy, garlic, coenzyme Q10, selenium, or chromium supplements have not been found to reduce CVD risk or prevent IHD mortality. (SOR **C**) **Enhanced external counterpulsation** (SOR **B**), **spinal cord stimulation** (SOR **C**), or **transmyocardial revascularization** (SOR **B**) may be considered to relieve anginal symptoms in those refractory to medical therapy. **Acupuncture** has not been found to be of benefit in either symptom or risk reduction. (SOR **C**)

B. **Unstable angina (UA)** manifests clinically as an abrupt onset of ischemic symptoms at rest or as an intensification or change in the pattern of ischemic symptoms as well as an increasing ease of provocation (symptoms at rest or with minimal effort). Acute management for UA as well as for NSTEMI includes **hospitalization; bed rest with continuous ECG monitoring; aspirin (ASA); NTG; supplemental oxygenation; morphine sulfate, if anginal symptoms persist despite NTG; and a beta-blocker, unless contraindicated**. Clopidogrel may be considered in patients with UA who have contraindications to ASA including hypersensitivity and gastrointestinal side effects. (SOR **A**) Anticoagulation may also be considered per the 2012 ACC guidelines.

1. **Initial invasive management.** The ACC 2012 guidelines for the management of UA/NSTEMI recommend **work-up via angiography and treatment with revascularization, if indicated, for high-risk patients**. High-risk patients are those who present with any of the following:

   a. Recurrent pain at rest or with minimal activity despite medical therapy
   b. Elevated troponin I or T
   c. New ST segment depression
   d. Angina with congestive heart failure symptoms, S_3 gallop, pulmonary edema, or new or worsening mitral regurgitation
   e. High-risk findings on noninvasive stress testing
   f. Ejection fraction of 40% or less
   g. Hypotension/hemodynamic instability
   h. Sustained ventricular tachycardia
   i. Percutaneous coronary intervention within the past 6 months
   j. Prior coronary artery bypass grafting
   k. Mild-to-moderate renal disease
   l. Type II diabetes mellitus
   m. An elevated risk stratification score (such as the thrombolysis in MI [TIMI]) (http://www.mdcalc.com/timi-risk-score-for-uanstemi/).

2. **Initial conservative management.** Patients without the above high-risk features and in consideration of patient and physician preferences are candidates for initial conservative management. This includes medication management and noninvasive procedures (i.e., echocardiogram, stress test) to further identify those who may benefit from angiography and possibly revascularization (recurrent ischemia at rest or on a noninvasive stress test).

C. **Revascularization.** Techniques of coronary revascularization include **coronary artery bypass graft (CABG) surgery and percutaneous coronary interventions (PCIs)**. PCIs include percutaneous transluminal coronary angioplasty (PTCA) and stenting. **Indications** for CABG versus PCI depend on the anatomy involved, patient surgical or procedural risk, and the likelihood of a positive long-term outcome. Revascularization may be performed to improve survival or for symptomatic relief. Patients with <50% left main or <70% nonleft main stenosis should generally not be considered for revascularization. A more indepth discussion of the indications for revascularization are discussed in the ACC guidelines.

1. **CABG surgery** is indicated to improve survival in significant (≥50% stenosis) left main coronary artery disease, three-vessel disease (≥70% stenosis), or two-vessel disease with significant proximal left anterior descending involvement. (SOR ❸) CABG surgery may also be preferred over PCI for patients with diabetes and multivessel disease. (SOR ❸) Large randomized trials have shown that for patients in whom CABG is indicated, CABG surgery provides better symptom relief, improved exercise tolerance, and decreased need for antianginal medications at 5 years when compared with medication management. After CABG, patients also have fewer repeat revascularization procedures when compared with PCI.

   a. Development of atherosclerosis in the graft resulting in angina generally occurs within 5 to 10 years.

2. General indications for PCI include symptom improvement in patients with single- or double-vessel disease, excluding the proximal left anterior descending coronary artery. The survival benefit of PCI in proximal LAD, two- or three-vessel disease is uncertain. (SOR ❸) Restenosis after PTCA continues to be a complication; however, the long-term outcome after successful angioplasty has been reported to be excellent even when compared with patients undergoing bypass surgery. Stenting has become the most widely used PCI because of less associated closure and restenosis compared with PTCA.

   a. Use of antithrombotic medications such as IIb/IIIa inhibitors and antiplatelet P2Y12 inhibitors (i.e., clopidogrel) has improved short- as well as long-term outcomes following PCI.

V. **Prognosis**

A. **Severity** of cardiac disease as determined by LV function, the amount of viable but jeopardized left ventricular myocardium, the percentage of irreversibly scarred myocardium, and the severity of underlying coronary atherosclerosis (location and degree of stenosis) are predictors of prognosis in conjunction with clinical patient characteristics. ETT has been used to establish the prognosis in patients with symptomatic IHD. The exercise parameters associated with poor outcome have been described earlier.

B. The **natural history** of IHD is one of slow disease progression cycling between asymptomatic, stable angina, worsening angina, and ACS phases. Multiple factors may be considered in estimating the risk of death or future nonfatal MI. Age is the strongest determinant of survival and functional limitation resulting from angina is second.

C. **Higher risk of complications** is seen in patients with cardiovascular risk factors (smoking, hypertension, dyslipidemia, a family history of premature CAD, sedentary lifestyle, and obesity) as well as coexisting medical conditions (type 2 diabetes mellitus, CKD, COPD, malignancy, peripheral artery disease, cerebrovascular disease, and heart failure).

D. Coexisting depression or anxiety in addition to poverty, stress, and lack of social support has also been implicated in worse prognosis.

E. Prior to the routine use of aspirin, beta-blockers, and aggressive risk factor modification, the average annual mortality for patients with stable IHD was 4%. **Annual mortality with optimal medical therapy and lifestyle changes** is 1% to 3% with a 1% to 2% rate of major ischemic events.

F. **CABG or PCI versus medical management**

   a. For patients who have undergone CABG surgery, approximately 75% can be predicted to be free from symptom recurrence, ischemic events, or sudden death after 5 years. Approximately 50% remain free after 10 years, and approximately 15% remain well after 15 years. Improved survival with CABG surgery versus medical therapy is seen only in the "sicker" subset of patients who are older and have more severe symptoms, particularly left main coronary artery disease, multivessel disease with left ventricular dysfunction or triple vessel disease including the left proximal LAD.

   b. The 2007 Clinical Outcomes Utilizing Revascularization and Aggressive Drug Evaluation (COURAGE) trial suggests that although PCI has been demonstrated to reduce death and MI in patients with ACS, for patients with chronic coronary artery disease, PCI does not reduce the incidence of death or MI compared to medical management alone.

SELECTED REFERENCES

Agency for Healthcare Research and Quality (AHRQ). *The Guide to Clinical Preventive Services: Recommendations of the U.S. Preventive Services Task Force.* Washington, DC: Agency for Healthcare Research and Quality; AHRQ Publication Number 06-0588; 2006.

Boden WE, O'Rourke RA, Teo KK, et al.; COURAGE Trial Research Group. Optimal medical therapy with or without PCI for stable coronary disease. *N Engl J Med.* 2007;356(15):1503–1516.

Bonow RO, Mann DL, Zipes DP, et al. *Braunwald's Heart Disease: a textbook of cardiovascular medicine.* 9th ed. Philadelphia, PA: Saunders; 2011.

Fihn S, Gardin JM, Abrams J, et al. 2012 ACCF/AHA/ACP/AATS/PCNA/SCAI/STS Guideline for the diagnosis and management of patients with stable ischemic heart disease. *J Am Coll Cardiol.* 2012; 60(24):e44–e164.

Levine G, Bates ER, Blankenship JC, et al. 2011 ACCF/AHA/SCAI Guideline for percutaneous coronary intervention: executive summary. *J Am Coll Cardiol.* 2011;58(24):2550–2583.

Longo DL, Fauci AS, Kasper DL, et al. *Harrison's Principles of Internal Medicine.* 18th ed. New York, NY: McGraw Hill; 2011.

Rogers PE, Green LA. Chest pain. In: PSloane PD, Slatt LM, Ebell MH, et al., eds. *Essentials of Family Medicine.* 6th ed. Philadelphia, PA: Lippincott, Williams & Wilkins; 2012:99–111.

Shu de F, Dong BR, Lin XF, et al. Long-term beta blockers for stable angina: systematic review and meta-analysis. *Eur J Prev Cardiol.* 2012;19(3):330–341.

Smith SC Jr, Benjamin EJ, Bonow RO, et al. AHA/ACCF Secondary prevention and risk reduction therapy for patients with coronary and other atherosclerotic vascular disease: 2011 updated. *J Am Coll Cardiol.* 2011;58(23):2432–2446.

---

80   Menopause

Linda M. Speer, MD, Tammy J. Lindsay, MD, & Mark Mengel, MD, MPH

KEY POINTS

- Menopause, and the perimenopausal period, is the natural transition from the reproductive years. It usually presents with a progressive lengthening of the menstrual cycle with irregular menses, hot flashes, and sleep disruption. Menopause is confirmed when no menses have occurred for 12 consecutive months. (SOR **C**)
- A person's cultural preconceptions in large part determine the general attitude, approach, and, therefore, smoothness by which this aging process occurs. (SOR **C**)
- Diagnostic testing is rarely indicated in women who are at an age when menopause is expected; however, in younger menopausal women and women on hormonal contraception, determination of a follicle-stimulating hormone (FSH) level may be warranted. (SOR **C**) Menopause is indicated by an FSH level of ≥30 mIU/mL.
- Menopause is associated with changes in many organ systems including the skin, reproductive system, and bones. (SOR **C**)
- In postmenopausal women with debilitating symptoms at menopause, short-term use (less than 5 years) of hormone therapy is appropriate, but long-term use to prevent chronic disease is no longer deemed acceptable. (SOR **A**)
- Certain drugs (e.g., clonidine, gabapentin, paroxetine, venlafaxine) have been shown to be modestly effective in reducing menopausal hot flashes. (SOR **B**)
- As women rapidly lose bone density once reproductive hormone secretion ceases, osteoporosis risk factor reduction, regular weight-bearing exercise, adequate intake of vitamin D and dietary calcium, and routine use of bone density testing are indicated. (SOR **A**)

I. Introduction

A. Definitions. Menopause is the permanent cessation of menstruation caused by a loss of ovarian function. This condition is traditionally defined in retrospect after 12 consecutive months of amenorrhea. **Perimenopause** is the transitional period between regular menstrual cycles and including the year after the last menstrual period when the condition is confirmed. **Postmenopausal** is the term applied to the stage of life that involves all of the years a woman spends after menopause. **Premature menopause** or primary ovarian insufficiency is menopause that occurs before the age of 40 years.

B. Epidemiology

1. Between 0.2% and 1% of visits made to primary care physicians are for menopausal symptoms.

2. The mean age of menopause is 51 years, with a range of 41 to 59 years. Current smoking is a risk factor associated with an earlier age of menopause. Other factors that may play an important role include a family history of early menopause, nulliparity, and having a history of heart disease or type 1 diabetes mellitus. By 55 years of age, 95% of women are menopausal.

3. Disabling symptoms attributable to a decline in estrogen production for which medical therapy is sought are estimated to occur in 10% to 15% of perimenopausal women. Current smoking and high body mass index are risk factors associated with the frequency and severity of hot flashes.

C. Pathophysiology. Menopause occurs with the depletion of ovarian follicles, which are the major source of estrogen production in women during their reproductive life. Levels of follicle-stimulating hormone (FSH) typically fluctuate during the years prior to menopause as do estrogen levels. After the last menstrual period, there is a sustained increase in FSH level to at least 30 mUI/mL, and often above 60 mUI/mL. Plasma estradiol declines to negligible levels after menopause. Many end-organ changes occur as a result of declining or absent circulating estrogen levels (Table 80–1).

II. Diagnosis

A. Symptoms and signs. Most women, in their late reproductive years, experience a gradual shortening of the menstrual cycle with lighter menses corresponding to a shortening of the luteal phase. Irregular periods, caused by anovulation, precede menopause for 1 to 7 years in most women. Bleeding may be heavy during this time.

1. **Vasomotor symptoms.** The hot flash and the flush are the two principal components of vasomotor symptomatology. Researchers believe that alterations in the

TABLE 80–1. END-ORGAN CHANGES RESULTING FROM ESTROGEN DEFICIENCY

Target Organ	Change or Symptom
Neuroendocrine organs (hypothalamus)	Hot flushes, flashes, or both Atrophy, dryness, pruritus
Skin/mucous membranes	Dry hair or loss of hair Facial hirsutism Dry mouth
Skeleton	Osteoporosis with related fractures Backache
Vocal cords	Lower voice
Breasts	Reduced size Softer consistency Drooping (loss of ligamentous support)
Heart	Coronary artery disease
Vulva	Atrophy, dystrophy, or both Pruritus vulvae
Vagina	Dyspareunia Vaginitis
Uterus/pelvic floor	Uterovaginal prolapse
Bladder/urethra	Cystourethritis Urethral prolapse (caruncle) Frequency and/or urgency Stress incontinence

Source: Adapted with permission from Utian WH. Overview on menopause. *Am J Obstet Gynecol.* 1987;156:1280.

hypothalamic set point because of estrogen withdrawal are responsible for the flush. Patients with such disorders as pheochromocytoma, hyperthyroidism, anxiety, excessive caffeine intake, hypoglycemia, and carcinoid syndrome usually present with vasomotor symptomatology in combination with other conditions such as hypertension, tachycardia, and diarrhea. The presence of such concomitant conditions suggests a nonmenopausal origin. When left untreated, vasomotor symptoms are usually most intense and frequent in the year following the last menstrual period before definitive diagnosis of menopause, after which severity gradually declines. On average, vasomotor symptoms will last 4 years. However, 25% of women report a duration of more than 5 years, and about 10% of women continue to have at least occasional symptoms for the rest of their lives.

    a. The **hot flash** is the sudden onset of warmth lasting 2 to 3 minutes. Experienced by 75% to 85% of menopausal women, the hot flash begins approximately 1 minute before the flush and lasts approximately 1 minute after its onset.

    b. The **flush** consists of visible redness of the upper chest, face, and neck and is followed by profuse sweating. The flush also lasts 2 to 3 minutes and is associated with a mean temperature elevation of 2.5°C (4.5°F).

    c. **Associated symptoms** commonly reported with the above vasomotor phenomena are heart palpitations, headache, throbbing in the head or neck, and nausea. Sleep disruption often occurs as a consequence because of the frequent nocturnal timing. Stressful situations are also a documented trigger for perimenopausal vasomotor symptoms.

2. Psychological symptoms. All of the following symptoms have been reported during the perimenopausal period: fatigue, insomnia, anxiety, and depression. Although dysphoria is associated with low estrogen states such as the days prior to menses and postpartum, studies do not support menopause causing depression. Sleep deprivation and possibly many life changes (children leaving, retirement, aging parents) likely contribute to the mood fluctuations more than menopause. (SOR ❸)

3. Lower genital symptoms

    a. **Vulvar pruritus** is common, especially in fair-skinned women.

    b. **Vaginal dryness and dyspareunia** from atrophy of vaginal mucosa are increasingly common over time after menopause. Symptoms also may include burning, leukorrhea, itching, and bleeding.

    c. **Urethral symptoms,** although less common, include frank urethritis, dysuria, urgency, and frequency. Urinary tract infection is more common during this life stage.

4. Signs. The physical examination is usually normal during the early perimenopausal period, with characteristic findings evident after the onset of menopause, when the estrogen loss becomes sustained.

    a. The **breasts** appear less firm and smaller, with a regression of glandular tissue and an increase in fatty tissue.

    b. The **pelvic examination** is most revealing in the postmenopausal period.

        (1) The **labia majora** are smaller and hair in the perivulvar area is thin.

        (2) The **vaginal epithelium** appears pale, thin, and dry, with a loss of rugae and secretions.

        (3) The **cervical os** is often smaller and may be stenotic. The cervical epithelium is thinner and more easily traumatized.

    c. **Uterine size** is diminished. Reduced collagen in the supporting ligamentous structures of the pelvis can lead to uterine prolapse and pelvic relaxation. This relaxation occurs especially when there is a history of multiparity, prior birth trauma, a family history of uterine prolapse or pelvic relaxation, or chronic pelvic stress from coughing, constipation, or heavy work. Pelvic laxity often contributes to urinary incontinence.

    d. The **ovaries** should not be palpable after menopause. Palpable ovarian enlargement in a menopausal woman suggests ovarian carcinoma until proven otherwise.

    e. **Urethral prolapse** can occur due to atrophy of the urethral mucosa. A prolapsed urethra or caruncle appears as a red, friable mass within the urethra itself.

    f. **Dry, wrinkled, and more easily traumatized skin** is attributable to both menopause and aging. Thinning of scalp hair and increased facial hair (hirsutism) may also be evident.

B. Laboratory tests. The presence of vasomotor symptoms, oligomenorrhea, and atrophy of the lower genital tract in women older than 45 years almost certainly confirms the onset of the perimenopausal period. Diagnostic testing (e.g., circulating estrogen and gonadotropin levels) is rarely, if ever, indicated in this circumstance.

1. **A complete evaluation for premature ovarian failure is warranted in any woman younger than 40 years experiencing signs and symptoms of menopause.** Specific causes of premature ovarian failure include genetic abnormalities, autoimmune disorders, and rare hormonal defects (see Chapter 3). FSH levels are the most sensitive indicator of ovarian failure. Menopausal status is suggested by FSH level ≥30 mIU/mL. As FSH levels are highly variable in the perimenopause, levels should be confirmed by a second test 1 to 3 months later. For women on cyclic oral contraceptives, testing should be performed at the end of the week off active pills. Alternatively, oral contraceptives (OCs) or extended cycle products can be stopped for at least 10 days prior to testing and an alternate means of birth control used.

2. Estradiol and progesterone are not reliably measured by single assays in perimenopausal women.

III. Treatment. The Women's Health Initiative (WHI) trial and Heart Estrogen/Progestin Replacement Study (HERS) findings have dramatically changed the use of hormone therapy (HT) in postmenopausal women. (The WHI was a primary prevention trial in postmenopausal women; the HERS was a secondary prevention trial in postmenopausal women with coronary artery disease.) Both studies showed that the long-term risks of oral synthetic estrogen/medroxyprogesterone as HT outweighed the benefits.

In a meta-analysis of nine studies, of which the largest were the WHI and HERS, investigators found that **for every 10,000 women treated per year,** there were more women with the following:

- **Women using combination HT,** *Harms:* Incontinence: 872 more; Dementia: 22 more; Gallbladder disease: 20 more; Deep vein thrombosis: 12 more; Pulmonary embolus: 9 more; Stroke: 9 more; Breast cancer: 8 more; and Lung cancer: 5 more. *Benefit:* 46 fewer fractures

- **Women using estrogen only,** *Harms:* Incontinence: 1271 more; Gallbladder disease: 33 more Stroke: 11 more; Deep vein thrombosis: 7 more. *Benefits:* Fractures: 56 fewer; Breast cancer: 8 fewer.

However, given that the average age of women in both the WHI and HERS trials was older than 60 years and that many had risk factors for coronary artery disease, it is likely that younger women without any risk factors would have less risk of harm. Therefore, in postmenopausal women with debilitating symptoms of menopause, short-term use of hormone replacement therapy is appropriate. (SOR **A**)

Protection from osteoporotic fractures is quickly lost after HT is stopped, which limits its use for that purpose. In addition, the risk–benefit ratio is better for other antiresorptive medications used to prevent and/or treat osteoporosis (see Chapter 83).

A. Indications for menopausal HT
1. Moderate to severe vasomotor symptoms.
2. Moderate to severe genital atrophy.
3. Diminished quality of life secondary to menopausal symptoms.

B. Contraindications to menopausal HT
1. Estrogen-dependent neoplasia (breast or endometrium).
2. Undiagnosed vaginal bleeding.
3. Past history of venous thromboembolism (deep venous thrombus, pulmonary embolus)
4. Past history of arterial thromboembolism (cerebral vascular accident or coronary artery disease).
5. Liver disease.
6. Caution, if several cardiovascular risk factors such as hypertension, hyperlipidemia, tobacco abuse, and diabetes mellitus are present.
7. Caution, if gallbladder disease is present.
8. Caution, if age is above 65 years.

C. Preparations available. Estrogen is available as an oral tablet, transdermal patch, topical gel and emulsion, and vaginal ring, cream, and tablet.
1. **Tablets.** The oldest available and most widely prescribed oral estrogen preparation is equine conjugated estrogen (Premarin), 0.30 to 2.5 mg orally every day. The typical starting dose is 0.625 mg; however, lower doses of 0.45 and 0.3 mg are proving to be effective for vasomotor symptoms in many women. (SOR **A**) Synthetic conjugated estrogen (Cenestin), 0.3 to 1.25 mg orally daily; esterified estrogen (Menest), 0.3 to 2.5 mg orally daily; micronized estradiol (Estrace and Gynodiol), 0.5 mg to 2 mg orally daily; ethinyl estradiol (Estinyl), 0.02 to 0.05 mg orally daily; and estropipate (Ogen or Ortho-Est), 0.75 to 3 mg orally daily, are also available. Many women

prefer the nonequine varieties of estrogen, fearing the effects of the metabolic breakdown products of that preparation.

2. **Transdermal patches.** Transdermal estradiol patches are available at a dose of 25 to 100 µg daily. Many preparations are available including Climara and Menostar (both one patch weekly), and Estraderm, Alora, Vivelle, Vivelle-Dot, and Esclim (all one patch twice weekly). Transdermal estrogen has been consistently associated with lower risk of thromboembolism. (SOR **B**) Unfortunately, approximately 24% of women who use this method have some form of skin irritation, which often can be managed by site rotation.

3. **Vaginal rings.** An estradiol acetate vaginal ring (Femring) is available in doses of 50 and 100 µg daily. Femring lasts for 90 days and has systemic effects. Estring is a vaginal ring that provides 7.5 µg/day of estradiol, a very low dose, and is used only for treating vaginal symptoms.

4. **Topical gel and emulsion.** Estradiol can also be given topically in a gel form (Estrogel 0.75 mg/pump or Divigel 0.25, 0.5 or 1.0 mg/g in 1g packets), applied to the arms, and in an emulsion form (Estrasorb), 2.5 mg/pouch, one pouch applied to each leg daily.

5. **Vaginal creams** are most useful for women with moderate-to-severe symptoms of atopic vaginitis, but who have mild vasomotor symptoms or prefer not to treat these symptoms with HT. Intravaginal creams, such as conjugated estrogen (Premarin), 0.625 mg/g, and estradiol (Estrace vaginal cream), 0.1 mg/g, can be helpful. For moderate-to-severe vaginal atrophy, the initial dose of vaginal cream is 2 to 4 g (contains 0.1 mg/g estradiol) vaginally daily for 1 to 2 weeks, gradually reduced to 50% of initial dose for 1 to 2 weeks. Maintenance of 1 g one to three times a week is adjusted to the dose needed to control symptoms. Intravaginal estrogen creams achieve some absorption resulting in systemic exposure, depending on the dose.

   a. **Vulvovaginal pruritus** may not respond to topical estrogens. Other treatments may be more helpful such as cotton underwear, adequate drying, loose fitting clothing, and steroid creams such as clobetasol propionate titrated to the lowest effective dose. (SOR **A**) Testosterone ointment is no longer recommended. (SOR **B**)

D. **Progestins** have been shown to relieve vasomotor symptoms in postmenopausal patients either alone or in combination with estrogens. They are also useful in preventing endometrial hyperplasia in women on HT. (SOR **A**)

1. **Progestin-only regimens.** Progestin-only treatment may be appealing for women with contraindications to estrogen therapy or who have experienced intolerable side effects such as breast tenderness, breakthrough bleeding, and nausea on estrogen therapy. Preparations include micronized progesterone (Prometrium) 100 to 200 mg daily, and norethindrone acetate (Aygestin). Caution with the use of medroxyprogesterone (Provera) due to an increased risk for breast cancer.

2. **Combination estrogen and progestin therapy.** Estrogen replacement alone may lead to endometrial hyperplasia in some women (fivefold increased risk after 3 years of use) that can progress to endometrial carcinoma. Maximal protection against endometrial hyperplasia occurs when a progestin is prescribed for at least 10 days of each calendar month. Because that regimen usually results in periods continuing, continuous low-dose daily combination therapy is often preferred.

   a. There are several options available. In tablet form, synthetic estrogen and medroxyprogesterone are combined in two different options, Prempro (continuous) and Premphase (cyclic). Prempro is available in multiple dosing options 0.3 to 1.5 mg, 0.45 to 1.5 mg, 0.625 to 2.5 mg, and 0.625 to 5 mg. Other options include ethinyl estradiol, norethindrone acetate (FemHRT), estradiol, norgestimate (Ortho-Prefest), and estradiol, norethindrone (Activella). Combination patch therapy is also available as estradiol, norethindrone acetate (CombiPatch), and estradiol, levonorgestrel (Climara Pro). Combined therapy using oral micronized progesterone is associated with no greater risk of breast cancer than in nonusers. (SOR **B**)

   b. All women with an intact uterus who use systemic estrogen should also be prescribed adequate progestin. A progestin is generally not indicated when estrogen therapy is administered intermittently (i.e., two to three times per week or less frequently) vaginally for vaginal atrophy or transdermally at the ultralow dose approved for the prevention of bone loss. Nonsystemic forms are low-dose vaginal cream, low-dose vaginal ring (Estring), and ultralow-dose Climara Pro Transdermal patch (0.045 mg per day 17-beta estradiol and 0.015 mg levonorgestrel); the ultralow-dose patch is not associated with endometrial hyperplasia.

    c. Progestin use for women who have had a hysterectomy and are receiving estrogen replacement therapy is not indicated. (SOR **Ⓐ**)

E. Effective nonhormonal treatments for menopausal symptoms. Given the results of the WHI and HERS studies noting adverse effects of HT, nonhormonal treatments for menopausal symptoms have become more popular. Women often discontinue these treatments, however, due to side effects.

    1. Treatments with some evidence for effectiveness include (SOR **Ⓑ** for all):

        a. Clonidine (Catapres), 0.1 to 0.2 mg per day

        b. Gabapentin (Neurontin), 300 mg orally three times daily

        c. Selective serotonin reuptake inhibitors (SSRIs) including paroxetine (Paxil), 10 to 25 mg orally daily; fluoxetine (Prozac), 20 mg orally daily; citalopram (Celexa), 10 mg orally daily; and sertraline (Zoloft), 50 mg orally daily

        d. Serotonin and norepinephrine reuptake inhibitors (SNRIs) venlafaxine (Effexor), 37.5 to 75 mg orally daily and desvenlafaxine (Pristiq), 100 mg orally daily

    2. In comparison to HT (estrogen-containing) which reduces hot flashes by 80% to 90%, gabapentin and the SSRIs and SNRIs have shown a reduction of about 60% compared to a placebo-response of 25%.

        a. The North American Menopause Society (NAMS) and American Congress of Obstetricians and Gynecologists both recommend the use of venlafaxine, paroxetine, and fluoxetine; venlafaxine and paroxetine appear to be more efficacious than fluoxetine and sertraline. Benefit can be seen after about 4 weeks of therapy.

        b. Paroxetine and fluoxetine, both potent inhibitors of CYP2D6, are **contraindicated** for women using tamoxifen as they reduce the production of the active metabolite of tamoxifen and can decrease its benefit in cancer protection.

F. Selective estrogen-receptor modulators. Raloxifene, 60 mg orally every day, a drug that has both estrogen-agonist effects on the bone, liver, and heart and estrogen-antagonist effects on the breast and uterus has been shown to reduce risks of breast cancer and osteoporosis in postmenopausal women. These effects make raloxifene an attractive alternative for those women concerned with estrogen's potential for cancer proliferation. Unfortunately, raloxifene has no effect on genital atrophy and may worsen the vasomotor symptoms of hot flashes and sweats. Like estrogen, the incidence of thrombophlebitis is increased compared with placebo.

G. Complementary and alternative medicine treatments

    1. Black cohosh has been demonstrated **not** to work in a well-designed randomized controlled trial but has limited side effects. (SOR **Ⓑ**)

    2. Soy and isoflavones studies have had conflicting results.

    3. Regular exercise has proven ineffective in one well-designed trial for hot flash prevention. (SOR **Ⓑ**) However, exercise should be recommended for peri- and postmenopausal women for its established health benefits.

    4. Dong quai, red clover, and ginseng have been demonstrated to be ineffective. (SOR **Ⓑ**) Wild yams are promoted as a "natural" precursor to hormones, but are not converted to reproductive hormones in the human body and have not proven more effective than placebo in one small trial. (SOR **Ⓑ**)

    5. Bioidentical hormone replacement. "Antiaging" advocates sometimes promote the use of bioidentical or natural estrogen, progestin, and testosterone replacement, with the belief that natural hormone replacement lacks the risks and side effects of synthetic hormone replacement. Saliva testing is often recommended to titrate dosing. However, compounded estrogen and progesterone have not been shown to be more effective or to have fewer side effects than other commercially available products, and saliva levels are not well correlated with serum hormone levels. The NAMS "does not recommend custom-compounded products over well-tested, government-approved proved products for the majority of women, and does not recommend saliva testing to determine hormone levels." (SOR **Ⓒ**)

IV. Management Strategies

    A. Patient education. For many women, the worst thing about menopause is not knowing what to expect. Thorough evaluation of the woman's understanding of menopause and accurate education directed at identification of symptoms and management options will greatly reduce anxiety in many postmenopausal women. Many myths surround menopause, including that menopause signals the end of a woman's sexual experience and that menopause is associated with a high incidence of mental health problems, cancer, and heart disease. Risk factor reduction for heart disease and cancer, a discussion

TABLE 80–2. KEY QUESTIONS TO UNCOVER SEXUAL PROBLEMS DURING THE PERIMENOPAUSAL AND POSTMENOPAUSAL PERIODS

Are you sexually active?
Do you have a partner at the present time?
Has there been any change in your interest in or desire for sexual activity?
Is intercourse pleasurable?
Do you experience any discomfort during intercourse?
Have you noticed any change in lubrication when you become aroused?
Do you reach orgasm satisfactorily?
Does your partner have any problems with your sexual relationship?

Source: Adapted with permission from Iddenden DA. Sexuality during the menopause. *Med Clin North Am.* 1987; 71:87.

of the patient's sexual interest and activities, and pertinent patient education are a good starting point (Table 80–2; the final two references are available online and are a part of a growing body of patient-oriented, web-based information).

B. Patient follow-up

1. Start **HT** with low-dose therapy and titrate upward if needed to control symptoms. **Periodic follow-up visits** are needed to monitor women on HT. Women should be specifically questioned on known side effects of HT at every visit. HT should be stopped as soon as possible. It is suggested that attempts to taper or discontinue therapy be made at 3- to 6-month intervals. Unfortunately, symptoms frequently return and titration has not been shown to prevent return of symptoms. It is recommended that treatment be limited to 3–5 years. (SOR **A**) The newer black box warnings associated with HT should be reviewed with the patient. Dementia risk may go up after 4 to 5 years of therapy in women older than 65 years. (SOR **B**) Most risks and benefits of HT disappear within 3 years after cessation of treatment. Risk for coronary heart disease is not increased among women treated with combination therapy who are less than 10 years postmenopause.

2. For women started on **antidepressants or other medications,** monitor for adverse effects; for antidepressants, these include constipation, weight gain, sexual dysfunction, sedation, and insomnia. If SSRIs/SNRIs are used for more than 4 weeks, taper by reducing the dose by 25% every 1 to 2 weeks when discontinuing to avoid discontinuation syndrome (gastrointestinal distress, lethargy, headache, paresthesias, and irritability).

3. **Endometrial biopsy.** Vaginal bleeding in a woman on HT requires evaluation with either an endometrial biopsy or vaginal ultrasound measuring the endometrial stripe. If the endometrial stripe on ultrasound is less than 5 mm, endometrial cancer is rare. Biopsies every 2 to 3 years for women at particularly high risk for endometrial cancer, even if asymptomatic, have been suggested as prudent.

4. **Osteoporosis management.** Women rapidly lose bone density once reproductive hormone secretion ceases. Risk factor reduction, weight-bearing exercise, adequate intake of vitamin D and dietary calcium, and routine use of bone density testing are all indicated (see Chapter 83).

SELECTED REFERENCES

Aiello EJ, Yasui Y, Tworoger SS, et al. Effect of a yearlong, moderate-intensity exercise intervention on the occurrence and severity of menopause symptoms in postmenopausal women. *Menopause.* 2004;11(4):382–388.

Canonico M, Plu-Bureau G, Lowe GD, Scarabin PY. Hormone replacement therapy and risk of venous thromboembolism in postmenopausal women: systematic review and meta-analysis. *BMJ.* 2008;336(7655):1227–1231.

Carroll DG. Nonhormonal therapies for hot flashes in menopause. *Am Fam Physician.* 2006;73:457–464, 467.

Carroll DG, Kelley KW. Use of antidepressants for the management of hot flashes. *Pharmcotherapy.* 2009;29(11):1357–1374.

Freeman R, Lewis RM. The therapeutic role of estrogens in prostmenopausal women. *Endocrinol Metab Clin N Am.* 2004;33:771–789.

Fournier A, Berrino F, Clavel-Chapelon F. Unequal risks for breast cancer associated with different hormone replacement therapies: results from the E3N cohort study. *Breast Cancer Res Treat.* 2008; 107(2):307–308.

Grady D. Management of menopausal symptoms. *N Engl J Med.* 2006;355:2338–2347.

Harris D. *Menopause Guidebook.* 6th ed. Cleveland, OH: The North American Menopause Society; 2006.

Heiss G, Wallace R, Anderson GL, et al. Health risks and benefits 3 years after stopping randomized treatment with estrogen and progestin. *JAMA.* 2008;299(9):1036–1045.

Imai A, Matsunami K, Takagi H, Ichigo S. New generation nonhormonal management for hot flashes 2013. *Gynecol Endocrinol.* 2013;29(1):63–66.

Loprinzi C. Extinguishing hot flash therapy. *Menopause.* 2013;20(3):248–249.

Nelson HD, Walker M, Zakher B, Mitchell J. Menopausal hormone therapy for the primary prevention of chronic conditions: a systematic review to update the U.S. Preventive Services Task Force recommendations. *Ann Intern Med.* 2012;157(2):104–113.

Newton KM, Reed SD, LaCroix AZ, et al. Treatment of vasomotor symptoms of menopause with black cohosh, multibotanicals, soy, hormone therapy, or placebo: a randomized trial. *Ann Intern Med.* 2006;145(12):869–879.

North American Menopause Society. Estrogen and progestogen use in peri- and postmenopausal women: March 2007 position statement of The North American Menopause Society. *Menopause.* 2007;14(1):1–17.

North American Menopause Society. The role of soy isoflavones in menopausal health: report of The North American Menopause Society/Wulf H. Utian Translational Science Symposium in Chicago, IL (October 2010). *Menopause.* 2011;18(7):732–753.

Nelson HD, Haney E, Humphrey L, et al. *Management of Menopause-Related Symptoms. Summary, Evidence Report/Technology Assessment No. 120.* (Prepared by the Oregon Evidence-based Practice Center, under Contract No. 290-02-0024.) Rockville, MD: Agency for Healthcare Research and Quality; 2005. AHRQ Publication No. 05-E016-1.

Rossouw JE, Anderson GL, Prentice RL, et al. Risks and benefits of estrogen plus progestin in healthy postmenopausal women: Principal results from the Women's Health Initiative randomized controlled trial. *JAMA.* 2002;288(3):321–333.

Rossouw JE, Prentice L, Manson JE, et al. Postmenopausal hormone therapy and risk of cardiovascular disease by age and years since menopause. *JAMA.* 2007;297(13):1465–1477.

Schierbeck LL, Reinmark L, Tofteng CL, et al. Effect of hormone replacement therapy on cardiovascular events in recently postmenopausal women: randomized trial. *BMJ.* 2012;345:e6409.

Shumaker SA, Legault C, Thal L, et al. Estrogen plus progestin and the incidence of dementia and mild cognitive impairment in postmenopausal women: The Women's Health Initiative Memory Study: a randomized controlled trial. *JAMA.* 2003;289(20):2651–2662.

U.S. Preventive Services Task Force. Postmenopausal hormone replacement therapy for the primary prevention of chronic conditions. Recommendations and rationale. *Am Fam Physician.* 2003;67(2):358.

Women's Health Initiative Steering Committee. Effects of conjugated equine estrogens in postmenopausal women with hysterectomy. *JAMA.* 2004;291:1701–1712.

Yates J, Barrett-Connor E, Barlas S, et al. Rapid loss of hip fracture protection after estrogen cessation: evidence from the National Osteoporosis Risk Assessment. *Obstet Gynecol.* 2004;103(3):440–446.

---

81   Obesity

Radhika R. Hariharan, MD, MRCP (UK), Brian C. Reed, MD, &
Sarah R. Edmonson, MD, MS

KEY POINTS

- Obesity is diagnosed when the body mass index is ≥ 30 kg/m^2. (SOR **G**)
- The primary goal of treatment should be weight loss of at least 10% of initial body weight. Maintenance of this new weight is the next priority. (SOR **G**)
- Strategies for weight loss include a low-calorie diet (SOR **A**), which is the cornerstone of management, along with exercise (SOR **A**), behavioral therapies (SOR **B**), and medications. (SOR **A**)
- Drug therapy is indicated when other therapies fail after 3 to 6 months of trial or when there is medical comorbidity indicating a need for more aggressive weight loss. (SOR **B**)
- Drug therapy should be viewed as long term and the risks should be carefully considered in the individual patient. (SOR **G**)
- Bariatric surgery is an appropriate alternative for patients who have failed conventional therapy. (SOR **A**) Long- and short-term risks should be discussed carefully before considering surgery. (SOR **G**)

TABLE 81-1. WORLD HEALTH ORGANIZATION'S CATEGORIZATION OF OBESITY

Body Mass Index (kg/m²)	
Normal	18.5–24.9
Overweight	25–29.9
Obesity class I	30–34.9
Obesity class II	35–39.9
Obesity class III	≥40

I. Introduction
A. Definitions
1. **Obesity** is a disorder of excess body fat resulting in an increased risk for adverse health conditions. It is defined as a BMI of 30 or greater.
2. **Body mass index (BMI).** In 1997, the World Health Organization's International Obesity Task Force recommended adoption of BMI as a standard for the assessment of body fat. (SOR **G**) BMI is calculated by dividing a person's weight in kilograms by one's height in meters squared. Based on these guidelines, one is considered **overweight** at a BMI between 25.0 and 29.9 kg/m². A BMI ≥30 kg/m² meets the criteria for **obesity** (see Table 81–1).

B. Epidemiology
1. **Prevalence.** Over 97 million adults in the United States are overweight or obese. Data from the National Health and Nutrition Examination Survey (NHANES) conducted in 2003 and 2004 revealed that the prevalence of obesity among adults aged 20 years or older in the United States was 32.2%. The percentage of overweight adults in the United States is 66.3%. About 34% of adults and 17% of children in the United States are obese and the numbers continue to increase.
2. **Health effects.** Obesity causes or exacerbates many disorders. It is associated with the development of diabetes mellitus; coronary heart disease; congestive heart failure; obstructive sleep apnea; gallbladder disease; breast, colon, and prostate cancers; osteoarthritis of large and small joints; and premature death. In the Framingham Heart Study, the risk of death within 26 years increased by 1% for each extra pound increase in weight between the ages of 30 and 42 years, and by 2% for those between 50 and 62 years.
3. **Risk factors**
   a. **Race.** The most recent NHANES survey revealed that higher percentages of non-Hispanic blacks and Mexican Americans are either obese or overweight when compared to non-Hispanic whites in similar age categories. Among non-Hispanic blacks, 76.1% of individuals older than age 20 meet the criteria for being overweight and 45.0% meet the criteria for being obese. Data revealed that 75.8% of Mexican Americans met the criteria for being overweight and 36.8% of Mexican American adults met the criteria for being obese. Of non-Hispanic whites older than 20 years, 64.2% meet the criteria for being overweight and 30.6% meet the criteria for being obese. The highest rates of obesity are in black women (50%) and Hispanic women (43%).
   b. **Age.** The prevalence of obesity increases with age and is particularly apparent between the ages of 40 and 60 years.
   c. **Inactivity.** The relative risk of obesity among children in the United States is 5.3 times greater for children who watch television for 5 or more hours a day compared with those who watched television for ≤2 hours. This relationship is valid even after correcting for a wide range of socioeconomic variables.
   d. **Socioeconomic status.** In industrialized countries, a higher prevalence of obesity is seen in those with lower educational levels and low income.
   e. **Marital status.** A tendency to increase weight after marriage and parity exists.

C. Etiology
1. Obesity represents a heterogeneous group of conditions with multiple causes. By definition, it results from imbalance between energy intake and expenditure. Energy expenditure is primarily derived from the resting metabolic rate and physical activity.
2. **Environmental factors.** Migrant studies attest to the critical role of environment in the development of obesity. A marked change in BMI is frequently observed when populations with a common genetic heritage live under new circumstances of plentiful

food and little exercise. Pima Indians in the United States, for example, are on average approximately 25 kg heavier than Pima Indians in Mexico.

3. **Genetic factors**
   a. Evidence from several twin and adoption studies shows a strong genetic predisposition for obesity. Recently, specific mutations causing human obesity have been found in those rare children with extreme obesity, with clear evidence for monogenic inheritance. Genetic syndromes associated with severe obesity include Prader-Willi, Bardet-Biedl, Cohen, Alstrom, and Klinefelter syndromes.
   b. The discovery of leptin, a novel adipocyte hormone, which is deficient in the obese ob/ob mouse, has significantly advanced the understanding of the neurobiology of obesity. Several mutations in leptin and leptin receptor have also been shown to cause monogenic human obesity.
   c. Genetic studies in the more common forms of obesity have shown a region of chromosome 2 that influences obesity-related phenotypes in several different racial groups. This region contains the pro-opiomelanocortin gene.

4. **Gene–environment interaction.** Body weight is determined by an interaction between genetic, environmental, and psychosocial factors. Although obesity runs in families, the influence of genotype may be modified by nongenetic factors. The genetic influences seem to operate through susceptibility genes, which increase the risk of developing obesity. The susceptible gene hypothesis is supported by findings from twin studies, in which pairs of twins were exposed to varying energy balance. The differences in the rate, proportion, and site of weight gain showed greater similarity within pairs than between pairs of twins.

5. **Other causes.** Medical conditions and some medications such as long-term corticosteroid use, phenothiazines, and antidepressants can also result in obesity, but such causes account for ≤1% of cases. Hypothyroidism and Cushing syndrome are the most common diseases that cause obesity. Diseases of the hypothalamus can also result in obesity, but these are quite rare. Major depression, which usually results in weight loss, can occasionally present with weight gain. Consideration of these causes is particularly important when evaluating recent weight gain.

II. **Diagnosis**
   A. **Assessment** of an obese patient involves evaluation of **three key measures: BMI, waist circumference, and an individual's risk factors for diseases and conditions associated with obesity** (Table 81–2).
      1. **Assessing waist circumference** is important because excess abdominal fat is an independent predictor of disease risk. Android obesity (excess fat located primarily in the abdomen or upper body) places an individual at a greater risk for congestive heart disease, hypertension, lipid disorders, and type 2 diabetes mellitus, whereas gynoid obesity (excess fat located primarily in the lower extremities or hips) does not. A waist circumference of ≥40 inches in men and ≥35 inches in women signifies increased risk in those who have a BMI of 25 to 34.9.
         a. Waist circumference is measured with a measuring tape placed around the abdomen at the level of the iliac crest.

TABLE 81–2. RISK ASSESSMENT IN OBESITY

	Normal/ Overweight	Obesity Class I	Obesity Class II	Obesity Class III
Waist circumference ≤40 inches (male) or ≤35 inches (female)	Low risk	Moderate risk	Moderate risk	High risk
Waist circumference ≥40 inches (male) or ≥35 inches (female)	Moderate risk		High risk	
Presence of comorbidities such as osteoarthritis, gallstones, stress incontinence, and menstrual irregularities		High risk		
Presence of comorbidities such as established coronary artery disease, other atherosclerotic disease, type 2 diabetes mellitus, and sleep apnea	High risk			

2. Gross calculation of BMI is not an effective estimation of risk in the following subgroups:

a. In children and adolescents, the appropriate ratio of weight to height differs from that for infants and toddlers; this ratio must be assessed using an age- and gender-specific table. Excessive calorie intake in children will usually manifest itself in additional height as well as excess weight. As such, children who demonstrate exceptional height should be evaluated for lifestyle factors that put them at risk for obesity.

b. Individuals who are ≤4 feet tall, or ≥7 feet tall, cannot be evaluated with a BMI. For these individuals, secondary measures can be used such as body fat analysis or fitness testing.

c. Competitive athletes and bodybuilders may have misleadingly high BMI levels. These patients often have low total body fat and excellent cardiovascular fitness. Although long-term survival data about this subgroup of patients are sparse, it seems likely that their excess muscle mass does not represent the same risk as in other overweight patients.

d. Pregnant women should not use BMI to evaluate risk, particularly in the second or third trimester.

B. Screening for medical conditions that may promote obesity should be performed.

1. Endocrine disorders that promote weight gain such as thyroid disease, hyperandrogenism or polycystic ovarian syndrome, and hypercortisolism are generally accompanied by global symptoms such as skin changes, hair loss and hair distribution changes, abnormal menstrual cycles, mood and energy derangement, gastrointestinal distress, and atypical fat distribution. In patients who demonstrate some or all of these symptoms, laboratory evaluation should precede weight-loss efforts.

2. Many **medications** are associated with weight gain including corticosteroids, antidiabetic drugs (i.e., sulfonylureas, thiazolidinediones, insulin and insulin secretagogues), antiepileptics (e.g., valproic acid and carbamazepine), anxiolytics, antidepressants (e.g., amitriptyline, imipramine, doxepin), the selective serotonin reuptake inhibitor (SSRI) paroxetine, and antipsychotics. Weight-loss plans are not necessarily contraindicated for patients on these drugs. However, changing therapy when possible will increase the patient's chance of successful weight loss.

3. Assessing the patient for the presence of comorbid **psychiatric disease** that could affect their ability to understand and follow a dietary plan can also be helpful.

C. Assess comorbidities

4. High-risk comorbidities include established coronary artery disease, other atherosclerotic disease, type 2 diabetes mellitus, and sleep apnea. Patients with these conditions should be offered aggressive weight management.

5. Osteoarthritis, gallstones, stress incontinence, and menstrual irregularities, while also associated with obesity, are less life-threatening.

6. Other conditions that may increase mortality risk in association with obesity include hypertension, smoking, hyperlipidemia, elevated fasting glucose, and increased age.

D. Dietary history should include information about both typical daily intake and deviations from this routine. Information should be collected about family events, celebratory behavior, and binge eating behavior. The frequency and type of atypical behavior should be noted. Specifically inquire about fast food intake and high-calorie beverages such as soda, juice, and milk. Alcohol intake should be noted and quantified.

E. Exercise history should include type, intensity, duration, and frequency. Encourage the patient to list informal physical activity at work or home in addition to deliberate attempts to exercise. The nature of work should also be explored for the number of hours of sedentary activity.

F. The physical examination of the obese patient can be difficult due to excessive adiposity. Particular attention should be paid to breast and pelvic examinations, which are often missed in this high-risk group. The cardiac examination may be facilitated by having the patient lean forward or, in the recumbent patient, having the arms raised to spread out chest wall tissue.

G. Laboratory evaluation. To rule out secondary causes and assess for comorbid conditions, an initial laboratory evaluation should be ordered including a lipid profile, fasting chemistry panel including blood glucose, and a thyroid-stimulating hormone test.

III. Treatment. The aim of a treatment program should be to reduce weight and maintain lowered weight. The goals of treatment should be tailored to the individual. In general, the primary goal is a 10% reduction from the initial weight at a rate of 0.5 to 1 kg (1–2 lbs) per week during a 6-month period. Successful weight loss should be regarded as a loss of more than 5% of the initial weight while very successful weight loss would be that of greater than 20% of initial body weight. A loss of 10% of body weight is of major clinical benefit with associated changes such as lowered blood pressure, lowered total cholesterol and triglycerides, an increase in high-density lipoprotein cholesterol, and a significant improvement in diabetic control. One appropriate treatment algorithm is shown in Figure 81–1.

A. Dietary interventions

   1. Diet control is the cornerstone of obesity management and its primary role should be emphasized to the patient. In order to successfully lose weight, one must create a deficit of 500 to 1000 kcal per day below what is needed to maintain weight. There are several dietary approaches to achieve this goal.

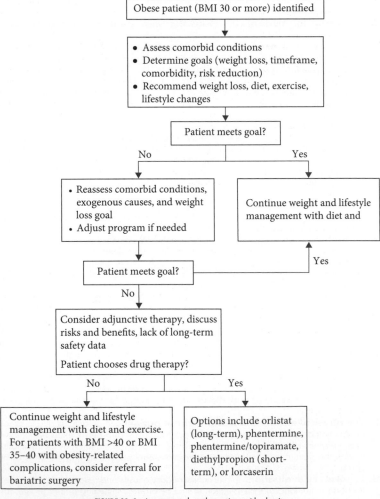

FIGURE 81–1. An approach to the patient with obesity.

    a. Low-calorie diets consisting of approximately 1000 to 1200 kcal per day have been successfully demonstrated to result in weight loss and decreases of abdominal fat. (SOR **A**)

    b. Very low-calorie diets that only permit 400 to 800 kcal per day promote initial weight loss between 13 and 23 kg. However, randomized controlled trials (RCTs) have shown that very low-calorie diets do not result in greater long-term weight loss when compared to low-calorie diets after 1 year. (SOR **A**)

2. In addition to the total caloric intake, the patient may benefit from changes in the **composition of the diet**. No specific diet, however, has consistently been shown to be superior to others on long-term outcomes.

    a. Lower-fat diets promote weight loss by limiting the percentage of daily calories from fat to 20% to 30%. Because dietary fat intake has been associated with cholesterol levels, heart disease, and increased risks for certain cancers, this approach may be desirable for patients with multiple comorbid conditions.

    b. Low-carbohydrate diets such as the South Beach or Atkins diet and the Zone diet are based upon the theory that overweight and obese people are efficient at converting excess carbohydrates into fat. Low-carbohydrate diets advocate restricting total daily carbohydrates to between 40 and 100 g per day. Currently, there is insufficient evidence to make recommendations for or against such low-carbohydrate diets.

        (1) The **South Beach diet** distinguishes itself from the Atkins diet by using the glycemic index of foods to distinguish between "good" and "bad" carbohydrates and permitting moderate consumption of carbohydrates after the first 2 weeks. The South Beach diet seeks to also lower cholesterol and triglycerides by promoting heart healthy fats and whole grains.

        (2) The **Zone diet** attempts to keep insulin levels at a steady state by adhering to a diet that consists of meals that are 40% carbohydrates, 30% protein, and 30% fat.

B. Behavioral therapy refers to the application of psychological techniques to treatment of obesity. Behavioral therapy is now an accepted treatment modality. Behavioral weight-loss programs seek to alter lifestyle and environment in order to effect a change in weight. They encourage the patient to become more aware of eating behavior and physical activity and to focus on changing the behaviors that influence them. The chief feature of this form of treatment is that it emphasizes personal responsibility for the initiation and maintenance of treatment.

    1. Behavioral therapy is best achieved by a therapist trained in this technique and in combination with other modalities.

    2. Behavior therapy is usually presented in an organized and comprehensive format and includes several components including stimulus control, self-reward, and cognitive restructuring.

    3. Although the degree of weight loss achieved with behavioral techniques alone is modest, averaging less than 10 kg in most studies, the advantages include the lack of side effects and the low-attrition rate. (SOR **A**) In a recent systematic review, behaviorally based treatment resulted in 3 kg greater weight loss in the intervention vs. control group after 12 to 18 months.

C. Exercise. While exercise alone results in only modest weight loss, RCTs consistently show the maintenance of weight loss for 2 years, especially at a level of 60 to 90 minutes per day. (SOR **A**) A combination of diet and exercise generally produces more weight loss than diet alone. Regular exercise results in reduction in blood pressure and improvements in lipid profiles, glycemic control, and cardiovascular fitness. Persuading an obese patient to participate and maintain an exercise program is difficult. Less vigorous forms of activity such as brisk walking and swimming may also provide significant improvement in metabolic profiles.

D. Pharmacotherapy of obesity

    1. Indications. Antiobesity medications may be useful additions in adults who have failed lifestyle modification and have a BMI ≥30 or a waist circumference ≥35 for women or ≥40 for men. They may also be useful in patients with a BMI of 27 to 30 and the presence of an additional risk factor for obesity-related disease (e.g., hyperlipidemia, diabetes, or hypertension) or for those awaiting bariatric surgery.

    2. General considerations. The choice of antiobesity drug(s) should be individualized, weighing potential risks and benefits of the agent and the presence of comorbidities.

    a. While all agents are effective in RCTs, there are a few trials of head-to-head comparisons and many of the existing trials have serious limitations in study design.

    b. Orlistat is the preferred medication for initial therapy due to its efficacy and long-term safety record. Weight loss with this agent is about 2.7 kg (95% confidence interval: 2.3–3.1 kg) over placebo and about 12% achieve a weight loss of 10% or greater. (SOR **Ⓐ**) Lorcaserin is an effective alternate with similar efficacy and fewer side effects. However, long-term safety data on the latter are limited.

    c. Combination medications such as phentermine–topiramate may be a good option for obese individuals without hypertension or coronary artery disease. While its efficacy may be greater than that of orlistat or lorcaserin, its side effect profile is also greater.

3. Goals of therapy

    a. Weight loss of 10% to 15% using drugs and behavioral modification is considered very good in drug trials. Weight loss of >15% is considered excellent.

    b. The maximal duration of therapy prescribed is about 4 years for orlistat. Little data are available for efficacy and safety beyond that timeframe.

    c. Drug therapy is not curative. When maximal therapeutic benefit is achieved, weight loss stops. If the drug is stopped, weight gain ensues.

    d. In patients with diabetes, depression, and cardiovascular disease, therapy of these conditions should consist of medications that do not cause weight gain.

4. Mechanism of action

    a. Drugs altering fat digestion (orlistat). Orlistat alters fat digestion by inhibiting pancreatic lipases. It is available for long-term treatment. The recommended dose is 120 mg three times daily. Side effects occur in 15% to 30% of users and include intestinal borborygmi, cramps, flatus, fecal incontinence, oily spotting, liver injury, and oxalate-induced acute renal injury. The absorption of fat soluble vitamins may also be affected. In a systematic review, the addition of orlistat to behavioral intervention resulted in 3 kg more weight loss than placebo at 1 year.

    b. Serotonin agonists (lorcaserin). Lorcaserin is a selective agonist of the serotonin 2C receptor. Unlike nonselective agents like fenfluramine and dexfenfluramine, lorcaserin does not appear to significantly increase the risk of serotonin-associated valvular heart disease. It was approved by the Food and Drug Administration (FDA) in 2012 as an adjunct to lifestyle modification in the treatment of obesity. It has a similar efficacy to orlistat with fewer side effects. Little long-term safety data currently exist. Side effects include headache, upper respiratory infection, dizziness, and nausea. It may also increase symptomatic hypoglycemia in patients with diabetics. The recommended dose is 10 mg twice daily with or without food. The response should be evaluated by the 12th week and the agent discontinued if there is no loss of at least 5% of body weight. It is contraindicated in pregnancy and renal failure.

    c. Sympathomimetic drugs are a heterogeneous group of agents and are approved for short-term (<12 weeks) use only. They reduce oral intake by causing early satiety and have a high potential for side effects and abuse. They are contraindicated in patients with coronary artery disease, hypertension, and hyperthyroidism. Side effects include increased heart rate and blood pressure, constipation, insomnia, and dry mouth. This category includes (1) medications that stimulate release of norepinephrine or inhibit its reuptake into the nerve terminals (phentermine, diethylpropion, benzphetamine, and phendimetrazine), (2) agents that block serotonin and norepinephrine update (sibutramine—withdrawn), and (3) agents that act on adrenergic receptors directly (phenylpropanolamine—withdrawn). Phentermine is the most widely used weight loss agent. Ephedrine stimulates weight loss by increasing thermogenesis and decreasing food intake. It has been withdrawn.

    d. Antidepressants (bupropion). Bupropion is a relative of diethylpropion and acts through the modulating effect of norepinephrine. It is an antidepressant and used in the prevention of weight gain in smokers. It has been used in trials in the dose of 300 to 400 mg per day.

    e. Antiepileptic drugs

        (1) Topiramate is approved for use in treating seizures and migraines and is associated with weight loss. While its monotherapy is not recommended at this time in obesity, it may be used in combination with phentermine. Side effects include paresthesias, somnolence, and decreased concentration.

   (2) Zonisamide has both serotoninergic and dopaminergic activities and inhibits sodium and calcium channels. It is associated with significant weight loss. Its use in obesity is not recommended at this time. Side effects include gastrointestinal, central nervous system, and psychiatric symptoms.

  f. Diabetic drugs. Metformin is useful in people with diabetes who are overweight, but does not produce enough weight loss to qualify as a anti-obesity agent. **Pramlintide** is associated with modest weight loss, but must be given by subcutaneous injection. It is a polypeptide hormone secreted by beta cells of the pancreas that slows gastric emptying. **Exenatide** is a long-acting synthetic peptide that is a GLP-1 receptor agonist. It inhibits gastric emptying and is administered subcutaneously twice daily. **Liraglutide** is another GLP-1 analog available for use in the United States and Europe. It is administered subcutaneously once daily. The role of these agents in patients with obesity without diabetes is unknown.

  g. Combination drugs are believed to work by combining different mechanisms of action. In 2012, the FDA approved phentermine and topiramate extended-release combination (qsymia) for use in obesity. This combination has been shown to increase weight loss in the first year of use. (SOR **B**) A bupropion–naltrexone combination has also been evaluated, but is not commercially available.

E. Dietary supplements for obesity management

  1. Agents such as chitosan, green tea, chromium picolinate, conjugated linoleic acid, guar gum, and garcinia cambogia have been promoted for weight loss. Although some of these substances have mechanisms of action that could lead to weight loss, there are insufficient data at this time regarding safety and efficacy.

  2. Ephedrine, an adrenergic agent with thermogenic and appetite suppressant properties, has been found in controlled studies to promote weight loss. Short-term randomized double-blind, placebo-controlled studies with herbal products containing ephedra alkaloids and caffeine have shown efficacy in promoting weight loss. Dietary supplements with ephedra (ma huang) have unpredictable and unstandardized amounts of active ingredients and are not recommended. Side effects may be serious and include hypertension, arrhythmias, myocardial infarcts, seizures, stroke, and sudden death. In April 2004, the FDA prohibited the sale of weight loss supplements that contain ephedrine.

F. Surgical treatment of obesity is very effective for a carefully selected group of morbidly obese adults. (SOR **A**) Recent advances have made these procedures safer and possibly more effective. RCTs and cohort studies comparing bariatric surgery and other nonsurgical techniques have found that surgery results in dramatic and a sustained loss of weight and leads to improvement in obesity-related comorbidities. Laparoscopic approaches have reduced the complication rates of bariatric surgery, which has increased the popularity of these procedures in recent years.

  1. Secondary effects. Bariatric surgery improves insulin sensitivity, blood pressure, left ventricular ejection fraction, cholesterol and triglyceride levels, sleep apnea, fertility, menstrual irregularity, and urinary stress incontinence. These procedures have also been postulated to affect neuroendocrine feedback loops associated with satiety and food-seeking behavior as well as maintenance of metabolic rate, with variable results on long-term hunger levels and specific food cravings.

  2. Selection criteria

    a. Bariatric surgery is indicated for well-motivated, well-informed patients capable of participating in long-term follow-up, whose BMI is ≥40 or ≥35 and experiencing significant obesity-related comorbid diseases such as type 2 diabetes mellitus or severe obstructive sleep apnea. (SOR **C**) Patients should have failed at nonsurgical attempts at weight reduction and have acceptable operative risks.

    b. Bariatric surgery is contraindicated in patients with significant psychiatric disease or instability, alcohol or drug abuse, cardiac or other medical conditions that lead to a high risk of intraoperative mortality, presence of endocrine disorders that promote obesity, and inability to understand risks and benefits of surgery. Surgery is also contraindicated in children and pregnant women.

    c. Mechanism of action. Surgical treatment involves restriction of size of the stomach and malabsorption of consumed calories due to bypassing sections of the bowel.

3. **Types of surgery.** The most commonly performed procedure is the **Roux-en-Y gastric bypass** (about 65%), followed by laparoscopic adjustable band procedure (around 25%), vertical banded gastroplasty (about 5%) and biliopancreatic diversion (around 5%).

   a. **Procedures that limit intake** include adjustable **gastric banding** and **stapled gastroplasty**. In adjustable gastric banding, a diameter-limiting prosthetic device is placed about the gastric body; this device may be adjusted in size through a subcutaneous reservoir. Stapled gastroplasty involves a partitioning of the stomach close to the gastroesophageal junction and creation of a small-caliber gastric outlet to the small intestine. Because of the reduced gastric capacity, the patient reaches satiety earlier in the meal and presumably eats fewer calories.

      (1) **Risks.** Immediate postoperative complications include surgical infection or wound dehiscence. Patients may develop severe gastroesophageal reflux or vomiting, chronic abdominal pain, obstructive disease, and incisional hernias. Up to 20% of patients may require reoperation for surgical correction of severe dysfunction including stomal outlet stenosis. Gastric banding may cause foreign body reactions or gastric body erosions leading to emergency surgery.

      (2) **Outcomes.** Early weight-loss results from these procedures can be up to 60% of the preoperative excess weight. (SOR **Ⓐ**) Many patients regain a substantial proportion of their lost weight within 5 years of surgery. In one longitudinal cohort study of 3227 patients following laparoscopic adjustable gastric banding, there was a durable mean excess weight loss at 15 years of 47%. However, there was a 40% revision rate for proximal gastric enlargements in the first 10 years. Results of these authors' systematic review showed similar success. In a 10-year follow-up of one randomized trial of laparoscopic adjustable gastric band surgery (92.5% of original subjects available) versus nonsurgical therapy (62.5% of original subjects available), the surgical group had a mean weight loss of 14.1 kg (63.4% of excess weight loss), compared with the nonsurgical group 0.4 kg.

   b. **Procedures that promote malabsorption** include gastric bypass procedures that not only reduce the size of the stomach pouch but also bypass a portion of the small intestine, causing variable amounts of caloric malabsorption. The most popular procedure is the Roux-en-Y bypass, in which a small stomach pouch is anastomosed to the mid-jejunum; the bypassed sections of duodenum and jejunum are all or partially left as a blind-ended pouch. More recent techniques vary the anatomic arrangement of bypassed sections in order to maximize caloric malabsorption while preserving absorption of important nutrients. Other gastric bypass techniques include the biliopancreatic bypass, the distal Roux-en-Y, and the duodenal switch.

      (1) **Risks.** Perioperative complications, such as pulmonary embolus and gastrointestinal leakage, may be as high as 15% with a 1% mortality rate. Long-term morbidity is strongly linked to malabsorptive syndromes, including anemia, fat-soluble vitamin deficiencies, and protein-calorie malnutrition. Diarrhea is typical after these surgeries. Some patients may develop dumping syndrome, an intense physiologic reaction when poorly digested food is deposited lower in the digestive tract. Dumping syndrome causes nausea, bloating, diarrhea, colic, lightheadedness, palpitations, and sweating.

      (2) **Outcomes.** Initial weight-loss results are excellent, with a mean loss of 75% to 80% of excess weight. (SOR **Ⓐ**) Longer-term efficacy is less well established, but appears to be better than volume restriction procedures.

4. **Long-term outcomes of bariatric surgery.** The Swedish Obese Subjects (SOS) study reports metabolic and cardiovascular effects of bariatric surgery up to 10 years after the procedure, in a nonrandomized prospective sample. This and other long-term studies provide the basis for predicting long-term outcomes of surgically induced weight loss. (SOR **Ⓑ**)

   a. **Respiratory.** The majority of observed subjects had long-term improvement in symptoms of asthma and obstructive sleep apnea.

   b. **Cardiovascular.** Bariatric surgery has been demonstrated to result in short-term improvement of hypertension, hyperlipidemia, and hypertriglyceridemia. These improvements appear to diminish over time and are indistinguishable from control groups at 10 years postsurgery.

c. **Endocrine.** Bariatric surgery recipients have a reduced chance of developing insulin resistance and diabetes. Long term, the degree of protection correlates with how well the weight loss is maintained.

d. **Digestive.** After bariatric surgery, patients have a long-term increased risk of digestive problems including stenotic changes, fistula formation, bowel obstruction, incisional hernias, dumping syndrome, and chronic diarrhea. Patients may also develop nutritional deficiencies as a result of the disrupted digestive process.

G. **Complications of weight loss.** Weight loss, particularly rapid loss, has been associated with a variety of medical sequelae.

1. **Biliary complications.** Rapid weight loss is associated with an increased prevalence of gallstones and cholecystitis. This complication has been observed with both low- and high-fat diets. Dietary supplementation with ursodeoxycholic acid has been proposed as a preventative tactic for this problem, but very little data support its efficacy.

2. **Ketosis.** Insufficient carbohydrate intake can promote production of large numbers of ketone bodies in the bloodstream. The long-term health impact of this phenomenon is controversial; speculation centers on the potential for renal damage or kidney stone formation in people following ketotic diets. Such complications have been well documented in children placed on ketotic diets for epilepsy control.

3. **Dietary deficiencies.** Caloric restriction can lead to insufficient intake of vitamins, minerals, essential fatty acids, or protein. Long term, this can cause protein-calorie malnutrition, vitamin deficiency, or osteoporosis. Twice yearly monitoring of vitamin D, calcium, parathyroid hormone, alkaline phosphatase, ferritin, vitamin B_{12}, and folate is recommended after the Roux-en-Y procedure for at least 2 years. Bone density is also recommended yearly till stable.

4. **Cosmetic issues.** Weight loss, particularly when rapid, may cause striae formation and loose skin, which may be cosmetically offensive to the patient.

5. **Psychiatric changes.** Slow or dramatic changes in body habitus may affect the patient's interaction with family, friends, and coworkers, as well as his own body image. Such changes are not always positive and may cause significant emotional distress.

IV. **Management Strategies**

A. Obesity management should be an individually tailored approach (Figure 81–1).

B. Although the goal of treatment is a 10% reduction from initial weight, weight loss of as little as 5% should be regarded as successful as there is considerable improvement in associated risk factors.

C. Weight maintenance after initial weight loss is often difficult and requires an ongoing program of diet, exercise, and behavioral therapy.

D. Regular physician contact is important to sustain maintenance efforts.

SELECTED REFERENCES

Adams TD, Gress RE, Smith SC, et al. Long-term mortality after gastric bypass surgery. N Engl J Med. 2007;357(8):753–761.

Bray GA, Ryan DH. Medical therapy for the patient with obesity. Circulation. 2012;125(13):1695–1703.

Leblanc ES, O'Connor E, Whitlock EP, et al. Effectiveness of primary care-relevant treatments for obesity in adults: a systematic evidence review for the U.S. Preventive Services Task Force. Ann Intern Med. 2011;155:434–447.

Li Z, Maglione M, Tu W, et al. Meta-analysis: pharmacologic treatment of obesity. Ann Internal Med. 2005;142(7):532–546.

Lyznicki JM, Young DC, Riggs JA, Davis RM. Obesity: assessment and management in primary care. Am Fam Physician. 2001;63:2185–2196.

Maciejewski ML, Livingston EH, Smith VA, et al. Survival among high risk patients after bariatric surgery. JAMA. 2011;305(23):2419–2526.

Maggard MA, Shugarman LR, Suttorp M, et al. Meta-analysis: surgical treatment of obesity. Ann Intern Med. 2005;142(7):547–559.

Mango VL, Frishman WH. Physiologic, psychologic, and metabolic consequences of bariatric surgery. Cardiol Rev. 2006;14(5):232–237.

National Institutes of Health. The Practical Guide: Identification, Evaluation and Treatment of Over-weight and Obesity in Adults. Bethesda, MD: National Institutes of Health, National Heart, Lung, and Blood Institute, and North American Association for the Study of Obesity; 2000 NIH publication 00-4084.

O'Brien PE, Brennan L, Laurie C, Brown W. Intensive medical weight loss or laparoscopic adjustable gastric banding in the treatment of mild to moderate obesity: long-term follow-up of a prospective randomised trial. Obes Surg. 2013;23(9):1345–1353.

O'Brien PE, MacDonald L, Anderson M, et al. Long-term outcomes after bariatric surgery: fifteen-year follow-up of adjustable gastric banding and a systematic review of the bariatric surgical literature. *Ann Surg.* 2013;257(1);87–94.

Ogden CL, Carroll MD, Curtin LR, et al. Prevalence of obesity and trends in obesity among U.S. adults 1999–2004. *JAMA.* 2006;295:1549–1555.

Palamara KL, Mogul HR, Peterson SJ, Frishman WH. Obesity: new perspectives and pharmacotherapies. *Cardiol Rev.* 2006;14(5):238–258.

Silk AW, McTigue KM. Reexamining the physical examination for obese patients. *JAMA.* 2011;305(2): 193–194.

Snow V, Barry P, Fitterman N, et al; Clinical Efficacy Assessment Subcommittee of the American College of Physicians. Pharmacologic and surgical management of obesity in primary care: a clinical practice guideline from the American College of Physicians. *Ann Intern Med.* 2005;142(7):525–531.

Yanovski SZ, Yanovski JA. Obesity. *N Engl J Med.* 2002;346:591–602.

---

82   Osteoarthritis

Charles Kodner, MD

KEY POINTS

- Osteoarthritis (OA) is no longer considered a normal process of aging and "wear and tear" on joints, but is a physiologically complex disorder involving physiologic and mechanical initiating events, joint and cartilage damage, synovial inflammation, and an imbalance of cartilage repair and destruction. (SOR ⓒ)
- Diagnosis is primarily on clinical grounds, emphasizing typical aching joint pain, crepitus, osteophyte formation, worsening pain with activity, and joint instability. Characteristic radiographic findings of joint space narrowing, osteophytes, irregular joint surfaces, and sclerosis of subchondral bone may assist in the diagnosis. (SOR ⓒ)
- Disease management should emphasize nonpharmacologic interventions, including regular exercise, physical therapy, weight loss, smoking cessation, physical pain relief modalities, gait support and other assistive devices, and patient education. (SOR ⓒ; SOR ⓐ for exercise and bracing in the knee)
- Pharmacologic treatment should be initiated with adequate, scheduled doses of acetaminophen, starting at 500 mg twice daily up to 1 g four times daily. (SOR ⓐ)
- Other medication options include nonsteroidal anti-inflammatory drugs (NSAIDs), and other analgesics such as tramadol and narcotic analgesics. (SOR ⓐ) Details are available in Table 82–1, with a list of the most common medications and dosages including herbal compounds and other treatment options.
- The COX-2-selective NSAID celecoxib provides as effective pain relief as other NSAIDs with reduced gastrointestinal toxicity compared to traditional NSAIDs (SOR ⓐ), but should be used in selected patients in light of evolving concerns about cardiovascular risks.
- Many patients require chronic opioid therapy for more advanced disease, and will require appropriate management of long-term opioid treatment. (SOR ⓒ)
- Topical capsaicin or oral glucosamine and chondroitin supplements may also provide pain relief. (SOR ⓑ)
- Joint injection with corticosteroids has been shown to be helpful in patients who have failed other treatment options or who are at risk of complications from NSAIDs or other therapy, though overall evidence for benefit is limited. (SOR ⓑ)
- Surgical joint replacement for hip or knee arthritis, or other surgical treatment options, should be considered for patients with disabling pain who have failed other treatment interventions. (SOR ⓒ)

I. Introduction

A. Definition. Osteoarthritis (OA) is characterized by slowly progressive joint pain, cartilage destruction, and functional instability, with typical radiographic findings of osteophytes and other characteristic changes. OA is the most common cause of disability among adults in the United States and carries a tremendous potential for reduced quality of life as the disease progresses. OA can be classified as primary (or idiopathic), involving the hands, feet, knees, hips, spine, and other joints; or secondary to trauma, obesity, congenital abnormalities affecting the limbs, other arthropathies (e.g., tophaceous gout, rheumatoid arthritis, etc.), metabolic disorders (e.g., hemochromatosis), disorders of collagen, or other medical conditions. Some patients with rheumatoid arthritis, systemic lupus erythematosus, gout, or other inflammatory conditions may develop degenerative changes in the joints that cause chronic symptoms without evidence of acute or active joint inflammation.

B. **Epidemiology.** OA is the most commonly encountered cause of joint pain and disability. Data from 2007 to 2009 suggest that approximately 1 in 5 or 50 million Americans have physician-diagnosed OA. OA increases with age, and the prevalence of OA is expected to increase dramatically as the US population ages. The growing epidemic of obesity can be expected to further increase the prevalence of OA as well. Many more people have radiographic or clinical evidence of OA than have symptomatic disease, with radiographic changes of knee OA present in approximately half of the population older than 65 years. OA is the indication for 95% of Medicare-funded knee and hip replacement surgeries and is the fourth most frequent primary diagnosis at hospital discharge. Knee and hip replacements for OA cost an estimated $42 billion in 2009.

C. **Risk factors** for OA include systemic susceptibilities and factors resulting in excessive mechanical stress on the joints. Mechanical stressors include obesity or overweight as well as local factors such as malalignment, muscle weakness, occupational factors, or joint damage including ligament disruption. Systemic risk factors include older age and obesity. Ethnicity, gender, hormonal status, genetic factors, bone density, and nutritional factors all have unproven associations with risk for, and severity of, osteoarthritis.

D. **Pathophysiology.** OA is historically thought of as a result of ongoing stress or "wear and tear" on aging joints related to activities, positioning, weight-related joint stresses, or other factors. While these factors do play an important role, OA is increasingly recognized as a complex disorder involving all joint structures. Physical stresses act as disease initiating or aggravating factors, but the disorder primarily involves an imbalance between joint tissue breakdown and repair, causing progressive joint failure, pain, and disability. The key pathophysiologic steps include damage to articular cartilage and meniscal degeneration, subchondral bone changes, synovial inflammation, bone and cartilage overgrowth, and central pain processing.

1. **Degeneration and destruction of the articular and meniscal cartilage** appears to be due to triggering factors for OA including excessive force applied to the joint, repetitive impact loading, or a genetic or metabolic defect in the articular cartilage or underlying subchondral bone. As a result of these triggering factors, chondrocytes multiply and become metabolically active, initially overproducing articular cartilage to compensate for the triggering factors and maintain joint function. Over time, these factors lead to production of altered proteoglycans and collagen in the articular cartilage, which becomes subject to erosions, cracks, and other damage typical of OA.

2. **Subchonral bone changes** such as new bone formation on trabeculae in the subchondral bone is one of the first pathologic signs of joint involvement in OA. Articular cartilage damage is associated with subchondral bony changes such as subchondral sclerosis, development of osteophytes, and formation of cyst-like bone cavities.

3. **Synovial inflammation** appears to play an active role in the progression of OA, even though OA is generally considered a noninflammatory arthritis. Synovitis can lead to joint swelling and effusion, stiffness, pain, and other manifestations of OA. Established synovial inflammation eventually leads to production of cytokines and other agents that cause further degradation of articular cartilage.

4. **Metabolically active chondrocytes** appear to signal subchondral bone osteoblasts, which begin to form new bone tissue around the edges of the joints. The resulting "bone spurs" or osteophytes are characteristic clinical or radiographic findings and contribute to joint pain, instability, and loss of function as well as possible gross joint deformity in later stages of OA.

5. **Central pain processing,** identified on various imaging studies as areas of the brain associated with aversive conditioning and motivation, is increasingly recognized as an important component of the pain syndrome associated with OA, beyond the pain expected from peripheral joint damage. Central pain perception changes explain the potential role of various nonanalgesic medications that can be used in treating OA-related pain.

II. Diagnosis. In OA, the findings from the history and physical examination are key to the diagnosis and guide the intensity and nature of therapy. The pain of OA is typically deep, aching, and poorly localized, is associated with reduced range of motion and functional impairment, and is slowly progressive.

There is no gold standard for diagnosing OA, and clinical guidelines for diagnosis currently focus on typical pain symptoms, radiographic features, and lack of evidence of inflammatory arthropathies. The American College of Rheumatology (ACR) criteria for the diagnosis of OA in commonly affected joints (available at http://www.hopkinsarthritis.org/physician-corner/education/arthritis-education-diagnostic-guidelines/) are based on typical pain symptoms, age >50 years, morning joint stiffness <30 minutes, absence of synovial warmth, and the presence of crepitus, bony tenderness, or bony enlargement. However, these criteria were developed primarily for the purpose of clinical trials or epidemiologic studies, and they perform poorly in a general clinical setting to diagnose OA, particularly in earlier stages.

A. Symptoms. OA characteristically produces pain and stiffness in the joints, with the stiffness worsened by immobilization and resolving quickly with movement (generally in ≤30 minutes after arising in the morning). The pain is typically dull and aching in character and is aggravated by cold or damp weather and by increased activity. If activity-associated pain is present, it usually starts quickly when the joint is used, but may last for hours after the activity has stopped. Often the history includes some minor injury leading to exacerbation of symptoms, though the true onset of OA symptoms is insidious in nature. Eventually, the pain becomes constant and wakes the patient from sleep.

    1. Many patients complain of **joint instability** or "giving way" in the case of OA involving the hips or knees. These patients may have difficulty climbing or descending stairs. Some patients may actually fall as a result of knee or hip joint instability.

    2. Symptoms of **crepitus**—grinding, popping, catching, and clicking—may also be present.

    3. OA of the hands commonly affects the base of the thumb (first carpometacarpal joint) and this may be a useful diagnostic clue.

B. Signs

    1. On physical examination, clinicians should assess the patient for features typical of OA, examine for evidence of other arthropathies, and assess the functional status of the joint. Specific findings to elicit include inspection for joint enlargement including osteophytes or nodules; examination for signs of inflammation including erythema, warmth, or "bogginess" of the joint; palpation for crepitus with passive range of motion; focal tenderness; and observation of instability with gait, squat-rise, or other movements.

        a. On examination of a **normally mobile joint,** crepitus may be noted when the joint is passively moved, and there may be localized tenderness. The range of movement of an osteoarthritic joint is limited.

        b. In weight-bearing joints, it is important to assess joint stability and the status of the supporting musculature, which has therapeutic significance.

    2. Joint-specific signs and symptoms. In addition to the above general findings on history and physical examination, OA involving specific joints may have additional clinical findings.

        a. Knees. In the knees, crepitus may be marked, with limitation of flexion and extension. Patients may complain of pain in the thighs, calves, or popliteal area related to compensatory muscle spasm. Osteophytes are sometimes actually palpable in the knee, and commonly, there are effusions.

        b. Hips. In the hip, OA manifestations include changed gait with a characteristically flexed, externally rotated hip, with the gait "sparing" the painful side. There may be limb shortening because of subluxation of the head of the femur. The pain from OA of the hip is often referred, with pain being felt in the groin, the buttocks, or even the knee. The first sign of OA in the hip is loss of rotation (since the hip is a ball-and-socket joint); this loss should be tested for in all older patients. Ultimately, there is limitation of all movements of the joint.

        c. Hands. In the hands, typical joints affected by OA include the distal interphalangeal (DIP) joints, proximal interphalangeal (PIP) joints, and first carpometacarpal (CMC) joints. Heberden nodes are a characteristic finding; these are firm, tender nodes on the dorsal aspect of the DIP joints, representing bony enlargement or osteophyte formation. Bouchard nodes are similar lesions that occur over the PIP joints. Pain in the hands is worsened by fine motor or physical activities such as gardening, sports, and hobbies. Destructive joint changes are possible, but are not as common as in rheumatoid arthritis.

d. Cervical spine. Chronic neck pain from OA in the cervical spine may be related to work posture, repetitive athletic injuries, or other factors. Osteophytes in the spinal vertebrae can produce nerve root pressure, with resulting radicular symptoms.

e. Lumbar spine. OA is common in the lumbar spine, but findings on examination or radiography do not correlate well with clinical symptoms. It is unclear whether degenerative changes per se, facet joint changes, muscle spasm, disk herniation, soft tissue changes, or all of these account for the lower back pain experienced.

f. Other joints. A number of other joints can be affected by OA, including the joints of the feet and ankles, the temporomandibular joint (TMJ), the true joint of the shoulder as well as the acromioclavicular joint, and the sternoclavicular joints. OA should be included in the differential diagnosis of pain in these areas, though other diagnoses (e.g., TMJ dysfunction, rotator cuff tendinitis) need to be considered.

C. Laboratory tests. The diagnosis of OA rests on clinical grounds; laboratory testing should be used selectively to rule out other diagnoses or to help guide treatment decisions.

1. Blood tests. There are no specific blood tests to order as part of the routine diagnosis of OA. Tests for inflammatory disorders (sedimentation rate, antinuclear antibody testing, rheumatoid factor, or anti-citrullinated protein antibody testing) should be used only when there is a strong suspicion for systemic lupus, rheumatoid arthritis, or other conditions, given the low predictive value and high false-positive rate for these tests in a general population of patients with arthralgias. These tests should not be ordered as a "screening panel" in patients with arthralgias, and positive results in low-risk patients should be interpreted carefully. Complete blood counts, uric acid levels, chemistry profiles, and other tests may be required to evaluate for septic arthritis, gout, renal osteodystrophy, or other disorders as the clinical picture dictates; these tests may also be useful before initiating treatment with anti-inflammatory drugs, particularly in patients who are older or have other chronic illnesses.

2. Joint aspiration. When joint effusion is present, joint aspiration is usually desirable to provide symptomatic relief. Diagnostically, joint aspiration is indicated in a patient with a moderately inflamed, tender, and swollen joint with effusion, where it is important to rule out septic arthritis, gout, pseudogout, or other disorders. Patients with septic arthritis may not present with characteristic findings of toxic appearance, fever, and marked joint tenderness and inflammation, but may only have focal joint inflammation early in the disease process. Joint fluid analysis is generally not indicated to confirm the diagnosis of OA.

3. Arthroscopy has a place in the diagnosis of arthritis, particularly in a joint that is "locking." Through the arthroscope, fragments of tissue can be removed and the fibrillar changes in the cartilages, which can contribute to early symptoms, can be planed off. The arthroscopic procedure itself is temporarily disabling, with a close risk/benefit balance, and should not be undertaken lightly. In one RCT, arthroscopic surgery with surgical lavage and debridement for knee OA provided no additional benefit compared to optimized physical and medical therapy.

D. Radiographic findings. A number of radiographic features are common in OA, but especially in disease of the spine and hips, there may be relatively poor correlation between observed radiographic changes and symptoms. Approximately half of patients with radiographic changes of OA of the knees complain of persistent pain. Radiographic studies are generally normal early in the course of OA, and the absence of radiographic findings does not rule out symptomatic OA. Likewise, the presence of typical radiographic findings of OA does not guarantee that OA is the source of a patient's current knee or hip pain; other diagnoses such as bursitis or other periarticular disorders may contribute to new or worsening pain symptoms.

1. Plain X-rays. Typical findings consistent with OA on plain radiographs include joint space narrowing because of destruction of articular cartilage, including narrowed intravertebral disk space or narrowed knee joint space; osteophyte formation at the margins of affected joints; irregular joint surfaces; sclerosis of subchondral bone; and bony cysts.

2. Computerized tomography (CT) and magnetic resonance imaging (MRI) are increasingly used, but have little role in diagnosing OA. These imaging modalities provide good visualization of soft tissues and subchondral bone changes, as well as of ligament and meniscal damage, and may be most useful to rule out other disorders causing joint pain, such as rotator cuff tear, avascular necrosis, osteochondritis dissecans, knee ligament disruption, and lumbar disk herniation.

3. **Musculoskeletal ultrasound (MSUS)** is increasingly investigated as a means of assessing articular cartilage damage, bone changes, joint inflammation, and adjacent soft-tissue lesions such as bursitis. MSUS can also be used to guide therapeutic joint aspiration.

III. **Treatment.** OA should be managed as any other chronic illness, with consideration of the patient's disease location and progression, the phase of the patient's illness, and attention to routine health maintenance and other medical comorbid conditions. Management of chronic pain can easily consume the time allotted to an outpatient office visit, and it is vital not to neglect these other management needs. The **goals of therapy for OA** include pain relief; improved or maintained joint function and mobility; prevention of destructive joint changes; minimization of disability and preserved functionality; and improved overall quality of life. An additional therapeutic goal is to educate patients and their families about the illness and enlist them as active participants in the management of the patient's illness.

A. **Physical interventions.** Nonpharmacologic interventions should be considered as primary therapy in OA, to accomplish the therapeutic objectives listed earlier.

1. **Exercise.** At-home or supervised exercise programs have been shown to provide benefits in pain control, functionality, overall well-being, and prevention of disability, primarily for OA of the knees (SOR Ⓐ) and hips (reduced pain only) (SOR Ⓑ). Exercise of weight-bearing joints must be of low impact, with avoidance of torsion, prolonged standing, and kneeling. Patients can be instructed in performing appropriate exercise by their physician or can be referred to a physical therapist for instruction or supervision.

a. **Types of exercise programs** include range-of-motion and flexibility exercises; instructions in joint positioning and posture and correction of joint malalignment; aerobic exercises, especially aquatic aerobics; fitness walking; and strength training, particularly quadriceps strengthening since quadriceps weakness is common in OA. Nonweight-bearing exercise is preferred, and impact on the knees can be spared by shoes and surfaces that cushion the limb while walking; an indoor skiing machine can be very helpful in OA of the knees.

2. **Physical therapy.** The physical therapist can be helpful in instructing patients in the above exercises, supervising correct and safe performance of exercises, and monitoring therapeutic response. (SOR Ⓒ) Therapists can also be helpful to assess patients' muscle weakness and gait, assist with the use of pain-control modalities, and assess patients for assistive devices. Occupational therapy evaluation can also provide support or assistive devices for activities of daily living for patients with OA of the hands.

3. **Gassistive devices.** The use of canes (held in the hand contralateral to the affected knee or hip joint), crutches, walkers, or other devices may be helpful for some patients but should not supplant the role of muscle-strength training, range-of-motion exercises, and other measures to improve functionality. Shoe orthotics, especially lateral wedges, may also be helpful to preserve joint positioning and help prevent joint damage.

4. **Pain control modalities.** Persistent pain, particularly nerve root pain, may be relieved by methods such as transcutaneous electrical nerve stimulation (TENS), ultrasonography, and other physical therapy techniques.

5. **Knee braces.** Some patients find relief of pain and improvement of joint stability by the use of knee bracing, patellar taping, or similar interventions. (SOR Ⓐ) These can be helpful in the short term, but also should not replace measures to maintain joint function and muscle strength. Neoprene knee braces with patellar cutouts may be most helpful in patients with early knee OA. Viscoelastic shoe inserts may also provide most relief early in the illness. Dynamic knee braces may be most helpful in patients with more advanced, or unicompartmental, knee OA. (SOR Ⓒ) The evidence supporting all these intervention is limited.

6. **Foot care.** When the feet are affected by OA or other conditions that affect gait and knee or hip joint function, attention to the shoes and to podiatric health is vital. Orthotic devices can be of considerable help in correcting chronic foot deformities, which predispose to other musculoskeletal pain, not only in the feet themselves but also in the knee, hip, or lumbar spine. The use of cushioned athletic shoes may be beneficial. Women used to high heels who move rapidly to "flats" (including sneakers) may develop Achilles tendinitis and other problems.

7. **Activities of daily living.** In all forms of arthritis of the hand, it is important to pay attention to the patient's routine tasks. Devices can assist in opening containers that require torsion strength and grip, functions that can chronically exacerbate and acutely precipitate arthralgia. Other methods of reducing joint stress and improving functionality, such as a raised toilet seat, grab bars, and tub seats or shower seats, can also reduce accidents.

B. **Behavioral interventions**

1. **Weight loss.** Obesity and overweight are important contributing factors to symptomatic OA in weight-bearing joints. Patients should be enrolled in dedicated weight-loss programs where possible, or advised regarding diet, exercise, and the role of weight-loss interventions if such programs are not available. Simple topics to address regarding diet include limiting portion size, avoiding high-carbohydrate drinks and snacks, and increasing the fruit and vegetable content of the diet. Aquatic aerobic exercises can be valuable in obese patients in limiting the weight applied to the knees. Sustained weight loss has been shown to improve OA symptoms.

2. **Smoking cessation.** Cessation of tobacco use is important in improving patients' overall sense of well-being, reducing the risks of NSAID-induced gastropathy, maintaining joint blood flow and tissue healing, and reducing the risk of cardiovascular disease and other comorbidities. Patients who smoke should specifically be counseled regarding cessation methods as part of the overall management of their OA.

C. **Oral medications.** Most patients with OA use pharmacologic treatment for pain relief, though there is no evidence that treatment alters the natural history of the disease. Medications should be seen as adjuncts to preventive and protective therapy, as aforementioned, rather than the primary focus of intervention. The evidence for benefit from any class of pharmacologic agent for treating OA is limited, implying that treatment decisions should be highly individualized based on severity of pain, response to analgesics, side effects, and comorbid chronic health conditions.

1. **Analgesics.** Simple analgesics remain the first-line treatment for patients with mild-to-moderate OA and represent the best efficacy and safety profile for such patients (see Chapter 71).

a. **Acetaminophen** remains first-line therapy for OA. (SOR **Ⓐ**) Recent meta-analyses indicate that its efficacy is significantly superior to placebo, though somewhat less than NSAIDs in terms of pain relief; likewise, some surveys and measures of quality-of-life scores indicate that patients prefer NSAIDs. However, the safety profile and low cost for acetaminophen support its use as initial therapy in patients with OA.

(1) Patients should be instructed that pain is best managed with **daily, scheduled dosing** rather than as-needed administration, as is the case with most pain-control regimens. Treatment should be initiated at 1 to 2 g total daily dose divided twice daily, with a maximum dose of 3 to 4 g daily divided into four doses (e.g., 1 g four times daily).

(2) **Potential safety issues** with acetaminophen include hepatotoxicity with overdose or in patients with liver disease, or prolongation of the half-life of warfarin; the greatest concern for toxicity is not the therapeutic dosage used, but rather additional inadvertent sources of acetaminophen such as nonprescription cold medications, concurrent use of combined acetaminophen-opioid medications, as well as concurrent use of alcohol. Patients on chronic acetaminophen should be counseled regarding other medications and about not drinking alcohol when taking acetaminophen.

b. **Topical analgesics.** Capsaicin cream is more effective than placebo for pain relief, especially for disease localized to the knee or hand, but requires four times daily application, which may limit its continued use by patients. (SOR **Ⓑ**) Nonprescription topical salicylates, and prescription topical lidocaine patches, may be effective alternatives in some patients, but there is little available evidence to guide their routine clinical use. (SOR **Ⓒ**)

c. **Tramadol hydrochloride,** a synthetic opioid, is another analgesic option for treating OA. Tramadol is not a controlled substance and is approved for moderate-to-severe pain in OA and may be equivalent to moderate-strength narcotics such as codeine. It may be particularly useful in older patients or other patients at a high risk for NSAID toxicity (see Table 71–1).

      d. Narcotics. Many patients with advanced OA do not respond adequately to acetaminophen, tramadol, NSAIDs, protective measures or braces, or corticosteroid injections. Such patients can safely and effectively be treated with chronic opiates, including codeine, oxycodone, hydrocodone, and morphine (see Table 71–1). Some patients require opiates only for short-term management of disease flares, though many will require chronic treatment with opiates, possibly as part of chronic medical management to defer joint replacement. See Chapter 71 for information on narcotic use for persistent pain.

  2. Anti-inflammatory medications. A variety of anti-inflammatory medications can be used to treat pain in patients who do not respond adequately to acetaminophen. (SOR **A**) These agents are effective in pain relief and are preferred to acetaminophen by many patients, highlighting the role of inflammation in OA. Issues to consider in prescribing NSAIDs include medication selection, dosage, and prevention of acute or chronic side effects (see Chapter 71).

      a. Selecting a medication. Meta-analyses have not shown any consistent difference in efficacy among the many available NSAIDs, including older nonacetylated agents as well as newer selective COX-2 inhibitor agents. Selection of agents should therefore be based primarily on individual patient analgesic effect, cost, availability, side effects, and ease of dosing. For unknown reasons, some patients seem to find relief with different classes of NSAIDs, whereas other agents are less effective; if patients find one NSAID ineffective, it may be appropriate to switch to a medication in a different class. However, once two or three NSAID classes have been tried and failed, other treatment options should be explored. A selection of anti-inflammatory agents by class, including typical dosing regimens, is provided in Table 82–1. For reasons of ease of administration, efficacy, low cost, and lack of proven differences in side effects, older NSAIDs such as ibuprofen are usually recommended for patients at a low risk for gastrointestinal (GI) or other side effects.

TABLE 82–1. SELECTED ANTI-INFLAMMATORY ANALGESICS

Drug Class	Generic Name	Usual Effective Dose
Nonacetylated salicylates	Aspirin[a, b,c]	325–650 mg every 4–6 h up to 3 g daily
	Diflunisal[a] (Dolobid)	250–500 mg twice daily
	Salsalate[a,c] (Disalcid)	1500 mg twice daily
Propionic acids	Ibuprofen[a,b] (Motrin, Advil)	200–800 mg three times daily
	Naproxen sulfate[a,b,c] (Naprosyn)	250–500 mg twice daily
	Ketoprofen[a,c] (Orudis, Oruvail)	50–75 mg three to four times daily OR 100–200 mg daily of ER formulation
	Oxaprozin[a] (Daypro)	1200–1800 mg once daily
	Flurbiprofen[a,c] (Ansaid)	200–300 mg/d divided two to four times daily
Acetic acids	Indomethacin[a,c] (Indocin)	25–50 mg two to three times daily OR 75 mg once to twice daily of ER formulation
	Sulindac[a] (Clinoril)	150 mg twice daily
	Diclofenac sodium[a] (Voltaren) 1% gel	50 mg two to three times daily OR 100 mg once to twice daily of ER formulation Apply 2–4 g to upper/lower extremities four times daily
	Tolmetin[a] (Tolectin)	200–600 mg three times daily
	Etodolac[a,c] (Lodine)	300–1000 mg two to three times daily OR 400–1000 mg daily of ER formulation
Oxicams	Piroxicam[a] (Feldene)	20 mg once daily
	Meloxicam[a] (Mobic)	7.5–15 mg daily
Naphthylalkanone	Nabumetone[a] (Relafen)	1000 mg once or twice daily
COX-2-selective agents	Celecoxib (Celebrex)	100–200 mg daily

[a]Available as generic.
[b]Available as nonprescription.
[c]The dose should be reduced in the elderly, usually to the lowest dose indicated.

  b. Dosage. As with other analgesic regimens, it is appropriate to recommend that NSAIDs be dosed on a **scheduled basis** rather than "as needed" to best affect the pain cycle for a disorder that is chronic in nature. Dosing should therefore begin at low doses and titrated upward for therapeutic effect, given the high risk of toxicity with prolonged NSAID use.

  c. Preventing side effects. The common side effects for the NSAIDs are GI upset (nausea, gastroesophageal reflux, constipation, diarrhea, gas, abdominal pain), dizziness, headache, rash, fluid retention/edema, and tinnitus. More serious side effects are GI bleeding, potentiation of renal insufficiency, and inhibition of platelet aggregation with prolongation of bleeding times. For the latter two complications, it is important to minimize the use and dosage of NSAIDs as much as possible in older patients or those with other chronic medical conditions; specific risk factors for worsening renal function because of NSAIDs include age older than 65 years, hypertension, congestive heart failure, concomitant use of diuretics or angiotensin-converting enzyme inhibitors, or existing renal insufficiency. Hypersensitivity reactions and hepatotoxicity are also recognized NSAID side effects. However, the selection of agents is guided most by the effort to prevent GI bleeding.

  (1) Among patients older than 65 years, approximately 25% of hospitalizations and deaths due to peptic ulcer disease are attributable to NSAIDs. The American College of Gastroenterology has high-, moderate-, and low-risk profiles as shown in Table 82–2. While not included in their risk profile, tobacco use and alcohol use are also risk factors for GI bleeding and should be considered before starting chronic NSAID therapy. In patients at a low risk for NSAID-induced gastropathy, there is no proven difference in safety profiles among the various anti-inflammatory medications. In these patients, drug selection should be based on cost, efficacy, and other factors, and physicians should attempt to minimize the dose, use, and duration of NSAID therapy. All patients should be advised to take NSAIDs following a meal or a snack and to limit or cease use of alcohol and tobacco products.

  (2) In patients at high risk, options to limit the risk of adverse GI events include the use of COX-2 specific agents or use of a gastroprotective medication. In high-risk patients, COX-2 specific medications have a significantly lower incidence of GI complications. In patients requiring additional medications for prevention of ulcers or gastritis, proton pump inhibitors are the preferred agents, though histamine H_2 receptor antagonists, misoprostol, or Carafate (cost may be prohibitive) are other options (see Chapter 84 for dosages). Topical NSAID preparations are also available and may be appropriate for higher-risk patients.

  (3) The uncertainty regarding the **cardiovascular risks of the COX-2 specific agents** necessitates additional care in using these agents for long-term management of OA. These agents should probably be reserved for patients who are at a higher risk for GI complications, lower risk of cardiovascular events, and do not improve with nonselective NSAIDs.

  (4) Drug interactions. NSAIDs have multiple interactions including those with large groups of common medications: anticoagulants/antiplatelet agents,

TABLE 82–2. RISK FACTORS FOR NSAID-INDUCED GASTROPATHY

High risk
History of a previously complicated ulcer, especially recently
Multiple (>2) risk factors

Moderate risk (one or two risk factors)
Age older than 65 yr
High-dose NSAID therapy
Concurrent use of aspirin (including low-dose), glucocorticoids, or anticoagulants
A previous history of uncomplicated ulcer

Low Risk
No risk factors

selective serotonin receptor inhibitors, serotonin norepinephrine reuptake inhibitors, ginkgo (risk of bleeding); antihypertensives (decreased antihypertensive efficacy) and in combination with angiotensin receptor blockers and potassium-sparing diuretics (risk of nephrotoxicity); sulfonylureas (risk of hypoglycemia); and quinolone antibiotics (risk of seizures).

3. Herbal preparations. Glucosamine (1500 mg per day in three divided doses) and chondroitin (800–1200 mg per day in three divided doses) may provide some pain relief, but Cochrane authors found that only the Rotta preparation of glucosamine was of benefit over placebo and the benefit is less clear when only higher quality studies are considered. (SOR **B**) Patients should be advised that these agents are available without a prescription and that different formulations may use lower doses, which may be ineffective. Patients may be reluctant to continue paying directly for these agents over the long term, but a trial of therapy for efficacy may be appropriate. Other herbal agents that may have some benefit include S-adenosylmethionine (SAMe), 200 mg three times daily, (SOR **B**) and avocado/soybean unsaponifiables, 300 mg per day. (SOR **C**)

D. Joint injection

1. In the presence of knee joint effusion and inflammation, **corticosteroid injection** has been shown to provide pain relief over 1 to 2 weeks, but is not effective for long-term pain relief. (SOR **A**)

2. Viscosupplementation via intra-articular injection of hyaluronic acid may be an option for patients who do not respond to medical therapy or who are at a high risk for NSAID-induced gastropathy, narcotic addiction or side effects, or other complications. Patients with persistent pain and functional limitations who are not surgical candidates may also benefit. The ideal candidate for injection therapy has not been defined and the overall benefit is described as "small and clinically irrelevant" in a recent meta-analysis, which concluded that the benefits do not outweigh the risks. (SOR **A**) Weekly injections are given for 3 to 5 weeks, and this regimen may be repeated only twice per year. The cost of these medications may be prohibitive for some patients (approximately $600 for a treatment course).

E. Acupuncture may provide relief in some patients with knee and hip OA, but has not been directly compared to other treatment modalities. (SOR **A**) The benefit of acupuncture, however, is small and may not be clinically significant.

F. Surgical management. Surgical options for OA of the knee include arthroscopic debridement, distal femoral osteotomy, unicompartmental knee replacement or hemiarthroplasty, patellofemoral arthroplasty, or total knee arthroplasty. Indications for surgical intervention include pain, instability, or disability uncontrolled with physical and medical management. Given the likelihood of prosthesis loosening and the need for subsequent reoperation after approximately 10 years, it is usually appropriate to defer surgical intervention using conservative measures until patients are older and have more limited activity requirements. There is only limited evidence, as noted earlier, to support arthroscopic debridement for knee OA and this treatment should not be recommended as routine treatment.

IV. Management Strategies. It is very important for the family physician to manage the "whole patient" and not to focus solely on medications and formal physical therapy in treating OA. Patient-focused management includes educating the patient (and the caregiver if relevant) in the many techniques that can reduce symptoms by reducing the stress on diseased joints and addressing other social and medical dimensions of their care. These techniques thus reduce the impact of the arthritis on the patient's life and help address not only pain but also total quality of life.

A. Patient education and support. Patients and families must be educated about the pathophysiology of OA and should be able to identify significant symptoms and recognize inflammatory phases and other symptoms that may necessitate modifications in management. An understanding of the disease process may be especially important in younger patients with OA, who are forced to begin management of a chronic illness. Patients and families should be directed toward organizations such as the Arthritis Foundation (www.arthritis.org/), which has local chapters and extensive educational and support activities.

1. In older patients, arthritis and its many consequences (which can be devastating to the patient's overall health and function) are often tolerated as "normal" accompaniments of aging, and patients should understand the nature of their illness and the breadth of management options available. Some patients may benefit from more frequent, scheduled visits than from "follow-up as needed" to continue patient education and address other aspects of disease management. Topics for anticipatory counseling should include sexuality, including finding comfortable sexual positions; posture, including chair height and style; toileting and bathing needs; exercise and activity habits; and driving, including entering and exiting the car.

B. Depression often accompanies chronic joint pain and then interferes with motivation and compliance as well as increasing the patient's awareness of the pain itself. Good clinical management thus involves seeing patients and their families in the entire context of their lives, functionality, and the rest of their health, since movement and everyday activities are inevitably affected by these illnesses. Counseling and medical treatment for depression may be needed in depressed patients (Chapter 94); use of tricyclic antidepressants, if otherwise appropriate, may provide additional benefit in terms of pain relief and help with sleep.

C. Disability assessments. Patients with chronic pain and self-assessed disability often request assistance from their physicians in applying for disability benefits. Assessing for true disability in terms of overall "whole patient" disability or isolated disabilities of specific limbs and joints is complex. Rational disability assessment is further complicated by issues of credibility, secondary gain, and effort on the part of the patient, and lack of expertise or familiarity on the part of the physician. Guidelines on disability determination are available (http://www.ssa.gov/disability/determination.htm), and consultation with a physician trained in occupational medicine is recommended. Patients in general should not be determined to be fully disabled without a more thorough assessment of their functional capacity.

D. Mobility assessments. Many patients with OA of the knees and/or hips have activity-limiting pain or joint instability that interferes with normal gait and mobility. Primary care clinicians are often asked to help patients in their application process for motorized wheelchairs or scooters, or other mobility assistive devices. Medicare covers these devices in qualified patients, but a significant paperwork burden often accompanies this process. Physicians should be prepared to assist patients in their effort to secure appropriate mobility assist devices. However, some patients do not qualify for such devices or can achieve adequate mobility and pain relief using other means, and physicians should emphasize this to patients and not recommend mobility devices based solely on patient request. Mobility assessments include the "get up and go" test (http://www.hospitalmedicine.org/geriresource/toolbox/pdfs/get_up_and_go_test.pdf) and the performance-oriented mobility assessment (http://www.hospitalmedicine.org/geriresource/toolbox/pdfs/poma.pdf).

E. Chronic narcotic therapy management. Routine management of patients who are on chronic narcotic therapy is probably one of the most challenging aspects of primary care chronic illness management, due to the balance of patient benefit versus societal obligation that it entails. While many patients derive great benefit and pain relief from chronic opiate therapy, many other patients are at a high risk for opiate overdose including death, and some may misuse or divert (sell) such medications leading to harm in others. As described in the Institute of Medicine "Relieving Pain in America" report of 2011, increased efforts are necessary by both physicians and society to provide appropriate pain relief in an effective, safe, and patient-focused manner.

1. Chronic opiate therapy management should be approached from an **office system perspective** and includes the following: documentation of a diagnosis that justifies chronic opiate therapy; documentation that other reasonable measures have failed; discussion of risks and benefits of such therapy with patients; explanation of appropriate drug use and refill patterns (obtain medications from only one physician and one pharmacy; take medications as prescribed; no early refills on medications will be given; medications will be discontinued if there is evidence of substance abuse; and patients need to follow up with their physician as instructed); periodic urine drug testing to help evaluate for drug diversion; and assessment for "doctor-shopping" or other evidence of drug addiction or "drug-seeking." Many physicians prefer to refer to specialists in pain management or to use "narcotic contracts" signed by the patient to address these requirements (see Chapter 71).

2. Management of patients on chronic opioids may require additional work and office protocols to ensure appropriate use of these medications and to prevent drug diversion; however, this management is well within the scope of practice for most family physicians, and management resting on an accurate diagnosis, an overall management plan, and appropriate monitoring and documentation is unlikely to lead to licensing or regulatory problems. With the growing population of elderly and obese patients, primary care clinicians are increasingly called upon to manage chronic pain conditions including OA, including chronic opiate management, and pain specialists do not exist in sufficient number to manage all these patients. As noted earlier, physiologic tolerance or dependence is distinct from drug addiction, which is rare in patients with chronic pain who do not have a history of substance abuse.

F. Referral criteria. In general, patients with OA can be effectively managed by primary care clinicians. Referral to physical therapists or occupational therapists is common, and joint management with therapists can be effective in overall patient care. Referral to rheumatologists may be necessary to confirm the diagnosis of rheumatoid arthritis or other conditions, and referral to orthopedic surgeons should be undertaken when surgical intervention is required, or if the primary care physician is uncomfortable performing joint injections. Referral to pain management specialists, as aforementioned, may be helpful in patients requiring long-term narcotic therapy.

V. Prognosis. Symptoms of OA can be expected to worsen over time, although improving muscular support and general fitness and continual attention to mobility and range of motion can keep symptoms at bay for years. Major interventions in OA, such as joint replacement (particularly the knee or hip), can be seemingly "curative" of that particular joint, provided that the patient can fully collaborate in the necessary rehabilitative process.

SELECTED REFERENCES

Bennell KL. Management of osteoarthritis of the knee. *BMJ.* 2012;345:e4934.

Brouwer RW, van Raaij TM, Jakma TT, et al. Braces and orthoses for treating osteoarthritis of the knee. *Cochrane Database Syst Rev.* 2005;(1):CD004020.

Fransen M, McConnell S, Hernandez-Molina G, Reichenbach S. Exercise for osteoarthritis of the hip. *Cochrane Database Syst Rev.* 2009;(3):CD007912.

Fransen M, McConnell S. Exercise for osteoarthritis of the knee. *Cochrane Database Syst Rev.* 2008;(4):CD004376.

Garstang SV. Osteoarthritis: epidemiology, risk factors, and pathophysiology. *Am J Phys Med Rehab.* 2006;85(11):S2–S10.

Hunter DJ. In the clinic. Osteoarthritis. *Ann Intern Med.* 2007;ITC8-1–ITC8-16.

Kirkley A, Birmingham TB, Litchfield RB, et al. A randomized trial of arthroscopic surgery for osteoarthritis of the knee. *N Engl J Med.* 2008;359(11):1097–1107.

Lo V. When should COX-2 selective NSAIDs be used for osteoarthritis and rheumatoid arthritis? *J Fam Pract.* 2006;55(3):260–262.

Manheimer E, Cheng K, Linde K, et al. Acupuncture for peripheral joint osteoarthritis. *Cochrane Database Syst Rev.* 2010;(1):CD001977.

Murphy L. The impact of osteoarthritis in the United States: a population-health perspective. *Am J Nursing.* 2012;112(3):S13–S19.

Nicholson B. Responsible prescribing of opioids for the management of chronic pain. *Drugs.* 2003; 63(1):17–32.

Reid MC. Pharmacologic management of osteoarthritis-related pain in older adults. *Am J Nursing.* 2012;112(3):S38–S43.

Sisto SA. Osteoarthritis and therapeutic exercise. *Am J Phys Med Rehab.* 2006;85(Suppl 11):S69–S78.

Sofat N. What makes osteoarthritis painful? The evidence for local and central pain processing. *Rheumatology.* 2011;50:2157–2165.

Stitik TP. Pharmacotherapy of osteoarthritis. *Am J Phys Med Rehab.* 2006;85(Suppl 11):S15–S28.

Towheed T, Maxwell L, Anastassiades TP, et al. Glucosamine therapy for treating osteoarthritis. *Cochrane Database Syst Rev.* 2005;(2):CD002946.

van Dijk GM. Course of functional status and pain in osteoarthritis of the hip or knee: a systematic review of the literature. *Arthritis Rheum.* 2006;55(5):779–785.

Yonclas PP. Orthotics and assistive devices in the treatment of upper and lower limb osteoarthritis. *Am J Phys Med Rehab.* 2006;85(Suppl 11):S82–S97.

Additional references are available online at http://langetextbooks.com/fm6e

83   Osteoporosis

William T. Manard, MD, FAAFP, & Richard O. Schamp, MD, CMD, CHCQM

KEY POINTS

- Osteoporosis is a multifactorial disease causing fractures which lead to significant morbidity. (SOR **C**)
- Screening for osteoporosis and treatment in women aged 65 years or older, and in younger women with a 10-year fracture risk equal to or greater than women of this age, may reduce fracture occurrence. (SOR **B**)
- Numerous treatment options are available for osteoporosis, from daily oral or nasal medications to an annual injection. (SOR **C**) Results of treatment trials are strongest for prevention of vertebral fractures with bisphosphonates, parathyroid hormone, denosumab, raloxifene, and estrogen. (SOR **A**)
- Clinical conditions other than advanced age and female sex may lead to secondary osteoporosis and should be treated accordingly. (SOR **C**)

I. Introduction

A. Osteoporosis is a systemic skeletal condition characterized by severe bone mineral loss and disruption of skeletal microarchitecture leading to enhanced bone fragility. This is chiefly manifested by atraumatic fractures of the vertebral column, upper femur, distal radius, proximal humerus, pubic rami, and ribs.

B. Bone constantly remodels through the process of resorption and formation, which allows for bone growth and repair. This process occurs at age-related rates, ranging from complete renewal of all bones in the first year of life to renewal of 15% to 30% of the skeleton per year in adults. Loss of bone mineral density (BMD) alone explains only approximately 60% to 80% of the variation in bone strength. Trabecular bone architectural changes contribute significantly to fracture risk, but are not easily assessed clinically.

C. Bone mass reaches a peak by 35 years, with age-related bone loss beginning by 40 years in both sexes. After menopause, the rate of bone resorption exceeds the rate of bone formation. Over her lifetime, a woman loses 35% of her cortical bone and 50% of her trabecular bone. Men lose only two-thirds of the bone that women lose as muscle mass decreases.

D. Three major types of osteoporosis are recognized, although most commonly osteoporosis is simply considered as primary or secondary.

1. **Postmenopausal (type I)** is the most common form, especially in Caucasian and Asian women, because of acceleration of trabecular bone resorption in the first decade or two following menopause.

2. **Involutional (type II)** occurs in both men and women older than 70 years and is because of a subtle, prolonged imbalance between rates of bone resorption and formation. Type II weakens cortical bone more than type I. Mixtures of types I and II are common, with additive effects.

3. **Secondary (type III)** generally occurs in response to other diseases or drugs, such as those outlined in Table 83–1. Treatment of these conditions generally arrests bone loss and may reverse bone demineralization.

E. Osteoporosis affects approximately 28 million people in the United States (≥15 million symptomatic cases) and thus is commonly seen in adult primary care practices. Seven percent of ambulatory postmenopausal women older than 50 years have osteoporosis. A 50-year-old white woman has lifetime risks of fracture of the spine, hip, and distal radius of 32%, 16%, and 15%, respectively. These risks greatly exceed her risk of developing endometrial or breast cancer combined. Age is a strong predictor of osteoporosis, which is five times more common in women older than 65 years than in women younger than 65 years.

F. Risk factors for osteoporosis are listed in Table 83–2. Factors associated with decreased risk for osteoporosis included higher body mass index, African-American heritage, estrogen use, thiazide diuretic use, moderate exercise, and moderate alcohol consumption. Clinical risk factors have poorly validated roles in predicting fractures and

TABLE 83–1. RISK FACTORS FOR OSTEOPOROSIS

Caucasian or Asian race
Excessive alcohol, caffeine, or tobacco use
History of falls (and reasons for falls such as hypotension, low vision, or poor balance)
Family history of osteoporosis or osteoporotic fracture
Increasing age
Low body weight (under 127 lbs or 58 kg, or body mass index [BMI] <20)
Low calcium or vitamin D intake
Low level of physical activity
Menstrual status: amenorrhea, early menopause, late menarche
Personal history of fracture

in determining who should have BMD measurement; however, use of a comprehensive calculator such as the FRAX tool can help stratify risk of fracture.

II. Screening and Prevention

   A. The United States Preventive Services Task Force (USPSTF) recommends **screening for osteoporosis in all women 65 years of age or older, and in younger women who have a risk** of osteoporotic fracture of at least that of a 65-year-old white woman with no additional risk factors. (SOR **B**) Risk is determined using a tool such as FRAX (http://www.shef.ac.uk/FRAX/).

   1. Screening for osteoporosis is done using a 2-site DEXA scan. (SOR **B**)

   B. The USPSTF concluded that evidence was insufficient for recommending screening in men. (SOR **C**) However, the American College of Physicians recommends screening **men at increased risk** (using FRAX tool) and who are candidates for pharmacotherapy. (SOR **B**) Recommendations from other organizations regarding screening of men are highly variable.

   C. Methods to prevent osteoporosis include regular weight bearing exercise, adequate dietary calcium and vitamin D, avoidance of heavy alcohol use, avoidance of smoking, and avoidance of glucocorticoid therapy.

   D. Patients with a likely fragility fracture and those receiving long-term glucocorticoid therapy or other agents known to cause osteoporosis should be screened for osteoporosis. (SOR **C**)

III. Diagnosis

   A. Osteoporosis is usually defined as a BMD T-score ≥2.5 standard deviations (SDs) below the young adult mean, or a fracture resulting from minimal trauma (fragility fracture).

TABLE 83–2. CAUSES OF SECONDARY OSTEOPOROSIS

Cancer	Multiple myeloma
	Bony metastases
	Lymphoma, leukemia
Chronic disease	Inflammatory arthritis (SLE, rheumatoid)
	Inflammatory bowel disease
	Chronic kidney disease
	Paget disease
Genetic disorders	Osteogenesis imperfecta
	Ehlers–Danlos syndrome
	Homocystinuria
Hormonal	Cushing syndrome
	Hyperthyroidism
	Hypogonadism
Medication use	Aluminum-containing antacids
	Anticonvulsants
	Cancer agents (anastrozole, letrozole, exemestane, goserelin, leuprolide)
	Corticosteroids
	Heparins
	Loop diuretics
	Proton pump inhibitors
Other	Inactivity or immobilization
	Malnutrition/eating disorders

SLE, Systemic lupus erythematosus.

BMD refers to the amount of mineral matter per square centimeter of bone. **Osteopenia** is defined as a BMD T-score between −1.0 and −2.5.

B. Other clinical features that may lead a clinician to suspect osteoporosis include unexplained back pain, unexplained low energy fractures, loss of height of 2 cm or more (or 6 cm below young adult height), poor dentition, or mechanical deformity of the spine. The presence of these conditions should prompt consideration of formal BMD determination. Height loss can be related to aging changes in the bones, muscles, and joints. People typically lose about 1 cm (0.4 inches) every 10 years after age 40 years. Height loss is even more rapid after age 70 years.

C. Laboratory tests

1. For patients likely to have primary postmenopausal osteoporosis, routine laboratory screening is not generally indicated.

2. Testing of presumed healthy patients with osteoporosis may reveal bone and mineral metabolism disorders, so clinicians should be alert to other signs and symptoms such as kidney stones (e.g., hypercalciuria, hyperparathyroidism), medication history (e.g., exogenous hyperthyroidism or steroid use), or abdominal striae and moon facies (Cushing disease). Tests might include serum calcium, alkaline phosphatase, creatinine, phosphate, and thyroid-stimulating hormone, which should be normal in patients with primary osteoporosis. (SOR ☻)

3. Consider 25-hydroxyvitamin D for at-risk populations (home-bound, institutionalized, or other sunlight-deprived circumstances). Other tests include intact parathyroid hormone (iPTH), serum protein electrophoresis (SPEP), testosterone (men), estradiol (women), and 24-hour urinary calcium excretion tests to rule out other secondary causes (Table 83–2). (SOR ☻)

4. Consider tests of bone metabolism in uncertain cases: (SOR ☻)

a. Urine calcium/creatinine ratio (elevated in hypercalciuria)

b. Tubular reabsorption of **phosphorus** (used to assess pathologic conditions associated with hypophosphatemia)

c. Bone-specific alkaline phosphatase (marker of bone formation)

d. Osteocalcin (biomarker of bone formation)

5. Bone biopsy is rarely needed and requires a nondecalcified bone specimen with tetracycline labeling and a specialized laboratory for interpretation.

6. Bone marrow aspiration and biopsy can be used to rule out multiple myeloma, metastatic carcinoma, and lymphoma, if clinically indicated.

D. Imaging studies

1. X-rays. By the time osteoporosis is evident on x-ray, 20% to 40% of bone is lost. The following changes can be seen on plain x-ray of the vertebral column: increased lucency, cortical thinning, increased density of end plate, anterior wedging and biconcavity of vertebrae, and loss of horizontal trabeculae.

2. BMD testing. The decision to order BMD testing in the patient with suspected or established osteoporosis entails several considerations:

a. Chief among these is whether the results will change treatment. Patients who are at sufficiently high risk for osteoporotic fracture (e.g., those older than 70 years with multiple risk factors) will not likely benefit from BMD testing if treatment is indicated on clinical grounds regardless. (SOR ☻)

b. Deciding which patients to consider for BMD measurement requires weighing risk factors on an individual basis. (SOR ☻)

c. Some clinicians will order serial studies to follow the effects of treatment on BMD, but there is little evidence to support this or to guide frequency of reassessment. (SOR ☻)

d. Three imaging modalities are commonly available: dual-energy x-ray absorptiometry (DXA), quantitative computed tomography (QCT), and calcaneal ultrasonography. DXA measurements are the basis for WHO criteria, with other techniques being useful for screening in certain circumstances.

e. DXA is the most precise technique, is used most widely for measuring BMD, and correlates best with the WHO criteria. Measurements are typically taken from the lumbar spine and the proximal femurs.

f. QCT results are less likely to be affected by degenerative spinal changes than spine DXA scanning. Also, unlike DXA, QCT allows for selective assessment of trabecular bone, which may show metabolic changes earlier. QCT can predict spinal fracture similarly to DXA scanning, but the costs and radiation exposure are higher.

g. Ultrasonography measures the speed of sound (related to bone density) and broadband ultrasonic attenuation (related to bone architecture) of the calcaneus, typically. Fracture risk prediction is equivalent to that of DXA, especially for hip fracture. Ultrasound is available for in-office use and is portable, making evaluation in the long-term care facility feasible. Lower precision makes this technique not recommended for serial measurements. (SOR **C**)

h. Deciding which bone imaging modality depends upon availability, age, site of interest, and costs. For example, vertebral fractures are of greater concern than hip fractures in women who are within 15 years of menopause. Any of the imaging modalities may be appropriate, especially those that include imaging of the spine. In women older than 65 years, hip fractures become more of a concern, so DXA of the hip or calcaneal ultrasound might be appropriate.

IV. Treatment

A. The continuous distribution of BMD and current available evidence preclude an absolute "fracture risk threshold" to initiate treatment. Other factors such as skeletal architecture (presently difficult to measure), fall risk, exercise patterns, life expectancy, medication adverse side effects, patient preferences, and the constellation of risk factors (Table 83–1) must be considered in a manner analogous to the management of hyperlipidemia or hypertension, in which treatment thresholds depend on other risk factors as well as lipid levels or blood pressure. An evidence-based, validated algorithm for the treatment of osteoporosis that includes patient-specific risk factors for fracture and BMD measure does not currently exist. Thus, current management has to be individualized.

B. Primary prevention includes patients with osteopenia. Although the majority of osteoporotic fractures occur in individuals with osteopenia, the use of antiosteoporotic medication in this group, based on T-score alone, is not advisable. Reasons include a high number needed to treat (NNT >100 vs. 10–20 for patients with osteoporosis) and lack of demonstrated treatment benefit from randomized clinical trials.

1. Lifestyle. Factors that can decrease calcium absorption, increase bone resorption, or impair bone formation such as smoking, excessive alcohol intake, and medications associated with osteoporosis should be avoided. (SOR **C**)

2. Weight-bearing exercise. Exercise should be weight bearing and skeletal stressing. Prolonged low-to-moderate physical activity is associated with higher BMD than either sedentary lifestyle or endurance-trained athletic activity. (SOR **B**)

3. Calcium supplements. The average American consumes ≤800 mg per day of calcium. Recommendations for calcium intake vary by age; adults aged 19 to 50 years and men until age 70 years should consume 1000 mg of calcium daily; women aged 51 years and older and those over age 70 years should consume 1200 mg of calcium daily. Calcium alone can prevent bone loss and fractures. (SOR **B**)

a. Estimating calcium intake. An estimation of the patient's dietary intake can be made quickly and easily using the rule of 300: the basal diet contains 300 mg of calcium, and each serving of dairy products, such as 8 oz milk, 8 oz yogurt, 1.5 oz cheese, or two cups cottage cheese, provides 300 mg of calcium. Excellent sources of nondairy calcium include calcium-fortified orange juice or calcium-fortified soy milk (200–400 mg/cup), sardines (372 mg in 3 oz), 1 cup of cooked spinach (240 mg), 3 oz of almonds (210 mg); 1 cup cooked broccoli (180 mg), 3 oz of canned pink salmon including the bones (167 mg), and baked beans (1 cup = 142 mg).

b. General information. There is little evidence favoring specific calcium supplements for efficacy in preventing osteoporotic fractures. Absorption is improved with doses ≤500 mg and when taken with food. Calcium supplements can interfere with absorption of other minerals and many drugs (e.g., iron, zinc, quinolones, bisphosphonates, tetracycline) (Table 83–3).

c. Calcium carbonate is usually derived from oyster shells, is the least expensive oral form of calcium supplement available, and requires the fewest tablets per day. It is also the form most commonly studied in clinical trials. It may cause more gastrointestinal upset (constipation, bloating, and gas) than other preparations. Stomach acid is required for absorption, which may limit effectiveness in patients who are elderly, taking proton pump inhibitors or H2-blockers, or have achlorhydria. Excessive dosing, or consuming milk plus antacids (calcium carbonate or sodium bicarbonate) together over time, can cause milk–alkali syndrome.

TABLE 83–3. PREVENTION AND TREATMENT OPTIONS FOR OSTEOPOROSIS

Drug[a]	Dose[b]	Common Side Effects	Contraindications	Drug Interactions
Primary Prevention				
Calcium[a]	Calcium carbonate: 500 mg twice daily Calcium citrate (250–315 mg) three to four tablets daily; each dose ≤500 mg	Constipation, gas, bloating	Hypercalcemia, hypercalciuria, hypophosphatemia	Lansoprazole, levothyroxine, phenytoin, quinolone antibiotics, tetracycline, ticlopidine propranolol, some antiretrovirals (↓ drug absorption—space apart)
Vitamin D[a]	Vitamin D$_3$ (cholecalciferol)[c] 600–800 IU daily; Vitamin D$_2$ (ergocalciferol) 50,000 IU weekly for 8–12 wk	Hypercalcemia	Hypercalcemia, hyperphosphatemia, sarcoidosis, renal osteodystrophy	Cimetidine, orlistat (↓ vitamin D levels)
Bisphosphonates				
Alendronate (Fosamax)[a]	70 mg orally weekly 35 mg orally weekly (prevention—osteopenia)	Indigestion, abdominal pain, diarrhea, constipation, headache, fever	Esophageal abnormalities or stricture, inability to sit or stand for at least 30 min, achalasia of esophagus, jaw osteonecrosis, CrCl <35 mL/min, hypocalcemia Caution with dysphagia, Barrett esophagus, GI ulcers	All medications, minerals, and foods interact with bisphosphonates and decrease absorption—these should not be taken until at least 30 min after the dose (60 min for ibandronate)
Risedronate (Actonel)[a] Risedronate ER (Atelvia)	35 mg orally weekly	Indigestion, abdominal pain, diarrhea, constipation, backache, UTI, flu-like illness, rash	See alendronate	See alendronate Risedronate ER is taken immediately after breakfast, but medications should not be taken for at least 30 min after the dose Calcium, magnesium, iron, and antacids should ideally be taken later in the day
Ibandronate (Boniva)[a]	150 mg orally monthly or 3 mg intravenously quarterly	Indigestion, abdominal pain, diarrhea, headache, backache, limb pain, bronchitis/URI, hypertension	See alendronate	See alendronate; food and medications should not be taken for at least 60 min following the dose
Zoledronic acid (Reclast)	5 mg intravenously annually	Indigestion, abdominal pain, diarrhea, headache, backache, limb pain, arthralgia, peripheral edema, asthenia, fatigue	Hypocalcemia, CrCl <35 mL/min, dehydration Pregnancy (category D)	None known

(continued)

TABLE 83–3. PREVENTION AND TREATMENT OPTIONS FOR OSTEOPOROSIS (*Continued*)

Drug[a]	Dose[b]	Common Side Effects	Contraindications	Drug Interactions
Other				
Raloxifene (Evista)	60 mg daily	Hot flashes, leg cramps	VTE, severe hot flashes Pregnancy (category X) Breastfeeding	Cholestyramine (↓ raloxifene absorption and effect), warfarin (loss of anticoagulation control)
Calcitonin nasal (Miacalcin)[c]	200 IU (one spray) daily; alternate nostrils	Nausea, flushing, rhinitis	None	Lithium (↓ lithium levels and efficacy)
Estrogen replacement therapy[a]	Varies	Nausea, abdominal pain, headache, breast pain, depression	Prior VTE, estrogen-dependent neoplasia, endometrial hyperplasia, undiagnosed genital bleeding, MI, protein C/S deficiency	**Multiple Interactions** Rifampin, phenytoin, carbamazepine, topiramate, griseofulvin, antiretroviral agents (↓ serum hormone concentration); cyclosporine (cyclosporine toxicity); tranexamic acid (risk of VTE); warfarin (altered anticoagulant effect)
Teriparatide (Forteo)	20 μg subcutaneously daily	Arthralgia, muscle spasm, GI distress, dizziness, cough, sweating, hypotension	Hypercalcemia, Paget bone disease, bone malignancy, recent urolithiasis, unexplained ↑ alkaline phosphatase	Digoxin (digoxin toxicity)
Denosumab (Prolia)	60 mg subcutaneously every 6 mo	Nausea, diarrhea, backache, limb pain, arthralgia, asthenia, headache, fatigue, nasopharyngitis, URI, cystitis, ↑ cholesterol, serious infection	Hypocalcemia Pregnancy (category X)	None known

[a]Available as generic medication.
[b]Dose for calcium in stated in milligrams of elemental calcium.
[c]Higher doses may be used for known vitamin D deficiency/low serum vitamin D level.
CrCl, creatinine clearance; GI, gastrointestinal; MI, myocardial infarction; URI, upper respiratory infection; UTI, urinary tract infection; VTE, venous thromboembolic event including deep vein thrombosis, pulmonary embolus, and stroke.

    d. Calcium citrate is best absorbed, has fewest side effects, need not be taken with meals in order to maximize absorption, and costs more than calcium carbonate. If carbonate forms are poorly tolerated, this option can be helpful. Calcium citrate is recommended for patients taking proton pump inhibitors and H2-blockers. Theoretically, lower doses may be effective because more is absorbed, but this has not been well studied. (SOR **C**)

    e. Absorption of all calcium products is improved with adequate vitamin D, with supplemental magnesium salts, and with thiazide diuretics. Sodium restriction reduces urinary excretion of calcium, but has unclear effects on bones.

4. Vitamin D is traditionally recommended in supplemental form since dietary intake or endogenous production is frequently suboptimal. This vitamin is manufactured variably in the skin following direct exposure to sunlight. Exposure of 10 to 15 minutes for the hands, arms, and face three times per week is often enough for young fair-skinned persons. Vitamin D production is decreased by dark skin, use of sunscreens, window glass, clothing, air pollution, aging, and lack of sun exposure (northern latitude, homebound persons, or cultural dressing habits).

    a. In combination with adequate calcium intake, supplemental vitamin D can reduce fractures significantly, up to 50% in nursing home patients. (SOR **B**) Recommended dose for ages 1 to 70 years is 600 IU/day and for over 70 years is 800 IU/day (Table 83–3).

    b. Potential (3%–5%) for hypercalcemia exists with high doses of vitamin D. The recommended upper level of intake is 4000 IU per day. Excessive vitamin D cannot be obtained from food (except cod liver oil) or sunlight exposure.

    c. Calcium and vitamin D together are strongly recommended for all patients taking long-term corticosteroids. (SOR **B**)

5. Secondary causes of osteoporosis should be sought and treated if possible, including use of drugs with adverse effects on BMD (Table 83–2).

6. Risks factors for fracture, such as orthostatic hypotension, lower limb dysfunction, and visual impairment especially in the frail, elderly patient, should be sought and reduced (Table 83–1). A home safety evaluation should be considered to prevent falls.

C. Secondary prevention attempts to detect disease early and minimize the risks in patients discovered to have asymptomatic osteoporosis, usually through screening or clinical suspicion. **Primary prevention strategies remain in force.** Drug therapy is often indicated. Agents shown to prevent vertebral fractures in postmenopausal women include alendronate, risedronate, ibandronate, zoledronic acid, teriparatide (parathyroid hormone), raloxifene (selective estrogen receptor modulator), estrogen, and denosumab (monoclonal antibody) (Table 83–3). (SOR **A**) Data are less robust for prevention of non-vertebral fractures and only support use of alendronate, risedronate, zoledronic acid, estrogen, denosumab, and teriparatide. Large trials with fracture outcomes are lacking regarding calcitonin.

1. Bisphosphonates inhibit bone resorption and have the best evidence for efficacy. (SOR **A**)

    a. Caution. Because calcium supplements or food taken at the same time as a bisphosphonate reduces already low (0.5%–1%) absorption of the drug, immediate release products should be taken on an empty stomach (before breakfast after an overnight fast) with a full glass of water and without eating, taking other medications, or lying down for 30 minutes (60 minutes for ibandronate).

    b. Adverse effects. Common side effects are shown in Table 83–3. There is also evidence of a rare atypical femoral shaft fracture (0.13% in the subsequent year for women with at least 5 years of treatment) and jaw osteonecrosis (0.7 per 100,000 patient-years with oral bisphosphonate therapy).

    c. Specific agents

        (1) Alendronate (Fosamax), 70 mg orally once weekly, has an NNT of 37 to 91 over 3 years for symptomatic fracture prevention in women with known osteoporosis (with previous fractures). Alendronate prevents bone density loss after discontinuation of hormone therapy (HT).

        (2) Risedronate (Actonel), 35 mg orally once weekly, has an NNT of 15 to 77 over 3 years for fracture prevention in women with preexisting vertebral fracture. Risedronate is also available as a sustained-release formulation (Atelvia), which is also administered as a 35-mg weekly dose. The sustained-release formulation is taken immediately after breakfast.

    (3) Ibandronate (Boniva), 150 mg orally once monthly, has NNT of 30 over 3 years for prevention of clinical vertebral fracture. It is also available as intravenous therapy, 3 mg administered once every 3 months; this form, however, has only been shown to improve BMD without fracture reduction.

    (4) Zoledronic acid (Reclast), 5 mg infused intravenously annually, has been shown to reduce both hip and vertebral fractures. The convenience of administration may make this a good choice for those unable to routinely take oral bisphosphonates. It has an NNT of 29 to 91 over 3 years for both primary and secondary prevention of fracture. There is an association between infusions of zoledronic acid and serious atrial fibrillation (absolute risk about 0.6% over placebo).

  d. Duration of treatment. Consider discontinuation of a bisphosphonate after 4 to 5 years of stability (some recommend after 3 years for zoledronic acid) or after 10 years of stability for high-risk patients. Treatment can be reinstituted if BMD declines substantially, bone turnover markers increase, or a fracture occurs.

    (1) After withdrawal of bisphosphonate treatment, benefits on BMD and bone turnover persist for about 2 to 3 years for alendronate and 1 to 2 years for ibandronate and risedronate. The benefits on BMD for zoledronic acid persist for at least 3 years after discontinuation.

    (2) Continuation of bisphosphonates without the need for further BMD evaluation is recommended for high-risk individuals. When bisphosphonates are continued, review treatment adherence and adverse effects, including renal function evaluation, every 5 years.

    (3) If bisphosphonates are discontinued, fracture risk should be reevaluated after every new fracture, or after 2 years if no new fracture occurs.

2. Raloxifene (Evista) is a selective estrogen receptor modulator (SERM). This agent may provide the beneficial effects of estrogen therapy on lipids and bone without some of its potentially serious side effects (e.g., endometrial and breast cancer), especially in those women with a history of breast cancer. (SOR **Ⓐ**)

  a. Raloxifene reduces risk of recurrent vertebral fracture in postmenopausal women with known osteoporosis (NNT 29/3 years). The benefit of preventing hip fractures is yet unproven.

  b. Adverse effects include venous thromboembolism (NNH 440/year) and hot flashes. It is a pregnancy category X agent and is contraindicated during breastfeeding.

  c. No increased risk of heart disease or breast cancer mortality is reported with raloxifene.

3. HT. Estrogen alone or in combination with progestin has been prescribed for prevention of postmenopausal osteoporosis. Accumulated evidence is variable regarding the fracture benefits of this practice (NNT ranges from 132/year to 1429/year for vertebral fracture prevention and NNT 2000/year for hip fracture prevention). The risks of estrogen supplementation must be considered with regard to cancer, heart disease, and other conditions. Estrogens and combined estrogen–progestin products should only be considered as a preventive strategy for women with significant risk of osteoporosis that outweighs the risks of the drug (SOR **Ⓑ**) or in those women who cannot take bisphosphonates. (SOR **Ⓒ**)

4. Teriparatide (Forteo) is an *N*-terminal fragment (1–34) of recombinant human PTH and the first Food and Drug Administration (FDA)-approved agent that stimulates new bone formation for osteoporosis in postmenopausal women and men with primary or hypogonadal osteoporosis. Use is limited to 2 years over a lifetime.

  a. Unlike other agents, teriparatide increases BMD. In high-risk patients with established osteoporosis, it prevents new vertebral fracture (NNT 10–11), new nonvertebral fractures (NNT 30), and new nonvertebral fragility fractures (NNT 35). So, teriparatide may be more effective than bisphosphonates. (SOR **Ⓐ**)

  b. It is supplied as an injector pen that supplies 20 μg for 28 days of dosing; doses are given subcutaneously into the thigh or abdominal wall once daily. The pen must be kept refrigerated at all times.

  c. The FDA boxed warning states that teriparatide should not be used if there is an increased baseline risk for osteosarcoma, Paget disease of bone, unexplained alkaline phosphatase elevations, open epiphyses, prior radiation therapy of skeleton, metastases, history of skeletal malignancies, metabolic bone diseases (other than osteoporosis), or preexisting hypercalcemia.

   d. Adverse effects include pain, arthralgia, asthenia, nausea, rhinitis, dizziness, headache, hypertension, increased cough, pharyngitis, constipation, diarrhea, and dyspepsia.

   e. Teriparatide is more costly than other options previously mentioned, which limit its use for routine osteoporosis care to those who have failed other therapies or are at particularly high risk for fracture.

5. **Denosumab** (Prolia) is a monoclonal antibody that binds the receptor activator of nuclear factor kappa-B ligand (RANKL). It is approved for reduction of fracture in women at a high risk for osteoporotic fracture. (SOR **Ⓐ**) It is dosed at 60 mg subcutaneously every 6 months.

   a. In women with osteoporosis, denosumab reduces vertebral fracture (NNT 21 over 3 years) and nonvertebral fracture (NNT 67 over 3 years).

   b. Adverse effects include eczema, cellulitis, and excessive flatus. Denosumab may increase risk of malignancies and serious infections as RANKL is involved in function of the immune system.

   c. Denosumab has not been proven superior in fracture reduction to any bisphosphonate therapy. (SOR **Ⓑ**)

6. **Calcitonin (Miacalcin, Fortical)** intranasally one nasal puff (200 IU) every day, alternating nostrils, is shown to reduce bone loss and decrease radiographic vertebral fracture risk (NNT 10 over 5 years). (SOR **Ⓑ**) No studies are available on clinical or nonvertebral fractures.

   a. Calcitonin appears to preserve bone mass in steroid-induced osteoporosis, but fracture prevention is not established.

   b. The drug must be kept refrigerated until use begins as it is stable at room temperature only for about 1 month.

   c. Decreased bone pain in acute vertebral fracture is reportedly because of the increase in endorphins stimulated by calcitonin.

   d. The intranasal form has largely replaced use of subcutaneous calcitonin 100 to 200 IU three times per week, although the subcutaneous form prevents more bone loss than intranasal calcitonin. The subcutaneous form is associated with nausea and occasional allergic reaction.

7. **Fluoride** therapy

   a. Use is highly controversial, due to a potential increase in risk of nonvertebral fracture at higher therapeutic doses (over 20 mg per day). Some form of fluoride may have a role in osteoporosis therapy in the future. (SOR **Ⓒ**)

8. **Ipriflavone** is a synthetic flavonoid (isoflavone) available as a supplement. Ipriflavone promotes the incorporation of calcium into bone and inhibits bone resorption.

   a. Isoflavones are approved in some European and Asian countries for osteoporosis prevention and treatment. It does not possess intrinsic estrogenic activity and behaves more like a SERM without significant adverse side effects. Studies are controversial regarding efficacy, but ipriflavone appears to prevent postmenopausal bone loss. No studies yet show a reduction in fracture rates. (SOR **Ⓒ**)

   b. Unregulated manufacture of supplement products in the United States limits the reliability of supplement product purity and potency (nonprescription drugs are monitored by the FDA).

9. **Hydrochlorothiazide** in low doses (up to 25 mg per day) was associated with preservation of BMD in one randomized trial. In doses of 50 mg per day, thiazides may be beneficial in treating the high urine calcium of patients with idiopathic hypercalciuria via improving gastrointestinal absorption of calcium. Thiazides should be used only in conjunction with other therapies for osteoporosis. (SOR **Ⓒ**)

D. **Tertiary prevention** involves the care of established symptomatic osteoporosis, with attempts made to restore to highest function, minimize the negative effects of disease, and prevent disease-related complications. Since the disease is now established, primary prevention activities may have been unsuccessful. Early detection through secondary prevention may have minimized the impact of the disease.

1. **Pain relief** is of primary importance in the patient with acute fracture and often will require hospital or nursing home admission. The nature of the fracture will guide specific therapeutic options.

2. **Treatment.** Vertebral compression fractures are commonly treated with bed rest, prevention of further injury and, occasionally, spinal bracing (see Chapter 28). (SOR **Ⓒ**)

   a. A long period of therapeutic exercises may be required to regain full function.

b. As stated earlier, calcitonin may reduce pain in an acute fracture. (SOR **B**) Analgesics can be used as liberally as the clinical situation dictates. Nonsteroidal anti-inflammatory drugs (NSAIDs) are often suitable if no contraindications exist. Caution should be exercised in using analgesics and NSAIDs in the elderly, however.

c. If bed rest is prolonged, consider venous thromboembolism prophylaxis.

3. Percutaneous procedures

    a. In **vertebroplasty,** polymethylmethacrylate cement is injected into the compressed vertebral body. Balloon kyphoplasty uses a balloon inflated inside the compressed vertebral body before the cement is injected.

        (1) Vertebroplasty and kyphoplasty are associated with reduced pain and improved function in uncontrolled studies. (SOR **C**)

        (2) These procedures, typically performed by orthopedic surgeons, interventional radiologists, and pain management specialists, are becoming more widely used. Long-term outcomes remain uncertain because of lack of good studies and inability to adequately control/blind to intervention.

V. Management Strategies

A. Patient education

    1. Counseling should be offered to all women regarding universal preventive measures related to fracture risk, calcium and vitamin D intake, weight-bearing exercise, smoking cessation, fall prevention, avoidance of excess alcohol intake, and the risks and benefits of HRT. (SOR **C**)

    2. The National Resource Center on Osteoporosis is a federally funded clearing house for the latest risks, prevention, and treatment of and information on osteoporosis (National Osteoporosis Foundation; http://www.nof.org). A fact sheet on osteoporosis is also available at http://www.womenshealth.gov/publications/our-publications/fact-sheet/osteoporosis.cfm.

B. Compliance with pharmacotherapy is improved when patients are given BMD testing. (SOR **C**) This may be due to the objectification of the disease when viewed as a laboratory report.

C. Follow-up after diagnosis or fracture includes the following:

    1. Schedule office visits bimonthly initially, then every 6 months. (SOR **C**)

    2. Promote periodic multiphasic screening, annual physical examination, and preventative screenings. (SOR **C**)

    3. Every 2 or 3 years, obtain BMD using the same technique and the same facility if possible. (SOR **C**)

    4. Repeat x-rays for acute pain or suspected fractures. (SOR **C**)

    5. Follow-up for patients on bisphosphonates, and following their discontinuation, is discussed in Section IV.C.1.d.

VI. Prognosis

A. Fracture risk

- 1 vertebral fracture at baseline = fivefold risk of more vertebral fractures.
- ≥1 vertebral fracture at baseline = 12-fold risk of more vertebral fractures.
- 1 symptomatic vertebral fracture at baseline = twofold risk of hip fracture.
- 1 SD decrease in hip BMD = twofold to threefold increase in hip fracture.

B. Life expectancy. Following a hip fracture, half of patients never fully recover and 25% require long-term care.

SELECTED REFERENCES

American Medical Directors Association (AMDA). *Osteoporosis and Fracture Prevention in the Long-Term Care Setting.* Columbia, MD: AMDA; 2009.

Eriksem EF. Treatment of osteoporosis. *Rev Endocr Metab Disord.* 2012;13(3):209–223.

Institute for Clinical Systems Improvement (ICSI). *Diagnosis and Treatment of Osteoporosis.* Bloomington, MN: ICSI; 2011. www.guideline.gov. Accessed October 30, 2013.

Iqbal MM. Osteoporosis: epidemiology, diagnosis, and treatment. *South Med J.* 2000;93(1):2–18.

Kanis J. FRAX WHO Fracture Risk Assessment Tool. www.shef.ac.uk/FRAX. Accessed October 30, 2013.

Osteoporosis. www.dynamed.com, updated October 24, 2013. Accessed October 31, 2013.

Qaseem A, Snow V, Shekelle P, et al; Clinical Efficacy Assessment Subcommittee of the American College of Physicians. Screening for osteoporosis in men: a clinical practice guideline from the American College of Physicians. *Ann Intern Med.* 2008;148(9):680–684.

Sweet MG, Sweet JM, Jeremiah MP, Galazka SS. Diagnosis and treatment of osteoporosis. *Am Fam Physician.* 2009;79(3):193–200.

Tannenbaum C, Clark J, Schwartzman K, et al. Yield of laboratory testing to identify secondary contributors to osteoporosis in otherwise healthy women. *J Clin Endocrinol Metab.* 2002;87:4431–4437.

University of Michigan Health System. *Osteoporosis: Prevention and Treatment.* Ann Arbor, MI: University of Michigan Health System; 2011. www.guideline.gov. Accessed October 30, 2013.

U.S. Preventive Services Task Force. Screening for osteoporosis: U.S. preventive services task force recommendation statement. *Ann Intern Med.* 2011;154(5):356–364.

World Health Organization. *Prevention and Management of Osteoporosis: Report of a WHO Scientific Group.* WHO Technical Report Series, 921. Geneva, Switzerland: WHO; 2003. http://whqlibdoc. who.int/trs/WHO_TRS_921.pdf. Accessed October 30, 2013.

Yimin Y, Zhiwei R, Wei M, Jha R. Current status of percutaneous vertebroplasty and percutaneous kyphoplasty—a review. *Med Sci Monit.* 2013;19:826–836.

84   Peptic Ulcer Disease

Carol Stewart, MD, FAAFP, Nancy Tyre, MD, & Lesley D. Wilkinson, MD

KEY POINTS

- Peptic ulcer disease (PUD) is primarily caused by *Helicobacter pylori* infection or by nonsteroidal anti-inflammatory drug (NSAID) use. (SOR **C**)
- Many patients present with epigastric pain. Most have gastroesophageal reflux disease (GERD) or functional dyspepsia; generally 15% or less have PUD. Initial endoscopy is reserved for patients with "alarm" symptoms (weight loss, anemia, bleeding, dysphagia or odynophagia, prior PUD, persistent vomiting, age over 55 years at first presentation), suggesting bleeding, perforation, or cancer. (SOR **C**)
- Patients at a higher risk for *H. pylori* should be considered for a "test-and-treat" approach. (SOR **A**) Many younger patients can be empirically treated with acid suppression alone. (SOR **A**) Rarely, one needs to consider more obscure causes such as Zollinger–Ellison syndrome. (SOR **C**)
- The first step in treatment is stopping NSAIDs or aspirin, starting acid-blocking medication, and initiating treatment for *H. pylori* if infection is present. (SOR **A**)

I. Introduction

A. Definitions. PUD is present when acid–peptic injury to the gastrointestinal mucosa results in defects (ulcerations) through the epithelial layer. GERD is usually defined as predominant or frequent (at least once a week) heartburn or acid regurgitation. Dyspepsia is chronic or recurrent pain or discomfort in the upper abdomen.

B. Pathophysiology. PUD is predominantly due to one or both of two underlying causes—*H. pylori* infection or use of NSAIDs. Less common causes are idiopathic and acid hypersecretory conditions (e.g., Zollinger–Ellison syndrome). A small but growing percentage of disease is now associated with non-NSAID medication use including potassium chloride, nitrogen-containing bisphosphonates, and immunosuppressants. Infrequently, PUD is caused by Crohn disease, systemic mastocytosis, alcoholism, malignancy, viral infections (herpes simplex, cytomegalovirus), tuberculosis, syphilis, and cocaine use. Acid is necessary, but not sufficient by itself, to develop PUD lesions.

1. ***Helicobacter pylori*** is a gram-negative microaerophilic, urease-producing bacterium that has adapted to the environment of the gastric mucosa. It causes persistent inflammation in the stomach with a vigorous immune response that rarely eliminates *H. pylori.* (Children clear the infection up to 20% of the time.) *Helicobacter pylori* gastritis is variable in clinical expression and is often asymptomatic. The lifetime risk of PUD in a patient infected with *H. pylori* is 3% in the United States and 25% in Japan. *Helicobacter pylori* should also be considered in the evaluation of gastric lymphoma (mucosa-associated lymphoid tissue [MALT] lymphoma), iron-deficiency anemia, idiopathic thrombocytopenic purpura (ITP), and vitamin B_{12} deficiency.

2. NSAIDs have a different mechanism of ulceration. They do not cause a diffuse gastritis. They primarily induce mucosal injury by disrupting prostaglandin-mediated cell protection and proliferation. Gastroprotective mechanisms that are disrupted include inhibition of acid secretion, bicarbonate production, gastric mucus production, and promotion of mucosal growth and repair. Many NSAIDs are also weak acids themselves and directly injure epithelial cells in the acid stomach environment.

C. Epidemiology. PUD results in approximately 3 million patient visits per year in the United States, with a current lifetime prevalence of up to 10%. US mortality due to PUD is approximately 3500 per year.

    1. Patients usually present with dyspepsia (epigastric pain), not "PUD." Dyspepsia accounts for 2% to 5% of all symptomatic ambulatory care visits in the United States. Up to 15% of patients with dyspepsia have PUD. Of the remainder, 1% to 2% have cancer, 6% to about 25% have GERD, and more than 60% have functional dyspepsia with normal endoscopies. **Most patients with dyspepsia do not have PUD.**

    2. The diagnosis and treatment of PUD have been transformed over the last 30 years by the development of medications that suppress acid formation and by the discovery that one of the primary etiologies of PUD is a curable infectious disease—*H. pylori*.

        a. *Helicobacter pylori* is the most common chronic bacterial infection in humans, with conservative estimates of infection rates at 50% worldwide. It is extremely common in the developing world (prevalence more than 80%), but rates in the industrialized world have been dropping as hygiene and public health have improved. Infection occurs almost exclusively before age 10 years in the industrialized world, so current prevalence rates by age reflect a cohort effect. The adult infection rate is approximately 0.5% per year.

        b. *Helicobacter pylori* is transmitted by fecal/oral or oral/oral routes. Its prevalence correlates strongly with socioeconomic conditions. Risk factors in the United States include birth in another country, older age, lower socioeconomic status, domestic crowding, and unsanitary conditions; these conditions are currently more common in nonwhite populations. US *H. pylori* prevalence in individuals younger than 30 years is <10%, so the incidence and etiology of PUD have already begun changing, and will be shifting more in the future.

    3. NSAIDs are a major cause of PUD, primarily because of the large number of patients utilizing them. At least 30 billion nonprescription tablets and 70 million prescriptions for NSAIDs per year are purchased in the United States. Nearly 40% of elderly Americans are prescribed NSAIDs each year, and NSAID use is gradually increasing because of the aging of the population and increasing use of aspirin prophylaxis. Since symptoms cannot reliably point to PUD with NSAIDs, it is important to be aware of preexisting risk factors for PUD when initiating NSAID treatment (Table 84–1).

    4. A small number of cases, currently 1% to 5%, are now attributed to other factors. This is an emerging list, explaining some of the previous idiopathic cases. This list is likely to take on increasing importance as the incidence of *H. pylori* continues to decline.

II. Prevention. The American College of Gastroenterology has identified risk factors for PUD that should be considered when starting someone on an NSAID. These include

- Prior history of a gastrointestinal event (ulcer, hemorrhage)
- Age >60 years
- High NSAID dosage
- Concurrent use of glucocorticoids
- Concurrent use of anticoagulants

TABLE 84–1. **RISK FACTORS FOR NSAID GASTROINTESTINAL COMPLICATIONS**

Helicobacter pylori infection, even if asymptomatic
Older age increases the risk, especially for women
History of peptic ulcer disease
Alcoholism
Poor health
Smoking
Use of steroids, chemotherapy, anticoagulation, SSRI, or alendronate
High dose or prolonged course of NSAID use, or both

NSAID, nonsteroidal anti-inflammatory drug; SSRI, selective serotonin reuptake inhibitor.

A. Use of a proton pump inhibitor (PPI) for prophylaxis should be considered for patients with the above risk factors, especially if more than one risk factor is present and if NSAID use will be longer term. (SOR ❻) Which NSAID is employed makes a small difference in the risk of PUD, but the dosage and length of use are more important factors.
B. Concurrent *H. pylori* infection is a risk factor for PUD with NSAIDs, so testing and treating for *H. pylori* in older patients or those otherwise at a higher risk for *H. pylori* infection is also appropriate when starting long-term NSAID therapy, particularly if a patient has a history of PUD. (SOR ❹)
C. There is evidence of an association between PUD and selective serotonin reuptake inhibitor (SSRI) use, particularly at higher doses of SSRIs and in high-risk patients, such as those on NSAIDs. Some studies show a 12- to 15-fold increase in upper gastrointestinal bleeding (UGI) bleeding with the combined use of NSAIDs and SSRIs, but more studies are needed. In the meantime, high-risk patients such as the elderly and patients with a history of PUD may benefit from a course of PPIs with their NSAIDs and antidepressants. (SOR ❻)

III. Diagnosis

A. History. Epigastric distress is the most common presentation of PUD. Patients usually describe this as a midline gnawing discomfort or feeling of hunger. Sometimes, it is painful with aching or burning, or a patient may have nausea with or without actual emesis. An acid taste is more common with GERD. The discomfort typically occurs 1 to 3 hours postprandial and overnight, classically between 1 and 2 AM. Food, antacids, or vomiting may relieve the symptoms within minutes. Minor weight loss may occur in up to 50% of patients with benign gastric ulcers. Significant weight loss is a red flag for malignancy. Patients with duodenal ulcers who eat to control their pain are more likely to present with weight gain.
   1. Alarm symptoms may indicate complicating diagnoses (Table 84–2). The presence of alarm symptoms is an indication for immediate endoscopy in the patient with dyspepsia. (SOR ❻)
B. The **physical examination** is usually nonspecific; epigastric tenderness is the most common finding.
C. Tests
   1. Definitive diagnosis of PUD requires endoscopy. Barium studies can also confirm the diagnosis, but do not allow for biopsy. Treatment with PPIs significantly decreases the sensitivity of endoscopy. Ideally, endoscopy should take place prior to treatment, or PPIs should be discontinued for at least 4 weeks before endoscopy. Even cancer may partially heal with PPI treatment despite its malignant nature, and it can be deceptive even for skilled endoscopists.
   2. Hemoglobin/hematocrit should be checked if there is any concern about a bleeding ulcer. Concerns about acute bleeding should prompt stool guaiac testing and gastric aspiration.
   3. Histology of tissue from at least two different sites remains the gold standard for the diagnosis of *H. pylori* infection, but many other methods are available (Table 84–3). Serology is the most common method used for diagnosis, but is unsuitable for assessing *H. pylori* eradication. **Stool antigen tests and urea breath tests** are accurate in detecting active infection, but generally revert to negative 1 month after effective treatment. If *H. pylori* breath test or fecal antigen test results are negative in a patient not taking NSAIDs, peptic ulcer disease is virtually excluded. The sensitivity of all *H. pylori* testing is decreased in the setting of PPI use and active GI bleeding.
D. Differential diagnosis. As noted earlier, most patients with PUD symptoms actually have functional dyspepsia or GERD. The differential diagnosis includes serious illnesses

TABLE 84-2. ALARM SYMPTOMS FOR PEPTIC ULCER DISEASE

Age older than 55 yr (incidence of cancer increases with age, <1% younger than 50 yr)
Unintentional weight loss or anorexia/early satiety
Anemia (iron deficiency)
Gastrointestinal bleeding (either hematemesis or hematochezia)
Dysphagia (difficulty swallowing) or odynophagia (pain on swallowing)
Jaundice
Vomiting (persistent)
Epigastric mass
Prior gastric surgery or peptic ulcer disease
Family history of gastric cancer
Severe or penetrating pain, or both

TABLE 84-3. DIAGNOSTIC TESTS FOR *Helicobacter pylori*

Test	Sensitivity	Specificity	Comments
Nonendoscopic Tests			
Serologic tests	85–94	80–95	• Least expensive of all tests • Positive may reflect old infection, so not good for confirming active infection or eradication
Urea breath tests	90–96	90–98	• Can be false-negative in people on PPIs, recent antibiotics, or bismuth ingestion
Stool antigen tests	88–95	90–98	• Technically challenging for patients
Endoscopic Tests			
Bacterial culture	80–94	100	• Sensitivity varies based on staff and facilities
Urease tests	88–95	95–99	• Can be false-negative in people on PPIs, recent antibiotics, or bismuth ingestion
Histology	93–96	97–99	• Need trained staff

PPI, proton pump inhibitor.
Source: Data from Smoot DT, Go MF, Cryer B. Peptic ulcer disease. *Prim Care.* 2001;28(3):487–503; and McColl KE. *Helicobacter pylori* infection. *NEJM.* 2010;362:1597–1604.

that require a high index of suspicion to diagnose: bleeding ulcer, perforated ulcer, gastric or esophageal cancer (duodenal ulcer is almost never malignant), severe GERD with stricture, as well as pancreatitis, cholecystitis, and cardiac or pulmonary etiologies.

IV. **Treatment.** An approach to the patient with dyspepsia can be found in Chapter 19, Figure 19–1.

   A. **Test and treat.** Current expert consensus is that patients presenting with dyspepsia, but NO alarm symptoms, should first be managed with either acid suppression or a "test and treat" approach, without obtaining a definitive biopsy-proven endoscopic diagnosis. (SOR **Ⓐ**) Patients can be considered for treatment without testing for *H. pylori* if they are young (<55 years) and not in a group or family suggestive of increased *H. pylori* risk, such as immigrants from high-prevalence countries (less than 10% prevalence cutoff for empiric treatment; SOR **Ⓒ**). Noninvasive testing (stool antigen, urea breath test) for *H. pylori* should be performed if needed and treatment initiated if positive. If the patient is on an NSAID, it should be stopped if possible. Treatment with acid suppression should begin. If these treatments fail to control symptoms, referral for endoscopy is indicated.

   B. **Acid suppression** promotes ulcer healing, and *H. pylori* treatments require higher pH to be successful. An empiric trial of 4 to 8 weeks of acid suppression is indicated for young people with low *H. pylori* risk. (SOR **Ⓐ**) If symptoms are not controlled, then the "test-and-treat" approach is indicated, with endoscopy if it also fails. If initial treatment is successful but symptoms recur after medication is discontinued, then a repeat trial of acid suppression is acceptable before any testing. (SOR **Ⓒ**)

     1. **PPIs are the most effective medications.** (SOR **Ⓐ**) They significantly raise gastric pH by disabling active hydrogen (proton) pumps in the parietal cells. It takes 3 to 4 days to reach full activity because all the pumps are not normally turned on at one time. All PPIs are similarly effective, but differ somewhat in drug interactions (Table 84–4).

     2. H_2 receptor antagonists (H_2 blockers) quickly decrease acid secretion by blocking histamine stimulation of parietal cell activity (Table 84–5). They are effective, but tolerance develops, and they are not as potent as PPIs for acid suppression or healing. They are second-line treatment for PUD in the United States.

     3. All other drugs are inferior at acid suppression and healing (Table 84–5). Patients can use antacids for symptom relief. Sucralfate is helpful, but is inferior to H_2 blockers. Misoprostol (Cytotec) is fairly effective at preventing NSAID-induced ulceration, but has a high (up to 30%) rate of diarrhea, is very expensive, and is inferior to PPIs.

   C. **Therapy for *H. pylori***

     1. **All patients diagnosed with *H. pylori* should be treated** (even if PUD is ultimately ruled out). A drug regimen of at least two antibiotics and an acid suppressor is required (Table 84–6). Multiple regimens have been tried because none is ideal; all are associated with potential side effects, potential poor adherence, expense, and significant failure rates. There is also significant antibiotic resistance of approximately 40% to metronidazole and approximately 10% to clarithromycin.

     2. To confirm eradication after *H. pylori* treatment for PUD, the patient should ideally be retested for active *H. pylori* 4 to 8 weeks after treatment, with either the urea breath

TABLE 84–4. MEDICATIONS FOR TREATMENT OR PREVENTION OF PEPTIC ULCER DISEASE, PART I

Drug[a]	Dose (Oral)	Notes	Drug Interactions
Proton Pump Inhibitors (PPIs)[b]			
Dexlansoprazole (Dexilant)	30 mg daily for GERD; 60 mg daily for erosive esophagitis	Not FDA approved for PUD; ♀ B	Methotrexate (methotrexate toxicity), digoxin (digoxin toxicity), warfarin (bleeding), iron (decreased absorption)
Esomeprazole magnesium (Nexium)	20–40 mg daily	Maintenance: 20 mg daily; ♀ B	As above; clopidogrel (risk of clotting), citalopram (QT prolongation)
Lansoprazole[a] (Prevacid)	DU: 15 mg daily GU: 30 mg daily Nonprescription 15 mg	Maintenance: 15 mg daily for DU Hypersecretory conditions: 60 mg daily, adjust up to max. 90 mg twice daily; ♀ B	See dexlansoprazole; antacids (decreased lansoprazole bioavailability)
Omeprazole[a] (Prilosec)	DU: 20 mg daily GU: 40 mg daily Nonprescription 20 mg	Maintenance: 20 mg daily Hypersecretory conditions: 60 mg daily, adjust up to max 120 mg three times daily; ♀ C; more potential drug interactions than other PPIs[b]	See esomeprazole; carbamazepine (carbamazepine toxicity); disulfiram (disulfiram toxicity); phenytoin (phenytoin toxicity); St. John's wort, ginkgo (decreased efficacy of omeprazole)
Omeprazole/ bicarbonate[a] (Zegerid)	Capsule DU/GERD/esophagitis: 20/1100 mg daily GU: 40/1680 mg daily	Also available in powder form 20/1100 mg and 40/1680 mg Do not substitute two doses of the 20 mg form due to bicarb dose[c]; ♀ C	See above
Pantoprazole sodium[a] (Protonix)	40–80 mg once daily	Maintenance: 40 mg daily Hypersecretory conditions: 40 mg twice daily, adjust up to max. 240 mg daily; ♀ B	Methotrexate (methotrexate toxicity), citalopram (QT prolongation), warfarin (bleeding), iron (decreased absorption)
Rabeprazole sodium (Aciphex)	20 mg daily after morning meal, swallow whole	Maintenance 20 mg daily Hypersecretory conditions: 60 mg daily, adjust max up to 100 mg daily or 60 mg twice daily; ♀ B	See pantoprazole; clopidogrel (risk of clotting), digoxin (digoxin toxicity)

[a]Available as a generic.
[b]FDA has issued warning about long-term PPI use and higher rates of osteoporosis and fractures.
[c]20 mg and 40 mg capsules contain the same amount of sodium bicarbonate (1100 mg); two capsules of 20 mg are not equivalent to one capsule of 40 mg.
DU, duodenal ulcer; GU, gastric ulcer; ♀, pregnancy class.

test or stool antigen test. Treatment failure requires a second regimen, generally quadruple therapy with alternative antibiotics, or sequential therapy if not previously used. A second treatment failure requires specialty referral with endoscopy, and culture for sensitivities. Salvage therapy with levofloxacin may be appropriate. It is fairly common for patients to resolve their *H. pylori* and PUD, but still require symptomatic PPI treatment for GERD or functional dyspepsia.

   D. Therapy for NSAID-related ulcers. The primary treatment is to stop the NSAID if at all possible and initiate acid suppression, usually with a PPI. Generally, treatment is rapid and effective if the NSAID can be stopped. Unfortunately, many patients need continuing NSAID treatment or aspirin prophylaxis. Under those circumstances, the NSAID dose should be minimized, and concomitant therapy begun with a PPI. Treatment with PPI while continuing low-dose ASA or NSAID results in a healing rate of 80% at 8 weeks. Use of COX-2-specific NSAIDs in these patients has decreased in popularity since the increased risk of cardiovascular side effects with these agents has become more apparent. If a patient requiring long-term NSAIDs also tests positive for *H. pylori*, treatment of the infection alone will not reduce their risk of PUD; these patients will require ongoing PPI therapy. (SOR Ⓐ)

   E. Relapse. If NSAIDs are discontinued and *H. pylori* is cured but the patient clinically relapses, then referral to a specialist is indicated, and PPIs should be reinitiated. Consider

TABLE 84–5. MEDICATIONS FOR TREATMENT OR PREVENTION OF PEPTIC ULCER DISEASE, PART II

Drug[a]	Dose (Oral)	Notes	Drug Interactions
H₂ Blockers (all available in generic form)			
Cimetidine[a] (Tagamet)	300 mg four times daily OR 800 mg nightly; nonprescription 200 mg OR 400 mg twice daily (DU only)	Maintenance 400 mg nightly Hypersecretory conditions: 300 mg four times daily up to 2400 mg daily May induce confusional states, particularly in the elderly; ♀ B	Multiple Interactions: Metformin (increased metformin levels); citalopram (QT prolongation); chloroquine (chloroquine toxicity); morphine, fentanyl (opiate toxicity); labetalol, propranolol (bradycardia, hypotension); warfarin (bleeding)
Famotidine[a] (Pepcid)	40 mg nightly OR 20 mg twice daily; Nonprescription 10 mg	Central nervous system adverse effects reported with moderate to severe renal insufficiency; ♀ B	Cyclosporine (decreased cyclosporine concentrations)
Nizatidine[a] (Axid)	300 mg nightly OR 150 mg twice daily Nonprescription 75 mg	Maintenance 150 mg nightly False-positive for urobilinogen with Multistix; ♀ B	None (with common medications)
Ranitidine[a] (Zantac)	150 mg twice daily OR 300 mg nightly for DU Nonprescription 75 mg	Maintenance 150 mg nightly Hypersecretory conditions: 150 mg twice daily up to 6 g daily; ♀ B	Fentanyl (opiate toxicity); warfarin (bleeding); glipizide (increased glipizide effect); triazolam (increased triazolam effect)
Other Medications for PUD Treatment/Prevention			
Misoprostol[a] (Cytotec)	200 µg four times daily, or if not tolerated, 100 µg four times daily	For prevention DU or NSAID-induced ulcers in patients at risk. ♀ X	None
Sucralfate[a] (Carafate)	1 g four times daily, with meals and bedtime (DU) OR 2 g twice daily (DU)	Maintenance (DU or GU): 1 g twice daily on empty stomach, adheres to ulcer crater; ♀ B	Quinolone antibiotics, warfarin, digoxin (decreased efficacy)

[a]Available as generic.
NSAID, nonsteroidal anti-inflammatory drug; ♀, pregnancy class.

unusual causes, particularly acid hypersecretory states. A fasting gastrin level is indicated in the presence of multiple ulcers, ulcers resistant to therapy, ulcers associated with severe esophagitis, and for patients awaiting surgery or with a family history of similar ulcer problems or other endocrine tumors.

F. Idiopathic PUD. If all treatable etiologies for PUD are ruled out, then treatment focuses solely on acid suppression. The percentage of idiopathic ulcers is increasing as the percentage of all ulcers from *H pylori* is decreasing.

G. Surgery. Operative treatment is indicated for patients with acute complications or refractory PUD. Rates of surgery for PUD have plummeted.

V. Management Strategies. The goal of ulcer therapy is complete healing without relapse. Prior to the appreciation of the role of *H. pylori,* many lifestyle issues were thought to be important in the pathogenesis and treatment of PUD. Now, they are largely understood to be secondary or even unrelated.

A. Smoking promotes ulcerogenesis, at least in patients with *H. pylori* infection. Smoking adversely affects ulcer development, healing, and complications. However, if *H. pylori* is eradicated, smokers do not appear to be at continued increased PUD risk. It is considered appropriate to recommend smoking cessation to all patients who smoke, but primary treatment remains that which is appropriate for the primary ulcer etiology (e.g., *H. pylori* or NSAIDs).

TABLE 84–6. TREATMENT OPTIONS FOR *Helicobacter pylori*

Regimen	PPI	Antibiotic #1	Antibiotic #2	Bismuth	Number of Days	Efficacy (%)
Triple therapy—usual initial regimen	PPI[a] twice daily	Amoxicillin 1 g twice daily (If PCN allergic: metronidazole 500 mg twice daily or / quadruple therapy)	Clarithromycin 500 mg twice daily (If macrolide allergic: metronidazole 500 mg twice daily or / quadruple therapy)	N/A	14	70–85
Sequential therapy—acceptable alternative, especially with clarithromycin resistance	PPI[a] twice daily	**Days 1–5** Amoxicillin 1 g twice daily	**Days 6–10** Clarithromycin 500 mg twice daily PLUS Tinidazole 500 mg twice daily	N/A	10	85–90
Quadruple therapy—for resistant infections or primary therapy in allergic patients or those recently exposed to triple component antibiotics	PPI[a] bid (H₂ blocker possible if must) / Tetracycline 500 mg qid	Tetracycline 500 mg four times daily	Metronidazole 500 mg four times daily	Bismuth subsalicylate[b] 525 mg four times daily	14	75–90
Salvage therapy for continued infection after treatment with first or second line regimen—no studies in USA[c]	PPI[a] bid / $	Amoxicillin 1 g twice daily	Levofloxacin 500 mg daily	N/A	10	87%

[a]Any PPI can be used: omeprazole (Prilosec), 20 mg; esomeprazole (Nexium), 20 mg; lansoprazole (Prevacid), 30 mg; pantoprazole (Protonix), 40 mg; rabeprazole (AciPhex), 20 mg, see Table 82–4.

[b]Pepto-Bismol.

[c]PPI, proton pump inhibitor.

Source: Data adapted from Chey WD, Wong BCY. American College of Gastroenterology guideline on the management of *Helicobacter pylori* infection. *Am J Gastroenterol.* 2007; 102(8):1808.

B. Alcohol has long been considered a cause of PUD. In fact, moderate alcohol intake is usually not a significant contributor. However, in large doses, alcohol damages the stomach epithelium directly. In patients who consume more than 20 drinks a week, ulcer rates are significantly increased, especially in the presence of cirrhosis.

C. Emotional stress can affect ulcer frequency to some extent. Severe societal stressors (such as major earthquakes) cause an increase in PUD rates in the affected areas. Severe physiologic stressors (such as surgery or intensive care unit admissions) are well known to predispose patients to ulcers. Emotional stress may be one of the factors that causes patients exposed to *H. pylori* or NSAIDs to become part of the small percentage that actually develop an ulcer. However, emotional strain does not interfere with treatment. Although conventional wisdom is that all ulcers are directly caused by "stress," reduction in stress is not necessary for adequate healing. Treatment should be directed at the primary etiology.

D. Diet does NOT contribute to PUD, and no special diets are needed during treatment. Patients may perceive diet as significant because it can affect symptoms of dyspepsia, but it does not affect ulcer healing.

E. Alternative treatments for PUD are unproven. Listed are a few of the most common strategies.
1. Acupuncture may decrease epigastric pain, acid secretion, or both.
2. Chinese herbal treatments include Xao Yao Wan dosed at eight tablets three times daily for soothing stress and gastric upset.
3. Naturopathic remedies include aloe vera juice one to two tablespoons twice daily or "stomach formula" as directed.
4. Individualized homeopathic remedies can be tried.

VI. Prognosis. The prognosis of PUD has improved dramatically. Although the mortality of acute upper GI bleed is approximately 5%, PUD can usually be cured or controlled for most of the patient population.

A. NSAIDs. Up to 4% of patients with NSAID users develop serious complications such as frank PUD with bleeding or perforation each year. Between 5% and 20% of long-term NSAID users have peptic ulcers at any given time. Of NSAID users with PUD, there is a 400% to 500% increase in complications. However, even for patients who must continue NSAIDs, continuous treatment with PPIs causes relapse rates for PUD to decrease to 5%.

B. *Helicobacter pylori*. Eradication of *H. pylori* dramatically alters the natural history of PUD. Previously, the natural history of PUD was chronic and relapsing, with more than 75% recurrence of ulcers. Now patients cured of *H. pylori* often require no further treatment, with relapse rates for PUD decreased to 5%.

VII. Patient Education
- Acid suppression medication is key to initial symptom treatment and may be needed long term.
- Symptoms such as vomiting blood, blood seen in the stool, or an abrupt increase to severe pain should be considered emergencies and patients should be instructed to contact their primary care provider or seek care in the emergency department immediately.
- Uncomplicated ulcers are almost exclusively due to NSAIDs or *H. Pylori*, so the key to resolution is avoiding NSAIDs and/or curing *H. Pylori*.
- Medication regimens for *H. Pylori* can be very challenging to take, but are crucially important if indicated.
- If NSAIDs cannot be avoided, including aspirin for cardioprotection, then strong acid-suppression medication must be continued indefinitely.
- Lifestyle factors, including diet, are minor for most ulcers; smoking and excessive alcohol should be avoided.

SELECTED REFERENCES

Chey WD, Wong BCY. American College of Gastroenterology guideline on the management of *Helicobacter pylori* infection. *Am J Gastroenterol.* 2007;102(8):1808–1825.

Malfertheiner P, Megraud F, O'Morain CA, et. al. Management of *Helicobacter pylori* infection—the Maastricht IV/ Florence Consensus Report. *Gut.* 2012;61:646–664.

McColl KE. *Helicobacter pylori* infection. *NEJM.* 2010;362:1597–1604.

Nimish V. Peptic ulcer disease. In: *Sleisenger and Fordtran's Gastrointestinal and Liver Disease.* 9th ed. Philadelphia, PA: Saunders; 2010;52:861–868.

Smoot DT, Go MF, Cryer B. Peptic ulcer disease. *Prim Care.* 2001;28(3):487–503.

Talley NJ, Vakil N. The Practice Parameters Committee of the American College of Gastroenterology. Guidelines for the management of dyspepsia. *Am J Gastroenterol.* 2005;100:2324–2337.

85   Premenstrual Syndrome

Heather R. Pickett, DO, FAAFP, Abby L. Harris, MD, & Michael Michener, MD

KEY POINTS

- Premenstrual syndrome is a group of symptoms sharing many features of depression and anxiety disorders, but is characterized chiefly by its occurrence exclusively in the luteal phase of the menstrual cycle. (SOR ⓒ)
- Premenstrual dysphoric disorder is characterized by more severe psychological symptoms that significantly interfere with daily functioning and interpersonal relationships. (SOR ⓒ)
- Symptoms occur approximately 2 weeks before the onset of menses, improve a few days after the onset of menses, and become minimal or absent in the week post-menses. (SOR ⓒ)
- Symptoms may include one or more of the following clusters: (SOR ⓒ)
  - Anxiety, irritability, or mood swings.
  - Weight gain, swelling, bloating, or breast tenderness.
  - Appetite change, food cravings, and fatigue.
  - Depression, sleep disturbance, or cognitive difficulty.
  - Pain, including headache and general muscular pains.
- Major depressive disorder with suicide risk must be ruled out, and medical conditions such as hypothyroidism that can present with some of the same symptoms should be considered. (SOR ⓒ)
- Education and cognitive therapy may improve symptoms. (SOR Ⓑ)
- Medications including selective serotonin reuptake inhibitors and oral contraceptive pills may improve symptoms. (SOR Ⓑ)

I. Introduction

A. Definition. Premenstrual syndrome (PMS) is the cyclic recurrence in the luteal phase of the menstrual cycle of a combination of distressing physical, psychological, and behavioral changes that can result in deterioration of interpersonal relationships or interference with normal activities. **Premenstrual dysphoric disorder (PMDD)** is a more severe variant of PMS that has primarily psychiatric symptoms with specific DSM-5 criteria (see Section II.B). For the purposes of this chapter, the term PMS will be used unless there is a specific variant in diagnosis or management between the two requiring differentiation.

B. Epidemiology. Most women report at least some minor physical and emotional symptoms in the postovulatory phase of the menstrual cycle. Thirty to forty percent have symptoms of moderate intensity, and it is estimated that 3% to 5% of women of reproductive age have PMS of an intensity that is temporarily disabling.

1. Age. Symptoms of PMS may occur at any age in the reproductive years; incidence of presenting for care peaks in the mid-30s. Some women experience cyclic symptoms even after menopause.

2. Social class. No clinically useful differences have been identified.

3. Race. PMS is reported to occur in all ethnic groups. Cultural variation in the prevalence rates and patterns of symptoms occur, but no clinically useful diagnostic or therapeutic differences have yet emerged.

4. Reproductive factors. Women with regular (ovulatory) menstrual cycles, as well as those with longer cycles and heavier menstrual flow, report symptoms of swelling, mood swings, and depression more than other women. PMS may occur in spontaneous anovulatory cycles and following oophorectomy or hysterectomy. More than half of patients with severe PMS have a history of preeclampsia or postnatal depression.

5. Genetics. A majority of studies have supported a strong genetic component to PMS and PMDD.

C. Pathophysiology. No single theory currently accounts for all clinical and pathophysiologic features of PMS. The similarity of PMS to depressive illness, as well as its response to antidepressant therapy, suggests shared metabolic abnormalities. However, metabolic differences between the two entities have been found. The interaction of several pathways may result in the development of PMS. Research points toward an interaction of hormones, neurotransmitters (serotonin being the most often implicated), nutrients, and behavioral or environmental factors in the development of significant symptoms. Because of the differences in response to treatment for women with similar symptoms, subtypes of PMS have been postulated. Multiple physiologic alterations may coexist that yield the same symptomatic outcomes; correction of single abnormalities without normalizing others (as is likely to happen in a clinical trial) may explain the variability in reported effectiveness of various treatments in different studies.

    1. One study concluded that the symptoms of PMS represent an abnormal response to normal cyclic hormone changes. Twenty women with PMS and twenty without PMS were given leuprolide versus placebo for 3 months. Women in the leuprolide arm had a significant decrease in symptoms compared to no change for the control women. Leuprolide responders were then given estradiol and progesterone, which were associated with a return of symptoms.

    2. Cyclic fluctuations in estrogen and progesterone can have effects on the serotonin system. Patients with PMS have lower blood serotonin levels. A twin study concluded there could be a genetic predisposition and other studies have suggested increases in aldosterone and plasma renin activity that could account for the bloating and fluid retention manifestations of PMS.

  D. Screening and prevention. There are no recommended screening guidelines or prevention strategies for PMS.

II. Diagnosis. For women who present with PMS symptoms, begin the diagnostic process with an open-ended inquiry. A recent multicountry study showed that when women were asked about PMS symptoms, they typically reported abdominal cramps and bloating, irritability, breast tenderness, and joint or back pain.

  A. Commonly reported PMS symptoms include
- Depressed mood, feelings of hopelessness, or self-deprecation
- Anxiety
- Affective lability
- Irritability or anger
- Difficulty concentrating
- Decreased energy
- Change in sleep
- Change in appetite
- Feelings of being out of control
- Bloating
- Breast tenderness
- Muscle or joint aches
- Headache

    1. The National Institute of Mental Health recommends that for a diagnosis of PMS there must be a **marked change in intensity (at least 30%) of symptoms measured from cycle days 5 to 10 compared to the 6-day interval prior to menses for at least two consecutive cycles.** The symptoms must be present for the week before menses and begin to remit the week after menses. According to the DSM-5 criteria, symptoms should begin to remit a few days after the onset of menses and become minimal or absent in the week post-menses.

    2. Once an overview of symptoms has been obtained, the patient's symptoms can be rated to establish a baseline, and other essential information can be requested, including: Is there a previous diagnosis of PMS?, What criteria were used to make the diagnosis?, Have the symptoms changed over time?, and What previous treatments have been successful or unsuccessful? Many patients will self-diagnose PMS from information found in the lay literature.

    3. In some studies, up to half of women presenting to PMS clinics did not meet diagnostic criteria for that disorder, but instead were assigned another diagnosis: most frequently, major depression, followed in frequency by dysthymia, anxiety disorder, menopause, or another gynecologic or medical disorder (e.g., hypothyroidism). "PMS" may be a diagnosis that is more acceptable to the patient than is depression or anxiety. By starting the evaluation in an unstructured manner, the clinician can avoid a premature (and possibly erroneous) diagnosis.

  B. DSM-5 criteria for PMDD include more severe psychological symptoms (depression, anxiety, emotional lability, and anger) that seriously interfere with work or usual social

Name: _____ Month: _____

Write the date in the first row, starting with today. Circle the days of your menstrual period.
Each day, rate the severity of your symptoms: 1 = no symptoms; 2 = mild symptoms; 3 = moderate symptoms; 4 = severe symptoms.

Date																															
Day of the month	1	2	3	4	5	6	7	8	9	10	11	12	13	14	15	16	17	18	19	20	21	22	23	24	25	26	27	28	29	30	31
Irritability or tension																															
Anger or short temper																															
Anxiety or nervousness																															
Depression or sadness																															
Crying or tearfulness																															
Relationship problems																															
Tiredness or lack of energy																															
Insomnia																															
Changes in sexual interest																															
Food cravings or overeating																															
Difficulty concentrating																															
Feeling overwhelmed																															
Headaches																															
Breast tenderness or swelling																															
Back pain																															
Abdominal pain																															
Muscle and joint pain																															
Weight gain																															
Nausea																															
Other (please specify)																															
Other (please specify)																															

FIGURE 85–1. Premenstrual syndrome symptom diary. A minimum of two symptomatic cycles must be included to establish the diagnosis.

activities or relationships. These symptoms should not be merely an exacerbation of the symptoms of another disorder, such as major depression, panic disorder, dysthymia, or a personality disorder (although it may be superimposed on any of these). The symptoms must not be attributed to a substance or another medical condition. The criteria must be confirmed by prospective, daily self-ratings (Figure 85–1) during at least two cycles and must not be present at other times in the menstrual cycle.

1. As many as 10% of women with PMS may report suicidal ideas and death wishes and thoughts.
2. More than half of women with major depression (see Chapter 94) will have an exacerbation of symptoms in the premenstrual phase, including increased severity of usual symptoms or the appearance of new symptoms such as increased aggression, suicidal tendencies, or depersonalization.

C. **PMS should be differentiated from symptoms arising from other chronic disorders,** but which are exacerbated during the premenstrual phase of the cycle (premenstrual magnification). Some patients experience exacerbation or precipitation of other medical problems, such as asthma, migraine, epilepsy, or bipolar illness just prior to menstruation. In addition, PMDD should be differentiated from other psychiatric disorders such as bipolar disorder.

D. **Associated health problems**
  1. **Mental health disorders.** Women with PMS are more likely to have lifetime histories of depression, anxiety disorder, suicide attempts, panic disorder, and substance abuse. While PMS, by definition, is not present during pregnancy, **postpartum depression** is frequently seen in women with PMDD.
  2. Women who **smoke** are more likely to experience PMS symptoms.
  3. Up to 40% of patients diagnosed with PMS have a **history of sexual abuse**.
E. **Symptom clusters.** PMS symptoms may fall into "clusters," which may be helpful in choosing therapy. Some women experience more anxiety, irritability, or mood swings. For some, the primary symptoms are weight gain, swelling, and bloating; for others, changes in appetite or cravings, fatigue, and headache are most troublesome. Still others have depression, sleep disturbance, or cognitive difficulties. Some women experience any or all of these, with some variations in severity and symptoms from cycle to cycle. However, for individual women, symptoms tend to be consistent from month to month.
F. **Timing of symptoms.** Patients should be encouraged to keep a prospective calendar of symptoms experienced relative to phase of the menstrual cycle (Figure 85–1) to help confirm that they are indeed premenstrual; (SOR **Ⓐ**) some women experience erratic symptom patterns and incorrectly attribute them to PMS. Basal temperature measurements can help rule out disorders of ovulation and provide further confirmation of the premenstrual timing of symptoms.
G. **Physical examination.** General physical and pelvic examinations are indicated to exclude disorders such as rheumatologic disease, anemia, neoplasms, endometriosis, or menopause that can present with similar symptoms.
H. **Laboratory tests.** There are no specific laboratory tests for PMS at this time. Other laboratory or physiologic tests may be necessary in individual cases to rule out other potential causes of symptoms such as electrolyte imbalance. Tests that are *not* likely to be useful in the diagnosis of PMS include follicle-stimulating hormone, luteinizing hormone, estrogen, progesterone, or testosterone unless other conditions are suspected. Tests to consider include
  1. **A complete blood cell count** if there is chronic fatigue or menorrhagia (anemia).
  2. **Chemistry profile** if there is chronic fatigue or suspicion of electrolyte disorder.
  3. **Thyroid-stimulating hormone** (unless done within the last 3 months), as the prevalence of thyroid disease is high for women in this age group.
  4. **Serum prolactin** in patients with galactorrhea, an irregular menstrual cycle, history of infertility, decreased libido, or atypical presentations of mastalgia.
  5. **Chlamydia and gonorrhea testing** if there is high-risk behavior, cervicitis, or pain upon pelvic examination.

III. **Treatment.** The goal of treatment should be symptomatic relief.
A. **Symptomatic treatments**
  1. For overall health, encourage a **proper diet** with adequate composition according to the current US Recommended Daily Allowances and Dietary Guidelines for healthy adults. Instruct the patient to follow the USDA Choose My Plate recommendations (www.eatright.org or www.choosemyplate.gov) with specific emphasis on avoiding salt, high loads of refined sugar, and animal fats. This will often provide symptom relief and potentially confer general health benefits as well. A diet high in complex carbohydrate-rich foods may improve mood symptoms and reduce food cravings. (SOR **Ⓒ**)
  2. **Dietary supplements.** Data support the use of calcium and vitamin B_6 for PMS. (SOR **Ⓑ**) Supplementation to ensure adequate amounts of calcium (1000 mg of elemental calcium per day) and vitamin B_6 (50–100 mg per day daily) should be considered. Higher doses of vitamin B_6, however, have been linked to peripheral neuropathy. Some benefit has been shown for vitamin D and vitamin E, but evidence is insufficient for recommending these for PMS. (SOR **Ⓒ**)
  3. **Regular aerobic exercise,** smoking cessation, and limiting alcohol use may improve PMS. (SOR **Ⓒ**)
  4. Teaching women to take control of symptoms through reduction of negative emotions by cognitive restructuring, improving problem-solving skills, and developing responsible assertiveness to deal with discomforts has been shown to provide significant relief of both physical and emotional symptoms.

5. If there is suboptimal improvement after 2 to 3 months of the treatments described earlier or if symptoms are severe, secondary treatment modalities displayed in Table 85–1 and discussed later can be considered:

   a. Anxiety, irritability, and mood swings. Many selective serotonin reuptake inhibitor (SSRI) antidepressants have been found effective for both the depressive as well as the anxiety symptoms of PMS. (SOR **Ⓐ**) These include fluoxetine, paroxetine, sertraline, fluvoxamine, and citalopram. Fluoxetine, paroxetine, and sertraline have been the most extensively studied and are FDA approved for the treatment of PMDD. SSRIs reduce both the physical and behavioral symptoms of PMS, and according to a recent Cochrane review are equally effective if prescribed continuously or intermittently (during luteal phase only).

   (1) The recommended doses for SSRIs are shown in Table 85–1. Paroxetine was made pregnancy category D in 2005 because of concern for cardiac malformations if exposed in the first trimester. Serotonin norepinephrine reuptake inhibitors, such as venlafaxine, can be considered, but have not been adequately studied.

   (2) If SSRIs are ineffective or cannot be used, **buspirone** for 12 days prior to menses is effective not only for social dysfunction but also for fatigue, cramps, and general aches and pains. (SOR **Ⓑ**) The anxiolytic alprazolam has been shown to be effective for some patients who meet the strict criteria of PMDD; (SOR **Ⓑ**) however, side effects and risk for addiction limit its use to a second-line therapy. Tricyclic antidepressants, monoamine oxidase inhibitors, and lithium are not effective in treating PMS/PMDD.

   b. Weight gain, swelling, and bloating. Spironolactone has produced significant reduction in somatic and affective symptoms. (SOR **Ⓐ**) Diuretic therapy should only be prescribed after two or three cycles of restriction of intake of simple sugars and salt, as the edema from these is diuretic-resistant, and other benefits may accrue from their restriction.

   c. Changes in appetite, cravings, and fatigue. Adherence to dietary guidelines, achievement of adequate sleep, and management of the environment to minimize exposure to added stress may offer some mitigation of symptoms.

   d. Depression, sleep disturbance, and cognitive difficulty. Antidepressant therapy with SSRIs has been shown to be significantly more effective than placebo. (SOR **Ⓐ**)

   e. Pain syndromes. Isolated headaches and general muscular pains are treated with simple analgesics, such as acetaminophen and ibuprofen. Migraine headaches occurring as part of PMS may be alleviated by daily treatment with a nonsteroidal anti-inflammatory drug, beginning approximately 10 days prior to menstruation.

B. Treatments based on presumed hormonal cause

   1. Progesterone. Not an effective treatment.

   2. Contraceptives. Combination oral contraceptives (OCs) may reduce physical symptoms of PMS. (SOR **Ⓑ**) A shortened pill-free interval (4 days instead of 7) may be helpful. Studies have shown efficacy for the OC Yaz (ethinyl estradiol and drospirenone), and it is the first FDA-approved OC for PMDD. The only randomized controlled trials (RCTs) that document effectiveness of OCs in treating PMDD have evaluated the continuous OCs containing drospirenone and ethinyl estradiol. Studies involving OCs have also shown a high placebo effect and further studies are needed to solidify the evidence for OCs.

   3. Gonadotropin-releasing hormone analogs. Leuprolide is effective in reducing symptoms of PMS, but causes side effects and sequelae of menopause (bone loss, vaginal dryness), which may be equally as or more troubling than PMS. GnRH agonists are not considered to be the first-line treatment of PMS, but if used are often combined with low-dose estrogen and progesterone to lessen side effects. (SOR **Ⓑ**)

   4. In the rare refractory case of severe PMDD, **surgery** (usually a bilateral salpingo-oophorectomy with hysterectomy) can be considered and has been shown to be effective in multiple observational studies. (SOR **Ⓒ**) Strict guidelines should be followed for selecting a patient who may be appropriate for surgical therapy.

C. Complementary and alternative medicine (CAM) therapies. A meta-analysis of CAM approaches, including 27 trials, and several systematic reviews evaluating herbs, vitamins, and minerals found limited evidence for recommending CAM therapies for PMS. Conclusions could be reported for the following:

TABLE 85–1. MEDICATIONS AND SUPPLEMENTS TO BE CONSIDERED FOR TREATMENT OF PMS

Medication or Supplement[a]	Dose	Major Side Effects	Contraindications or Cautions	Drug Interactions
Spironolactone[a]	25 mg daily to four times daily	Gynecomastia, hyperkalemia, agranulocytosis, renal failure, menstrual irregularities	Renal impairment hyperkalemia	Potassium-sparing diuretics, eplerenone, sulfamethoxazole/trimethoprim, ACEI (hyperkalemia); lithium (lithium toxicity); NSAID (↓ diuretic efficacy, nephrotoxicity)
Alprazolam[a]	0.25 mg three times daily	Sedation, memory impairment, irritability, dry mouth, constipation, change in appetite	Avoid abrupt withdrawal	Azole antifungals (↑ sedation); digoxin (digoxin toxicity); HIV protease inhibitors (prolonged sedation); barbiturates, opioid analgesics (respiratory depression); clarithromycin (ataxia, lethargy)
Buspirone[a]	5–10 mg three times daily	Dizziness, somnolence, headache, nausea, anxiety	MAOIs	SSRI, SNRI, amitriptyline, fentanyl, trazodone, tramadol, (serotonin S); ginkgo (mental status change); linezolid, MAOIs (hypertensive crisis
NSAID[a]	Drug dependent	Nausea, heartburn, dizziness, gas, rash, GI bleeding, PUD, nephrotoxicity, pancytopenias	Asthma/urticarial reaction to aspirin, other NSAID, renal impairment, CABG post-op, PUD/GI bleed, third trimester pregnancy	Cyclosporine (nephrotoxicity); anticoagulants, antiplatelet agents SSRIs, venlafaxine, ginkgo (bleeding); antihypertensives (↓ antihypertensive effect); lithium (lithium toxicity); sulfonylureas (hypoglycemia)
Fluoxetine[a] (Prozac)	20–60 mg daily	**Increased suicidality in teens,** diaphoresis, rash, nausea, dry mouth, dizziness, insomnia, somnolence, anxiety, tremors, rhinitis, QT prolongation, hyponatremia, seizure, depression, serotonin S, neuroleptic malignant S	Use within 14 days of MAOI therapy, concomitant pimozide, use within 5 weeks of thioridazine	**Multiple Interactions** Metoclopramide (extrapyramidal reactions); MAOI, triptans, trazodone, ginkgo (serotonin S); anticoagulants, antiplatelet agents, NSAIDs (bleeding); propranolol (heart block); tramadol (seizures and serotonin S); digoxin (digoxin toxicity); lithium (lithium toxicity); carbamazepine (carbamazepine toxicity); cyclobenzaprine, TCAs (QT prolongation)

Name	Dose	Side Effects	Contraindications	Drug Interactions
Sertraline (Zoloft)[a]	25–200 mg daily	Constipation, N/V, diarrhea, indigestion, dizziness, headache, insomnia, tremor, reduced libido, fatigue, abnormal bleeding, SiADH secretion	Same as fluoxetine and concurrent use with disulfiram	See Fluoxetine
Citalopram (Celexa)	20–40 mg daily	Same as fluoxetine, QT prolongation	As above	As above
Combined oral contraceptives[a]	Drug dependent	Nausea, bloating, depression, edema, amenorrhea, break-through bleeding	Thromboembolism, hepatic adenoma, stroke, MI, >35 years with CAD, gallbladder disease, estrogen/progesterone-dependent cancer, hepatic tumors, smokers	Rifampin, antiretroviral therapy, isotretinoin, St John's wort, griseofulvin, modafinil, carbamazepine, phenytoin, topiramate (↓ contraceptive efficacy); broad-spectrum antibiotics (possible ↓contraceptive efficacy)
Vitamin B$_6$ (pyridoxine)[a]	50–100 mg daily	No major		Levodopa (↓↓ levodopa effectiveness); altretamine (↓ altretamine efficacy)
Calcium carbonate[a]	1000–1200 mg daily	Constipation, nausea, gas, bloating		Levothyroxine (↓ levothyroxine absorption); quinolone antibiotics (space apart, ↓ antibiotic absorption)
Chasteberry	20–40 mg daily	GI upset, headache, rash, irregular menstrual bleeding, insomnia, weight gain	Hormone-sensitive cancers or conditions, in vitro fertilization	Oral contraceptives (possible ↓ contraceptive efficacy)

[a]Available in generic.

ACEI, angiotensin enzyme inhibitor; CAD, coronary artery disease; MAOI, monoamine oxidase inhibitor; MI, myocardial infarction; NSAID, nonsteroidal anti-inflammatory drug; S, syndrome; SiADH, syndrome of inappropriate antidiuretic hormone; SSRIs, selective serotonin reuptake inhibitors; SNRIs, serotonin norepinephrine reuptake inhibitors; TCA, tricyclic antidepressant.

1. There is no evidence of benefit for use of evening primrose oil or magnesium oxide. (SOR **B**)
2. There is limited evidence in support of ginkgo biloba, saffron, *Sillix Donna®*, and soy. (SOR **C**)
3. There is evidence supporting the use of **Vitex agnus castus** (chasteberry; also called Vitex), 20 to 40 mg per day, (SOR **A**) which appears to ameliorate PMS better than placebo. Vitex is somewhat more effective for physical symptoms such as breast tenderness, swelling, cramps, and food cravings compared with fluoxetine; the latter being more effective for psychological symptoms such as depression, irritability, insomnia, nervous tension, and feeling out of control. As Vitex may have estrogen and progestin activity and can suppress prolactin, it should not be used by women taking OCs or who have estrogen/hormone-sensitive medical conditions.
4. There is conflicting information on St. John's wort, with one meta-analysis concluding that the use for PMS was no different than placebo.
5. **Massage therapy** has been shown to decrease general pain symptoms in women with PMS or dysmenorrhea.
6. **Acupuncture** may be effective for PMS. (SOR **C**)

D. **Seasonal and nonseasonal PMDD** have been shown to improve with **phototherapy**. (SOR **B**)

E. **Negative studies.** Evening primrose oil (SOR **A**), free fatty acids, and ginkgo biloba have not been shown to be effective treatments for PMS. However, since most of these treatments have minimum side effects, if a woman finds relief from any of them, she can be reassured that they are safe.

IV. **Management Strategies**

A. **Patient education.** Patients are exposed to information about PMS from many medical and nonmedical sources and may have strong convictions about the condition and its treatment. Some express the fear that their symptoms represent an untreatable condition. Uncertainties about PMS causes in the literature notwithstanding, the likelihood of successful treatment of PMS is high, and reassurance of this fact is the first step to successful treatment. Empathy and affirmation are particularly useful in dealing with women who have PMS.

1. Patient education alone may lead to a dramatic reduction in symptoms during the 3 months when the patient is completing the symptom diary. In addition, such general advice builds patient's self-esteem and ability to cope with symptoms. In controlled trials of PMS treatment, the placebo response rate is sometimes as high as 50%, emphasizing the significant therapeutic value of discussing symptoms with a caring clinician. (SOR **C**)

2. **Helpful patient education handouts** can be printed and given to patients from FamilyDoctor.org (http://familydoctor.org/familydoctor/en/diseases-conditions/premenstrual-syndrome-pms.html).

V. **Prognosis.** PMS symptoms cease in most patients after menopause, although cyclical hormone replacement can trigger the re-expression of symptoms. Many therapies have been found to provide significant relief to a many patients; therefore, the prognosis for improvement of symptoms in PMS is excellent. The medical team must be empathetic, creative, patient, and persistently willing to try different or multiple therapies. Other comorbid conditions, such as memory of past trauma, may surface during treatment for PMS and indicate the need for further treatment or referral.

SELECTED REFERENCES

ACOG Practice Bulletin No. 110: noncontraceptive uses of hormonal contraceptives. Clinical Management Guidelines for Obstetrician-Gynecologists. 2010 (reaffirmed 2012).

Allen LS, Lam CAN. Premenstrual syndrome and dysmenorrhea in adolescents. *Adolesc Med State Art Rev.* 2012;23(1):139–163.

American Psychiatric Association (APA). *Diagnostic and Statistical Manual of Mental Disorders.* 5th ed. Arlington, VA: APA; 2013.

Armstrong C. ACOG guidelines on noncontraceptive uses of hormonal contraceptives. *Am Fam Physician.* 2010;82(3):288–295.Biggs WS, Demuth RH. Premenstrual syndrome and premenstrual dysphoric disorder. *Am Fam Physician.* 2011;84(8):918–924.

Casper RF, Yonkers KA. Treatment of premenstrual syndrome and premenstrual dysphoric disorder. www.uptodate.com. Accessed August 8, 2013. Online version 4.0.

Condon JT. The premenstrual syndrome: a twin study. *Br J Psychiatry.* 1993;162:481–486.

Dante G, Facchinetti F. Herbal treatments for alleviating premenstrual symptoms: a systematic review. *J Psychosom Obstet Gynaecol.* 2011;32(1):42–51.

Dennerstein L, Lehert P, Heinemann K. Epidemiology of premenstrual symptoms and disorders. *Menopause Int.* 2012;18(2):48–51.

Ford O, Lethaby A, Roberts H, Mol BWJ. Progesterone for premenstrual syndrome. *Cochrane Database Syst Rev.* 2012;(3):CD003415.

Freeman EW, Halbreich U, Grubb GS, et al. An overview of four studies of a continuous oral contraceptive (levonorgestrel 90 mcg/ethinyl estradiol 20 mcg) on premenstrual dysphoric disorder and premenstrual syndrome. *Contraception.* 2012;85(5):437–445.

Halbreich U. Selective serotonin reuptake inhibitors and initial oral contraceptives for the treatment of PMDD: effective but not enough. *CNS Spectr.* 2008;13(7):566–572.

Lopez LM, Kaptein AA, Helmerhorst FM. Oral contraceptives containing drospirenone for premenstrual syndrome. *Cochrane Database Syst Rev.* 2012;(2):CD006586.

Marjoribanks J, Brown J, O'Brien P, Wyatt K. Selective serotonin reuptake inhibitors for premenstrual syndrome. *Cochrane Database Syst Rev.* 2013;(6):CD001396.

National Guideline Clearinghouse. Premenstrual syndrome. www.guidelines.gov. Current as of January 2010. Accessed July 20, 2013.

Rosenfeld R, Livne D, Nevo O, et al. Hormonal and volume dysregulation in women with premenstrual syndrome. *Hypertension.* 2008;51(4):1225–1230.

Schellenberg R. Treatment for the premenstrual syndrome with agnus castus fruit extract: prospective, randomized, placebo controlled study. *BMJ.* 2001;322:134–137.

Schmidt PJ, Nieman LK, Danaceau MA, et al. Differential behavioral effects on gonadal steroids in women with and in those without premenstrual syndrome. *N Engl J Med.* 1998;338:209–216.

Stevinson C, Ernst E. Complementary/alternative therapies for premenstrual syndrome: a systematic review of controlled trials. *Am J Obstet Gynecol.* 2001;185:227–235.

Whelan AM, Jurgens TM, Naylor H. Herbs, vitamins and minerals in the treatment of premenstrual syndrome: a systematic review. *Can J Pharmacol.* 2009;16(3):407–429.

Yonkers KA, Casper RF. Clinical manifestations and diagnosis of premenstrual syndrome and premenstrual dysphoric disorder. www.uptodate.com, online version 8.0. Accessed August 8, 2013.

---

86   Renal Failure

Terrence T. Truong, MD

KEY POINTS

- Prerenal disease can be distinguished from ischemic or nephrotoxic acute tubular necrosis by the recovery of renal function within 24 to 72 hours after fluid repletion. (SOR **C**)
- For patients with systolic heart failure, inotropic agents and a vasodilator should be initiated when serum creatinine and blood urea nitrogen rise with diuretic therapy (see Chapter 73). Calcium channel blocker or β-adrenergic blockers are indicated if diastolic heart failure is present. (SOR **B**)
- Treatment of hypertension in patients with polyarteritis nodosa and renal disease may require a calcium channel blocker if an angiotensin-converting enzyme (ACE) inhibitors worsen renal function. (SOR **C**)
- ACE inhibitors and angiotensin II receptor blockers are efficacious in treating hypertension and confer renal protection in patients with benign hypertensive nephrosclerosis. (SOR **A**) However, thiazide diuretics provide greater cardioprotective effects. (SOR **A**)
- Radiocontrast media-induced renal failure may be prevented by the use of lower dose low- or iso-osmolal nonionic agents, maintenance of normovolemia, and avoidance of concomitant use of nonsteroidal anti-inflammatory drugs. (SOR **B**)
- Bladder catheterization, performed to rule out bladder neck obstruction, can also be therapeutic in bladder and urethral obstruction. (SOR **C**)

I. Introduction

A. Definition. Renal failure is a syndrome describing disturbances in renal function resulting in impaired or loss of maintenance of extracellular homeostasis, systemic and renal hemodynamics, calcium and bone metabolism, and erythropoiesis. **Acute kidney injury** is defined as an increase in serum creatinine concentration of 0.3 mg/dL or higher within 48 hours; or increase in serum creatinine concentration 1.5 times or higher than baseline within the prior 7 days; or urine volume <0.5 mL/kg/h for 6 hours. Acute renal failure may occur in patients with previously normal renal function or preexisting stable renal impairment. **Chronic kidney disease** is defined as presence of kidney structural damage or reduced renal function, GFR <60 mL/minute, for >3 months.

B. **Etiology.** Renal diseases can be characterized by the anatomic location primarily affected by the underlying pathology.

1. **Prerenal disease** occurs with glomerular hypoperfusion secondary to decreased circulating volume or relative hypotension, leading to acute decline of glomerular filtration rate. Etiologies include acute hemorrhage; gastrointestinal, urinary, or cutaneous fluid losses; congestive heart failure; hepatorenal syndrome; sepsis; and shock.

2. **Vascular disease** can cause acute or chronic kidney disease.
   a. **Acute.** Malignant hypertension, thromboemboli, scleroderma, and systemic vasculitides cause acute disease.
   b. **Chronic.** Hypertensive nephrosclerosis and bilateral renal artery stenosis are the major causes of chronic kidney disease.

3. **Glomerular disease** is caused by entities that result in focal nephritis, diffuse nephritis, or nephrosis. Overlap of these patterns may occur.
   a. **Focal glomerulonephritis.** Etiologies include postinfectious glomerulonephritis, Henoch–Schönlein purpura, IgA nephropathy, thin basement membrane disease, hereditary nephritis, mesangial proliferative glomerulonephritis, and systemic lupus erythematosus.
   b. **Diffuse glomerulonephritis.** Etiologies include postinfectious glomerulonephritis, membranoproliferative glomerulonephritis, rapidly progressive glomerulonephritis, vasculitides, and fibrillary glomerulonephritis.
   c. **Nephrotic syndrome** is a nonspecific kidney disorder in which there is increased permeability of the capillary walls of the glomerulus leading to proteinuria, hypoalbuminemia, and edema. Etiologies include diabetic nephropathy, IgA nephropathy, minimal change disease, focal glomerulosclerosis, mesangial proliferative glomerulonephritis, and membranous nephropathy.

4. **Tubular or interstitial disease** refers to damage to structures outside the glomerulus and can lead to acute or chronic kidney disease.
   a. **Acute.** Acute tubular necrosis, acute tubular nephritis, and cast nephropathy are the major causes of acute renal failure. Etiologies include hypersensitivity reactions, infections, immunologic diseases, and acute transplant rejection.
   b. **Chronic.** Polycystic kidney disease, vesicoureteral reflux, autoimmune disorders, and analgesic abuse cause chronic disease. Other etiologies include neoplasia such as myeloma and leukemia, heavy metal exposure, immunologic diseases, and metabolic diseases.

5. **Obstructive uropathy** may occur due to urinary flow obstruction anywhere along the urinary tract.
   a. **Adults.** Prostatic disease, urinary calculus, and pelvic or retroperitoneal neoplasm are major causes in adults. Bilateral obstruction is obligatory to produce renal impairment in patients with otherwise normal renal functions.
   b. **Children.** Urethral valves and strictures and ureterovesicular and ureteropelvic stenosis are major causes in children.

II. **Diagnosis**

A. **Symptoms and signs**

1. **Prerenal disease.** Symptoms and signs are related to fluid loss and the resultant electrolyte abnormalities. Response to fluid administration with recovery of renal function within 24 to 72 hours is highly suggestive, though not diagnostic, of prerenal disease.

2. **Vascular disease**
   a. **Acute.** Aside from characteristic systemic symptoms, systemic vasculitides produce renal function impairment and hypertension. Patients with thromboemboli typically present with flank pain, nausea, vomiting, fever, and hypertension. Renal atheroemboli, in contrast, may present with acute marked renal impairment, progressive renal impairment interspersed with episodes of relatively stable function over periods of weeks, or chronic stable renal impairment. Typically, there is preceding aortic or other large artery manipulation.

b. Chronic. Patients with benign hypertensive nephrosclerosis have no specific symptoms. They present with slowly progressive, worsening renal function, and mild proteinuria with a history of preexisting mild-to-moderate hypertension. Chronic kidney disease due to bilateral artery stenosis should be considered in patients who have systemic atherosclerosis, hypertension that is severe or refractory, elevation of serum creatinine with ingestion of an angiotensin-converting enzyme (ACE) inhibitor, or asymmetric renal size.

3. Glomerular disease

a. Patients with **focal nephritic disease** may be asymptomatic. They have normal blood pressure and no edema. They typically have hematuria and proteinuria with no significant renal impairment.

b. Patients with **diffuse nephritic disease** have hypertension, edema, and usually decreased kidney function.

c. Patients with **nephrotic syndrome** may present with malaise, anorexia, edema, weight gain, and frothy urine. By definition, nephrotic syndrome requires the presence of proteinuria of 3 g per day or more, serum albumin <3.0 g/dL, and peripheral edema.

4. Tubulointerstitial disease

a. Acute tubular necrosis typically produces no specific symptoms or signs. There is usually a history of exposure to a nephrotoxic agent or medical conditions leading to ischemia. Differentiating acute tubular necrosis from prerenal acute renal failure can be difficult and may require serial blood urea nitrogen (BUN) and serum creatinine measurements.

b. Acute interstitial nephritis, most commonly induced by medications such as nonsteroidal anti-inflammatory drugs (NSAIDs), antibacterials such as penicillins, and sulfonamides, occurs within 3 days to months after exposure to the offending agent. Symptoms and signs include fever and skin rash associated with an acute rise in the serum creatinine concentration related to drug exposure, generalized aches and pains, or history of recent infection. Additionally, signs of Fanconi syndrome may be observed including proteinuria, glycosuria, and hyperuricosuria leading to dehydration, growth failure, and osteomalacia.

c. Cast nephropathy occurs with multiple myeloma and is due to tubular injury and intratubular cast formation and obstruction. Symptoms and signs of the underlying multiple myeloma include weakness, bone pain, anemia, lytic bone lesions, and hypercalcemia. Renal failure can be acute or chronic. Radiocontrast media exposure can precipitate acute kidney injury in this setting.

5. Postrenal disease. Obstructive uropathy may cause acute injury or chronic kidney disease. Pain may or may not be present, depending on the location and rate of the developing obstruction. Normal urine volume is maintained except in complete bilateral obstruction and shock. Hypertension may also be present. Bladder catheterization should be performed to rule out bladder neck obstruction.

B. Laboratory tests

1. Serum creatinine concentration estimates glomerular filtration rate. A rise in serum creatinine concentration represents a reduction in glomerular filtration rate.

2. Creatinine clearance is obtained from a 24-hour urine collection. It is more accurate than serum creatinine concentration in estimating glomerular filtration rate. Creatinine clearance may be estimated by the Cockcroft–Gault equation in patients with stable serum creatinine concentration.

a. The equation for creatinine clearance is [(140 − age) × ideal body weight in kg]/ (serum creatinine in mg/dL × 72) (× 0.85 for women). For men, the ideal body weight is 50 kg + 2.3 kg for each inch over 5 feet. For women, the ideal body weight is 45.5 kg + 2.3 kg for each inch over 5 feet. Web-based calculators are available (e.g., http://www.mcw.edu/calculators/creatinine.htm).

(1) If the actual body weight is less than the ideal body weight, use the actual body weight for calculating the creatinine clearance.

(2) If the actual body weight is 25% greater than the ideal body weight, use an adjusted body weight calculated by the ideal body weight + 0.3 (actual body weight − ideal body weight).

3. Urinalysis is an essential test to evaluate renal failure. Urinary sediment patterns may be indicative of the underlying renal disease.

      a. Normal or near-normal with a few cells and little or no cast indicates prerenal disease, obstruction, hypercalcemia, multiple myeloma, acute tubular necrosis, or vascular disease.

      b. Hematuria with red cell casts and heavy proteinuria indicates glomerular disease or vasculitis.

      c. Renal tubular epithelial cells with granular and epithelial cell casts indicate acute tubular necrosis.

      d. Pyuria with white cell and granular or waxy casts and no or mild proteinuria indicates tubular or interstitial disease or obstruction.

      e. Hematuria and pyuria with no or variable casts or proteinuria indicates glomerular disease, vasculitis, infection, obstruction, renal infarction, or acute, usually drug-induced, interstitial nephritis.

      f. Hematuria alone indicates vasculitis or obstruction.

  4. Urinary sodium concentration is useful in differentiating acute tubular necrosis from volume depletion as the cause of renal failure.

  5. Fractional excretion of sodium eliminates the effect of urine output on urinary sodium concentration.

C. Entity-specific tests

  1. Prerenal disease. An elevated BUN to serum creatinine ratio, often greater than 20:1, occurs in the absence of increased urea production. However, a normal ratio may be observed with concomitant liver disease or decreased protein intake. Urinalysis is normal, though hyaline casts may be present. Urinary sodium concentration is typically <20 mEq/L, with fractional excretion of sodium <1% and urinary osmolality >500 mOsm/kg.

  2. Vascular disease

    a. Acute.

      (1) Systemic vasculitides. Urinalysis reveals an active sediment with red cells, red cell and granular casts, and non-nephrotic range proteinuria. Classic polyarteritis nodosa, on the other hand, may only produce glomerular ischemia, and thus, a relatively normal urinalysis. Renal biopsy with histologic, immunofluorescence, and electron microscopic evaluation would be confirmatory.

      (2) Thromboemboli. One-third of patients have gross or microscopic hematuria. Serum lactate dehydrogenase levels are often elevated with no significant change of serum transaminases. Radioisotope renogram is confirmatory.

      (3) Renal atheroemboli. Urinalysis reveals a few cells or casts. Proteinuria is usually in the non-nephrotic range. Eosinophilia, eosinophiluria, and hypocomplementemia may be present.

    b. Chronic

      (1) Hypertensive nephrosclerosis. Proteinuria is typically minimal unless an underlying renovascular disease is also present. Urinary sediments are relatively normal. Renal biopsy is rarely indicated, except in instances when there is no clear history of hypertension preceding the development of proteinuria and renal function impairment.

      (2) Bilateral renal artery stenosis. Serum creatinine is increased with exposure to an ACE inhibitor. Renal size may be asymmetric. Doppler ultrasonography may be confirmatory.

  3. Glomerular disease

    a. Focal nephritic. Urinalysis reveals red cells, occasionally red cell casts, and proteinuria <1.5 g per day. Renal function is preserved. Light microscopy reveals inflammatory lesions in less than half of the glomeruli.

    b. Diffuse nephritic. Urinalysis is similar to that of focal nephritic disease, although proteinuria may be in nephrotic range. Light microscopy reveals lesions in most or all of the glomeruli.

    c. Nephrotic syndrome. A few cells or casts are observed in the urine. Proteinuria is at least 3 g per day and serum albumin <3.0 g/dL. Hyperlipidemia and hyperlipiduria may also be present.

  4. Tubulointerstitial disease

    a. Acute tubular necrosis. The BUN-to-serum creatinine ratio remains normal, with the rate of rise of serum creatinine >0.3 to 0.5 mg/dL/d. Additionally, urinary sodium concentration is >40 mEq/L. Fractional excretion of sodium is >2% in the absence of chronic prerenal states such as cirrhosis. Urine-to-serum creatinine concentration is <20. Muddy brown, granular, and epithelial cell casts and free, epithelial cells are usually, though not universally, present on urinalysis. Urinary osmolality, usually <450 mOsm/kg, and urine flow rate are of limited value in distinguishing acute tubular necrosis from prerenal disease.

   b. Acute interstitial nephritis. Eosinophilia and eosinophiluria are also present except in NSAID exposure in which there is no fever, rash, or eosinophilia. Urinalysis reveals pyuria, hematuria, and white cell casts. Minimal proteinuria (<1 g per day) is present except in elderly patients who can excrete up to 3 g per day and NSAID-exposure cases in which nephrotic syndrome can be concurrent. Renal biopsy is the only definitive diagnostic tool.

   c. Cast nephropathy. Urinalysis reveals minimal or no albumin by dipstick, though it is markedly positive with sulfosalicylic acid testing, indicating the presence of light chains. Diagnosis is confirmed by bone marrow examination.

5. **Postrenal disease.** Urinalysis may be normal. Plain film x-ray of the abdomen, renal ultrasonography, or computerized tomography (CT) scanning is diagnostic in most cases. Intravenous pyelogram is of limited value except when staghorn calculus or multiple renal or parapelvic cysts are suspected, when CT scan cannot identify the level of obstruction, and when an obstructing calculus is suspected in the absence of collecting system dilatation.

D. Staging of chronic kidney disease involves recognizing the cause of the disease and categorizing the degree of impairment based on glomerular filtration rate and albuminuria (Table 86–1). Staging, along with comorbid conditions, affects kidney-specific outcomes, complications, and overall prognosis.

III. Treatment. Careful history-taking and physical examination with judicious use of the laboratory will frequently identify the processes that require prompt intervention. Supportive measures are initiated to correct fluid balance and electrolyte abnormalities and to maintain optimum nutritional status. Medications are reviewed and withdrawn or adjusted accordingly. Dialysis is indicated when fluid overload, acidosis, or electrolyte imbalance develops despite medical therapy, or when uremia ensues.

A. Prerenal disease

1. **Hypovolemia.** Fluid repletion is necessary to restore circulating volume. The tonicity of the fluid is dependent on the serum sodium concentration. Blood transfusion is required if the underlying abnormality is acute hemorrhage.

2. **Hypotension.** As hypotension may occur with hypovolemia, cardiac dysfunction, or sepsis, treatment is directed at the underlying entity. Additionally, hypotension may be the result of therapy for chronic severe hypertension. Unless an ACE inhibitor is given in the presence of underlying bilateral renal artery stenosis, renal function will improve without discontinuing the antihypertensive agent.

3. **Heart failure** (see Chapter 73). Enhancing cardiac output will improve renal function. Diuretic therapy reduces pulmonary and peripheral edema, thus increases

TABLE 86–1. CHRONIC KIDNEY DISEASE CATEGORIES BY GFR AND ALBUMINURIA

Stage	GFR mL/min/1.73 m^2	Description
G1	>90	Normal or high
G2	60–89	Mildly decreased
G3a	45–59	Mildly to moderately decreased
G4	30–44	Moderately to severely decreased
G5	15–29	Severely decreased
G 6	<15	Kidney failure

Stage	AER (mg/24 hr)	Description
A1	<30	Normal to mildly increased
A2	30–300	Moderately increased
A3	>300	Severely increased

GFR, glomerular filtration rate; AER, albumin excretion rate.

cardiac output. However, when serum creatinine and BUN levels rise with diuresis, inotropic agents and vasodilators should be started unless there is underlying diastolic dysfunction, in which case the nondihydropyridine calcium channel blockers, verapamil and diltiazem, or β-adrenergic blockers would be indicated to improve ventricular filling (Table 86–2). Verapamil or diltiazem can be started at 120 to 240 mg orally every day or in divided doses. Atenolol or metoprolol can be initiated at 12.5 to 25 mg orally every day. Carvedilol, a nonselective β-receptor and α₁-antagonist receptor with an evidence of decreased cardiovascular mortality (SOR **B**), is given 12.5 mg orally twice daily. Careful monitoring for hemodynamic compromise and drug accumulation is mandatory with titration.

   4. **Cirrhosis** (see Chapter 72). Hepatorenal syndrome treatment is aimed at reversing hepatic failure to recover renal function. Medical therapy and shunting procedures only provide short-term benefits. (SOR **B**) Definitive treatment is liver transplantation.

B. **Vascular disease**
   1. **Acute**
      a. **Vasculitides.** Corticosteroids and immunosuppressive agents are used in the treatment of the underlying disease. Treatment of hypertension in polyarteritis nodosa may require the use of a calcium channel blocker such as amlodipine, at 2.5 to 5 mg orally every day, if ACE inhibitors worsen renal function (Table 86–2).
      b. **Thromboemboli.** Intravenous heparin and oral warfarin are the standard treatment. Thrombolytic therapy may be beneficial if treatment is instituted within 2 hours. Treatment of hypertension, which may be transient, can be with ACE inhibitors such as captopril at 12.5 to 25 mg orally twice daily; enalapril (5 mg) or lisinopril (10 mg) orally every day (Table 86–2). Monitoring for first-dose hypotension is advisable for patients who have not been previously exposed to ACE inhibitors or who are currently on diuretics.
      c. **Atheroemboli.** There is no effective medical therapy. Surgical therapies include bypass grafts, angioplasty, and extracorporeal arterial reconstruction, but these may not be successful if the atheroembolism source is in the suprarenal part of the aorta.
   2. **Chronic**
      a. **Hypertensive nephrosclerosis** (see Chapter 77). Blood pressure control is essential and may necessitate utilization of multiple agents from different classes. ACE inhibitor and angiotensin II receptor blockers are drugs of choice for renal protection (Table 86–3). However, thiazide diuretics, such as hydrochlorothiazide (12.5–25 mg orally every day), effective when glomerular filtration rate is above 30 mL/min, provide greater cardioprotective effects. (SOR **A**)
      b. **Bilateral renal artery stenosis.** ACE inhibitors can control blood pressure in most patients. However, revascularization, whether by renal artery bypass grafting or percutaneous angioplasty, would be indicated with severe or refractory hypertension and progressive renal function decline.

C. **Glomerular disease.** Treatment involves corticosteroids and immunosuppressive agents directed at the underlying pathology.

D. **Tubulointerstitial disease**
   1. **Acute tubular necrosis.** As the process is short-lived, supportive measures are instituted and any offending agent is discontinued. Radiocontrast media-induced kidney injury may be prevented by the use of lower-dose, low- or iso-osmolal nonionic agents, maintenance of normovolemia, and avoidance of concomitant use of NSAIDs. Treatment includes hydration with normal saline.
   2. **Acute interstitial nephritis.** Withdrawal of the responsible agent in drug-induced cases is the primary treatment. Corticosteroids may also be indicated.
   3. **Cast nephropathy.** Vigorous hydration, corticosteroids, and cyclophosphamide decrease light-chain production. Loop diuretics may be administered if hypercalcemia is present. Plasmapheresis (SOR **C**) and dialysis are other modalities that can be considered.

E. **Postrenal disease.** Treatment, directed at restoration of urinary flow by relieving the underlying obstruction, may include bladder catheterization, percutaneous nephrostomy, lithotripsy, ureteral stenting, and urethral stenting.

IV. **Management Strategies.** Effective management of renal failure begins with the evaluation and diagnosis of the underlying disease process. Proper management includes preventing, monitoring for, and treating complications, and maintaining nutritional support with protein restriction.

TABLE 86–2. ANTIHYPERTENSIVE AGENTS: CALCIUM CHANNEL BLOCKERS AND β-BLOCKERS

Agent Name	Oral Starting/ Max Dosage	Renal Impairment Dose	Side Effects/ Benefits/Notes
Calcium Channel Blocker			
Amlodipine (Norvasc)	5 mg daily/10 mg		Jaundice, elevated LFTs 2.5 mg daily in hepatic dysfunction
Diltiazem (Cardizem CD)	Cardizem CD: 120 mg daily/480 mg Cardizem LA:180 mg daily/540 mg		Elevated LFTs
Felodipine (Plendil)	5 mg daily/10 mg		Elevated level in elderly and hepatic dysfunction
Isradipine (DynaCirc CR)	5 mg daily/20 mg		Elevated level in elderly and hepatic dysfunction
Nicardipine (Cardene SR)	30 mg twice daily/ 120 mg		Maximum BP effect 2–6 h after dose
Nifedipine (Procardia XL, Adalat CC)	30 mg daily/120 mg		Giddiness, heat sensation, muscle tremor, positive Coombs'
Nisoldipine (Sular)	20 mg daily/60 mg		Elevated level in elderly and hepatic dysfunction
Verapamil (Calan SR)	180 mg daily/480 mg		Elevated LFTs
B-Adrenergic Blocker			
Acebutolol (Sectral)	400 mg daily/1200 mg	Reduce dose 50% if GFR <50, 75% if GFR <25	Selective β_1-receptor blocker
Atenolol (Tenormin)	50 mg daily/100 mg	Max 50 mg/d GFR <35 Max 25 mg/d GFR <15 Hemodialysis: 25 to 50 mg post-HD	Indicated for angina pectoris
Carvedilol (Coreg)	6.5 mg twice daily/50 mg		Decreased mortality with CHF, overall mortality
Labetalol (Normodyne, Trandate)	100 mg twice daily/ 2400 mg		Nonselective β- and α_1-receptor blocker Jaundice, elevated LFTs Elevated levels in elderly and hepatic dysfunction
Metoprolol (Lopressor, Toprol XL)	Succinate: 25 to 100 mg daily/400 mg Tartrate: 100 mg daily/450 mg		Long-acting agent decreased mortality in CHF Indicated for angina pectoris
Nadolol (Corgard)	40 mg daily/320 mg	Dosage interval: every 24 to 36 h if GFR 50 or less; every 24 to 48 h if GFR 30 or less Every 40 to 60 hours if GFR 10 or less	Nonselective β-receptor blocker Indicated for angina pectoris
Propranolol (Inderal, Inderal LA)	Extended release: 80 mg daily/640 mg Immediate release: 40 mg twice daily/640 mg		Nonselective β-receptor blocker Reduction of CV mortality and reinfarction Indicated for angina pectoris
Timolol (Blocadren)	10 mg twice daily/60 mg		Nonselective β-receptor blocker Reduction of CV mortality and reinfarction

BP, blood pressure; CHF, congestive heart failure; CV, cardiovascular; GFR, glomerular filtration rate; LFTs, liver function tests.

TABLE 86–3. ANTIHYPERTENSIVE AGENTS: ANGIOTENSIN-CONVERTING ENZYME INHIBITORS (ACEIs) AND ANGIOTENSIN RECEPTOR BLOCKERS (ARBs)

Agent Name	Oral Starting/ Max Dosage	Renal Impairment Dose	Side Effects/ Benefits/Notes
Angiotensin-Converting Enzyme Inhibitor			
Benazepril (Lotensin)	10 mg daily/80 mg	Initial 5 mg/d if CrCl <30 mL/min; max 40 mg	Reduces progression to renal failure
Captopril (Capoten)	25 mg two to three times daily/450 mg	Reduce initial dose	Neutropenia, nephritic syndrome, rash Reduces mortality in MI Slows progression of diabetic nephropathy
Enalapril (Vasotec)	5 mg daily/40 mg	2.5 mg/d if CrCl <30 mL/min	Reduces mortality in NYHA II–IV CHF Reduces renal function decline in type 2 diabetics
Fosinopril (Monopril)	10 mg daily/80 mg	Initial dose 5 mg daily	Impaired LFT increases unchanged plasma level Lower risk of MI, CVA than amlodipine
Lisinopril (Prinivil, Zestril)	10 mg daily/80 mg	Initial dosing: 5 mg/d if CrCl 10–30 mL/min 2.5 mg/d if CrCl <10 mL/min	Reduces mortality in MI Reduces renal function decline in type 2 diabetics
Moexipril (Univasc)	7.5 mg daily/60 mg	3.75 mg/d if CrCl ≤40 mL/min; max dose 15 mg	Food decreases bioavail-ability Dosage reduction in hepatic dysfunction
Perindopril (Aceon)	4 mg daily/16 mg	2 mg/day if CrCl 30 or more with renal dysfunc-tion; max dose 8 mg Not recommended for CrCl <30	Safety not known if CrCl <30 mL/min
Quinapril (Accupril)	10 mg daily/80 mg	5 mg/d if CrCl 30–60 mL/min 2.5 mg/d if CrCl 10–30 mL/min	Reduces tetracycline absorption Not removed by dialysis
Ramipril (Altace)	2.5 mg daily/20 mg	1.25 mg/d CrCl <40 mL/min 5 mg/d maximum (HTN) or 2.5 mg (CHF)	Impaired LFT increases unchanged plasma level Reduces mortality in MI with CHF; CVA, CVD, MI and mortality in patients at high risk for CVD
Trandolapril (Mavik)	1 mg daily (non-Blacks) or 2 mg daily (Blacks)/ 8 mg	0.5 mg/d CrCl <30 mL/min	Reduce dosage to 0.5 mg/d in hepatic cirrhosis No data on removal by hemodialysis
Angiotensin Receptor Blocker			
Candesartan (Atacand)	16 mg daily/32 mg		Reduces microalbuminuria in type 2 diabetes mellitus Reduces CHF death or hospitalization
Eprosartan (Teveten)	600 mg daily/800 mg	Moderate to severe renal impairment: max 600 mg/d	
Irbesartan (Avapro)	150 mg daily/300 mg	Hemodialysis: start at 75 mg daily	Reduces rate of progression in Type 2 DM nephropathy

TABLE 86–3. ANTIHYPERTENSIVE AGENTS: ANGIOTENSIN-CONVERTING ENZYME INHIBITORS (ACEIs) AND ANGIOTENSIN RECEPTOR BLOCKERS (ARBs) *(Continued)*

Agent Name	Oral Starting/ Max Dosage	Renal Impairment Dose	Side Effects/ Benefits/Notes
Losartan (Cozaar)	50 mg daily/100 mg		Decreased CHF morbidity and mortality Decreased CHF morbidity and mortality after MI
Olmesartan (Benicar)	20 mg daily/40 mg		Delays onset of Type 2 DM microalbuminuria; increased risk of fatal CV event in patients with CAD
Telmisartan (Micardis)	40 mg daily/80 mg		Reduces rate of progression in Type 2 DM nephropathy
Valsartan (Diovan)	80 mg daily/320 mg		Reduces CV mortality
Azilsartan (Edarbi)	80 mg daily/80 mg		post-MI with LV failure

CHF, congestive heart failure; HTN, Hypertension; CrCl, creatinine clearance; CVA, cerebrovascular accident; CVD, cardiovascular disease; LFTs, liver function tests; LV, left ventricular; MI, myocardial infarction; NYHA, New York Heart Association.

A. **Acute renal failure.** Prerenal disease and acute tubular necrosis are the most common etiologies in the inpatient setting. If there is difficulty in differentiating between the two, fluid replacement may be initiated in the absence of heart failure and hepatorenal syndrome, and potentially offending agents are withheld while the workup is ongoing. Recovery of renal function in the ensuing 24 to 72 hours would point to prerenal disease. Other acute causes will have their characteristic history, physical findings, or urinalysis findings. Their management is specific to the underlying pathology.

B. **Chronic kidney disease.** While treatments for chronic kidney disease are determined by the primary diagnosis, supportive measures and treatment of hypertension are initiated to prevent further deterioration of renal function. Additionally, monitoring for, preventing and managing metabolic, fluid balance, hematologic, and nutritional complications are of paramount importance.

    1. **Metabolic surveillance** should include periodic assessment of serum potassium, calcium, phosphorus, albumin, acidemia, and when appropriate, parathyroid hormone level.

    2. **Nephrology consultation** is beneficial to assist in diagnosis of the renal disease, comanage complications, initiate dialysis, and prepare the patient for kidney replacement as indicated. Comprehensive patient care consists of clear communication and concise coordination of care with the nephrologist and other specialists during the predialysis, dialysis, and transplantation period.

    3. **Hypertension** is common once chronic kidney disease develops (see Chapter 77). Often, blood pressure responds well to ACE inhibitors or angiotensin II receptor blockers (Table 86–3). The goal blood pressure is <130/80 mm Hg.

        a. In the ACE inhibitor naïve or frail patient, captopril, with its short half-life and thus quicker clearance once discontinued should class-related side effects be detected, may be initiated at 6.25 mg orally two to three times daily, and titrated up to 50 mg orally three times daily. Alternatively, longer-acting agents such as enalapril, 5 mg, or lisinopril, 10 mg orally once daily, with titration up to 40 mg orally daily, may improve compliance without incurring significant cost.

        b. For patients who cannot tolerate an ACE inhibitor, losartan (50 mg) or irbesartan (150 mg) orally daily can also be used, with target doses of 100 mg and 300 mg orally daily, respectively. No dosage reduction for renal impairment is necessary. However, patient cost for these agents may be greater. Up to a 35% increase in serum creatinine is acceptable in the course of therapy, unless hyperkalemia develops. Once glomerular filtration rate drops below 30 mL/min, increased doses of loop diuretics and the addition of other classes of medications are typically necessary to control blood pressure.

    4. **Potassium metabolism**

        a. **Hyperkalemia** occurs commonly due to decreased tubular secretion, medications, volume depletion, dietary intake, and hypoinsulinemia. Specific treatments are dependent on the severity of hyperkalemia and may include removing offending medications, restoring fluid balance, maintaining a strict low-potassium dietary regimen, initiating thiazide or loop diuretics, and using sodium polystyrene sulfonate (Kayexalate) 15 g orally one to four times daily or 30 to 50 g rectally every 6 hours.

b. Hypokalemia results from diuresis or renal disease itself. Each mEq/L decrease represents a 200 mEq reduction in total body potassium. Oral replacement with potassium chloride, 40 to 100 mEq per day may be initiated for mild hypokalemia. Intravenous replacement is reserved for severe cases. Judicious replacement, 10 mEq/h, is coupled with frequent assessment of serum levels.

5. Calcium metabolism

   a. Hypocalcemia is observed with renal disease when glomerular filtration rate is <30 mL/min or when there is secondary hypoparathyroidism or hypoalbuminemia. Serum-ionized calcium and mathematical correction for hypoalbuminemia confirm hypocalcemia. Elemental calcium, 500 mg to 2 g, is given three to four times daily with meals. Replacement strategy, utilizing carbonate or acetate salt, is contingent on the presence of hyperphosphatemia. Calcium carbonate contains 40% elemental calcium. Though more expensive, calcium acetate, containing 25% elemental calcium, is preferred over calcium carbonate when serum phosphorus is >4.5 mg/dL.

   b. Hypercalcemia in renal failure occurs with multiple myeloma, malignancy, sarcoidosis, and calcium replacement therapy. Treatment is targeted at the underlying pathology. Calcium replacement is halted or decreased. When calcium × phosphate product exceeds 70, aluminum hydroxide, 300 to 600 mg orally three times daily with meals, can be used for no more than 10 days.

6. Phosphorus metabolism is impaired in renal failure. Phosphate retention leads to hyperphosphatemia and consequently secondary hyperparathyroidism. Treatment begins with dietary restriction to 0.8 to 1.2 g per day of phosphorus (for food list, see http://www.nephinc.com/food-lists.asp#Phosphorus). Binders such as calcium carbonate or calcium acetate are then added if hyperphosphatemia persists. Aluminum hydroxide, 1.9 to 4.8 g orally two to four times daily, can also be used for short duration, though not concurrent with citrate-based binders.

7. Serum albumin and prealbumin, though of limited value in the presence of inflammation, can be used to estimate nutritional status. Dialysis patient mortality increases with decreasing albumin levels.

8. Metabolic acidosis exists in renal failure due to the accumulation of organic acids and impaired renal acidification. Treatment, aimed at raising serum bicarbonate level to 20 mEq/L, is effected by providing 0.5 mEq/kg/d of bicarbonate in divided doses. Each 650-mg tablet provides 7.6 mEq of bicarbonate.

9. Volume overload commonly occurs with chronic kidney disease due to progressive renal impairment, excess salt load, inadequate diuresis, and medication side effects. Treatment initially includes weight monitoring and dietary salt restriction. A loop diuretic is then administered daily or twice daily if euvolemia is not achieved. A thiazide diuretic may be added if twice daily loop diuretic therapy is unsuccessful. Refractory volume overload is best treated with dialysis.

10. Anemia is defined by the World Health Organization as hemoglobin <11 g/dL in children aged 6 to 59 months or pregnant women, <11.5 g/dL in children aged 6 to 11 years, <12 g/dL in children aged 11 to 14 years and in women aged 15 years and older, and >13 g/dL in men aged 15 years and older. Evaluation should include iron studies, reticulocyte count, red blood cell indices, and occult stool blood test. Gastrointestinal blood loss is treated in consultation with a gastroenterologist (see Chapter 35).

   a. Oral iron replacement therapy, ferrous sulfate (325 mg orally three times daily without food or other medicines), begins when ferritin is <200 ng/mL and is maintained for 6 months or until iron-deficiency anemia resolves. Intravenous iron, iron dextran, may be given if ferritin is <100 ng/mL or transferrin saturation is <20%.

   b. If hemoglobin remains <10 g/dL despite identification and adequate treatment of all causes of anemia, epoetin alfa should be considered. Treatment then should be coordinated with a hematologist/oncologist and a nephrologist. Red blood cell transfusions are necessary for patients with severe symptomatic anemia or those with epoetin resistance and chronic blood loss.

11. Nutritional imbalance is common in renal failure. Nutritionist consultation should be arranged early in the course of the disease. Assessment should include evaluation of general nutritional and energy status, electrolyte modification requirements, and lipid status. The daily caloric requirement is 35 kcal/kg body weight for patients younger than 60 years, and 30 to 35 kcal/kg body weight for those older than 60 years. A low-protein diet, 0.6 g/kg/d, may slow the progression of renal impairment. (SOR **B**) A very low-protein diet, 0.3 g/kg, supplemented by 10 g per day of essential amino acids, is even more efficacious (http://depts.washington. edu/pku/PDFs2/ModifyingRecipesFoodList.pdf). (SOR **B**) However, compliance may be an issue. Additionally, this must be balanced with protein malnutrition that may result from adherence to a very low-potassium-restricted diet in the treatment of persistent hyperkalemia.

   12. Dialysis indications include metabolic derangement unresponsive to medical therapy, refractory volume overload, uremic symptoms unmanageable by dietary manipulation, or advanced uremia.

V. Prognosis. Generally, the prognosis for recovery of renal function depends on the underlying pathology, presence of coexisting diseases, and complications associated with renal failure.

   A. Prerenal disease. Recovery of renal function is generally expected when there is prompt resolution of glomerular hypoperfusion. Residual impairment may persist with prolonged ischemia. Patients with hepatorenal syndrome tend to have a poor prognosis overall.

   B. Vascular disease. The prognosis is contingent on response to treatment of the underlying vascular disease. Patients with atheroembolic disease tend to have a very poor prognosis, though this may be related to the severity of the associated cardiac and vascular disease.

   C. Glomerular disease. The prognosis depends on the underlying pathologic process. Children with poststreptococcal glomerulonephritis typically recover fully from the initial renal failure. Some, however, may develop hypertension, proteinuria, and renal insufficiency later in life.

   D. Tubulointerstitial disease

   1. Acute tubular necrosis. Recovery of function occurs within 3 weeks except in those with preexisting renal disease and repeated ischemia or exposure to nephrotoxic agents.

   2. Acute interstitial nephritis. Though renal function may not return to baseline, most patients recover after withdrawal of the offending agent or treatment of the underlying infection.

   3. Cast nephropathy. The prognosis is dependent on tumor mass and light-chain production rate. Improvement is expected in treated individuals.

   E. Postrenal disease. Recovery of renal function is inversely related to the severity and duration of the obstruction, as well as the presence of any preexisting renal disease and infection. Full recovery is expected in complete obstruction of <1 week's duration. It is much more variable in incomplete obstruction.

SELECTED REFERENCES

ALLHAT Officers and Coordinators for the ALLHAT Collaborative Research Group. The Antihypertensive and Lipid-Lowering Treatment to Prevent Heart Attack Trial. Major outcomes in high-risk hypertensive patients randomized to angiotensin-converting enzyme inhibitor or calcium channel blocker vs. diuretic: the Antihypertensive and Lipid-Lowering Treatment to Prevent Heart Attack Trial (ALLHAT). *JAMA.* 2002;288:2981–2997.

Chobanian AV, Bakris GL, Black HR, et al. The Seventh Report of the Joint National Committee on Prevention, Detection, Evaluation, and Treatment of High Blood Pressure: The JNC 7 Report. *JAMA.* 2003;289(19):2560–2572.

James PA, Oparil S, Carter BL, et al. 2014 evidence-based guideline for the management of high blood pressure in adults: report from the panel members appointed to the eight Joint National Committee (JNC-8). *JAMA.* 2013;284427. Published online December 18th, 2013

Kidney Disease Outcomes Quality Initiative (K/DOQI). K/DOQI clinical practice guidelines on hypertension and antihypertensive agents in chronic kidney disease. *Am J Kidney Dis.* 2004;43:5(suppl 1):S1.

Kidney Disease: Improving Global Outcomes (KDIGO) Acute Kidney Injury Work Group. KDIGO clinical practice guideline for acute kidney injury. *Kidney Int Suppl.* 2012;2:1–138.

Kidney Disease: Improving Global Outcomes (KDIGO) CKD Work Group. KDIGO 2012 Clinical practice guideline for the evaluation and management of chronic kidney disease. *Kidney Int Suppl.* 2013;3:1–150.

Palevsky PM. Acute renal failure. *Neph SAP.* 2003;2(2):41–76.

Veterans Health Administration, Department of Defense. *VHA/DoD Clinical Practice Guideline for the Management of Chronic Kidney Disease and Pre-Esrd in the Primary Care Setting.* Washington, DC: Department of Veterans Affairs (U. S.), Veterans Health Administration; 2001.

87 Seizure Disorders

Mindy A. Smith, MD, MS, Shawn H. Blanchard, MD, & William L. Toffler, MD

KEY POINTS

- A seizure is a clinical sign of an underlying condition and does not necessarily warrant treatment acutely. (SOR **C**)
- Epilepsy is a condition of recurrent seizures that requires definitive diagnosis and treatment. (SOR **A**)
- Status epilepticus is an acute state of continued or frequent seizures for 5 or more minutes without a return to consciousness or alertness and requires emergent treatment. (SOR **A**)
- Should the patient be seizing, ensure airway, breathing and circulation, protect the patient from physical harm, and ascertain the duration of the seizure. (SOR **B**)
- A seizure continuing past 5 minutes warrants medication intervention, usually starting with intravenous lorazepam. (SOR **B**)
- Treat seizures with antiepileptic drugs based on the type of seizure, using monotherapy as the preferred approach. (SOR **C**)

I. Introduction

A. Definition. An epileptic seizure is a sudden change in cortical electrical activity, manifested by motor, sensory, or behavioral changes, with or without an alteration in consciousness. A nonepileptic seizure presents with transient symptoms, but without electrical disturbance in the brain.

B. Classification and organizational schemes. A seizure can be initially classified as an epileptiform (convulsive) seizure and a nonepileptiform seizure (NES). The terminology and organization of seizures was revised in 2010 by the International League Against Epilepsy (ILAE) Commission on Classification and Terminology. There were no changes in the elements for specific types of electroclinical syndromes, but the list has been simplified; neonatal seizures are no longer regarded as a separate entity, myoclonic absence seizures and eyelid myoclonia are now recognized as types of absence seizures, the distinction between different types of focal seizures such as complex partial seizures has been eliminated, and spasms are now included under the classification of epileptic spasms.

    1. Epileptiform seizures or electroclinical syndromes are further classified as generalized seizures, focal seizures, and unknown type. There appears to be a preferential propagation pattern for a given seizure type. However, an individual patient can have more than one seizure type.

        a. Generalized seizures involve alteration of consciousness and, while originating at some discrete point, rapidly involve both hemispheres including cortical and subcortical structures. This classification includes tonic-clonic; absence seizures which are further subdivided into typical, atypical, and absence with special features (myoclonic absence seizures and eyelid myoclonia); myoclonic (including myoclonic atonic and myoclonic tonic); clonic; tonic; and atonic seizures.

        b. Focal seizures occur without loss of consciousness and are conceptualized as originating within one hemisphere; this may be within a subcortical structure. These may have motor, sensory, psychic, and autonomic characteristics and may progress to a generalized seizure. Focal seizures are further described by the degree of impairment during the seizure:

            (1) Without impairment of consciousness or awareness. This category can be further described as seizures with observable motor or autonomic components (roughly corresponding to the previous classification of simple partial seizure) or involving subjective sensory or psychic phenomena only.

            (2) With impairment of consciousness or awareness. This category roughly corresponds to the previous classification of complex partial seizure.

            (3) Evolving to a bilateral convulsive seizure.

    c. Unknown including epileptic spasm.

  2. Organization of forms of epilepsy can also be divided by specificity into electroclinical syndromes as above, nonsyndromic epilepsies with structural–metabolic causes, and epilepsies of unknown cause.

  3. Natural classes can also be used to classify seizures based on patient characteristics such as underlying cause, age at onset, or associated seizure type. One scheme that may be particularly helpful for the primary care clinician divides seizures into **nonepileptic seizures, provoked seizures, and unprovoked seizures**. Provoked seizures come from an underlying disease (e.g., neurologic disorder) or event (e.g., head injury, stroke, drugs or toxins) that disrupts brain circuitry or metabolic homeostasis. Unprovoked seizures have no known trigger, although up to one-third may result from a remote brain injury or preexisting neurologic disorder.

  C. NES are further classified as physiologic NES and psychogenic NES. In physiologic NES, seizure activity is seen on electroencephalogram (EEG) without the clinical findings associated with convulsive epilepsy; this condition requires acute evaluation and treatment with respect to the root cause (see Table 87–1). Psychogenic NES, formerly called pseudoseizures, require psychotherapy and possibly pharmacotherapy with antidepressant and/or anxiolytic drugs (SOR ❸) (see Table 87–1).

  D. Febrile seizures are one or more generalized seizures occurring between 3 months and 5 years of age associated with fever and that are without evidence of any other apparent cause (see Chapter 50).

  E. Status epilepticus is a neurologic emergency involving repetitive generalized seizures without return to consciousness between seizures. The Neurocritical Care Society defines it as 5 or more minutes of continuous clinical and/or electrographic seizure activity or recurrent seizure activity without recovery in between. It is also classified as convulsive and nonconvulsive.

II. Epidemiology

  A. Each year four million people in the United States have at least one seizure. The incidence increases with age to more than 100 cases per 100,000 persons in those over age 70 years. The risk of recurrence after a single unprovoked seizure is approximately 35%.

  B. Between two and four million people, or roughly 1% of the US population, have a diagnosis of epilepsy. The incidence of unprovoked seizures ranges from 41 to 63 cases per 100,000 person-years.

  C. Seizure risk increases to 10% for children with mental retardation, or cerebral palsy, and to 50% with both conditions.

TABLE 87–1. CLASSIFICATION OF NONEPILEPTIC SEIZURES

Physiologic	Psychogenic
Cardiac arrhythmias	Misinterpretation of physical symptoms
Complicated migraines	Psychopathologic processes
Dysautonomia	Anxiety disorders
Effects of drugs and toxins, overdose, and withdrawal	Posttraumatic stress disorder
Hypoglycemia, Natrena	Conversion disorder
Movement disorders	Dissociative disorder
Sleep disorders	Hypochondriasis
Syncopal episodes	Psychoses
Transient ischemic attacks	Somatization disorders
Vestibular symptoms	Reinforced behavior patterns in cognitively impaired patients
Hyperthyroidism	Response to acute stress without evidence of psychopathology
Hypoglycemia	Panic attacks
Nonketotic hyperglycemia	
Hyponatremia	
Uremia	
Porphyria	
Hypoxia	

D. There is no significant difference in prevalence between genders.

E. Approximately 1 in 15 children will have a seizure during their first 7 years of life. The prevalence of seizures in children delivered breech is 3.8% when compared with a prevalence of 2.2% in children delivered vertex.

F. Febrile seizures occur in 3% to 4% of all children. Fifty percent of febrile seizures occur during the second year of life and almost 90% before the third birthday. Sixty-four percent of children with febrile seizures will have only one episode. The earlier the age of onset, the more likely the child is to have more febrile seizures. No evidence exists that would suggest recurrent febrile seizures increase the risk of epilepsy.

G. Among 714 patients suffering a first stroke, forty-five patients (6.3%) presented with acute symptomatic seizures in one multicenter Italian study.

H. More than 10,000 episodes of status epilepticus occur in the United States each year.

III. Diagnosis. A systematic approach to diagnosing the cause of a first seizure includes a history, often obtained from a family member, a physical examination focusing on cardiac, neurologic, and mental status (including a developmental assessment in children) and individualized supporting laboratory data and imaging.

  A. Symptoms. The patient's history should include details regarding the episode such as antecedent events, auras, progression, duration, ictal period, and any prolonged neurologic impairment.

  B. The possible causes of a seizure can be grouped into the following categories; the age of the patient may help find a cause (Table 87–2).

TABLE 87–2. POSSIBLE CAUSES OF RECURRENT SEIZURES BASED ON AGE

Age at Onset (yr)	Most Likely Causes
Infancy (0–2)	Perinatal hypoxia Birth injury Congenital abnormality Metabolic Hypoglycemia Hypocalcemia Hypomagnesemia Vitamin B_{12} deficiency Phenylketonuria Acute infection Febrile seizure Idiopathic
Childhood (2–10)	Acute infection Trauma Idiopathic
Adolescent (10–18)	Trauma Drug and alcohol withdrawal AV malformations Idiopathic
Early adulthood (18–25)	Drug and alcohol withdrawal Tumor
Middle age (25–60)	Drug and alcohol withdrawal Trauma Tumor Vascular disease
Late adulthood (older than 60)	Vascular disease, atrioventricular disease Tumor Degenerative disease Metabolic Hypoglycemia Uremia Hepatic failure Electrolyte abnormality Drug and alcohol withdrawal

1. **Genetic.** Disorders such as tuberous sclerosis or malformation of cortical development.
2. **Structural/metabolic**
   a. **Focal brain disease,** including cerebrovascular events (e.g., stroke), head trauma, and neoplasm.
   b. **Infection,** such as meningitis, encephalitis, and abscess.
   c. **Chronic disorder** such as cancer, diabetes, cirrhosis or renal failure causing uremia, hyponatremia, or hypoglycemia, and deficiency states such as phenylketonuria.
3. **Subacute conditions,** such as Creutzfeldt–Jakob disease and subacute sclerosing panencephalitis.
4. **Drug-related causes,** such as cocaine, amphetamines, and alcohol withdrawal.
5. **Toxins,** such as lead poisoning (especially in children) and mercury poisoning in adults.
6. **Asphyxia** from hypoxia, carbon monoxide poisoning, or birth injury.
7. **Psychogenic** seizures account for approximately 20% of cases referred to epilepsy clinics. Clues to this diagnosis include resistance to antiepileptic drugs (AEDs); multiple seizures per day on most days; and comorbid depression, anxiety, or other psychiatric diagnoses.
8. **Misdiagnosed syncope as seizure,** including vasovagal episodes, postural hypotension, and arrhythmias.
9. **Unknown,** in which no clear etiology is found.

C. **Signs**
1. **Fever** may indicate an infectious cause such as meningitis or encephalitis, or it may directly trigger a febrile seizure.
2. **Focal neurologic findings** may indicate a possible tumor or a localized injury to the brain.
3. **Papilledema** indicates increased intracranial pressure that may be caused by an intracranial hemorrhage or tumor.
4. **Hemorrhagic eye grounds** suggest underlying high blood pressure and may be a cause of seizure associated with hypertensive intracranial bleeding.
5. **Stiff neck (meningismus)** may be present with inflamed meninges.
6. **Headache** is a nonspecific complaint compatible with infection or hemorrhage.

D. **Laboratory tests**
1. The following laboratory tests should be considered for all patients with a new seizure and for those with recurrent seizures if indicated by the history and physical examination:
   a. **Serum** glucose and sodium generally should be ordered. Additional tests may include a comprehensive metabolic panel and ammonia level for a patient with cirrhosis; pregnancy test for women of childbearing age; potassium, calcium, phosphorus, magnesium, and blood urea nitrogen in clinical situations associated with dehydration, nausea, vomiting, altered consciousness, or drug ingestion.
   b. **AED levels.** The most common cause of recurrent seizures in children as well as in many adults is a subtherapeutic AED level. Drug levels should be evaluated in all individuals taking an AED who present with recurrence of their underlying seizure disorder.
   c. **Drug, alcohol level, and toxic screens** may be indicated if an adequate history cannot be obtained.
   d. **A complete blood count** may assist in the evaluation of a possible underlying infection.
   e. **A serum prolactin** obtained 10 to 20 minutes after the seizure can be useful for distinguishing epileptiform seizure from NES. A level that is twice normal is moderately sensitive and highly specific for generalized tonic–clonic seizures and focal seizures with altered consciousness. This test is not recommended for the routine diagnosis of epilepsy.

E. **Lumbar puncture (LP).** Indicated if there is suspicion of a central nervous system infection after obtaining a negative CT scan. In infants younger than 12 months, an LP should be strongly considered because clinical seizures and symptoms of meningitis may be subtle.

F. **Brain imaging** is useful in adults unless the physician can confidently attribute the seizure to a metabolic cause. The yield of neuroimaging for detecting abnormalities that change management in adult patients in nonemergency settings after first seizure is about 10%. The American College of Radiology recommends the following:

1. **Adults, new onset. A head magnetic resonance imagining (MRI) without and with contrast or head MRI without contrast** should be obtained for those with new onset seizure unrelated to trauma, alcohol, and/or drugs. **In the emergency room setting, a head computed tomography (CT) scan** may be the study of choice and is helpful in detecting mass effect or hemorrhage.

2. **Adults, medically refractory epilepsy, surgical candidate and/or surgical planning.** A head MRI without or without and with contrast and fluorine-18-2-fluoro-2-deoxy-D-glucose positron emission tomography (FDG-PET)/CT head. Other options include functional head MRI, head CT with contrast, or magnetoencephalography/magnetic source imaging to provide information about the ictal onset zone or for guidance in placement of invasive electroencephalogram grids.

3. **Child, nonfebrile seizure.** The yield of neuroimaging after a first nonfebrile seizure in children is much lower than for adults, particularly for children who are neurologically normal. In addition, caution should be used in administration of gadolinium-based contrast agents, particularly in children with underlying severe renal dysfunction, as this can result in nephrogenic systemic fibrosis, a disorder with a scleroderma-like presentation that can result in death.

   a. **Neonatal seizures. Ultrasound and MRI of the head without contrast** (particularly for children with hypoxic ischemic encephalopathy and congenital malformations).

   b. **Post-traumatic seizure. Head CT without contrast;** consider MRI of the head without contrast.

   c. **Partial seizures. MRI of the head without contrast or head CT without and with contrast if MRI is unavailable or contraindicated.** For recurrent seizures, consider FDG-PET/CT head or single-photon emission computed tomography (SPECT) of the head.

   d. **Generalized seizures (neurologically abnormal). MRI of the head without contrast and/or CT of the head without contrast;** consider MRI without and with contrast to clarify an abnormality on the non-contrast MRI or if considering infection or inflammation.

   e. **Intractable or refractory seizures. MRI of the head without contrast.** Add contrast to clarify an abnormality on the noncontrast MRI or if considering infection or inflammation; consider FDG-PET/CT head or SPECT head.

G. **Additional tests.** The following tests are usually ordered in consultation with a specialist:

1. **Electroencephalogram (EEG).** The National Institute for Health and Clinical Excellence recommends a 12-lead EEG for all adults with suspected epilepsy. For children and adolescents, a 12-lead EEG should be considered in cases of diagnostic uncertainty. The EEG, ideally performed 24 to 58 hours after a seizure, is positive in 29% of adults and 59% of children with new-onset seizures. The sensitivity, specificity, and predictive value of this test depend on the underlying cause and anatomic location of a seizure focus. EEG and video EEG are becoming increasingly valuable in diagnosing epilepsy, particularly in patients having difficulty with monotherapeutic control. (SOR **B**)

   a. **Delta waves** (less than three waveforms per second) are an indication of a disturbance of cerebral function.

   b. **Generalized slowing** is related to an acute disturbance such as encephalitis, encephalopathy, anoxia, a metabolic disturbance, or drug effect. Generalized slowing may occur with hyperventilation, sleep, and drowsiness and is more common in young patients.

   c. **Focal slowing** implies acute local disturbance, such as contusion, stroke, local infection, or tumor. Focal slowing may occur as a postictal phenomenon that may last hours or days after a focal seizure. Slowing also varies with age and state of arousal.

   d. **Spikes** generally represent an old disturbance seen after brain damage, but they may take years to develop. Spikes are less of an indication for further evaluation than focal slowing. A spike wave, defined as three spikes per second, is noted in absence seizures.

TABLE 87-3. STATUS EPILEPTICUS MANAGEMENT

1. Ensure airway—intubate and/or assist ventilation, if necessary; administer oxygen.
2. IV with normal saline; If systolic blood pressure <90 mm Hg, give vasopressor support; give thiamine.
3. Check glucose level by finger stick, or give 50 mL of 50% dextrose solution after thiamine is administered.
4. Lorazepam IV (preferred) or diazepam IV; may need to repeat in 5–10 min (see Table 87–4 for doses).
   Alternatives: midazolam is the drug of choice for intramuscular (IM) administration or rectal diazepam can be given when there is no IV access and IM administration of midazolam is contraindicated.
5. Perform neurologic examination, evaluating for mass lesion or acute intracranial process.
6. If seizures continue, try a second agent such as phenobarbital IV; preferred over phenytoin especially in very young children.
7. Urinary catheter and continuous electroencephalogram.
8. General anesthesia can be considered and given.
9. Treatment should continue until clinical seizures (SOR **Ⓐ**) and electrographic seizures (SOR **Ⓑ**) are halted.
10. Pursue diagnostic testing (see Text).
11. A period of 24–48 h of electrographic control is recommended prior to slow withdrawal of continuous infusion AEDs for RSE (SOR **Ⓒ**)

Source: Data from Brophy GM, Bell R, Claassen J, et al, Neurocritical Care Society Status Epilepticus Guideline Writing Committee. Guidelines for the evaluation and management of status epilepticus. *Neurocrit Care.* 2012;17(1):3–23.

   2. 24-hour ambulatory EEG may be very helpful in identifying "events" and is useful in separating psychogenic NES from epileptic seizures, especially where the two coexist.
   3. Video monitoring may be coupled with a continuous EEG. It may be useful in localizing seizures such as a frontal seizure or a temporal seizure, when the physician is considering surgical correction. This method may also be useful in evaluating suspected psychogenic NES and other paroxysmal behaviors. The evaluation is generally performed with the patient as an inpatient.
IV. Treatment
   A. Acute treatment
   1. The patient's airway must be protected.
   2. Medication is usually not necessary.
   3. If seizure activity persists longer than 5 minutes, intravenous medication should be given (Table 87–3). Lorazepam is more effective than diazepam or phenytoin alone for cessation of status epilepticus and carries a lower risk of seizure continuation.
   4. In children, rectal paraldehyde can be considered; in one case series, the drug terminated prolonged convulsion in 33 of the 53 episodes.
   B. Drug therapy
   1. Initially, only one drug should be prescribed (see Table 87–4). Approximately 50% to 70% of patients can be maintained on one AED. With the older AEDs used as monotherapy, fewer than 50% of patients become seizure free. A specific side effect, such as decrease in cognitive function, might lead the physician to select a particular drug (e.g., phenytoin over phenobarbital) in certain circumstances.
   2. Dosage should be increased as tolerated to achieve a therapeutic blood level. However, clinical response is a more reliable therapeutic indicator than blood levels. (SOR **Ⓒ**)
   3. Based on Cochrane reviews, pregabalin may be less effective than lamotrigine for newly diagnosed focal (partial) seizures and oxcarbazepine and carbamazepine appear similarly effective for this indication. No differences in efficacy were found between carbamazepine versus phenytoin monotherapy or between carbamazepine versus phenobarbital monotherapy for epilepsy. Data remain sparse for comparing other agents.
   4. If the therapeutic goal is not achieved with monotherapy, an alternate single AED can be tried. Only after failure of several single agents should combination therapy be considered. If a second AED is added, it should have a different mechanism of action from the first, although there is no clear evidence in humans to support this approach. (SOR **Ⓒ**)
   5. Because therapy is continued for many years (often a lifetime), chronic side effects must be considered. If the patient is overly sedated or develops other significant side effects, some seizure control may have to be sacrificed to improve function. The

TABLE 87-4. MEDICATION OPTIONS FOR SEIZURES

Drugs for Particular Type of Seizure[a]	Dose (Adult: Usual Dose in mg/d; Peds: mg/kg/d)[b]	Adult Starting Dose	Side Effects	Therapeutic Range (µg/mL)	Drug Interactions
Generalized—Tonic–Clonic					
Valproic acid (Depakene) (Divalproex, extended release [ER])	Adult: 1000–3000 (30–60 mg/kg/d) Peds: 10–60	250 mg three times daily (once daily dosing for ER)	Sedation, nausea, loss of appetite, weight gain, hair loss, dizziness, tremor, insomnia, edema, GI and hematologic toxicity, thrombocytopenia Pregnancy Category X	50–100	**Multiple Interactions** Carbapenem antibiotics (loss of seizure control); warfarin (bleeding); SSRIs, SNRIs, TCA, trazodone (serotonin S)
Lamotrigine (Lamictal)	**Adult: 100–400** Peds: 0.15–1.2 depending on other drugs coadministered	25 mg daily or every other day if also taking valproic acid	Vision changes, poor coordination, skin rash, tremor, GI distress, headache, insomnia	—	Divalproex (lamotrigine toxicity, life-threatening rash); OCs, rifampin, ritonavir (↓ lamotrigine effect); sertraline (lamotrigine toxicity); escitalopram (myoclonus)
Carbamazepine (Tegretol) CR recommended	Adult: 600–1200 Peds: 20–30	200 mg two to three times daily	Dizziness, nausea, sedation, diplopia, ataxia, dry mouth, constipation, aplastic anemia, hypo-osmolality	4–12	**Multiple Interactions** Nefazodone, fluconazole, fluoxetine, (carbamazepine toxicity); MAO-I, trazodone (serotonin S); anti-retroviral therapy (failure of antiretrovirals); tramadol (seizures)
Levetiracetam (Keppra)	Adult/Peds 12 yr plus: 1500 twice daily (ER given once daily) Peds: 4–12 yr, 60 mg/kg/d; 6 mo to 4 yr, 50 mg/kg/d	500 mg twice daily (adult)	Somnolence, depression, headache, irritability, asthenia, infectious disease, pancytopenia, alopecia, behavioral change	—	Carbamazepine (carbamazepine toxicity): ginkgo (↓ anticonvulsant efficacy)
Topiramate (Topamax)	Adult: 200 mg twice daily [b]Peds: 5–9 (focal seizures)	25 mg twice daily	Somnolence, loss of appetite and weight, memory impairment, Metabolic acidosis, abnormal bicarbonate level, behavioral problems, kidney stones, diabetes, rash, speech changes	—	Metformin (acidosis); citalopram (QT prolongation); oral contraceptives (loss of contraceptive efficacy); HCTZ (topiramate toxicity, decreased potassium levels); ginkgo (↓ anticonvulsant efficacy)

Generalized—Absence

Ethosuximide (Zarontin)[a]	Adult: 250–1000 (20–30 mg/kg) Peds: 20	250 mg twice daily	Nausea, vomiting, lethargy, dizziness, hiccups, headache, blood dyscrasias	40–100	Phenytoin (phenytoin toxicity); phenobarbital, carbamazepine (↓ ethosuximide efficacy); valproic acid (ethosuximide toxicity); ginkgo (↓ anticonvulsant efficacy)
Valproic acid (Depakene)[a]	Adult: 1000–3000 Peds: 10–60	250 mg three times daily	See valproic acid above	50–100	See above
Lamotrigine (Lamictal)[c]	Adult: 100–400 Peds: 0.15–1.2 depending on other drugs coadministered	25 mg daily or every other day if taking valproic acid	See lamotrigine above	—	See above
Generalized—Myoclonic					
Valproic acid (Depakene)[a]	See above	250 mg three times daily	See valproic acid above	50–100	See above
Levetiracetam (Keppra)[c]	See above[b]	500 mg twice daily	See levetiracetam above	—	See above
Topiramate[c] (Topamax)	See above[b]	25 mg twice daily	See topiramate above	—	See above
Focal Seizures					
Carbamazepine (Tegretol)[a]	See above	See above	See above	See above	See above
Lamotrigine (Lamictal)[a]	See above	See above	See above	—	See above
Levetiracetam (Keppra)	See above	See above	See above	—	See above
Oxcarbazepine (Trileptal)	Adult: 1200 twice daily max (1200 mg/d if adjunct) Peds: 8–10 in two divided doses[b]	300 mg twice daily	Hyponatremia, rash, dizziness, visual changes, GI distress, ataxia, dizziness, headache, abnormal vision, fatigue, speech impairment, behavioral changes	—	Sertraline (serotonin S); citalopram (QT prolongation); simvastatin (↓ simvastatin efficacy); OCs (loss of contraceptive efficacy); ginkgo (↓ anticonvulsant efficacy)
Valproic acid (Depakene)	See above	See above	See above	See above	See above

(continued)

TABLE 87–4. MEDICATION OPTIONS FOR SEIZURES (Continued)

Drugs for Particular Type of Seizure[a]	Dose (Adult: Usual Dose in mg/d; Peds: mg/kg/d)[b]	Adult Starting Dose	Side Effects	Therapeutic Range (µg/mL)	Drug Interactions
Primidone[c] (Mysoline)	Adult: 750–2000 Peds: 10–25	100–125 mg/day in divided doses	Vertigo, ataxia	6–12	**Multiple Interactions** Valproic acid, fentanyl (severe CNS depression); benzodiazepines, methocarbamol (respiratory depression); apixaban, rivaroxaban, warfarin (↓ anticoagulant effect); ginkgo (↓ anticonvulsant efficacy)
Topiramate[c] (Topamax)	See above[b]	See above	See above	See above	See above
Gabapentin[c] (Neurontin)	Adult: 300–600 mg three times daily (1200 mg three times daily max.) Peds: 3–4 yr, 40; 5–12 yr, 25–35	300 mg daily	Rash, thrombocytopenia, leucopenia, dizziness, edema, blurred vision, headache, somnolence, ataxia, nystagmus, hostility, viral illness, edema		Morphine (gabapentin toxicity); antacids (↓ gabapentin efficacy); ginkgo (↓ anticonvulsant efficacy)
Status epilepticus[d]					
Lorazepam (Ativan)	Adult/Peds: 0.1 mg/kg IV up to 4 mg/dose; may repeat in 5–10 min	Up to 2 mg/min IV push	Respiratory depression, sedation, somnolence, dizziness, ataxia		**Multiple Interactions** Barbiturates, opioids, methocarbamol (respiratory depression); sedating agents (additive sedation)
Diazepam (Valium)	Adult: 0.15 mg/kg IV to 10 mg/dose; may repeat in 5 min Peds, PR: 2–5 yr, 0.5 mg/kg; 6–11 yr, 0.3 mg/kg; 12 plus yr, 0.2 mg/kg	Up to 5 mg/min IV push	See lorazepam		See lorazepam
Midazolam (Versed)	Adult: 0.2 mg/kg IM up to 10 mg/dose Peds: 5 mg IM 13–40 kg; 10 mg IM >40 kg OR 0.2 mg/kg intranasally or 0.5 mg/kg buccal		See lorazepam; hiccoughs; long-lasting memory deficits, respiratory depression, sedation, hypotension		Oral azole antifungals, antiretroviral agents (midazolam toxicity); see lorazepam

Phenobarbital	Adult/Peds: 20 mg/kg IV, may give additional 5–10 mg/kg	50–100 mg/min IV	See lorazepam	15–40	**Multiple Interactions** Benzodiazepines (respiratory depression); Warfarin (↓ anticoagulant effect)
Phenytoin (Dilantin)	Adult/Peds: 20 mg/kg IV, may give additional 5–10 mg/kg	Adult: 3–6 mg/kg/min; Peds: 1.5–3 mg/kg/min	Decrease in cognitive function, sedation, ataxia, diplopia, rash	10–20	**Multiple Interactions** Fluvastatin, sertraline (phenytoin toxicity); apixaban, (↓ anticoagulant effect); atorvastatin (↓ statin efficacy); cyclophosphamide, methotrexate (cyclophosphamide, methotrexate toxicity);

[a]Recommended as first choice by the National Institute for Health and Clinical Excellence guideline (2012).

[b]Pediatric doses are in mg/kg/d except where indicated; drug doses in this table are representative doses only. Actual doses vary by drug product used, age, type of seizure, and whether an agent is being used as monotherapy or adjunct therapy. Dosing should be checked before use for individual patients.

[c]Recommended as adjunctive medication in refractory seizure; prior to dosing, a baseline serum bicarbonate level is recommended and in patients at high risk for renal impairment (older age, or comorbid diabetes mellitus, hypertension, or autoimmune disease) obtain an estimated GFR.

[d]For additional drugs used for this purpose, see Brophy GM, Bell R, Claassen J, et al, Neurocritical Care Society Status Epilepticus Guideline Writing Committee. Guidelines for the evaluation and management of status epilepticus. *Neurocrit Care.* 2012;17(1):3–23.

GI, gastrointestinal; IM, intramuscular; IV, intravenous; MAOI, monoamine oxidase inhibitor; OC, oral contraceptive; PR, per rectum; S, syndrome; SSRI, selective serotonin reuptake inhibitor; SNRI, serotonin norepinephrine receptor inhibitor; TCA, tricyclic antidepressant.

patient should be involved in deciding what balance between frequency of seizures and the occurrence of side effects is most appropriate. The newer AEDs offer alternatives for balancing seizure frequency and drug side effects.

C. Treatment during pregnancy
1. Drug metabolism may be drastically altered during pregnancy.
2. There is about a twofold risk of congenital malformation (predominantly facial cleft and neural tube defects) in mothers who take anticonvulsants to control seizures. Malformations are most strongly associated with valproic acid.

D. Converting from polytherapy to monotherapy
1. The single drug most likely to be successful should be chosen. The dosage of the preferred drug should be slowly increased while the undesirable drug is slowly withdrawn. Long-acting drugs should be discontinued slowly over 1 to 3 months by halving the dose once per week. (SOR **B**)
2. The plan, including the alternatives and the risks, should be fully discussed with the patient. It should be modified if control of seizures is diminished.

E. Febrile seizures. In general, anticonvulsants are not indicated for a patient with febrile seizures (see Chapter 50).

F. Surgical and other treatments
1. **In patients with drug-resistant temporal lobe epilepsy,** resective surgery (anteromedial temporal resection) plus medication treatment resulted in a lower probability of seizures during year 2 of follow-up than continued AED treatment alone in one randomized controlled trial (RCT). (SOR **B**) Trigeminal nerve stimulation may also be effective in reducing monthly seizure frequency. (SOR **C**) Based on a meta-analysis of 11 studies, anterior temporal lobectomy is associated with better outcomes than selective amygdalohippocampectomy for postoperative seizure control in patients with temporal lobe epilepsy. (SOR **A**)
2. **For patients with refractory seizure,** vagus nerve stimulation appears useful. (SOR **A**)
3. **Cognitive-behavioral therapy** can be considered for patients with NES, based on one RCT. (SOR **B**)
4. **A ketogenic diet** could improve seizure control for those with poorly controlled seizures, but tolerability is poor.
5. Data do not support use of acupuncture for epilepsy.

V. Management Strategies are dependent on the type of seizure the patient has experienced.
A. Seizures beginning early in life may be caused by developmental defects, perfusion defects of the brain, intrauterine hypoxemia, or fetal infection. Assisting the patient with developmental problems such as learning deficits is as important as controlling the seizures.
B. In 80% of childhood seizures, no clear cause is found despite an exhaustive workup. If the seizures are controlled, normally no impairment in development occurs. If seizures are poorly controlled, difficulties with scholastic, emotional, and social development may arise.
C. New onset of seizures in adolescence generally has no adverse effect on the patient's development as long as the seizures are controlled. Compliance with treatment may prove a significant problem in this age group.
D. New onset of seizures in adults may indicate serious disease, including alcoholism or drug abuse. Patients in early adulthood or middle age must be screened carefully regarding the use of alcohol and "recreational" drugs, as well as the appropriate use of prescription drugs. Identification and intervention may prevent an extensive workup.
E. Onset of seizures late in life indicates possible cerebral vascular disease or tumor. If the cause of the seizures is not investigated, a potentially correctable problem may be missed and control of the seizures may be difficult to achieve.

VI. Prognosis
A. Based on one study, patients who began an AED within 6 months after a first seizure had an unadjusted risk of recurrence in the next 12 months of 14% (95% confidence interval [CI], 10%–18%). This was somewhat less than for patients not started on drug therapy (18%; 95% CI, 13%–23%). Nearly all patients (92%) with nonfebrile unprovoked first seizure achieve 2-year remission within 5 years.
B. With time, seizure activity may become quiescent. Some patients eventually can discontinue AED therapy. Withdrawal of therapy can be considered after the patient has been

seizure-free for 2 years. The relapse rate of patients who have been medication-free for 3 years is approximately 33%. Relapse is related to seizure type. Patients with complex partial seizures with generalization have the worst prognosis, and those with partial seizures without generalization have the best prognosis. Patients with risk factors for recurrence such as abnormal EEG or prior brain injury or brain lesion should probably continue on treatment. (SOR **G**)

   C. Prognosis also is dependent on the cause of the seizure and whether the patient can change their seizure-provocative behavior.
   D. After ICU admission for convulsive status epilepticus, authors in a study of 177 patients found severe functional impairments at 90 days in half of the survivors; 42 patients (18.8%) died. Longer seizure duration, cerebral insult, and refractory convulsive status epilepticus were strongly associated with poor outcomes.
   E. Sudden unexpected death in epilepsy occurs 20 times more frequently than unexpected death in the general population; risk is increased among men, patients with long-duration epilepsy, and those on antiepileptic polytherapy.

SELECTED REFERENCES

Alsaadi Taoufik M, Marquez Anna V. Psychogenic nonepileptic seizures. *Am Fam Physician.* 2005; 72:849–856.

Berg AT, Berkovic SF, Brodie MJ, et al. Revised terminology and concepts for organization of seizures and epilepsies: Report of the ILAE Commission on Classification and Terminology, 2005–2009. http://www.ilae.org/Visitors/Centre/ctf/documents/ClassificationReport_2010_000.pdf. Accessed October 2013.

Bonnett LJ, Tudur-Smith C, Williamson PR, Marson AG. Risk of recurrence after a first seizure and implications for driving: further analysis of the Multicentre study of early Epilepsy and Single Seizures. *BMJ.* 2010;341:c6477.

Brophy GM, Bell R, Claassen J, et al.; Neurocritical Care Society Status Epilepticus Guideline Writing Committee. Guidelines for the evaluation and management of status epilepticus. *Neurocrit Care.* 2012;17(1):3–23.

Engel J Jr, McDermott MP, Wiebe S, et al. Early surgical therapy for drug-resistant temporal lobe epilepsy: a randomized trial. *JAMA.* 2012;307(9):922–930.

Englot DJ, Chang EF, Auguste HI. Vagus nerve stimulation for epilepsy: a meta-analysis of efficacy and predictors of response. *J Neurosurg.* 2011;115(6):1248–1255.

Gelb DJ. *Introduction to Clinical Neurology.* 2nd ed. Woburn, MA: Butterworth-Heinemann; 2000: 129–151.

Glauser TA, Cnaan A, Shinnar S, et al.; Childhood Absence Epilepsy Study Team. Ethosuximide, valproic acid, and lamotrigine in childhood absence epilepsy: initial monotherapy outcomes at 12 months. *Epilepsia.* 2013;54(1):141–155.

Goldstein LH, Chalder T, Chigwedere C, et al. Cognitive-behavioral therapy for psychogenic nonepileptic seizures: a pilot RCT. *Neurology.* 2010;74(24):1986–1994.

Josephson CB, Dykeman J, Fiest KM, et al. Systematic review and meta-analysis of standard vs selective temporal lobe epilepsy surgery. *Neurology.* 2013;80(18):1669–1676.

National Institute for Health and Clinical Excellence (NICE). The epilepsies: the diagnosis and management of the epilepsies in adults and children in primary and secondary care. http://www.guideline. gov/content.aspx?id=36082&search=seizure. Accessed October 2013.

National Institute for Clinical Excellence (UK). Newer drugs for epilepsy in adults, full guidance. Technology appraisal guidance 76; 2004. www.nice.org.uk/guidance/TA76. Accessed August 15, 2008.

Prasad K, Al-Roomi K, Krishnan PR, Sequeira R. Anticonvulsant therapy for status epilepticus. *Cochrane Database Syst Rev.* 2005;(4):CD003723.

Reuber M, Elger C. Psychogenic nonepileptic seizures: review and update. *Epilepsy Behav.* 2003; 4(3):205–216.

Schachter SC. Seizure disorders. *Med Clin North Am.* 2009;93(2):343–351.

Shorvon S, Tomson T. Sudden unexpected death in epilepsy. *Lancet.* 2011;378(9808):2028–2038.

Wilden JA, Cohen-Gadol AA. Evaluation of first nonfebrile seizures. *Am Fam Physician.* 2012; 86(4):334–340.

Additional references are available online at http://langetextbooks.com/fm6e

88   Stroke

Michael P. Temporal, MD

KEY POINTS

- Rapid evaluation (including noncontrast computed tomography of the head or diffusion-weighted magnetic resonance imaging) and use of intravenous recombinant tissue plasminogen activator within 3 hours of onset of symptoms of ischemic stroke can improve outcome. (SOR **A**)
- Immediate stroke management should include monitoring of oxygen and cardiac rhythm status as well as management of fever, agitation, and glucose control. (SOR **C**)
- Blood pressure (BP) control during the acute ischemic stroke syndrome may be detrimental. BP should be treated only if systolic BP is ≥220 mm Hg or diastolic BP is ≥120 mm Hg. (SOR **B**)
- Secondary prevention should be based on stroke etiology and may include warfarin (for cardiac embolic source or intracranial disease), (SOR **A**) aspirin, (SOR **A**) or another antiplatelet agent (clopidogrel, 75 mg per day, or aspirin/dipyridamole twice daily) for stroke with an atherosclerotic etiology. (SOR **B**)
- Chronic anticoagulation is indicated in patients with a stroke caused by cardiogenic emboli. (SOR **A**)
- Modification of risk factors including smoking cessation, BP control, limiting alcohol consumption, reduction of elevated cholesterol, and diabetes management are important to decrease future stroke risk. (SOR **C**)

I. Introduction

A. Stroke is a clinical syndrome consisting of the sudden or rapid onset of a constellation of neurologic deficits that persist for more than 24 hours due to a vascular event. "Brain attack" is a term used to alert health care providers, patients, and their families and friends of the emergency condition that threatens the life and function of irreplaceable brain tissue.

B. Stroke and cerebrovascular disease is the third leading cause of death in the United States, the most common cause of disability, and the most frequently cited reason for patients needing long-term care. Nearly 500,000 Americans have new (75%) or recurrent (25%) stroke each year. Although one-third of stroke survivors will have permanent disability requiring help to care for themselves, up to one-half of the 4.4 million survivors of stroke have little or no disability.

C. Transient ischemic attacks (TIAs) are reversible neurologic defects and should prompt the clinician to aggressively evaluate. Following a first TIA, 10% to 25% of patients will have a cerebrovascular accident (CVA) in the next 90 days; up to half of these within the 48 hours following the TIA.

D. Types of stroke. In adults, 80% of strokes are **ischemic,** including atheroembolic/atherothrombotic stroke (60%–70% of strokes), cerebral embolic, and lacunar (small-vessel occlusive). The rest of strokes in adults are **hemorrhagic** and are classified by location as intracerebral or subarachnoid.

E. The **differential diagnosis for stroke** includes mass lesions (e.g., subdural hematoma or neoplasm), metabolic abnormalities (e.g., hypoglycemia, hyponatremia, or hypernatremia), infectious processes (e.g., meningitis or cerebral abscess), inflammatory processes (e.g., temporal arteritis), and idiopathic processes (e.g., epilepsy, migraine headache). Arrhythmia, syncope, or acute cardiac events may also present like a stroke (see Chapters 48, 57, and 79). Illicit drug use may be a consideration (see Chapter 90).

II. Diagnosis.
The presentation of stroke represents a continuum from TIA (with quickly resolving neurologic deficit) to acute stroke syndrome with progression (worsening deficits, most common with large vessel thrombosis, lacunes, or emboli) to completed stroke (static neurologic deficits). Early presentation, rapid imaging, and prompt treatment are key goals for health care providers and the communities they serve. Evaluation and management in dedicated stroke centers can improve outcomes. (SOR **A**)

TABLE 88-1. CLINICAL PRESENTATION OF STROKE

Stroke Type/Artery or Site Involved	Clinical Presentation	Special Considerations
Atherothrombotic stroke Internal carotid artery (mostly extracranial) Vertebral artery (mostly intracranial) Basilar artery	Stuttering onset, can occur upon waking; cerebellar infarction causes severe edema/brain stem compression	Preceded by TIA in 50% of cases
Embolic stroke Middle cerebral artery Anterior cerebral artery Posterior cerebral artery	Sudden onset of maximal deficit	
Lacunar infarction (penetrating arteries) Middle cerebral perforator–lenticulostriate Posterior cerebral perforator Basilar artery perforating branches	Develops suddenly or over several hours; headache, loss of consciousness, and emesis do not occur	Lacunar syndromes: pure motor hemiparesis, pure sensory loss, crural paresis, and ataxia/dysarthria (clumsy hand syndrome)
Intracerebral hemorrhage Deep cerebral hemisphere (putamen) Subcortical white matter (lobar intracranial hemorrhage) Cerebellar Thalamic Midbrain	Smooth onset, although can be sudden; emesis and loss of consciousness do occur	Selective surgical clot evacuation; unpredictable course in cerebellar ICH; most midbrain ICHs improve with supportive care
Subarachnoid hemorrhage (ruptured aneurysm) Circle of Willis Internal carotid artery Anterior communicating artery Middle cerebral artery	Sudden onset ("brutal" headache, emesis, loss of consciousness then awakening with headache and stiff neck); *note:* aneurysms are rarely symptomatic before rupture	Complications: re-rupture, obstruction of spinal fluid flow (communicating hydrocephalus), vasospasm 3–14 d postevent

ICH, intracerebral hemorrhage; TIA, transient ischemic attack.

A. **Symptoms** and **signs** of stroke reflect the cerebrovascular territory affected by the stroke process. The vessels most often involved are listed in Table 88-1. Sudden onset of weakness, numbness, or problems with speech or vision or the sudden development of dizziness, trouble walking, or headache are early warning signs of stroke. $ABCD^2$ is a tool that can predict the risk of stroke in 2 days following a TIA (Table 88-2).

The initial history should document time of symptom onset, associated activities or trauma, other neurologic symptoms (headache, seizure, vomiting, alteration of consciousness) as well as present and past illnesses and surgeries, medications taken, illicit drug use, and allergies. Identifying stroke risk factors and contraindications to thrombolytic therapy is also essential.

B. **Physical examination.** The NIH Stroke Scale **(NIHSS) (Table 88-3)** provides a rapid and relatively comprehensive neurologic assessment that can facilitate communication among health care professionals. (SOR **B**) The NIHSS score can have prognostic value: patients with a mild stroke (<5) may have very good recovery; a score >25 would be an exclusion to recombinant tissue plasminogen activator (rtPA) after 3 hours of onset of symptoms. The general physical examination should identify trauma, infection, or comorbid cardiac, respiratory, and abdominal disorders.

C. **Brain imaging studies** are used to detect the presence of hemorrhage and exclude other causes (tumor, abscess, or subdural hematoma). The initial study should be obtained and interpreted within 60 minutes of presentation to an emergency setting to facilitate decisions on thrombolytic therapy. (SOR **A**) Advances in brain imaging offer early distinction of the core area of ischemic tissue with severely compromised cerebral blood flow (CBF) from the "penumbra," that is, the surrounding rim of moderately

TABLE 88–2. ABCD² SCORE RISK ASSESSMENT TOOL^a

Risk Factor	Score
Age 60 yr or older	1 point
Blood pressure: systolic ≥140 mm Hg **OR**	1 point
diastolic ≥90 mm Hg	
Clinical features of TIA (choose one):	2 points
Unilateral weakness with or without speech impairment **OR**	1 point
Speech impairment without unilateral weakness	
Duration:	2 points
TIA duration ≥60 min	1 point
TIA duration 10–59 min	
Diabetes	1 point

^aTotal Score 0–7 points; Score 0–3, 2-day stroke risk 1.0%, hospital observation may be unnecessary without another indication (e.g., new atrial fibrillation); Score 4–5, 2-day stroke risk 4.1%, hospital observation justified in most situations; Score 6–7, 2-day stroke risk 8.1%, hospital observation worthwhile.
Source: ©2014 National Stroke Association. Content provided by permission of National Stroke Association. www.stroke.org for stroke education resources.

ischemic brain tissue with impaired electrical activity but preserved cellular metabolism and viability.

1. **Computed tomography (CT)** gives reliable differentiation of hemorrhagic from ischemic stroke with scanning obtained during the first 72 hours of the stroke. All rtPA-administration protocols call for pretreatment noncontrast CT scan within 3 hours of onset of symptoms, and ideally within 45 minutes of presentation to the emergency room, to rule out hemorrhagic events. CT scan will show a subarachnoid hemorrhage with 95% sensitivity if performed within 5 days of the event. Normal CT scans are frequently obtained in lacunar or brain stem infarctions when the lesions are small. Early in the course of an ischemic infarction, plain CT scan can show loss of gray–white matter differentiation and cerebral edema.

   a. If there is no delay in obtaining or interpreting the study, the addition of spiral CT angiography can help identify large-vessel occlusion or a possible mechanism for ischemia. Spiral CT angiography can rapidly and noninvasively evaluate the intracranial and extracranial vasculature in the acute, subacute, and chronic stroke setting. (SOR **A**)

   b. Whole brain perfusion CT can identify regions of hypoattenuation and may differentiate thresholds of reversible and irreversible ischemia. Dynamic perfusion CT can be used to measure blood flow and blood volume, but provides incomplete visualization of selected vascular territories

2. **Magnetic resonance imaging (MRI)** is the preferred imaging study, if time allows, within the window of opportunity for rtPA and if a patient presents outside the 3–4.5 hours from onset of symptoms.

   a. **MRI or diffusion-weighted imaging (DWI)** has emerged as the most sensitive and specific technique for acute infarct, with sensitivity (88%–100%) and specificity (95%–100%) far better than those of CT or any other MRI sequence.

   b. **Advantages** of MRI include the ability to identify small or deep cortical lesions of an acute or chronic nature as well as identify potentially reversible areas of ischemia, the penumbra. Intracranial MR angiography (MRA) provides additional information for acute proximal large-vessel disease that may be amenable to acute intervention. Limitations to MRI/MRA include availability, time to obtain, patient tolerability, and motion artifact.

   D. **Laboratory tests.** The following blood tests are recommended for all patients with a suspected acute ischemic stroke: **basic metabolic panel, glucose, complete blood count and platelets, prothrombin time (PT) and international normalized ratio (INR), and cardiac enzymes.** (SOR **B**) In selected patients, additional acute tests may include liver function tests, toxicology and blood alcohol level, pregnancy test, thyroid stimulating hormone, and arterial blood gas.

   Subsequent tests can be helpful after the acute stroke including a lipid profile and specific coagulation factors (proteins C, S, and antithrombin III). (SOR **B**) Elevated homocysteine levels have been associated with increased stroke risk and may be improved with vitamin B complex supplementation. (SOR **C**)

TABLE 88–3. NATIONAL INSTITUTES OF HEALTH STROKE SCALE

Item	Description	Scoring Response
1A	Level of Consciousness	0—alert 1—drowsy 2—obtunded 3—coma/unresponsive
1B	Orientation Questions (2)	0—answers both correctly 1—answers one correctly 2—answers neither correctly
1C	Response to Commands (2)	0—performs both tasks correctly 1—performs one task correctly 2—performs neither correctly
2	Gaze	0—normal horizontal movements 1—partial gaze palsy 2—complete gaze palsy
3	Visual Fields	0—no visual field defect 1—partial hemianopia 2—complete hemianopia 3—bilateral hemianopia
4	Facial Movements	0—normal 1—minor facial weakness 2—partial facial weakness 3—complete unilateral palsy
5	Motor Function (arm) R (score each) L	0—no drift 1—drift before 5 s 2—drift before 10 s 3—no effort against gravity 4—no movement
6	Motor Function (leg) R (score each) L	0—no drift 1—drift before 5 s 2—drift before 10 s 3—no effort against gravity 4—no movement
7	Limb Ataxia	0—no ataxia 1—ataxia in 1 limb 2—ataxia in 2 limbs
8	Sensory	0—no sensory loss 1—mild sensory loss 2—severe sensory loss
9	Language	0—normal 1—mild aphasia 2—severe aphasia 3—mute or global aphasia
10	Articulation	0—normal 1—mild dysarthria 2—severe dysarthria
11	Extinction or Inhibition	0—absent 1—mild (loss 1 sensory modality) 2—severe (loss 2 sensory modalities)

Source: Available at http://www.ninds.nih.gov/doctors/NIH_Stroke_Scale.pdf. Accessed September 2013.

E. Additional studies

1. An initial electrocardiogram is obtained in all patients presenting with stroke to identify arrhythmia or other cardiac conditions. Routine **chest radiographs** are indicated only if underlying lung pathology is suspected. (SOR **B**)

2. Imaging of the extracranial and intracranial vessels. Plain CT and MRI can show signs of large-vessel occlusion, but noninvasive imaging of intracranial vasculature can help identify other areas of vasculature lesions and establish possible mechanisms of ischemia to prevent subsequent episodes. Either helical CT angiography or MR angiography can be obtained acutely, and should be performed soon following the acute event.

   a. Transcranial Doppler (TCD) ultrasonography is used to detect middle cerebral and distal (intracranial) internal carotid artery stenosis, with a sensitivity of 92% and a specificity of 100%. However, this technique is insufficient to detect stenosis or occlusion in the posterior circulation, and the middle cerebral artery cannot be seen in up to one-fourth of patients. TCD is capable of detecting microembolic material of both gaseous and solid states within intracranial cerebral arteries.

   b. Carotid Doppler ultrasound criteria for stenosis may vary by institution and is limited in imaging proximal or distal to the carotid bifurcation.

3. **Cerebral angiography,** the gold standard of vascular imaging, is performed on a case-specific basis, primarily when surgical intervention is considered or when angiographic confirmation of stenosis detected by other techniques is required. Evaluation by **CT or MR angiography** offers the best sensitivity and specificity as well as delineation of lesions of the extracranial vessels.

   a. Digital subtraction angiography is another technique that allows visualization of carotid and vertebral arteries and information of collateral flow.

   b. Oculoplethysmography offers an indirect measure of carotid arterial blockage by measuring arterial pulsations in the retinal artery.

4. **Echocardiography** (transthoracic or transesophageal) and **24-hour Holter monitoring** are performed when an embolic process is suspected, when surgical intervention is planned, or when the patient with stroke has significant risk factors for emboli (e.g., atrial fibrillation, suspected infective endocarditis, prosthetic heart valve, dilated cardiomyopathy, or recent anterior myocardial infarction [MI]).

5. A **lumbar puncture** is useful when brain imaging is normal and subarachnoid hemorrhage or meningitis is suspected. Although cerebrospinal fluid is usually bloody in ventricular extension of a hypertensive hemorrhage, vascular malformation, and ruptured aneurysm, a clear tap does not guarantee absence of hemorrhage. Leukocytosis in the cerebrospinal fluid suggests infection.

6. **Electroencephalography** may show slow waves in strokes involving the cortex and is performed when seizure activity has occurred or is suspected.

III. **Treatment**

   A. **Immediate management.** Acute stroke is a medical emergency. The first step is patient education directed at encouraging patients to seek medical care as soon as symptoms develop. Initiation of diagnosis and treatment within the first few hours of onset enhances the chances for minimizing irreversible ischemic damage and thus improve outcomes. Care in specialized stroke units has been shown to improve outcomes. (SOR **Ⓐ**) Attention to rehabilitation goals begins as soon as possible after the acute event.

   1. **Stabilization of the patient** involves blood pressure (BP) control, arrhythmia detection and treatment, airway protection, and, if needed, ventilatory assistance. Supplemental oxygen is only needed to correct hypoxemia and to maintain oxygen saturation >94%. (SOR **Ⓒ**)

   a. Identification and treatment of **hyperthermia** to maintain normothermia may be indicated, but the role of routine induced hypothermia has not been determined. (SOR **Ⓒ**)

   b. Position. Lying flat in the supine or side position may help cerebral perfusion, but a 15- to 30-degree elevation of the head may be better tolerated or necessary to maintain oxygenation. Proper positioning may be needed to avoid pressure sores.

   c. Additional measures. Diligent correction of metabolic disturbances and skilled monitoring of stroke progression via repeated neurologic examinations are important. Continuous cardiac monitoring during the first 24 hours is advised because of the high risk of cardiac arrhythmias.

   2. **BP control.** The prevention of neurologic and cardiovascular compromise caused by BP extremes poses a unique clinical challenge in the patient with stroke. Post-stroke BP elevation usually declines spontaneously by approximately 10% in the first 24 hours. In fact, elevated BP can be a physiologic response to acute brain ischemia. Normalization of BP often occurs when specific effects of stroke are controlled: pain, nausea, agitation, bladder distention, increased intracranial pressure (ICP), stress of stroke, and underlying hypertension. Furthermore, exaggerated responses

to antihypertensive drugs can cause sudden drops in BP that compromise cerebral perfusion and thus worsen neurologic status.

a. **Pharmacologic therapy for hypertension associated with ischemic stroke** is only used for specific indications (e.g., MI or arterial dissection) or for systolic BP ≥220 mm Hg or diastolic BP ≥120 mm Hg on repeated measurements over a 30- to 60-minute period. (SOR **B**) Bringing the BP to below 180/110 mm Hg is needed to qualify for intravenous rtPA, and maintenance following rTPA to below 180/105 mm Hg is used to decrease the risk of intracranial hemorrhage.

b. **Treatment options** include intravenous labetalol (10–20 mg, may repeat once), or nicardipine infusion (5 mg/h titrated by 2.5 mg/hour every 5 to 15 minutes to a maximum of 15 mg/hour). Other agents (e.g., hydralazine, enalaprilat, nitropaste) may be considered when appropriate.

c. **The approach** to BP control must take into account whether the pre-event BP was known to be normotensive or not. Additionally, patients with **hemorrhagic stroke, after thrombolysis and in the postoperative period** (e.g., carotid endarterectomy or hematoma removal) **require more aggressive treatment of hypertension**. Long-term antihypertensive therapy can be considered 24 hours after the acute event. (SOR **C**)

3. **Intravenous fluids** are used for correction of hypovolemia or for maintenance at 30 mL/kg body weight. Use of 0.9% saline is less likely to exacerbate ischemic brain edema than dextrose 5% or 0.45% saline solutions. (SOR **C**)

4. **Glucose control** may include correction of hypoglycemia (blood glucose <60 mg/dL) and maintenance of blood glucose in the range of 140 to 180 mg/dL. (SOR **C**) Tight glucose control, in one meta-analysis, was associated with lower infection rates and improved neurologic outcomes in critically ill neurologic and neurosurgical patients, but did not affect mortality.

5. **Reperfusion** therapy aimed at recanalization of the affected vessel(s) in acute stroke includes pharmacologic, angioplastic, and surgical recanalization options.

a. **Pharmacologic agents.** Thrombolytic therapy is associated with a reduction in the combination endpoint of death or dependency at 3 to 6 months following ischemic stroke. (SOR **A**) However, there is an increased risk of death at 3 to 6 months (odds ratio [OR] 1.31, 95% confidence interval [CI] 1.14–1.50) and symptomatic intracranial hemorrhage (OR 3.49, 95% CI 2.81–4.33) with thrombolytic therapy versus the control group. Drugs tested in treatment trials included urokinase, streptokinase, rtPA, recombinant pro-urokinase, and desmoteplase. A discussion of all the drugs is beyond the scope of this chapter, so only rtPA will be discussed as this drug is commonly used.

The US Food and Drug Administration (FDA) has approved **rtPA** for treatment of CT-proven nonhemorrhagic stroke within the first 3 hours of onset of symptoms and within 4.5 hours in selected patients. Studies show that the sooner the intervention, the greater the chance of a good outcome. Uncontrolled BP ≥185/110 mm Hg is a contraindication to rtPA.

(1) After evaluation for inclusion or exclusion criteria for its use (Table 88–4), rtPA is administered at 0.9 mg/kg (up to 90 mg) intravenously. Intra-arterial administration of rtPA is recommended for patients with occlusions of the internal carotid, main stem middle cerebral, and basilar arteries. Intravenous rtPA is best for patients with intracranial circumferential branch artery occlusions.

(2) The greatest risk of thrombolysis in acute stroke is intracerebral hemorrhage (ICH). Intensive care unit monitoring after thrombolysis includes attention to signs of ICH: decreased consciousness, headache, nausea, vomiting, and increased neurologic focal deficits. The risk of ICH is decreased by lowering BP (treat for systolic ≥185 mm Hg and diastolic ≥110 mm Hg). Neither aspirin nor anticoagulation is given for the initial 24 hours after thrombolysis, and neither is initiated after that until a repeat CT scan shows no hemorrhage. CT scans are usually repeated after 24 hours if the patient will continue on anticoagulant or antiplatelet therapy or at any time there is a worsening of neurologic condition.

b. **Other endovascular interventions** are under evaluation and show favorable outcomes. All of these have been in association with intra-arterial thrombolytic therapy and limited to comprehensive stroke centers.

TABLE 88-4. RECOMBINANT TISSUE PLASMINOGEN ACTIVATOR (rtPA) USE IN PATIENTS WITH STROKE

Inclusion criteria
   Diagnosis of ischemic stroke causing measurable neurologic deficit
   Onset of symptoms <3 h before beginning treatment
   Aged ≥18 yr

Exclusion criteria
   Recent major surgery or trauma in past 14 d
   Significant head trauma or prior stroke in previous 3 mo
   Symptoms suggest subarachnoid hemorrhage
   Arterial puncture at noncompressible site in previous 7 d
   History of previous intracranial hemorrhage
   Intracranial neoplasm, arteriovenous malformation, or aneurysm
   Recent intracranial or intraspinal surgery
   Elevated blood pressure (systolic >185 mm Hg or diastolic >110 mm Hg)
   Active internal bleeding
   Acute bleeding diathesis, including but not limited to
   Platelet count <100,000/mm^3
   Heparin received within 48 h, resulting in abnormally elevated aPTT greater than the upper limit of normal
   Current use of anticoagulant with INR >1.7 or PT >15 s
   Current use of direct thrombin inhibitors or direct factor Xa inhibitors with elevated sensitive laboratory tests
       (such as aPTT, INR, platelet count, and ECT; or appropriate factor Xa activity assays)
   Blood glucose concentration <50 mg/dL (2.7 mmol/L)
   CT demonstrates multilobar infarction (hypodensity >1/3 cerebral hemisphere)

Relative exclusion criteria
   Only minor or rapidly improving stroke symptoms (clearing spontaneously)
   Pregnancy
   Seizure at onset with postictal residual neurologic impairments
   Major surgery or serious trauma within previous 14 d
   Recent gastrointestinal or urinary tract hemorrhage (within previous 21 d)
   Recent acute MI (within previous 3 mo)

rtPA may be considered between 3 and 4.5 h of onset of symptoms if
   Age <80 yr
   NIHSS score <25
   Not taking any anticoagulant regardless of INR
   No history of both diabetes and prior ischemic stroke
   Intra-arterial needle-sticks in noncompressible sites
   Computerized tomography (CT) results showing involvement of more than one-third of the distribution of the
       major carotid artery
   Infective endocarditis
   Seizure at onset of stroke
   Any evidence of blood on CT imaging
   Abnormal platelet counts (≤100,000/mm^3)
   Elevated International normalized ratio (≥1.7) or partial thromboplastin time (PTT)
   Administration of heparin in the past 24 h
   Chest compression
   Gastrointestinal or urinary tract hemorrhage in past 21 d
   Recent MI
   Recent lumbar puncture in past 7 d
   Pregnancy
   Uncontrolled hypertension: systolic ≥185 mm Hg; diastolic ≥110 mm Hg

    (1) Angioplasty with stenting may be considered in the higher risk surgical candidate. Emergency angioplasty with stent in conjunction with intra-arterial thrombolysis has been helpful. (SOR ⓒ)

    (2) Mechanical clot disruption of the middle cerebral artery and the internal carotid artery can improve the success of recanalization. (SOR ⓒ) Mechanical clot disruption/extraction systems include the Merci Retrieval System and the Penumbra System, Solitaire FR, and Trevo thrombectomy devices which include a coil retriever or an aspirator, a filter, and a reperfusion catheter.

  6. Acute anticoagulation. There is no standard of care for the use of **heparin** in the acute phase of stroke. Heparin should not be a substitute for patients otherwise eligible for thrombolytic therapy. Studies from the International Stroke Trial showed that while the risk of early recurrent stroke was lowered, excess major bleeding complications negated any benefits. (SOR **B**) Likewise, trials using low-molecular-weight heparins or danaparoid for acute stroke have not demonstrated benefit. (SOR **A**) Heparin as an adjunctive therapy should not begin within 24 hours of thrombolytic therapy. (SOR **B**) Emerging trials using direct thrombin inhibitors are under clinical review.

B. Subsequent management

1. **Carotid endarterectomy (CEA)** for ipsilateral severe (70%–99%) carotid artery stenosis in symptomatic patients with recent nondisabling carotid artery ischemic events (TIA or stroke) is clearly beneficial. The NASCET (North American Symptomatic Carotid Endarterectomy Trial) demonstrated benefit for severe lesions and for moderate (50%–69%) stenosis in recurrent ischemic events compared to medical therapy. (SOR **A**)

   a. Recommendation for prophylactic CEA in **asymptomatic** patients, based on the AHA guidelines for CEA, is related to surgical risk. The surgeon's specific morbidity and mortality statistics are a significant factor in estimating this risk. Patient selection and postoperative management of modifiable risk factors should be considered as well.

   b. For asymptomatic patients with a life expectancy of at least 5 years and a surgical risk ≤6%, ipsilateral CEA is considered a proven benefit when stenosis is greater than 59%, regardless of plaque characteristics (e.g., ulceration), contralateral carotid status, or antiplatelet therapy. (SOR **B**) Unilateral CEA is acceptable at the time of indicated coronary artery bypass grafting in asymptomatic patients whose ipsilateral carotid artery stenosis is ≥59%. Those whose surgical risk is ≤3% have no proven indication. (SOR **B**)

2. **Cerebral edema** is a leading cause of death in the first week of stroke. Treat or avoid conditions that tend to increase ICP: fever, pain, hypoxia, agitation, fluid overload, hypercarbia, and drugs that dilate intracranial vessels. Corticosteroids are ineffective in managing brain edema secondary to stroke. The two medical modalities used to treat cerebral edema are **osmotherapy** (e.g., mannitol and glycerol) and **hyperventilation therapy** in patients with markedly increased ICP. (SOR **C**) Surgical intervention (e.g., decompression hemicraniectomy) is sometimes necessary to control increasing ICP. (SOR **B**)

3. **Nimodipine** is a dihydropyridine calcium channel blocker that affects mainly the central nervous system vasculature. Approved for treating cerebral ischemia associated with subarachnoid hemorrhage, nimodipine is initiated within 96 hours of bleeding at a dosage of 60 mg orally every 4 hours for 21 days (the period of time during which neurologic deficit from vasospasm is most likely). (SOR **B**)

C. Prevention of stroke recurrence through secondary risk reduction is key to continued reduction of morbidity and mortality of stroke.

1. Nonmodifiable risk factors for stroke include age (risk doubles each decade beyond 55 years), family history, male gender, and ethnicity (African-American and Hispanic). The greatest risk factor, however, is previous stroke: Stroke begets stroke.

2. **Modifiable risk factors.** General lifestyle modification that should be encouraged includes healthy weight, smoking cessation, and moderate alcohol consumption. (SOR **C**) **Weight** goal is a body mass index between 18.5 and 24.9 kg/m². Moderate intensity **physical activity** of at least 30 minutes almost daily is desirable. **Tobacco** and street drug use is highly discouraged. Moderate alcohol consumption (≤2 drinks per day) is not associated with increased risk but binge drinking, particularly in young adults, has been associated with increased stroke risk. **Diabetes** control is glycohemoglobin ≤8% to reduce mortality risk, (SOR **B**) although the optimal glucose control following stroke is unknown.

3. **Antihypertensive treatment** is associated with a 30% to 40% stroke risk reduction. (SOR **A**) The benefit of treatment should be considered for all patients following TIA and the acute stroke period, both with or without a history of hypertension. (SOR **B**)

   a. **BP goal** should aim for below 130/80 mm Hg with at least an average reduction of 10/5 mm Hg. (SOR **B**) Lifestyle modification is always encouraged (see Chapter 77).

   b. The optimal **drug regimen** should be individualized to the patient, but can reasonably begin with a diuretic or diuretic/angiotensin-converting enzyme inhibitor (ACEI). (SOR **B**) A meta-analysis demonstrated significant reduction of recurrent stroke with the use of diuretics and diuretics combined with ACEIs. The same reduction was not seen using beta-blockers or ACEI alone, but this finding may have been related to the degree of BP reduction achieved. (SOR **B**)

    c. Angiotensin II blockade has been helpful for protecting against vascular occlusive disease. The Heart Outcomes Prevention Evaluation (HOPE) study demonstrated an absolute risk reduction for any stroke of 1.5% and death from any cause of 1.8% with the use of ramipril. (SOR **B**) The Perindopril Protection Against Recurrent Stroke Study (PROGRESS) used a flexible regimen of perindopril plus indapamide if necessary, versus placebo; active treatment reduced the absolute rates of ischemic stroke from 10% to 8%. (SOR **B**)

    d. The Losartan Intervention for endpoint Reduction in Hypertension (LIFE) study showed a favorable (25%) relative risk reduction for stroke compared to atenolol. (SOR **B**)

4. Cholesterol management should follow the 2013 American College of Cardiology/American Heart Association Guideline on the Treatment of Blood Cholesterol to Reduce Atherosclerotic Cardiovascular Risk in Adults. (see Chapter 76). Adults ≤75 years should be placed on high intensity statin therapy to lower low density cholesterol by approximately 50% or more. Moderate intensity statin therapy is recommended for those over age 75 or who are not a candidate for high intensity therapy. (SOR **B**) Even those with no preexisting indication for statins are reasonable candidates for treatment with statins to reduce the risk of vascular events. (SOR **B**)

5. The role of **CEA** has been discussed in Section III.B.1.

6. Anticoagulation therapy with warfarin may be indicated for ischemic strokes caused by cardiogenic emboli.

    a. For patients with persistent or paroxysmal **atrial fibrillation,** anticoagulation with warfarin, dabigatran (a direct thrombin inhibitor, FDA-approved in 2010), or rivaroxaban (a factor Xa inhibitor, FDA-approved in 2011) is recommended to prevent first or recurrent stroke. (SOR **A**) (see Chapter 48) There are no data showing that one is superior to the other as head-to-head trials are lacking. Drug selection, therefore, should be based on risk factors, cost, tolerability, patient preference, potential for drug interactions, and other clinical characteristics.

    b. Apixaban, another factor Xa inhibitor, received FDA approval in December 2012 and has been recommended by the American Heart Association/American Stroke Association Scientific Advisory on use of the new oral antithrombotic agents to prevent stroke in patients with nonvalvular atrial fibrillation (see Chapter 48).

    c. If unable to take oral anticoagulants, aspirin 325 mg per day is recommended. (SOR **A**)

    d. In the setting of **acute MI and left ventricular thrombus,** anticoagulation is used for at least 3 months and up to 12 months. (SOR **B**) Concomitant enteric coated aspirin for coronary artery disease should be used. (SOR **A**)

    e. Patients with **dilated cardiomyopathy** may be offered warfarin or antiplatelet therapy. (SOR **C**) For patients with **rheumatic mitral valve disease,** warfarin is reasonable. Routine addition of concomitant enteric coated aspirin is not recommended, but 81 mg per day may be added if there is recurrent embolism on warfarin. (SOR **C**)

    f. Likewise, for patients with **prosthetic heart valves** who have ischemic stroke on warfarin, aspirin 81 mg per day is reasonable. (SOR **B**)

7. Antiplatelet therapy. For patients with noncardioembolic ischemic stroke or TIA, antiplatelet agents rather than oral anticoagulation are recommended to reduce the risk of recurrent stroke and other cardiovascular events. (SOR **A**) In meta-analyses, a 28% relative odds reduction in nonfatal strokes and a 16% relative reduction in fatal strokes has been demonstrated.

    a. Aspirin 325 mg per day for secondary prevention following stroke can begin 24 to 48 hours after the acute event. (SOR **A**) While the acute initiation of aspirin or the glycoprotein IIb/IIIa inhibitors may be helpful in acute coronary syndromes, they are not recommended in the management of acute stroke outside of clinical trials. (SOR **B**)

    b. Clopidogrel (Plavix), 75 mg per day, is a potent, noncompetitive inhibitor of adenosine diphosphate-induced platelet aggregation. It can be used in patients allergic to aspirin. The Clopidogrel versus Aspirin in Patients at Risk of Ischemic Events (CAPRIE) trial included patients with stroke, MI, or peripheral vascular disease; clopidogrel was shown to be marginally better than aspirin for stroke risk reduction. (SOR **B**) It may have relatively more stroke risk benefit in those with diabetes and MI. The combination of aspirin plus clopidogrel offers no additional benefit and increases the risk of bleeding. (SOR **A**) Diarrhea and rash are common side effects, and while neutropenia is not a problem, thrombotic thrombocytopenic purpura has been reported.

c. **Extended-release dipyridamole/aspirin** (Aggrenox), 200 mg/25 mg twice daily, also inhibits platelet activation and aggregation. The combination has been shown to decrease the risk of stroke by 37% compared to aspirin (18%) or dipyridamole (18%) alone in the European Stroke Prevention Study (ESPS-2). (SOR **B**) Headache is the most common side effect; no additional bleeding risk compared to that by aspirin was noted.

IV. **Management Strategies.** Stroke indicates generalized vascular disease; it is one event in a prolonged and ongoing process. Management strategies center on prevention of further manifestations of the disease and maximization of poststroke function during the three stages of stroke.

A. **Stage I.** The **acute stage** of stroke spans the first week. Attention to evaluation, maintenance, and return of function includes passive range of motion of extremities, proper positioning, frequent turning, and maintenance of good hygiene. (SOR **C**) Evaluation of swallowing function should be done before starting eating and drinking. (SOR **B**)

B. **Stage II.** The **subacute stage** of stroke usually lasts 3 months. Return of neurologic function is greatest during this interval.

a. **Rehabilitation** involves interdisciplinary assessment and treatment by a team of nurses, physical therapists, occupational therapists, speech therapists, a dietitian, and the physician to maximize functional return and independence. Measurement tools like the Barthel Index (Table 88–5) or the Functional Independence Measure (http://www.dementia-assessment.com.au/symptoms/FIM_manual.pdf) are useful

TABLE 88–5. BARTHEL INDEX

A score above 60 usually means that ≤2 h of personal care assistance is required each day. A score of 60 or less indicates that 4 or more h of personal care assistance is needed daily. A score of 0 is given when a criterion cannot be met.

Functional activity

1. Feeding
  5—Dependent
  10—Independent
2. Transfer from bed to wheelchair, back to bed (includes sitting up in bed)
  5—Assisted out of bed only
  10—Needs some help/cueing
  15—Independent
3. Grooming (wash face; comb hair; shave, including preparing razor; clean teeth; and apply own make-up if worn)
  0—Dependent
  5—Independent
4. Toileting (transfer on/off toilet, handling clothing, wiping, and flushing)
  5—Dependent
  10—Independent
5. Bathing (tub, shower, or complete sponge bath)
  0—Dependent
  5—Independent
6. Ambulation, 50 yards, level surface
  0—Totally dependent
  5—Dependent on wheelchair but able to propel
  10—Able to walk with assistive device
  15—Able to walk without assistive device
7. Ascending/descending stairs (mechanical assistive devices allowed)
  5—Dependent
  10—Independent
8. Dressing (includes tying shoes and donning assistive devices; excludes nonprescribed girdles or bras)
  5—Dependent
  10—Independent
9. Bowel continence (suppository, enema allowed)
  5—Dependent
  10—Independent
10. Urinary continence
  5—Dependent
  10—Independent

Source: Modified with permission from Mahoney FI, Barthel DW. Functional evaluation: the Barthel index. *MD State Med J.* 1965;14:61.

for categorizing the degree of impairment and improvement and the need for additional services. Selection of the site of rehabilitation (e.g., a formal rehabilitation unit, a skilled nursing home, the patient's home with home health care agency coordination, or outpatient facilities) depends on the patient's medical condition, the family situation (supports and weaknesses), financial considerations, and available resources.

(1) To benefit from any kind of rehabilitation, the patient must be able to communicate (verbally or nonverbally), follow a two- to three-step command, and remember what is learned.

(2) Rehabilitation units require that a patient's cardiopulmonary endurance allows 2 to 3 hours of intense therapy daily. Patients with marked dementia, severe chronic obstructive pulmonary disease, marked limitation of cardiovascular reserve, or severely debilitating multiple joint disease are not likely to benefit from acute inpatient rehabilitation, although such patients may receive benefit from skilled or subacute care in the immediate posthospitalization period.

C. **Stage III.** The **chronic stage** of stroke recovery begins after 3 months. Neurologic return may continue for as long as 1 year after an event and functional recovery can occur for as long as 2 years afterwards. Maintenance of the functional gains achieved in the subacute stage is important.

1. **Involvement of the family or caregiver** in the acute and intermediate phases of stroke care enhances their knowledge and expectations regarding the patient's condition. Careful coordination of patient and family involvement, including discharge planning, and involving the family or caregiver in teaching sessions with the patient and with each of the patient's regular therapists and team nurse is helpful.

2. **Home health care agency involvement** allows for smooth transition and capable problem solving as the patient returns home.

3. **Monitoring of the patient by the physician** at regular intervals is important to assess and promote risk management strategies, identify and treat complicated illness (e.g., depression), evaluate recurrence of symptoms, assess functional status (e.g., Barthel index; Table 88–5), negotiate potential blocks to maintenance of function, and facilitate the patient's acceptance of disability.

V. **Prognosis.** Overall, the vast majority of initially alert patients survive the acute phase of stroke. Acute-phase deaths are generally due to cerebral causes related to irreversible failure of vital function of the brain stem. Pulmonary embolism and cardiac events contribute to early mortality in stroke patients. Systemic causes (e.g., pneumonia, pulmonary embolism, ischemic heart disease, or recurrent stroke) are the usual causes of death in the subacute and chronic phases. The risk of recurrence of stroke is substantial.

A. **The major complications** of stroke are aspiration, infection (e.g., urinary tract infection or pneumonia), pressure sores, corneal abrasion, and depression. Third-nerve palsy (signaling uncal herniation), increased age of the patient, and hemorrhagic events are associated with grave immediate prognoses.

B. **In hemorrhagic events,** the prognosis following total unilateral motor deficit and coma is poor. Brain stem infarctions such as pontine hemorrhages have an extremely poor prognosis. Lacunar infarctions involve subcortical small vessels and have the lowest mortality rate of all strokes.

SELECTED REFERENCES

Furie KL, Kasner SE, Adams RJ, et al. Guidelines for prevention of stroke in patients with ischemic stroke or transient ischemic attack. *Stroke.* 2011;42:227–276.

Furie KL, Goldstein LB, Albers GW, et al. Oral anti fibrillation: a science advisory for healthcare professionals from the American Heart Association/American Stroke Association. *Stroke.* 2012;43:3442–3453.

Jauch EC, Saver JL, Adams HP, et al. Guidelines for the early management of patients with acute ischemic stroke. *Stroke.* 2013;44:870–947.

Johnston SC, Rothwell PM, Huynh MN, et al. Validation and refinement of scores to predict very early stroke risk after transient ischemic attack. *Lancet.* 2007;369:283–292.

Latchaw RE, Alberts MJ, Lev MH, et al. Recommendations for imaging of acute stroke. *Stroke.* 2009;40:3646–3678.

Ooi tC, Daqi TF, Maltenfort M, et al. Tight glycemic control reduces infection and improves neurological outcome in critically ill neurosurgical patients. *Neurosurgery.* 2012;71(3):692–702.

Wardlaw JM, Murray V, Berge E, del Zoppo GJ. Thrombolysis for acute ischemic stroke. *Cochrane Database Syst Rev.* 2009;(4):CD000213.

ELECTRONIC RESOURCES

http://www.ninds.nih.gov/ is the Web site for the National Institute of Neurologic Disorders and Stroke with links to multiple organizations. Accessed September 11, 2013.

http://stroke.ahajournals.org/ is the Web site of the American Heart Association with links to consensus statements and journal articles. The parent site is www.strokeassociation.org. Accessed September 11, 2013.

http://www.stroke.org is the Web site of the National Stroke Association with excellent resources for patients, providers, and caregivers. Accessed September 11, 2013.

http://www.strokecenter.org is the clinical Web site of Washington University in St. Louis also with clinical updates and useful tools. Accessed August 15, 2008.

---

89   Thyroid Disease

Jeri R. Reid, MD, & Angela R. Wetherton, MD

KEY POINTS

- A sensitive thyroid-stimulating hormone assay is the best single screening test for both hypothyroidism and hyperthyroidism. (SOR **C**)
- Levothyroxine is usually begun at full estimated replacement dose (1.6 μg/kg) in patients younger than 65 years without cardiac disease and is the treatment of choice for hypothyroidism. (SOR **B**)
- Radioactive iodine (^{123}I) uptake (RAIU) scanning can help clarify hyperthyroidism of uncertain etiology. (SOR **C**)
- Oral radioactive iodine (RAI) is the treatment of choice for most patients with hyperthyroidism in the United States, but antithyroid drugs and surgery are appropriate in selected patients. (SOR **C**)
- The evaluation of a thyroid nodule usually begins with TSH, ultrasound and a fine-needle aspiration biopsy. (SOR **C**)

I. Introduction

   A. Physiology. Thyrotropin-releasing hormone, secreted by the hypothalamus, stimulates the anterior pituitary to produce thyroid-stimulating hormone (TSH). The major hormone released by the thyroid gland in response to TSH is thyroxine (T_4), which is converted peripherally to triiodothyronine (T_3), a more potent hormone. T_4 and T_3 are both highly but reversibly bound to plasma thyroid-binding globulin and, to a lesser extent, to albumin and prealbumin. Only the minute unbound (free) fractions are metabolically active. The most sensitive indicator of thyroid status is the level of TSH, which is controlled in classic negative-feedback fashion by the concentration of unbound thyroid hormones.

   B. Screening for thyroid disease in the asymptomatic general population, except newborns, is controversial. The American Thyroid Association recommends that women and men >35 years of age should be screened every 5 years. The American Association of Clinical Endocrinologists states that older patients (age not specified), especially women, should be screened. The American Academy of Family Physicians recommends that patients ≥60 years of age should be screened. However, the United States Preventive Services Task Force and Royal College of Physicians of London found insufficient evidence for or against screening. (SOR **C**)

   C. Diagnostic evaluation. Tables 89–1 and 89–2 list the most common symptoms and signs of hypothyroidism and hyperthyroidism, respectively.

   1. The single **most important diagnostic test** for the evaluation of thyroid disease is the highly sensitive serum **TSH**. The accepted range of normal TSH is between 0.45 and 4.5 mIU/L.

TABLE 89-1. COMMON SIGNS AND SYMPTOMS OF HYPOTHYROIDISM[a]

Signs or Symptoms	Affected Patients (%)
Weakness	99
Skin changes (dry or coarse skin)	97
Lethargy	91
Slow speech	91
Eyelid edema	90
Cold sensation	89
Decreased sweating	89
Cold skin	83
Thick tongue	82
Facial edema	79
Coarse hair	76
Skin pallor	67
Forgetfulness	66
Constipation	61

[a]Only signs and symptoms that occur in 60% or more of patients with hypothyroidism are listed in this table.
Source: Adapted with permission from Larsen PR, Davies TF, Hay ID. The thyroid gland. In: Wilson JD, Foster DW, Kronenberg HM, Larsen PR, eds. *Williams Textbook of Endocrinology.* 9th ed. Philadelphia, PA: Saunders; 1998:461. Copyright © Elsevier.

2. **Free thyroxine (FT₄)** is commonly used for the diagnostic evaluation of thyroid disease including hypothyroidism, subclinical hypothyroidism, hyperthyroidism, and subclinical hyperthyroidism.
3. **Total triiodothyronine (TT₃),** measured directly, is also available and used for the evaluation of hyperthyroidism and subclinical hyperthyroidism.
4. **Antithyroid peroxidase antibody (anti-TPOAb)** measurements may be useful when evaluating subclinical hypothyroidism. The presence of positive TPOAb predicts an increased risk of developing overt hypothyroidism.
5. **Radioactive iodine uptake (RAIU)** is performed when the etiology of hyperthyroidism is unclear.

TABLE 89-2. COMMON SIGNS AND SYMPTOMS OF HYPERTHYROIDISM

Signs and Clinical Symptoms	Patients Older Than 70 yr (%)	Patients Younger Than 50 yr (%)	P Value
Tachycardia	71	96	.01
Fatigue	56	84	.01
Weight loss	50	51	.87
Tremor	44	84	<.001
Dyspnea	41	56	.20
Apathy	41	25	.20
Anorexia	32	4	<.001
Nervousness	31	84	<.001
Hyperactive reflexes	28	96	<.001
Weakness	27	61	.01
Depression	24	22	87
Increased sweating	24	95	<.001
Polydipsia	21	67	<.001
Diarrhea	18	43	.02
Confusion	16	0	.01
Muscular atrophy	16	10	.52
Heat intolerance	15	92	<.001
Constipation	15	0	.01
Increased appetite	0	57	<.001

Source: Trivalle C, Doucet J, Chassagne P, et al. Differences in signs and symptoms of hyperthyroidism in older and younger patients. *J Amer Geriatr Soc.* 1996;44(1):50–53. With permission from Wiley-Blackwell Publishing, Ltd.

6. **Thyroid ultrasound** is useful for evaluating palpable thyroid nodules or multinodular goiters.

7. **Fine-needle aspiration (FNA)** biopsy plays an integral role in the evaluation of thyroid nodules.

II. **Hypothyroidism**

A. **Types of hypothyroidism**

1. **Primary hypothyroidism,** most commonly from chronic autoimmune (Hashimoto thyroiditis), radioactive iodine therapy, or surgery, accounts for the overwhelming majority of cases in the United States. It results from insufficient production of thyroid hormones. Overt hypothyroidism is found in 0.3% to 0.4% of the general population. It is more common in women and increases progressively with age.

2. **Secondary hypothyroidism** results from decreased pituitary secretion of TSH. This condition is usually accompanied by other manifestations of pituitary hyposecretion. Causes include postpartum pituitary necrosis (Sheehan syndrome) and pituitary tumors.

3. **Subclinical hypothyroidism** is an early stage of thyroid dysfunction. It is found in 4.3% to 8.5% of the general population. The risk of developing subclinical hypothyroidism increases with age. Subclinical hypothyroidism has been linked to adverse cardiac events, elevations in total and low-density lipoprotein cholesterol, and the development of systemic and neuropsychiatric symptoms.

B. **Diagnosis** (Figure 89–1)

1. **Primary hypothyroidism.** In a patient with suggestive signs and symptoms, a high TSH (>4.5 mIU/mL) and a low FT_4 are diagnostic of primary hypothyroidism.

2. **Secondary hypothyroidism.** In the setting of signs and symptoms of hypothyroidism, a TSH that is normal or only mildly elevated suggests secondary hypothyroidism. Concurrent amenorrhea, galactorrhea, postural hypotension, loss of axillary and pubic hair, and visual field deficits may be present to suggest a central cause. If secondary hypothyroidism is suspected, assessment of other pituitary hormones as well as neuroimaging should be performed.

3. **Subclinical hypothyroidism** is distinguished by an elevated TSH, a normal FT_4, and a few, if any, symptoms of hypothyroidism. TPOAb measurements should be considered when evaluating these patients because if positive, overt hypothyroidism occurs at a rate of 4.3% per year versus 2.6% per year when antithyroid antibodies are negative. Transient forms of hypothyroidism should be excluded by repeating a TSH and FT_4 within 2 to 12 weeks.

C. **Treatment**

1. **Primary hypothyroidism**

a. **Levothyroxine** is preferred for routine replacement therapy. Interchangeability studies of levothyroxine products have not shown significant fluctuations in hormone levels when switching among name-brand or generic preparations. (SOR **B**) Current evidence does not support the use of combinations of levothyroxine and T_3 for replacement therapy. (SOR **C**)

(1) Adults require approximately **1.6 µg/kg/day for full replacement.** Therapy is usually initiated with the full replacement dose in young healthy adults. (SOR **B**) Patients older than 50 to 60 years without coronary heart disease can be started on 50 µg per day. The usual starting dose for patients with known coronary heart disease is 12.5 to 25 µg per day. The dose is then gradually titrated as indicated. (SOR **C**)

(2) Pregnant women with hypothyroidism often require increased thyroid hormone replacement so it is important to measure a TSH as soon as possible and monitor throughout pregnancy to avoid adverse outcomes affecting the fetus and the mother.

(3) Levothyroxine should be taken with water 30 to 60 minutes before eating or at bedtime 4 hours after the last meal. It is important to note that multiple medications including proton pump inhibitors, bisphosphonates, calcium salts, cholestyramine, ferrous sulfate, and H_2 receptor antagonists can interfere with levothyroxine absorption. Other drugs such as carbamazepine, rifampin, and phenytoin can accelerate levothyroxine metabolism, necessitating higher replacement doses.

2. **Secondary hypothyroidism.** The American Association of Endocrinologists and the American Thyroid Association recommend consultation with an endocrinologist for patients with pituitary disorders.

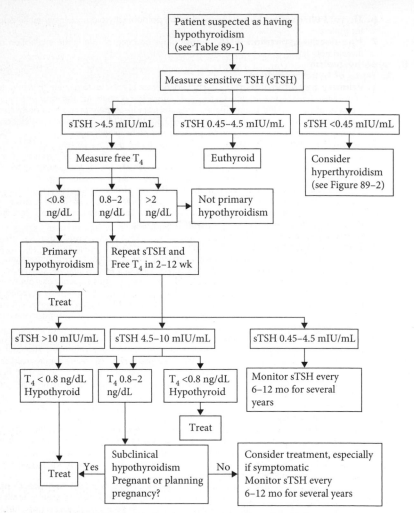

FIGURE 89-1. Approach to the patient with hypothyroidism. T_4, thyroxine.

3. Subclinical hypothyroidism
   a. Levothyroxine is recommended for patients with **TSH levels above 10 mIU/L** because these patients are at an increased risk for heart failure and cardiovascular mortality. A trial of levothyroxine for symptomatic patients with TSH between 4.5 and 10 mIU/L can be considered, but medication should be discontinued if symptoms do not improve. Patients usually do not require the full replacement dose.
   b. Treatment with levothyroxine should be **considered in women who are pregnant** or contemplating pregnancy.
D. Management strategies
   1. Primary hypothyroidism. Patients should have TSH assessed at 4- to 8-week intervals until the levothyroxine dose has been titrated to produce a normalized TSH. Once the appropriate dose has been determined, TSH should be measured after 6 months and then at least annually or as clinically indicated.

2. **Secondary hypothyroidism.** Consultation with an endocrinologist is recommended.
3. **Subclinical hypothyroidism**
   a. If a decision is made to treat, the management is similar to primary hypothyroidism. Care should be taken to avoid overtreatment which is a risk factor for the development of atrial fibrillation and osteoporosis when TSH is below 0.1 mIU/L.
   b. If a decision is made not to treat, the patient should be monitored clinically and biochemically every 6 to 12 months for evidence of progressive thyroid dysfunction. (SOR **Ⓒ**)

III. Hyperthyroidism
A. **Introduction.** Hyperthyroidism results from elevated levels of thyroid hormones and is less common than hypothyroidism in the general population. In the United States, the prevalence of hyperthyroidism is 1.2% with 0.5% overt disease and 0.7 % with subclinical disease. Graves disease (GD) accounts for approximately 50% to 80% of hyperthyroidism.
B. **Types of hyperthyroidism.** Hyperthyroidism encompasses a heterogeneous group of disorders.
   1. **GD** is an autoimmune disease that results from the action of thyrotropin receptor antibodies (TRAbs) on thyroid gland TSH receptors causing increased thyroid hormone production. It demonstrates a familial predisposition. **Graves ophthalmopathy** develops in up to 50% of patients and its course is independent of the thyroid disease.
   2. **Toxic multinodular goiter (TMNG; Plummer disease),** the most common cause of hyperthyroidism in those older than 40 years, occurs when a patient with nontoxic multinodular goiter develops one or more autonomous hyperfunctioning nodules.
   3. **Toxic adenoma (TA),** the least common cause of hyperthyroidism, is produced by one or more hyperfunctioning thyroid adenomas capable of functioning independently of TSH or other thyroid stimulators.
   4. **Thyroiditis** may produce transient hyperthyroidism as hormone leaks from an inflamed gland. Transient hypothyroidism often follows as the intrathyroidal stores of hormone are depleted.
   5. **Subclinical hyperthyroidism** is much less common than subclinical hypothyroidism and is more common in women, in the elderly, and in patients with low-iodine intake.
      a. Excessive thyroid hormone replacement is the most common cause (14%–21%). Other important causes include nodular thyroid disease, subclinical GD, thyroiditis, and ingestion of iodine-containing drugs such as amiodarone.
C. **Diagnosis.** The history and the physical examination are critical to distinguish among the causes of hyperthyroidism (Table 89–3).
   1. A diagnostic approach to patients who present with signs and symptoms of hyperthyroidism is summarized in Figure 89–2. A **suppressed TSH and elevated FT₄ level** are diagnostic of hyperthyroidism. In a clinically hyperthyroid patient with a suppressed TSH and a normal free T_4 level, TT_3 should be measured to evaluate for possible T_3 thyrotoxicosis.
   2. **Subclinical hyperthyroidism** is distinguished by a **low or undetectable TSH (<0.45 mIU/L) and normal FT₄ and TT₃**. The patient may be asymptomatic or display signs and symptoms of hyperthyroidism. Factors that can suppress TSH levels, such as severe illness, high-dose glucocorticoids, dopamine, and pituitary dysfunction should be excluded. Laboratory findings consistent with subclinical hyperthyroidism can be a normal variant in the elderly.
   3. **Radioactive iodine (^{123}I) uptake (RAIU)** can help clarify hyperthyroidism of uncertain origin. Diffuse increase in RAIU is consistent with GD, whereas nodular concentration indicates TA or multinodular goiter. (SOR **Ⓒ**) If RAIU is decreased, a serum thyroglobulin measurement can distinguish between exogenous (factitious) hyperthyroxinemia (thyroglobulin decreased) and thyroiditis (thyroglobulin increased).
      When RAIU is unavailable or contraindicated, or when the diagnosis of GD is clinically apparent (symmetrically enlarged thyroid gland, recent onset of ophthalmopathy, and moderate-to-severe hyperthyroidism), the diagnosis can be confirmed by an elevated TRAb and/ or a TT_3 to total T_4 ratio of >20. (SOR **Ⓒ**)
D. **Treatment**
   1. **Antithyroid drugs (ATDs)** are the preferred first-line treatment for GD in Europe, Japan, and Australia. They are not recommended for the treatment of TMNG or TA.

TABLE 89–3. COMMON ETIOLOGY AND CLINICAL DIAGNOSIS OF HYPERTHYROIDISM

Cause	Pathophysiology	Gland Size[a]	Nodularity	Tenderness
Toxic adenoma	Autonomous hormone production	Decreased	Single nodule	Nontender
Toxic multinodular goiter	Autonomous hormone production	Increased	Multiple nodules	Tender
Subacute thyroiditis	Leakage of hormone from gland	Increased	None	Tender
Lymphocytic thyroiditis, postpartum thyroiditis, medication-induced thyroiditis	Leakage of hormone from gland	Moderately increased	None	Nontender
Graves disease (thyroid-stimulating antibody)	Increased glandular stimulation (substance causing stimulation)	Increased	None	Nontender
Iodine-induced hyperfunctioning of thyroid gland (iodide ingestion, radiographic contrast, amiodarone [Cordarone])	Increased glandular stimulation (substance causing stimulation)	Increased	Multiple nodules or no nodules	Nontender
Functioning pituitary adenoma (TSH); trophoplastic tumors (human chorionic gonadotropin)	Increased glandular stimulation (substance causing stimulation)	Increased	None	Nontender
Factitial hyperthyroidism	Exogenous hormone intake	Decreased	None	Nontender
Struma ovarii; metastatic thyroid cancer	Extraglandular production	Decreased	None	Nontender

[a]In most cases.
Source: Reproduced with permission from Reid JR, Wheeler SF. Hyperthyroidism: diagnosis and treatment. Am Fam Physician. 2005;72:623–630.

a. **Methimazole (MMI) and propylthiouracil (PTU),** the two agents available in the United States, work by inhibiting thyroid hormone synthesis. PTU also inhibits peripheral conversion of T_4 to T_3. ATDs lead to remission in up to 30% of patients in the United States with GD treated for 12 to 18 months. Remission rates are higher (over 50%) in patients with **mild disease, small goiters, and negative TRAb**. Therapy past 18 months has not been shown to improve remission rates. (SOR **A**)

   (1) **MMI** is the drug of choice in nonpregnant patients because of its lower cost, longer half-life, and lower incidence of hematologic side effects. (SOR **B**) The starting dose is 15 mg (mild) or 30 to 40 mg (moderately severe) or 60 mg (severe) orally daily in three divided doses 8 hours apart. **PTU is the preferred treatment for pregnant women** because MMI has been associated with a rare congenital anomaly. The starting dose is 300 to 400 mg per day orally in divided doses every 8 hours. (SOR **C**)

   (2) Once euthyroidism is achieved, as measured by normalized FT_4 and/or TT_3 (usually within 6–8 weeks), the dose can be titrated down to maintain euthyroidism. TSH will remain suppressed for several months so it cannot be used to monitor for initial euthyroidism. Typical maintenance doses are 5 to 15 mg daily for MMI and 100 to 150 mg orally in two to three divided doses for PTU. (SOR **C**)

   (3) Most clinicians treat patients for 18 to 24 months before attempting to withdraw antithyroid therapy. Before discontinuing therapy, the patient should be clinically and biochemically euthyroid. **Relapse is more likely to occur in smokers, patients with large goiters, and patients with persistently elevated TRAb levels.** Relapse is more likely in the first 3 to 6 months after ATD discontinuation; it is recommended that the patient should be monitored every 1 to 3 months for 6 to 12 months. (SOR **A**)

   (4) **Major side effects of ATDs** include polyarthritis (1%–2%) and agranulocytosis (0.1%–0.5%). Agranulocytosis usually occurs within 3 months of starting therapy. PTU has a higher dose-related risk of this reaction, and it is very rare with MMI doses less than 30 mg daily. **Baseline complete blood counts**

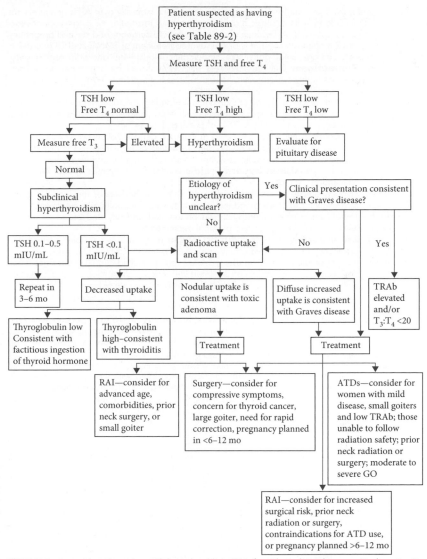

FIGURE 89-2. Approach to the patient with hyperthyroidism. TSH, thyroid-stimulating hormone; T_4, thyroxine; T_3, triiodothyronine; TRAB, thyroid receptor antibody; ATD, antithyroid drug; RAI, radioactive iodine; GO, Graves ophthalmopathy.

and liver profiles are recommended. Patients should be warned to discontinue the drug and come in for a complete blood count if they experience a sudden fever or sore throat. Patients taking PTU should have liver function testing if they experience a pruritic rash, jaundice, light-colored stools, dark urine, abdominal pain anorexia, nausea, or fatigue. (SOR Ⓖ)
  2. **Radioactive iodine (RAI, ¹³¹I),** usually administered orally, concentrates in the thyroid gland, where it destroys follicular cells. Most physicians in the United States

prefer this treatment for GD. Factors that favor this modality over ATDs or surgery for GD include increased surgical risk, previous neck irradiation or surgery, prior reaction or relapse with ATDs, lack of access to thyroid surgeon, and desired pregnancy >6 to 12 months after RAI. It is also a favored treatment of TMNG and TA in patients of advanced age, small goiter size, significant comorbidities, and prior neck surgery.

    a. Pretreatment with beta-blockers and MMI should be considered in patients who are highly symptomatic, have a FT_4 two to three times normal, are elderly, or have significant comorbidities. (SOR **C**)

    b. An ablative RAI dose, rather than a lower gland-specific dosage, is recommended, especially in the elderly or in patients with heart disease, and results in permanent remission in approximately 75% of patients. (SOR **C**)

    c. RAI exerts its full effect over a 2- to 6-month period. Follow-up at 4- to 6-week intervals to measure FT_4 and TT_3 and to assess clinical response is appropriate until thyroid function stabilizes within the normal range or hypothyroidism ensues.

    d. If there is **persistent hyperthyroidism** after 3 to 6 months, repeat RAI is recommended. (SOR **C**)

    e. Hypothyroidism is less likely in patients with toxic nodules or multinodular goiter because the rest of the gland may start to function normally after treatment.

    f. Thyroid replacement therapy should be initiated and adjusted based on the FT_4 level, clinical symptoms, and physical examination.

    g. RAI is contraindicated during pregnancy and it is usually advised that pregnancy be postponed 6 to 12 months following therapy. Otherwise, there are no contraindications to the use of RAI in women of child-bearing age, since it has not been shown to cause cancer, infertility, or to produce ill effects in subsequent children of those so treated. **Breastfeeding** women should avoid RAI because it appears in breast milk. The use of RAI in **children** is controversial, but is becoming more accepted as data emerge about its long-term safety.

    h. RAI therapy can exacerbate **ophthalmopathy** in 15% of patients with GD, especially smokers. This exacerbation can be prevented or improved in two-thirds of patients by administration of prednisone (40–80 mg per day, with the dose tapered over a period of 3 months). Although it is controversial, some physicians substitute ATDs or lower-dose RAI to treat patients with active eye disease, since post-treatment hypothyroidism has been associated with worsening Graves ophthalmopathy. Aggressive treatment with **high-dose glucocorticoids, in consultation with an ophthalmologist** experienced in the treatment of orbital disease, can also be considered for progressive and severe ophthalmopathy.

3. Surgery for hyperthyroidism has declined in popularity because of the effectiveness of ATDs and RAI. Near-total or total thyroidectomy should be performed for GD and TMNG. Thyroid lobectomy or isthmusectomy is appropriate for TA.

    a. Factors that favor surgical treatment include compressive symptoms, large goiters, suspected malignancy, moderate-to-severe Graves ophthalmopathy, and pregnancy planned in <4 to 6 months.

    b. Patients should be rendered euthyroid with ATDs and/or iodides preoperatively to avoid thyrotoxic crisis.

    c. Complications include hypocalcemia due to temporary or permanent hypoparathyroidism. Prophylactic calcium supplementation should be given and adjusted based on postoperative parathyroid hormone (PTH) and serum calcium levels. Permanent hypoparathyroidism occurs in <2% of patients undergoing thyroidectomy by a high volume surgeon. Recurrent laryngeal nerve injury occurs in <1% and mortality is between 1 in 10,000 and 5 in 1,000,000.

    d. Recurrent hyperthyroidism occurs in 8% of patients who are treated with subtotal thyroidectomy. Permanent hypothyroidism occurs in 25% of patients undergoing subtotal thyroidectomy. Total thyroidectomy is 100% effective, but carries a 100% risk of permanent hypothyroidism. (SOR **A**)

4. Adjunctive medical therapies are useful for relieving symptoms in patients undergoing definitive therapy with other agents or in those with transient forms of hyperthyroidism.

    a. β-Adrenergic antagonists provide prompt symptomatic relief of the hyperadrenergic manifestations of hyperthyroidism and should be considered in all patients with symptoms of hyperthyroidism. They should also be considered in the elderly with resting heart rates above 90 bpm. (SOR **A**) Propranolol is the most widely used beta-blocker for this purpose. Initial doses of 10 to 30 mg four times daily are adjusted to control tachycardia and symptoms. In most cases, a dose of 80 to 120 mg per day is sufficient.

  b. Calcium channel blockers such as diltiazem or verapamil may be used in patients who cannot tolerate, or have contraindications to, beta-blockers.

  c. Thyroiditis (subacute, lymphocytic, and postpartum) can produce a transient hyperthyroidism that usually resolves within 8 months. Treatment focuses on symptom control with beta-blockers and other adjunctive medical therapies such as nonsteroidal anti-inflammatory drugs. Severe symptoms respond to prednisone, 20 to 40 mg per day. Transient hypothyroidism may follow the initial hyperthyroid phase and can be symptomatic enough to warrant levothyroxine therapy.

E. Management strategies. The successful treatment of hyperthyroidism requires an accurate diagnosis followed by appropriate therapy after a detailed discussion with the patient about the risks and benefits of each modality. The physician needs to give careful consideration not only to the patient's comorbidities but also to their preferences.

  1. ATDs, RAI, and surgery have been shown to be equally effective as initial treatment of GD and result in similar long-term quality of life. (SOR **Ⓐ**)

  2. RAI and surgery are effective and relatively safe treatments for TMNG and TA. (SOR **Ⓑ**)

  3. ATDs may be preferred by patients with GD who do not want the exposure to RAI or the risk of surgery and do not mind long-term monitoring for relapse (or remission).

  4. RAI may be chosen by patients with GD, TMNG, or TA seeking definitive control of hyperthyroidism and/or more rapid resolution of symptoms. Patients with TMNG may choose this option since there would be a possibility of becoming euthyroid without thyroid hormone replacement.

  5. A patient might prefer surgery for GD, TMNG, or TA if they desire definitive control but want to avoid radiation exposure (and/or side effects of ATDs in GD). Patients with TA may consider this option due to the possibility of becoming euthyroid after surgery.

  6. Subclinical hyperthyroidism often disappears, and progression to overt hyperthyroidism is uncommon in patients with a sensitive TSH between 0.1 and 0.45 mIU/L. However, in patients with a TSH lower than 0.1 mIU/L, the risk of developing overt hyperthyroidism is 1% to 2% per year. The condition has been associated with atrial fibrillation and other cardiac abnormalities and with increased cardiac mortality in patients older than 60 years. The incidence of atrial fibrillation is increased by threefold in patients with TSH <0.1 mIU/L. Bone density is also decreased with prolonged subclinical hyperthyroidism but no link to increased fractures has been demonstrated.

    a. If excessive hormone replacement is the cause, the dose should be reduced.

    b. If subclinical hyperthyroidism is associated with nodular thyroid disease, subclinical GD, heart disease, and osteoporosis or is found in patients older than 60 years, antithyroid treatment should be seriously considered. (SOR **Ⓒ**)

    c. In patients not meeting the above criteria, careful follow-up is acceptable.

  7. Once euthyroidism is achieved, life-long annual follow-up is recommended to detect remission in those treated with RAI, ATDs or subtotal thyroidectomy and to manage hypothyroidism in those treated with RAI and total thyroidectomy. (SOR **Ⓒ**)

IV. Thyroid Nodules

  A. Introduction. Palpable nodules are present in 3% to 7% of adults in North America. However, physical examination is relatively insensitive, and, with the increase in the use of ultrasonography over the past 20 years, thyroid nodules are now estimated to occur in 20% to 76% of the general population. In addition, many patients with solitary nodules on examination are found to have multiple nodules on ultrasound. Approximately 5% of all thyroid nodules are carcinomas.

  1. Thyroid nodules are found more commonly in the elderly, in women, and in patients with iodine deficiency or exposure to radiation. Prior radiation exposure increases the rate of development of both benign and malignant new nodules to approximately 2% per year. Peak incidence is 15 to 25 years after exposure.

  2. Since similar frequencies of cancer have been found in patients who have solitary or multiple nodules on palpation, dominant nodules in multinodular glands should also be considered for diagnostic evaluation.

B. Diagnosis
   1. A thorough **history** and **physical examination** should focus on the following thyroid cancer risk factors:
      a. A family history of benign or malignant thyroid disease, especially medullary thyroid carcinoma, multiple endocrine neoplasia 2, or papillary thyroid carcinoma.
      b. A personal history of prior head and neck radiation exposure. Childhood exposures increase thyroid cancer risk 10-fold.
      c. Physical findings suggestive of cancer are progressive or rapid growth, firmness, fixation to surrounding structures, local lymphadenopathy, and persistent hoarseness, dysphonia, dysphagia, or dyspnea.
      d. Other risk factors include age younger than 14 years or older than 70 years and male gender.
   2. High-resolution ultrasound with **Doppler capability** should be performed in all patients with thyroid cancer risk factors, regardless of physical examination findings. Ultrasound should also be part of the workup of all palpable thyroid nodules or multinodular goiter. Ultrasound and color-flow Doppler criteria such as margins, shape, vascularity, content, and echogenicity are used to stratify the malignant potential of a nodule. (SOR **C**)
   3. Serum **TSH** identifies patients with unsuspected thyroid dysfunction. If the TSH is normal, no further laboratory testing is warranted. An elevated TSH should prompt testing of FT_4 levels and TPOAb to rule out hypothyroidism. Decreased TSH levels should be followed by testing of FT_4 and TT levels to rule out hyperthyroidism. Basal serum calcitonin is indicated only if there is a family history of medullary thyroid cancer or multiple endocrine neoplasia 2.
   4. FNA biopsy plays an integral role in the evaluation of thyroid nodules. Ultrasound-guided FNA (UGFNA) is more accurate than direct FNA and is recommended in the following situations (SOR **B**):
      a. A nodule >1 cm diameter and hypoechoic on ultrasound (US).
      b. A nodule of any size in a patient with risk factors of prior radiation exposure, family or personal history of thyroid malignancy, or increased calcitonin levels.
      c. A nodule <1 cm that has two or more suspicious US features.
      d. Toxic nodules (those that show increased uptake on RAIU) should not be biopsied.
   5. Biopsy specimens should be interpreted by an experienced cytopathologist. **Cytologic diagnosis** is broken down into five categories:
      a. Class 1 is a **nondiagnostic** specimen with insufficient cells, or inadequate preparation.
      b. Class 2 is a **benign** lesion consistent with a colloid nodule, a hyperplastic nodule, thyroiditis, or a cyst.
      c. Class 3 are **follicular lesions** that include follicular neoplasm, Hürthle cell lesions and the follicular variant of papillary thyroid carcinoma.
      d. Class 4 are **suspicious lesions** that do not meet all of the malignancy criteria.
      e. Class 5 are **malignant lesions**.
C. Treatment
   1. Class 1. UGFNA should be repeated after a nondiagnostic sample is obtained. Suspicious, malignant, or repeatedly nondiagnostic specimens are an indication for surgery. If ultrasound characteristics are favorable, the nodule could be followed closely.
   2. Class 2. Cytologically benign nodules should be followed clinically and with US in 6 to 18 months. Repeat USFNA should be performed if there is an >50% increase in nodule size or a 20% increase in at least two dimensions of a solid nodule. (SOR **C**) **Thyroid hormone suppression** is not recommended in most cases of nodular thyroid disease. It may be considered in iodine-deficient patients, young patients with small nodules, or those with nodular goiters with no evidence of functional autonomy. However, clinically significant reduction in nodule volume with suppressive therapy is rare and the risks of prolonged subclinical hyperthyroidism must be included in the risk–benefit analysis. (SOR **B**) Surgery, embolectomy, or thermal ablation may be considered for nodules causing pressure symptoms or cosmetic issues.
   3. Classes 3, 4, 5. Surgical treatment is recommended.
D. Management strategies
   1. A patient with a benign (Class 2) lesion, and no growth on repeat US done 6 to 18 months after USFNA, can have repeat US follow-up in 3 to 5 years. (SOR **C**)

2. The use of genetic marker testing and PET scanning has shown promise in stratifying Class 2 and 3 lesions and avoiding unnecessary surgery.

SELECTED REFERENCES

Bahn RS, Burch HB, Cooper DS, et al. Hyperthyroidism and other causes of thyrotoxicosis: management guidelines of the American Thyroid Association and American Association of Clinical Endocrinologists. *Thyroid.* 2011;21(2):593–646.

Col NF, Surks MI, Daniels GH. Subclinical thyroid disease: clinical applications. *JAMA.* 2004; 291(2):239–243.

Garber JR, Cobin RH, Gharib H, et al. Clinical practice guidelines for hypothyroidism in adults. The American Association of Clinical Endocrinologists and the American Thyroid Association. *Thyroid.* 2012;22(12):1200–1235.

Gharib H, Papini E, Pascke R, et al. American Association of Clinical Endocrinologists, Associazione Medici Endocriologi, and European Thyroid Association medical guidelines for clinical practice for the diagnosis and management of thyroid nodules. *Endocrine Pract.* 2010;16(Suppl 1):1–43.

Popoveniuc G, Jonklaas J. Thyroid nodules. *Med Clin N Am.* 2012;96:329–349.

90   Alcohol and Drug Abuse

Robert Mallin, MD, & Kristen Hood Watson, MD

KEY POINTS

- The diagnosis of substance use disorders most typically begins with a screening test that identifies a user at risk. Screening adults in primary care settings, including pregnant women, is recommended. (SOR **B**)
- Substance abuse is a pattern of misuse during which the patient maintains control, whereas in substance dependence, control over use is lost. Physiologic dependence, evidenced by a withdrawal syndrome, may exist in either state. (SOR **C**)
- The primary means by which the diagnosis of substance abuse or dependence is made is by careful history. Although substance-disordered patients may be consciously less truthful in their history, more often the defense mechanism of denial is what prevents the patient from seeing the connection between substance use and consequences. (SOR **C**)
- Biochemical markers can support the diagnostic criteria gathered in the history or can be used as a screening mechanism to consider patients for further evaluation. (SOR **C**)
- There is a strong relationship between the time and intensity spent in alcohol and drug treatment and success at remaining abstinent. (SOR **B**)

I. Introduction

A. The prevalence of alcohol and drug disorders in primary care outpatients is between 23% and 37%. The high prevalence of these disorders suggests that family physicians are confronted with these problems daily. These disorders rarely present overtly, however. Patients often deny the connection between their substance use and its consequences, frequently minimize the amount of use, and often do not seek assistance for their substance abuse problem. Excessive alcohol use is the third leading cause of lifestyle-related mortalities in the United States.

B. The epidemiology of alcohol and drug disorders has been well studied. Lifetime prevalence rates for **alcohol disorders** from the Epidemiologic Catchment Area (ECA) Program survey data of the National Institute of Mental Health were 13.5%; 23.8% for men and 4.7% for women. The National Comorbidity Survey revealed lifetime prevalence of alcohol abuse without dependence to be 12.5% for men and 6.4% for women. Lifetime prevalence of alcohol dependence was higher, at 20.1% in men and 8.2% in women. The ECA data yield an overall prevalence of **drug-use disorders** of 6.2%. As with alcohol use disorders, drug use disorders occur more frequently in men (lifetime prevalence 7.7%) than in women (4.8%).

Characteristics known to influence the epidemiology of substance use disorders include gender (men have higher risk), age (less frequent with increasing age), family history (alcoholism risk for the child of an alcoholic is approximately 50%), marital status (single persons at higher risk vs. married), employment status (unemployed at higher risk), and occupation/educational status (less educated at higher risk).

C. The Diagnostic and Statistical Manual of Mental Disorders (DSM) V defines **substance abuse and dependence** as a maladaptive pattern of substance use, leading to clinically significant impairment or distress, as manifested by two (or more) of the following occurring at any time within a 12-month period: (1) Recurrent substance use resulting in failure to fulfill major role obligations at work, school, or home (e.g., repeated absences or poor work performance related to substance use; neglect of children or household); (2) recurrent substance use in situations in which it is physically hazardous (e.g., driving an automobile or operating a machine); (3) a craving or a strong desire or urge to use the substance, (4) continued substance use despite having persistent social or interpersonal problems caused or exacerbated by the effects of the substance (e.g., arguments with spouse about consequences of intoxication, physical fights); 5) tolerance defined by

TABLE 90–1. CAGE QUESTIONS ADAPTED TO INCLUDE DRUGS

1. Have you felt you ought to **C**ut down on your drinking or drug use?
2. Have people **A**nnoyed you by criticizing your drinking or drug use?
3. Have you felt **G**uilty about your drinking or drug use?
4. Have you ever had a drink, or used drugs first thing in the morning to steady your nerves or to get rid of a hangover or to get the day started? (**E**ye-opener)

Two or more yes answers indicate a need for a more in-depth assessment. Even one positive response should raise a red flag about problem drinking or drug use.
Source: Data from Schulz JE, Parran T, Jr. Principles of identification and intervention. In: Graham AW, Shultz TK, eds. *Principles of Addiction Medicine.* 2nd ed. Chery Chase, MD: American Society of Addiction Medicine; 1998:249.

either a need for markedly increased amounts of the substance to achieve intoxication or the desired effect or markedly diminished effect with continued use of the same amount of the substance; (6) withdrawal, as manifested by either a characteristic withdrawal syndrome for the substance or the same (or closely related) substance is taken to relieve or avoid withdrawal symptoms; (7) the substance is often taken in larger amounts or over a longer period than was intended; (8) there is a persistent desire or unsuccessful efforts to cut down or control substance use; (9) a great deal of time is spent in activities necessary to obtain the substance, use the substance, or recover from its effects.

When patients become dependent (addicted), they no longer have full control of their drug use. The brain has been "hijacked by a substance that affects the mechanism of control over the use of that substance." This addiction is far more than physical dependence. The need to use the drug becomes as powerful as the drives of thirst and hunger.

1. The evidence that the brains of addicted individuals are different from those of non-addicted persons is compelling. Many of these abnormalities predate the use of the substance and are thought to be inherited. In genetically predisposed individuals, substances of abuse cause changes in the dopaminergic mesolimbic system that result in a loss of control over substance use. These changes are mediated by a number of neurotransmitters: dopamine, γ-aminobutyric acid (GABA), glutamate, serotonin, and endorphins.

The different classes of substances of abuse act through one or more of these neurotransmitters, ultimately affecting the level of dopamine in the mesolimbic system (known as the reward pathway). These changes in the brain are permanent and are the primary reason for relapse in the addicted patient trying to maintain abstinence or control of use.

II. Screening for substance abuse disorders of adults and pregnant women in the primary care setting is recommended by the USPSTF. (SOR **B**) There is no one screening tool that is superior to another.

1. The CAGE questionnaire (Table 90–1) is perhaps the most widely used screening tool for the identification of patients at risk for substance use disorders. When answering yes to two or more questions on the CAGE, the sensitivity is 60% to 90% and the specificity 40% to 60% for substance use disorders. (SOR **B**)

2. Because a screening test is more predictive when applied to a population more likely to have a disease, clinical clues (Table 90–2) to substance use disorders can be useful for determining which patients to screen. Once a patient screens positive for a substance use problem, the question becomes: Is it abuse or dependence (see earlier)?

III. Diagnosis

A. Differential diagnosis. Substance abuse is a behavioral disorder and there is a high comorbidity of substance use disorders with psychiatric disorders. Approximately 50% of psychiatric patients have a substance use disorder. (SOR **A**) When one looks at patients with addictions, however, the rates of psychiatric disorders are similar to those in the general population. Problems, such as substance-induced mood disorders (frequently noted in alcohol, opiate, and stimulant abuse) and substance-induced psychotic disorders (most frequently associated with stimulant abuse), complicate differentiating the primary psychiatric disorders from those that are primarily substance use disorders. Most clinicians agree that psychiatric disorders cannot be reliably assessed for patients who are currently or recently intoxicated. Thus, detoxification and a period of abstinence are necessary before evaluation for other psychiatric disorders can effectively be completed. (SOR **B**)

TABLE 90–2. CLINICAL CLUES TO ALCOHOL AND DRUG PROBLEMS

Social History	Medical History
Arrest for driving under the influence	History of addiction to any drug
Loss of job or sent home from work for alcohol or drug reasons	Withdrawal syndrome
	Depression
Domestic violence	Anxiety disorder
Child abuse/neglect	Recurrent pancreatitis
Family instability (divorce, separation)	Recurrent hepatitis
Frequent, unplanned absences	Hepatomegaly
Personal isolation	Peripheral neuropathy
Problems at work/school	Myocardial infarction age <30 yr (cocaine)
Mood swings	Blood alcohol level >300 or >100 without impairment
	Alcohol on breath or intoxicated at office visit
	Tremor
	Mild hypertension
	Estrogen mediated signs (telangiectasias, spider angiomas, palmer erythema, muscle atrophy)
	Gastrointestinal complaints
	Sleep disturbances
	Eating disorders
	Sexual dysfunction

B. **Symptoms and signs.** The symptoms and the signs of substance abuse are varied and often subtle. Most patients do not recognize their substance use as the cause of their problems and are often quite resistant to that interpretation. Several questionnaires have been used to screen for alcohol-use disorders. The CAGE (Table 90–1) is frequently used by primary care providers to assess the need for further investigation. Another, screening tool the Alcohol Use Disorders Identification Test (AUDIT) can be used but has varying sensitivity and specificity depending on the population. The CAGE appears to be more beneficial in assessing alcohol abuse/dependence and the AUDIT better suited for identifying heavy drinkers.

Signs, such as those described in Table 90–2 as potential clues to substance abuse, should lead the clinician to obtain a full substance use history (Table 90–3). While physical dependence is not always seen with substance abuse, its presence suggests abuse unless the patient is on long-term, prescribed addictive medicines.

C. **Symptoms and signs of withdrawal.** In dealing with sedative hypnotic, alcohol, or opiate withdrawal, assessment of the degree of withdrawal is important to determine appropriate use and dose of medication to both reduce symptoms and, in the case of sedative hypnotic drugs including alcohol, prevent seizures and mortality. The Clinical Institute Withdrawal Assessment Scale (Table 90–4) allows quantification of the symptoms and signs of withdrawal in a predictable fashion that allows clinicians to discuss the severity of withdrawal for a given patient and thus choose intervention strategies that are effective and safe. (SOR **B**)

D. **Laboratory tests**
   1. **γ-Glutamyl transferase (GGT).** GGT is an enzyme produced in the liver and induced by heavy alcohol consumption. In addition, damage to the hepatic cells during chronic heavy alcohol consumption results in leakage of GGT into the serum. It has a high sensitivity but low specificity secondary to nonalcoholic liver disease, diabetes, pancreatitis, hyperthyroidism, heart failure, and anticonvulsant and anticoagulant use—all of which may cause it to be elevated. (SOR **C**)
   2. Other **liver function tests** that may be elevated during heavy alcohol consumption include aspartate aminotransferase (AST) and alanine aminotransferase (ALT). These markers are also elevated as the result of hepatic cellular damage caused by heavy alcohol consumption. Sensitivity of these markers is low because there must be significant liver damage before these markers rise. Specificity is compromised because nonalcoholic liver disease also causes increases. Differences in the ratio of AST/ALT can help to distinguish between alcohol and nonalcohol-related liver disease. A ratio of >2 is highly suggestive of alcohol-related liver disease. (SOR **C**)

TABLE 90–3. ELEMENTS OF THE SUBSTANCE USE HISTORY

1. Determine the type, frequency, route of administration, and amount of substance use
   a. Alcohol
   b. Tobacco
   c. Other drugs (e.g., cocaine, marijuana)
2. Determine consequences of substance use; ask about
   a. Legal problems
      i. Arrests (driving under the influence, public intoxication, disorderly conduct, etc.)
      ii. Civil suits for financial problems, bankruptcy, etc.
   b. Social problems
      i. Social isolation
   c. Family problems
      i. Marital problems
      ii. Parenting problems
      iii. Domestic violence
      iv. Family members with depression
      v. Divorce
   d. Work or school problems
      i. Frequent absences
      ii. Poor performance
      iii. Frequent job changes
   e. Financial problems
      i. Significant debt
      ii. Selling personal possessions
      iii. Stealing and selling possessions of others
   f. Psychological problems
      i. Agitation
      ii. Irritability
      iii. Anxiety
      iv. Panic attacks
      v. Mood swings
      vi. Hostility
      vii. Violence
      viii. Sleep disturbance
      ix. xi. Sexual dysfunction
      x. Depression
      xi. Blackouts
   g. Medical problems
      i. Gastritis
      ii. Peptic ulcer
      iii. Abdominal pain
      iv. Hypertension
      v. Peripheral neuropathy
      vi. Nasal septum perforation
      vii. Vasospasm
      viii. Dysrhythmias
      ix. Weight loss
      x. HIV
      xi. Skin abscesses
      xii. Trauma

3. **Carbohydrate-deficient transferrin (CDT).** CDT has become available in clinical settings as a blood test to screen for excessive alcohol consumption. Consumption of four to seven drinks daily for at least a week results in a decrease in the carbohydrate content of transferrin. Sensitivity and specificity of CDT are high, higher than both MCV and GGT, with regard to differentiating heavy drinkers from those who drink very little or not at all. Additionally, the sensitivity increases by combining the results of all three tests. When used in larger, more heterogeneous populations, it appears less sensitive. (SOR **C**)
4. **Urine drug screening** is a sensitive test for common substances of abuse. Knowledge of drug half-life and the importance of confirmation of positive tests by gas chromatography are essential for interpretation of results. A number of substances

TABLE 90–4. CLINICAL INSTITUTE WITHDRAWAL ASSESSMENT SCALE

Patient_____ Date _____ Time ____ BP___/___
Age_____ Race/Sex ___ Drugs of choice (Primary) ____ Other____

1. Autonomic hyperactivity
Pulse rate/minute

0	<80
1	81–100
2	101–110
3	111–120
4	121–130
5	131–140
6	141–150
7	>150

Sweating (observation)

0	No sweating
1	Barely perceptible sweating, palms moist
2	
3	
4	Beads of sweat obvious on forehead
5	
6	
7	Drenching sweats

2. Hand tremor: arms extended and fingers spread apart:
Observation

0	No tremor
1	Not visible
2	
3	
4	Moderate with patients arms extended
5	
6	
7	Severe, even with arms not extended

3. Anxiety: Ask, "Do you feel nervous or anxious?"
Observation

0	No anxiety, at ease
1	Mildly anxious
2	
3	
4	Moderately anxious
5	
6	
7	Severe equivalent to panic

Total Score ___ Max Score = 56
Rater's initials ___

4. Transient tactile auditory or visual disturbances: Ask, "Do you have any itching, pins, and needle sensations, any burning or numbness, or do you feel bugs crawling on or under your skin?, Are you more aware of sounds around you and are they harsh?, Are you hearing things that you know are not there?, Does the light appear too bright?, Does it hurt your eyes?, Are you seeing anything that is disturbing to you?"
Observation

0	Not present
1	Present but minimal
2	
3	Moderate
4	Frequent
5	
6	
7	Hallucinations almost continuous

5. Agitation:
Observation

0	Normal activity
1	Somewhat more than normal activity
2	
3	
4	Moderately fidgety and restless
5	
6	
7	Paces back and forth during most of the interview, or constantly thrashes about

6. Nausea or vomiting: Ask, "Do you feel sick to your stomach or have you vomited?" Include recorded vomiting since last observation
Observation

0	Not present
1	Very mild
2	
3	
4	Moderate
5	
6	
7	Severe

7. Headache: Ask, "Does your head feel full? Does it feel like there is a band around your head?" Don't rate for lightheadedness.
Otherwise rate severity

0	Not present
1	Very mild
2	
3	
4	Moderate
5	
6	
7	Severe

can cause false-positive results (e.g., false-positive for opiates with dextromethorphan, poppy seeds, quinine, quinolones, and rifampin), so attention to the drug and food ingestion history is important.

5. Ethyl glucuronide testing of the urine (EtG). EtG has recently become a popular test for detecting recent alcohol consumption. Unlike CDT, the presence of EtG in the urine only confirms that the patient has recently consumed alcohol, and says nothing about the level of the consumption. Consequently, its greatest usefulness is in the monitoring of those patients who are committed to abstinence from alcohol. (SOR **C**)

IV. Treatment. Many substance-use disorders resolve spontaneously or with brief interventions on the part of physicians or other authority figures in the workplace, legal system, family, or society. This resolution often occurs because the patient with a substance-abuse disorder continues to maintain control over their use so that when the consequences of that use outweigh the benefits of the drug, they choose to quit. Patients with substance dependence disorders, on the other hand, have impaired control by definition and rarely quit without assistance.

Substance-use disorders can be treated successfully. Brief interventions and outpatient, inpatient, and residential treatment programs reduce morbidity and mortality associated with substance abuse and dependence. (SOR **B**) Detoxification, patient education, identification of defenses, overcoming denial, relapse prevention, orientation to 12-step recovery programs, and family services are goals of substance abuse treatment.

A. Formal process. The traditional intervention for alcohol or drug addiction is a formal process, best accomplished by an addiction specialist trained in this process. This approach is often effective, resulting in positive results in approximately 80% of cases. (SOR **B**) Although effective, the traditional, formal model of intervention is often less than ideal for the primary care provider. Specialist involvement and orchestration of significant relationships with the patient is sometimes difficult to achieve. In addition, if the intervention fails, the physician's relationship with the patient may become difficult if not impossible to continue.

B. Brief interventions. This highly effective approach to intervention is based on the work of Miller and Rollnick on motivational interviewing and Prochaska and DiClementi's work on stages of change. Presenting the diagnosis of a substance use disorder by itself can be viewed as a brief intervention. As many as 70% of patients are in the precontemplation or contemplation stage when presented with the diagnosis. The resistance associated with these stages tends to force the clinician into one of two modalities, that of avoiding the diagnosis or confronting and arguing with the patient; generally both futile approaches. The SOAPE glossary (Table 90–5) provides positive suggestions to use when talking to patients about their addiction. Even when the patient is in the precontemplation stage at presentation of the diagnosis, continued use of the brief intervention strategy will ultimately reduce the amount of drug use if not result in abstinence.

1. Brief interventions should include some of the elements of motivational interviewing. These elements include offering empathetic, objective feedback of data, meeting patient expectations, working with ambivalence, assessing barriers and strengths, reinterpreting past experience in light of current medical consequences, negotiating

---

TABLE 90–5. SOAPE GLOSSARY FOR PRESENTING THE DIAGNOSIS

Support: Use phrases such as "We need to work together on this," "I am concerned about you and will follow-up closely with you," and "As with all medical illnesses, the more people you work with, the better you will feel." These words reinforce your physician–patient relationship, strengthen the collaborative model of chronic illness management, and help convince the patient that the physician will not just present the diagnosis and leave.

Optimism: Most patients have controlled their alcohol or drug use at times and may have quit for periods of time. They may expect failure. By giving a strong optimistic message, such as "You can get well," "Treatment works," and "You can expect to see improvements in many areas of your life," the physician can motivate the patient.

Absolution: By describing addiction as a disease and telling the patients that they are not responsible for having an illness, but that now only they can take responsibility for their recovery, the physician can lessen the burden of guilt and shame that often is a barrier to recovery.

Plan: Having a plan is important to the acceptance of the illness. Using readiness to change categories can help you design a plan that takes the patient's willingness to move ahead. Indicating that abstinence is desirable, but recognizing that all patients will not be able to commit to that goal immediately, can help prevent a sense of failure early in the process. Ask "What do you think you will be able to do at this point?"

Explanatory model: Understanding your patient's beliefs about addiction may be important. Many patients believe this is a moral weakness and that they lack willpower. An explanation that willpower cannot resolve physical illnesses like diabetes mellitus, hypertension, or alcoholism may go a long way to reassure the patient that recovery is possible.

TABLE 90–6. TREATMENT REGIMENS FOR ALCOHOL WITHDRAWAL

Using the Clinical Institute Withdrawal Assessment (CIWA) for monitoring
Do CIWA scale every 4 h until the score is below 8 for 24 h
For CIWA >10
Give Chlordiazepoxide 50–100 mg (every 2–4 h to a maximum of 300 mg/d)
or   Diazepam 2–10 mg (twice to four times daily based on symptom severity)
or   Lorazepam 2 mg every 6 h (for four doses) then 1 mg every 6 h (for eight doses)
or   Oxazepam 15–30 mg (three to four times daily)
Repeat CIWA 1 h after dose to assess need for further medication.
Nonsymptom-driven regimens

For patients likely to experience withdrawal:
Chlordiazepoxide, 50 mg every 6 h for four doses, followed by 50 mg every 8 h for three doses, followed by
   50 mg every 12 h for two doses, and finally by 50 mg at bedtime for one dose.
Other benzodiazepines may be substituted at equivalent doses.
Patients on a predetermined dosing schedule should be monitored frequently for breakthrough withdrawal symptoms
   as well as excessive sedation.

a follow-up plan, and providing hope. While these techniques have not been shown to be effective in women, men receiving one to four interventions from their primary care provider tend to have reduced alcohol consumption and decreased morbidity from injuries related to alcohol. (SOR **B**)

C. **Detoxification.** Detoxification, treatment of withdrawal, and any medical complications have first priority. Alcohol and other sedative hypnotic drugs share the same neurobiologic withdrawal process. Chronic use of this class of drugs results in downregulation of the GABA receptors throughout the central nervous system (GABA is an inhibitory neurotransmitter). Abrupt cessation of sedative hypnotic drug use results in an upregulation of GABA receptors and a relative paucity of GABA for inhibition. The result is stimulation of the autonomic nervous system.

1. **Withdrawal seizures.** These are a common manifestation of sedative hypnotic withdrawal. They occur in 11% to 33% of patients withdrawing from alcohol. Alcohol withdrawal seizures are best treated with benzodiazepines and by addressing the withdrawal process. Lorazepam is a good choice because it can be given intravenously or intramuscularly, 2 to 4 mg every 1 to 4 hours as needed for seizure activity. Patients should be on a cardiac monitor and sometimes require intubation to protect their airway if seizure activity is persistent. Long-term treatment for alcohol withdrawal seizures is not recommended, and phenytoin should not be used to treat seizures associated with alcohol withdrawal. (SOR **A**)

2. **Other withdrawal symptoms.** The cornerstones of treatment for alcohol withdrawal syndrome are the benzodiazepines. All drugs that provide cross-tolerance with alcohol are effective in reducing the symptoms and sequelae of alcohol withdrawal, but none has the safety profile and evidence of efficacy of the benzodiazepines (see Table 90–6 for recommendations in the treatment of alcohol withdrawal).

3. **Opiate/cocaine/stimulant withdrawal.** While not life-threatening, symptoms can be significant enough that without supportive treatment most patients will not remain in treatment (see Table 90–7 for recommendations for the treatment of opiate withdrawal). The symptoms of cocaine and other stimulant withdrawal are somewhat less predictable and much harder to manage. Despite multiple studies with many different drug classes, no medications have been shown to reliably reduce the symptoms and craving associated with cocaine withdrawal.

D. **Patient education.** Patient knowledge and understanding of the nature of substance use disorders is key to recovery.

1. For patients still in control of their use, education about appropriate substance use will help them to choose responsibly if they continue to use.

2. For patients who meet the criteria for **addiction,** abstinence is the only safe option. Once having made the transition to addiction, one can never use addictive substances reliably again. The neurobiologic changes in the brain are permanent, so loss of control is unpredictable and can occur at any time that the brain is presented with an addictive substance. Consequently, addicted patients may find that they can

TABLE 90-7. TREATMENT FOR OPIOID WITHDRAWAL

Methadone: A pure opioid agonist restricted by federal legislation to inpatient treatment or specialized outpatient drug treatment programs. Methadone 20–30 mg once. Maintenance dose of 5–10 mg can be given 2–4 h later if needed. Adjust dose based on control of withdrawal 2–4 h post dose. Usual dose is 80–120 mg/d.

Clonidine: An α-adrenergic blocker 0.1 mg three times daily to relieve symptoms of withdrawal may be effective; titrate to symptoms. Hypotension is a risk and sometimes limits the dose. It can be continued for 10–14 d and tapered by the third day by 0.2 mg/d.

Buprenorphine and Buprenorphine/naloxone (Suboxone): Buprenorphine is a partial μ receptor agonist and naloxone is a μ receptor antagonist given sublingually. Dosing on days 1 and 2 is with buprenorphine alone as 8 mg and 16 mg, respectively. From day 3 onward, buprenorphine/naloxone is used at the same buprenorphine dose as day 2. The recommended target dose is 16 mg/4 mg once daily. Adjust the dose in increments of 2–4 mg for the management of opioid withdrawal symptoms (likely range of buprenorphine is 4–24 mg/d).

Naltrexone/clonidine: A rapid form of opioid detoxification involves pretreatment with 0.2–0.3 mg of clonidine followed by 12.5 mg of naltrexone (a pure opioid antagonist). Naltrexone is increased to 25 mg on the day 2, 50 mg on day 3, and 100 mg on day 4, with clonidine given at 0.1–0.3 mg three times daily.

use a drug (or alcohol) for a variable period of time with control. This sense of control gives them the false impression that they were never addicted or perhaps have been cured. Invariably, if they continue to use addictive substances, they will lose control of their use and begin to experience consequences at or above the level that they did before. Understanding addiction as a chronic disorder for which there is remission but no cure becomes essential. The question then becomes not if one should remain abstinent, but rather how one remains abstinent.

E. **Identification of defenses/overcoming denial.** During this phase of treatment, patients typically work in a group therapy setting and are encouraged to look at the defenses that have prevented them from seeking help sooner. Denial can best be defined as the inability to see the causal relationship between drug use and its consequences. Thus, the patients who believe they drank because they lost their job can be encouraged to consider that they lost their job because they drank.

F. **Pharmacologic treatment of addiction.** These drugs act through one of the several mechanisms: (1) sensitizing the body's response to result in a negative or aversion reaction to ingesting the drug (e.g., disulfiram and alcohol); (2) reducing the reinforcing effects of a drug (e.g., naltrexone or acamprosate in alcoholism); (3) blocking the effects of a drug by binding to the receptor site (e.g., naltrexone for opiates); (4) saturating the receptor sites by agonists (e.g., methadone in opioid maintenance therapy); and (5) using unique approaches such as the creation of an immunization to cocaine. Drug therapy to prevent relapse is seen as adjunctive. No drug alone has sufficient power to prevent relapse to addictive behavior. Still, in some patients, use of medication can provide the edge needed to move closer to recovery.

1. Disulfiram is a drug that is not often initiated by family physicians but is frequently continued and monitored in the primary care setting. The usual dose is 250 to 500 mg every morning. Disulfiram works as a deterrent causing a severe negative reaction following ingestion of any form of alcohol; manifestations include flushing, nausea, and vomiting. Efficacy in achieving abstinence is mixed and is enhanced by taking the medication while observed. (SOR ❸) Disulfiram is contraindicated in patients who are hypersensitive to its use, those who have consumed alcohol in the past 12 hours, or those with psychosis or severe coronary artery disease.

2. Naltrexone, an opiate antagonist, has been shown to reduce the craving to drink in alcoholics. It does not increase overall abstinence rates but has moderate efficacy in decreasing the amount and frequency of alcohol consumption. At doses of 50 mg daily, this medication may reduce the patient's desire to drink. It is contraindicated with opiate use, liver failure, or acute hepatitis. This medication is less effective when not accompanied by a comprehensive recovery program. (SOR ❸)

3. Acamprosate, recently released and FDA approved for alcoholism treatment, has been shown to be effective in reducing the craving to drink alcohol. Studies have shown significant effects in reducing drinking and increasing the length of abstinence.

(SOR **Ⓑ**) Currently, it is prescribed at 333 mg three times daily. It is not likely to be effective in the absence of a comprehensive recovery program.

4. Buprenorphine is a partial mu-opioid receptor agonist used in the treatment of opioid addiction. This medication can only be prescribed by a DEA-licensed physician after completing an 8-hour course. It can be prescribed alone (Subutex) or in combination with the opioid antagonist naloxone (Suboxone). Side effects of the medication include sedation, headache, insomnia, anxiety, and depression.

The use of buprenorphine in managing withdrawal consists of three phases: induction (3–7 days), stabilization (1–2 months), and maintenance (indefinitely).

  a. The induction phase begins when withdrawal symptoms begin. The initial dose of buprenorphine/naloxone is 4/2 mg (2 mg of buprenorphine alone) and should not exceed 8/12 mg. Buprenorphine alone can be used on day 1, but later it is recommended to use buprenorphine/naloxone. The dose on day 2 should not exceed 16 mg and the maximum Suboxone dose for the rest of induction is 32/8 mg.

  b. During stabilization, the lowest dose that minimizes withdrawal symptoms and side effects from the medication is chosen. Typically, the dose of Suboxone in this stage is 12/3 mg to 24/6 mg.

  c. The maintenance dose is also chosen with the goal of maximizing benefit and reducing symptoms for an undefined period of time.

V. Management Strategies

  A. Relapse prevention. Once patients receive education about the nature of their disease and have identified destructive defense mechanisms, relapse prevention becomes the primary goal. Identification of triggers for alcohol and drug use, avoidance of opportunities to relapse, and finding new ways to deal with problems help patients to maintain their abstinence.

  1. In most treatment programs, a relapse prevention plan will be developed and individualized for each patient. The most effective way that the family physician can support relapse prevention is to be aware of the relapse prevention plan that the patient has developed in treatment and reinforce its application. For example, it is useful, when seeing the patients who are new to recovery, to ask them about their 12-step meeting attendance, sponsor contacts, and whether they have been able to remain abstinent since your last meeting.

  2. For patients who have not had the benefit of treatment, identification of triggers followed by cognitive strategies to avoid these triggers may enhance their recovery. These are usually relatively simple to create. For example, for patients who report that they drink after an argument with their spouse, consideration of alternative means of coping such as calling a friend, exercising, or engaging in relaxation techniques may be helpful. (SOR **Ⓑ**)

  B. Orientation to 12-step recovery. Despite millions of dollars in research, and the efforts of a large segment of the scientific community, there has been no treatment, medication, or psychotherapy that is more effective than the 12 steps of Alcoholics Anonymous (AA) (see Table 90–8). (SOR **Ⓑ**) There is often confusion about what AA does and does not do. AA is not treatment, although many treatment programs have 12-step recovery fellowships; these fellowships, however, are not affiliated with treatment centers by design.

  Other important 12-step programs for patients with substance use disorders include Al-Anon, for friends and family of alcoholics; Narcotics Anonymous, for those with drug problems other than alcohol; and Cocaine Anonymous, for those with cocaine addiction. At the heart of each of these fellowships is the program of recovery outlined in the 12 steps.

  1. AA and related 12-step programs are spiritual, not religious, in nature. No one is told they must believe in anything, including God. Agnostics and atheists are welcome in AA and are not asked to convert to any religious belief.

  2. Newcomers in AA are encouraged to go to meetings regularly (daily is wise initially), get a sponsor, and begin work on the 12 steps. A sponsor is someone of the same gender who is in stable recovery and has worked the steps. The sponsor helps guide the newcomer through the steps and provides a source of information and encouragement.

  3. At meetings, members share their experience, strength, and hope around topics of their recovery. In this fashion, storytelling often becomes the means by which information about strategies for recovery is relayed.

TABLE 90-8. THE TWELVE STEPS OF ALCOHOLICS ANONYMOUS

We:

1. Admitted we were powerless over alcohol—that our lives had become unmanageable;
2. Came to believe that a Power greater than ourselves could restore us to sanity;
3. Made a decision to turn our will and our lives over to the care of *God as we understood Him;*
4. Made a searching and fearless moral inventory of ourselves;
5. Admitted to ourselves, and to another human being the exact nature of our wrongs;
6. Were entirely ready to have God remove all these defects of character;
7. Humbly asked Him to remove our shortcomings;
8. Made a list of all persons we had harmed, and became willing to make amends to them all;
9. Made direct amends to such people wherever possible, except when to do so would injure them or others;
10. Continued to take personal inventory and when we were wrong promptly admitted it;
11. Sought through prayer and meditation to improve our conscious contact with God as we *understand Him,* praying only for knowledge of His will for us and the power to carry that out;
12. Having had a spiritual awakening as the result of these steps, we tried to carry this message to alcoholics, and to practice these principles in all our affairs.

Source: Reproduced with permission from Alcoholics Anonymous World Service.

4. AA meetings vary in their composition and structure, given that one of the traditions of AA is that each group is autonomous. Consequently, if a patient feels uncomfortable at one meeting, another may be more acceptable. There are meetings for women or men only, for young people, and for physicians or lawyers; virtually, any special-interest group is represented in large cities.

C. **Effectiveness of AA.** From multiple sources, it appears clear that AA and other 12-step recovery programs are among the most effective tools we have to combat substance disorders. Approximately 6% to 10% of the population has been to an AA meeting during their lives. This number doubles for those with alcohol problems. Although, one-half of those who come to AA drop out; of those who stay for a year, 67% stay sober; of those who stay for 2 years, 85% stay sober; and of those who stay sober for 5 years, 90% remain sober indefinitely.

   1. Outcome studies of 8087 patients treated in 57 different inpatient and outpatient treatment programs showed that those attending AA at 1 year were 50% more likely to be abstinent than those not attending. (SOR **B**) Adolescents studied were found to be four times more likely to be abstinent if they attended Alcoholics Anonymous/Narcotics Anonymous, when compared to those who did not.

   2. In an effort to identify which groups attending AA did better than others, studies of involvement in AA (defined as service work, having a sponsor, leading meetings, etc.) found that those who were involved, as compared to those just attending meetings, did better at maintaining abstinence. (SOR **C**)

D. **Contacts.** Having a list of AA members willing to escort potential new members to meetings is a powerful tool for physicians to help patients into recovery. Generally, in every AA district, there is a person identified as the chair of the Cooperation with Professional Community Committee who can help physicians identify people willing to perform this service. Al-Anon and Narcotics Anonymous have similar contacts. The telephone numbers for most of these 12-step groups can be found in the telephone book. These contacts can often supply the physician with relevant literature to help dispel some of the myths patients may hold regarding 12-step recovery. Patients will often use these myths as excuses for why AA will not work for them.

VI. **Prognosis.** Alcohol causes approximately 100,000 deaths yearly and is associated with motor vehicle accidents, other accidents, homicides, cirrhosis of the liver, and suicide. Injection drug use is responsible for the fastest-growing population of human immunodeficiency virus infection. See Table 90-9 for common medical complications from substance abuse.

   1. It is unknown what the rate of relapse is overall. Being male, young, and having fewer social supports are related to higher rates of relapse.

   2. The prognosis for professionals who participate in a monitoring program after treatment is better than for nonprofessionals. (SOR **B**)

TABLE 90–9. MEDICAL COMPLICATIONS OF SUBSTANCE ABUSE

Drug	Medical Complication
Alcohol	Trauma
	Cardiovascular: Hypertension
	Cardiomyopathy
	Dysrhythmias
	Ischemic heart disease
	Hemorrhagic stroke
	Gastrointestinal: Esophageal reflux
	Barrett's esophagus
	Mallory–Weiss tears
	Esophageal cancer
	Acute gastritis
	Pancreatitis
	Chronic diarrhea malabsorption
	Alcoholic hepatitis
	Cirrhosis
	Hepatic failure
	Hepatic carcinoma
	Neurologic: Headache
	Sleep disorders
	Memory impairment
	Dementia
	Sexual dysfunction
	Substance-induced mood disorders
	Substance-induced psychotic disorders
	Other: Immune disorders
	Nasopharyngeal malignancy
Cocaine (other stimulants)	Chest pain
	Congestive heart failure
	Cardiac dysrhythmias
	Cardiovascular collapse
	Seizures
	Cerebrovascular accidents
	Headache
	Spontaneous pneumothorax
	Noncardiogenic pulmonary edema
	Nasal septal perforations
Injection drug use	Hepatitis C, B
	HIV infection
	Subacute endocarditis
	Soft-tissue abscesses

SELECTED REFERENCES

American Psychiatric Association Highlights of Changes from DSM-IV-TR to DSM V. p.16. http://www.dsm5.org/Documents/changes%20from%20dsm-iv-tr%20to%20dsm-5.pdf. Accessed June 2013.

Beich A, Thorsen T, Rollnick S. Screening in brief intervention trials targeting excessive drinkers in general practice: Systematic review and meta-analysis. *BMJ*. 2003;327:536–542.

Bradley KA, Bush KR, McDonnell MB, et al. Screening for problem drinking: Comparison of CAGE and AUDIT. *J Gen Intern Med*. 1998;13:379–389.

Cayley WE Jr. Effectiveness of acamprosate in the treatment of alcohol dependence. *Am Fam Physician*. 2011;83:522–524.

Donaher PA, Welsh C. Managing opioid addiction with buprenorphine. *Am Fam Physician*. 2006; 73(9):1573–1578.

Enoch MA, Goldman D. Problem drinking and alcoholism: diagnosis and treatment. *Am Fam Physician*. 2002;65(3):441–448. [Summary in *Am Fam Physician* 2002;65(3):449–450; PMID: 11858628].

Gomez A, Conde A, Santana JM, et al. Diagnostic usefulness of brief versions of Alcohol Use Disorders Identification Test (AUDIT) for detecting hazardous drinkers in primary care settings. *J Stud Alcohol.* 2005;66:305–308.

Hock B, Schwarz M, Domke I, et al. Validity of carbohydrate-deficient transferrin (%CDT), gamma-glutamyl transferase (gamma-GT) and mean corpuscular erythrocyte volume (MCV) as biomarkers for chronic alcohol abuse: a study in patients with alcohol dependence and liver disorders of non-alcoholic and alcoholic origin. *Addiction.* 2005;100:1477–1486.

Jonas DE, Garbutt JC, Amick HR, et al. Behavioral counselling after screening for alcohol misuse in primary care: a systematic review and meta-analysis for the U.S. Preventive Services Task Force. *Ann Intern Med.* 2012;157(9):645–654.

Kaner EF, Beyer F, Dickinson HO, et al. Effectiveness of brief alcohol interventions in primary care populations. *Cochrane Database Syst Rev.* 2007;CD004148.

Kenna GA, McGeary JE, Swift RM. Pharmacotherapy, pharmacogenomics, and the future of alcohol dependence treatment, part 1. *Am J Health Syst Pharm.* 2004;61:2272–2279.

Saitz R. Clinical practice. Unhealthy alcohol use. *N Engl J Med.* 2005;352:596–607.

USPSTF. Screening and behavioral counseling interventions in primary care to reduce alcohol misuse: Recommendation statement. *Ann Intern Med.* 2004;140:554–556.

Yancey JR, Lumbad J. Opioid antagonists for the treatment of alcohol dependence. *Am Fam Physician.* 2011;84:990–992.

91 Anxiety

John C. Rogers, MD, MPH, MEd, & Alicia A. Kowalchuk, DO

KEY POINTS

- Anxiety disorders are the most common class of mental disorders in the general population with a lifetime prevalence of 15%. (SOR **C**)
- The three most common clinical conditions are phobias, general anxiety disorder, and panic disorder. (SOR **C**)
- Cognitive-behavioral therapies are useful treatments for a majority of patients with anxiety disorders. (SOR **A**)
- Medications typically used to treat patients with anxiety disorders are antidepressants, benzodiazepines, and buspirone (see Table 91-1 for prescribing information). (SOR **A**)

I. Introduction

A. Anxiety is exaggerated worry and tension over everyday events and decisions. One or more fearful experiences prime a person to respond excessively to situations in which most people would experience no fear or only moderate nervousness. Deeply etched memory results in hypervigilance, making it hard to focus and leading to feelings of anxiety in many situations.

1. Recent research suggests that anxiety disorders are associated with activation of the amygdala. Studies also suggest that memories stored in the amygdala are relatively indelible. Researchers are attempting to develop therapies that increase cognitive control over the amygdala so that the "act now, think later" response can be interrupted.

2. Cognitive factors play a significant role in the onset of anxiety disorders. People at risk tend to be overly responsive to potentially threatening stimuli.

3. Evidence points to genetics as a factor in the origin of anxiety disorders. Studies of twins found that genes play a role in panic disorder and social phobia.

B. Generalized anxiety disorder (GAD) is a syndrome of excessive or unrealistic anxiety or worry about two or more life circumstances for 6 months or longer.

1. GAD is the fourth most common mental health disorder, following substance abuse, major depressive disorder, and phobias. Two to five percent of the US population exhibits this disorder in any given year.

    a. The mean age at onset of symptoms is in the mid-20s, with most cases developing between the ages of 16 and 40 years. The mean duration of symptoms before treatment is about 5 years.

    b. In the general medical care setting, the female-to-male ratio is 2–3:1, but among psychiatric patients, the sex ratio is 1:1. First- and second-degree relatives of a person affected by GAD have at least a threefold increased risk of being affected.

    c. Comorbidity with depression is frequent (just over 50% of depressed patients have concurrent GAD).

C. Panic disorder is the recurrence of episodic periods of intense fear or apprehension accompanied by at least four somatic symptoms, such as diaphoresis, dyspnea, faintness, paresthesias, or flushing. These episodes or attacks strike unexpectedly and repeatedly for no apparent reason.

    1. Panic disorder occurs in 1.4% of the US population.

        a. The mean age at presentation is 25 years, with onset generally between ages 17 and 30 years.

        b. The female-to-male ratio is 2.5–3:1. This disorder has a familial tendency, with first-degree relatives having a twofold increased risk of being affected compared with control subjects.

        c. Comorbidity with depression occurs (nearly 10% of depressed patients have panic disorder) and leads to more frequent and severe symptoms.

D. A phobia is a persistent fear of an object, an activity, or a situation that is out of proportion to the objective danger.

    1. Phobia is the most common anxiety disorder. Fifteen to twenty percent of the US population is affected by phobias.

        a. Social phobia is fear of extreme embarrassment when interacting with others and usually begins during the early to late teens. Simple phobias, fear of an object or situation, can begin at any age, however, depending on typical exposure to the object or situation. The most common objects of simple phobia are, in descending order and frequency, animals, storms, heights, illness, and death.

        b. Social phobia is reportedly more frequent in men than in women, whereas simple phobias are more frequent in women than in men.

        c. Comorbidity with depression and substance abuse is common (over 20% of depressed patients have concurrent phobia).

E. Posttraumatic stress disorder (PTSD) is a reaction to a terrifying event that keeps returning in the form of frightening, intrusive memories and brings on hypervigilance and deadening of normal emotions. PTSD develops after an individual experiences emotionally or physically distressing events that are outside the range of usual human experience and would be extremely traumatic for virtually any person. Examples include combat experience, natural catastrophes, assault, rape, serious threat or harm to one's family members, or sudden destruction of one's home or community.

    1. The cause of this disorder is related to the severity of the stressor, the social environment of the victim and availability of social supports, the personality traits of the victim, and the victim's premorbid biologic vulnerability such as previous psychiatric illness, history of childhood learning disorder, or traumatic brain injury. PTSD affects 0.5% of men and 1.2% of women in the general population. Onset can be at any age, but because of the types of precipitating situations that are most common, this disorder is most common in young adults. The initiating trauma for men is usually combat experience. The initiating trauma for women is most often assault or rape.

    2. PTSD is also very common in military veterans. Between 2004 and 2009, 21% of all veterans treated by the Veterans Administration were diagnosed with PTSD. PTSD is also common in Vietnam War veterans.

II. Diagnoses

    A. GAD diagnostic criteria include the following (per DSM V):

        1. Excessive anxiety and worry occurring on the majority of days for at least 6 months.

        2. The person finds it difficult to control the anxiety.

        3. The anxiety and worry are associated with three or more of the following symptoms:

            a. Restlessness

            b. Fatigue

            c. Difficulty with concentration

            d. Irritability

            e. Muscle tension

            f. Sleep disturbance

        4. The focus of the anxiety is not focused on one thing in particular.

        5. The symptoms cause clinically significant distress or impairment in function.

6. The anxiety is not caused directly by the physiologic effects of a substance or a medical disorder.

B. Diagnoses that must be ruled out for patients suspected of having GAD include substances (e.g., caffeine intoxication; stimulant abuse; withdrawal from alcohol, sedatives, or hypnotics), medical conditions (e.g., thyrotoxicosis, paroxysmal atrial tachycardia, mitral valve prolapse), hyperventilation, or mental disorder (e.g., panic disorder, phobias, obsessive–compulsive disorder, adjustment disorder with anxious mood, depression, dysthymia, somatization disorder, and schizophrenia).

C. Panic disorder. Panic attacks, which are spontaneous, unexpected episodes that occur in the absence of any apparent precipitant, generally last no more than 20 to 30 minutes, with attacks of 1 hour being rare. Fear without any apparent source and an impending sense of death and doom are characteristic. Such mental thoughts are associated with somatic symptoms typically tachycardia, palpitations, dyspnea, and sweating. Syncope during panic attacks is experienced by as many as 20% of patients. Panic disorder is diagnosed in the absence of agoraphobia.

Diagnostic criteria for panic disorder, based on the DSM V, are:

1. Both recurrent, unexpected panic attacks with at least one of the attacks followed 1 month (or more) by one or more of the following:

    a. Persistent concern about having additional attacks.

    b. Worry about the implications of the attack or its consequences (e.g., losing control, having a heart attack, or "going crazy").

    c. A significant change in behavior related to the attacks.

D. Diagnoses that must be ruled out for patients suspected of having panic disorder include substances and medical conditions (as above) or mental disorders such as social phobia (e.g., occurring upon exposure to feared social situations), specific phobia (e.g., on exposure to a specific phobic situation), obsessive–compulsive disorder (e.g., upon exposure to dirt in someone with an obsession about contamination), PTSD (e.g., in response to stimuli associated with a severe stressor), or separation anxiety disorder (e.g., in response to being away from home or close relatives)

E. Phobia. Diagnostic criteria include the following (based on DSM V):

1. Persistent fear that is significant and unreasonable in response to a specific stimuli.

2. Exposure to the stimuli provokes an immediate anxiety response.

3. The person recognizes that the fear is unreasonable.

4. The phobic stimulus is avoided or is endured with intense anxiety or distress.

5. The avoidance, anticipation, or distress of the phobic stimuli interferes with the person's normal daily routine, functioning, or relationships.

F. The most common biomedical **disorders confused with phobia** are intoxication with hallucinogens, sympathomimetics, and other drugs of abuse; small cerebral tumor; and cerebrovascular accidents. The most common mental disorders in the differential diagnoses are depression, schizophrenia, obsessive–compulsive disorder, and personality disorders (schizoid, avoidance, or paranoid).

G. PTSD. In DSM V, PTSD is included in the trauma and stress-related disorders section instead of the anxiety section. Diagnostic criteria include the following.

1. The person has been exposed to a traumatic event in which he/she witnessed an event that involved serious threat and their response involved intense fear, helplessness, or horror.

2. The traumatic event is repeatedly re-experienced by recurrent and intrusive thoughts, recurrent dreams, feeling like the traumatic event is happening again, intense psychological distress at any reminder of the event, or physiologic reaction to any reminder of the event.

3. Avoidance of stimuli associated with the traumatic event including efforts to suppress or avoid any thoughts, activities, or people that remind the person of the event.

4. May be associated with decreased interest in participating in certain activities, feelings of detachment toward others, or inability to form attachments or see a future.

5. Symptoms of increased arousal including difficulty with sleep, concentration, increased irritability, hypervigilance, or exaggerated startle response.

6. Duration of symptoms is more than 1 month and is considered acute if the duration of symptoms is less than 3 months and chronic if the duration is more than 3 months.

H. Biomedical conditions to be ruled out in patients suspected of having PTSD include head injury and alcohol and drug abuse. Psychiatric conditions in the differential diagnosis include GAD, panic disorder, depression, adjustment reaction, factitious disorder, malingering, borderline personality disorder, and schizophrenia.

III. Treatment

A. GAD treatment is directed toward reduction in symptoms so that patients can function in relationships and work. To achieve this goal, the physician must provide patience, realistic reassurance, education about the condition, and encouragement to socialize and assume work and family responsibilities. Interventions with the longest duration of effect are, in descending order: psychological therapy, pharmacologic treatment (antidepressants), and self-help. (SOR **A**)

1. Psychological therapy

   a. Cognitive behavioral therapy (CBT) should be used and delivered only by those trained in and following established treatment protocols. (SOR **C**) The hallmarks of CBT are evaluating apparent cause-and-effect relationships between thoughts, feelings, and behaviors as well as implementing relatively straightforward strategies to lessen symptoms and reduce avoidant behavior. Two-thirds of patients are clinically improved by 6 months. (SOR **A**)

   b. The optimal range of CBT is 16 to 20 hours (SOR **A**), typically 1 to 2 hours per week over 4 months. (SOR **B**)

   c. Briefer CBT should be supplemented with information and tasks. (SOR **B**)

2. Pharmacologic therapy (see Table 91–1)

   a. Short-term treatment.

   (1) Benzodiazepines are appropriate pharmacologic treatment for immediate management of this disorder, (SOR **A**) but should not be used for more than 2 to 4 weeks. (SOR **B**) The pharmacologic properties of common benzodiazepines are displayed in Table 91–1. Patients respond best to anxiolytic agents with short half-lives; however, shorter-acting compounds have somewhat greater abuse liability because of more rapid and abrupt onset of withdrawal symptoms. Use of rapid-acting benzodiazepines as needed may be superior to routine dosing. Concerns with benzodiazepines are (1) 20% to 30% of patients fail to respond to these agents, (2) their potential for producing drug dependence (i.e., physiologic or behavioral symptoms after discontinuation of use), and (3) impaired alertness and increased risk of accidents. Four benzodiazepines widely prescribed for treatment of anxiety disorders are diazepam (starting dose, 2 mg two to four times daily); lorazepam (1 mg two to three times daily); clonazepam (0.25 mg twice daily); and alprazolam (0.25 mg three times daily). Each is available in generic formulations.

   (2) The sedating antihistamine **hydroxyzine** 50 mg per day is effective for immediate management as well (SOR **A**) and represents an alternative to benzodiazepines especially in patients with a history of addictive disorders.

   (3) Beta-blockers can be used to treat peripheral somatic symptoms such as tremor or palpitation. Propranolol can be started at 60 to 80 mg per day in divided doses and gradually increased to optimum response or a maximum dose of 240 mg per day. Combination beta-blocker and benzodiazepine therapy is more effective than a benzodiazepine alone.

   (4) Azapirones (buspirone) are superior to placebo but not benzodiazepines in the short-term. (SOR **A**) It is unclear if the azapirones are superior to antidepressants. Long-term effectiveness is not known. These medications act on the serotoninergic system and do not act through the γ-aminobutyric acid–benzodiazepine receptor complex, so problems of tolerance, dependence, and impaired alertness are avoided.

   Buspirone is most useful for treatment of GAD, particularly for those who have not been on a benzodiazepine, and is now frequently used as an adjunct to selective serotonin reuptake inhibitors (SSRIs) in long-term treatment. Buspirone takes 4 to 6 weeks to exert therapeutic effects, like antidepressants, and has little value for patients when taken on an "as-needed" basis. It should be started at 5 mg three times a day for 3 to 7 days and then increased to 10 mg twice or three times daily, the usual maintenance dose. The dose should not exceed 60 mg per day.

   b. Long-term treatment.

   (1) Antidepressants are first-line agents for long-term treatment. (SOR **A**) Most antidepressant medications have substantial antianxiety and antipanic effects in addition to their antidepressant action. Current practice guidelines

TABLE 91–1. TREATMENT OPTIONS FOR PATIENTS WITH ANXIETY DISORDERS

Drug[a]	Dose	Major Side Effects	Contraindications	Drug Interactions
Selective Serotonin Reuptake Inhibitors				
Fluoxetine[a] (Prozac)	Adult 20–80 mg once or divided twice daily Elderly 10–40 mg daily Pediatric (age 7 yr and older) 10–60 mg daily (OCD only)	**Increased suicidality in children, teens, and young adults,** appetite suppression, insomnia, anxiety, somnolence, rash, sweating, nausea, dry mouth, weakness, dizziness, rhinitis, pharyngitis, sexual dysfunction, hyponatremia, bleeding risk, serotonin syndrome, seizure, prolonged (↑) QT interval	Concomitant use within 14 days of MAOI therapy, metoclopramide (extrapyramidal reactions)	**Multiple Drug Interactions** Ticlopidine, aspirin, NSAIDs, warfarin (bleeding); clarithromycin (psychosis); TCAs, cyclobenzaprine, class IA antiarrhythmics (↑ QT); triptans, St. John's wort, duloxetine, tramadol, cyclobenzaprine, trazodone (serotonin S), carbamazepine (carbamazepine tox), dextromethorphan (dextromethorphan tox), tramadol (seizures)
Sertraline[a] (Zoloft)	Adult 20–200 mg daily Elderly consider lower/less frequent dosing Pediatric (age 6 yr and older) 25–200 mg daily (OCD only)	Same as fluoxetine, diarrhea, constipation, headache, tremor, rhabdomyolysis, Stevens–Johnson syndrome	Concomitant or use within 14 d of MAOI therapy, selegiline (CNS toxicity/serotonin syndrome), concomitant use of disulfiram	**Multiple Drug Interactions** Ticlopidine, aspirin, NSAIDs, warfarin (bleeding); triptans, St. John's wort, duloxetine, tramadol, TCAs, cyclobenzaprine, trazodone (serotonin S); phenytoin (phenytoin tox); dextromethorphan (dextromethorphan tox); tramadol (seizures)
Paroxetine[a] (Paxil)	Adult 12.5–75 mg daily controlled release; 20–60 mg/d immediate release Elderly 12.5–50 mg daily Pediatric—not approved	Same as fluoxetine, constipation, headache, palpitation, paresthesia, blurred vision, Stevens–Johnson syndrome	Same as fluoxetine	**Multiple Drug Interactions** Ticlopidine, aspirin, NSAIDs, warfarin (bleeding); triptans, St. John's wort, duloxetine, tramadol, TCAs, cyclobenzaprine, trazodone, lithium, dextromethorphan (serotonin S); lithium (lithium tox); tamoxifen (↓ tamoxifen concentration), dextromethorphan (dextromethorphan tox); cimetidine (paroxetine tox)
Fluvoxamine (Luvox)	Adult 100–300 mg extended release at bedtime Elderly titrate slowly Pediatric—not approved	Same as fluoxetine, Stevens–Johnson syndrome, agranulocytosis	Same as fluoxetine, tizanidine, cisapride	**Multiple Drug Interactions** Ticlopidine, aspirin, NSAIDs, warfarin (bleeding); triptans, St. John's wort, duloxetine, tramadol, TCAs, cyclobenzaprine, trazodone, lithium (serotonin S); propranolol (bradycardial); phenytoin (phenytoin tox)
Escitalopram[a] (Lexapro)	Adult 10–20 mg once daily Elderly 10 mg once daily Pediatric—not approved	Same as fluoxetine, headache, diarrhea, constipation	Same as fluoxetine	**Multiple Drug Interactions** Ticlopidine, aspirin, NSAIDs, warfarin (bleeding); triptans, St. John's wort, duloxetine, tramadol, TCAs, cyclobenzaprine, trazodone, lithium, dextromethorphan (serotonin S); dextromethorphan (dextromethorphan tox)

(continued)

TABLE 91–1. TREATMENT OPTIONS FOR PATIENTS WITH ANXIETY DISORDERS (*Continued*)

Drug[a]	Dose	Major Side Effects	Contraindications	Drug Interactions
Citalopram[a] (Celexa)	Adult 20–40 mg once daily Elderly 20 mg once daily Pediatric—not approved	Same as fluoxetine, diarrhea, constipation, QT prolongation, MI, CVA	Same as fluoxetine, fluconazole, cisapride	**Multiple Drug Interactions** Ticlopidine, aspirin, NSAIDs, warfarin (bleeding); triptans, St. John's wort, tramadol, cyclobenzaprine, duloxetine, trazodone, lithium, dextromethorphan (serotonin S); dextromethorphan (dextromethorphan tox); amiodarone, ondansetron, trazodone, cyclobenzaprine, PPIs, TCAs, methadone, itraconazole, salmeterol (↑ QT); lithium (lithium tox)
Azapirones Buspirone[a] (BuSpar)	Adult 7.5–30 mg twice daily Elderly 5–30 mg twice daily Pediatric—not approved	Dizziness, anxiety, nausea, headache, insomnia, somnolence, CHF, MI, CVA	Metabolic acidosis, concomitant MAOIs	Grapefruit, diazepam, diltiazem, verapamil, erythromycin, itraconazole, ketoconazole, ritonavir, rifampin, Phenobarbital, carbamazepine, cimetidine, warfarin, digoxin
Tricyclic Antidepressants Imipramine (Tofranil)	Adult 75–200 mg daily in divided doses Elderly 30–100 mg daily Pediatric (6–11 years) 25–50 mg daily Adolescents 25–75 mg daily	**Increased suicidality in children, teens and young adults,** dry mouth, constipation, blurred vision, somnolence, weakness, dizziness, headache, weight gain, urinary retention, orthostatic hypotension, cardiac arrhythmia, prolonged QT, agranulocytosis, seizure, decreased liver function, CVA	Concomitant or use within 14 days of MAOI therapy; MI, during acute recovery; Metoclopramide, cisapride,	**Multiple Drug Interactions** Quinidine (cardiotox); Clonidine (↓ efficacy); fluoxetine, cotrimoxazole, phenothiazines, ziprasidone, Quinolone and macrolide antibiotics, mifepristone, fluconazole, Class 1 antiarrhythmics, triptans, venlafaxine, solifenacin, ciprofloxacin, (↑ QT); sertraline, cyclobenzaprine, dextromethorphan, trazodone, (serotonin S); tramadol (seizures)
Desipramine (Norpramin)	Adult 100–300 mg daily Elderly 25–150 mg daily Pediatric (adolescents only) 25–150 mg daily	Same as imipramine	Same as Imipramine	Same as Imipramine
Beta-Blocker Propranolol[b] (Inderal)	Adult 40 mg two to three times daily (usual dose) or 10 mg 1 h prior to event; 10–20 mg two to three times daily may be as effective Pediatric 2–4 mg/kg/d twice daily	Dermatitis/pruritus, dizziness, fatigue, bronchospasm, CHF, heart block, erythema multiforme, Stevens–Johnson syndrome	Asthma, sinus bradycardia, second- to third-degree heart block, cardiogenic shock	Amiodarone, diltiazem, verapamil, cimetidine, (hypotension, bradycardial); clonidine (bradycardia); St John's wort (↓ efficacy of beta-blocker); warfarin (bleeding); sertraline (chest pain)

Drug	Dosing	Side Effects	Contraindications	Drug Interactions
Antihistamine				
Hydroxyzine[a] (Atarax, Vistaril)	Adult 50–100 mg four times daily; Elderly start at 50 mg four times daily; Pediatric 12.5–25 mg four times daily	Dry mouth, headache, somnolence	Early pregnancy, breast-feeding	Potentiates other sedatives
Benzodiazepines				**Multiple Drug Interactions**
Alprazolam (Xanax)	Adult 0.25–0.5 mg three times daily (max 4 mg/d); Elderly 0.25 mg two to three times daily, increase slowly; Pediatric—not recommended	Appetite suppression increased appetite, weight gain, constipation, dry mouth, cognitive impairment, incoordination, dysarthria, light headed, somnolence, irritability, sexual dysfunction, Stevens–Johnson syndrome, liver failure, drug dependence risk benzodiazepine withdrawal (seizure)	Pregnancy (evidence of human fetal risk); lactation; Concomitant use with ketoconazole or itraconazole.	Opioids, alcohol, barbiturates (additive respiratory depression); fluconazole, indinavir, clarithromycin, fluoxetine (alprazolam tox); digoxin (dig tox); St. John's wort (↓ benzodiazepine effect); sertraline (psychomotor impairment)
Clonazepam (Klonopin)	Adult 0.25–2 mg twice daily; Elderly titrate slowly; Pediatric—not approved	Ataxia, dizziness, somnolence, problem behavior (impaired academic performance, social anxiety, worsening attention with ADHD), URI		Opioids, alcohol, barbiturates (additive respiratory depression); St. John's wort (↓ benzodiazepine effect); amiodarone (clonazepam tox)
Diazepam (Valium)	Adult 2–10 mg two to four times daily; Elderly 2–2.5 mg daily or twice daily, increase slowly; Pediatric 1–2.5 mg three to four times daily increase slowly	Hypotension, muscle weakness, ataxia, somnolence, neutropenia		Opioids, alcohol, barbiturates (additive respiratory depression); St. John's wort (↓ benzodiazepine effect); itraconazole, isoniazid, erythromycin (diazepam tox); phenytoin (↓ phenytoin concentration)
Lorazepam (Ativan)	Adult 1–5 mg twice daily; Elderly 0.5–1 mg twice daily, titrate slowly; Pediatric—not recommended	Weakness, dizziness, sedation, ataxia, delirium, acidosis		Opioids, alcohol, barbiturates (additive respiratory depression); St. John's wort (↓ benzodiazepine effect)
Oxazepam (Serax)	Adult 10–30 mg three to four times daily; Elderly 10–15 mg three to four times daily; Pediatric (<12 yr)—not recommended	Dizziness, headache, somnolence		Same as lorazepam

[a]Available as generic.

ADHD, attention deficit and hyperactivity disorder; CVA, cerebrovascular accident; MAOI, monoamine oxidase inhibitor; MI, myocardial infarction; NSAID, nonsteroidal anti-inflammatory drug; OCD, obsessive compulsive disorder; PPI, proton pump inhibitor; S, syndrome; TCA, tricyclic antidepressant; tox, toxicity; URI, upper respiratory infection.

rank the tricyclic antidepressants below the SSRIs for treatment of anxiety dis-orders because of the SSRIs' more favorable tolerability and safety profiles. (SOR **Ⓐ**) Other antidepressants are effective as well: serotonin norepineph-rine reuptake inhibitors (SNRIs), serotonin antagonist and reuptake inhibi-tors, and noradrenergic and serotonin selective antagonists. When effec-tive in treating anxiety, antidepressants should be maintained for at least 6 months and then tapered slowly to avoid discontinuation-emergent activation of anxiety symptoms. (SOR **Ⓒ**)

SSRIs should be offered first unless there are other considerations. (SOR **Ⓑ**) Number-needed-to-treat is approximately 5. The SSRI paroxetine is effective compared with placebo, as is the SNRI venlafaxine. (SOR **Ⓐ**) Nefazodone (serotonin antagonist and reuptake inhibitor) and mirtazapine (noradrener-gic and serotonin selective antagonist) are also effective. (SOR **Ⓑ**) Imipramine can also be used. (SOR **Ⓒ**) Imipramine dosing starts at 50 to 75 mg per day and is increased every 2 weeks, depending on response, to a maximum of 150 mg per day in divided doses.

(2) Self-help
    (a) Bibliotherapy based on CBT should be offered. (SOR **Ⓐ**)
    (b) Regular exercise can help reduce symptoms. (SOR **Ⓑ**) Elimination of caf-feine and other stimulants may help as well.

B. Panic disorder treatment is directed toward control of symptoms so that the patient can be as functional as possible.
    1. Interventions with evidence of longest duration of effect in descending order are psy-chological treatment, pharmacologic treatments, and self-help.
        a. Psychological treatments. CBT is the psychological treatment of choice. (SOR **Ⓐ**) Combined psychological and pharmacologic therapy in acute treatment is superior to either treatment alone. After acute active treatment, combined treat-ment is better than antidepressant treatment alone and equal to psychological treatment. Either psychological or pharmacologic are acceptable as first-line treat-ments. (SOR **Ⓐ**)
        b. Pharmacologic treatments
            (1) SSRIs are considered the first-line pharmacologic treatment. (SOR **Ⓐ**) They are as effective as benzodiazepines in improving anxiety, have fewer side effects than the alternatives, show no interference with CBT, and provide treatment of concurrent depression. Fluoxetine, 5 to 40 mg per day, is rec-ommended as a single morning dose. The starting dose is 5 mg (2 mg if there is significant insomnia or agitation) with increases weekly. The dose for sertraline is 25 mg per day to start, with a maximum of 200 mg per day. The starting dose for paroxetine is 10 mg per day, with a maximum of 50 mg per day. Fluvoxamine starts at 25 mg twice a day, with a maximum of 150 mg twice a day. The dose of escitalopram is most often 10 mg per day. The starting dose of citalopram is 20 mg per day, with a maximum of 60 mg per day. Full response occurs after a minimum of 4 weeks and can take up to 8 to 12 weeks. Relapse is common. (SOR **Ⓐ**) Treatment should continue for at least 6 months (SOR **Ⓐ**) and up to 12 to 24 months (SOR **Ⓑ**) with slow discontinuation over 4 to 6 months.
            (2) The tricyclic antidepressants, imipramine and clomipramine, are effective agents. (SOR **Ⓐ**) Imipramine, 150 to 00 mg per day, is recommended as a single bedtime dose. The starting dose is 50 to 100 mg per day, which can be increased every 2 weeks until an optimum response or maximum dose is reached. Desipramine is sometimes better tolerated by patients than imipramine.
            (3) Benzodiazepines can be useful for acute, short-term symptom control. Alprazolam and clonazepam provide effective rapid relief, but relapse is high when discontinued. (SOR **Ⓐ**) Benzodiazepines produce long-term out-comes that are less effective than those of the antidepressants and should not be prescribed routinely. (SOR **Ⓐ**) Other disadvantages of using benzodiaz-epines are that nearly half of patients with panic disorder have concurrent major depression that is not helped by benzodiazepines; benzodiazepines have a high abuse potential, and are more difficult to taper than are tricyclic antidepressants. Gradual tapering of the dose is recommended when discon-tinuing treatment. (SOR **Ⓑ**) CBT may facilitate tapering. (SOR **Ⓑ**)

(a) Self-help
    (1) Bibliotherapy based on CBT principles is effective. (SOR **A**)
    (2) Exercise may help control symptoms. (SOR **B**)
C. Treatment of phobia requires commitment on the part of the patient and clear identification of the phobic object or situation.
    1. Behavioral treatment techniques are the most effective, with systematic exposure therapy to the feared situation/object. (SOR **A**) A cognitive strategy of suggesting new ways of thinking about the phobic object or situation may be used in addition to muscle relaxation techniques. CBT, exposure to feared situation, and group approaches are effective for social phobia. (SOR **A**)
    2. Pharmacologic therapy
        a. Beta-blockers such as propranolol can be useful for specific performance anxiety (SOR **B**) just prior to direct challenge to the phobic situation. Propranolol, 10 to 20 mg 45 to 60 minutes before exposure to the phobic object, or up to 40 mg, is usually effective.
        b. SSRIs are effective first-line treatments for social phobia (SOR **A**) with paroxetine the most studied. Fluvoxamine and sertraline may be of use, particularly in patients with social phobia.
D. PTSD treatment consists primarily of psychotherapy, but there is growing evidence for a role of pharmacotherapy when the patient has symptoms of depression or a panic-like disorder. Consider psychiatry referral for these patients.
    1. Trauma-focused CBT, stress management, and group trauma-focused CBT are effective (SOR **A**) and should be continued for 6 months. (SOR **A**) Treatment should not be initiated and continued only in the primary care setting. (SOR **C**) Time-limited psychotherapy uses cognitive and supportive approaches to minimize the risk of dependency and chronicity. The patient is encouraged to garner support from friends and relatives; to review emotional feelings associated with the event; to consciously re-enact the event through imagination, words, or actions; and to plan for future recovery. Group and family therapies have been particularly effective.
    2. SSRIs are effective (SOR **A**) and should be continued at least 12 months. (SOR **A**)
IV. Management Strategies
    A. GAD. Patient education about the disorder and the scheduling of frequent, short office visits are the physician's primary responsibilities. Listening carefully to the patient's account of problems is very beneficial. Specific management techniques include being supportive of patient choices, expanding coping strategies, normalizing symptoms through reassurance, encouraging confrontation of anxiety-provoking situations, and being available for brief clinical encounters.
    B. Panic disorder. Patients with panic disorder should be reassured that they have a treatable condition. The patient's somatic symptoms should be discussed in such a way as to avoid the attachment of any stigma to the patient. Eliciting the patient's explanation of the symptoms and goals for treatment is crucial. Panic-focused CBT and medications are effective treatments for panic disorder. There is no evidence that one is superior to the other so the choice between psychotherapy and pharmacotherapy depends on the efficacy, benefits, risks, and the patient's personal preferences.
    C. Phobias. The goal of therapy is for the affected person to discover that the feared situation is not as much of a threat as previously thought. Avoidance should be discouraged, and behavioral techniques should be used until the phobic object or situation has been fully confronted. Hypnosis may be used as an adjunct method of relaxation and as a method of offering alternative cognitive appraisals of the phobic object. Family therapy may be particularly useful in this condition.
    D. PTSD. Physicians caring for patients with this disorder must deal effectively with suspicion, paranoia, and mistrust on the part of the patient. Gentle confrontation is necessary to overcome the patient's denial of the traumatic event and to encourage the individual to remain in the treatment program of therapy and medications. Groups of individuals suffering similar events, such as assault self-help groups, can also be useful. Hospitalization may be necessary if the patient is suicidal or a danger to others.
V. Prognosis
    A. GAD is a chronic condition with a typical duration of illness just over 10 years. Affected individuals usually respond to treatment, but relapse after withdrawal of treatment may occur in as many as 80% of patients, nearly 25% of whom may go on to develop panic disorder.

B. Panic disorder is a chronic, remitting, and relapsing condition that is often precipitated by stressful life events. In one study, at 5-year follow-up, 30% of affected patients were moderately to severely impaired, and 50% were mildly impaired; at 20-year follow-up, 15% had moderate-to-severe symptoms, and 70% had mild symptoms with no disability. Between 30% and 70% of patients experience a major depressive disorder subsequent to the onset of the panic attacks. These individuals are at an increased risk for suicide, alcohol and drug dependence, and obsessive–compulsive disorder. Once an effective drug dose is achieved, the medication should be continued unchanged for 6 to 12 months. At that time, medication is slowly tapered. Drug treatment should be reinstituted if symptoms return. Patients with good function prior to development of symptoms of brief duration tend to have a better prognosis.

C. Phobias beginning in childhood can resolve without treatment, but others may become chronic. Those that are chronic in nature seem to increase after middle age. Most affected individuals experience little disability, since the phobic object or situation can usually be easily avoided.

D. PTSD. The full syndrome can develop from 1 week to as long as 30 or more years after the traumatic event. Symptoms fluctuate with exacerbations during periods of stress. Individuals with a good prognosis usually have rapid onset of symptoms, symptoms of less than 6 months' duration, good functioning before the onset of the syndrome, strong social support, and the absence of any other medical or emotional disorders. Over time, 10% of affected patients remain unchanged or become worse, 20% have moderate symptoms, 40% have mild symptoms, and 30% recover.

SELECTED REFERENCES

American Psychiatric Association (APA). *Diagnostic and Statistical Manual of Mental Disorders.* 5th ed. Arlington, VA: APA; 2013.

Bisson J, Andrew M. Psychological treatment of post-traumatic stress disorder (PTSD). *Cochrane Database Syst Rev.* 2005;(2):CD003388.

Chessick CA, Allen MH, Thase ME, et al. Azapirones for generalized anxiety disorder. *Cochrane Database Systematic Rev.* 2006;(3):CD006115.

Congressional Budget Office. The Veterans Health Administration's treatment of PTSD and traumatic brain injury among recent combat veterans. 2012. http://www.cbo.gov/sites/default/files/cbofiles/attachments/02-09-PTSD.pdf. Accessed May 2013.

Furukawa TA, Watanabe N, Churchill R. Combined psychotherapy plus antidepressants for panic disorder with or without agoraphobia. *Cochrane Database Syst Rev.* 2009;(1):CD004364.

Gillies D, Taylor F, Gray C, et al. Psychological therapies for the treatment of post-traumatic stress disorder in children and adolescents. *Cochrane Database Syst Rev.* 2012;(12):CD006726.

Hambrick JP, Weeks JW, Harb GC, Heimberg RG. Cognitive-behavioral therapy for social anxiety disorder: supporting evidence and future directions. *CNS Spectr.* 2003;8(5):373–381.

Kapczinski F, Lima MS, Souza JS, et al. Antidepressants for generalized anxiety disorder. *Cochrane Database Syst Rev.* 2003;(2):CD003592.

Lepola U, Arató M, Zhu Y, Austin C. Sertraline versus imipramine treatment of comorbid panic disorder and major depressive disorder. *J Clin Psychiatry.* 2003;64(6):654–662.

Marchesi C. Pharmacological management of panic disorder. *Neuropsychiatr Dis Treat.* 2008; 4(1):93–106.

McHugh RK, Smits JA, Otto MW. Empirically supported treatments for panic disorder. *Psychiatr Clin North Am.* 2009;32(3):593–610.

McIntosh A, Cohen A, Turnbull N, et al. *Clinical guidelines for the management of anxiety. Management of anxiety (panic disorder, with or without agoraphobia, and generalised anxiety disorder) in adults in primary, secondary and community care.* London, UK: National Institute for Clinical Excellence (NICE); 2004: 165p. [151 references].

Quilty LC, Van Ameringen M, Mancini C, et al. Quality of life and the anxiety disorders. *J Anxiety Disord.* 2003;17(4):405–426.

Resick PA, Nishith P, Griffin MG. How well does cognitive-behavioral therapy treat symptoms of complex PTSD? An examination of child sexual abuse survivors within a clinical trial. *CNS Spectr.* 2003; 8(5):340–355.

Rose S, Bisson J, Churchill R, Wessely S. Psychological debriefing for preventing post traumatic stress disorder (PTSD). *Cochrane Database Syst Rev.* 2002;(2):CD000560.

Singapore Ministry of Health, National Medical Research Council. *Anxiety Disorders.* Singapore: Singapore Ministry of Health; 2003: 69p. [74 references].

Solvason HB, Ernst H, Roth W. Predictors of response in anxiety disorders. *Psychiatr Clin North Am.* 2003;26(2):411–433.

Stein DJ. Algorithm for the pharmacotherapy of anxiety disorders. *Curr Psychiatry Rep.* 2003; 5(4):282–288.

Stein DJ, Ipser JC, Seedat S. Pharmacotherapy for post traumatic stress disorder (PTSD). *Cochrane Database Systematic Rev.* 2006;(1):CD002795.

CLINICAL GUIDELINES

American Psychiatric Association (APA). *Practice guideline for the treatment of patients with panic disorder.* Washington, DC: American Psychiatric Press; 1998: 86p. [273 references].

Institute For Clinical Systems Improvement (ICSI). Major depression, panic disorder and generalized anxiety disorder in adults in primary care. Institute For Clinical Systems Improvement (ICSI) (Bloomington, Minnesota); 2002;55p. [108 references].

Work Group on Panic Disorder. American Psychiatric Association (APA). Practice guideline for the treatment of patients with panic disorder. *Am J Psychiatry.* 1998;155(5 suppl):1–34. [273 references].

WEB SITES

http://www.cdc.gov/mentalheealth/basics/burden.htm
http://www.nlm.nih.gov/medlineplus/anxiety.html
http://www.nlm.nih.gov/medlineplus/panicdisorder.html
http://www.nlm.nih.gov/medlineplus/phobias.html
http://www.nlm.nih.gov/medlineplus/posttraumaticstressdisorder.html
http://www.surgeongeneral.gov/library/mentalhealth/chapter4/sec2.html

---

92   Attention Deficit Hyperactivity Disorder

H. Russell Searight, PhD, MPH, Jennifer Gafford, PhD, & Stephanie L. Evans, PharmD, BCPS

KEY POINTS

- Attention deficit hyperactivity disorder (ADHD) has three core symptom clusters: inattention, hyperactivity, and impulsivity. (SOR **C**)
- Among US children, current prevalence rates are 6% to 8%. (SOR **C**)
- Approximately 80% of children diagnosed with ADHD continue to manifest symptoms in adolescence, with 60% meeting diagnostic criteria in adulthood. (SOR **B**)
- Common comorbid psychiatric conditions include oppositional defiant and conduct disorder. (SOR **C**)
- Evaluating suspected ADHD includes a history and physical examination, detailed clinical interview, behavioral ratings, and on occasion, referral for specialized assessment. (SOR **C**)
- Stimulant pharmacotherapy continues to be the most common treatment. (SOR **A**) However, there are several nonstimulant medication options.

I. Introduction

A. Overview of condition. Attention deficit hyperactivity disorder (ADHD) is a common neurobehavioral disorder beginning in childhood that typically continues through adulthood and is characterized by chronic, pervasive inattention, hyperactivity–impulsivity, or both, that is inconsistent with the patient's developmental level. ADHD adversely affects cognitive, academic, behavioral, emotional, and social functioning.

    1. The initial diagnosis is typically made between the ages of 6 and 10 years, when symptoms of hyperactivity and impulsivity tend to peak. Inattention remains stable through the lifespan.

    2. Although children may begin to develop ADHD symptoms as early as age 3 years, diagnoses of ADHD made during preschool years are unreliable. Approximately half of these individuals will no longer meet criteria by age 5 years while fewer than 10% of nondiagnosed 3-year-olds manifest the condition 2 years later. However, diagnoses made between ages 4 and 6 years, particularly of more severe forms of the condition, are associated with persistent symptoms later in childhood. The clinical practice guideline of the American Academy of Pediatrics states that primary care providers should initiate an evaluation for ADHD for any child 4 to 18 years of age who presents with academic or behavioral problems and symptoms of inattention, hyperactivity, or impulsivity. (SOR **Ⓑ**)

3. Approximately 60% to 75% of children with ADHD continue to exhibit symptoms into adulthood.

4. ADHD is often comorbid with other conditions including learning disabilities, speech and language disorders, oppositional defiant disorder, conduct disorder, mood disorders, anxiety disorders, sleep disorders, and Tourette syndrome. Adolescents and young adults with ADHD are at particular risk for substance abuse.

5. ADHD is frequently associated with substantial impairments such as low self-esteem, rejection by peers and adults, workplace difficulties, elevated risk of accidental injury, and academic underachievement.

B. Epidemiology. ADHD is among the leading reasons school-age children in the United States are referred to mental health practitioners. As one of the most widespread childhood psychiatric disorders, the rate of ADHD in the general population is estimated to be 9% of males and 3% females. Rates vary, however, depending on the population studied, the geographic region under investigation, the definition of ADHD employed, and the degree of agreement required among parents, teachers, and professionals. In fact, prevalence estimates range between 1% and 20% depending on these factors. The Center for Disease Control and Prevention (CDC) data indicate fairly substantial increases (e.g., 30% to 40%) in reported prevalence in the past 10 years. As discussed later, the change in symptom onset and reduced number of symptoms evident in two or more settings defined in the fifth edition of the Diagnostic and Statistical Manual of Mental Disorders (DSM-5) is likely to lead to further increases in prevalence rates.

1. ADHD occurs two to four times more commonly in boys than in girls for the predominantly inattentive and predominantly hyperactive-impulsive subtypes, respectively. In clinical populations, the ratio of males to females is estimated to be as high as 9:1 because of referral biases.

2. Based on recent epidemiologic data, prevalence rates of ADHD in adults is approximately 4%.

3. Rates of ADHD appear to vary as a function of socioeconomic status (SES), with women from lower-SES groups having a slightly higher incidence of ADHD in their offspring.

4. Compared with children of white European background, African-American and Hispanic children exhibiting comparable levels of inattention and overactivity are less likely to be diagnosed with ADHD. Explanations for these differences vary and include economic disadvantage, health care access, and racial bias. Studies of school teachers indicate that the explanatory label of ADHD is more likely to be applied to overactive white children while Hispanic and African-American children exhibiting hyperactivity are seen as experiencing parenting problems or cognitive impairment.

C. Etiology. While there is considerable evidence of a neurophysiologic etiology, at the specific biologic mechanisms are not entirely clear. Children born to parents with at least six genes influencing dopamine, serotonin, and norepinephrine along with several novel candidate genes have a hereditary predisposition. Neuroanatomical findings include reduced gray matter volume and a smaller corpus callosum. In some patients, sustained stimulant therapy is associated with normalization of these structures. Allergens and environmental toxins do not appear to play a role in the development of the disorder.

D. Risk factors. A number of risk factors have been identified for the development of ADHD. Immunizations, however, are not associated with the risk of developing ADHD.

1. A family history of ADHD is a major risk factor. The mean heritability for ADHD among children was found to be 77% with corresponding figures of 40% for adolescents and 30% for adults.

2. Pre- and perinatal risk factors include younger maternal age, smoking and/or alcohol use during pregnancy, premature delivery, low birth weight, and other delivery complications. Parental factors include maternal depression and paternal antisocial behavior.

3. Children with ADHD who are very active and demanding, coupled with maternal psychological distress and family dysfunction, exhibit symptoms of ADHD that are more persistent into later childhood and often comorbid with oppositional behaviors.

II. Diagnosis

A. Primary features of ADHD include inattention, hyperactivity, and impulsivity (behavioral disinhibition). Deficient rule-governed behavior and variability in sustained-task performance can be considered core features as well.

1. Inattention refers to problems with alertness, arousal, selectivity, attention, and distractibility, which tend to be most evident in situations in which individuals are required to sustain attention to repetitive and monotonous tasks. Children and adolescents with attentional problems are commonly described by parents and teachers as "not listening to instructions," "off task," "daydreaming," and "becoming bored easily." Adults may be perceived by spouses and coworkers as forgetful, disorganized, unmotivated, or irresponsible because of chronic issues with lateness, missed deadlines, or careless errors.

2. Hyperactivity across multiple settings is the most classic, distinguishing feature of ADHD. Described by parents and teachers as "in constant motion," "driven by a motor," and "extremely talkative," children and adolescents with ADHD are thought to be deficient in their ability to regulate their activity level to the particular setting or task demands. While the motor activity may become less obvious in adolescence and adulthood, restlessness, fidgeting and excessive speech and interrupting conversations often persist. Hyperactivity tends to be the most socially problematic feature for children with ADHD because it tends to be disruptive in situations such as the classroom.

3. Impulsivity, or behavioral disinhibition, is also socially problematic for individuals with ADHD, especially in situations in which patience, cooperation, and restraint are required. Poor planning and impulsivity often persist into adulthood. Clinically, these individuals appear to respond quickly to situations without waiting for instructions or considering consequences. Adults may make important decisions without considering long-term implications. As children, adolescents, or adults, these individuals are characterized by poor delay of gratification, poor behavioral inhibition, and high risk-taking behavior.

B. Other core features

1. Difficulty with rule-governed behavior may be another primary deficit of individuals with ADHD. Failing to follow through with instructions or to comply with rules is a common problem, particularly in situations in which directions are not explicit or supervision is limited. Individuals with ADHD do not necessarily refuse to follow rules and directions; it is more a problem of behavioral self-regulation or sustaining response to rules or commands.

2. Individuals with ADHD also tend to show high variability in task performance, particularly during childhood and adolescence. While a certain amount of behavioral inconsistency is not uncommon, individuals with ADHD exhibit this fluctuation to a much greater degree.

C. ADHD tends to be associated with a variety of other problems in addition to the primary features of inattention, hyperactivity, and impulsivity.

1. Children and adolescents with ADHD often exhibit behavior problems such as noncompliance, argumentativeness, and temper outbursts.

2. Emotional functioning tends to be impaired in individuals with ADHD including low self-esteem, reduced tolerance for frustration, and symptoms of depression or anxiety (or both).

3. Interpersonal relationships are affected as well. Children and adolescents with ADHD may be neglected or rejected by peers, and adults can experience increased interpersonal conflict. Family relationships may be complicated by frequent discord and negative interactions.

4. Academic performance as well as cognitive and language abilities represent other areas of difficulty for children and adolescents with ADHD. They are typically underachievers in school and frequently exhibit learning disabilities with reading difficulties being the most common. As a whole, children and adolescents with ADHD score lower on standardized intelligence tests compared with normal controls and exhibit more difficulty on complex problem solving tasks. Adults with ADHD have histories of attaining less formal education as well as poorer occupational performance and lower employment status and attendance. (SOR **Ⓑ**)

5. Children and adolescents with ADHD tend to experience medical and health problems more commonly than normal controls. These include physical injuries, minor physical anomalies, sleep disturbances, and ear and respiratory infections. (SOR **Ⓑ**) Traffic accidents and violations are more frequent in adolescents and adults with ADHD than in the general population. (SOR **Ⓑ**)

D. DSM-5 criteria for ADHD require that six or more symptoms of inattention, hyperactivity–impulsivity, or both, are present for at least 6 months, and that the symptoms are inconsistent with developmental level. For individuals 17 years and older, the symptom requirement is reduced to five, or for the combined presentation, 10. There must be clear evidence that the symptoms interfere with, or reduce the quality of, social, academic, or occupational functioning. Several symptoms must be present before the age of 12 years and noted in two or more settings. The symptoms should not be better accounted for by another mental disorder, nor should they solely reflect a manifestation of oppositional behavior, defiance, hostility, or failure to understand tasks and activities.

1. Inattention

   a. Often fails to give close attention to details or makes careless mistakes in schoolwork, at work, or during other activities (e.g., overlooks or misses details, work is inaccurate).

   b. Often has difficulty in sustaining attention in tasks or play activities (e.g., has difficulty remaining focused during lectures, conversations, or lengthy reading).

   c. Often does not seem to listen when spoken to directly (e.g., mind seems elsewhere, even in the absence of any obvious distraction).

   d. Often does not follow through on instructions and fails to finish schoolwork, chores, or duties in the workplace (e.g., starts tasks but quickly loses focus and is easily sidetracked).

   e. Often has difficulty organizing tasks and activities (e.g., difficulty managing sequential tasks; difficulty keeping materials and belongings in order; messy, disorganized work; has poor time management; fails to meet deadlines).

   f. Often avoids, dislikes, or is reluctant to engage in tasks that require sustained mental effort (e.g., schoolwork or homework; for older adolescents and adults, preparing reports, completing forms, reviewing lengthy papers).

   g. Often loses things necessary for tasks or activities (e.g., school materials, pencils, books, tools, wallets, keys, paperwork, eyeglasses, mobile telephones).

   h. Is often easily distracted by extraneous stimuli (for older adolescents and adults, may include unrelated thoughts).

   i. Is often forgetful in daily activities (e.g., doing chores, running errands; for older adolescents and adults, returning calls, paying bills, keeping appointments).

2. Hyperactivity–impulsivity

   a. Often fidgets with or taps hands or feet or squirms in seat.

   b. Often leaves seat in situations when remaining seated is expected (e.g., leaves his or her place in the classroom, in the office or other workplace, or in other situations that require remaining in place).

   c. Often runs about or climbs excessively in situations in which it is inappropriate (Note: in adolescents or adults, may be limited to feeling restless).

   d. Often unable to play or engage in leisure activities quietly.

   e. Is often "on the go," acting as if "driven by a motor" (e.g., is unable to be or uncomfortable being still for an extended time as in restaurants or meetings; may be experienced by others as being restless or difficult to keep up with).

   f. Often talks excessively.

   g. Often blurts out answers before a question has been completed (e.g., completes other people's sentences; cannot wait for their turn in conversation).

   h. Often has difficulty in awaiting his or her turn (e.g., while waiting in line).

   i. Often interrupts or intrudes on others (e.g., butts into conversations, games, or activities, starts using other people's things without asking or receiving permission; for adolescents and adults, may intrude into or take over what others are doing).

E. ADHD diagnoses in the DSM-5 are also specified according to the severity of current symptoms, remission of symptoms, and symptom presentation.

   1. Severity specifiers are a new feature of the DSM-5, a relevant distinction in terms of clinical outcomes among individuals with ADHD.

   a. Mild. A few, if any, symptoms in excess of those required to make the diagnosis are present and symptoms result in no more than minor impairments in social or occupational functioning (e.g., ADHD, combined presentation, mild).

   b. Moderate. Symptoms or functional impairment between "mild" and "severe" are present (e.g., ADHD, combined presentation, moderate).

   c. Severe. Many symptoms in excess of those required to make the diagnosis, or several symptoms that are particularly severe, are present or the symptoms result in marked impairment in social or occupational functioning (e.g. ADHD, combined presentation, severe).

2. **In partial remission** is specified when full criteria were previously met, fewer than the full criteria have been met for the past 6 months, and current symptoms still result in impairment in social, academic, or occupational functioning (e.g., ADHD, combined presentation, in partial remission).

3. **Symptom presentation**

   a. **ADHD, combined presentation** represents the most common ADHD diagnosis, accounting for 50% to 75% of ADHD individuals. Youths with the combined type have features of both inattention and hyperactivity–impulsivity; they also exhibit more co-occurring psychiatric and substance abuse disorders and are the most impaired overall compared to the other subtypes. Children with this subtype are commonly diagnosed at 6 to 7 years of age when symptoms of hyperactivity and impulsivity begin to peak.

   b. **ADHD, predominantly inattentive presentation** is the next most common group, accounting for 20% to 30% of individuals with ADHD. Symptoms of inattention are present without associated hyperactivity and impulsivity. This diagnosis is often made somewhat later, at the age of 9 or 10 years, when symptoms of inattention typically become more noticeable. The age of onset criteria has been increased from 7 to 12 years in the DSM-5 compared to the DSM-IV, allowing these individuals to be more easily captured diagnostically. Compared with the other subtypes, individuals with predominant inattention are more likely to be female and have fewer other emotional and behavioral problems. However, they tend to have greater academic impairment than those with only hyperactivity-impulsivity.

   c. **ADHD, predominantly hyperactive-impulsive presentation** accounts for <15% of ADHD diagnoses and describes a subset of individuals with symptoms of hyperactivity and impulsivity without inattention. Children with this subtype are also often diagnosed at approximately 6 to 7 years of age.

F. **Changes from the DSM-IV to the DSM-5**

   1. **Maximum age of onset was increased** from 7 to 12 years in the DSM-5; a systematic research review did not support use of age 7 years as a cutoff.

   2. **More developmentally sensitive examples,** particularly for adults, were provided in the DSM-5 criteria, and the **required symptoms were reduced** from 6 to 5 for each presentation. A major difficulty with the former criteria was that they were most applicable to children between the ages of 7 and 12 years, and there was little evidence supporting the requirement of six symptoms for a diagnosis in adolescence and adulthood. (SOR **C**)

   3. A diagnosis of ADHD in the DSM-5 requires the **presence of some features (rather than 6) in each of two or more settings**. Determining whether symptoms are present in two or more settings is often difficult because of different interpretations of behavioral characteristics by different observers. Inter-rater agreement coefficients for behavior ratings between parents and teachers, for example, are often <0.50. Ratings between parents differ as well, with coefficients typically <0.6 or 0.7.

   4. The diagnostic process reflected in the DSM-5 **better addresses the issue of functional impairment by requiring severity specifiers**. The former diagnostic process was heavily weighted toward meeting a specified number of symptoms with far less attention paid to the degree of functional impairment. As a result, patients demonstrating long-standing, pervasive inattention and distractibility that substantially impairs social and work relationships, but having no other symptoms, would not, by DSM-IV standards, have received the diagnosis of ADHD.

   5. **Greater attention is given to comorbidity** versus differential diagnoses in the DSM-5. Symptoms of ADHD overlap with many other disorders, often making it difficult to determine whether symptoms of other disorders are mimicking ADHD or comorbid with ADHD.

   6. **DSM-5 contains an altered NOS category** including three separate distinctions for ADHD symptoms that are clinically significant but do not meet full criteria. It is not yet clear how this change will affect the rate of atypical diagnoses from the DSM-IV to the DSM-5.

      a. Other Specified ADHD, with Insufficient Inattention Symptoms applies when symptoms of inattention predominate and significantly interfere with adaptive behavioral functioning but do not meet full criteria for the disorder.

    b. Other Specified ADHD, with Insufficient Hyperactivity/Impulsivity Symptoms applies when hyperactive-impulsive features predominate but the clinical picture does not meet full criteria for diagnosis.

    c. Unspecified ADHD is applied when there is insufficient information available to make a diagnosis, but features of inattention and/or hyperactivity-impulsivity cause clinically significant impairment in functioning.

G. Variations in symptom presentation through the lifespan. Symptoms of inattention, hyperactivity, and impulsivity peak at different ages, decline with age at different rates, and manifest differently depending on the individual's level of development. As a result, ADHD presents differently from preschool through adulthood.

    1. Preschool. Many children begin to exhibit symptoms of ADHD in preschool, as early as 3 to 4 years of age. However, it is often difficult to differentiate ADHD in preschool children from other discipline problems at this age; some children have simply never learned limits or experienced appropriate and consistent consequences for misbehavior. Preschool children with ADHD tend to show predominantly features of hyperactivity and impulsivity. Symptoms of inattention tend to peak several years later and are less apparent during the preschool years.

    2. Late childhood/adolescence. By adolescence, features of hyperactivity have declined steadily while symptoms of inattention and impulsivity continue to be problematic. Individuals with the predominantly inattentive subtype may have only recently been diagnosed with ADHD because of the later symptom expression.

        Comorbidity increases dramatically in adolescents with ADHD, to the extent that "pure" ADHD may be the exception rather than the rule by this age. (SOR ❸) Problems that tend to be associated with ADHD include poor academic performance, affective disorders, school suspensions, expulsions, cigarette and alcohol use, illicit drug use, aggressive behavior, and conduct problems. Adolescents with ADHD who are untreated, poorly supervised, and in an environment in which alcohol and other illicit substances are readily available appear to be at the highest risk for negative outcomes. (SOR ❻)

    3. Adults. The symptom picture is likely to be more subtle in adults than in children. Deficits in executive function tend to be most salient, including poor organization, poor time management, and memory disturbance, which can be associated with academic and occupational failure. The "hyperactivity" of childhood may be replaced by experiences of restlessness, difficulty relaxing, and feeling chronically "on edge." Patients with impulsivity or behavioral disinhibition may be unable to prevent immediate responding and have deficits in their capacity for monitoring their behavior and modulating emotional intensity.

H. Differential diagnosis

    1. Medical conditions. While psychiatric conditions are more common differential diagnoses, some medical conditions can present with ADHD-like symptoms. Vision and hearing should be routinely screened among children.

        a. An audiologic condition that may appear similar to the inattentive subtype of ADHD-inattentive type is **auditory processing disorder (APD)**. APD, typically diagnosed by audiologists, is a deficit in comprehending or tracking information presented through auditory channels despite normal hearing. APD can arise from deficits in underlying functions such as auditory discrimination, pattern recognition, and management of competing input.

        b. Cognitive deficits such as mental retardation and fetal alcohol or drug syndrome can be confused with ADHD. Elevated lead levels can also be associated with cognitive impairment and hyperactivity.

        c. Thyroid disturbance may affect activity and secondarily, attention, and concentration.

        d. Drugs. Cognition and motor activity can be altered pharmacologically. For example, anabolic steroids commonly used by athletes are associated with impulsive aggression while the anticonvulsant, phenytoin, often results in cognitive inefficiency.

        e. Seizure disorders, particularly convulsive status epilepticus, produce cognitive impairment similar to the inattention seen in ADHD.

        f. Sleep disorders. Among adolescents and adults, obstructive sleep apnea may impair attention, concentration, and short-term recall. Adults with other sleep disorders such as narcolepsy and idiopathic hypersomnia commonly report impaired attention. Further complicating the picture is that children and adults with ADHD have a particularly high incidence of sleep disorders.

TABLE 92–1. DIFFERENTIAL DIAGNOSIS OF PEDIATRIC ADHD

Condition	Commonly Shared Features	Distinctive Features
Conduct disorder	Disruptive, impulsive behavior	Severe rule violations, illegal acts, significant aggression
Oppositional defiant disorder	Disruptive behavior annoying to others, noncompliant with adult requests	Argumentative, negativistic, irritable
Learning disabilities	Poor academic performance; may appear off task in classroom	Academic skills significantly below level expected for IQ
Major depression	Impaired attention and concentration, initial insomnia	Hypersomnia/terminal insomnia, appetite/weight disturbance, pervasive dysphoric/irritable mood, suicidal ideation
Bipolar disorder	High activity level, distractibility cyclic mood variation	Delusions, pronounced insomnia, widely fluctuating mood
Disruptive Mood Dysregulation Disorder	Severe and frequent temper outbursts, irritability	Frequency and intensity of explosive behavior, persistent irritability or anger

2. **Psychiatric conditions.** Many pediatric and adult psychiatric conditions feature impulsivity and impaired attention, concentration, and impaired short-term memory as commonly associated symptoms. The diagnosis of ADHD is complicated by conditions appearing similar to ADHD that also are part of the differential diagnosis. These psychiatric disorders are challenging because they are often comorbid with ADHD. Pediatric and adult patients will be discussed separately.

   a. **Pediatric conditions.** Table 92–1 summarizes common psychiatric conditions that are part of the differential diagnosis of childhood ADHD, including features shared with ADHD as well as distinguishing symptoms.

   (1) Childhood ADHD is a risk factor for developing other psychiatric conditions. More than 40% of children with ADHD have at least one other disorder, with approximately 30% having two comorbid psychiatric conditions. Developmentally, rates of comorbidity increase with age. For example, up to 40% of ADHD adolescents may also have oppositional defiant or conduct disorder.

   (2) Conversely, while controversial, up to 90% of children diagnosed with bipolar disorder have comorbid ADHD. DSM-5 has introduced a new diagnosis, disruptive mood dysregulation disorder, which is believed to be more a valid syndrome for children exhibiting bipolar features.

   b. **Adult conditions.** While the differential diagnosis of adult ADHD (Table 92–2) includes some of the same conditions as in childhood, symptoms of both ADHD

TABLE 92–2. DIFFERENTIAL DIAGNOSIS OF ADULT ADHD

Condition	Commonly Shared Features	Distinctive Features
Major depression	Subjective report of poor concentration, attention, and memory (often not supported by objective data), difficulty with task completion	Enduring dysphoric mood or anhedonia, sleep and appetite disturbance
Bipolar disorder	Hyperactivity, difficulty with maintaining attention; distractibility	Enduring dysphoric or euphoric mood, insomnia, delusions
General anxiety	Fidgetiness, difficulty concentrating	Exaggerated apprehension and worry, somatic symptoms of anxiety
Substance abuse or dependence	Difficulties with attention, concentration, and memory; mood swings	Pathologic pattern of substance use with social consequences, physiologic and psychologic tolerance and withdrawal
Personality disorders, particularly borderline and antisocial personality	Impulsivity, affective lability	Arrest history (antisocial personality), repeated self-injurious or suicidal behavior (borderline personality), lack of recognition that behavior is self-defeating

Source: Data adapted from Searight HR, Burke JM, Rottnek F. Adult AD/HD: evaluation and treatment in family medicine. *Am Fam Physician.* 2000;62:2077, 2091.

TABLE 92–3. EVALUATION PROCESS FOR SUSPECTED ADHD

Typically, at initial office visit
1. Diagnostic interview
2. Medical history and physical examination
3. Any indicated laboratory tests
4. Behavioral rating forms to teachers, parents, other collateral informants, and with adults, to patients themselves
5. Review of behavior ratings and other relevant documents (e.g., report cards)

Typically, at follow-up office visit
6. Mental status evaluation (possible continuous performance testing)
7. If indicated, referral for specialized psychological or educational testing
8. If ADHD, institute treatment
9. If other conditions are present, refer for mental health or educational intervention (or both)

and other psychiatric syndromes vary with age. Adult ADHD symptoms are more subtle than those in children. While some adults with ADHD will have an established diagnosis from early childhood, many patients will be seeking assistance for the first time as adults. Up to two-thirds of adults self-referred for inattention, distractibility, and impulsivity actually have a different primary psychiatric condition.

I. Process of diagnosis in primary care (Table 92–3)

  1. Thorough diagnostic interview. Parents should be encouraged to describe their concerns about their child in an open-ended manner. Physicians should carefully listen for core symptoms of ADHD versus those of other psychiatric conditions. Examples of specific behavior concerns should be elicited. The duration and degree of functional impairment should also be assessed. Parents should be asked when they initially noticed symptoms. Fluctuation or variability in symptoms according to time of day or setting should also be noted. A detailed developmental history is also important, with particular attention to specific milestones and the initial appearance and course of ADHD symptoms.

  2. Medical history and physical examination. A history of ADHD symptoms in all biologic relatives should be elicited. ADHD risk factors are discussed in Section I.D. During the physical examination, the physician may note multiple scars and abrasions among children with ADHD because of their impulsivity.

  3. Laboratory tests. Blood chemistry should be obtained with particular attention to abnormal thyroid function and elevated serum lead levels. While most children with ADHD have normal laboratory results, these tests can exclude other causes for symptoms.

  4. Behavioral rating forms. Standardized behavioral rating forms should be given to the parents and teachers to complete. Commonly used pediatric scales are classified into broadband measures, assessing a number of psychiatric conditions, versus narrowband instruments, assessing only externalizing behavioral problems such as ADHD, oppositional defiant disorder, and conduct disorder. Because adult ADHD symptoms, when taken individually, are nonspecific and can be associated with a range of medical and psychiatric conditions, these rating scales should be used with caution. While these measures have high sensitivity, their specificity is relatively modest. Physicians should use these completed scales as a guide for the clinical interview.

    a. The Child Behavior Check List (CBCL) and the longer Conners Parent and Teacher Rating Scales assess a wide range of psychiatric symptoms. More narrowly focused instruments include the Conners-Short Forms, the Disruptive Behavior Disorder (DBD) Scale, and the NICHQ Vanderbilt Assessment Scale. The parent and teacher forms of the Vanderbilt Assessment Scale are included in the National Initiative for Children's Healthcare Quality (NICHQ) ADHD toolkit. In addition to the ADHD features, the Vanderbilt scales include disruptive behavioral symptoms, anxiety and depressive symptoms, and questions about academic performance.

    b. With adults, the following questions are often helpful as an initial screen for ADHD: *Were you ever diagnosed with ADHD as a child?, Do any first-degree members of your family have ADHD?, and Do you have a lifelong history of chronic distractibility, inattention, and/or disorganization?* If the patient responds yes to any of these questions, a more formal screening measure is recommended.

      (1) The Conners' Adult ADHD Rating Scale (CAARS) and the Adult Self Report Scale (ASRS-v1.1) are used to assess current symptoms. The CAARS is a self-report measure but can also be administered to a collateral informant such as a spouse, parent, or close friend. The CAARS assesses hyperactivity, impulsivity, emotional lability, attention/memory, and self-concept. The ASRS, developed through the World Health Organization, assesses the 18 DSM-IV-TR ADHD symptoms. A six-item version, intended for brief screening in primary care, was derived from the items most predictive of an ADHD diagnosis.

   c. In reviewing completed rating scales, the physician should distinguish core symptoms of ADHD such as inattention, distractibility, and impulsivity from other problem behaviors. Extreme ratings, particularly when they suggest significant levels of broadband symptomatology, should be viewed with caution. While these extreme profiles suggest a significant degree of disruptive behavior, they may have limited value in making a specific diagnosis.

   Comparing teacher and parent ratings may be helpful. Agreement rates are likely better with narrowband versus broadband instruments. In general, when parent ratings suggest high levels of perceived problems at home with a few symptoms reported at school, a diagnosis of ADHD is less likely. (Sources for scales are provided at the end of the reference section. Most of the instruments are proprietary.) In terms of adult assessments of ADHD, patients' retrospective accounts of their childhood symptoms may have limited validity.

5. **Office mental status examination.** Brief cognitive screening conducted in the office, focusing on short-term memory and attention and concentration, while not adequate for diagnosis, does provide useful clinical data. Immediate recall and attention may be assessed by orally presenting progressively longer strings of random digits and asking the patient to repeat them. Attention can also be assessed through vigilance tasks such as asking the patient to hold up a finger whenever the physician says the letter "A" in a series of random letters. A slightly more demanding task involving a higher level of concentration and attentional focus is asking patients to repeat digits in reverse order or the serial sevens test from the mini-mental status examination. Both children and adults can be asked to remember four words and queried about their recall at 5, 10, and possibly 15 minutes. Adolescents' and adults' short-term recall can be further assessed by reading them a short paragraph and asking them to verbally present it back to the examiner.

6. **Continuous performance tasks.** There are several computer-based tests of attention, concentration, and ability to manage distractions such as the Gordon Diagnostic System, the Test of Variable Attention (TOVA), and the Conners Continuous Performance Task. These tests are brief and provide a useful source of data that can be obtained in a standard office visit. The computer program typically calculates the number of omission errors (an index of inattention) and commission errors (a measure of impulsivity). While these tests provide useful information, there is no single task that is diagnostic of ADHD.

7. **Diagnosis and referral.** The evaluation process typically leads to one of four outcomes:

   a. **ADHD is not present.** Symptoms are attributable to another medical or psychiatric condition.

   b. **Clear, unequivocal evidence of ADHD.** Pharmacotherapy will likely be initiated.

   c. **Diagnosis of ADHD and a comorbid condition.** The physician initiates pharmacotherapy for ADHD and refers the patient to a mental health provider for further assessment and treatment of comorbid conditions, such as oppositional defiant disorder or learning disability.

   d. **Diagnosis remains unclear.** In cases of an ambiguous diagnostic picture, the patient can be referred for more in-depth testing. For example, when a learning disability is suspected, the physician may refer the patient to the school district for a psychoeducational evaluation. Concerns about APD would lead to referral to a clinical audiologist. In an adult with possible sleep apnea, a sleep study would be conducted. The results of these consultations may lead the physician to exclude ADHD or diagnose ADHD with a comorbid condition or ADHD alone.

III. **Treatment.** The goal of treatment is to decrease the core symptoms of ADHD—inattentiveness, hyperactivity, and impulsiveness—without causing adverse effects.

   A. **Pharmacotherapy** (Table 92–4). Medication use should be based on the child's age. In the treatment of preschool age children (4–5 years old), methylphenidate (MPH) is preferred

TABLE 92-4. PHARMACOTHERAPY OPTIONS FOR PATIENTS WITH ADHD

Generic Name	Brand Name	Daily Dose	Major Side Effects	Contraindications	Drug Interactions[a]
Stimulants					
Mixed amphetamine salts	Adderall[b] Adderall XR[b]	2.5–40 mg once to twice 5–40 mg once	Poor appetite and weight loss, abdominal pain, N, headache, sleep disturbances, ↑ blood pressure, anxiety	Concomitant use of MAOIs or use within 2 weeks of MAOI, agitation, glaucoma, moderate-to-severe hypertension, hyperthyroidism, history of drug abuse. Caution: tics or family history of Tourette's, psychosis, CV conditions (HF, recent MI, arrhythmias), seizure disorder	MAOIs (hypertensive crisis); Antihypertensives (↓ antihypertensive effect); warfarin (bleeding, only with methylphenidate); citalopram, venlafaxine, trazodone (serotonin S), TCA (HTN, cardiac effects)
Dextroamphetamine	Dexedrine[b] Dextrostat[b] Dexedrine Spansule[b]	2.5–40 mg two to three times 5–40 mg once to twice			Antacids
Lisdexamfetamine	Vyvanse	30–70 mg once			
Methylphenidate	Concerta[b]	18–54 mg (<13 yr) once 18–72 mg (≥13 yr) once			
	Daytrana	10–30 mg once			
	Metadate CD	20–60 mg once			
	Methylin[b], Ritalin[b]	5–60 mg two to three times			
	Methylin ER[b]	10–60 mg once			
	Quillivant XR	20–60 mg once			
	Ritalin LA[b]	20–60 mg once			
	Ritalin SR[b]	20–60 mg once to twice			Antacids
Dexmethylphenidate	Focalin[b] Focalin XR	2.5–20 mg twice 5–30 mg once			Antacids
Non stimulants					
Atomoxetine[c]	Strattera	10–50 mg once to twice <70 kg: 0.5 mg/kg/d Max. dose: 1.4 mg/kg/d or 100 mg/d (whichever is less) >70 kg: 40 mg/d (initial dose); Max. dose: 100 mg/d	Children: ↓ appetite, N/V, fatigue, dyspepsia, dizziness, mood swings, weight loss, constipation Adult: dry mouth, insomnia, N, ↓ appetite, sinus headache, constipation, erectile disturbances, dysmenorrhea, dizziness, ↓ libido, liver injury	MAOIs, narrow angle glaucoma, pheochromocytoma, Severe CV disorders, liver disease	MAOIs, albuterol (↑ heart rate, blood pressure), antihypertensives (↓ antihypertensive effectiveness), vasopressors (↑ heart rate, blood pressure)
Extended-release guanfacine	Intuniv	1–4 mg once	Somnolence, fatigue, N, dizziness, hypotension, ↓ heart rate, headache, dry mouth, insomnia (Guanfacine)	Children with preexisting cardiac or vascular disease (both guanfacine and clonidine)	Strong CYP3A4 inhibitors and inducers (dosage adjustments), CNS depressant (↑ somnolence)
Extended-release clonidine	Kapvay	0.1–0.4 mg once to twice			

[a]See text for more information.
[b]Available as generic.
[c]Black-box warning suicidal ideation (see text).
MAOI, monoamine oxidase inhibitor; TCA, tricyclic antidepressant; SSRI, selective serotonin reuptake inhibitor; N/V, nausea and vomiting; CV, cardiovascular; CNS, central nervous system; S, syndrome.

after behavioral interventions. (SOR **B**) For children aged 6 to 11 years and adolescents aged 12 to 18 years, stimulant medication is preferred as first-line treatment. (SOR **A**) If there are contraindications or the family is concerned about diversion or abuse, alternative nonstimulant medications such as atomoxetine or extended-release α_2-adrenergic agonists (clonidine and guanfacine) are considered first-line agents. (SOR **A**).

1. **Stimulants** reduce symptoms of hyperactivity, impulsivity, and inattentiveness. Inhibition of dopamine and norepinephrine reuptake is the principal mechanism. Children and adolescents demonstrate a response rate of approximately 70% for a specific stimulant, and approximately 90% will respond if a second stimulant is tried. One stimulant agent is not preferred over another, but if a child does not respond to one stimulant medication, then another one may be tried. Currently, there is no method to predict which stimulant a patient will respond to best. Long-acting agents may improve adolescent driving performance compared to short-acting agents. Short-acting stimulants are the preferred treatment in very small children (<16 kg). Stimulant medication doses can be titrated every 3 to 7 days. The medication should be titrated until maximum dosage is reached, symptoms of ADHD subside, or intolerable adverse effects occur, whichever occurs first. A positive response to a stimulant is not diagnostic of ADHD since children with comorbid conditions such as narcolepsy and depression may show a positive response as well. Additionally, children and adults without ADHD who ingest stimulants demonstrate improvement in attention, concentration, and memory tasks.

   a. **MPH** preparations are available in various dosages and delivery systems, including a transdermal patch, solution, chewable tablet, and suspension. Metadate CD and Ritalin LA are extended-release (ER) capsules with a bimodal release profile. Metadate CD's capsules contain a mixture of IR and ER beads in a 30:70 ratio, whereas Ritalin LA's capsules are in a 50:50 ratio. Both capsules' contents may be emptied and sprinkled over a spoonful of applesauce. Concerta is dosed once daily and uses osmotic pressure to deliver MPH at a constant rate. Daytrana is the first transdermal system introduced for ADHD treatment; it provides several advantages to oral medications: patients who have difficulty taking oral medications may prefer the patch, caregivers can visually monitor compliance, and therapy can be tailored to the patient. Daytrana provides a constant release of medicine, yet can be removed early to minimize adverse effects late in the day. The patch should be placed 2 hours before an effect is needed, and it is applied to alternating hips daily for a period of 9 hours. A medication effect continues for approximately three more hours after a patch is removed. Quillivant XR is the first extended-release MPH oral suspension. It is dosed once daily and is stable for 4 months at room temperature after reconstitution.

   b. **Dexmethylphenidate (Focalin)** is composed of the d-threo-enantiomer of MPH. It is available as an IR and ER formulation. Focalin XR is a 50:50 mixture containing one-half the dose as IR beads and the other one-half as enteric coated, delayed-release beads. As with Ritalin LA and Metadate CD, Focalin XR can be sprinkled over applesauce. When converting a patient from MPH to dexmethylphenidate, only one-half of the total daily MPH dose is used (e.g., MPH IR 5 mg twice daily is equivalent to dexmethylphenidate 2.5 mg twice daily).

   c. **Dextroamphetamine** (Dexedrine) is also available in IR and ER forms. It is as effective as MPH, but may be preferred for those who do not tolerate or do not respond to MPH. When switching a patient from MPH to dextroamphetamine, approximately one-half of the MPH total daily dose is used.

   d. **Mixed amphetamine salts (Adderall)** have a longer half-life than IR MPH, but not as long as the Dexedrine Spansule. Adderall XR is a capsule composed of IR and delayed-release beads in a ratio of 50:50 and may be sprinkled over food.

   e. **Lisdexamfetamine (Vyvanse)** is the first stimulant prodrug introduced for the treatment of ADHD. It is pharmacologically inactive until it is absorbed in the gastrointestinal (GI) tract where it is converted to D-amphetamine. It was designed to reduce the potential for abuse, overdose toxicity, and drug tampering. The capsule's contents may be opened and dissolved in water for ease in administration.

   f. **Adverse effects.** Common adverse effects are shown in Table 92–4. Less common side effects include social withdrawal, nervousness, irritability, and tics. In recent studies, MPH has not been shown to increase or worsen motor tics in patients with or without comorbid tic disorders and ADHD. In some cases,

TABLE 92–5. HOW TO MANAGE ADVERSE EFFECTS OF STIMULANT MEDICATIONS

Adverse Effect	Management
Anorexia	Bedtime snack
	Reduce dose
Dyspepsia	Take with food
Insomnia	Add clonidine or diphenhydramine
	Eliminate last dose or adjust time last dose of medication given (IR formulations)
	Take off patch earlier (Daytrana)
	Recommend sleep hygiene protocol
	If enuresis, add imipramine
Emotional lability, nervousness, irritability	Reduce or adjust dose
	Switch to another medication
Tics	Switch to another medication
	Add α_2-agonist

however, stimulants can exacerbate tics. While there has been concern about how stimulants affect the growth rate of children, it appears that reduced growth rates may only occur during the first 2 years of treatment and seem to attenuate over time. The effect of stimulants on ultimate adult height is unknown. The transdermal patch can also cause application site irritation. Table 92–5 presents possible management strategies for adverse effects caused by stimulants.

g. Drug interactions (Table 92–4).

h. Cardiovascular concerns. Patients with preexisting structural cardiac abnormalities or other serious heart problems should generally not be prescribed stimulant medication. Patients with known structural cardiac abnormalities, cardiomyopathy, serious cardiac arrhythmias, coronary artery disease, or other serious cardiac problems should obtain a cardiology consult before using stimulant medications. Sudden death, stroke, and myocardial infarction have been reported in patients taking stimulant drugs for ADHD; however, current evidence does not support a higher risk of sudden cardiac death with stimulant medications when compared with the general population. Even though a causal relationship has not been established, prescribers should be aware of the risk when prescribing this class of drugs. There is an online screening tool that can be used to identify sudden death cardiac risk factors among children starting stimulant medication (www.icsi.org/_asset/60nzr5/ADHD-Interactive0312.pdf#page73).

i. Abuse of stimulants. Currently, all available stimulant medications for ADHD are a schedule II controlled substance. While it is true that these drugs may be abused or diverted, prescription stimulants fail to produce a euphoric sensation via the oral route. Abuse or diversion is more common with IR preparations that can be crushed and snorted rather than with ER forms.

(1) Reports have shown that treating ADHD in adolescents actually decreases the risk of substance abuse compared to individuals with ADHD who are untreated. Perhaps more common than recreational use of stimulants, high school and college students may share stimulants when completing papers, tests, and final examinations as a "study drug" to boost performance and should be cautioned against this practice.

(2) Alternatives for prescribers who have patients and/or patient's family members with a history of substance abuse include using the ER formulations, atomoxetine, the MPH patch, or lisdexamfetamine. ER formulations can be used to prevent diversion since it can be taken once daily at home and not taken to school. The transdermal patch has limited abuse potential since it is difficult to extract MPH from the patch and is difficult to reapply a used patch. Lisdexamfetamine is a prodrug that is not therapeutically active until it is metabolized in the body, thus limiting its abuse potential.

2. Nonstimulant medications, such as atomoxetine and extended-release selected α_2-adrenergic agonists, should be considered when stimulants have failed, patients have contraindications or significant adverse effects to stimulants, or there is concern about diversion or abuse. Atomoxetine, extended-release guanfacine, and extended-release clonidine have demonstrated benefit for all three core ADHD symptoms—hyperactivity, inattention, and impulsivity. Maximum responses with these medications will not be seen as fast as with stimulants. Maximum response can be seen after 4 to 6 weeks with atomoxetine and 2 to 4 weeks with extended-release guanfacine and clonidine.

   a. Atomoxetine is the first nonstimulant medication to be approved by the Food and Drug Administration (FDA) for treatment of both children and adults with ADHD. Similar to stimulants, atomoxetine inhibits norepinephrine reuptake. Advantages of atomoxetine include low risk for diversion or abuse, no known adverse effects on tic disorders, and no known long-term effects on growth suppression.

     (1) Adverse effects (Table 92–4). It is recommended to start with one-half the recommended treatment dose the first week to decrease initial somnolence and GI symptoms. Because it increases norepinephrine levels, atomoxetine can increase blood pressure and heart rate.

     (2) Drug interactions (Table 92–4). Atomoxetine is a CYP-2D6 substrate; therefore, its levels may increase when used in patients who are taking CYP-2D6 inhibitors such as fluoxetine and paroxetine. For patients using atomoxetine concomitantly with strong CYP-2D6 inhibitors, atomoxetine should only be increased up to 1.2 mg/kg/d after 4 weeks if the patient weighs <70 kg and only increased to 80 mg per day after 4 weeks if the patient weighs >70 kg.

     (3) Cardiovascular concerns. As with stimulant medications for ADHD, sudden death has been reported in adults, children, and adolescents with structural cardiac abnormalities or other serious heart problems. In adults, stroke and myocardial infarction have also been reported. In patients with known structural cardiac abnormalities, cardiomyopathy, serious heart rhythm abnormalities, or other serious cardiac problems, atomoxetine is generally not recommended because of the additive risk of cardiac adverse effects. Patients with known structural cardiac abnormalities, cardiomyopathy, serious cardiac arrhythmias, coronary artery disease, or other serious cardiac problems should obtain a cardiology consult before using atomoxetine.

     (4) Severe liver injury. There have been postmarketing reports of severe liver injury in patients treated with atomoxetine. Based on these reports, the FDA has mandated a bolded warning to be added to the package insert to warn prescribers of the potential danger. The medication should be discontinued in patients who develop jaundice or laboratory evidence of liver injury. Atomoxetine should not be restarted in these patients. Currently, routine liver enzyme testing is not recommended.

     (5) Suicidal ideation in children and adolescents. There is a black-box warning concerning atomoxetine and the possibility of suicidal ideation, but given the evidence, this concern should not be overstated. In short-term studies, an increased risk of suicidal ideation in children and adolescents was reported. While no suicides occurred, the average risk was 0.4% (5 of 1357 patients) in patients treated with atomoxetine compared to 0% in placebo-treated patients. The number of patients affected was low but physicians, parents, and caregivers should closely monitor patients during the initial months of treatment and after any dose change. Occurrences of agitation, irritability, unusual changes in behavior, and any suicidal ideation should be reported to the provider immediately. All events occurred during the first month of treatment. A similar analysis of adult patients with ADHD using atomoxetine did not reveal an increased risk of suicidal ideation.

   b. α_2-Adrenergic agonists, extended-release **clonidine** and **guanfacine,** are the only two nonstimulant medications FDA approved for use as adjunctive therapy with stimulants. α_2-Agonists do not worsen tics and can be used with a stimulant to help decrease unwanted tics. α_2-Agonists should not be used in children with preexisting cardiac or vascular disease without consultation with a cardiologist. Blood pressure and pulse should be measured when initiating therapy, increasing the dose, and periodically while taking the medication. Upon discontinuation of therapy, doses of clonidine and guanfacine should be tapered every 3 to 7 days to avoid rebound hypertension.

     (1) Adverse effects (Table 92–4).

(2) Drug interactions (Table 92–4). Dosage adjustments should be made when extended-release guanfacine is administered with strong CYP3A4 inducers (e.g., rifampin) and inhibitors (e.g., clarithromycin). The maximum dose is 2 mg per day when a strong CYP3A4 inhibitor is used and 8 mg per day is the maximum dose when a strong CYP3A4 inducer is used. Medications that can affect sinus node function or AV nodal conduction (e.g., digoxin, calcium channel blockers, and beta-blockers) should be used with caution.

B. Discussing pharmacotherapy with patients and families

1. Listen to the parents' concerns and dispel any myths. Reassure parents that the child will not become addicted to the stimulant medication and that stimulant safety and efficacy have been demonstrated in numerous studies and years of clinical practice. Set realistic behavioral goals with the parent and child. Review potential benefits of treatment (decreased hyperactivity, improved concentration, impulse control, and decreased disruptive behavior). Educate the parents about the potential consequences of untreated ADHD, such as poor school performance, grade retention, relationship difficulty, and increased risk of adolescent substance use, psychiatric disorders (major depression and personality disorders), traffic violations, and delinquency.

2. Educating the parents about the most common adverse effects of stimulants such as appetite suppression (with weight loss), sleep difficulties, rebound moodiness, and irritability will reduce their anxiety if these symptoms occur and increase the likelihood of adherence. Parents should periodically assess their child's nutritional status. It may be helpful to have the child eat breakfast before taking their morning dose. Children who eat little at lunch will usually eat a hearty snack in the afternoon as their medication is wearing off. Difficulty falling asleep can be addressed by delaying the child's bedtime to after 9 PM or adding a sedating medication such as clonidine. Recent research suggests that children with ADHD fall asleep more quickly when a sleep hygiene protocol is implemented. (SOR ❸) Rebound moodiness and irritability may occur for approximately 30 to 60 minutes as the medication is wearing off. Adding a small, short-acting dose immediately after school or allowing the child some quiet time before beginning homework may help alleviate these symptoms.

3. Between 50% and 75% of individuals diagnosed with ADHD as a child will continue to have symptoms persisting into adulthood. As in other chronic health conditions, pharmacotherapy may be lifelong.

4. Although drug holidays have been advocated in the past, many children will require drug therapy year-round to maintain attention and decrease hyperactivity—symptoms that frequently disrupt family, recreational, and social activities.

5. While response to stimulants is typically rapid, several dosage titrations may be required to obtain optimal clinical response. Therefore, frequent follow-up is suggested for at least the first 6 to 12 months. Similar to other chronic health conditions, patients treated for ADHD benefit from having a consistent medical home.

6. Children who have been responding well to medication treatment for many months may return to the physician due to complaints by parents and teachers that the medication is no longer "working." Tolerance does seem to develop over the first 6 to 12 months but then plateaus, suggesting that medications may need to be increased during this period to maintain effectiveness and relatedly adherence. While adjustment of medication dosages may in fact be indicated, other causes should be considered as well. The physician should specifically inquire about the types of behavior that are of concern. Issues such as lying, talking back, and angry outbursts may reflect development of comorbid conditions. Adults' point of reference for the child may have unconsciously shifted over time. Initially, children treated with medication are compared with themselves prior to medication initiation. However, over time this reference point may change and the child may be implicitly compared to school-aged peers or siblings. Goals for treatment should include 50% remission of symptoms; most children with ADHD continue to manifest some symptoms of the disorder even when on an optimal medication regimen. When questions of medication effectiveness arise, a new set of behavioral ratings may clarify the clinical picture.

7. Neurotoxicity. Stimulants represent the largest single class of psychotropic medication prescribed to children in the United States, with 9% of boys and 4% of girls receiving these medications for treatment of ADHD. As a result, the long-term safety of stimulant medications has been a focus of research in neuroanatomic studies. The

fear of neurotoxicity has diminished over the past 10 years, with the focus of more recent research on the neuroprotective effects of stimulants on cortical development in children and adolescents with ADHD. Indeed, results have been favorable, suggesting that stimulant and nonstimulant therapy seems to support developmental normalization and/or compensation of brain alterations in patients with ADHD, especially during sensitive phases of neuronal plasticity.

8. Medication adherence has been linked to a number of factors including practical aspects of medication administration, side effects, socioeconomic factors, and ethnicity. Nonadherence with stimulant treatment is a significant issue, with some studies indicating rates below 50% within 6 months of treatment initiation. (SOR **B**) Moreover, in the treatment of children and adolescents, parents do not appear to be accurate reporters of their child's adherence. Positive treatment alliance, education regarding the risks and benefits of the medication, and regular follow-up improve adherence.

C. Special issues in pharmacotherapy across the lifespan. Because of the instability of the diagnosis among preschoolers, parent behavioral management has been recommended as the initial treatment for 4- and 5-year olds exhibiting mild-to-moderate symptom levels. Compared with older children, there are suggestions that 3- to 5-year olds are more likely to experience adverse effects of stimulants. Evidence to date suggests that substance abuse is significantly more likely among adolescents and adults with ADHD. Because of this risk, careful assessment of substance use should be conducted before initiating stimulant pharmacotherapy. For adults who do not respond to stimulants or have contraindications for their use, bupropion, TCAs, and atomoxetine are suitable alternatives. Bupropion and TCAs are used more often in adults and can be beneficial in patients with comorbid psychiatric conditions.

D. Nonpharmacologic treatment for children and adolescents with ADHD.

1. Pharmacotherapy is the treatment of choice for ADHD among school-aged children, adolescents, and adults, and is beneficial for the vast majority of patients. In head-to-head comparisons with behavioral therapies, medications demonstrate a greater effect on problem behavior. (SOR **A**)

2. Nevertheless, two psychosocial treatments have received empirical support: behavioral parent training and behavioral modification in the classroom. These are superior to no-treatment conditions and can be helpful for children with ADHD who cannot tolerate medication or who do not respond well. (SOR **A**) Additionally, some evidence exists that combining systematic behavior therapy with well-delivered medication can yield better outcomes than medication alone. (SOR **B**)

    a. Behavioral parent training typically involves 8 to 30 sessions in which the therapist guides the parents through a structured behavioral program designed to enhance the parents' understanding of ADHD and of behavioral principles. The therapist teaches the importance of specifying target behaviors, providing consistent and regular rewards for positive behavior, involving teachers in the behavioral plan, and generalizing the skills to a variety of situations.

    b. Clinicians perform **behavioral modification in the classroom** by teaching the regular- or special-education teachers how to implement the behavioral strategies that are taught in parent training (e.g., specific target behaviors and regular rewards), with modifications for classroom settings. Teachers can do any or all of the following: seat the child with ADHD closer to the front of the classroom; encourage attention through prompting; implement a reward system; and complete a daily behavioral report card.

3. Additional psychosocial treatments include psychoeducation, special education services, and child interventions.

    a. Psychoeducation provides the child, parents, family, and school with information about ADHD, its treatment, and its impact on learning, behavior, self-esteem, social skills, and family functioning. Educating the family also allows the physician an opportunity to correct misperceptions. For example, the child may feel that he/she is "dumb" or the parents may fear that the child is going to become a "drug addict" as a result of the stimulant medication. Family physicians should inform families of appropriate sources for ADHD information such as Children and Adults with Attention Deficit/Hyperactivity Disorder (CHADD) (www.chadd.org), National Instituites of Heath (http://www.nlm.nih.gov/medlineplus/attention deficithyperactivitydisorder.html), and the American Academy of Child and Adolescent Psychiatry (AACAP) (http://www.aacap.org/iMIS/ContentManagement/ Search.aspx?SearchTerms=ADHD).

    b. Special education services are often important in the treatment and monitoring of ADHD symptoms.

        (1) ADHD is included as a disability under the Individuals with Disabilities Education Act (IDEA [PL-101-476]). Therefore, children with ADHD may qualify for special education services or appropriate accommodations within the regular classroom setting under Section 504 of the Rehabilitation Act of 1973. Patients may also be eligible for reasonable accommodations in secular private schools and postsecondary education under The Americans with Disabilities Act.

        (2) Classroom accommodations can include changes in the child's educational programming such as tutoring, resource room support, extended time to complete tasks, and decreased workload.

    c. Most **child interventions** for ADHD such as social skills training, cognitive behavioral therapy (CBT), and study/organizational skills do not have solid empirical support as primary treatment of ADHD, and the gains achieved in the treatment setting typically do not transfer into the classroom or home settings. However, child interventions may be indicated when there are comorbid conditions such as major depression, anxiety, and obsessive-compulsive disorders that are also the focus of treatment.

E. Psychotherapy, organizational skills, and environmental modification for the ADHD adult. CBT is a beneficial adjunct to medication and improves ADHD symptoms and global symptom severity to a greater extent than medication alone. (SOR **B**) CBT has also proven beneficial for comorbid depressive symptoms. In addition, the following strategies can be helpful:

    1. To foster **self-management skills,** organizers such as calendars, day planners, and specialized applications for i-phone and android (http://www.healthline.com/health-slideshow/top-adhd-android-iphone-apps#13), when consistently employed, may prompt recall and improve personal organizational skills.

    2. Reducing distractions in the workplace is helpful. For adults with ADHD, flexible work times and going into work before most coworkers arrive is valuable. This "quiet time" may help with getting organized and accomplishing tasks before distractions increase. Similarly, this strategy of early awakening is also useful in managing a household. The patient's immediate workplace itself should be free of clutter and other distractions such as family photos and personal mementos.

    3. For adults in an ongoing relationship, conjoint counseling can address communication issues and help educate both spouses about the impact of ADHD in their daily lives.

    4. For adults involved in a formal educational program such as college or professional school, accommodations may be available. Examples include **extended time for tests and the option of taking tests alone** in a special resource room rather than in a traditional classroom with other students. Formal documentation of an ADHD diagnosis is typically required.

F. Complementary and alternative medicines. Complementary and alternative treatments are used by up to 60% of parents for their children with ADHD. Until more controlled studies are done to determine efficacy of complementary and alternative treatments, proven pharmacologic therapies should remain first line.

    1. Neurofeedback is believed to improve attentiveness and impulsivity. While it may have some success in reducing symptoms, the long-term effects are not known.

    2. Attention training often uses laboratory vigilance tasks in which children receive reinforcement for correct responses. While children with ADHD demonstrate improvement on laboratory tasks, there has not been consistent evidence of improved attention and reduced hyperactivity in daily functioning.

    3. Progressive relaxation and meditation have demonstrated some benefit for reducing hyperactivity; however, the clinical significance and durability of this improvement have, so far, been limited.

    4. Minerals: Iron supplements are based on the belief that children with ADHD have an iron deficiency. If iron deficiency is suspected, hematologic testing should be performed; otherwise, routine use of iron supplementation should not be used in nondeficient children. **Zinc deficiencies** have been associated with impaired cognitive functioning. Zinc supplementation may augment the benefits of MPH.

    5. Diet for children has been altered in several different ways to attempt to decrease the symptoms of ADHD. Despite popular myths, sugar does not exacerbate or cause hyperactivity. Elimination of food dye from food and drinks has yielded inconclusive evidence.

6. **Homeopathic** treatments such as Cina and *Hyoscyamus niger* have been used to decrease symptoms. Despite potential use for these products, additional evaluation is needed to determine efficacy and place in therapy.

7. **Herbal medicines,** such as ginkgo, evening primrose, valerian, lemon balm, and more have been used to decrease symptoms of hyperactivity. Parents should be reminded that herbal medications are not regulated by the FDA and may not contain standardized doses.

8. **Dietary supplements.** There is no evidence to support that children with ADHD benefit from megadoses of vitamins. Omega-3 and omega-6 supplements have shown a significant, yet modest, effect for ADHD symptoms. (SOR **C**)

IV. **Prognosis.** ADHD is a chronic neurologic condition with many symptoms persisting into adolescence and adulthood in up to 70% of diagnosed children. Developmentally, specific symptoms may change with marked reductions in hyperactivity and impulsivity beginning at age 9 years. However, inattention typically persists through adolescence and into adulthood.

A. The relatively few prospective ADHD studies suggest that adolescents and adults with ADHD histories are **at risk for legal problems, traffic accidents, noncompletion of formal education, substance abuse, and other psychiatric disorders**. However, in counseling parents about the prognosis for children with ADHD, available research has several limitations. Diagnostic standards have changed during the past 15 years, with recent DSM-IV and DSM-5 criteria identifying milder forms of ADHD than previously. These changing diagnostic criteria are likely to be a factor in recent increased ADHD prevalence rates among adults than previously reported. Adults with ADHD, if diagnosed as children, were likely to have had particularly severe symptoms.

B. ADHD's longitudinal course is further complicated by increased comorbidity through the lifespan. Comorbidity rises to at least 50% during adolescence and may be as high as 70% in adulthood. A consistent research finding is the particularly poor psychiatric and legal outcomes for ADHD with comorbid conduct disorder.

C. With these caveats, adolescents with an ADHD history are two to four times more likely to be arrested, two to four times more likely to be diagnosed with antisocial personality, and four times more likely to have non-alcohol substance abuse problems. While severity of substance use is greater for ADHD with comorbid conduct disorder, young adults with ADHD alone are more likely than non-ADHD controls to become regular smokers. Primary care risk counseling should be particularly thorough teenagers with ADHD.

D. Among adults, an ADHD history is associated with a greater likelihood of receiving both inpatient and outpatient psychiatric treatment. These adults are more likely to be fired from or quit jobs and have lower SES than adults without ADHD. ADHD is also a risk factor for relationship conflict including separation and divorce.

E. While data are scarce, ADHD treatment during childhood appears to reduce the incidence of later adverse outcomes. A common parental fear is that stimulant pharmacotherapy during childhood may lead to substance abuse. Several studies suggest that stimulant treatment may actually protect against late adolescent and young adult drug and alcohol abuse.

SELECTED REFERENCES

Adler L, Mattingly G. Optimizing clinical outcomes across domains of life in adolescents and adults with ADHD. *J Clin Psychiatr.* 2011;72(7):1008–1014.

American Academy of Pediatrics. ADHD: clinical practice guideline for the diagnosis, evaluation, and treatment of attention-deficit/hyperactivity disorder in children and adolescents. *Pediatrics.* 2011; 128(5):1–16.

American Psychiatric Association. *Diagnostic and Statistical Manual of Mental Disorders.* 5th ed. Washington, DC: American Psychiatric Association; 2013.

Barkley R, Murphy K, Fischer M. *ADHD in Adults: What the Science Says.* New York, NY: Guilford; 2008.

Boomsma D, Saviouk V, Hottenga J, et al. Genetic epidemiology of Attention Deficit Hyperactivity Disorder (ADHD index) in adults. *PLoS One.* 2010;5(5):e10621.

Centers for Disease Control. http://www.cdc.gov/Features/dsADHD/. Accessed June 2013.

Charach A, Ickowicz A, Schachar R. Stimulant treatment over five years: adherence, effectiveness, and adverse effects. *J Am Acad Child Adolesc Psychiatry.* 2004:43(5):559–567.

Charach A, Carson P, Fox S, et al. Interventions for preschool children at high risk for ADHD: A comparative effectiveness review. *Pediatrics.* 2013;131(5):1584–1604.

Dobie C, Donald WB, Hanson M, et al. Institute for Clinical Systems Improvement. Diagnosis and Management of Attention Deficit Hyperactivity Disorder in Primary Care for School-Age Children and Adolescents. Agency for Health Care Research and Quality. http://www.qualitymeasures.ahrq.gov/content.aspx?id=36859. Updated March 2012. Accessed June 2013.

Duval-Harvey J, Rogers, K. Attention-deficit/hyperactivity disorder. In: Hampton R, Gullotta T, Eds. *Handbook of African-American Health.* New York, NY: Guilford; 2010:375–418.

Faraone S, Biederman J, Morley C, Spencer T. Effect of stimulants on height and weight: a review of the literature. *J Am Acad Child Adolesc Psychiatry.* 2008;47(9):994–1009.

Faraone SV, Biederman J, Spencer T, et al. Diagnosing adult attention deficit hyperactivity disorder: are late onset and subthreshold diagnoses valid? *Am J Psychiatry.* 2006;163(10):1720–1729.

Galera C, Cote S, Bouvard M, et al. Early risk factors for hyperactivity-impulsivity and inattention trajectories from age 17 months to 8 years. *Arch Gen Psychiatry.* 2011;68(12):1267–1275.

Gizer IR, Ficks C, Waldman ID. Candidate gene studies of ADHD: a meta-analytic review. *Hum Genet.* 2009;126:51.

Hazell P. 8-year follow-up of the MTA sample. *J Am Acad Child Adolesc Psychiatry.* 2009;48(5):461–462.

Hines J, King T, Curry W. The Adult ADHD Self-Report Scale for screening for adult attention deficit-hyperactivity disorder (ADHD). *J Am Board Fam Med.* 2012;25:847–853.

Osterloo M, Lammers GJ, Overeem S, et al. Possible confusion between primary hypersomnia and adult attention-deficit/hyperactivity disorder. *Psychiatry Res.* 2006;143:293–297.

Pappadopulos E, Jensen P, Chait A, et al. Medication adherence in the MTA. *J Am Acad Child Adolesc Psychiatry.* 2009;48(5):501–510.

Perrin J, Friedman R, Knilans T; The Black Box Working Group, the Section on Cardiology and Cardiac Surgery. Cardiovascular monitoring and stimulant drugs for attention-deficit/hyperactivity disorder. Cardiovascular monitoring and stimulant drugs for attention-deficit/hyperactivity disorder. *Pediatrics.* 2008;451–453.

Rothenberger A, Rothenberger L. Updates on treatment of attention-deficit/hyperactivity disorder: facts, comments, and ethical considerations. *Curr Treat Options Neurol.* 2012;14(6):594–607.

Searight HR, Robertson K, Smith T, et al. Complementary and alternative therapies for pediatric attention deficit hyperactivity disorder. *ISRN Psychiatry.* 2012;2:1–8.

Shaw P, Gilliam M, Liverpool M. Cortical development in typically developing children with symptoms of hyperactivity and impulsivity: support for a dimensional view of attention deficit hyperactivity disorder. *Am J Psychiatry.* 2011;168:143.

Shaw P, Sharp S, Morrison M, et al. Psychostimulant treatment and the developing cortex in attention deficit hyperactivity disorder. *Am J Psychiatry.* 2009;166:58–63.

Solanto M, Marks D, Wasserstein J, et al. Efficacy of meta-cognitive therapy for adult ADHD. *Am J Psychiatry.* 2012;167:958–968.

Toomey S, Sox C, Rusinak D, Finkelstein JA. Why do children with ADHD discontinue their medication? *Clin Pediatr.* 2012;51(8):763–769.

Zwi M, Jones H, Thorgaard C, et al. Parent training interventions for Attention Deficit Hyperactivity Disorder (ADHD) in children aged 5 to 18 years. *Cochrane Database Syst Rev.* 2011;(12):CD003018.

SOURCES FOR RATING SCALES

Adult Self Report Scale (ASRS v1.1). http://webdoc.nyumc.org/nyumc/files/psych/attachments/psych_adhd_screener.pdf. Accessed May 2014.

Child Behavior Checklist (CBCL). http://www4.parinc.com/Search.aspx?q=child%20behavior%20checklist. Accessed June 14, 2013.

Conners Rating Scales. http://www.pearsonassessments.com/tests/crs-r.htm. Accessed June 14, 2013.

Disruptive Behavior Disorders Rating Scale. Comprehensive Treatment for Attention Deficit Disorder. http://ccf.buffalo.edu/pdf/DBD_rating_scale.pdf. Accessed June 14, 2013

National Initiative for Children's Healthcare Quality. Vanderbilt Parent and Teacher Scales. American Academy of Pediatrics. http://www.nichq.org/toolkits_publications/complete_adhd/04VanAssesScaleTeachInfor.pdf (Teacher Informant). Accessed June 14, 2013.

National Initiative for Children's Healthcare Quality. Vanderbilt Parent and Teacher Scales. American Academy of Pediatrics. http://www.nichq.org/toolkits_publications/complete_adhd/03VanAssesScaleParent%20Infor.pdf (Parent Informant). Accessed June 14, 2013.

93   Family Violence: Child, Intimate Partner, and Elder Abuse

F. David Schneider, MD, MSPH, Nancy D. Kellogg, MD, &
Melissa A. Talamantes, MS

KEY POINTS

- Know the laws in your state regarding mandatory reporting of family violence, including child abuse, intimate partner violence, and elder abuse. (SOR ❸) Most states have mandatory reporting laws for both those younger than 18 years and older than 64 years.
- Ask about family violence as a routine part of your history taking, especially for women of childbearing age. (SOR ❸) This gives patients permission to talk about it when they feel comfortable.
- Assess the situation for lethality—use of guns or knives by the perpetrator or escalating violence may require immediate intervention by police. (SOR ❸)
- Learn about your community resources for support of victims of family violence and use them when appropriate with your patients. (SOR ❸)

I. **Introduction.** Family violence encompasses violence and abuse within families and other interpersonal relationships and includes child abuse and neglect, intimate partner violence (IPV), and elder abuse and neglect. Its effects on peoples' lives are far reaching, ranging from social dysfunction to health effects such as mental health issues such as anxiety, depression, and post traumatic stress disorder (PTSD) and physical health issues such as hypertension, cancer, and heart disease. The costs are estimated to be in the billions of dollars annually in the United States. The role that providers can play is crucial to our patients' ability to overcome these effects. This chapter is divided into the three types of family violence: Child abuse and neglect, IPV, and elder abuse and neglect. However, it should be stated that these divisions are artificial and there is much overlap between these types of violence.

II. **Child Abuse**

   A. **Definitions.** Types of child abuse include neglect and physical, sexual, and emotional abuse.

      1. **Neglect** can be defined as a failure to provide adequate nutrition, shelter, medical/dental care and/or basic needs, or as a failure to protect. Medical neglect occurs when the caretaker ignores important medical or dental treatment plans. Supervision neglect occurs when a parent fails to protect a child from a dangerous environment, such as leaving an 8-month-old on a bed they can crawl off of, or engages in behavior that compromises their ability to protect their child, such as illicit drug use. Neglect is most common of the four types and comprises about 73% of the total.

      2. **Child physical abuse** is any intentional injury resulting in tissue damage, including bruises, burns, lacerations, fractures, and organ or blood vessel rupture. In addition, any inflicted injury that is visible for more than 24 hours constitutes significant injury. Physical abuse comprises approximately 14% of the four types of abuse and neglect.

      3. **Child sexual abuse** encompasses a variety of interactions that adults or adolescents use to take advantage of vulnerable children in a sexual manner, including both sexual contact and exploitation for pornography or prostitution. Another form of sexual abuse involves solicitation through the computer; almost one in five children who go "online" regularly is approached by strangers for sex. More recently, "sexting," or sending/receiving nude or nearly nude images through social media has been identified as a criminal activity that involves minors in the United States. Approximately 7% of maltreated children are sexually abused.

      4. **Emotional abuse** includes rejecting a child's worth or needs, constant berating or belittlement, or making the child engage in destructive behavior. Children who are only emotionally abused comprise about 6% of abuse cases, but emotional abuse is commonly associated with physical abuse, sexual abuse, and neglect.

   B. **Epidemiology.** There are more than 3 million reported cases of child abuse and neglect in the United States annually; about 1500 children die of abuse or neglect each year. Eighty percent of child abuse fatalities occur in children younger than 5 years, and 40% occur during a child's first year of life. Neglect most often involves the youngest, more dependent infants and children, whereas sexual abuse tends to be reported during school age and adolescent years. Despite large numbers of reported cases, child abuse and neglect remains an under-detected and under-reported problem. It has been estimated that 20% of children will sustain an abusive injury and 14% to 40% of females will be sexually abused before reaching adulthood.

C. Diagnosis

1. **Barriers to diagnosis.** Child abuse injuries are frequently subtle and often missed. Detection is compromised by other factors: the child or family may deem injuries as acceptable if inflicted for reasons of discipline; clinicians typically rely on a caretaker's history, which may be untruthful if abuse has occurred; victims may be too young to explain how they were injured; verbal victims may be reluctant to disclose abuse out of fear, guilt, or shame; and injuries may be old, indistinct, or nonexistent.

   a. Once abuse is suspected, many clinicians are reluctant to report because they think reporting would harm or provide no benefit for the child and family, or they think child protective services is ineffective. It is important for a clinician to remember that reporting is a legal obligation and child protective services rely on information from several sources in assessing referrals. The role of the clinician is to ensure that investigators understand the characteristics (location, type, approximate age, etc.) of the injury, the likely mechanisms that explain the injury(s) and the likelihood of abuse or neglect based on the medical assessment.

2. **Physical abuse.** The diagnosis of physical abuse and neglect typically begins with "what you see." Bruises are the most common manifestation of physical abuse, yet it is important to remember that most bruises of childhood are accidental rather than inflicted. Location of bruises (e.g., buttocks or ears) as well as characteristics (petechial or patterned bruising) and size (large bruises) help distinguish abusive from accidental causes. The developmental capability of the child is key in evaluating the plausibility of accidental trauma: "if you don't cruise (developmental milestone achieved around 8 months of age), you don't bruise." Table 93–1 lists injuries and conditions that are suspicious for abuse and neglect.

   a. Explanation consistency. Once a suspicious injury or condition is identified, the clinician should gather a careful detailed history and determine whether the history (from the child or caregiver) reasonably explains the characteristics (shape, size, location, type, severity) of the injury. It is not unusual for children with inflicted injuries (such as patterned belt marks) to provide a false history of a benign accident to explain the injuries. Children (generally, 4 years and older) and caretakers should be questioned separately.

   (1) Information gathered should include when the injury occurred; what the child was doing before, during, and after the injury; any symptoms of pain or injury and when these were noted; and any witnesses to the injury. A developmental history can assist in assessing the plausibility of a described accident (e.g., a 6-month-old child may roll off a bed but would not be able to climb out of a crib with the rails up). Whenever abuse is suspected, the child should be examined carefully for signs of neglect; a feeding history should be obtained as well as plotting the weight, height, and head circumference should also be obtained.

   (2) Clinicians should remain emotionally neutral, unbiased, and cautious in sharing diagnostic assessments when talking with caregivers or children who are suspected victims. When talking to children, it is critical not to ask questions that express bias or suggest the clinician thinks the child was (or was not) abused: "What happened to your arm?" is preferable to "Who hurt your arm?" or "Did Daddy hurt you?"

   b. Tests. Some injuries may warrant further laboratory and radiologic testing to assess the possibility of coagulopathies, bone disorders, and other conditions that may mimic abuse. Depending on the age and severity of the injury, the clinician may also assess the child for other signs of trauma or abuse such as occult liver (liver function tests), bone (skeletal survey), and intracranial (magnetic resonance imaging or computerized tomography [CT] of the head) injuries.

   (1) In children with intracranial injuries, a dilated ophthalmologic examination may reveal retinal hemorrhages; severe retinal hemorrhages are associated with abusive head trauma.

TABLE 93-1. INJURIES (BRUISES, BURNS, AND FRACTURES) THAT SHOULD BE CAREFULLY EVALUATED FOR PHYSICAL ABUSE

1. Age 0–6 mo: *Any injury.*
2. Age 6 mo or older:
   a. Bruises, lacerations, or burns to protected, fleshy, or flexor surfaces—*for example,* the inner thighs, lateral/posterior arms, thorax, abdomen, neck, face (other than frontal prominence), pinna, and genitalia.
   b. Bruises, lacerations, or burns showing an object pattern—*for example,* belt loop, cigarette burn, and curling iron.
   c. Oral injuries, *especially* frenula and palate lacerations.
   d. Third-degree burns or large second-degree burns, *especially* scald burns.
   e. Fractures, *especially* metaphyseal fractures, complex or wide skull fractures, rib fractures, spiral fractures of humerus or femur, and scapula fractures.
   f. Significant head injury, *especially* subdural hematoma, retinal hemorrhage, avulsed hair, complex, or wide skull fracture. Head injury should be considered whenever a child presents with vomiting or altered consciousness, or bloody spinal fluid is found on lumbar puncture, but an infectious process cannot be readily diagnosed.
   g. Intra-abdominal injury, *especially* rupture or hematoma of hollow organs.
3. Positive urine or blood screen for alcohol or drugs of abuse.

Findings that should be carefully evaluated for *sexual abuse*:
1. Injuries to the genitalia (*especially* to the hymen or vestibule in girls) or anus.
2. Identification of an STD: Chlamydia, gonorrhea, HSV, HPV, HIV, HBV, HCV, *Trichomonas*, syphilis (note that perinatally acquired HPV may delay in clinical presentation for up to 3 years).
3. Positive pregnancy test.
4. Any history or statement or witnessed incident consistent with sexual abuse.

Findings that should be carefully evaluated for *neglect*:
1. Weight or length/height crossing 2 or more percentile lines/channels over time; weight that is 80% of expected weight-for-height.
2. Lack of medical care for a significant health problem—*for example,* no medications for asthma and diabetes and no care of severe dental caries.
3. Lack of normal bonding with parent/guardian.
4. Disregard of one or more basic child care needs—*for example,* soft drink in baby bottle, child found in street, and failure to place child in auto safety seat or belt.

Note: A child may have findings suggesting more than one form of abuse or neglect.
HBV, hepatitis B virus; HCV, hepatitis C virus; HIV, human immunodeficiency virus; HPV, human papilloma virus; HSV, herpes simplex virus; STD, sexually transmitted disease.
Source: Excerpted with permission from the Texas Pediatric Society Committee on Child Abuse. Clinical Practice Resource for Hospitals and Emergency Departments.

(2) When abuse is strongly suspected in a child younger than 2 years, a repeat skeletal survey 2 weeks after the initial evaluation is recommended; when abuse is suspected in an infant, a head CT is recommended, regardless of the sentinel injury.

(3) In evaluating suspected nutritional neglect, complete electrolyte and hematologic profiles may establish the severity and chronicity of malnutrition. However, the diagnosis of failure to thrive usually relies on a comprehensive history, including social and family factors, as well as gathering and plotting the weights, lengths/heights, and head circumference on a growth chart (see Chapter 24).

3. **Sexual and emotional abuse.** The detection of sexual and emotional abuse generally depends on "what you hear." More than 90% of child sexual abuse is first discovered when the child tells someone about the abuse. Emotional abuse is typically detected when a child's behaviors or emotions cause concern and questioning confirms suspicion of abuse.

   a. **The medical diagnosis of sexual abuse** relies primarily on the history from the child. Forensic materials, genital or anal injury, and sexually transmitted infections (STIs) are not seen or recovered in the significant majority of victims. Recovery rates for forensic evidence decline rapidly within hours of an assault, and factors such as eating, bathing, and urinating further decrease yield. Acute genital injuries are seen in up to 30% of female victims that present within 3 days of an assault, and most injuries heal completely within a week; healed injuries are observed in fewer than 10% of children and adolescents who are examined more than 3 days after sexual contact. While most examinations are normal, "normal" does not mean "nothing happened"; in one study only 2 of 36 pregnant adolescents had confirmed healed tears of the hymen.

   b. Comprehensive descriptions of injuries on a body map or photodocumentation of physical or sexual abuse injuries, as well as visible signs of neglect, are considered standards of care for abuse evaluations.

   c. While most children and adolescents do not have STIs, increased rates of detected gonorrhea and chlamydia infections are attributed to broader use of nucleic acid amplification tests which have improved sensitivities over culture techniques.

D. Treatment strategies and intervention. Once a child is medically stable and a provider has established that abuse or neglect is suspected, laws in all 50 states require reporting to child protective or law enforcement agencies. Failure to report suspected abuse is a criminal offense; the provider is not required to prove that abuse has occurred to report.

   1. The decision to inform the family of reporting depends on whether sharing such information could potentially jeopardize the child's safety until reporting agencies can intervene; healthcare insurance portability and accountability act (HIPAA) exempts the clinician from sharing verbal or written information with a legal guardian if the child could be endangered by such.

   2. Many areas have established **specialized child abuse assessment programs** that include trained medical professionals, and in some cases, board certified Child Abuse Pediatricians. A primary care clinician may opt to conduct a limited medical assessment once abuse is suspected and refer such cases to these programs, when available. Children's Advocacy Centers and Sexual Assault Nurse Examiner programs are found in most states and can provide assistance to clinicians regarding resources, services, and assessments for abused children.

E. Prognosis. Abused children are at a greater risk for psychiatric disorders, learning disabilities, eating disorders, and low school functioning. Abused and neglected children are also more likely to become teenage mothers, substance abusers, runaways, and delinquents. Affective, anxiety, and personality disorders often persist into adulthood. Obesity, posttraumatic stress disorder, and chronic pelvic pain are frequently seen in adult survivors of child sexual abuse. Child abuse and neglect clearly compromise children's abilities to become productive, healthy adults. In addition, without effective intervention, child abuse becomes an **intergenerational cycle**. An abused child is more likely to become an abuser, an adult partner of a child abuser, or an abused adult.

III. Intimate Partner Violence

A. Definition. Wife or spouse abuse is often used interchangeably with domestic violence or **IPV**. IPV is used more often today because it is more inclusive of all kinds of intimate relationships including dating, sex partners, and same-sex relationships. IPV includes verbal harassment or threats, sexual assault, financial or physical isolation of the victim, and physical attacks. The battering syndrome, which includes all of these forms of abusive behavior, is used to gain control of the victim's behavior. Examples of these forms of abuse include:

   1. Verbal or emotional abuse ranges from repeated insults or insinuations up to threats to hurt or kill the victim or loved ones.

   2. Sexual assault is any form of nonconsensual sexual activity including rape, forced sex against one's will, or engagement (attempted or completed) in sexual activity with a person who is unable to comprehend the nature of the activity, or who is unable to decline participation.

   3. Physical abuse includes harming an intimate partner by punching, kicking, choking, use of a knife or a gun, use of physical restraints, or any other method.

B. Epidemiology. A minimum of 2 to 4 million women are abused annually by their male partners. More than 1.8 million of these women are seriously assaulted. The abuse can become lethal; domestic violence causes one-third of the female murders in the United States. Ninety percent of these cases are the result of males violently assaulting their female partners. Although mutual battering exists, studies have shown that men are more likely than women to perform more severe acts of violence. Men who admit to acts of violence often cite a desire to control or alter their victim's behavior. On the other hand, women who admit to violence indicate that they are often responding to a perceived threat.

C. Violent relationships. Within an abusive relationship, there is usually a typical pattern of tension building, violence, and reconciliation. This cycle has been deemed "the cycle of violence." Over the duration of an abusive relationship, this cycle recurs many times, often with the violence increasing in severity and frequency.

1. **Tension building.** The tension building phase is characterized by frequent hostile verbal attacks, heightened surveillance of the victim, and escalating demands. This part of the cycle is actually the most destructive to the woman's ego and self-esteem. She feels like she is walking on eggshells, not knowing what will set her partner off.

2. **Outburst.** Violence occurs after a build-up of days or months of increasing tension. This can be precipitated by a particular event or can come without warning. Some women have been awakened by beatings.

3. **Reconciliation/honeymoon.** The reconciliation phase quickly follows. The attacker is often remorseful and promises never to be physically abusive again. This is often followed by a "honeymoon" period during which the relationship is calm, however, the cycle most often repeats.

4. **Power and control.** Abusive partners exert control over their partners using many common techniques: financial control, isolation, coercion and threats, intimidation, male privilege, guilt, shame, and using their children.

D. Diagnosis

1. **Awareness.** The key to identification by the primary care clinician is the realization that anyone could be a victim of IPV. Stereotypes regarding poor, uneducated, minority women, or the woman who somehow "provokes" her partner to attack her must be dispelled. A heightened awareness is necessary to consider IPV when evaluating women. Victims of abuse commonly present with multiple somatic complaints including headache, abdominal pain, muscle aches, joint pain, fatigue, vaginal or pelvic complaints, anxiety disorders, depression, or a host of other symptoms often seen in the primary care office. Victims of IPV often go from clinician to clinician and are frequently identified as "difficult patients." Feelings of guilt, shame, and low self-esteem, and patients' perceptions that clinicians do not want to know about abuse are the primary reasons that many battered women are hesitant to discuss abuse.

2. **Screening versus case finding.** This is a controversial issue with respect to IPV. Most professional medical organizations recommend that clinicians should ask about abuse routinely as part of any history and physical examination. The United States Preventive Health Services Task Force recently reviewed IPV screening and recommends that clinicians screen women of childbearing age for IPV and refer or provide intervention services to women who screen positive. (SOR **B**)

   a. Asking about abuse lets the patient know that the clinician is approachable and willing to help. Battered women who do not reveal abuse at an initial visit may discuss it later if they feel safe and that their clinician is receptive. A nonjudgmental statement such as "I often see depression in women who have been hurt by someone close to them. Has this ever happened to you?" is a good screening question for partner abuse. Additionally, placing literature in a safe place, such as the restroom, gives the patients the knowledge that their clinician is open to discussing IPV.

   b. **There are several validated tools to screen for IPV** in a medical setting including HITS (http://www.orchd.com/violence/documents/HITS_eng.pdf), the Partner Violence Screen (http://www.medicine.uiowa.edu/uploadedFiles/Departments/FamilyMedicine/Content/Research/Research_Projects/partner.pdf), and the Woman Abuse Screening Tool (http://www.fmpe.org/en/documents/doc_aids/aid_spabuse.pdf). The Conflict Tactics Scale is used in research but is too long to be useful in a primary care setting.

E. Management strategies. Clinicians are often reluctant to elicit a history of abuse because they are unsure about how to proceed if abuse is reported.

1. **Acknowledge the abuse.** The therapeutic process has already begun when the patient talks to the clinician about the abuse. The clinician needs to convey:

   a. There are many women who have had similar experiences.

   b. It is not their fault.

   c. Abuse is wrong.

   d. They are not crazy.

   It is normal for victims to feel overwhelmed and in need of support. It is also important that the patient understands that her symptoms are a reaction to the abuse. Reassurance helps decrease the sense of isolation and helplessness.

2. **Assess for potential lethality.** The level of continuing danger must be assessed. If there is imminent danger of serious harm or death, arrangements for a shelter should be made before the patient leaves the office. It is important to ask about the following indicators of potential lethality:
   a. Change in severity/frequency of violence
   b. Drug or alcohol use
   c. Possession of a firearm
   d. Threats of suicide/homicide
   e. Recent break-up
   f. Threats or assault with weapon
   g. Attempted strangulation
   h. Stalking behavior
   If children are directly involved in the abuse, by law, this must be reported to your state's child protection agency. In some states (e.g., Utah), domestic violence **in the presence** of children constitutes child abuse. Every clinician should be aware of their state's laws concerning abuse. Most police agencies have a Victims Assistance Unit or equivalent.

3. **Provide resources.** The patient needs to know what resources are available, even if she/he is not yet ready to leave an abusive relationship. Group sessions with survivors of abuse who have had similar experiences are especially helpful. The patient should be given the telephone number of a women's shelter or other resources in the area before she leaves the office. There are often no shelter services available for men including gay, bisexual, or transgender men. Instead, men may be given a hotel voucher if shelter is needed.

4. **Documentation.** Objective documentation including as many details as possible in the history and physical examination is very helpful. Drawing figures or diagrams depicting exact areas of ecchymosis, swelling, lacerations, and other injuries further documents the abuse. Taking photographs may contribute evidence if this were to go to court and is helpful to the victim. Record the name and badge number of any police officer who comes to your office, and any legal action that ensues.

5. **Remember your role.** The clinician may feel frustrated because the patient cannot or will not leave an abusive relationship. The clinician cannot make this decision for the patient. The role of clinician is that of facilitator, helping the patient work through the process of recovery.

F. **Prognosis.** Effects on the victim vary, but certain emotional and behavioral sequelae are commonly seen in an abused partner.

1. **Depression** is one of the most common manifestations suffered by battered women. Depression can come from anger at the abuser turned inward and feelings of guilt or self-blame for "allowing the abuse to happen." Additionally, survivors of abusive relationships often end up lacking financial resources, which adds to their depression. Suicide attempts are not uncommon. Depression can persist after the victim has left the abusive relationship.

2. **Anxiety disorders and PTSD.** Living in an abusive relationship produces high levels of anxiety, and even after the relationship has terminated, many women will still have environmental triggers that can provoke panic attacks. Anxiety, posttraumatic stress disorder, and depression are common ways battered women will present to the primary care clinician. Victims and survivors are often substance abusers, self-treating their undiagnosed psychiatric disorders. Other self-destructive behavior is common and can manifest as smoking or failure to use safety items such as seat belts.

3. **Somatic complaints and chronic pain,** such as abdominal or pelvic pain, headaches, or chronic musculoskeletal pain are also common in patients with histories of victimization. Patients' understanding of this connection often helps ameliorate pain severity.

G. **Prevention** of family violence is rooted in our patients' understanding of positive relationships and nonviolent means of resolving conflict. Asking about relationships and risk factors for violence and our patients' means of resolving conflict provides an opportunity to educate our patients about maintaining nonviolent lifestyles. Questioning about these issues should be part of a comprehensive history with all patients.

1. **Risks for violence** include a history of childhood adversities such as
   • History of abuse (physical, sexual, or emotional) or neglect as a child
   • Witnessing domestic violence during childhood
   • Loss of a parent during childhood (through separation or divorce)

- Household substance abuse or mental illness
- Criminal behavior by a household member

2. Other risk factors for IPV include
- A history of IPV
- Conduct problems and histories of aggression in either partner
- Depression
- Substance abuse

IV. Elder Abuse

A. Definitions. The term *elder abuse* is used interchangeably with *elder mistreatment* and includes many types of abuse against older adults. The National Aging Resource Center on Elder Abuse (NARCEA) (http://www.ncea.aoa.gov/) has developed working definitions for elder abuse and neglect. The types of elder abuse include physical, psychological, and sexual abuse; psychological and physical neglect; violation of rights; and financial or material exploitation. Neglect, physical, and psychological abuse may also be self-inflicted.

1. Physical abuse is the act of causing physical pain or injury resulting in bruising, fractures, dislocations, abrasions, burns, welts, lacerations, and other multiple injuries. Physical abuse can be intentional or unintentional and includes at least one act of violence including beating, slapping, burning, cutting, inappropriate use of physical restraints, and intentional overmedicating.

2. Physical neglect is the failure of a caregiver to meet care obligations such as providing goods and services including food, clothing, shelter, medical, and personal care. Indicators of neglect may include malnutrition, dehydration, decubitus ulcers, poor hygiene, and lack of caregiver compliance with medical regimens.

3. Psychological neglect is the failure of a caregiver to provide a dependent elder with meaningful social contact or stimulation. Examples of this type of neglect include isolating or ignoring the elder for long periods. This commonly results in depression, anxiety, extreme withdrawal, or agitation.

4. Psychological abuse includes the infliction of mental anguish through intimidation, threats, verbal assaults, berating, deprivation, infantilization (treating the older adult like an infant), humiliation, or the provocation of internal fear. The end result of this type of abuse is similar to that of psychological neglect in which the elder is depressed, withdrawn, or fearful and can present with symptoms of "failure to thrive."

5. Sexual abuse is defined as molestation or forced sexual activity. Although this type of abuse is the most underreported, it may occur more often than previously suspected.

6. Violation of personal rights includes preventing elders from making their own decisions regarding housing arrangements; financial matters; and personal decisions such as marriage, divorce, and medical treatment. Physicians and other healthcare providers can observe for signs of violation of personal rights through observation of the caregiver–elder interaction. Does the caregiver insist on being present for the examination? Does the caregiver interrupt the elder's conversation, never allowing the elder to respond to the clinician's questions? Does the caregiver deny the elder the right to make health-care decisions?

7. Material or financial abuse refers to the illegal exploitation of monetary or material assets. This type of abuse includes control of the elder's income and assets by the caregiver; coercion in signing contracts or making changes in a will or durable power of attorney; or the theft of money or property. Specific indicators include a caregiver's refusal to release funds to purchase needed care or patient complaints that they have inadequate funds to buy medication.

8. Self-neglect refers to the behavior of an elderly person that threatens his/her own health or safety. Self-neglect occurs when an older person refuses or fails to provide himself/herself with adequate food, water, clothing, shelter, personal hygiene, medication (when required), and safety precautions.

   a. Signs and symptoms of self-neglect include but are not limited to dehydration, malnutrition, untreated or improperly attended medical conditions, and poor personal hygiene; hazardous or unsafe living conditions/arrangements (e.g., improper wiring, lack of indoor plumbing, heat, or running water); unsanitary or unclean living quarters (e.g., animal/insect infestation, fecal/urine contamination, or odor); inappropriate and/or inadequate clothing, lack of the necessary medical aids (e.g., eyeglasses, hearing aids, and dentures); and grossly inadequate housing or homelessness.

    b. Self-neglect excludes any situations whereby a mentally competent older person makes a conscious and voluntary decision to engage in acts that threaten his/her health or safety as a matter of personal choice.

B. Epidemiology

1. Prevalence and incidence. The NARCEA estimates that between 1.5 and 2 million older adults in the United States suffer from physical abuse or neglect annually. Elder abuse occurs in all communities, regardless of gender, ethnicity or race, socioeconomic status, or religious affiliation. Because of the variation in state reporting requirements, it is difficult to determine the actual rate of elder abuse; however, the majority of state adult protective and regulatory agencies responsible for the identification, investigation, and prevention of elder abuse report an increase in reported cases over the last decade. Because of the absence of a nationalized tracking system for elder mistreatment, prevalence and incidence figures are based on individual researchers and various statewide studies. Estimates on the frequency of elder mistreatment range from 2% to 10% based on various sampling methods and case studies.

2. Identity and background of the perpetrators. Physical abuse is perpetrated most often by spouses with acute or chronic health problems or responsibilities for providing companionship, financial resources, or property maintenance for their dependent spouse. Adult children may psychologically abuse and neglect their parents as well as financially exploit them. These children are often financially dependent on the parent and have a history of mental illness or substance abuse. Many perpetrators are financially dependent on their victims or depend on them for housing.

3. Risk factors for abuse. Increased life expectancy, functional or psychological dependency, learned helplessness, poor physical health, and stress and burnout experienced by the caregiver are primary risk factors for abuse. Other risk factors include living arrangements, caregivers with mental illness or substance abuse, or a family history of violence. Potential predictors of elder mistreatment include poverty, race, and cognitive impairment.

C. Diagnosis

1. A physical examination assessing the patient's general appearance, hygiene, functional status, and mannerisms should be part of the preliminary assessment phase followed by examining skin for bruising, lesions, abrasions, decubitus ulcers, bite marks, and dehydration. Examination of the head and neck areas for trauma, scalp hematomas, traumatic alopecia, or other evidence of direct physical violence should be part of the physical examination. An examination of the musculoskeletal system should reveal any new or old fractures, lesions on wrists or ankles, gait difficulties, cigarette, or other burns. In the genitourinary tract area, attention should be paid to poor hygiene, vaginal or rectal bleeding, inguinal rash, and impaction of feces or infestations. Thorough neurologic/psychiatric evaluation to assess mental status, depressive symptoms, anxiety, or other psychiatric symptoms including hallucinations or delusions is essential in the evaluation process. Cognitive impairment and depression have been shown to be risk factors for elder mistreatment.

2. Based on clinical findings, specific laboratory tests should include albumin, blood urea, nitrogen, creatinine levels, toxicologic screening, and assessment for other deficiencies.

D. Management.
The American Medical Association (AMA) recommends that all clinicians ask their patients about family violence regardless of whether there is clinical evidence or suspicion of abuse or neglect. However, the USPSTF found inconclusive evidence for routine screening of elderly or vulnerable adults (physically or mentally dysfunctional) for abuse and neglect.

1. If the elderly patient is not cognitively impaired, a thorough interview, separate from the caregiver, should occur to assess whether the patient is safe. Nonthreatening questions should be asked, such as (1) "Do you feel safe in your home?," (2) "Who helps you with your personal care, such as bathing, taking your medications, and preparing your meals?," (3) "What happens if your family member becomes tired or cannot help you?," (4) "What happens if you have a disagreement?," and (5) "Who helps you pay your bills?" If the patient has cognitive impairment, history and screening questions must be obtained from the caregiver or family member if available.

    2. If the elder does not feel safe and accepts clinician intervention, hospitalization should be considered. If hospitalization is not an option, the clinician should discuss other placement options with Adult Protective Services (APS). APS has several emergency, court-ordered options available, and can facilitate this process. The following approach with the caregiver facilitates the interview process and reduces some of the tension that may exist: "It must be very difficult to care for your mother with this type of illness. Do you find yourself feeling tired, frustrated, and unable to deal with the situation?" Advising the family member that you will be making a report to APS to help reduce some of the stress that the caregiver may be experiencing may be less threatening to the caregiver. The caregiver should be informed of available resources such as adult day care, respite care, home health care, senior companion programs, caregiver support groups, and individual counseling.

E. Ethical and legal obligations. Clinicians play a critical role in the assessment of elder abuse and neglect, as well as in the intervention process. In long-term clinician–patient relationships in which trust has been established, the process may be easier to facilitate.

    1. Clinicians have a legal responsibility to report suspected cases of abuse or neglect. Mandatory reporting laws exist in most states. Designated state agencies are responsible for conducting investigations and interventions. APS is the agency assigned to investigate and intervene with elder abuse cases. Persons who are licensed, registered, or certified to provide health care, education, and social, mental health, and other human services are required to report abuse. Anonymous reports can be made. Clinicians are usually granted immunity from civil suits in reporting cases of suspected abuse or neglect. Failure to report suspected abuse can result in civil liability and fines for any subsequent damages that may occur. Failure to follow state guidelines for reporting abuse may result in criminal prosecution, professional delicensure, or other penalties.

SELECTED REFERENCES

Adams JA. Evolution of a classification scale: medical evaluation of suspected child sexual abuse. *Child Maltreat.* 2001;6:31–36.

Bonnie RJ, Wallace RB, Eds. *Elder Mistreatment: Abuse, Neglect and Exploitation in an Aging America.* Washington, DC: National Research Council Panel to Review Risk and Prevalence of Elder Abuse and Neglect. National Academies Press; 2003.

Child Maltreatment 2010 report (Child Welfare Board). http://www.acf.hhs.gov/programs/cb/stats_research/index.htm#can. Accessed July 2013.

Christian CW, Lavelle JM, De Jong AR, et al. Forensic evidence findings in prepubertal victims of sexual assault. *Pediatrics.* 2000;106(1):100–104.

Dong XQ. Advancing the field of elder abuse: future directions and policy implications. *JAGS.* 2012;60:2151–2156.

Johannesen M, LoGiudici D. Elder abuse: a systematic review of risk factors in community-dwelling elders. *Age Aging.* 2013;42:292–298.

Kellogg ND; American Academy of Pediatrics Committee on child abuse. The evaluation of child sexual abuse. *Pediatrics.* 2005;116:506–512.

Kellogg ND; American Academy of Pediatrics Committee on Child Abuse. The evaluation of suspected child physical abuse. *Pediatrics.* 2007;119:1232–1241.

Lachs MS, Pillemer K. Elder abuse. *Lancet.* 2004;364:1192–1263.

Langhinrichsen-Rohling J, Capaldi DM. Clearly we've only just begun: developing effective prevention programs for intimate partner violence. *Prev Sci.* 2012;13:410–414.

Moyer VA. Screening for intimate partner violence and abuse of elderly and vulnerable adults: U.S. Preventive Services Task Force recommendation statement. *Ann Intern Med.* 2013;158(6):478–486.

National Center on Elder Abuse. http://www.elderabusecenter.org/default.cfm. Accessed July 12, 2013.

Shugarman LR, Fries BE, Wolf RS, Morris JN. Identifying older people at risk of abuse during routine screening practices. *J Am Geriatr Soc.* 2003;51:24–31.

Reilly JM, Gravdal JA. An ecological model for family violence prevention across the life cycle. *Fam Med.* 2012;44:332–335.

Rolling ES, Brosi MW. A multi-leveled and integrated approach to assessment and intervention of intimate partner violence. *J Fam Viol.* 2010;25:229–236.

Whitfield CL, Anda RF, Dube SR, Felitti VJ. Violent childhood experiences and the risk of intimate partner violence in adults. *J Interpersonal Viol.* 2003;18:166–185.

94 Depression

Rhonda A. Faulkner, PhD, & Luis T. Garcia, MD, A.B.F.M.

KEY POINTS

- Depression is the most common psychological disorder that primary care clinicians will encounter. (SOR **C**)
- Most adults with major depression never see a mental health professional and will receive most or all of their care through primary care clinicians. (SOR **C**)
- Depressed patients frequently present to their primary care provider with somatic complaints as opposed to complaining of depressed mood. (SOR **C**)
- Approximately 1% of patients with depression may have bipolar disease so the family clinician should be alert for manic episodes that might be precipitated by treatment with an antidepressant. (SOR **C**)
- Selective serotonin reuptake inhibitors (SSRIs) offer simpler dosing schedules and fewer side effects than some of the older antidepressants. (SOR **B**) The combination of antidepressant medications with psychotherapy demonstrates the best outcomes in treatment of depression. (SOR **A**)
- Patients starting a course of antidepressant therapy should be advised that symptoms will not subside for 2 to 6 weeks, with a trial of 6 to 8 weeks at maximum dose necessary to confirm treatment success or failure. (SOR **B**)
- In order to prevent the risk of relapse, a treatment period of 6 to 9 months is recommended. (SOR **A**)
- No one particular antidepressant agent has proven superior over another in regards to efficacy; therefore, side effect profiles, presence of medical and psychiatric comorbidities, and prior treatment response are used as guidelines in selecting antidepressant medications. (SOR **A**)
- Patients treated with antidepressants should be closely monitored for potential worsening of depression or suicidal ideation at the onset of therapy and during any change of dosage. (SOR **C**)

I. Introduction. Depression is the seventh most common outpatient diagnosis in family medicine and is often undiagnosed and under-treated.

A. Definitions

1. Major depressive disorder (MDD), the most severe form of depression, is a mood disorder characterized by at least 2 weeks of five or more of the following symptoms: (1) depressed mood; (2) loss of interest or pleasure in daily activities; (3) weight loss or gain; (4) insomnia or hypersomnia; (5) psychomotor agitation or retardation; (6) fatigue or loss of energy; (7) feelings of guilt or worthlessness; (8) inability to concentrate; and (9) thoughts of death or suicidal ideation.

2. Persistent depressive disorder in the DSM V (previously called **Dysthymia** in the DSM IV) is a milder, chronic disorder that is diagnosed when patients experience depressed mood for at least 2 years. Patients with dysthymia may be thought of as having a depressive personality or character style. Although depressive symptoms in dysthymia are not as severe as those of major affective disorder, they are too prolonged to be thought of as adjustment responses. While antidepressants have been found somewhat less efficacious in treatment of dysthymic disorder as compared to MDD, a substantial proportion of patients will respond to antidepressants and psychotherapy. (SOR **B**)

3. Adjustment disorder with depressed mood is a type of mood disorder readily attributable to a recent psychosocial stressor such as a loss of a loved one or employment and should resolve as the stressor decreases. It is distinguished from MDD by its milder severity and shorter time course. Some bereaved patients manifest primarily psychological symptoms and seek counseling, while others develop somatic symptoms and seek medical attention. Unfortunately, many individuals with MDD have stressors that may be identified as the cause of their depression, and thus their illness may be overlooked.

4. **Depressive disorder not otherwise specified (NOS)** is a depressive illness that lasts longer than 6 months. This diagnosis is used to describe mixed states of anxiety and depression that do not meet the criteria for other anxiety or depressive diagnoses.

5. **Mood disorder due to a general medical condition (or substance).** This condition is diagnosed when a prominent mood disturbance can be attributed to a direct physiologic consequence of a general medical condition (i.e., hypothyroidism, AIDS), substance abuse (i.e., alcohol withdrawal), or medication (i.e., beta-blockers, levodopa, steroids, reserpine, and oral contraceptives).

6. **Bipolar disorder** (also known as manic-depressive illness), a condition with a strong genetic predisposition, occurs in approximately 1.2% of the population. These patients experience symptoms of depression along with mania.

7. **Other psychiatric disorders.** Depressive symptoms may also be present in other psychiatric disorders, although they are not predominant. In particular, depression and anxiety are highly comorbid conditions. Therefore, the evaluation of depressive symptoms should include a psychiatric history and a brief review of systems, looking for psychotic features, phobias, panic attacks, somatization, and personality disorders.

B. **Epidemiology.** At any one time, at least 5% of the US population suffers from chronic depression. The lifetime prevalence of major depression in the United States is 16.2%, with approximately 5% to 10% of primary care patients meeting old DSM V criteria for major depression and 3% to 5% for dysthymia. The prevalence of major depression is estimated at 20% to 40% among patients with medical illness such as diabetes and heart disease. Major depression is the leading cause of disability in the United States for individuals aged 15 to 44 years.

1. A depressive disorder can begin at any age, but the average age of onset is the late 20s. Psychosocial events or stressors can play a significant role in precipitating the first or second episode of MDD, but may play little or no role in subsequent episodes.

2. Multiple studies support the finding that major depression is more common in women than in men. This gender difference is found in community samples and is not the result of higher rates of help-seeking behavior by women. Recent studies have disproved the belief that the incidence of depression in women increases during menopause. Prevalence rates for MDD are not related to race, education, or income.

3. Certain individuals are at an increased risk for depression, including alcohol and drug abusers, patients with somatization disorders (see Chapter 96), patients with a life-threatening disease such as a stroke or myocardial infarction, individuals recovering from major surgery, women in the postpartum state, and patients with a family history of depression. Screening for postpartum depression is particularly important, as recent data demonstrate that between 50% and 80% of women experience this reaction within 1 to 5 days after childbirth, lasting up to 1 week. This condition should be distinguished from postpartum psychosis, which occurs in 0.5% to 2% of women, with symptoms beginning 2 to 3 days after delivery.

C. **Etiology**

1. **Genetic factors.** A combination of biologic and environmental factors causes depression. Multiple lines of research point to a genetic or inherited predisposition for MDD that may be activated or precipitated by psychosocial or physiologic stressors. The general understanding of how these stressors interact with a genetic predisposition to produce clinical depression is limited.

2. **Psychosocial factors.** Psychosocial stressors such as death of a spouse, divorce, or developmental life course transitions (e.g., empty nest syndrome) may make patients more vulnerable to experiencing depression. The presence of social support is a mitigating factor for depression; therefore, primary care clinicians should assess social support and facilitate mobilization of these resources.

3. The interaction among these environmental and genetic factors is postulated to culminate in the final common pathway of limbic–hypothalamic dysfunction, which is clinically manifested as a depressive illness. It was originally believed that depletion of neurotransmitters, including norepinephrine, serotonin, and γ-aminobutyric acid, in hypothalamic centers of the brain contributed to the symptom complex of depression. More recent studies suggest a dysregulation hypothesis rather than depletion of a single neurotransmitter.

II. Screening for depression can improve outcomes, particularly when screening is coupled with system changes that ensure adequate treatment and follow-up.

    A. The United States Preventive Services Task Force (USPSTF) **recommends screening adults for depression** when staff-assisted depression care supports are in place to assure accurate diagnosis, effective treatment, and follow-up (SOR **B**) and even when such supports are not in place. (SOR **C**) The USPSTF found insufficient evidence to support a recommendation for routine screening of child and adolescent patients, although primary care clinicians should use their clinical judgment about screening their younger patients.

        1. Screening can be performed by asking the following two simple questions regarding mood and anhedonia: (1) "Over the past 2 weeks, have you felt down, depressed, or hopeless?" and (2) "Over the past 2 weeks, have you felt little interest or pleasure in doing things?" Additionally, eight of the DSM V symptoms (all but depressed mood) can be readily recalled using the mnemonic "SIG: E CAPS" (i.e., "prescribe energy capsules") to assess Sleep, Interest, Guilt, Energy, Concentration, Appetite, Psychomotor, and Suicide.

    B. The American College of Obstetricians and Gynecologists note that screening for depression has the potential to benefit a woman and her family and should be strongly considered; women who screen positive require follow-up evaluation and treatment if indicated. At this time, however, there is insufficient evidence to support a recommendation for universal antepartum or postpartum screening.

III. Diagnosis. Recent studies have documented improvements in the recognition and treatment of MDD in primary care settings, with two-thirds of patients recognized and nearly half prescribed antidepressants.

    A. Symptoms and signs

        1. The clinical diagnosis of depression depends on recognition of an identifiable cluster of signs and symptoms suggesting the disorder.

            a. Five (or more) of the following symptoms have been present during the same 2-week period and represent a change from previous functioning; at least one of the symptoms is either (1) depressed mood or (2) loss of interest or pleasure.

            Note: Do not include symptoms that clearly result from a general medical condition or mood-incongruent delusions or hallucinations.

- Depressed mood most of the day, nearly every day, as indicated by either subjective report (e.g., feels sad or empty) or observation made by others (e.g., appears tearful). **Note:** In children and adolescents, can be irritable mood
- Markedly diminished interest or pleasure in all, or almost all, activities most of the day, nearly every day (as indicated by either subjective account or observation made by others)
- Significant weight loss when not dieting or weight gain (e.g., a change of >5% of body weight in a month) or decrease or increase in appetite nearly every day. **Note:** In children, consider failure to make expected weight gains
- Insomnia or hypersomnia nearly every day
- Psychomotor agitation or retardation nearly every day (observable by others, not merely subjective feelings of restlessness or being slowed down)
- Fatigue or loss of energy nearly every day
- Feelings of worthlessness or excessive or inappropriate guilt (which may be delusional) nearly every day (not merely self-reproach or guilt about being sick)
- Diminished ability to think or concentrate, or indecisiveness, nearly every day (either by subjective account or as observed by others)
- Recurrent thoughts of death (not just fear of flying), recurrent suicidal ideation without a specific plan, or a suicide attempt or a specific plan for committing suicide

            b. Any of the symptoms listed may represent the leading edge of a cluster of depressive symptoms. For example, a recent study found that 80% of patients with the chief complaint of fatigue go on to be diagnosed with an affective disorder. The DSM V requires that five or more symptoms be present during the same 2-week period and that at least one be either a depressed mood or loss of interest or pleasure. It is not uncommon for a depressed patient to deny feeling sad, but instead admit to "not caring anymore."

        2. Although the DSM V is useful in evaluating the possibility of depression in a patient, it was designed primarily by and for psychiatric researchers and was validated on a psychiatric population. DSM V criteria may not be as applicable to a primary care population.

3. Age-specific features in the diagnosis of depression.
   a. Elderly patients with psychomotor retardation, slow thinking, and indecisiveness may be misdiagnosed as having dementia (see Chapter 74).
   b. Prepubertal children often present with somatic complaints, irritable mood, or a psychomotor agitation that manifests itself as a **marked drop in school performance**.
   c. In adolescents, similar findings can occur. Antisocial behavior, restlessness, agitation, **substance abuse,** aggression, poor school performance, withdrawal from social activities, and increased emotional sensitivity are also common. Children and adolescents are often unable to recognize these changes or to associate them with depression.
   d. Patients with depression may present with vague physical symptoms without organic diseases or with symptoms out of proportion to the physical examination. Complaints such as fatigue and dizziness that result in multiple visits without a specific diagnosis should alert the clinician to consider depression.

B. Laboratory tests
   1. The clinical interview remains the most effective method for detecting depression. No reliable biochemical markers for depression exist. Only a limited number of laboratory tests should be conducted to detect potential general medical causes of depressive symptoms. No standard "screening" workup can be used to rule out potential underlying organic causes for depressive symptoms. The evaluation should be directed by demographic and historical clues. For example, hypothyroidism should be considered in an older patient who presents with depressive symptomatology. Medications known to be associated with depressive symptoms (e.g., beta-blockers, antabuse, anticonvulsants, benzodiazepines, barbiturates, estrogen, opiates) should be stopped, especially if recently prescribed.
   2. Several **self-administered questionnaires and depression screening tools** are available for use across the lifespan and are designed to help identify patients with depressive symptomatology (http://www.aafp.org/afp/20020915/1001.html). These tests, which are more useful than as screening tests, possess sensitivities in the 70% range and specificities in the 80% range. They are easily administered and well accepted by patients. Widely used tests include the following:
      a. Beck Depression Inventory, including the short-form version with 13 items (http://www.cawt.com/Site/11/Documents/Members/Evaluation/BeckDepressionInventory1.pdf).
      b. The Zung Self-Rating Depression Scale (SDS), which also has 20 items (http://healthnet.umassmed.edu/mhealth/ZungSelfRatedDepressionScale.pdf).
      c. The nine-item Patient Health Questionnaire (PHQ-9) (http://www.integration.samhsa.gov/images/res/PHQ%20-%20Questions.pdf).

IV. Treatment. Primary care clinicians treat most patients with symptoms of depression. The goals of treatment are (1) to resolve signs and symptoms of the depressive syndrome, (2) to restore occupational and psychosocial functioning to baseline, and (3) to reduce the likelihood of relapse and recurrence. Treatment can be divided into three phases: acute, continuation, and maintenance.

A. Acute phase treatment. In primary care, the most common acute treatment modalities are medication, psychotherapy or counseling, or a combination of medication and psychotherapy. **Mild depression can be treated effectively with either medication or psychotherapy, while the combination approach of medication and psychotherapy together yields best treatment outcomes for moderate-to-severe depression.** (SOR **A**)
   1. Medications have been shown to be effective in all forms of MDD and should be considered first-line therapy in moderate-to-severe MDD. (SOR **A**)
      a. Medication selection should be based on side effect profile; history of prior response; and patient symptoms, concurrent medical conditions, and concurrently prescribed medications (Table 94–1).
         (1) Although there are no clinically significant differences in the effectiveness of antidepressant medications, selective serotonin reuptake inhibitors (SSRIs) are usually preferred over tricyclic antidepressants (TCAs) and monoamine oxidase inhibitors (MAOIs) due to simpler dosing schedules and fewer side effects. No single medication results in remission for all patients.

TABLE 94–1. ANTIDEPRESSANTS

Drug[a]	Starting Dose	Daily Dose	Adverse Effects				
			Sedation	Anticholinergic	Orthostatic Hypotension	Cardiac Conduction	Insomnia
Tricyclics							
Amitriptyline[a] (Elavil)	50 mg at bedtime[b]	75–300 mg	High	High	Moderate	High	Very low
Doxepin[a] (Sinequan)	50 mg at bedtime[b]	75–300 mg	High	Moderate	Moderate	Moderate	Low
Imipramine[a] (Tofranil)	50 mg daily[b]	75–300 mg	Moderate	Moderate	High	High	Very low
Nortriptyline[a] (Pamelor)	25 mg daily[b,c]	40–200 mg	Moderate	Moderate	Low	Moderate	Low
Desipramine[a]	25 mg daily	25–300 mg	Low	Low	Low	Low	Low
Heterocyclics							
Bupropion[a] (Wellbutrin)	100 mg twice daily[d]	200–450 mg	Moderate	Moderate	Very low	Very low	Moderate
Trazodone[a] (Desyrel)	150 mg bedtime[b]	75–300 mg	High	Low	Moderate	Very low	Very low
Selective Serotonin Reuptake Inhibitors							
Citalopram[a] (Celexa)	20 mg daily	20–60 mg	Low	Very low	Very low	Very low	Very low
Escitalopram[a] (Lexapro)	10 mg daily	20 mg	Very low	Very low	Very low	Very low	Very low
Fluoxetine[a] (Prozac)	10–20 mg in am	10–80 mg	Very low	Very low	Very low	Very low	High
Paroxetine[a] (Paxil)	10–20 mg daily	10–60 mg	Low	Low	Very low	Very low	Low
Sertraline[a] (Zoloft)	50 mg daily	50–200 mg	Very low	Low	Very low	Very low	Low
Vilazodone[a] (Viibryd)	10 mg daily	10–40 mg	Very low	Very low	Very low	Very low	Low
Serotonin/Norepinephrine Reuptake Inhibitors							
Desvenlafaxine (Pristiq)	50 mg daily	50–100 mg	Very low	Very low	Very low	Very low	Moderate
Duloxetine Hydrochloride (Cymbalta)	20 mg twice daily	40–60 mg	Very low	Low	Low	Low	Moderate
Venlafaxine[a] (Effexor)	37.5 mg twice daily	75–300 mg	Very low	Low	Very low	Very low	Moderate
Other Antidepressants							
Mirtazapine[a] (Remeron)	7.5–15 mg at bedtime	30–45 mg	High	Moderate	Moderate	Low	Low
Trazodone[a] (Desyrel)	50 mg at bedtime	100–300 mg twice daily	High	Low	Moderate	Low	Low

[a]Available as generic.
[b]May be better tolerated if given in divided doses.
[c]Begin at lower dose in the elderly, titrate to serum level of 50–150 ng/mL.
[d]Not to exceed 150 mg/dose to minimize seizure risk.

(2) In 2007, the Food and Drug Administration (FDA) issued a **black-box warning on all antidepressants** (36 listed) approved for use in patients younger than 25 years to include increased risks of suicidality. The meta-analysis that raised this awareness did not show evidence of completed suicide in young patients taking SSRIs despite the increased suicidality.

b. In order to be proficient in the treatment of depression, the primary care clinician should learn how to use at least three or four antidepressants well and become familiar with dosages, side effects, and serum levels. The chosen medications should have varying side effect profiles and be applicable to different types of presenting symptomatologies.

c. Suggested guidelines for selection include the following:

(1) If the patient has insomnia and early morning awakening, a more sedating medication (e.g., a TCA such as amitriptyline or imipramine) should be chosen.

(2) If the patient's symptoms are characterized by an excessive need for sleep, then a more stimulating and less sedating medication should be selected. Patients with hypersomnia and motor retardation may benefit from bupropion or venlafaxine and should avoid using mirtazapine.

(3) If anxiety is a major component of the symptom complex, then a medication with a lower index of insomnia or agitation side effects is recommended. For patients with generalized anxiety and insomnia, citalopram, escitalopram, and mirtazapine are good choices.

(4) For patients in whom weight gain is a goal, mirtazapine is a good choice.

(5) For patients in whom smoking cessation is also a goal, bupropion can work well.

(6) Elderly patients are especially sensitive to the orthostatic and anticholinergic side effects of some antidepressants. As a result, the SSRIs have replaced TCAs as first-line therapy in the elderly. Careful observation of cardiac function, vital signs, cognitive functioning, and physical complaints will often help identify potential problems early.

(7) If the medication is relatively sedating, compliance can be improved by having the patient take the entire dosage either at bedtime or a few hours before.

(8) Tricyclic drugs do not seem useful for treating children before puberty and are of moderate benefit at best for adolescents. (SOR **B**)

(9) For pregnant woman with moderate-to-severe MDD, the clinician should consider an antidepressant. Consider continuing medication for pregnant women who have MDD that is in remission, are on maintenance medication, and are deemed to be at a high risk of a recurrence if the drug is discontinued. (SOR **B**) SSRIs are most commonly prescribed for pregnant women, but use in the third trimester has caused withdrawal symptoms in newborns (e.g., jitteriness, increased muscle tone, irritability, altered sleep patterns, tremors, difficulty eating) and may be associated with preterm birth and low birth weight. Changes in pharmacokinetics during pregnancy may require dose adjustment. Most antidepressants have an FDA Pregnancy Category C classification due to limited research.

d. Contraindications for specific antidepressants:

(1) Bupropion is contraindicated for patients with seizure disorder.

(2) For patients who have experienced sexual dysfunction prior to depression, SSRIs **should** be avoided.

(3) Hypertension is a relative contraindication to venlafaxine.

(4) Patients experiencing hypersomnia and motor retardation should avoid mirtazapine.

(5) For patients experiencing agitation and insomnia, bupropion and venlafaxine should be avoided.

(6) Mirtazapine and TCAs are **less** preferred for patients with obesity.

2. Psychotherapy

a. Studies have shown that the combination of medication with psychotherapy provides a better response than either form of treatment used alone. (SOR **A**)

b. Depression rarely occurs independent of psychosocial issues. It is vital that the patient begin to address these issues if true recovery is to occur. If relationships within the family, such as a poor marital relationship, prove to be a precipitating factor, then involvement of other family members in counseling may be important.

c. Psychotherapy alone may be preferable in patients with milder forms of MDD who do not desire medication, who have unacceptable side effects to medication, and who have medical conditions limiting medication options.

d. Clinicians may find it useful to use the **BATHE** technique in order to help focus the counseling encounter. The acronym "BATHE" stands for: B = *background:* "What is going on in your life?"; A = *affect:* "How do you feel about that?"; T = *trouble:* "What about this situation or problem troubles you the most?"; H = *handling:* "How are you handling that?"; and E = *empathy:* "That must be very difficult for you."

(1) Often, the patient needs only a sympathetic listener to be able to work through the conflicts he or she is experiencing.

(2) Encounters need not be lengthy. Ten or fifteen minutes is enough time to allow the patient to explore problems in a therapeutic way, with the clinician facilitating this process by asking open-ended questions.

(3) It is not important that the clinician produce a final answer to all of the patient's questions, doubts, or problems, but help the patient's to set goals and decrease negative thoughts about their life.

e. Many clinicians establish a good working relationship with a local psychiatrist, psychologist, or family therapist to whom they can refer patients for counseling or psychotherapy.

3. Patient education

a. A key element in acute phase treatment is the provision of adequate information to both the patient and his or her family about the condition. In addition, the provision of support, advice, reassurance, and hope is critical for depressed patients who are experiencing fatigue, low mood, and poor concentration. Several studies have found that patient education improves adherence to treatment in depressed outpatients. (SOR **B**)

b. An important point to make with many patients is that antidepressant medication is not habit-forming or addictive. Many patients are fearful of "nerve pills" because of friends or relatives who may have developed drug dependence.

c. Nearly half of all patients will stop taking their antidepressant medication within the first month of treatment. Patients should be educated in advance about the side effects of the medications, such as dry mouth, constipation, sexual side effects, and sedation. Patients should be reassured that most will resolve with time.

d. Patients should be told not to expect overnight results. It often takes 4 to 6 weeks for noticeable improvement to occur. It is often helpful to remind patients that their symptoms developed over a similar, if not longer, time interval. (SOR **C**)

4. Aerobic exercise is often promoted as an active strategy to prevent and treat depression and has been shown to be associated with decreased depression scores when compared to no intervention in a small number of treatment trials. While acupuncture, yoga, tai chi, and meditation are of interest to some patients, there is currently insufficient evidence to determine whether or not these modalities are effective in the management of depression.

5. Alternative treatment modalities. Studies indicate a growing preference among patients to pursue self-help and complementary/alternative therapies in the treatment of depression.

a. Herbal products. Many patients use herbal remedies, such as St. John's wort (*Hypericum perforatum*), for treatment of their depression without consulting their clinician. A systematic review found that St. John's wort was superior to placebo in treating depression and comparable to standard antidepressants. (SOR **B**) One drawback to St. John's wort is that it is dosed three times a day.

b. A meta-analysis has shown phototherapy to be associated with a significant reduction in symptom severity with effect sizes similar to pharmacotherapy trials for patients with mild depression. (SOR **B**)

6. Neuromodulation procedures. Many patients with unipolar major depression do not respond to standard treatment with pharmacotherapy and psychotherapy and are thus candidates for noninvasive neuromodulation procedures, including repetitive transcranial magnetic stimulation (TMS) and electroconvulsive therapy (ECT). While ECT has been proven more effective than repetitive TMS, this option may be preferable to patients, given it is better tolerated and does not require general anesthesia and induction of seizures. In a meta-analysis of 34 randomized trials, patients with major depression who did not respond to one or more trials of pharmacotherapy found significant improvement with rTMS treatment. (SOR **B**)

B. Continuation and maintenance treatment. The goal of continuation treatment is to decrease the likelihood of relapse (a return of the current episode of depression).

1. Patients who respond well to acute treatment should be **continued on the same dosage for at least 6 to 12 months after they have resolved their depressive symptoms**. There is very strong evidence that continuation of treatment for this time interval is effective at preventing relapse and recurrence. (SOR **A**)

   a. Patients who experience a second episode of depression will have an 80% chance of additional recurrences and should continue with antidepressant medications for 1 to 2 years. (SOR **B**)

   b. Patients experiencing a third episode of depression have a 90% chance for recurrence and will require indefinite treatment maintenance. (SOR **B**)

V. Management Strategies

A. Overcoming patient resistance. Depression can be difficult for the primary care clinician to treat because the diagnosis itself is often socially unacceptable and culturally invalid for many patients. A survey of 350 family practice physicians revealed that the major obstacle to treatment of depressed patients was patient resistance to the diagnosis.

1. Many clinicians find it useful to approach an explanation of the illness in terms that are better understood by the patient. Such an explanation often begins by explaining how the human body responds to stress and then defining the illness as an imbalance of chemical messengers in the nervous system.

   a. Patients are often more accepting of the diagnosis of depression and more willing to address the psychosocial precipitants, as well as use medication properly, when such an explanation is given.

2. It is often useful, if not crucial, to involve the family in such an explanation, since their support is vital to a successful outcome.

B. Suicide. Suicide potential and prevention must always be considered when the diagnosis of depression is made.

1. The fear that asking about suicide may precipitate a suicide attempt is unfounded. Evidence to date suggests that patients appreciate the concern demonstrated by such questioning.

   a. Some clinicians find it useful to ask a patient who has considered suicide to form a safety contract or agreement. The patient agrees to call the clinician or 911 or go immediately to the nearest Emergency Room before taking any action. No studies exist to support the efficacy of this arrangement, however. Additionally, there are no data to support that screening for suicide in primary care reduces mortality.

2. Individuals at highest risk for a suicide attempt are young females. These attempts are usually gestures and often not successful. Medication overdose is a common method of suicide in females. If suicide is judged to be a risk, it is prudent to limit the amount of medication prescribed at any one time.

3. Persons at highest risk for successful suicide are middle-aged to older men. Other high-risk factors include social isolation and substance abuse.

C. Referral or hospitalization. Even though most depressed patients who present to primary care settings can be managed as outpatients, some will need hospitalization in an inpatient psychiatric unit or referral to a psychiatrist.

1. **The patient who presents with suicidal ideation and specific suicide plans is at serious risk, and hospitalization should be strongly considered.**

2. The patient whose depression is severe enough to interfere with activities of daily living, such as dressing and feeding, should probably be hospitalized.

3. Referral should be considered if the patient has a history suggestive of bipolar disorder.

4. Referral should be sought if evidence of a thought disorder or psychotic features of the depression itself, such as fixed delusions, are present.

5. If the patient fails to respond to treatment after 3 months, referral to a psychiatrist should be considered.

D. Frequency of office visits

1. Follow-up should be scheduled at 2 weeks after the initial diagnosis for most patients with mild-to-moderate depression. Patients with more severe forms of MDD should be seen weekly for the first 4 to 6 weeks of treatment. Subsequent visits may be scheduled

at 4- to 12-week intervals, depending on the degree of response and the need for office counseling.

2. Therapeutic blood levels of antidepressant drugs have been established. Nortriptyline, imipramine, and amitriptyline have well-established minimal therapeutic blood levels. Drug levels should be obtained in the following instances:

    a. When an adequate response is not achieved on full therapeutic doses. Nonresponsiveness to a medication cannot be established unless the steady-state serum level is within the therapeutic range for 2 to 4 weeks.

    b. When serious side effects occur at normal doses. Similarities exist between depressive and toxic symptoms in patients who are clinically deteriorating.

VI. Prognosis

  A. Prognosis without treatment. An untreated episode of depression typically lasts 6 months or more. A remission of symptoms then occurs and functioning often returns to the premorbid level.

    1. Of those patients with recurrent episodes, 5% will have a manic attack at a later date, resulting in a change in their diagnosis to bipolar mood disorder.

    2. Half of all suicide victims are thought to have had an MDD. Suicide occurs in 1% of patients with an acute episode of depression and in 25% of patients with a chronic depression.

  B. Prognosis with treatment

    1. Randomized controlled trials demonstrate that antidepressants are effective in about 30% to 60% of patients with MDD. Patients who do not respond to one particular type of medication may respond well to another. Most patients will respond to at least one antidepressant medication. (SOR **A**) However, two large studies in primary care and psychiatric clinics found only 30% response rates.

    2. In severe cases of MDD, ECT has a high rate of therapeutic success, including speed and safety and may be the treatment of choice for the elderly or acutely suicidal patients. (SOR **A**) However, this is not administered as a first-line treatment and patients requiring this form of treatment should be referred for psychiatrist consultation.

SELECTED REFERENCES

American College of Obstetricians and Gynecologists Screening for depression during and after pregnancy. Committee Opinion No. 453. *Obstet Gynecol.* 2010;115:394-395.

American Psychiatric Association. *Practice Guideline for the Treatment of Patients with Major Depressive Disorder.* 3rd ed. In: *National Guideline Clearinghouse.* Rockville, MD: Agency for Healthcare Research and Quality. http://www.guideline.gov/content.aspx?id=24158. Accessed August 2012.

Feldman MD, Christensen JF: *Behavioral Medicine in Primary Care: A Practical Guide.* 2nd ed. New York, NY: McGraw-Hill; 2003.

Gartlehner G, Hansen RA, Morgan LC, et al. Comparative benefits and harms of second-generation antidepressants for treating major depressive disorder: An updated meta-analysis. *Ann Intern Med.* 2011;155:772-785.

Howland RH. Sequenced Treatment Alternatives to Relieve Depression (STAR*D). Part 2: Study outcomes. *J Psychosoc Nurs Ment Health Serv.* 2008;46(10):21-24.

Linde K, Berner MM, Kriston L. St John's wort for major depression. *Cochrane Database Syst Rev* 2008;(4):CD000448.

O'Connor EA, Whitlock EP, Bell TL, Gaynes BN. U.S. Preventive Services Task Force: screening for depression in adult patients in primary care settings: a systematic evidence review. *Ann Intern Med.* 2009;151:793-803.

Slotema CW, Blom JD, Hoek HW, Sommer IE. Should we expand the toolbox of psychiatric treatment methods to include Repetitive Transcranial Magnetic Stimulation (rTMS)? A meta-analysis of the efficacy of rTMS in psychiatric disorders. *J Clin Psychiatry.* 2010;71:873-874.

Stuart MR, Lieberman JA. *The Fifteen Minute Hour: Practical Therapeutic Interventions in Primary Care.* 3rd ed. Philadelphia, PA: Saunders; 2002.

Sutherland JE, Sutherland SJ, Hoehns JD. Achieving the best outcome in treatment of depression. *J Fam Pract.* 2003;52:201-209.

U.S. Food and Drug Administration. Antidepressant Use in Children, Adolescents, and Adults. http://www.fda.gov/Drugs/DrugSafety/InformationbyDrugClass/ucm096273. Accessed August 2012.

van der Lem R, van der Wee NJ, van Veen T, et al. Efficacy versus effectiveness: a direct comparison of the outcome of treatment for mild to moderate depression in randomized controlled trials and daily practice. *Psychother Psychosom.* 2012;81(4):226-234.

95 Eating Disorders

Brian C. Reed, MD

KEY POINTS

- Making the diagnosis of an eating disorder can be difficult as patients with eating disorders often have poor insight into their condition. Presenting complaints can include fatigue, dizziness, abdominal discomfort, sore throat, heartburn, amenorrhea, and change in their weight. (SOR **C**)
- Weight and cardiac status are the most important components of the physical examination of individuals with eating disorders. Individuals with abnormal vital signs or failure to gain weight in highly structured outpatient programs should be hospitalized. (SOR **A**)
- Psychotherapy and nutritional rehabilitation are the mainstays of treatment for eating disorders. (SOR **A**) An interdisciplinary team consisting of physicians, dietitians, behavioral health care professionals, and nursing should attempt to form a therapeutic relationship with the patient. (SOR **C**)
- Adjunctive treatment with antidepressants can provide additional benefit during the weight maintenance phase of treatment of patients with anorexia nervosa and may decrease binge eating behavior in patients with bulimia nervosa. (SOR **A**)

I. Introduction

A. Definition. Eating disorders are psychological disorders characterized by an altered perception of body weight or shape and serious disturbances in eating behavior. The Diagnostic and Statistical Manual of Mental Disorders (DSM-IV) criteria for diagnosis of eating disorders was used for the listed criteria below, but is due to be updated soon.

1. Anorexia nervosa. Individuals with anorexia nervosa display the following behaviors:

    a. Refusal to maintain body weight at or above a minimally normal weight for age and height (e.g., weight loss leading to maintenance of body weight less than 85% of that expected; or failure to make expected weight gain during period of growth, leading to body weight less than 85% of that expected). Individuals with this disorder typically weigh less than 85% of the normal weight for that person's age and height from the Metropolitan Life Insurance tables or have a BMI less than or equal to 17.5 kg/m^2.

    b. An intense fear of gaining weight or becoming overweight.

    c. Disturbance in the way in which one's body weight or shape is experienced, undue influence of body weight or shape on self-evaluation, or denial of the seriousness of the current low body weight.

    d. Amenorrhea in premenopausal females (i.e., the absence of at least three consecutive menstrual cycles. A woman is considered to have amenorrhea if her periods occur only with hormone administration.)

    e. Two subtypes of anorexia nervosa exist: restricting type and binge eating/purging type. An individual with the restricting type of anorexia nervosa accomplishes weight loss through dieting, fasting, or excessive exercise. An individual who has the binge eating type of anorexia nervosa regularly engages in binge eating and/or purging.

2. Bulimia nervosa. Individuals with bulimia nervosa display the following behaviors:

    a. Engage in binge eating characterized by both eating an amount of food that is larger than what most people would eat during a similar period of time (e.g., within any 2-hour period) and under similar circumstances AND have a sense of lack of control over eating during the episode.

    b. Recurrent inappropriate compensatory behaviors to prevent weight gain (e.g., self-induced vomiting; misuse of laxatives, diuretics, enemas, or other medications; fasting; or exercising excessively).

    c. The binge eating and inappropriate compensatory behaviors both occur, on average, at least twice a week for 3 months.

d. Self-evaluation is unduly influenced by body shape and weight.

e. The episode does not occur exclusively during episodes of anorexia nervosa.

f. As with anorexia nervosa, two subtypes of bulimia nervosa exist: purging type and nonpurging type. Individuals with the purging subtype regularly engage in self-induced vomiting, laxative abuse, and misuse of diuretics and enemas. A person with the nonpurging type of bulimia nervosa employs fasting or excessive exercise as a means of compensating for an episode of binge eating.

3. Eating disorder not otherwise specified. This category describes disorders of eating that fail to meet the criteria for either anorexia nervosa or bulimia nervosa. Examples include women who display all of the behaviors consistent with anorexia nervosa except that they have regular menstruation or someone who engages in binge eating and inappropriate compensatory behaviors at a frequency of less than twice a week for 3 months. Two conditions that fall within this category are:

a. Binge eating disorder

(1) Binge eating disorder features recurrent episodes of binge eating similar to bulimia nervosa.

(2) Since individuals with binge eating disorder do not regularly employ inappropriate compensatory behaviors such as purging or fasting, this disorder differs from bulimia nervosa.

b. Female athlete triad

(1) When associated with athletic training, the combination of disordered eating, amenorrhea, and osteoporosis is known as the female athlete triad.

(2) Usually, these athletes do not meet the criteria for anorexia nervosa.

(3) Amenorrhea in female athletes results from intense training, fluctuations in weight, imbalance between energy intake and expenditure, and low levels of estrogen.

(4) Prolonged low levels of estrogen can lead to osteoporosis and fractures.

B. Epidemiology

1. Anorexia nervosa

a. Prevalence. Studies estimate the lifetime prevalence of anorexia nervosa to be approximately 0.6% among women in the United States. Among men, the prevalence of anorexia nervosa is approximately one-tenth that among women. More than 90% of the individuals with anorexia nervosa are women.

b. Because of the typical age of onset, anorexia nervosa is most commonly encountered in adolescents and young women. Anorexia nervosa usually begins in mid-to-late adolescence (age 15–19 years). The disorder rarely occurs in women older than 40 years.

c. When comparing women of different ethnic origins, anorexia nervosa is more common among Caucasians, Native Americans, and Hispanic women and less common among African-American and Asian-American women in the United States.

2. Bulimia nervosa

a. Prevalence. Based upon the current criteria for definition of bulimia nervosa, the lifetime prevalence is approximately 1% among women in the United States. Similar to anorexia nervosa, the prevalence of bulimia nervosa among men is one-tenth that of women. Bulimia nervosa usually begins in late adolescence or early adulthood.

b. When comparing women of different ethnic origins, bulimia nervosa is most common among Caucasians. However, studies reveal that African-American women are more likely to develop bulimia nervosa than anorexia nervosa and are much more likely to engage in purging with laxatives instead of vomiting.

3. Eating disorder not otherwise specified (NOS) and binge eating disorder

a. Prevalence. The lifetime prevalence of binge eating disorder is approximately 2.8% among women in the United States.

b. The majority of patients with eating disorders are diagnosed with binge eating disorder or eating disorder NOS.

4. Risk factors

a. Cultural factors. Women and adolescents who are preoccupied with their weight and experience social pressure to be thin are at an increased risk for developing an eating disorder. Such societal pressures are found more commonly in industrialized nations such as the United States, Canada, Western Europe, and Japan.

    b. Familial factors. Studies reveal that a hereditary component in the development of eating disorders, especially anorexia nervosa, may exist.

        (1) First-degree female relatives of individuals with anorexia nervosa have higher rates of both anorexia nervosa and bulimia nervosa. They also have higher rates of eating disorders that do not fully meet the diagnostic criteria for anorexia or bulimia.

        (2) Studies of the identical twin siblings of individuals who have anorexia nervosa or bulimia nervosa reveal that they have a higher prevalence of eating disorders.

        (3) However, studies of first-degree relatives of patients with bulimia nervosa do not conclusively demonstrate a hereditary transmission of bulimia nervosa.

    c. History of sexual abuse. Differing studies report that 20% to 50% of individuals with anorexia nervosa and bulimia nervosa have been victims of sexual abuse.

    d. Psychiatric illness. High rates of comorbid psychiatric illness, such as major depression or dysthymia, have been reported to exist among 50% to 75% of individuals with anorexia nervosa and bulimia nervosa. The estimated prevalence of bipolar disorder among patients with anorexia or bulimia is between 4% and 6%. Reports indicate that obsessive–compulsive disorder has lifetime prevalence as high as 25% among patients with anorexia. Personality disorders are also common among patients with eating disorders.

C. Pathophysiology. Although a conclusive origin of eating disorders has yet to be discovered, several theories exist regarding their etiology.

    1. Some studies suggest a neuroendocrine etiology with researchers noting impaired serotonin transmission among individuals with eating disorders. Other studies have observed alterations in serum leptin levels, an important regulator of weight gain and loss.

    2. A genetic etiology has been postulated. Refer to Section I.B.4.b for further details.

    3. Cultural influences and a history of dieting are also thought to be a component in the development of eating disorders.

II. Diagnosis. One must meet the diagnostic criteria mentioned in Section I.A to have either anorexia nervosa or bulimia nervosa. See Table 95–1 for a suggested medical evaluation.

A. Symptoms and signs

    1. Patients with eating disorders can **present with nonspecific complaints** such as fatigue, dizziness, and general lack of energy. Additional complaints include symptoms associated with starvation or purging behaviors such as abdominal pain, constipation, amenorrhea, sore throat, and palpitations. Since patients with anorexia rarely possess insight into their illness, they rarely present with complaints about weight loss. Concerned family members and friends may bring patients with eating disorders for an office visit.

    2. When obtaining a history, it is important to **establish rapport and obtain a thorough diet history**. Questions should include inquiries about the number of diets used within the past year and the patient's perception of their weight.

    3. Weight and cardiac status are the most important components of the physical examination of individuals with eating disorders.

    4. During treatment, one must closely monitor the weight of patients. Patients with eating disorders sometimes wear extra layers of clothing, place weights in their pockets, and drink extra fluids prior to being weighed.

    5. Early in the disorder, the physical examination may be normal.

    6. As the severity of the eating disorder worsens or with increased duration, complications can cause several abnormal findings on physical examination as listed:

        a. Cardiac. Bradycardia, orthostatic hypotension, and acrocyanosis are among the cardiac abnormalities.

        b. Dental. Erosion of dental enamel and salivary gland enlargement are signs of purging behavior.

        c. Gastrointestinal. Patients may have significant abdominal distention secondary to decreased bowel motility.

        d. Skin. Patients can develop lanugo, dry skin, or loss of subcutaneous fat. Repeated induction of vomiting may cause calluses or scarring on the dorsum of the hand (Russell sign).

TABLE 95–1. SUGGESTED MEDICAL EVALUATION OF PATIENTS WITH EATING DISORDERS

Evaluation	Anorexia Nervosa Restricting Type	Binge/Purge Type	Bulimia Nervosa Purging Type	Nonpurging Type
Weight for height	X	X	X	X
Temperature, pulse, blood pressure	X	X	X	X
Physical examination	X	X	X	X
Dental examination		X	X	
Electrocardiogram	X	X	X	
Complete blood cell count	X	X	X	X
Urinalysis	X	X	X	X
Blood urea nitrogen				
Creatinine	X	X	X	X[a]
Amylase		X[a]	X[a]	X[a]
Electrolytes	X	X	X	X[a]
Magnesium	X	X	X[a]	
Calcium	X	X	X[a]	
Phosphate	X		X	X[a]
Albumin	X	X	X[a]	
Bone mineral densitometry[b]	X[a]	X[a]	X[a]	X[a]
LH/FSH/estradiol[b]	X[a]	X[a]	X[a]	X[a]
Liver enzymes	X	X	X	
TSH, T$_4$	X	X	X	X
Cholesterol	X	X	X	X
Glucose	X	X	X	X
Blood/urine screen for drugs/ alcohol, laxatives/diuretics	X[a]	X[a]	X[a]	X[a]

[a]May be indicated, depending on the patient's clinical circumstances.
[b]In patients with long-standing amenorrhea.
FSH, follicle-stimulating hormone; LH, luteinizing hormone; TSH, thyroid-stimulating hormone.

B. Laboratory findings

1. Among individuals with eating disorders, laboratory testing may be normal until complications (as mentioned earlier) develop.
2. Because of complications, testing can reveal abnormal electrolytes, renal functioning, complete blood cell counts, thyroid function test abnormalities, and osteopenia. See Section V.A (medical complications) for further details.

C. Differential diagnosis

1. **General medical conditions.** When evaluating an individual for anorexia nervosa or bulimia nervosa, one must consider other possible causes of weight loss and binge eating.
   a. Gastrointestinal disorders, endocrine diseases, occult malignancies, and acquired immunodeficiency syndrome (AIDS) are among the medical conditions that should be considered.
   b. Individuals with the neurologic disorder Kleine–Levin syndrome can experience binge eating similar to a person with bulimia nervosa.
   c. Patients who experience weight loss due to a medical condition usually do not experience the distortion of body image that individuals with anorexia nervosa display.
2. **Psychiatric disorders.** Several psychiatric disorders can cause severe weight loss.
   a. **Major depressive disorder** can cause decreased appetite and weight loss.
   b. Patients with **schizophrenia** may display odd eating behaviors and experience weight loss.
   c. **Social phobia** can provoke feelings of humiliation or embarrassment while eating in public.
   d. **Body dysmorphic disorder** can cause altered perception of body image.
   e. Some individuals with **obsessive–compulsive disorder** experience obsessions and compulsions related to food.

III. Treatment
A. Goals
1. **Anorexia nervosa.** Goals in the treatment of anorexia nervosa include the restoration of a healthy weight, management of physical complications, treatment of comorbid psychiatric conditions, restoration of healthy eating patterns, correction of maladaptive thoughts regarding food, building a support network, and prevention of relapse.
2. **Bulimia nervosa.** A reduction in binge eating and purging are the primary goals in the treatment of bulimia nervosa. Since most individuals with bulimia nervosa have a normal body weight, weight restoration is not a primary goal.

B. Treatment location (Table 95–2). Weight, cardiac complications, and metabolic status are the most important physical parameters in the determination of treatment location.
1. **Inpatient hospitalization**
   a. Indications for immediate hospitalization are marked orthostatic hypotension with an increase in pulse of >20 beats per minute or >20 mm Hg drop in standing blood pressure, bradycardia <40 beats per minute, tachycardia >110 beats per minute, or inability to sustain body core temperature. (SOR ❸)
   b. Severely underweight individuals (patients who weigh <75% of their individually estimated healthy weights) and adolescents and children with rapid weight loss also require 24-hour hospitalization. (SOR ❸)
   c. Failure of outpatient treatment, persistent weight loss, and declines in oral intake despite participation in outpatient treatment programs, and the presence of additional physical stressors such as concurrent viral illnesses or psychiatric disturbances are indications for inpatient treatment. (SOR ❷)
   d. Most patients with uncomplicated bulimia do not require inpatient hospitalization. Bulimic patients may require inpatient treatment if they have serious concurrent medical problems, suicidality, severe psychiatric disturbances, concurrent substance abuse, or have failed trials of outpatient therapy. (SOR ❷)
   e. Evidence suggests that patients with eating disorders have better outcomes when treated on inpatient units that specialize in the treatment of these disorders than when treated in general inpatient hospitals. (SOR ❹)
2. **Outpatient treatment**
   a. Highly structured outpatient programs are often necessary for individuals with anorexia nervosa who weigh <85% of their individually estimated healthy weight.
   b. The more successful programs require patients participate in treatment at least 8 hours a day for 5 days a week. (SOR ❹)
   c. Partial hospitalization and day hospital programs are being increasingly used in the treatment of eating disorders.

C. Nutritional rehabilitation
1. A program of nutritional rehabilitation should be established for those who are markedly underweight. The program should seek to restore weight, achieve normal eating patterns, correct maladaptive thoughts about hunger, and correct sequelae of malnutrition. (SOR ❹)
2. **Typical goals for weight gain are 2 to 3 lbs per week for patients in the inpatient setting and 0.5 to 1 lb per week in the outpatient setting.** Initial intake levels should begin at 30 to 40 kcal/kg/day and should be gradually advanced. During the weight-gain phase, daily food intake may be increased by 70 to 100 kcal/kg/day. (SOR ❸)
3. During refeeding, solid foods are preferable to liquid diets.
4. In life-threatening situations, nasogastric feeding and parenteral feedings may be necessary.
5. During nutritional rehabilitation or refeeding, medical monitoring of vital signs, electrolytes, edema, and volume overload is essential.
6. Since many patients with bulimia nervosa have a normal weight, restoration of weight is often not necessary. In these patients, nutritional counseling should focus on reducing dysfunctional eating behaviors and correcting nutritional deficiencies.

D. Psychosocial interventions
1. For patients with anorexia nervosa, the goals of treatment are to encourage patient cooperation during their physical and nutritional rehabilitation, change dysfunctional behaviors related to their eating disorder, address comorbid psychopathology, and improve social functioning.

TABLE 95–2. LEVEL-OF-CARE CRITERIA FOR PATIENTS WITH EATING DISORDERS

Characteristic	Level 1 Outpatient	Level 2 Intensive Outpatient	Level 3 Full-day Outpatient	Level 4 Residential Treatment Center	Level 5 Inpatient Hospitalization
Medical complications	Medically stable to the extent that more extensive monitoring as defined in levels 4 and 5 is not required			Medically stable (not requiring NG feeds, IV fluids, or multiple daily laboratories)	Adults: HR <40 beats/min; BP <90/60 mm Hg; glucose <60 mg/dl (3.3 mmol/L); K^+ <3 mg/dl (0.8 mmol/L); temperature <36.1°C (97°F); dehydration; renal, cardiovascular, or hepatic compromise. Children and adolescents: HR <50 beats/min; BP <80/50, orthostatic BP, hypokalemia, hypophosphatemia.
Suicidality	No intent or plan			Possible plan but no intent	Intent and plan
Weight, as percent of healthy body weight	>85%	>80%	>70%	<85%	Adults <75%. Children and adolescents: acute weight decline with food refusal.
Motivation to recover (cooperativeness, insight, ability to control obsessive thoughts)	Good to fair	Fair	Partial, preoccupied with ego-syntonic thoughts more than 3 h/d; cooperative.	Fair to poor; preoccupied with ego-syntonic thoughts 4–6 h/d; cooperative with highly structured environment.	Poor to very poor; preoccupied with ego-syntonic thoughts; uncooperative with treatment or cooperative only with highly structured environment.
Comorbid disorders (substance abuse, depression, anxiety)	Presence of comorbid condition may influence choice of level of care				Any existing psychiatric disorder that would require hospitalization.
Structure needed for eating/gaining weight	Self-sufficient		Needs structure to gain weight	Needs supervision at all meals or will restrict eating	Needs supervision during and after all meals, or NG/special feeding
Impairment and ability to care for self, ability to control exercise	Able to exercise for fitness; fitness; able to control obsessive exercise		Structure required to prevent excessive exercise	Complete role impairment, cannot eat and gain weight by self; structure required to prevent patient from compulsive exercise	Needs supervision during and after all meals
Purging behavior	Can greatly reduce purging in nonstructured settings; no significant medical complications such as ECG abnormalities or others suggesting the need for hospitalization			Can ask for and use support or skills if desires to purge	
Environmental stress	Others able to provide adequate emotional and practical support	Others able to provide at least limited support and structure	Severe family conflict, problems or absence so as unable to provide structured treatment in home, or lives alone without adequate support system and structure		
Treatment availability/living situation	Lives near treatment setting				Too distant to live at home

BP, blood pressure; ECG, electrocardiogram; HR, heart rate; IV, intravenous; K^+, potassium level; NG, nasogastric.

Source: Adapted with permission from Practice guideline for the treatment of patients with eating disorders (revision). American Psychiatric Association Work Group on Eating Disorders. *Am J Psychiatry.* 2000;157(Suppl 1):1–39.

2. Systematic trials, case series, and expert opinions suggest that a well-conducted regimen of psychotherapy helps improve symptoms of anorexia nervosa and prevent relapse. (SOR **Ⓐ**) One meta-analysis comparing behavioral psychotherapy programs to treatment with medication alone revealed that behavioral therapy resulted in more consistent weight gain and shorter hospital stays. Clinical consensus favors individual psychotherapy during the acute phase of treatment for anorexia nervosa.

3. Structured inpatient and partial hospitalization programs have produced good short-term therapeutic effects. These behavioral programs often employ nonpunitive reinforcers such as empathic praise and privileges for achieving weight goals.

4. Individual psychotherapy and family psychotherapy have proven to be helpful in the management of anorexia nervosa. (SOR **Ⓐ**)

5. Cognitive behavioral therapy is the single most effective intervention in the treatment of bulimia nervosa. (SOR **Ⓐ**)

6. Additionally, studies have demonstrated that group treatment, family therapy, and individual psychotherapy are helpful in the treatment of bulimia nervosa. (SOR **Ⓐ**)

E. Medications

1. Antidepressants. Although antidepressants do not augment the benefits of psychotherapy during the acute management phase of patients with anorexia, antidepressants are effective in the weight maintenance phase of treatment plans. (SOR **Ⓐ**) Additionally, antidepressants are effective in the acute treatment of bulimia nervosa. Studies have demonstrated 50% to 75% reductions in binge eating and vomiting with use of antidepressant medications. (SOR **Ⓐ**)

   a. Selective serotonin reuptake inhibitors (SSRIs) such as fluoxetine are commonly considered for patients with anorexia nervosa who have depressive, obsessive, and compulsive symptoms. Fluoxetine is typically dosed at 40 mg per day in the weight-maintenance phase of anorexia. Doses of fluoxetine up to 60 mg per day may help prevent relapse among patients with anorexia. Similarly, a 60- to 80-mg daily dose of fluoxetine is beneficial in the treatment of bulimia nervosa. Presently, fluoxetine (Prozac) is the only medication approved by the U.S. Food and Drug Administration (FDA) for the treatment of bulimia nervosa. (SOR **Ⓐ**)

   b. Bupropion. People with anorexia have a lowered seizure threshold so the use of bupropion (which can also lower the seizure threshold) is not recommended.

   c. Tricyclic antidepressants and MAOIs. Tricyclic antidepressants, bupropion, and MAOIs are effective in the treatment of bulimia nervosa. The MAOIs, phenelzine or isocarboxazid, dosed between 30 and 45 mg per day can reduce binge eating behavior in patients with bulimia. Dosing of the tricyclic antidepressants usually starts at 50 mg per day. MAOIs and tricyclic antidepressants should be avoided in malnourished patients because of greater risk of adverse reactions.

2. Psychotropic medications. Antipsychotic medications such as olanzapine, risperidone, and quetiapine have demonstrated some usefulness in patients with anorexia who have severe, unremitting resistance to gaining weight, severe obsessional thinking, and extreme denial. (SOR **Ⓒ**) Thus far, controlled studies have yet to demonstrate efficacy of other psychotropic medications such as neuroleptics in the treatment of anorexia nervosa or bulimia nervosa.

3. Other medications

   a. Treatment of osteoporosis. Calcium (500 mg two to three times daily), estrogen replacement, and bisphosphonates have been used in the treatment of patients with anorexia nervosa to prevent osteopenia and osteoporosis. Usually oral contraceptives are used as a means of hormone replacement and restoration of menstruation. Presently, no evidence has proven the effectiveness of these interventions.

   b. Management of abdominal pains. Metoclopramide, 10 mg with meals, has been used in the treatment of gastroparesis and early satiety.

IV. Management Strategies

A. Establish a therapeutic relationship. The idea of gaining weight for an individual with an eating disorder or discontinuing binge eating patterns can be anxiety provoking. Without patients having a trusting relationship with their physician, such goals will never be achieved.

B. Collaborate with other health professionals. Nutritional counseling, group psychotherapy, and medical consultation with specialists may be necessary to fully restore the health of an individual with bulimia nervosa or anorexia nervosa.

C. **Monitor dysfunctional eating behaviors.** The careful assessment of a patient's perceived food intake and the anxiety provoked by eating is necessary. Having a meal with a patient may allow the clinician further insight into the patient's disordered patterns of eating.

D. **Monitor the patient's general medical condition and psychiatric status.**

E. **Assess the family and provide treatment.** Parents often struggle with denial, feelings of guilt, anger, and feelings of rejection. Family assessment and family therapy are usually a significant part of comprehensive care.

V. **Prognosis**

A. **Medical complications.** Patients with anorexia nervosa and bulimia nervosa are susceptible to serious medical complications as a result of starvation and purging.

   1. **Cardiovascular complications** include orthostatic hypotension, palpitations, and arrhythmias such as bradycardia. Cardiomyopathy may result from low weight or syrup of ipecac abuse. Additionally, severe electrolyte imbalances can lead to sudden cardiac death.

   2. **Dental complications.** Multiple dental caries and dental enamel erosions can occur after several years of induced vomiting in anorexia or bulimia nervosa. Patients may also develop enlarged salivary glands.

   3. **Gastrointestinal complications.** Vomiting related to the compensatory purging behavior in patients with anorexia nervosa and bulimia nervosa can eventually cause gastritis, esophagitis, or Mallory–Weiss tears. Patients can develop esophageal dysmotility disorders such as gastroesophageal reflux. Individuals who repeatedly use laxatives as a means of purging can develop melanosis coli and other problems with colonic motility. Chronic constipation and bloating may occur in laxative abusers. Cases of rectal prolapse have been reported in the literature.

   4. **Endocrine complications.** Patients with anorexia nervosa can develop elevated serum cortisol levels and decreased levels of serum thyroxine (T_4) and triiodothyronine (T_3).

   5. **Hematologic complications.** Nutritional deficits and changes associated with starvation can cause normochromic normocytic anemia, neutropenia, and thrombocytopenia. Rarely, patients with anorexia nervosa experience clotting disorders.

   6. **Metabolic complications.** Because of starvation and purging, patients can develop serious electrolyte imbalances. Laxative abusers can develop a metabolic acidosis, hypomagnesemia, and hypophosphatemia. Metabolic alkalosis (elevated serum bicarbonate levels, hypochloremia, and hypokalemia) and hyperamylasemia can result from repeated induced vomiting.

   7. **Musculoskeletal complications** include osteoporosis and arrested skeletal growth. Young female athletes with amenorrhea and altered eating behaviors are particularly at risk for the development of stress fractures. Bone mineral density testing for osteoporosis and osteopenia should be considered in patients with chronic amenorrhea.

   8. **Renal complications.** Renal abnormalities are seen in up to 70% of patients with anorexia nervosa. Complications include decreased glomerular filtration rate, increased blood urea nitrogen, and pitting edema. Monitoring of renal function during treatment is strongly recommended.

   9. **Reproductive complications** include amenorrhea and infertility. Amenorrhea occurs in women due to low estrogen levels. Men with anorexia nervosa may have low serum testosterone levels. Both men and women with eating disorders can experience loss of libido and infertility. Adolescents and young women can experience arrest of sexual development or regression of secondary sexual characteristics.

   10. **Skin complications.** Repeated manual stimulation of the gag reflex to induce vomiting can cause callus development and scarring on the dorsum of the hand. This is known as Russell sign.

   11. **Suicide** is a major cause of death among patients with anorexia nervosa.

B. **Outcomes**

   1. **Anorexia nervosa**

      a. Approximately 44% of patients with anorexia nervosa fully recover and successfully restore their weight to within 15% of recommended weight for height. Approximately 24% of patients never restore their weight and between 2.5% and 5% of patients with anorexia nervosa die.

      b. Worse prognosis is associated with lower minimum weight, earlier age of onset, and disturbed family relationships.

    c. Follow-up studies conducted for more than 10 to 15 years reveal that it may take between 57 and 79 months to achieve full recovery.

2. Bulimia nervosa

    a. Approximately 25% to 30% of patients with bulimia demonstrate spontaneous improvement within 1 to 2 years.

    b. With interventions such as medication and psychosocial intervention, between 50% and 70% of patients have significant reduction in binge eating and purging.

SELECTED REFERENCES

American Psychiatric Association. *Diagnostic and Statistical Manual of Mental Disorders*. 4th ed., text revision. American Psychiatric Association; 2000:583–595.

American Psychiatric Association. Treatment of patients with eating disorders, 3rd ed. *Am J Psychiatry*. 2006;163(suppl 7):4–54.

Hobart JA, Smucker DR. The female athlete triad. *Am Fam Physician*. 2000;61(11):3357–3364, 3367.

The McKnight Investigators. Risk factors for the onset of eating disorders in adolescent girls: results of the McKnight Longitudinal Risk Factor Study. *Am J Psychiatry*. 2003;160(5):248.

Smink FR, Hoek HW. Epidemiology of eating disorders: incidence, prevalence and mortality rates. *Curr Psychiatry Rep*. 2012;14:406–414.

Williams PM, Goodie J, Motsinger CD. Treating eating disorders in primary care. *Am Fam Physician*. 2008;77(2):187–195.

---

96   Somatization

Juliet Bradley, MD, & Tracy R. Juliao, PhD

KEY POINTS

- More than 50% of patients presenting to outpatient medical clinics with a physical complaint do not have a medical condition. (SOR **C**)
- Diagnosis of somatization involves recognizing common symptoms and being aware that medical diseases and mental disorders may be comorbid. (SOR **C**)
- Treatment is multifaceted but relies most heavily on developing a trusting relationship with a single provider who engages in active listening, education, teaching self-regulation strategies, and developing a therapeutic contract that includes both supportive care and setting limits.

I. Introduction

    A. Definition. Somatization is a syndrome of distressing physical symptoms plus abnormal thoughts, feelings, and behaviors in response to these symptoms. Somatization symptoms may be caused or exacerbated by anxiety, depression, and interpersonal conflicts; it is common for somatization, depression, and anxiety to all occur together. The physical symptoms of somatization are not intentional, that is, under voluntary control. Somatization is associated with significant psychosocial impairment.

    B. Epidemiology

        1. Prevalence

        a. Somatization is extremely common. More than 50% of patients presenting to outpatient medical clinics with a physical complaint do not have a medical condition. Between 60% and 80% of healthy persons experience somatic symptoms in any given week, and 70% of patients with emotional disorders present a somatic complaint as the reason for their office visit.

        b. The prevalence of **somatic symptom disorder** is estimated to be 5% to 7% in the general population, with a higher prevalence in women. The DSM V emphasizes the presence of positive symptoms and signs (distressing somatic symptoms plus abnormal thoughts, feelings, and behaviors in response to these symptoms) rather than the absence of a medical explanation for them (Table 96–1).

TABLE 96–1. COMMON SYMPTOMS FOUND IN DISORDERS INVOLVING SOMATIZATION

- Essential feature includes a chronic history of unexplained symptoms for which the patient denies any psychological contribution
- Pain symptoms, focused or diffuse
- Gastrointestinal symptoms (e.g., nausea, abdominal pain, diarrhea)
- Cardiopulmonary symptoms (e.g., chest pain, shortness of breath, palpitations)
- Pseudoneurologic symptoms (e.g., fainting, muscle weakness, blurred vision, difficulty walking, amnesia)
- Reproductive organ symptoms (e.g., dysmenorrhea, burning in sex organs)
- General preoccupation with symptoms
- Multiple unexplained symptoms
- Lack of methods to ameliorate symptoms and/or unclear factors that exacerbate symptoms
- Lack of positive findings on physical examination
- Patients often elicit negative reactions from clinicians and are often perceived/labeled as "difficult patients"

    c. In primary care practice, the prevalence of **illness anxiety disorder,** a preoccupation with having or acquiring a serious illness, may be as high as 10% in the general population.

    d. Conversion disorder (functional neurologic symptom disorder) describes a syndrome in which various neurologic symptoms are clearly incompatible with neurologic disease. There may be one or more symptoms of various types. Motor symptoms include weakness, paralysis, abnormal movements, gait abnormalities, and abnormal limb posturing. Sensory symptoms include altered, reduced, or absent skin sensation, vision, or hearing. There may be episodes of abnormal limb shaking with apparent alteration of consciousness resembling epileptic seizures.

2. Risk factors

    a. Personal characteristics associated with somatization include female sex, older age, fewer years of education, lower socioeconomic status, unemployment, and recent experience of stressful life events. Childhood sexual abuse and recent exposure to sexual or physical violence are consistently associated with somatization in adult women.

    b. Cultural factors. Somatization occurs throughout the world, and the tendency to somatize does not vary from culture to culture. Although there are no significant cross-cultural differences in the rate of somatic symptom disorders, cultural differences in somatic presentations do exist. These differences have been described as "idioms of distress" because somatic symptoms may have special meanings in particular cultural contexts and may shape provider–patient relationships. Dizziness, burning in the head, and "too much heat in the body" are examples of symptoms that are common in some cultures but rare in others.

C. Pathophysiology. Multiple theories have been proposed to explain somatization (Table 96–2). Controversy exists about whether somatization is a purely psychiatric disorder, or whether it should be viewed as a syndrome of vague symptomatology complicating the presentation of a general medical condition. Somatic symptom disorder is associated with marked impairment of health status. The genetic basis for somatization is unclear; familial patterns have been inconsistently demonstrated. These patterns may be due to genetic or environmental factors, or both.

II. Diagnosis. Somatization is a complex, multifactorial process. It is perhaps best to think of somatization as a spectrum that ranges from occasional functional somatic symptoms to full-blown DSM V somatic disorder. A medical and psychosocial etiology for a patient's symptoms should be explored simultaneously so that the patient has confidence that their medical needs are being addressed. In addition, patients who present with a new illness

TABLE 96–2. THEORIES OF SOMATIZATION ETIOLOGY

- **Neurobiologic.** Abnormal central nervous system regulation of incoming sensory information leads to an impairment in attentional processing.
- **Psychodynamic.** Somatization is a defense mechanism.
- **Behavioral.** Somatization is a learned behavior in which environmental reinforcers maintain abnormal illness behavior.

episode may be more willing to discuss psychosocial concerns at the onset of their evaluation, rather than after all medical examinations have failed to identify a cause for their symptoms.

A. History. In taking a history, the clinician should pay attention to how the physical symptoms are related to the patient's emotions and social situation, and if any stressful personal events such as losses have occurred.

1. The patient should be asked about medications including nonprescription, prescription, and complementary medications. Additionally, patients should be questioned about substance use, including alcohol.

2. It is important to ask whether the patient has experienced **physical or sexual abuse,** whether the patient feels safe in his/her current relationships, and whether he/she feels threatened or afraid in any way, either at home or in other settings.

3. Past medical history is very important and may demonstrate a pattern of suspected ailments, which were not confirmed pathologically, or a pattern of symptom preoccupation in different organ systems. A history of multiple surgical procedures without pathologic confirmation of disease raises the likelihood of somatization. The patient may have a history of changing doctors frequently or leaving the hospital against medical advice.

B. Differential diagnosis

1. Poorly understood conditions in which somatization might play a role or which might be confused with somatization include **fibromyalgia, irritable bowel syndrome, premenstrual dysphoric disorder, dysphagia, chronic fatigue syndrome, idiopathic environmental intolerance** (multiple chemical sensitivity), and **temporomandibular joint dysfunction.**

2. Nonpsychiatric medical conditions with vague, diffuse, or episodic complaints may be mistaken for somatization, especially early in their clinical course. These conditions include hypothyroidism, multiple sclerosis, porphyria, systemic lupus erythematosus, and musculoskeletal and neuropsychiatric manifestations of Lyme disease.

3. Amplified symptoms of underlying organic disease may also be involved in somatization.

4. Psychiatric disorders in which somatization is not the primary process may be "masked" by an array of somatic complaints. These disorders include **major depression** (see Chapter 94), **alcohol and substance abuse** (see Chapter 90), and **generalized anxiety** and **panic disorders** (see Chapter 91). Somatization frequently occurs in depression, and clinicians should consider major depression and dysthymia whenever somatization is present. In an international multicenter study, 69% of those with major depressive disorder presented with only somatic symptoms and 50% had multiple unexplained symptoms.

5. Disorders including somatization. Diagnosis of these conditions is based on the fifth edition of the American Psychiatric Association Diagnostic and Statistical Manual of Mental Disorders.

a. Somatic symptom disorder.

- The presence of one or more somatic symptoms that are distressing or result in significant disruption of daily life.
- Excessive thoughts, feelings, or behaviors related to the somatic symptoms or associated health concerns as manifested by at least one of the following:
  - Disproportionate and persistent thoughts about symptom seriousness.
  - Persistently high anxiety level about health or symptoms.
  - Excessive time and energy devoted to these symptoms or health concerns.
- Although one somatic symptom may not be continuously present, the state of being symptomatic is persistent (typically for more than 6 months).
- *Specify* if:
  - **With predominant pain** (previously pain disorder): This specifier is for individuals whose somatic symptoms predominantly involve pain.
  - **Persistent,** characterized by severe symptoms, marked impairment, and duration of more than 6 months.
- *Specify* current severity:
  - **Mild:** Only one of the symptoms specified is fulfilled.
  - **Moderate:** Two or more of the symptoms is fulfilled.
  - **Severe:** Two or more of the symptoms specified are fulfilled, plus there are multiple somatic complaints (or one very severe symptom).

b. Conversion disorder (functional neurologic symptom disorder)
- Presence of one or more symptoms of altered voluntary motor or sensory function.
- Clinical findings provided evidence or incompatibility between the symptom and recognized neurologic or medical conditions.
  - The symptom or deficit is not better explained by another medical or mental disorder.
  - The symptom or deficit causes clinically significant distress or impairment in social, occupational, or other important areas of functioning or warrants medical evaluation.
  - *Specify* symptom type: With weakness or paralysis, with abnormal movement (e.g., tremor, dystonic movement, myoclonus, gait disorder), with swallowing symptoms, with speech symptoms (e.g., dysphonia, slurred speech), with attacks or seizures, with anesthesia or sensory loss, with special sensory symptoms (e.g., visual, olfactory, or hearing disturbances), or with mixed symptoms.

c. Illness anxiety disorder
- Preoccupation with having or acquiring a serious illness.
- Somatic symptoms are not present, or, if present, are only mild in intensity. If another medical condition is present or there is a high risk for developing a medical condition (e.g., a strong family history is present), the preoccupation is clearly excessive or disproportionate.
- There is a high level of anxiety about health, and the individual is easily alarmed about personal health status.
- The individual performs excessive health-related behaviors (e.g., repeatedly checks his or her body for signs of illness) or exhibits maladaptive avoidance (e.g., avoids doctor appointments or hospitals).
- Illness preoccupation has been present for at least 6 months, but the specific illness that is feared may change over that period of time.
- The illness-related preoccupation is not better explained by another mental disorder such as somatic symptom disorder, panic disorder, generalized anxiety disorder, body dysmorphic disorder, obsessive-compulsive disorder, or delusional disorder, somatic type.

d. Psychological factors affecting other medical conditions
- A medical symptom or condition (other than a mental disorder) is present.
- Psychological or behavioral factors adversely affect the medical condition in one of the following ways:
  - The factors have influenced the course of the medical condition as shown by a close temporal association between the psychological factors and the development or exacerbation of, or delayed recovery from, the medical condition.
  - The factors interfere with the treatment of the medical condition (e.g., poor adherence).
  - The factors constitute additional well-established health risks for the individual.
  - The factors influence the underlying pathophysiology, precipitating or exacerbating symptoms or necessitating medical attention.
- The psychological and behavioral factors are not better explained by another mental disorder (e.g., panic disorder, major depressive disorder, posttraumatic stress disorder).
- *Specify* current severity:
  - **Mild:** Increases medical risk (e.g., inconsistent adherence with antihypertensive treatment).
  - **Moderate:** Aggravates underlying medical condition (e.g., anxiety aggravating asthma).
  - **Severe:** Results in medical hospitalization or emergency room visit.
  - **Extreme:** Results in severe, life-threatening risk (e.g., ignoring heart attack symptoms).

e. Factitious disorder imposed on self
- Falsification of physical or psychological signs or symptoms, or induction of injury or disease, associated with identified deception.
- The individual presents himself or herself to others as ill, impaired, or injured.

- The deceptive behavior is evident even in the absence of obvious external rewards.
- The behavior is not better explained by another mental disorder, such as delusional disorder or another psychotic disorder.
- *Specify* if single episode or recurrent episodes (two or more events of falsification of illness and/or induction or injury).

   f. Factitious disorder imposed on another (previously factitious disorder by proxy)
   - Falsification of physical or psychological signs or symptoms, or induction of injury or disease, in another, associated with identified deception.
   - The individual presents another individual (victim) to others as ill, impaired, or injured.
   - The deceptive behavior is evident event in the absence of obvious external rewards.
   - The behavior is not better explained by another mental disorder, such as delusional disorder or another psychotic disorder.
   - *Specify* if single episode or recurrent episodes (two or more events of falsification of illness and/or induction or injury).

C. Symptoms and signs
   1. Symptoms favoring somatization are presented in Table 96–1. The presence of several of these characteristics strongly suggests somatization, even though evidence of organic disease may also be present. Recognition of these symptoms, particularly when clustered together, can help with the differential diagnosis. It is also important to recognize that the presence of a somatic disorder does not preclude the presence of a mental disorder or a medical condition.
   2. **Pain** is the most frequent single complaint, present in more than 80% of patients with somatization.
   3. **Three symptom clusters suggestive of somatization secondary to depression, anxiety, or panic disorder are**
      - Atypical chest pain, palpitations, tachycardia, or difficulty catching one's breath (sighing, not true dyspnea), or all of these.
      - Headache, dizziness, lightheadedness, presyncope, or paresthesias.
      - Dyspepsia, heartburn, "gas," flatulence, or other gastrointestinal symptoms, or all of these.

D. Laboratory tests. Laboratory and imaging studies serve only to rule out organic disease, although evidence of a disease entity does not exclude the diagnosis of somatization. Abnormalities unrelated to the patient's symptoms may be discovered with sophisticated diagnostic technology that are not particularly helpful and may even fuel the patient's belief that if more tests are ordered, or more specialists are consulted, the "true" cause of his/her symptoms will be revealed. For example, the presence of minimal mitral valve prolapse on echocardiography cannot explain an array of somatic symptoms. Avoid tests with low yields that may create new problems for the patient, such as increased anxiety or side effects from the procedure itself.

III. Treatment. Appropriate treatment for any underlying problems is the first priority. Treatment is not likely to be effective unless maintaining factors are addressed and minimized.
   A. Basic treatment principles. A list of general principles for treatment of somatization are displayed in Table 96–3. While there may be specific treatment recommendations for particular disorders involving somatization, these basic principles apply to all patients with somatization. It is important to encourage patients to develop a stable, trusting relationship with a single provider who oversees their care and manages collaborative efforts with other providers.
   1. Never say, "It's all in your head" or "There's nothing wrong with you." Avoid the debate of whether symptoms are primarily psychiatric or nonpsychiatric. Directly challenging the patient's belief that symptoms are caused by a medical condition may unintentionally undermine the relationship with the patient. It is more reasonable for the clinician to explain that there is no evidence of a life-threatening illness, but rather, the patient has a well-described, although not well-understood, condition that results in the set of symptoms.
   2. Give a clear explanation of symptoms presented in functional or physiologic terms. Explain the sympathetic nervous system's "fight-or-flight" stress response, the science of how emotions reside in the physical body, and the interaction (not cause)

TABLE 96–3. GENERAL TREATMENT PRINCIPLES FOR SOMATIZATION

- Establish a therapeutic alliance with the patient
- Establish importance of collaborative treatment approach, encouraging patient to be active participant in his/her care
- Schedule regular visits
- Evaluate and treat diagnosable medical disease and/or mental disorder
- Acknowledge and legitimize symptoms and associated suffering
- Limit diagnostic testing and referrals to specialists
- Reassure that serious medical diseases have been ruled out
- Communicate with other providers and be sure that same message is communicated to the patient by each provider
- Set explicit goal of treatment as improving functional abilities and developing coping skills
- Educate patients about coping with physical symptoms that may not be alleviated or eliminated
- Evaluate for and treat substance abuse and addiction

of cognitions and the body. The physician should describe the problem in terms the patient can understand and in a way that fits in with his or her belief system about health and illness. When you do not understand and cannot explain a symptom, tell the patient that with empathy. **Clinicians should acknowledge the patient's physical and emotional suffering, emphasize that they regard the symptoms as real, and should assure the patient that the presence of a psychiatric disturbance or disorder does not negate the reality of his or her suffering.** Acknowledgment of the patient's suffering may facilitate the patient's acceptance of a formal psychiatric intervention, if needed.

3. Initiate a well-defined treatment program: **Regular, brief appointments are often recommended over "as needed" appointments.** The frequency of appointments depends upon the individual patient. The goal is to find the appropriate frequency that leads to avoidance of unnecessary emergency room visits or unscheduled phone calls.

   a. **Treatment may consist of a combination of explanation, reassurance, observation, and symptomatic measures.** The clinician should provide relatively definite information about how to proceed, how long the symptoms might last, and what to do next. Ambiguity increases anxiety.

   b. Crises should be managed firmly so that chronic or recurrent symptoms do not lead to unnecessary evaluations, referrals, or tests that can be costly and often lead to reinforcement for the patient to seek additional support/treatment.

4. **Engage the patient's active participation**. Encourage the patient to keep a log or diary of factors that influence symptoms such as emotion, daily stressors, and activities they are involved in; this may serve to make the problem appear less unpredictable and out of control. General behavior change techniques also may be initiated. For example, an exercise program to enhance "muscle tone" or a diet for weight reduction, if successful, generally enhances the patient's sense of control and self-mastery. Specific, realistic, incremental, and measurable goals that include observable behavior encourage patients to be active participants in their care and enable them to witness progress in a tangible manner.

B. **Multifaceted treatment approach**
   1. **Pharmacotherapy.** There are no adequate clinical trials of drug treatment for primary somatization per se. However, drugs may be effective in the following situations:

      a. Specific intractable symptoms such as headaches, myalgias, and other forms of chronic pain may be ameliorated by **selective serotonin reuptake inhibitors (SSRIs)** or **tricyclic antidepressants** (see Chapter 94). (SOR **B**)

      b. Even when DSM V criteria for depression are not present, patients who demonstrate somatic symptoms of depression often benefit from adequate doses of SSRIs. Likewise, anxious patients may experience relief of somatic symptoms in response to benzodiazepine therapy, even though they do not fulfill DSM V criteria for panic or anxiety disorders (see Chapter 91). (SOR **B**)

      c. Because patients who somatize often have a low tolerance for medication side effects, symptomatic medications (e.g., analgesics or antispasmodics) should be used sparingly and in the minimal effective doses. (SOR **C**)

      d. There is rarely, if ever, a place for opioids in treating somatization symptoms. (SOR **C**)

2. Consultation with a psychiatrist or psychologist. While integrated care or collaborative care in which a psychologist is a part of the primary care team is ideal, this does not always work out practically.

   a. Consultation or referral to behavioral medicine programs, psychiatry, or cognitive behavior therapy has been shown to be effective with this population. Psychiatric consultation has been shown over 1 year to be effective in reducing hospitalizations and overall medical costs of patients with somatization disorder. (SOR **B**) In one study, a single consultation report to the primary physician was associated with a 12% reduction in costs.

   b. A course of **cognitive behavioral therapy** has been associated with improvements in functioning and decreases in healthcare utilization for up to 18 months. (SOR **B**)

   c. Many patients with somatization are skeptical of referrals to mental health professionals. Therefore, care should be taken to explain that their suffering is "real" and that this is a "part" of their treatment plan, not a "physician replacement" or rejection of future treatment.

3. Patients with severe chronic somatization may benefit from intensive, multidisciplinary treatment programs that include individual, group, and family therapy; educational programs; physical and occupational therapy; biofeedback; and vocational rehabilitation.

IV. Management Strategies. Optimal management of somatizing patients requires relief of symptoms, treatment of underlying medical or psychiatric disorders, and avoidance of the pathologic cycle of intervention (medical treatment, temporary improvement, renewal of symptoms, disappointment, and patient and physician anger).

A. The **therapeutic contract** should be emphasized and its parameters defined. While recognizing the reality of the patient's symptoms, one should attempt to develop a broader framework for physician–patient interaction by following these guidelines:

   1. Tolerate symptoms and scale down the goals of therapy. Speak in terms of reduction, lessening, and coping, rather than complete symptom alleviation. Evaluate new symptoms as they occur, but do so conservatively in a stepwise fashion. Openly discuss the risks of medication side effects and the possibility of complications with invasive procedures.

   2. Discuss psychiatric or psychosocial issues not as direct causes of symptoms, but rather as possible aggravating factors or as unfortunate results of physical symptoms.

   3. Promote stability in the physician–patient relationship by scheduling office visits at regular intervals, thereby diminishing the patient's need for a "ticket of admission." Increase the length of office visits to allow relatively unrushed attention. Schedule visits at times when interruptions will be minimal, not on "emergency-prone" days such as Mondays or Fridays.

   4. Explicitly discourage dependent behaviors, such as unscheduled phone calls or drop-in visits. Prearranged follow-up phone calls or emails may allow a reduction in the frequency of office visits. Ask the patient not to "doctor shop" or to seek specialist care without consulting the primary care physician.

B. Somatization may be a sign of **family dysfunction** in which the identified patient's symptoms may serve to stabilize a pathologic family situation. It may be necessary to enlist family members in behavioral strategies to "wean" the patient from secondary gain (e.g., using somatization to avoid household tasks, to require special meals, or to excuse irritability and angry outbursts).

C. While remaining supportive of the symptomatic person, the physician should attempt to avoid certifying the person as **permanently and totally disabled**. The label of *disability* can be viewed as another "medical intervention" with adverse consequences as well as benefits. Nonetheless, the physician should realize that severe and chronic somatization is a disabling condition. Chronic pain syndrome, for example, may qualify under Medicare guidelines as a cause of total disability. While perhaps not desirable in terms of "curing" the somatization, disability may, in certain cases, for economic and social reasons be the best palliative option.

D. Physicians often develop a great deal of **anger** and **frustration** when treating patients who somatize. To maintain equanimity, the physician can use the following strategies:

   1. Make the diagnosis of somatization and modify treatment objectives accordingly, rather than wallowing in frustration over the absence of objective findings of disease.

   2. Set up firm and explicit guidelines as described earlier and review them frequently with the patient. Arrange office appointments so that somatizers are not clustered together.

3. Develop an informal relationship with a psychiatrist or a psychologist to whom feelings about these patients can be ventilated and with whom treatment problems can be discussed.

V. Prognosis

    A. A large proportion of patients with functional somatic symptoms recover without specific intervention. Favorable prognostic factors include acute onset and short duration of symptoms, younger age, higher socioeconomic class, absence of organic disease, and absence of personality disorder.

    B. The long-term prognosis for patients with somatization disorder is guarded, and usually lifelong supportive treatment is required. If somatization is a mask for another psychiatric disorder, its prognosis depends on that of the primary problem. In one study of patients with psychiatric disorders presenting with a recent onset of physical symptoms, 40% subsequently developed chronic somatoform disorders.

    C. Discrete conversion symptoms have a better prognosis. They may resolve spontaneously when no longer "required" or may respond to specific psychotherapy.

SELECTED REFERENCES

American Psychiatric Association. *Diagnostic and Statistical Manual of Mental Disorders.* 5th ed. Arlington, VA: American Psychiatric Publishing; 2013.

Coulehan JL, Block MR. Seal up the mouth of outrage: interactive problems in interviewing, Chapter 12. In: *The Medical Interview: Mastering Skills for Clinical Practice.* Philadelphia, PA: FA Davis; 2001:195–219.

Deary V, Chalder T, Sharpe M. The cognitive behavioural model of medically unexplained symptoms: a theoretical and empirical review. *Clin Psychol Rev.* 2007;27:781–797.

Dickinson WP, Dickinson LM, deGruy FV, et al. The somatization in primary care study: a tale of three diagnoses. *Gen Hosp Psychiatry.* 2003;25:1–7.

Dinwiddle SH. Somatization disorder: past, present, and future. *Psychiatric Ann.* 2013;43:78–83.

Escobar JI, Hoyos-Nervi C, Gara M. Medically unexplained symptoms in medical practice: a psychiatric perspective. *Environ Health Perspect.* 2002;110(suppl 4):631–636.

Hiller W, Fichter MM, Riet W. A controlled treatment study of somatoform disorders including analysis of healthcare utilization and cost-effectiveness. *J Psychosomatic Res.* 2003;54:369–380.

Hoedeman R, Blankenstein AH, van der Feltz-Cornelius CM, et al. Consultation letters for medically unexplained physical symptoms in primary care. *Cochrane Database Syst Rev.* 2010;(12):CD006524.

Kroenke K. Efficacy of treatment for somatoform disorders: a review of randomized controlled trials. *Psychosom Med.* 2007;69:881–888.

Maynard CK. Assess and manage somatization. *Nurse Pract.* 2003;28:20–29.

Oyama O, Paltoo C, Greengold J. Somatoform disorders. *Am Fam Physician.* 2007;76:1333–1338.

Simon GE, Von Korff M, Piccinelli M, et al. An international study of the relation between somatic symptoms and depression. *N Engl J Med.* 1999;341(18):1329–1335.

Smith JK, Jozefowicz RF. Diagnosis and treatment of somatoform disorders. *Neurol Clin Pract.* 2012: 94–102.

Stanley IM, Peters S, Salmon P. A primary care perspective on prevailing assumptions about persistent medically unexplained physical symptoms. *Int J Psychiatry Med.* 2002;32:125–140.

SECTION IV. Reproductive Health

Grant M. Greenberg, MD, MA, MHSA, Nell Kirst, MD,
& Margaret Dobson, MD

KEY POINTS

- More than half of all pregnancies in the United States are unintentional, as are 92% of pregnancies in adolescents aged 15 to 19 years. Unintentional pregnancies occur because contraceptives are not used, because they are used sporadically or incorrectly, or due to failure of the contraceptive method despite proper use.
- Knowledge of contraceptive failure rates, risks, benefits, and acceptability allows the provider to "match" the contraceptive method to the needs and desires of the patient.
- Hormonal methods of birth control are the most commonly used reversible method; however, at 1 year, only about two-thirds of women continue their use.
- Long-acting reversible contraceptive (LARC) methods such as IUDs and implants can be used by women of all ages and are two of the most efficacious contraceptive methods available. An increase in use of LARC can be helpful in reducing unintended pregnancy.
- Condoms are the only method that offer some protection against sexually transmitted infections.
- Emergency contraception (postcoital contraception) is available as levonorgestrel 1.5 mg single dose; available as a nonprescription product and ulipristal a 30 mg single dose prescription medication. Levonorgestrel provides about a 75% reduction in risk of pregnancy while ulipristal reduces pregnancy risk by 85%. Ulipristal is more effective especially at >72 hours after unprotected intercourse.

I. Introduction. Contraception is an important topic to discuss with all sexually active men and women of childbearing age.
  A. More than half of all pregnancies in the United States are unintentional, as are 92% of pregnancies in adolescents aged 15 to 19 years. Unintentional pregnancies occur because contraceptives are not used, because they are used sporadically or incorrectly, or due to failure of the contraceptive method despite proper use.
  B. Numerous contraceptive options are available, so the choice of a particular option should take place after a review of the risk and benefits of all appropriate choices, and education on the option chosen so correct use is assured.
  C. The only 100% effective method of birth control is abstinence. Correct use of any contraceptive device does not guarantee protection. Many women who experience unintended pregnancy use their selected methods consistently and properly; pregnancy rates also depend on the efficacy of the method in a typical user (see Table 97–1).
  D. Long-acting reversible contraceptive (LARC) methods, primarily intrauterine devices (IUDs), are contributing to an increase in contraceptive effectiveness in the United States. The proportion of US women using the IUD and implant increased from 2.4% in 2002 to 8.5% in 2009, more than offsetting decreases in sterilization. These LARC methods require little intervention on the part of the user and do not interfere with sex.
II. Choosing a Birth Control Method. Consideration of the following factors will help patients make the best possible choices: accessibility, efficacy, safety, and acceptability. It is important to take the time also to educate patients about the risks and benefits of their birth control options. Studies have found that many women who begin using a contraceptive method stop using it within the first year of use. Less than half of women using spermicides alone, withdrawal, sponge, or condoms are still using them at 1 year; just over half continue use of Depo-Provera or diaphragms, and about two-thirds continue use of combined hormonal contraceptives. Rates of continued use are higher with IUDs and implants (78%–84%). Providing more complete information about the method may prevent discontinuation and can help women be knowledgeable about other options.
   Desirable properties of contraceptives are a high rate of effectiveness, prolonged duration of action, reversibility for those desiring future fertility or permanence for those who

TABLE 97–1. CONTRACEPTIVE OPTIONS AVAILABLE IN THE UNITED STATES IN 2012

| Method | Unintended Pregnancies with 1 yr of Use (%) | | Noncontraceptive Benefits | Use with Breastfeeding |
	Typical Use	Theoretical		
None	85	85	—	—
Spermicide	29	18	None	Yes
Withdrawal	27	4	None	Yes
Periodic abstinence (fertility awareness)	25	3–5	None	Yes
Diaphragm with spermicide	16	6	None	Yes
Female condom	21	5	Prevents STDs	Yes
Male condom	15	2	Prevents STDs	Yes
Oral contraceptive pills (OCPs)–combined and progestin-only	8	0.3	Regulation of menstrual cycle and dysmenorrhea, possible decrease in ovarian and endometrial cancer risk, acne	No
Contraceptive patch	8	0.3	Same as OCPs	No
Vaginal ring	8	0.3	Same as OCPs	No
Depo-Provera	3	0.3	Same as OCPs	Yes
Copper-containing IUD	0.8	0.6	None	Yes
Levonorgestrel IUD	0.2	0.2	Regulation of menstrual cycles and dysmenorrhea	Yes
Female sterilization	0.5	0.5	None	Yes
Male sterilization	0.15	0.10	None	Yes
Etonogestrel implant	0.05	0.05	Same as OCPs	Safety conditional

Source: Trussell J. Contraceptive efficacy. In Hatcher RA, Trussell J, Nelson AL, Cates W, Stewart FH, Kowal D, Policar M, eds. *Contraceptive Technology.* 20th rev ed. New York, NY: Ardent Media; 2011:827–1010; Herndon EJ, Zieman M. New contraceptive options. *Am Fam Physician.* 2004;69:853–860; Herndon EJ, Zieman M. *Improving Access to Quality Care in Family Planning: Medical Eligibility Criteria for Contraceptive Use.* 2nd ed. Geneva, Switzerland: Reproductive Health and Research, World Health Organization, 2000. http://whqlibdoc.who.int/publications/2004/9241562668.pdf. Accessed July 4, 2006; Speroff L, Fritz MA. *Clinical Gynecologic Endocrinology and Infertility.* 7th ed. Philadelphia, PA: Lippincott Williams & Wilkins; 2005.

wish to have no future fertility, privacy of use, protection against sexually transmitted infections (STIs), safety, and acceptable or minimal side effects. To support informed contraceptive decision-making, healthcare professionals should realize that a woman's view of a method's ease of use is more important than perceived efficacy, tolerability, health benefits, or risks.

A. Efficacy

1. **Theoretical efficacy rates** are defined as the rate of unintended pregnancies per 100 women estimated to occur during the first year of use of a given contraceptive method assuming correct and consistent use.

2. **Actual efficacy rates** reflect the actual rate of unintended pregnancies per 100 women during the first year of use of a given contraceptive method if they do not stop using the method for any other reason. The efficacy of a given contraceptive method is influenced by many factors including fertility, the frequency of intercourse, the ability of the patient to use the method properly, and the theoretical efficacy rate of the method.

3. **Safety concerns** include risks of morbidity and mortality as well as noncontraceptive safety benefits (see Table 97–2), such as protection from STIs or resolution of menstrual problems.

4. **Acceptability** of a method depends on a number of subjective factors:
   a. **Cost.** What is the out of pocket cost to the individual using the method? Cost will vary based on health insurance coverage, retail pricing of nonprescription

TABLE 97–2. NONCONTRACEPTIVE HEALTH BENEFITS OF CONTRACEPTIVE METHODS

Agent	Benefits
Combined hormonal contraceptives	Decreased dysmenorrhea Decreased menstrual blood loss and anemia Possible reduction of premenstrual syndrome (PMS) Decreased risk of ectopic pregnancy Decreased risk of endometrial and ovarian cancer Decreased risk of pelvic inflammatory disease Reduction of acne
Progesterone-only contraceptives	Decreased dysmenorrhea Amenorrhea May reduce dysfunctional uterine bleeding in women who are overweight Decreases risk of endometrial and ovarian cancer Decreases risk of pelvic inflammatory disease Can decrease the number/severity of crises in patients with sickle-cell anemia Can decrease frequency of seizures, does not interact with antiepileptic medications Reduces risk of uterine leiomyomata formation
Levonorgestrel IUD	Decreases menstrual blood loss Decreased dysmenorrhea
Male/female condom	Decreased risk of STI transmission including HIV

methods, and should consider time off work for surgical or irreversible methods.

    b. Individual preferences. Does the patient have any ethical or religious concerns regarding the method? Do they have a preference based on frequency (or lack) of menstrual cycles or based on noncontraceptive benefits of a particular method?

    c. Duration. How long after initiation of the method is it considered effective? For what duration can the method be used and be considered effective?

    d. Reversibility. For reversible methods: after discontinuation how long until the patient is able to conceive? For permanent methods, is irreversibility desired?

    e. Privacy. Does the method afford the patient enough privacy? This includes having to purchase a nonprescription contraceptive at a retail store, having to store the contraceptive in a private location, taking time to see a healthcare provider for an injection, the visibility of a subdermal implant, or even a scar from a surgical procedure.

    f. Availability. Does the method require office visits, a prescription, or any other special situation to obtain?

    g. Convenience. Is it easy to use the method when needed? Does it require an intentional action to apply or is it available when needed without additional effort?

B. Patient education. Providing clear instruction on proper use, expected side effects and how to minimize them, and potential risks of any contraceptive method is important. Pointing the patient to on-line educational resources such as www.womenshealth.gov can facilitate better understanding of options, side effects, and proper use.

III. Hormonal Contraception. This method works by suppressing ovulation and follicle maturation, thickening cervical mucus so that sperm are less effective, and making the endometrium less receptive to embryo implantation.

A. Oral contraception—combination of estrogen–progestin pills. This birth control method is used by an estimated 28% of reproductive-aged women and is the most popular form of reversible contraception in the United States. Oral contraceptives (OCs) contain different doses and two types of estrogen (ethinyl estradiol and mestranol, a prodrug converted to ethinyl estradiol) and different doses and types of progestin. Biphasic

TABLE 97–3. CHOOSING AMONG ORAL CONTRACEPTIVES (OCPs)

Patient Characteristics	Preferred Type of Oral Contraceptive	Generic Examples (Brand Name) Estrogen Content and Comments
Acne	Less androgenic activity pills: those containing third-generation progestins: norgestimate, desogestrel or drospirenone, or low-dose norethindrone	Norgestimate (Ortho Tri-Cyclen[a], Ortho-Cyclen, Sprintec); desogestrel (Desogen/Ortho-Cept, Apri, Mircette, Kariva, Ortho Tri-Cyclen Lo, Cyclessa); low-dose norethindrone (Ovcon 35, Brevicon, Modicon), norethindrone acetate (Estrostep[a]), drospirenone (Yaz, Beyaz, Yasmin, Safyral)
Nausea or breast tenderness when taking OCPs	Progestin-only or lower (20 mcg) estrogenic activity pills	Progestin-only: see above 20 mcg pills (Alesse, Loestrin 1/20, Aviane, Yaz)
No prior use of OCPs	Lower-dose pills minimize side effects	20 mcg pills, see above 30 mcg pills (Desogen, Ortho-Cept, Apri, Yasmin, Levlen, Levora, Loestrin 1.5/30, Lo/Ovral, Cryselle) 35 mcg pills (Ortho Novum 1/35, Ovcon 35, Demulen 1/35, Zovia 1/35E, Brevicon, Modicon, Neocon 0.5/35, Ortho-Cyclen, Sprintec, Norinyl 1+35, Necon 1/35, Tri-Norinyl, Ortho Novum 7/7/7)
Nursing women	Progestin-only pills will not interrupt milk supply	Norethindrone (Ovrette, Micronor)
Scanty or absent withdrawal bleeding	Build up endometrium	Increase estrogen dose or lower progestin dose/potency
Spotting/break-through bleeding (BTB)	Stabilize endometrium	Explore reasons for spotting: missing pills, erratic timing, drug interactions Reassure women that BTB is common during the first several month of OC use. Changing estrogen dose or type of progestin does not alter bleeding rates. Do not use progestin-only pills for women concerned about BTB (SOR Ⓑ)
Use of rifampin, phenytoin, barbiturates or other liver enzyme-inducing medications	Use an alternative contraceptive (preferred; increased side effects of 50 mcg dose, uncertain contraceptive efficacy of higher estrogen dose) or increase estrogen to 50 mcg/tablet.	50 mcg pills (Ovral, Ovcon 50, Demulen, Ortho-Novum 1/50, Norinyl 1/50)

[a]FDA-approved for the treatment of acne.

and triphasic OCs contain different amounts of hormone throughout the menstrual cycle in an attempt to more closely mimic natural hormone production. However, there is insufficient evidence to support any clear benefit of multiphasic over monophasic formulations. Choosing among the many OCs can be done on the basis of characteristics of both the patient and the OC. See Table 97–3 for common characteristics and recommendations for use.

1. **Failure rate for typical use** is 9 pregnancies expected per 100 women per year; **correct use** <1 pregnancy per 100 women per year.
2. **Risks** include dizziness, nausea, breast tenderness, elevated blood pressure, thromboembolic disease, and change in menstruation and mood. It should be noted that the risk of deep vein thrombosis (DVT) or pulmonary embolus (PE) with any of these methods is significantly lower than that for pregnancy.
    a. **Contraindications.** For a complete list of conditions where the health risks likely outweigh the benefits of use or for which there are unacceptable health risks, the reader is referred to the Centers for Disease Control and Prevention at http://www.cdc.gov/reproductivehealth/UnintendedPregnancy/PDF/effectiveness_of_contraceptive_methods.pdf. OCs should not be used in the following cases:
    (1) Women older than 35 years who smoke more than 15 cigarettes per day.

(2) Women with cardiovascular problems, such as a history of thromboembolic disease or thrombogenic conditions, uncontrolled hypertension (>stage 2), cerebrovascular disease, and ischemic heart disease.

(3) Any woman who has migraine headaches with aura or any woman over age 35 years with migraine, due to an increased risk for stroke.

(4) Women <1 month postpartum because OCs can diminish breast milk production in the first month postpartum and increase risk for thromboembolic disease in the first 21 days postpartum. Progestin-only pills are acceptable. The American Academy of Pediatrics advises against the use of OCs as long as the woman is exclusively breastfeeding; women can begin OCs as soon as supplemental nutrition is part of the infant's diet.

(5) Known or suspected pregnancy is a contraindication; although these medications have no proven teratogenic potential, there is clearly no benefit for pregnant women.

(6) Women with other conditions including breast cancer, liver tumor, and cirrhosis of the liver.

3. Benefits

  a. Reduction in risk of endometrial and ovarian cancers. (SOR **B**)

  b. More regular and less painful menstrual periods with less bleeding and iron-deficiency anemia. Premenstrual syndrome may be less common and less severe in women using OCs, as are benign breast disease and benign ovarian cysts, endometriosis, acne, hirsutism, and anovulatory bleeding. (SOR **B**)

4. Acceptability

  a. Convenience. Must be taken daily.

  b. Availability. Current FDA regulations require a prescription.

5. Extended use of combined OC pills. Three agents are FDA approved for extended use. *Seasonale* and *Seasonique* contain 84 days of active tablets and seven placebo tablets, and *Lybrel* contains a full year of active tablets with no placebos. These agents are equally effective as more traditional monthly cycling, but have a greater risk for breakthrough bleeding during the first few months of use. Other monophasic combined OCs can be dosed for extended use, but are not FDA approved for this purpose. If doing so, typically, active tablets of three pill packs are used consecutively (63 tablets) followed by a 7-day placebo or no pill period.

B. Oral contraception—progestin-only pills. These medications contain only progestin and are most often used when combinations pills are contraindicated. They work by reducing and thickening cervical mucus, decreasing tubal motility and suppressing ovulation to prevent fertilization and by making the endometrium less receptive to embryo implantation. The only progestin-only pill available in the United States is norethindrone 0.35 mg, which is taken daily throughout the entire month with no week off for a menstrual period.

1. Failure rate for typical use is 9 pregnancies expected per 100 women per year; **correct use** <1 pregnancy per 100 women per year.

2. Risks include irregular bleeding, acne, and breast tenderness.

  a. Contraindications. This method should not be used in women with breast cancer. Known or suspected pregnancy, current DVT or PE, active hepatitis, severe cirrhosis, or benign/malignant liver tumors are also contraindications.

3. Benefits include the ability to use the methods during lactation, reduced risk of endometrial and ovarian cancers, and the fact that the progestin-only pill does not carry the cardiovascular and thromboembolic risks of combination OCs.

4. Acceptability

  a. Convenience: Must be taken daily. Due to relatively short duration of action and short half-life of medication, it must be taken at the same time every day for maximum efficacy. Because of compliance issues and increased rates of breakthrough bleeding compared with combined OCs, the progestin-only contraception pill is generally recommended only in breastfeeding women or for women who have a contraindication to estrogen use.

  b. Availability. Daily contraceptive agent requires a prescription. Progestin-based emergency contraceptive agents (see section III.G) are available as nonprescription products in the United States.

C. Injectable hormones. Depo-medroxyprogesterone acetate (Depo-Provera; DMPA) is a widely used contraceptive that is given as either a deep intramuscular injection of

150 mg or a subcutaneous injection of 104 mg every 12 weeks. The slower rate of absorption of the subcutaneous formulation allows for a lower dose of DMPA.

1. **Failure rate for typical use** is 6 pregnancies expected per 100 women per year; **correct use** <1 pregnancy/100 women/year.
2. **Risks include** irregular bleeding, weight gain, breast tenderness, headaches, and potentially delayed return of fertility (may be delayed as long as 10–18 months).
    a. **Contraindications.** This method should not be used in women with breast cancer or known or suspected pregnancy and used with caution in women at an increased risk for osteoporosis. There is considerable controversy over DMPA's effect on bone. Bone loss does occur and is greater with increasing duration of use. Most studies have shown that bone loss is reversible once a woman stops DMPA; however, especially in teenagers who have not reached their maximum bone density, clinical implications are unclear. Most experts agree that it is safe to use DMPA for over 2 years if it is the best contraceptive option available. All women on DMPA should be counseled about the potential risk of bone loss and should make sure to get adequate calcium and vitamin D intake. Prescribing oral estrogen supplementation may mitigate bone loss. There is insufficient evidence to support screening bone mineral density in long-term users.
3. **Benefits include amenorrhea** in addition to reduction in menorrhagia, dysmenorrhea, and iron-deficiency anemia. **Lactation is not adversely affected;** trace amounts are detectable in breast milk without apparent adverse effects to infants.
4. **Acceptability**
    a. **Convenience.** One injection every 3 months.
    b. **Availability.** Must have a prescription and access to a facility with the ability to administer the injection appropriately.
D. **Transdermal hormonal patch. Norelgestromin and ethinyl estradiol (Ortho Evra)** is a combination contraceptive that is provided in a transdermal system. Patches containing 6.00 mg norelgestromin and 0.75 mg ethinyl estradiol are placed on the skin of the buttocks, abdomen, upper torso, or upper outer arms weekly. Each patch releases 150 µg of norelgestromin and 20 µg of ethinyl estradiol daily. The patch functions similarly to combination OCs, but provides higher cumulative doses of estrogen, whereas pills have higher peak doses.
1. **Failure rate for typical use** is 9 pregnancies expected per 100 women per year; **correct use** <1 pregnancy per 100 women per year.
2. **Risks** are similar to combination OCs; however, the patch may be associated with an increased risk of blood clotting compared with OCs, based on early European studies. (SOR **B**) Some women experience skin irritation and/or difficulty with getting the patches to stick to the skin for an entire week.
    a. **Contraindications.** Same as those for combination OCs.
3. **Benefits** are the same as for OCs. The patch is more convenient in a transdermal route for some women.
4. **Acceptability** is enhanced over that of OCs because of the weekly transdermal route of administration.
    a. **Convenience.** The patch is applied once a week for 3 weeks. Patch is not worn during the fourth week, and women have a menstrual cycle during that week.
    b. **Availability:** Must have a prescription.
E. **Vaginal ring. A flexible silicone ring impregnated with etonogestrel and ethinyl estradiol (Nuvaring)** is another alternative route of administration for combination hormonal contraceptives. It delivers 0.120 mg of etonogestrel and 0.015 mg ethinyl estradiol daily. The ring is placed in the posterior fornix of the vagina; the exact position of the ring is not important for contraceptive function. Because of the "local" administration of hormones, lower doses can be used.
1. **Failure rate for typical use** is 9 pregnancies expected per 100 women per year; **correct use** <1 pregnancy per 100 women per year.
2. **Risks** include vaginal discharge and irritation; otherwise similar to combination OCs.
    a. **Contraindications** are the same as those for combination OCs.
3. **Benefits** are similar to those of OCs. May be associated with less prolonged bleeding or spotting.
4. **Acceptability.** It does not require daily administration and is a good choice for women who desire a lower dose of hormones.

    a. Convenience. Inserted by the woman, the ring remains in place for 3 weeks and is then removed for 1 week. If out of place for more than 3 hours, an alternative method is required for 7 days after reinsertion.

    b. Availability. Must have a prescription.

F. Subdermal Implant of etonogestrel is a long-term hormonal contraceptive available under the brand name "Nexplanon," which replaced the previous implant "Implanon." The implant is a 40 mm × 2 mm semirigid, radio-opaque plastic rod containing 68 mg of etonogestrel released over 3 years (initially 60–70 mcg per day, falling to 25–30 mcg per day at the end of the third year). As a progestin-only method, mechanisms of action are similar to those of the progestin-only contraceptive pill.

    1. Failure rate is <1 for both "typical" and "correct" use. There may be decreased contraceptive efficacy in obese women.

    2. Risks include unscheduled bleeding, especially in the first 3 months of use which decreases during the first year. Other side effects are headache, weight gain, acne, and breast tenderness.

        a. Contraindications. Should not be used in women with breast cancer, a history of breast cancer, or known or suspected pregnancy.

    3. Benefits. No action required for contraceptive efficacy once placed.

    4. Acceptability. Because unscheduled bleeding is commonly experienced; however, the discontinuation rate does not appear to be higher for this method.

        a. Convenience. Must be placed by a physician via minor surgery. May remain in place for up to 3 years, and requires removal by a physician.

        b. Availability. Must have a prescription.

G. Postcoital contraceptives (emergency contraceptives). The hormones that make up the medication appear to inhibit ovulation if it has not occurred. Two formulations are available in the United States, "Plan B One-Step," Next Choice One-Step" and My Way (levonorgestrel 1.5 mg single dose), and "Ella" (ulipristal 30 mg single dose). In addition, OCs containing levonorgestrel or norgestrel can be used as an emergency contraceptive (Yuzpe regimen). When OCs are used as an emergency contraceptive, it is necessary to give two doses 12 hour apart. Each dose must contain the number of OC tablets needed to provide at least 100 mcg of ethinyl estradiol and at least 0.5 mg of levonorgestrel or 1 mg of norgestrel. The Yuzpe regimen is less effective than levonorgestrel or ulipristal and is associated with more side effects as it contains estrogen. However, it may be available as an option when the other agents are not.

    1. Failure rate. Best taken as soon after unprotected sex as possible for highest effectiveness. About 75% reduction in risk of pregnancy for a single act of unprotected sex for levonorgestrel products and 85% for ulipristal. Ulipristal is more effective especially at >72 hours after unprotected intercourse.

    2. Risks include nausea, vomiting, abdominal pain, fatigue, and headache. Ulipristal should not be administered more than once in a menstrual cycle due to lack of safety data. In addition, because it binds to progesterone receptors, ulipristal may affect the efficacy of OCs. Barrier contraceptives should be used in addition to the OC for the remainder of a cycle in which ulipristal has been taken.

        a. Pregnancy. No specific contraindications to its use. The levonorgestrel emergency contraceptives do not have an adverse fetal effect if inadvertent exposure occurs during early pregnancy. A pregnancy test should be obtained prior to use of ulipristal as it is not known if it will harm a fetus. **None of the emergency contraceptives disrupt an established pregnancy.**

    3. Benefits. Only contraceptive available for emergency postcoital use.

    4. Acceptability

        a. Convenience. Levonorgestrel should be taken within 72 hours of unprotected intercourse, but may be effective up to 120 hours after unprotected intercourse. Ulipristal should be taken within 120 hours of unprotected intercourse. The earlier these methods are used, the more effective. (SOR **B**)

        b. Availability. Levonorgestrel 1.5 mg (Plan B One-Step) has recently been approved by the FDA for over-the-counter sale to anyone regardless of age. Next Choice One-Step and My Way are only available to women over age 17 years without a prescription. Ulipristal is only available by prescription.

    5. Special note. Clinicians should provide information on Emergency contraceptions (ECs) when prescribing a non–long-acting contraceptive. It is also important to discuss this method of contraception with female victims of sexual assault.

6. Administration. Levonorgestrel 1.5 mg and ulipristal are both administered as a single oral dose taken as soon after unprotected intercourse as possible. Women should be counseled to expect their menses within 3 weeks of taking emergency contraception; if not, they should obtain a pregnancy test.

IV. Barrier Methods. These methods prevent conception by providing a mechanical barrier to sperm. Avoid using oil-based lubricants and medications (e.g., vaginal antifungals) because they can cause latex condoms to deteriorate. (SOR **Ⓒ**) Polyurethane and plastic condoms are not adversely affected by non–water-based lubricants or vaginal antifungals.

A. Male condoms are made of latex, the cecum of lambs (skins), or polyurethane (for latex-sensitive individuals). Most condoms have a shelf-life of 5 years if stored properly in a cool place.

   1. Failure rate is 18 pregnancies expected per 100 women per year. Condoms with lubrication and a receptacle end (to hold the ejaculate) are less likely to tear or split.

   2. Risks. Irritation, allergic reactions, and unintended devise failure. Condoms with spermicidal lubrication are higher in cost, have a shorter shelf-life, and are associated with a greater risk of urinary tract infections among female partners.

   a. Contraindications. Latex condoms should not be used if one or both partners are allergic to latex.

   3. Benefits include some (but not 100%) protection from STIs for latex and polyurethane condoms; skin condoms are too porous to provide this benefit.

   4. Acceptability. Limited if a couple finds using condoms distracting or embarrassing.

   a. Convenience. Applied before intercourse, one time use.

   b. Availability. No prescription needed.

B. Female condom. This is made of polyurethane and provides coverage of the external genitalia and lines the vagina entirely. It can be inserted 6 hours before intercourse.

   1. Failure rate is 21 pregnancies expected per 100 women per year.

   2. Risks. Irritation and allergic reaction.

   3. Benefits. Some protection from STI.

   4. Acceptability.

   a. Convenience. Inserted before intercourse, one time use.

   b. Availability. No prescription needed, but it is more expensive than male condoms.

C. Diaphragms are dome-shaped, rubber cups with arching or coiled rims. This device is used in conjunction with spermicide applied to the inner cup and around the rim. Additional spermicide can be inserted before repeated intercourse.

   1. Failure rate is 12 pregnancies expected per 100 women per year.

   2. Risks. Irritation and urinary tract infection.

   a. Contraindications. A history of toxic shock syndrome.

   3. Benefits. Possible protection against some STIs, reduced cervical cancer, and privacy of use.

   4. Acceptability

   a. Convenience. Inserted up to 6 hours prior to intercourse and left in place at least 6 hours following intercourse. The diaphragm can be left in place for 24 hours with additional spermicide inserted vaginally for repeated intercourse. May be difficult for some women to insert easily.

   b. Availability. Must have a prescription and fitting managed by an experienced provider.

D. Cervical cap: Soft rubber cup with a round rim, which fits snugly around the cervix; used with spermicide.

   1. Failure rate (number of pregnancies expected per 100 women per year): prentif Cap 17, FemCap 23.

   2. Risks include irritation, abnormal Pap test, and toxic shock.

   3. Benefit. Privacy.

   4. Acceptability.

   a. Convenience. May be difficult to insert, can remain in place for 48 hours without reapplying spermicide for repeated intercourse.

   b. Availability. Must have a prescription and fitting managed by an experienced provider.

E. Sponge. One-size polyurethane foam single-use device containing spermicide. Mechanism of action includes physical blockage and absorption of sperm and spermicidal effect (see later).

1. **Failure rate for typical use** (number of pregnancies expected per 100 women per year): nulliparous women 12, parous women 24.
2. **Risks** include increased risk of vaginal infection, urinary tract infection, and toxic shock. The sponge should not be used by menstruating women (increased risk of toxic shock syndrome).
3. **Benefit.** Protection against some STIs lasts 24 hours including for multiple acts of intercourse and privacy of use.
4. **Acceptability**
   a. **Convenience.** Additional spermicide does not need to be added for additional act(s) of intercourse. The sponge should be removed within 24 hours and may be difficult to remove.
   b. **Availability.** No prescription needed.
V. **Spermicide.** These methods inactivate sperm by destroying the sperm cell membrane and interfering with motility. Spermicides are available in the form of gels, creams, foams, tablet, suppositories, and film.
   A. **Failure rate for typical use** is 28 pregnancies expected per 100 women per year.
      1. **Risks** include irritation, allergic reaction, and urinary tract infection. High rate of unintended pregnancy occurs when used as a solitary agent.
      2. **Benefits.** Privacy of use. Best when used in combination with a barrier method such as condom, diaphragm, and cervical cap.
      3. **Acceptability**
         a. **Convenience.** Inserted between 5 and 90 minutes before intercourse and usually left in place at least 6 to 8 hours later.
         b. **Availability.** No prescription needed.
VI. **Intrauterine Devices.** IUD use in the United States is on the rise as it is recognized as a highly effective, long-acting, and safe form of reversible contraception. The mechanism of action of IUDs is not entirely clear, but the foreign body effect of the IUD is thought to immobilize sperm and therefore prevent fertilization of ova. Levonorgestrel IUDs also create a thick cervical mucus and, in some women, inhibit ovulation. The common misperception that IUDs function by preventing fertilized ovum from implantation has not been proven. (SOR **B**)

There are three types of IUDs approved for use in the United States. All are T-shaped; the ParaGard T380A has copper wound around the base, and LNg20 Mirena and LNg14 Skyla are impregnated with levonorgestrel. All three have fine, nylon tails that hang through the cervix, which allows women to check for the presence of the IUD.
   A. **Failure rate** is <1 pregnancy expected per 100 women per year.
   B. **Risks.** Cramping, bleeding, and rarely (<1 in 1000) perforation of the uterus during placement. IUDs do not increase the risk of pelvic inflammatory disease.
   C. **Contraindications.** Known anatomic uterine anomaly such as bicornuate uterus or large distorting fibroids or pregnancy. Abnormal bleeding should be investigated before placing an IUD.
      1. Preexisting severe dysmenorrhea may become worse with the copper IUD and will likely improve with levonorgestrel IUDs. Use of a levonorgestrel IUD is not recommended in women who have had breast cancer.
   D. **Benefits.** The levonorgestrel IUDs decrease the volume of menstrual blood and dysmenorrhea in symptomatic women. All IUDs are long acting and not coital dependent.
   E. **Acceptability**
      1. **Convenience.** Once in place, provides reliable long-term contraception (10 years for the copper T, 5 years for Mirena, and 3 years for Skyla). IUD string check by a provider is recommended 4 to 8 weeks after placement, and then annually.
      2. **Availability.** Must have a provider with procedural experience in placing IUDs.
   F. **Special notes.** Always read the manufacturer's instructions for the specific kind of IUD to be used. Both the insertion and the removal of an IUD are office procedures. A consent form should be signed and lot number of the device recorded. Pregnancy testing should be performed and documented as negative immediately prior to placement. In addition, age- and risk-appropriate testing for chlamydia and gonorrhea should be completed either before or at the time of IUD placement.
      1. The IUD can be placed in both nulliparous and parous women dependent on depth of the uterine cavity.
      2. One dose of a nonsteroidal anti-inflammatory drug is helpful to reduce discomfort from cramping if taken 1 hour prior to insertion or removal.

3. Insertion is easiest during menses because the cervix is slightly dilated, although the incidence of expulsion is slightly higher if the IUD is inserted at this time. Any time during the cycle is acceptable for insertion. The IUD may be removed at any time during the cycle.

4. Insertion can also be performed in the immediate postpartum period (10 minutes after the placenta is delivered) although expulsion rate with this timing is quite high (58%).

5. Leave a tail of at least 3 cm to allow the patient to check for expulsion of her IUD and to allow for later trimming if needed and easy removal. Let her feel the remnant of string so that she knows what to feel for monthly after her menses.

6. IUD removal is not required in the setting of STI. Treatment of the STI should be performed, and removal of the IUD only considered in the setting of more severe pelvic inflammatory disease. (SOR **B**)

7. There is an immediate return to fertility upon IUD removal. Hence, appropriate counseling regarding contraceptive options is recommended upon removal.

8. Placement of a copper IUD is an alternative, recognized method of emergency contraception. (SOR **A**) The copper IUD is extremely effective, more effective than the oral emergency contraceptives. Women using the copper IUD had pregnancy rates of 0.09% compared to women using an oral emergency contraceptive who had pregnancy rates of 1% to 2%. The IUD must be inserted within 5 days after unprotected intercourse.

VII. **Natural Family Planning**

A. **Periodic abstinence** depends on avoidance of intercourse during fertile days. Fertile days can be determined by many different methods. The Billings method of family planning relies on changes in cervical mucus. Other methods use the length of past menstrual cycles or a combination of basal body temperature and cervical mucus changes (sympotothermal method). These methods rely heavily on motivated patients, but can enhance awareness of a woman's body and cycles. Other methods which have been described are the Creighton model NaProEducation system and the Standard Days Method. Abstinence is usually required for 6 to 9 days during the cycle. Some couples use barrier methods during the fertile time.

1. **Failure rate** is 24 pregnancies expected per 100 women per year.

2. **Risks**

   a. There are no contraindications to the use of natural family planning. The calendar method alone should not be used in women with irregular menstrual cycles (as in lactating or nearing menopause).

   b. Due to relatively higher rates of unintended pregnancy compared to other methods, the most significant risk of this method is unintended pregnancy.

3. **Benefits.** Self-knowledge of a woman's cycles, which can be helpful if desiring pregnancy as well. This information also enhances both partners' awareness and involvement in family planning.

4. **Acceptability.**

   a. **Convenience.** Requires frequent monitoring of body functions.

   b. **Availability.** Requires special instructions.

5. **Special notes.** Patient instructions are complex initially and take some time to master. A course with a trained instructor may be necessary. More information is available through American Pregnancy Association (http://americanpregnancy.org/preventingpregnancy/fertilityawarenessNFP.html), Couple to Couple League (http://www.ccli.org/nfp/), or Georgetown University Institute for Reproductive Health (http://irh.org/).

B. **Lactation amenorrhea method (LAM)** is based on the normal time of infertility after pregnancy. If a woman breastfeeds exclusively, the average length of infertility is 14 months. If a woman has given birth in the past 6 months, is exclusively breastfeeding (no solids, water, juice, or pacifier), and has not yet menstruated, she has approximately 98% effectiveness for breastfeeding alone. Increasing the time between feedings is the strongest factor leading to the return of fertility. Efficacy is limited to only those women who nurse exclusively on demand.

C. **Coitus interruptus, or the withdrawal method,** depends on withdrawal of the penis from the vagina before ejaculation occurs. Some ejaculate, however, is released before climax, and the failure rate is similar to the rate of pregnancy when using periodic abstinence or spermicide alone (Table 97–1).

VIII. Sterilization is a permanent form of birth control resulting from ligation/obstruction of the vas deferens in men (vasectomy) or ligation/obstruction of the fallopian tubes in women. It is the most prevalent form of birth control used in the United States.

    A. Vasectomy. Sealing, tying, or cutting the vas deferens inhibiting sperm travel.

        1. Failure rate is <1 pregnancy expected per 100 women per year.

        2. Risks. Swelling, bruising, pain, and hematoma epididymitis. There is no increased risk for testicular or prostate cancer in men receiving a vasectomy. (SOR **Ⓐ**)

        3. Benefits. The safest and most effective method for couples in a stable, monogamous relationship with no desire for future fertility. Irreversibility. Since this method involves the male partner, it facilitates avoidance of hormonal agents for women with potential contraindications for their use or who experience adverse effects.

        4. Acceptability

            a. Convenience. Outpatient surgical procedure.

            b. Availability. Widely available by trained physicians.

    B. Sterilization implants. Small metallic implant (essure) placed into the fallopian tubes through a hysteroscopic procedure. The device causes scaring blocking fallopian tubes.

        1. Failure rate is <1 pregnancy expected per 100 women per year.

        2. Risks. Pain and ectopic pregnancy.

        3. Benefit. Permanence.

        4. Acceptability

            a. Convenience. Outpatient surgical procedure.

            b. Availability. Trained physician with appropriate facilities and equipment. May require a follow-up hysterosalpingogram to document successful blockage.

    C. Transabdominal surgical sterilization. Fallopian tubes are blocked, so the egg and sperm cannot meet. This can be done in the immediate postpartum period prior to hospital discharge after a delivery, or at any time after 6 weeks postpartum.

        1. Failure rate is <1 pregnancy expected per 100 women per year.

        2. Risks. Pain bleeding, infection, surgical complications, and ectopic pregnancy.

        3. Benefit. Permanence.

        4. Acceptability

            a. Convenience. Operative procedure, often but not always performed laparoscopically.

            b. Availability. Surgical centers or hospitals with trained, credentialed surgeons with experience performing tubal ligations.

    D. Special notes

        1. Informed consent is critical for a surgical procedure and must describe the methods as irreversible, yet acknowledge a small risk of failure and pregnancy (possibly ectopic for the tubal ligation).

        2. Because of the permanence of these methods, it is important for patients to think carefully about whether any change such as death or separation from a partner or from a child would make them regret the choice. A good question to ask is "If anything were to happen to your current spouse and children, would you want to have another child?"

SELECTED REFERENCES

Birth Control Methods Fact Sheet. Nov 2011. Office on Women's Health, U.S. Department of Health and Human Services. Available at http://www.womenshealth.gov/publications/our-publications/fact-sheet/birth-control-methods.cfm. Accessed 8/1/13.

Center for Disease Control and Prevention. U.S. Selected Practice Recommendations for Contraceptive Use, 2013: adapted from the World Health Organization Selected Practice Recommendations for Contraceptive Use, 2nd Edition. *MMWR Recomm Rep.* 2013;62(RR05):1–46.

Centers for Disease Control and Prevention (CDC). U.S. medical eligibility criteria for contraceptive use, 2010: adapted from the World Health Organization medical eligibility criteria for contraceptive use, 4th edition. *MMWR Recomm Rep.* 2010;59(RR-4):1–86.

Egarter C, Frey Tirri B, Bitzer J, et al. Women's perceptions and reasons for choosing the pill, patch, or ring in the CHOICE study: a cross-sectional survey of contraceptive method selection after counseling. *BMC Womens Health.* 2013;13:9.

Schrager SB. DMPA's effect on bone mineral density: a particular concern for adolescents. *J Fam Pract.* 2009;58(5):E1–E8.

Van Vliet HAAM, Grimes DA, Lopez LM, et al. Triphasic versus monophasic oral contraceptives for contraception. *Cochrane Database Syst Rev.* 2011;(11):CD003553.

98   Infertility

Keith A. Frey, MD, MBA

KEY POINTS

- Infertility occurs in approximately 15% to 20% of couples, many of whom present to their primary care physician for initial evaluation. (SOR **C**)
- A thorough evaluation of both partners is necessary, as 25% of couples have more than one etiologic factor. (SOR **C**)
- Emotional support for the couple is an important aspect of their care. (SOR **C**)

I. Introduction

A. Definition. Infertility is defined as 1 year of unprotected heterosexual intercourse or 6 to 12 months of artificial insemination in which a pregnancy has not been achieved. Fifteen to twenty percent of couples in the United States are infertile. Evaluation of an infertile couple is indicated after a year of unsuccessful conception or after 6 months if the woman is over age 35 years.

B. Common diagnoses. The causes of infertility include abnormalities of any portion of the male or female reproductive system. Although infertility results from a single cause in the majority of couples, more than one factor contributes to infertility in as many as 25% of couples. "Unexplained" infertility, in which no specific cause is identified, occurs in approximately 25% of infertile couples. The following causes of infertility have been identified:

1. **Male factors** (25%)
2. **Ovulatory dysfunction** (20%)
3. **Tubal pathology** (15%)
4. **Other problems** including endometriosis, uterine, or cervical factors and unusual problems (15%)

C. Pathophysiology

1. **Male factors.** The most commonly encountered cause of male infertility is oligospermia or azoospermia secondary to varicocele. Other causes of male infertility include primary hypogonadism (e.g., congenital or acquired testicular disorders, orchitis), altered sperm transport (e.g., absent vas deferens), and secondary hypogonadism (e.g., androgen excess or pharmacologic effects). These disorders manifest as oligospermia or azoospermia, disorders of sperm function or motility (asthenospermia), and abnormalities of sperm morphology (teratospermia).

2. **Ovulatory dysfunction.** Ovulation disorders account for 40% of female factor infertility. Anovulation or inconsistent ovulation may be suggested by a history of irregular menses. The possible causes of anovulation can be grouped into the following major categories:

   a. Aging
   b. Diminished ovarian reserve
   c. Endocrine disorders (e.g., hypothalamic amenorrhea, hyperprolactinemia, thyroid disease, adrenal disease)
   d. Polycystic ovary syndrome (PCOS)
   e. Premature ovarian failure
   f. Tobacco use

3. **Tubal and pelvic pathology.** Infertility may be associated with tubal damage or adnexal adhesions. Tubal obstruction can result from scarring due to acute salpingitis, although many cases of tubal occlusion are encountered in which no episodes of salpingitis are recalled. Anatomic distortion of adnexal structures can also be caused by endometriosis. The chronic inflammation associated with endometriosis may disrupt normal conception by causing tubal damage or by secretion of toxic substances.

4. **Unusual problems.** Cervical mucus abnormalities occur if, at the time of ovulation, the mucus is either insufficient in quantity or poor in quality. Factors contributing to

the formation of such unreceptive cervical mucus include cervical infections, previous cervical surgery or cautery, and clomiphene therapy.

II. **Diagnosis.** The physician should arrange a meeting with the couple early in the diagnostic workup. This provides an important opportunity to review reproductive biology and the rationale for subsequent laboratory tests.

A. **Signs and symptoms.** Since infertility may arise from one or more areas of the reproductive system, it requires a comprehensive diagnostic evaluation. The initial assessment of both partners consists of a thorough history and physical examination. Specific areas requiring extra attention are noted in Table 98–1.

B. **Laboratory tests** (Tables 98–2 and 98–3). In addition to a comprehensive history and physical examination, each couple must be evaluated by a series of laboratory tests and appropriately timed studies to evaluate each major reproductive factor that may be the cause of infertility. This comprehensive diagnostic survey should be completed for most couples in 6 to 12 months. Each couple's evaluation should be individualized based on the findings of the history and the physical examination. However, an initial survey of each major reproductive factor is necessary in *all* couples and can be coordinated by the primary care physician.

1. **Male factors.** The man is evaluated with a complete blood count, urinalysis, and at least two semen analyses. Each semen analysis is performed on a fresh (within 2 hours), warm specimen obtained by masturbation after at least 2 days of abstinence. Evidence of oligospermia after two or more semen analyses will require further diagnostic evaluation.

   a. The initial evaluation includes blood levels for follicle-stimulating hormone (FSH) and testosterone. If the testosterone level is low, a pituitary etiology may be evaluated by luteinizing hormone (LH) and prolactin levels. Testicular biopsy may be required, particularly if azoospermia is discovered.

2. **Ovulatory dysfunction.** Anovulation or inconsistent ovulation is confirmed by an abnormally low serum progesterone level in the luteal phase, persistently negative home LH testing, or a flat basal body temperature chart.

TABLE 98–1. THE INFERTILITY WORKUP IN OUTLINE: HISTORY (MALE, FEMALE, OR BOTH)

Male Factors	
Adult Illnesses	**Surgery**
Acute viral or febrile illness in past 3 mo	Herniorrhaphy
Mumps orchitis	Retroperitoneal surgery
Renal disease	Vasectomy
Radiation therapy	**Drug Use**
Sexually transmitted disease	Alcohol, tobacco, marijuana, and cocaine
Stress and fatigue	Alkylating agents
Tuberculosis	Anabolic steroids
Childhood illness	Nitrofurantoin
Cryptorchidism	Sulfasalazine
Timing of puberty	Cimetidine

Female Factors	
Gynecology	**Surgery**
Contraceptive use	Female pelvic surgery
Diethylstilbestrol use by mother	**Review of Systems**
Menarche	Focus on endocrine conditions (diabetes, thyroid disorders)
Menses (regularity and flow)	
Mittelschmerz	

Both Male and Female Factors	
General History	**Occupation and Habits**
Duration of infertility	Exposure to radiation, chemicals, and excessive heat (saunas, hot tubs, etc.)
Fertility in previous relationships	
Frequency of intercourse	
Sexual potency and techniques	
Use of coital lubricants	

TABLE 98–2. THE INFERTILITY WORKUP IN OUTLINE: PHYSICAL EXAMINATION/ROUTINE LABORATORY TESTS (MALE AND FEMALE)

Male		Female	
Physical Examination	**Routine Laboratory Tests**	**Physical Examination**	**Routine Laboratory Tests**
Hair pattern	CBC, RPR	Breast formation	CBC, RPR, Rubella titer
Genitalia	Semen analysis[a]	Distribution of body fat	Pap smear
Meatus size and location	Results (normal)	Galactorrhea	Urinalysis and urine
Prostate and seminal	Volume: 2–5 mL	Hair pattern (virilization)	culture if indicated
vesicles	Liquefaction: complete	Height and weight	Day 3 FSH and Estradiol
Scrotum	within 30 min	Neurologic: anosmia,	(for age ≥30 yr)
Testicular size (≥4 cm in	Sperm count:	visual fields	TSH and prolactin (if
long axis)	>20 million/mL	Pelvic exam:	oligo- or anovulation)
Varicocele (standing and	Sperm motility: 50%	External genitalia	At-home ovulation test
Valsalva maneuver)	Morphology: 50% normal	Retrovaginal area (endo-	
Neurology	forms	metriosis)	
Anosmia	Repeat testing if	Uterus and adnexa	
Visual fields	azoospermia or severe	Vagina and cervix	
	oligospermia		
	Urinalysis and urine		
	culture if indicated		

[a]Collected following abstinence of at least 2 days with masturbation into sterile vessel and transferred to the laboratory (warm) within 2 hours.
CBC, complete blood cell count; RPR, rapid plasma reagin; TSH, thyroid-stimulating hormone.

  a. If the patient is not ovulating, further laboratory evaluation is needed (serum prolactin and thyroid-stimulating hormone [TSH]).
  b. Women with a diminished ovarian reserve (day 3 FSH >10) should be referred to an infertility specialist.
 3. Tubal factors. The woman must undergo an evaluation for tubal patency. If the history or physical examination shows no clear evidence of tubal damage, proceed with a hysterosalpingogram or refer the patient for laparoscopy (especially if there are other indications for laparoscopy, such as possible endometriosis).
III. Treatment. Generally, treatment should not be initiated until the diagnostic evaluation is completed. The partners should be treated as a couple whenever possible and therapy should proceed at a rate that the couple finds comfortable.
 A. Male factors. Specific antibiotics are used to treat infections such as prostatitis and epididymitis. Consultation with an urologist will generally be required to complete the evaluation and coordinate treatment. It should be noted that varicocele repair has been suggested to increase the likelihood of conception, although current findings are inconclusive. The estimate of the number needed to treat is 17.
 B. Ovulatory dysfunction. Underlying causes of ovulatory dysfunction such as thyroid abnormalities or hyperprolactinemia should be corrected. If anovulation is diagnosed, consider treatment with clomiphene.

TABLE 98–3. THE INFERTILITY WORKUP IN OUTLINE: FURTHER DIAGNOSTIC TESTS

Hysterosalpingography
Preferred test of tubal patency
Performed 2–6 d after cessation of menstrual flow
May enhance fertility temporarily

Laparoscopy
Performed if hysterosalpingography is unproductive
Permits examination of pelvic contents

Serum Progesterone
Sample drawn 5–7 d after supposed ovulation
Serum level ≥6 ng/mL is compatible with ovulation

1. **Clomiphene treatment.** Clomiphene citrate is an antiestrogen that has been available for over 30 years. A careful evaluation for galactorrhea and a prolactin level should precede treatment. Among the patients best suited for clomiphene are those with chronic anovulation and unexplained infertility. (SOR **B**) The usual starting dose is 50 mg per day orally on days 5 to 9 of the menstrual cycle. The dose can be increased to 100 mg per day in the second and third cycles. (SOR **C**)

   a. **Common side effects** include vasomotor flushes (10%), abdominal or pelvic discomfort (5.5%), nausea (2.2%), and breast tenderness (2%). Ovarian hyperstimulation and twinning (rates of 8% to 12%) can occur in patients who receive clomiphene therapy, especially with higher doses. Patients with PCOS are at the highest risk for these complications.

   b. Consider referral to an infertility specialist if pregnancy is not achieved within 6 months of clomiphene therapy or if doses of 100 mg per day do not achieve ovulation.

   c. **Expected results.** Ovulation should be expected 5 to 10 days after the last dose of clomiphene; ovulation should be confirmed by a positive ovulation predictor kit and an elevated level of serum progesterone on day 21. If ovulation does not occur despite clomiphene therapy, consultation with a reproductive endocrinologist is recommended.

2. **Metformin treatment.** Metformin has been found to increase the rate of ovulation in patients who have anovulation secondary to PCOS. However, there was no increase in the rate of pregnancy in women who received metformin alone. Clomiphene plus metformin can increase the rate of pregnancy in women with resistant PCOS compared to clomiphene alone. (SOR **A**)

C. **Tubal and pelvic pathology.** Tubal blockage or deformity may necessitate surgical correction. The management of endometriosis in a woman desiring to achieve pregnancy depends on the degree and location of endometrial deposits.

   1. Conservative surgical treatment can enhance fertility potential by destroying endometrial implants and endometriomas. Laparoscopic conservative surgical treatment should be considered as a treatment option for mild endometriosis-associated infertility.

   2. Patients with endometriosis may also benefit from ovulation induction with or without other assisted-reproduction techniques. (SOR **A**) For patients with more severe tubal and pelvic pathology, referral for assisted reproductive technologies is warranted.

D. **Unusual problems.** For cervical mucus abnormalities, antibiotics should be used to treat the specific bacterial cause of the problem. Low-dose estrogens can be used for poor cervical mucus that does not result from infectious causes. However, intrauterine insemination (IUI) is the best treatment option for a cervical factor.

E. **Assisted reproductive technology (ART).** The methods used to achieve pregnancy by artificial or partially artificial means are called ART. Such technologies may be necessary when the treatments outlined earlier fail to achieve pregnancy, or for fertile couples for genetic reasons or certain communicable diseases (e.g., AIDS). Examples of ART include IUI, in vitro fertilization (IVF), intracytoplasmic sperm injection (ICSI), and cryopreservation.

   1. IUI is a process whereby washed fresh or frozen sperm is injected into a woman's uterus at ovulation. IUI can be performed during a normal cycle or with ovulation induction (e.g., clomiphene or synthetic FSH). IUI achieves a pregnancy rate of about 15% per month in women under age 35 years.

   2. IVF is more successful at achieving pregnancy than IUI, with success rates of 30% or more per cycle. In IVF, a woman undergoes ovarian stimulation with synthetic FSH and surgical removal of the eggs. The eggs are then combined with sperm so that fertilization happens in the laboratory. The embryos are supported in their growth for 3 to 5 days. The embryos or blastocysts are then inserted into a woman's uterus.

   3. ICSI is a procedure whereby the sperm is injected directly into the egg during an IVF procedure to improve fertilization rates.

   4. Cryopreservation is now available for sperms, embryos, and eggs so that couples can have opportunities to achieve pregnancy at a later time.

IV. **Management Strategies.** The workup, diagnosis, and treatment of infertility can precipitate intense emotional reactions. The physician should discuss such emotions as anger, guilt, self-doubt, depression, and grief with the couple. The actions described later may also prove beneficial.

    A. Help the couple understand their motives for parenting, which may include desires (1) to parent, (2) to experience a pregnancy, (3) to meet the expectations of others, and (4) to promote genetic continuity.

    B. Assist the couple in the development of mutual support and an adaptive "couple-coping" style. Discuss sexual issues and encourage the couple to nurture their intimacy; they will need its strength to deal with the problems associated with infertility. Periodic meetings with the couple to review diagnostic progress provide further opportunity to reinforce coping skills.

    C. Help the couple broaden their support systems, including self-help groups, such as Resolve, Inc.

    D. The ART treatments are very expensive and not usually covered by health insurance. The primary care provider can assist the infertile couple in assessing their options for payment.

V. Prognosis. The exact prognosis of infertility is difficult to define because of the multiple potential causes. For most of these, conception will not be achieved without specific treatment. However, with specific therapy, subsequent pregnancy rates have been studied and results are favorable. Chances of a successful pregnancy decrease with increasing age of the woman and duration of the infertility.

    A. "Unexplained" infertility is the persistent inability to conceive after a comprehensive diagnostic assessment of the couple fails to establish a specific diagnosis. If a comprehensive diagnostic workup fails to identify a cause, or if the appropriate treatment is unsuccessful, the physician should discuss adoption options with the couple.

SELECTED REFERENCES

Frey KA. Male reproductive health and infertility. *Prim Care.* 2010;37:643–652.

Frey KA, Patel KS. Initial evaluation and management of infertility by the primary care physician. *Mayo Clin Proc.* 2004;79(11):1439–1443.

Hughes E, Brown J, Collins JJ, Vanderkerchove P. Clomiphene citrate for unexplained subfertility in women. *Cochrane Database Syst Rev.* 2010;(1):CD000057.

Jose-Miller AB, Boyden JW, Frey KA. Infertility. *Am Fam Physician.* 2007;75:849–856.

Kamel RM. Management of the infertile couple: an evidence-based protocol. *Reprod Biol Endocrinol.* 2010;8:21 (open access).

Kolettis PN. Evaluation of the subfertile man. *Am Fam Physician.* 2003;67:2165–2172.

Kroese ACJ, de Lange NM, Collins J, Evers JLH. Surgery or embolization for varicoceles in subfertile men. *Cochrane Database Syst Rev.* 2012;(10):CD000479.

Sinawat S, Buppasiri P, Lumbiganon P, Pattanittum P. Long versus short course treatment with metformin and clomiphene citrate for ovulation induction in women with PCOS. *Cochrane Database Syst Rev.* 2012;(10):CD006226.

The Practice Committee of the American Society for Reproductive Medicine. Diagnostic evaluation of the infertile female: a committee opinion. *Fertil Steril.* 2012;98(2):302–307.

ELECTRONIC RESOURCE

RESOLVE National Home Page. http://www.resolve.org.

---

99   Preconception and Prenatal Care

Kirsten Vitrikas, MD

KEY POINTS

- Preconception care that offers smoking cessation, folic acid supplementation, (SOR **A**) excellent glycemic control in patients with diabetes mellitus, (SOR **A**) monotherapy for seizures and avoidance of phenytoin and valproic acid, (SOR **B**) immunization against rubella, and alcohol cessation has been shown to improve subsequent pregnancy outcome.
- Clinicians should follow specific evidence-based protocols and monitor women for signs of obstetric emergencies, particularly late in pregnancy. Comprehensive prenatal care,

particularly if begun early in pregnancy, has been shown to improve pregnancy outcomes. (SOR **B**)
- Women older than 35 years should be offered genetic counseling and testing. All women who present for care prior to 20 weeks should be offered Down syndrome screening in the first trimester. (SOR **B**)
- To prepare for labor and delivery, women and their partners should be enrolled in prenatal classes which can have a positive effect on labor and delivery experience. (SOR **B**)

I. Introduction

   A. Antenatal care refers to a comprehensive approach to medical care and psychosocial support of the family that ideally begins prior to conception and ends with the onset of labor.

   B. Preconception care is the physical and mental preparation of both parents for pregnancy and childbearing prior to conception in order to improve pregnancy outcomes.

   C. Prenatal care formally begins with the initial diagnosis of pregnancy and includes ongoing risk assessment, education, and counseling to promote health as well as identification and management of problems.

II. Preconception Care

   A. Medical history. Nearly half of all pregnancies are unintended; therefore, all women of childbearing age, particularly those not using contraception effectively, are candidates for preconception evaluation. Identifying conditions and risks that could adversely affect a future pregnancy, followed by appropriate interventions and counseling to improve the outcome of pregnancy are the primary tasks of the preconception evaluation.

   1. **Chronic medical conditions** should be evaluated both for potential effects on pregnancy and for effects that pregnancy may have on the medical condition. Significant chronic illnesses include diabetes mellitus, hypertension, thyroid disorders, anemias, coagulopathies, seizure disorders, asthma, human immunodeficiency virus (HIV)/acquired immunodeficiency syndrome, and cardiovascular diseases. Also notable are a past history of recurrent urinary tract infections and phlebitis.

   2. Note **previous surgeries,** particularly abdominal and pelvic procedures.

   3. A thorough review of **prescription and nonprescription medications** currently being taken is helpful to anticipate and minimize adverse effects, particularly during the period of organogenesis from the 4th to the 10 weeks' gestation. The US Food and Drug Administration's Pregnancy Categories and other reviews such as the Teris database or Organization of Teratology Information Specialists' Web site (www.otispregnancy.org) are useful in determining risk, including teratogenic risk, versus benefit. Drugs clearly proven to have significant teratogenic risk in humans include alcohol, chemotherapeutic agents, anticonvulsants, androgens, warfarin, lithium, and isotretinoin.

   4. Note **allergies and sensitivities** to medications and anesthetics.

   5. **Current methods of contraception.** Ideally, methods should be discontinued several menstrual cycles prior to conception to assist with accurate dating.

   6. **Genetic risk assessment** performed in the preconception period, as opposed to the prenatal period, allows women and their partners to consider a greater number of options in family planning. The background incidence of congenital malformations is approximately 3%. Genetic causes account for approximately 20% of anomalies. Genetic counseling and further testing may be beneficial when the following conditions are identified: advanced maternal (older than 35 years) or paternal (older than 55 years) age; a family history of or previous child with neural tube defect (NTD), congenital heart disease, hemophilia, thalassemia, sickle cell disease, Tay–Sachs disease, cystic fibrosis, Huntington chorea, muscular dystrophy, mental retardation, Down syndrome, or other inherited disorders; maternal metabolic disorders; recurrent pregnancy loss (three or more); use of alcohol, recreational drugs, and medications; and environmental or occupational exposures.

   7. **Obstetric and menstrual history.** Review the number, date, length, and outcome of prior pregnancies. Record any history of significant pregnancy-related health concerns, such as gestational diabetes, intrauterine growth restriction (IUGR), preterm labor, or hemorrhage. Make note of any complications during labor and delivery. A detailed menstrual history is helpful, paying particular attention to irregular menses and infertility.

B. Psychosocial history. This is a critical area of the history, since significant risks may be identified that may be addressed prior to pregnancy. A potential pregnancy may also serve as an incentive to the patient to alter unhealthy habits including tobacco use, alcohol consumption, illicit drug use, and poor nutrition. Psychosocial risks include a past history of mental illness, inadequate personal supports and coping skills, high stress, exposure to intimate partner violence or abuse, single marital status, inadequate housing, low income, and less than high school education. A history of occupational or environmental exposure to potential teratogens should also be taken.

C. Immunization history. Rubella, varicella, and hepatitis B immunity are best addressed prior to conception.

D. Physical examination

1. Height and weight. Patients who weigh >200 lbs or <90 lbs may be at a greater risk for problems in pregnancy.

2. Blood pressure

3. Breast examination

4. Pelvic examination can include clinical pelvimetry (although pelvimetry is unlikely to affect the outcome of the pregnancy).

E. Laboratory tests

1. Recommended laboratory tests include hemoglobin or hematocrit, rubella titer, Pap smear (if due), screening for gonorrhea and chlamydia, hepatitis B surface antigen, and syphilis serology. Counseling regarding HIV testing should occur with all patients. Women should be assessed for evidence of varicella immunity.

2. Additional screening with the following may be appropriate for women who are identified to be at a greater risk: tuberculosis, toxoplasmosis, cytomegalovirus, herpes simplex, varicella, and hemoglobinopathies.

F. Health promotion

1. Optimize management of preexisting medical conditions such as diabetes mellitus, thyroid disease, and hypertension.

2. Administer appropriate immunizations (see Chapter 105). Women should avoid becoming pregnant for 1 month after live virus vaccinations.

3. The US Public Health Service recommends that all women of child-bearing age should consume 0.4 mg of folic acid per day to reduce the risk of NTDs. (SOR **Ⓐ**) Women with a prior fetus or baby with an NTD should consume 4 mg of folic acid beginning 1 month prior to conception.

4. Provide counseling and educate regarding the following topics:

a. Pregnancy planning. Accurate recording of menstrual cycles is helpful. Oral contraceptives should be discontinued and a barrier method should be used to establish regular cycles prior to attempting pregnancy.

b. Nutrition and weight correction, if necessary. Weight should be optimized prior to conception. Obese women (BMI >30) are at an increased risk for infertility and miscarriage in addition to adverse perinatal outcomes and operative complications. (SOR **Ⓐ**) They should be encouraged to lose weight prior to attempting pregnancy. Women who have undergone bariatric surgery should be assessed for inadequate vitamin absorption, particularly vitamin B_{12}.

c. Smoking cessation (SOR **Ⓐ**) **and avoidance of alcohol** (SOR **Ⓐ**) **and illicit drugs** (SOR **Ⓒ**).

d. Genetic risks, if any.

e. Avoidance of teratogens, including prescription and nonprescription medications, and occupational and environmental exposures.

f. Preparation of the family for pregnancy and enhancement of social support. Intimate partner violence may begin or escalate during pregnancy. It is more prevalent than any condition in pregnancy with the exception of preeclampsia. Providers should inquire about intimate partner violence and offer support and referral to appropriate agencies as needed.

g. Proper exercise. Current recommendations are for 30 minutes or more of exercise on most if not all days of the week in the absence of contraindications. (SOR **Ⓒ**)

III. Prenatal Care

A. Initial diagnosis of pregnancy

1. Symptoms include cessation of menses, breast tenderness and enlargement, nausea, fatigue, and frequent urination.

2. Signs such as uterine enlargement and a dark bluish coloring of the cervix and vaginal mucosa (Chadwick sign) are present.

   3. Urinary tests for elevated levels of β-human chorionic gonadotropin (β-hCG) are generally positive at about the time of the first missed menses and have a sensitivity of 98% and a specificity of 99%.

B. The **first prenatal visit** should occur before 8 weeks' gestation, as this is critical for determining an accurate delivery date, evaluating risk status, and providing essential patient education. The visit may be abbreviated if a recent preconceptual visit has occurred.

   1. Patient history (see Section II). A detailed menstrual history as well as the last contraceptive method used is important for establishing dates. The estimated date of delivery (EDD) should be established before 20 weeks' gestation, when techniques for dating are most accurate. The date of the start of the last menstrual period (LMP) is used to determine EDD. A first-trimester ultrasound can confirm gestational age within ±4 days and is considered more accurate than LMP, although routine use for dating is controversial as it does not improve maternal or neonatal outcomes. (SOR **Ⓐ**) In addition, a history of illnesses, medications, and exposures since the LMP should be obtained. A patient's questions concerning common symptoms in early pregnancy can be answered at this time.

   2. Physical examination. This should include evaluation of fetal heart tones (usually heard by hand-held Doppler between 11 and 13 weeks).

   3. Routine laboratory work. In addition to testing recommended during the preconception visit (see Section II.E), blood and Rh type, antibody screen, microscopic urinalysis, and urine culture are recommended. Women at a high risk for tuberculosis should be screened early in pregnancy. All pregnant women should be tested for HIV infection unless they decline. This is known as the opt-out approach.

   4. Patient education early in pregnancy is critical. Important issues to be addressed are described below:

      a. High-risk behaviors

         (1) Smoking has been associated with IUGR, prematurity, placenta previa, placental abruption, and preterm rupture of membranes. Brief counseling during visits has been shown to be effective in reducing the number of cigarettes smoked per day. (SOR **Ⓑ**) If nonpharmacologic therapy fails, nicotine replacement with patches or gum may be considered; however, the U.S. Preventive Services Task Force (USPSTF) has concluded that their use has not been sufficiently evaluated to determine their efficacy or safety during pregnancy.

         (2) Alcohol use is linked to fetal alcohol syndrome (craniofacial abnormalities, limb and cardiovascular defects, and growth and mental retardation) and other childhood behavioral problems such as learning disabilities and attention-deficit/hyperactivity disorder. There is no known safe amount of alcohol consumption during pregnancy.

         (3) Cocaine is associated with increases in spontaneous abortions, placental abruption, preterm labor and delivery, low birth weight, neonatal withdrawal syndromes, and central nervous system damage. To reinforce or encourage abstinence from illicit drugs, consider periodic questioning or random drug screens.

         (4) Opiates can cause IUGR, preterm delivery, and an increased rate of intrauterine hypoxemia and fetal distress.

         (5) Daily consumption of more than 300 mg of **caffeine** (about three cups of coffee) has been associated with an increased risk of IUGR and low birth weight.

      b. Nutrition and weight gain. Total weight gain of 25 to 35 lbs is recommended by the Institute of Medicine guidelines for women at an appropriate weight at the time of conception. Women with <90% or >120% of ideal body weight should gain 30 to 35 lbs or 15 to 25 lbs, respectively, to minimize risks. A weight gain of <10 lbs at 20 weeks' gestation is associated with increased complications.

         (1) The average pregnant woman needs approximately 1900 to 2750 kcal per day (300 kcal more than nonpregnant patients). The best clue to adequate caloric intake is maternal weight gain.

         (2) The diet should include increased amounts of calcium (1200 mg per day, equivalent to three to four milk servings), iron (27 mg elemental iron), vitamins C and D, and folic acid (0.4–0.8 mg per day) and consist of 50% to 60% complex carbohydrate, up to 20% protein, and no more than 30% fat. A prenatal multivitamin and mineral supplement is recommended when dietary intake is inadequate. Vegetarians require additional iron, vitamin B_{12}, and zinc.

(3) Women with iron-deficiency anemia require 60 to 120 mg of elemental iron daily. Excessive doses of vitamins, particularly vitamins A, C, and D, can be harmful to the fetus. DHA supplementation has not been shown to positively affect neurodevelopment.

(4) Fish are an excellent source of omega-e fatty acids, which are considered important for central nervous system development. To avoid ingesting the teratogen methylmercury, women should avoid eating large fish such as shark, tilefish, swordfish, and king mackerel. Up to 12 ounces a week of fish low in mercury such as shrimp, canned light tuna, salmon, pollock, and catfish is recommended. Women should follow local fish advisories.

(5) Pregnant women should not eat hot dogs or luncheon meat unless they are steaming hot to avoid risk of **listeria**. They should also avoid unpasteurized soft cheese. Listeriosis has been associated with preterm delivery.

  c. **Patient expectations,** the benefits of childbirth education classes, and family issues should be discussed.

  d. **Sexual intercourse** during pregnancy is contraindicated only for patients with placenta previa and for those at risk for abortions or premature labor.

  e. **Physical activity** should not be significantly increased during pregnancy; however, moderate intensity exercise for 30 minutes on most days of the week is recommended in the absence of contraindications. Exercise in pregnancy may be beneficial in the prevention of gestational diabetes. Contact sports, activities requiring repeated Valsalva maneuvers or rapid changes in direction, or those involving unpredictable risk should be discouraged.

  f. **Symptoms for which patients need to promptly contact their physician** should be clearly outlined. These include any vaginal bleeding or escape of fluids from the vagina, swelling of the face and fingers, severe continuous headache, dimness or blurring of vision, abdominal pain, persistent vomiting, chills or fever, dysuria, and change in frequency or intensity of fetal movements.

C. Additional prenatal care. Traditionally, prenatal visits occur every 4 weeks through the 28th week of pregnancy, every 2 to 3 weeks through the 36th week, and then weekly until delivery. The frequency of visits can be altered based on the risk status of the patient. Decreasing the frequency of visits has not been shown to affect maternal or fetal outcomes, but may decrease the satisfaction level of the patient. (SOR **Ⓐ**) Prenatal care provided in a group setting has similar outcomes to traditional care with increased patient satisfaction and some evidence for decreased rates of preterm labor.

Measurement of weight, blood pressure, and fundal height; assessment of edema; and documentation of fetal heart rate should occur at every visit. Most providers check a urine dipstick for protein and glucose at each visit. Other tests and interventions may be needed at specific times during pregnancy, as noted below.

1. Care prior to 14 weeks (first trimester). Initial care during the first trimester can prepare both clinician and patient for a healthy pregnancy.

  a. Review initial laboratory work and define maternal risk status more precisely.

  b. Counsel patients regarding the initial troubling symptoms of pregnancy such as nausea, fatigue, and emotional changes. Encourage good nutrition. Review signs of miscarriage. Inquire about the partner's adjustment.

  c. All patients who present for care before 20 weeks' gestation should be offered first trimester screening for Down syndrome. (SOR **Ⓑ**) Screening that assesses nuchal translucency in addition to serum markers is equivalent to the quadruple screen in detection of Down syndrome and allows for early intervention. There are several ways this can be accomplished:

  (1) **Integrated screening.** Measurement of nuchal translucency and serum pregnancy associated plasma protein A (PAPP-a) levels at 10 to 13 weeks combined with serum levels of hCG, estriol, AFP, and inhibin at 15 to 20 weeks.

  (2) **Serum integrated screening.** Serum testing as aforementioned with no nuchal translucency.

  (3) **Sequential screening.** First trimester testing as aforementioned with second trimester testing only in those with negative or at intermediate risk (contingent) based on calculations. Those at a high risk based on screening should be offered diagnostic testing in the first trimester.

    d. Offer early prenatal diagnostic studies to all patients with genetic risk factors (see Section II.A.6). Chorionic villus sampling (CVS) is performed between 9 and 12 weeks' gestation, which allows for earlier termination of pregnancy with less maternal morbidity if abnormalities are found. Amniocentesis is usually performed after 15 weeks, but can be done as early as 13 weeks' gestation. Unlike amniocentesis, CVS cannot be used for prenatal diagnosis of NTDs and may be associated with limb reduction defects. Amniocentesis carries a 0.5% to 1% risk of fetal loss. The risk from CVS is slightly higher. A detailed ultrasound scan performed in the second trimester can also assist in the evaluation of fetal anomalies, but is not recommended as a screening test.

    e. Fetal heart tones are first heard with Doppler ultrasound between 11 and 13 weeks' gestation and sometimes as early as 9 weeks in multigravidas.

2. Care between 14 and 28 weeks' gestation (second trimester). An obviously pregnant body and the first sensations of fetal movement often lead to an increased appreciation of being pregnant. The second trimester is an excellent time to schedule a joint visit with the patient and her partner to discuss expectations about parenting. In addition, enrollment in prenatal classes can better prepare women and their partners for childbirth, encourage a more active role on the part of the woman, and can have a beneficial effect on performance in labor and delivery. (SOR **B**)

    a. Confirmation of the estimated date of delivery. At approximately 20 weeks' gestation, the uterine fundus is at the level of the umbilicus, and fetal heart tones can usually be heard with a fetoscope. The sensation of fetal movement (quickening), which may first be a fluttering sensation, is usually felt at 16 to 20 weeks' gestation.

    b. Routine prenatal screening for NTDs and chromosomal abnormalities such as Down syndrome (trisomy 21) are offered during this time for women who do not present early enough for first trimester screening. NTDs occur in 4 per 10,000 live births. Screening involves measuring the **maternal serum α-fetoprotein (MSAFP)** between 16 and 18 weeks' gestation. Approximately 50 of 1000 women will have an elevated (>2.5 multiples of the median) MSAFP, indicating the possibility of an NTD. Most will be falsely positive, resulting from inaccurate dating, multiple gestations, or other anomalies. An elevated MSAFP in the absence of other anomalies is associated with poor pregnancy outcomes. A targeted anatomic ultrasound to confirm dates can detect 90% to 95% of NTDs in addition to other defects associated with elevated MSAFP (omphalocele, gastroschisis, and cystic hygroma).

        Reduced levels of MSAFP (<0.7 multiples of the median) indicate an increased risk of Down syndrome. An association with reduced levels of estradiol and elevated levels of hCG and inhibin-A (the quadruple screen) has a false-positive rate of 5% and will identify approximately 76% of cases. (The older "triple screen" has a similar false-positive rate, but a lower detection rate of 60%–69%.) Amniocentesis offers the only definitive diagnosis, once dating is confirmed by ultrasound. Parents should be carefully advised of the benefits and risks of these screening tests, with documentation of the discussion and their decision recorded in the chart.

    c. Universal screening for **gestational diabetes** between 24 and 28 weeks is widely recommended and practiced (see Table 99–1 for tests and results). (SOR **C**) Testing based on risk factors excludes only a few women. Recent evidence indicates that treatment of gestational diabetes decreases pregnancy complications such as macrosomia and subsequent birth trauma. (SOR **A**) Some physicians advocate earlier screening (prior to 24 weeks) for high-risk women. Risk factors include a past history of gestational diabetes or a macrosomic infant (>4000 g), a family history of type II diabetes, or a maternal weight >200 lbs.

TABLE 99–1. TESTING FOR GESTATIONAL DIABETES

1-h glucose tolerance test (50 g oral glucose load)	Positive if blood glucose 1 h after ingestion is >130–140 mg/dL

3-h glucose tolerance test (100 g oral glucose load) to be done fasting when 1-h test is positive	Normal levels:
	  Fasting <95 mg/dL
	  1 h <180 mg/dL
	  2 h <155 mg/dL
	  3 h <140 mg/dL

   d. The hemoglobin or hematocrit can be repeated at the same time as screening for diabetes, along with antibody screening for D (Rh)-negative women.

   e. **D (Rh)-negative** women should be given D (Rh) immune globulin (Rhogam) at 28 weeks' gestation if the antibody screening is negative. D (Rh) immune globulin should be given earlier if an event has occurred exposing the patient to fetal blood (e.g., CVS, amniocentesis, or significant trauma). A repeat dose given within 72 hours after delivery is also necessary.

   f. Influenza vaccine should be offered to all pregnant women during the flu season.

3. Care beyond 28 weeks' gestation (third trimester). This is often a period of increasing discomfort for the patient, with sleep disturbances, dyspnea, urinary frequency, and fatigue being common. The incidence of complications such as pre-eclampsia, maternal hypertension, and malposition of the fetus leads to a need for more frequent and intensive monitoring. Allow time to discuss expectations and wishes regarding labor and delivery, and review indications for calling the office. Prepared childbirth education can have beneficial effects on performance in labor. (SOR **Ⓐ**)

   a. **Blood pressure** should be carefully monitored. Systolic blood pressures ≥140 mm Hg or diastolic blood pressures ≥90 mm Hg are diagnostic of gestational hypertension and warrant further evaluation for preeclampsia, particularly when associated with proteinuria.

   b. **Fetal position** should be regularly assessed. Most babies are vertex by the final month of pregnancy. For other presentations, external version is often successful and increases the chances of a vaginal delivery.

   c. Testing for **sexually transmitted infections** in high-risk women, if appropriate, should be repeated at 36 to 38 weeks' gestation. Testing allows for treatment prior to delivery.

   d. The Centers for Disease Control and Prevention (CDC) revised guidelines for **screening for group B streptococcal (GBS) infection** in 2002 and reaffirmed them in 2010. These are based on findings that universal screening was >50% more effective in preventing GBS infection in newborns than basing treatment on risk factors. The CDC recommends that all pregnant women (except for those with a history of GBS bacteriuria or a past history of an infant with invasive GBS disease) be screened with vaginal and rectal swabs for GBS between 35 and 37 weeks' estimated gestational age. Intrapartum antibiotic prophylaxis is then offered to all women who test positive, as well as to women with a history of GBS bacteriuria in the current pregnancy or a past history of an infant with invasive GBS disease. Antepartum prophylaxis is not recommended.

   e. In 2013, the Advisory Committee on Immunization Practices advised that all pregnant women should receive TdAP vaccine to optimize prevention of pertussis in infants. This is ideally timed between 27 and 36 weeks' gestation, regardless of prior immunization status.

   f. Patients who wish a trial of labor after cesarean section (TOLAC) should be counseled on the risks and benefits.

   g. Women should be counseled on the nutritional and immunologic benefits of breastfeeding. (SOR **Ⓑ**)

D. Common symptoms

1. Nausea and vomiting, which usually begin at approximately 6 weeks and disappear by 14 to 16 weeks, are commonly worse in the morning and occur in up to 70% of pregnant women. Hyperemesis gravidarum occurs in 0.5% to 2% of pregnancies. Nonpharmacologic therapies include having frequent, small meals; avoiding greasy, spicy foods; having a protein snack at bedtime; eating dry crackers before getting out of bed in the morning; and avoiding drinking liquids on an empty stomach. (SOR **Ⓒ**) Purposeful stimulation of the P6 (Neiguan) acupuncture point located three fingerbreadths proximal to the distal wrist crease and between the two central flexor tendons of the forearm, via pressing firmly with the fingers for 5 minutes every 4 hours while awake or via use of Seabands, can be quite helpful. (SOR **Ⓑ**)

   Women who consume a daily multivitamin at the time of conception have reduced severity of nausea and vomiting. Ginger capsules have shown promise in alleviating symptoms. (SOR **Ⓑ**) The American Congress of Obstetricians and Gynecologists (ACOG) recommends pyridoxine (vitamin B₆) 25 mg two or three times daily in combination with doxylamine 10 mg as first-line pharmacologic treatment. (SOR **Ⓐ**) Diclegis (containing 10 mg of doxylamine and 10 mg of pyridoxine) is

FDA-approved for the management of pregnancy-associated nausea and vomiting and is Pregnancy category A (see http://www.diclegnis.com).

Other medications include promethazine 12.5 to 25 mg orally or rectally every 4 hours, dimenhydrinate 50 to 100 mg every 4 to 6 hours, metoclopramide 5 to 10 mg every 6 to 8 hours, or ondansetron 4 to 8mg orally every 8 hours. (SOR ❸) For severe cases, ondansetron or even steroid tapers may be considered. Early treatment is important to prevent progression to hyperemesis. Reassurance that symptoms may be related to higher levels of maternal estrogens and an associated improved pregnancy outcome may also be useful. If a woman is dehydrated, intravenous fluids in the office are helpful.

2. **Headache** is common before 20 weeks' gestation and is usually benign, although in most cases no specific cause can be found. This symptom can be safely treated with acetaminophen. Relaxation and use of warm compresses may help. The pattern of migraine may change during pregnancy. The physician must consider preeclampsia, particularly later in pregnancy.

3. **Gastrointestinal symptoms common during pregnancy**
   a. **Heartburn** occurs in approximately one-half of pregnant women at some time. This condition has been attributed to a number of factors including decreased tone in the lower esophageal sphincter, displacement and compression of the stomach by the uterus, and decreased gastric motility. Treatment consists of having frequent small meals and avoiding bending over or lying flat soon after eating. Low-sodium liquid antacids are helpful and safe; however, those agents that contain magnesium or aluminum hydroxides impair absorption of iron. Over-the-counter H_2-blockers such as ranitidine are also considered safe for use in the second and third trimesters.
   b. **Constipation** is common in pregnancy because of hormone-induced changes in bowel transit time. Dietary measures are the mainstay of treatment and include high-fiber foods, liberal consumption of water and other liquids, and regular, low-intensity exercise. Mild laxatives such as milk of magnesia, stool softeners, and bulk laxatives are safe and effective.
   c. **Abdominal pain** may occur during pregnancy and warrants evaluation. The physician should consider the same causes for abdominal pain that occur in the nonpregnant state. However, these conditions may present differently in pregnant women. Types of abdominal pain specific to pregnancy are described below:
      (1) Ectopic pregnancy should be ruled out in women with lower abdominal or pelvic pain early in pregnancy (see Chapter 50).
      (2) Preeclampsia may be associated with upper abdominal pains in the epigastrium or the right upper quadrant.
      (3) Placental abruption should be considered when pain is associated with bleeding, particularly in the third trimester.
      (4) Urinary tract infections (see Chapter 21).
      (5) Other, less significant causes include round ligament or broad ligament discomfort, which results from increased tension on these structures as the uterus enlarges.

4. **Urinary complaints,** such as increasing frequency and stress incontinence, are often noted, especially during the first and third trimesters, because of uterine pressure on the bladder. Decreasing nighttime fluid intake (without any overall restrictions) and Kegel exercises can be helpful. Infection, however, is common and should be considered when frequency is associated with dysuria. The USPSTF recommends that all pregnant women be screened for asymptomatic bacteriuria at 12 to 16 weeks or their first prenatal visit. (SOR ❹)

5. Increased **vaginal discharge (leukorrhea)** is common, often with no pathologic cause. This physiologic discharge is related to increased estrogen. Infectious causes should be ruled out (see Chapter 63) in the presence of associated symptoms of itching, burning, foul odor, or labial swelling.

6. **Vaginal bleeding** can occur at any time during pregnancy and should always be considered significant enough to warrant further evaluation, including pelvic examination, appropriate cultures, and pelvic ultrasound.
   a. Bleeding in the first trimester is a relatively frequent occurrence. Causes range from physiologic bleeding as a result of implantation to life-threatening conditions. Extrauterine pregnancy should be considered when bleeding occurs during this

time, even in the absence of pain. Any bleeding occurring in the first half of pregnancy, particularly with cramping, may be associated with spontaneous abortion.

   b. Bleeding in the latter half of pregnancy occurs less frequently and may be associated with cervical trauma during coitus. Painless bleeding may suggest placenta or vasa previa, whereas painful bleeding is classically associated with placental abruption.

7. Edema in the feet and the ankles is common, particularly during the third trimester. This edema is secondary to sodium and water retention combined with increased lower extremity venous pressure. Edema should raise concerns of preeclampsia when it is accompanied by hypertension and proteinuria. Benign edema normally responds to leg elevation, avoidance of long periods of sitting or standing, and use of support stockings.

8. Backache is relatively common during pregnancy and is partially related to increased joint laxity as well as compensatory postural changes that occur as the uterus enlarges. Avoiding excessive weight gain, wearing flat or low-heeled shoes, and improving posture may provide some relief. Chiropractic care may be effective and is safe during pregnancy.

9. Varicose veins are aggravated by pregnancy, prolonged standing, and advancing age. This condition usually worsens as pregnancy advances, because of increased femoral pressure. Treatment is limited to periodic rest with leg elevation and elastic stockings; more definitive treatment is delayed until after pregnancy.

10. Hemorrhoids are the result of increased pressure on hemorrhoidal veins by the uterus and by the tendency toward constipation during pregnancy. Effective treatments include sitz baths in warm water for 20 minutes followed by local application of witch hazel, topically applied anesthetics, and stool softeners (see Chapter 51).

E. Medications in pregnancy. Most drugs should be used only when benefits clearly outweigh risks, particularly in the first trimester. Patients need to understand that taking any medication during pregnancy involves some small degree of risk.

   1. Antihistamines are generally acceptable when used in normal therapeutic doses, with the possible exception of brompheniramine.

   2. Antiemetics may be used safely if other conservative measures are not effective.

   3. Decongestants. These medications should be avoided in the first trimester, as both pseudoephedrine and phenylephrine have been associated with malformations after use in early pregnancy. Pseudoephedrine (30 mg every 6 hours) is relatively safe to use for limited periods, but large doses should be avoided, as they may negatively influence uterine perfusion. Decongestants are contraindicated when uteroplacental insufficiency is suspected. Try recommending the substitution of saline nose spray or irrigation or limited (up to 3 days) use of topical decongestants.

   4. Oral analgesics and anti-inflammatory agents

   a. Acetaminophen is the drug of choice for mild analgesia and antipyresis. Continuous high doses may cause maternal anemia and fatal kidney disease in the newborn (case report).

   b. Low-dose aspirin has been used to lower the risk of preeclampsia in high-risk women. Although there is no clear consensus regarding the benefits related to preeclampsia, aspirin has proven to be a relatively safe drug when used in low doses, although there seems to be an increased risk of placental abruption. Chronic or intermittent high doses should be avoided (Pregnancy category D for all trimesters).

   c. Nonsteroidal anti-inflammatory drugs (NSAIDs), such as ibuprofen and naproxen, have a theoretical risk of prenatal closure of the ductus arteriosus when used near term. They also cause a reversible decrease in amniotic fluid levels. Indomethacin, if used after 34 weeks' gestation, can lead to persistent pulmonary hypertension of the newborn, inhibition of labor, and prolongation of pregnancy. NSAIDs have been shown to block blastocyst implantation and are associated with an increased risk of spontaneous abortion.

   d. Codeine is not absolutely contraindicated, although association with malformations has been reported. Neonatal withdrawal has been documented. Hydrocodone–acetaminophen combinations (Vicodin) may be safer in pregnancy than codeine.

   e. Tramadol when used continuously can cause withdrawal in neonates similar to narcotic analgesics and should be avoided in the third trimester.

5. Antibiotics

  a. Penicillins (with or without clavulanate) and cephalosporins are among the most effective and least toxic of available antibiotics and can be used at any time during pregnancy.

  b. Erythromycin has not been reported to be of harm to the fetus, except as the estolate salt, which is contraindicated in pregnancy. Other macrolides have limited data in humans, but are considered safe.

  c. Tetracyclines and quinolones are contraindicated in pregnancy because of adverse effects on developing teeth and bones.

  d. Sulfonamides may be used in the first two trimesters. Use near term and during nursing should be avoided since sulfonamides can cause significant jaundice or hemolytic anemia in the newborn.

  e. Oral metronidazole is considered safe, although some prefer to wait until after the first trimester for its use. (SOR ❻) Topical metronidazole is safe throughout pregnancy.

  f. Nitrofurantoin should be used with care in late pregnancy since it has the ability to induce hemolysis in neonatal red blood cells.

6. Antisecretory gastrointestinal agents

  a. H_2 receptor blockers such as ranitidine and cimetidine are generally considered safe in pregnancy.

  b. Proton pump inhibitors are considered to have low risk for associated birth defects in several epidemiologic reviews.

7. Antidepressants and benzodiazepines

  a. Tricyclic antidepressants should be used with caution in the first trimester. These medications have extensive clinical use and are generally considered safe in pregnancy.

  b. Selective serotonin reuptake inhibitors, particularly fluoxetine, have generally been proven relatively safe during pregnancy. However, epidemiologic studies found an association between paroxetine and congenital cardiac defects. Use in the third trimester for all drugs in this class requires caution, as there is some evidence of neonatal withdrawal that can include irritability and seizures in rare cases.

  c. Lithium is contraindicated during pregnancy.

  d. Benzodiazepines should be used cautiously, if at all, as there is some evidence of an increased risk of cleft palate or cleft lip.

IV. Depression is common in women of reproductive age. Infants of mothers who are depressed may have delayed development. Screening for and treating depression in mothers can improve mental and behavioral disorders in children. Specific scales such as the Edinburgh Postnatal Depression Scale, Postpartum Depression Screening Scale, and Patient Health Questionnaire-9 are highly sensitive in screening for depression and easily administered in the office (see Chapter 94).

V. Obesity is a looming problem in the United States. Rates in women of childbearing age are 20% to 30% based on self-reported BMI data gathered by the CDC. Obese women are more likely to suffer miscarriage or have infants with birth defects. In addition, these women are at risk for medical complications of pregnancy such as gestational diabetes and preeclampsia.

Additional baseline testing should be considered in obese women to screen for diabetes. Macrosomia is associated with pregravid maternal obesity in addition to excessive weight gain and development of glucose intolerance or gestational diabetes. Pregravid weight loss can decrease the incidence of large-for-gestational-age infants. Obese women are also at a higher risk of gestational hypertension and preeclampsia.

VI. Preterm Labor (PTL) is defined as regular uterine contractions accompanied by descent of the presenting part and progressive dilatation and effacement of the cervix occurring before 37 weeks' gestation. PTL complicates only 8% to 10% of pregnancies, but is responsible for more than 60% of all perinatal morbidity and mortality. Risk factors include occult maternal genitourinary tract infections, maternal smoking, high levels of stress, low socioeconomic status, maternal age younger than 18 years or older than 35 years, cervical dilatation >1 cm or cervical effacement >30% between 26 and 34 weeks' gestation, and uterine anomalies. Risk factors most likely are synergistic. Screening and treatment of bacterial vaginosis in high-risk women may decrease the incidence of preterm labor. (SOR ❸)

  A. Diagnosis. Early diagnosis is crucial, as tocolysis is most effective before 3 cm of cervical dilatation or 50% effacement. Symptoms suggestive of regular uterine contractions

TABLE 99–2. DIAGNOSIS OF PREECLAMPSIA

New onset of hypertension after 20 weeks' gestation with proteinuria

- Blood pressure >140/90 mm Hg on two occasions more than 6 h apart
- Proteinuria (>1+ on urine dipstick or >300 mg/24 h) present on two occasions more than 6 h apart

Edema is supportive of the diagnosis, but not required.

should be evaluated with serial examinations for cervical change and by external monitoring of uterine activity. Vaginal ultrasound to assess cervical length, along with fetal fibronectin measurements, can be helpful in predicting the likelihood of preterm birth.

B. Treatment. The risks of preterm delivery must outweigh the risks of tocolysis. Advancing gestational age clearly improves the preterm infant's prognosis until approximately 35 weeks, when delaying delivery has less overall effect. Survival increases to 90% at 29 weeks, mortality then decreases approximately 1% per week. The acuteness and severity of preterm labor suggest the type of treatment.

    1. Women with uterine irritability without significant cervical change may benefit from rest at home, intake of fluids, and treatment of causative factors such as urinary tract infection, if present.

    2. Tocolytic therapy is indicated in preterm labor if no contraindications, such as severe preeclampsia or chorioamnionitis, exist. All tocolytics have potentially severe side effects for both mother and fetus. Choices include β-sympathomimetics, magnesium sulfate, nifedipine, and indomethacin.

    3. Evaluation for possible triggers, particularly occult urinary tract infection, is indicated. Randomized controlled trials have found no clear benefit to the use of antibiotics in women with PTL with intact membranes on prolonging gestation or improving neonatal morbidity or mortality. (SOR **Ⓐ**) Treatment with **antenatal corticosteroids** given before 34 weeks' gestation and >24 hours but <7 days prior to delivery is of benefit in reducing the incidence and severity of respiratory distress syndrome and improving neonatal survival rates. (SOR **Ⓐ**) In addition, use of betamethasone has been associated with a 50% decrease in the incidence of periventricular malacia. (SOR **Ⓑ**)

VII. Hypertensive disorders of pregnancy are present in 6% to 8% of all pregnancies.

    A. Chronic hypertension in pregnancy is diagnosed when a woman has an elevated blood pressure (>140/90 mm Hg) prior to 20 weeks' gestation. Morbidity in chronic hypertension is from IUGR and superimposed preeclampsia. Growth ultrasounds should be performed every 4 weeks starting at 28 weeks in women with chronic hypertension.

    B. Gestational hypertension is diagnosed when a woman develops elevated blood pressure after 20 weeks without any proteinuria. Half of these women will develop preeclampsia.

    C. Preeclampsia is a life-threatening multisystem disorder that includes elevated blood pressures and proteinuria (Table 99–2). Calcium and low-dose aspirin are used to prevent preeclampsia in high-risk women. Consequences of severe preeclampsia include seizures, hepatic abnormalities, and coagulation disorders (Table 99–3). Delivery of the baby is the cure for preeclampsia. Magnesium sulfate is used to prevent seizures and either labetalol or hydralazine is used to control blood pressure.

TABLE 99–3. DIAGNOSTIC CRITERIA FOR SEVERE PREECLAMPSIA

In addition to elevated blood pressure and proteinuria, to be diagnosed with severe preeclampsia, women must also present with

- Headaches
- Visual disturbances
- Pulmonary edema
- Abnormal liver function tests
- Abdominal pain (usually right upper quadrant or epigastric)
- Evidence of renal dysfunction
- Thrombocytopenia or hemolysis

VIII. Fetal Assessment and Postdates Pregnancy

A. Fetal assessment. Several methods have been developed to assess fetal well-being when risk factors exist. Fetal assessment begins between 32 and 34 weeks' gestation or whenever the risk develops. Testing may begin as early as 26 to 28 weeks in particularly worrisome conditions. Major indications for antenatal testing include diabetes mellitus, hypertensive disorders, maternal substance abuse, third-trimester bleeding, IUGR, previously unexplained stillbirth, D (Rh) sensitization, oligohydramnios, multiple gestations, and decreased fetal movement as perceived by the mother. Fetal assessment techniques also are routinely applied when a pregnancy becomes postterm (42 weeks from the LMP). Testing is generally repeated weekly or biweekly until delivery. (SOR ❸)

1. Fetal movement counts. A quantitative method of counting fetal movements has been developed as a means of fetal assessment near term. The patient is asked to count fetal movements during a 2-hour period each day and report <10 movements during that period. A positive test (fewer than 10 movements) is an indication for additional fetal assessment. The advantages of this test are its low cost and maternal involvement. (SOR ❸)

2. Fetal heart rate testing

a. The **nonstress test** (NST) is a noninvasive method based on the premise that in a healthy fetus, acceleration of the heart rate occurs during fetal movement. An external monitor is used to record the fetal heart rate while the mother reports fetal movement. A reactive or normal test has two or more accelerations of more than 15 beats per minute, each lasting for 15 seconds, in a 20-minute period and in the absence of decelerations. If fetal movement does not occur in 20 minutes, abdominal palpation or vibroacoustic stimulation can be applied to awaken a sleeping fetus. A reactive NST accurately identifies a healthy fetus 98% of the time.

Evaluation of a nonreactive NST should include extending the testing period to 60 to 90 minutes when possible. Nonreactive NSTs and variable decelerations on reactive NSTs should prompt additional evaluation. It must be noted that 15% of fetuses younger than 32 weeks may have a nonreactive NST in the absence of fetal compromise. In gestations less than 32 weeks criteria for an adequate acceleration are an increase of 10 beats per minute persisting for 10 seconds.

b. The **contraction stress test** (CST) is a test of the fetal heart rate in response to uterine contractions. The uterus may be stimulated to contract through intermittent stimulation of one nipple or through intravenous infusion of low-dose oxytocin. A satisfactory test requires at least three contractions in 10 minutes. The test is interpreted as negative, or normal, if there are no decelerations and positive, or abnormal, if late decelerations follow 50% or more of contractions. A positive CST is highly suggestive of fetal distress and must be treated immediately with oxygen, positional changes, labor induction, or cesarean section. Equivocal results occur with intermittent late decelerations or significant variable decelerations and the CST should be repeated in 24 hours.

3. An **amniotic fluid index** is used to complement fetal heart rate testing. Ultrasonography is used for estimating amniotic fluid volume, which is an indirect measure of placental function. The largest anteroposterior fluid depth in each of four quadrants of the uterus is measured. The sum should exceed 5 cm.

4. The **biophysical profile** (BPP) is a quantitative score that combines the NST with ultrasonic observation of the fetus for up to 30 minutes and measurement of the amniotic fluid index. A score of 2 is given **for each normal result** (fetal breathing movements, gross body movements, tone, amniotic fluid index, and NST) and 0 for an abnormal condition. A total score of 8 to 10 is reassuring, 6 is equivocal, and 4 or less is worrisome. An equivocal test should prompt delivery if at term or be repeated in 12 to 24 hours. A score of 4 or less should be a consideration for delivery regardless of gestational age or further evaluation. A combination of NST and amniotic fluid evaluation known as a modified BPP is considered comparable to the biophysical profile in assessing fetal well-being.

5. Doppler ultrasonography of the umbilical artery has been used to assess resistance to blood flow in the placenta which may be present in intrauterine growth restriction. It should be used in conjunction with other measures of fetal well-being to guide timing of delivery and is not recommended for screening in the general population.

B. Postterm pregnancy. Defined as lasting longer than 42 weeks from the beginning of the LMP, approximately 3.5% to 12% of pregnancies are postdates. Prolonged pregnancy is one lasting longer than 41 weeks. Accurate dating is essential to avoid mislabeling a pregnancy as postterm. (SOR **Ⓐ**)

1. Chronic uteroplacental insufficiency leading to fetal compromise occurs in up to 20% of postterm pregnancies. Additional complications include oligohydramnios, meconium passage, and macrosomia, which may contribute to a higher cesarean section rate.

2. Evaluation. Fetal assessment testing should be performed in all postterm pregnancies. Perinatal morbidity and mortality increase past 41 weeks; therefore, monitoring the pregnancy with antepartum testing is common practice. (SOR **Ⓒ**)

3. Management. International randomized controlled clinical trials have shown a clear benefit to induction of labor at 41 to 42 weeks' gestation. The fetal mortality rate of 2 per 1000 at this gestational age is lowered to virtually zero and cesarean section rates are lowered. Elective induction with oxytocin, using prostaglandins before as needed for cervical ripening, is relatively safe and effective. Women with a favorable cervix are generally induced. (SOR **Ⓒ**) Women with an unfavorable cervix can be managed expectantly or with induction. (SOR **Ⓐ**) Delivery should be attempted if there is evidence of fetal compromise or oligohydramnios on testing. (SOR **Ⓐ**) Sweeping (stripping) of the membranes reduces the need for other methods of induction, but may cause discomfort for the patient. (SOR **Ⓐ**)

IX. Normal Labor and Delivery. Signs of labor include passage of the mucus plug, bloody show (small amount of blood-tinged mucoid vaginal discharge), regular uterine contractions, and spontaneous rupture of membranes. In the general population, approximately 90% of women should be able to have a healthy birth outcome without medical intervention. The great majority of women deliver in the hospital utilizing family-centered birthing focusing on safety for the mother and child and fostering a positive experience for the woman, her partner, and family.

SELECTED REFERENCES

Agency for Healthcare Research and Quality. Efficacy and safety of screening for postpartum depression. Rockville, MD: Agency for Healthcare Research and Quality; April 2013. http://www.ahrq.gov/research/findings/postpartumdep.html. Accessed May 2013.

American Academy of Pediatrics and the American College of Obstetricians and gynecologists. *Guidelines for Perinatal Care.* 7th ed. Elk Grove, IL: American Academy of Pediatrics; 2012.

American College of Obstetricians and Gynecologists. ACOG Practice Bulletin No 31, 2001 (Reaffirmed 2010). Assessment of risk factors for preterm birth.

American College of Obstetricians and Gynecologists. ACOG Practice Bulletin No. 52, 2004 (Reaffirmed 2009). Nausea and vomiting of pregnancy.

American College of Obstetricians and Gynecologists. ACOG Committee Opinion No. 402. Antenatal corticosteroid therapy for fetal maturation. *Obstet Gynecol.* 2008;99:871–873.

American College of Obstetricians and Gynecologists. ACOG Committee Opinion No. 267. Exercise during pregnancy and the postpartum period. *Obstet Gynecol.* 2002;99:171–173. (Reaffirmed 2009)

American College of Obstetricians and Gynecologists. ACOG Committee Opinion No 315. (Reaffirmed 2008). Obesity in pregnancy. *Obstet Gynecol.* 2005;106:671–675.

American College of Obstetricians and Gynecologists. ACOG Committee Opinion No. 316. Smoking cessation during pregnancy. *Obstet Gynecol.* 2005;106:883–888.

American College of Obstetricians and Gynecologists. ACOG Technical Bulletin No. 77, Jan 2007 (Reaffirmed 2008). Screening for fetal chromosomal abnormalities.

Briggs G, Freeman RK, Jaffe SJ. *Drugs in Pregnancy and Lactation: A Reference Guided to Fetal and Neonatal Risk.* 9th ed. Philadelphia, PA: Lippincott, Williams & Wilkins; 2011.

Centers for Disease Control and Prevention. Prevention of Group B streptococcal disease. *MMWR.* 2010;59(RR-10):1–32.

Centers for Disease Control and Prevention. Updated recommendations for use of tetanus toxoid, reduced diphtheria toxoid, and acellular pertussis vaccine (TdAP) in pregnant women. *MMWR.* 2013;62(07):131–135.

Doswell T, Carroli G, Duley L, et al. Alternative versus standard packages of antenatal care for low risk pregnancy. *Cochrane Database Syst Rev.* 2010;(10):CD000934.

100   Postpartum Care

Shami Goyal, MD, MS, & Jeannette E. South-Paul, MD

KEY POINTS

- Puerperal infections usually occur 2 to 5 days postpartum. First-line treatments are clindamycin, and gentamicin or cefoxitin. (SOR ⊙)
- The most common nonpuerperal infections that occur in the postpartum period are urinary tract infections and mastitis. (SOR ⊙)
- Other common postpartum complications include thromboembolic disease, postpartum hemorrhage, and postpartum depression. (SOR ⊙)
- Hospital discharge instructions include daily rest, sitz baths, instructions on when to resume sexual activity, encouragement of breastfeeding (and continuation of prenatal vitamins if doing so), and to return for the postpartum examination 6 to 8 weeks after birth. (SOR ⊙)

I. Introduction

A. Definition. The postpartum period, or puerperium, is the period of time that begins with the delivery of the placenta and ends with the resumption of ovulatory menstrual cycles. In nonlactating women, this usually occurs 6 to 8 weeks after delivery. Health care providers should be aware of the medical and psychological needs of the postpartum mother and sensitive to cultural differences that surround childbirth, which may involve eating particular foods and restricting certain activities.

B. Pathophysiology and epidemiologic data

  1. The **uterus** decreases in size dramatically following delivery (involution). The weight of the uterus decreases from approximately 1000 g immediately postpartum to 60 g 6 to 8 weeks later. This change is accompanied by a high level of uterine activity (contractions, afterpains) that diminishes smoothly and progressively after the first 2 hours postpartum. The placental implantation site sheds organized thrombi and obliterated arteries to prevent scar formation and preserve normal endometrial tissue.

  2. Cervix. The cervical os admits two fingers for the first 4 to 6 days postpartum, but constricts thereafter. The external os never resumes its pregravid shape; the small, smooth, regular circular opening of the nulligravida becomes a large, transverse, stellate slit after childbirth. Histologically, the cervix does not return to baseline for up to 3 to 4 months after delivery.

  3. Vagina. Large and smooth-walled following delivery, the vagina begins to develop rugae by the end of the fourth week. It regains its nonpregnant size by the end of the sixth to eighth week.

  4. Lochia. The uterine discharge, which is bright red at delivery, changes within a few days to the reddish-brown lochia rubra, composed of blood and decidual and trophoblastic debris. Lochia serosa, a more serious combination of old blood, serum, leukocytes, and tissue debris, appears 1 week postpartum and last for a few days. Lochia alba, a whitish-yellow discharge that contains serum leukocytes, decidua, epithelial cells, mucus, and bacteria, follows and continues until approximately 2 to 4 weeks postpartum. Up to 15% of women continue to pass lochia for 6 to 8 weeks.

  5. Urinary tract. Passage of the infant through the pelvis traumatizes the bladder. Trauma or conduction analgesia may also cause the bladder to be insensitive to changes in intravesicular pressure, resulting in an impaired urge to urinate. Symptoms of urinary incontinence increase with parity. Practice of pelvic muscle exercise by primiparas results in fewer urinary incontinence symptoms during late pregnancy and the puerperium. The glomerular filtration rate remains elevated during the first postpartum week.

  6. The **abdominal wall** begins to resume a nonparous condition in approximately 6 to 7 weeks. The skin remains lax, but the muscles regain substantial tone with proper exercise. Long-term sequelae may include low back pain, abdominal discomfort, and cosmetic concerns.

7. **Cardiovascular changes.** Cardiac output decreases to nonpregnant levels within 2 to 3 weeks postpartum. Lower-extremity varicosities and pelvic varices regress during this period. Plasma volume decreases more rapidly than do cellular components initially, so the hematocrit increases slightly during the first 72 hours postpartum.

8. **Weight change.** Weight gain during the first 20 weeks of pregnancy predicts postpartum retained weight. The influence of lactation on weight loss postpartum is unclear. Women lose approximately half of the average weight gain of pregnancy (25 lbs) in the first 2 weeks after delivery. The remainder is lost during the following weeks. Women should return to their nonparous weight in approximately 8 weeks.

9. **Breasts.** Milk production and engorgement begin within 3 days postpartum, following the decrease in estrogen and increase in prolactin produced by suckling. Suckling is the single most important stimulus for the maintenance of milk production.

10. **Hypothalamic–pituitary–ovarian function.** Forty percent of nonlactating women will resume menstruation within 6 weeks following delivery, 65% within 12 weeks, and 90% within 24 weeks. Approximately 50% of the first cycles are ovulatory. In nursing mothers, menstruation is resumed within 6 weeks in only 15% and within 12 weeks in only 45%. In 80% of these women, the first ovulatory cycle is preceded by one or more anovulatory cycles.

11. **Reproductive hormones.** Typically, HCG values return to normal nonpregnant levels 2 to 4 weeks after term delivery, but can take longer. The most serious concern in women with rising hCG levels postpartum is gestational trophoblastic disease.

    Gonadotropins and sex steroids are at low levels for the first 2 to 3 weeks postpartum. Women who breastfeed have a delay in resumption of ovulation postpartum. This is believed to be due to prolactin-induced inhibition of pulsatile gonadotropin-releasing hormone release from the hypothalamus.

12. **Skin and hair.** Striae, if present, fade from red to silvery, but are permanent. Chloasma resolves in the postpartum period. During pregnancy, there is an increase in the percentage of "growing" or anagen hair relative to the "resting" or telogen hair. This ratio is reversed in the puerperium. Telogen effluvium is the hair loss commonly noted 1 to 5 months after delivery. This is usually self-limited with restoration of normal hair patterns by 6 to 15 months after delivery.

II. **Diagnosis and Treatment of Postpartum Complications** (see Table 100–1)
  A. **Abnormalities of the puerperium**
    1. **Puerperal infection** is defined as infection of the genital tract that sometimes extends to other organ systems. Cesarean delivery is the most important risk factor for the development of postpartum endometritis. Onset is insidious and can occur 2 to 5 days postpartum. Nonspecific symptoms are malaise, anorexia, and fever. In many cases, a temperature of 38°C (100.4°F) or higher on any 2 of the first 10 days postpartum, exclusive of the first 24 hours, indicates a puerperal infection. The first 24 hours are excluded because low-grade fever during this period is common and often resolves spontaneously, especially after vaginal birth.
      a. **Differential diagnosis** of postpartum fever includes surgical site infection, mastitis/breast abscess, urinary tract infection (UTI), pneumonia, and pelvic vein thrombosis as well as other causes of fever unrelated to the postpartum state. Onset of fever after the 10th postpartum day is usually of a nonobstetric nature.
      b. **Puerperal infections are usually polymicrobial.** *Escherichia coli* and group B streptococci are the most common causative agents, but there has been some reemergence of infections secondary to group A β-hemolytic streptococci that can result in tissue damage, toxin-mediated shock, and multiple organ failure. Multiple bacteria of low virulence, common in the genitourinary tract, may become pathogenic as a result of hematomas and devitalized tissue. Cultures are of limited usefulness, since the same organisms are identified in patients with or without infections. (SOR **Ⓐ**)
      c. **Predisposing factors**
        (1) **Antepartum.** Premature or prolonged rupture of membranes, malnourishment, and anemia increase the likelihood of puerperal infections.
        (2) **Intrapartum.** Soft-tissue trauma, residual devitalized tissue, prolonged labor, and hemorrhage.
      d. **Specific puerperal infections**
        (1) **Endometritis** involves inflammation and leukocytic infiltration of the superficial layers of the endometrium or decidual layer. Endometritis may be

TABLE 100-1. POSTPARTUM COMPLICATIONS REQUIRING TREATMENT

Complications	Symptoms	Etiology	Predisposing Factors	Treatment
Puerperal infection	2–5 d postpartum, $T > 100.4°F$, anorexia	Polymicrobial—anaerobes and aerobes, *Escherichia coli*; Group B streptococci	Prolonged ROM, malnutrition; hemorrhage/anemia, soft-tissue trauma	Clindamycin 2.4–2.7 g/d in three to four doses + gentamicin 2 mg/kg load, then 1.5 mg/kg every 8 h IV OR ampicillin 2 g IV + sulbactam 1 g IV every 6 h OR cefoxitin or moxalactam
Endometritis/parametritis	Lethargy, $T > 100.4°F$, lower abdominal pain	Polymicrobial	Prolonged labor and ROM, prior gynecologic infections, hematomas, devitalized tissue, maternal age younger than 17 yr	Same as above
Urinary tract infections	Fever; abdominal pain; ± dysuria	Polymicrobial	Trauma-induced bladder hypotonicity; frequent catheterizations	Amoxicillin 500 mg orally three times daily × 10–14 d
Deep vein thrombosis	Deep vein tenderness, Homan sign, extremity swelling	Sluggish circulation, estrogen-induced hypercoagulability	Trauma to pelvic veins	Heparin 5000–10,000 U load to get PTT at 2× normal or enoxaparin 1 mg/kg SC twice daily followed by warfarin orally to maintain INR 2.0–3.0
Superficial thrombophlebitis	Palpable cords in lower extremities, tenderness, skin warmth		High estrogen state	Elastic support stockings, walking, leg elevation at rest, moist local heat
Pelvic vein thrombosis (right ovarian syndrome)	Abdominal pain, fever; tender, sausage-shaped mass in right mid-abdomen		High estrogen state	Heparin anticoagulation (as above)
Necrotizing fasciitis	3–5 d postpartum; symptoms as in other puerperal infections	Polymicrobial, especially anaerobes	Diabetes, immunocompromised state, status post c-section	Clindamycin 2.4 mg/kg in 4 doses + gentamicin 1.5 mg/kg every 8 h IV; surgical debridement
Toxic shock syndrome	$T > 102°F$; macular erythematous rash, especially on palms and soles	*Staphylococcus aureus* exotoxin-1	Prolonged tampon use	Hospitalization; fluid; electrolytes; PRBCs; coagulation factors; oxacillin or nafcillin or methicillin 1 g IV every 4 h or vancomycin 1 g every 6 h

INR, international normalized ratio; PRBCs, packed red blood cells; PTT, partial thromboplastin time; ROM, rupture of membranes; T, temperature.

accompanied by chills, extreme lethargy, lower abdominal pain, and fever. It is not necessarily associated with significant uterine tenderness by abdominal or vaginal palpation.

This type of infection is relatively uncommon following uncomplicated vaginal delivery with a prevalence of 1% to 2%. The prevalence approaches 6% in high-risk women: those with protracted labor and prolonged rupture of membranes, prior history of gynecologic infections, hematomas or devitalized tissue, postpartum anemia, maternal age younger than 17 years, and where there is manual removal of the placenta.

For patients undergoing cesarean delivery, antibiotic prophylaxis is recommended and spontaneous placental extraction in vaginal deliveries minimizes the risk of postpartum endometritis. (SOR **Ⓐ**) Treatment of postpartum endometritis is indicated for relief of symptoms and prevention of sequelae (Table 100–1).

- **(2) Group B streptococcal sepsis.** This is a major cause of puerperal infections usually presenting with fever within 12 hours of delivery accompanied by tachycardia and endomyometritis. **Group B streptococcal-positive mothers** (typically the distal vagina and anorectum are cultured between 35 and 37 weeks' gestation) **are administered antibiotics intrapartum** to produce a 30-fold risk reduction in the incidence of early-onset group B streptococcal sepsis infection. (SOR **Ⓐ**)
- **(3) Parametritis.** This infection involves the broad ligament adjacent to the uterus. Parametritis is usually associated with endometritis. In its most isolated mild form, it can follow cesarean section. Treatment is the same as for endometritis. (SOR **Ⓒ**)
- **(4) Perineal infection** is more likely in the presence of a small, unnoticed hematoma. Examination of the perineum reveals an edematous, erythematous lesion with purulent drainage. Sutures must be removed to enhance drainage.
- **(5) Mastitis** is a localized, painful inflammation in the breast that is associated with fever and malaise in breastfeeding women. Risks include mastitis with previous pregnancy, inadequate drainage of the breast, and breakdown of the nipples. Emptying the breast with either nursing or pumping, antibiotics directed at *Staphylococcus aureus*, and supportive care such as gentle massage or use of a warm washcloth over the affected breast prior to breastfeeding are successful in most cases. If an abscess develops, some women may need an incision and drainage.

2. **Nonpuerperal complications** (Table 100–1).
   a. **Urinary tract infections.** The high incidence of UTIs during the postpartum period is usually attributed to trauma-induced hypotonicity of the bladder. Several other factors have been implicated including catheterization, epidural anesthesia, and vaginal procedures. Cystitis usually results in local symptoms without fever. In contrast, the symptoms of pyelonephritis are more severe: flank pain, shaking chills, and fever to 40°C (104°F) are frequent accompaniments. Urinary catheters should be removed as soon as they are no longer needed.
   b. **Thrombophlebitis and thromboembolic disease.** These conditions occur in less than 1% of all parturients, but occur significantly more often in the parturient than in the nonpregnant woman. Increased rates are associated with c-section and pelvic infections.
      - **(1) Disorders of the deep veins** in the postpartum period have been attributed to sluggish circulation, trauma to pelvic veins due to pressure from the fetal head, estrogen-induced hypercoagulability, and pelvic infection. Deep vein thrombophlebitis is characterized by fever, deep vein tenderness, Homan sign, and extremity swelling secondary to venous obstruction (see Chapter 64).
      - **(2) Superficial thrombophlebitis** usually involves the saphenous system and is palpable on physical examination. Tenderness and increased skin warmth are also evident. Treatment is described in Table 100–1. (SOR **Ⓒ**)
      - **(3) Pelvic thrombophlebitis** is the term used to describe thrombophlebitis occurring in the ovarian veins and other pelvic vessels. The patient often complains of abdominal pain and fever. If no evidence of pelvic abscess

exists, and appropriate antibiotic therapy has resulted in no improvement in 72 hours in a patient with suspected endometritis, the diagnosis of ovarian vein syndrome should be considered. A sausage-shaped, tender mass may be palpated in the right mid-abdomen. Dramatic improvement usually results once **anticoagulation with heparin** is initiated, but defervescence may only occur after 4 to 5 days of heparin therapy, in doses similar to those used for the treatment of pulmonary embolism (see Chapter 64). (SOR **C**) Currently available imaging studies (computerized tomography scan and ultrasound) are poor in diagnosing this entity, so clinical suspicion is important.

   (4) Massive pulmonary embolism is characterized by the sudden onset of pleuritic chest pain, cough (with or without hemoptysis), fever, apprehension, and tachycardia. Friction rub, signs of pleural effusion and atelectasis, hypotension, diaphoresis, electrocardiographic signs of right heart strain, and increasing central venous pressure may all be present in severe cases (see Chapter 64).

3. Postpartum hemorrhage (PPH) is defined as an estimated blood loss of 500 mL or more after vaginal birth or of 1000 mL or more after cesarean delivery. PPH is also classified as primary or secondary: primary PPH occurs within 24 hours after delivery (also called early PPH) and secondary PPH occurs 24 hours to 12 weeks after delivery (also called late PPH).

   a. Uterine atony is the most common cause of PPH and can result from excessive uterine stretching secondary to polyhydramnios, multiple gestation, multiparity, prolonged labor, and certain general anesthetic agents. Initial management includes **fundal massage, removal of any remaining placental fragments,** and **oxytocin** (10 U intramuscularly [IM] every 4 hours, or 10–40 U intravenously [IV] diluted in 1000 mL of 0.5 normal saline titrated IV) to control atony. (SOR **C**) Methylergonovine maleate (0.2 mg IM every 4 hours for 48 hours) can be used instead of oxytocin. Prostaglandin analogs can also be used alone or in combination with other uterotonic agents (carboprost tromethamine, 0.25 mg IM every 15–90 minutes up to eight doses; misoprostol—1000 μg, single dose via rectal, vaginal, or buccal routes). (SOR **C**)

   b. Lacerations. Routine inspection of the cervix, vagina, and perineum immediately following delivery affords the opportunity for timely repair of extensions to the episiotomy or lacerations.

   c. Hematomas. Perineal pain and noticeable mass suggest hematomas, which usually occur at the sites of lacerations or episiotomy repair. If managed within the first 24 hours after delivery with incision, drainage, and ligation of bleeding vessels, the cavity can be closed with a figure-of-eight suture. (SOR **C**)

   d. Less common causes of PPH are placenta accreta, inverted uterus, coagulation defects (e.g., associated with amniotic fluid embolism or preeclampsia-eclampsia), retained placental fragments, or uterine rupture. Digital examination of the uterus and lower uterine segment upon delivery is necessary to detect uterine rupture, especially after a vaginal delivery following prior cesarean section.

4. Postpartum emotional disorders

   a. "Baby blues" or **"postpartum blues."** This transient depression is encountered in 70% to 80% of women during the first week postpartum, usually on the second or third day following delivery. This self-limited disorder usually presents with tearfulness and resolves within 3 to 7 days.

   b. Postpartum depression. Twelve percent of women will present with depressive disorders within 6 weeks postpartum, but 90% of these cases are associated with a situational or long-standing problem. Postpartum depression occurs between 2 weeks and 12 months postpartum. Risk factors for postpartum depression include a previous history of depression, depression during pregnancy, a family history of depression, and psychosocial stressors (including child care issues and social support).

   If the symptoms are severe enough to interfere with the new mother's ability to cope with ordinary daily tasks and activities, counseling and pharmacotherapy are advisable (see Chapter 94). (SOR **A**) Individual-based interventions are more effective than group-based interventions. Severe postpartum depression can also be associated with psychosis so the clinician needs to monitor closely.

III. Management Strategies

A. Immunizations

1. Non-isoimmunized D-negative women who deliver a D-positive infant should be given 300 mg of anti-D immune globulin (RhoGAM) shortly after delivery. (SOR **B**)
2. The postpartum hospitalization period is also an appropriate time for vaccination of women not already immune to rubella. It is also appropriate to give a tetanus toxoid booster injection prior to discharge unless it is contraindicated. (SOR **C**)

B. Discharge instructions

1. Periods of rest during the day are advisable for the **first month postpartum**. If vaginal bleeding increases upon resumption of activity, parturients should stop for 2 to 3 days to allow further uterine involution and then resume activity. (SOR **C**) The parturient may gradually increase her activity and exercise level as soon as 2 weeks following an uncomplicated delivery.
2. **Sitz baths,** basins designed to fit over the toilet seat and be filled with warm water and 1 oz of Betadine solution, or tub baths for 30 minutes two to three times daily, are helpful for painful episiotomies or lacerations. (SOR **C**)
3. **Sexual intercourse** can be resumed when bleeding has stopped and the woman is comfortable. Contraception should be discussed, if appropriate, and a method and back-up method should be selected prior to discharge from the hospital (see Chapter 97). Although intrauterine devices can be inserted immediately after delivery of the placenta, the usual practice in the United States is to wait until 6 weeks postpartum because of an increased risk of expulsion. Diaphragms, sponges, and foams are also not usually advised until 6 weeks after delivery. (SOR **C**)
4. **Breastfeeding.** Human milk is recognized as the optimal feeding for all infants because of its proven health benefits to infants and their mothers. The World Health Organization (WHO), American Academy of Pediatrics (AAP), American Congress of Obstetricians and Gynecologists (ACOG), and United States Preventive Services Task Force all recommend exclusive breastfeeding for the first 6 months of life.

   a. Components of milk

   (1) **Colostrum.** This liquid is secreted by the breasts for the first 5 days of parturition. It contains more protein (mostly globulin), minerals, and less sugar and fat than the more mature milk that is ultimately secreted. Host resistance factors, such as complement components, macrophages, lymphocytes, lactoferrin, lactoperoxidase, and lysozyme, as well as immunoglobulin, are present in colostrum and milk.

   (2) **Milk.** The major components are proteins (α-lactalbumin, β-lactoglobulin, and casein), lactose, water, and fat. All vitamins except vitamin K are present in human milk in variable amounts. Iron is present in low concentrations, and iron levels in breast milk do not seem to be influenced by maternal iron stores. The predominant antibody present is secretory immunoglobulin A. These antibodies are thought to act locally within the infant's gastrointestinal tract.

   b. Nursing

   (1) **Advantages**

   (a) Accelerates involution of the uterus via oxytocin release.

   (b) Gives ideal nourishment. Breast milk meets the nutritional needs of the infant.

   (c) Provides immunologic advantage. In addition, breastfed babies are less prone to respiratory and enteric infections than are bottle-fed babies.

   (d) Contributes to bonding. Nursing is generally well tolerated by infants.

   (e) Delays ovulation.

   c. Breast care. Cleanliness and attention to fissures on the nipples are important. Water and mild soap can be used to cleanse the areolae before and after nursing. Lanolin-containing cream is recommended for nipple protection during the initial weeks of breastfeeding to deter nipple chapping and cracking. Should severe nipple irritation occur, a nipple shield can be used for 24 hours or more.

5. **Suppression of lactation.** Women who do not wish to breastfeed should avoid all breast stimulation, suckling, manipulation, and showers, and should use a firm bra (rather than breast binding), and analgesia, if needed, for 1 week. Minor symptoms of tenderness and a sense of fullness are common. Neither parenteral Deladumone nor oral bromocriptine is currently recommended.

6. Postpartum examination. The postpartum visit is usually scheduled for 4 to 6 weeks after delivery, since most of the systemic signs of pregnancy have resolved by this time. (SOR ⊜) Following normal labor and puerperium, the postpartum evaluation should consist of blood pressure and weight determinations, palpation of the thyroid gland, a breast examination, a pelvic examination with cytologic examination of the cervix if indicated, evaluation of rectal sphincter tone, examination of abdominal wall tone, and urinalysis. Based on a Danish registry study, the prevalence of postpartum UTI was 2.8% after cesarean delivery and 1.5% after vaginal birth. Routine postpartum hematocrits are unnecessary in clinically stable patients with an estimated blood loss of <500 cc.

SELECTED REFERENCES

Dennis CL, Fung K, Grigoriadis S, et al. Traditional postpartum practices and rituals: a qualitative systematic review. *Womens Health (Lond Engl)*. 2007;3:487–502.
Halbreich U. The association between pregnancy processes, preterm delivery, low birth weight, and postpartum depressions—the need for interdisciplinary integration. *Am J Obstet Gynecol*. 2005;193: 1312–1322.
Resnik R. The puerperium. In: *Maternal Fetal-Medicine, Principles and Practice*. Creasy RK, Resnik R, eds. Philadelphia, PA: W.B. Saunders; 2004.
U.S. Preventive Services Task Force. Primary care interventions to promote breastfeeding: U.S. Preventive Services Task Force recommendation statement. *Ann Intern Med*. 2008;149:560–564.
World Health Organization. Global Strategy for Infant and Young Child Feeding (2003). www.who.int/nutrition/publications/infantfeeding/en/index.html. Accessed May 2013.

Additional references are available online at http://langetextbooks.com/fm6e

---

101   Sexual Dysfunction

Elizabeth H. Naumburg, MD, & Elizabeth J. Brown, MD, MPH

KEY POINTS

- Most people experience trouble with sexual response at some time in their life; determining sexual dysfunction is a collaboration between the patient and the clinician. (SOR ⊜)
- A simple question like "How are things going for you sexually?" can help physicians to discover patients' sexual concerns. People are willing to talk with their physicians about their sexuality but hesitate to raise the subject themselves. (SOR ⊜)
- Sexual dysfunction (e.g., erectile dysfunction in men and arousal disorder in women) may be the presenting sign or symptom of other serious underlying disorders (e.g., diabetes, atherosclerosis, depression, alcohol, or drug abuse). Therefore, a thorough biopsychosocial diagnostic evaluation is a necessary part of comprehensive management. (SOR ⊜)
- Psycho-educational treatments are the mainstays of care for most causes of sexual dysfunction, and can be used alone or in conjunction with medical therapies. (SOR ⊕)

I. Introduction. Sexual dysfunction is defined as a disturbance in desire or in the sexual response cycle that causes distress. It is important to note that the definition depends on the perception that the situation is causing a concern or problem for the person and not based on some objective measures of what is defined as normative. There is a wide range of normal.
  A. The Diagnostic and Statistical Manual (DSM) V requires sexual dysfunction to be present for at least 6 months and further classifies sexual dysfunctions as lifelong versus acquired, generalized versus situational, and due to psychological factors versus due to combined factors.
    1. To understand the common sexual dysfunction diagnoses, it is useful to be aware of the **sexual response cycle.** Initially described by Masters and Johnson based on male physiology (excitement, plateau, orgasm, resolution) and then revised by

Kaplan to include psychological components (desire, arousal, orgasm), it was most recently revised by Basson specifically for women to place sexuality in the context of relationships. The traditional scheme for sexual dysfunction follows a four-stage model of sexual response (desire, arousal, orgasm, resolution), but current understanding incorporates the biopsychosocial nature of sexual dysfunction.

2. There are **gender differences** in sexual function. These differences come from anatomic, physiologic, psychological, and cultural factors. A new, intimacy-based female sexual response cycle starts with emotional intimacy that motivates the sexually neutral woman to be responsive to sexual stimuli, leading to sexual arousal and desire, which eventually leads to emotional and physical satisfaction.

    a. The epidemiology and treatments of disorders vary by gender. However, it is important to remember that intragender differences are far greater than intergender differences. The spectrum of normal human sexuality is so broad that the areas of overlap mean that many men and women will have very similar patterns.

B. Sexual dysfunction is essentially a **biopsychosocial condition** that typically has a multifactorial basis and comorbid diagnoses. A problem with one part of an individuals' sexual function can affect other parts, amplifying the problem.

II. Prevention and Screening

A. Physicians should include a brief query about sexual relationships during routine well visits. They may bridge their conversation from the medical history to the sexual history with a statement such as, "Your sexual functioning is just as important to me as the rest of your body's functioning, so as a part of a complete history, I always ask a few questions about how things are going sexually."

B. **General case-finding questions** include queries such as "How are things going for you sexually?," "What questions or concerns do you have about your sexuality at this time?," or "How satisfying is your sex life for you?" Questions like these give patients "permission" to discuss their sexuality with the physician if they wish.

III. Common Diagnoses (Table 101–1)

A. **Sexual desire disorders (SDDs)** include two diagnoses, Hypoactive Sexual Desire Disorder (HSDD) and Sexual Aversion Disorder. The second disorder, defined as an aversion or avoidance of all genital sexual contacts with a partner, is rare and most often due to a problem with another aspect of sexual function (e.g., dyspareunia) or a psychological problem. The new DSM V has distinguished between genders in classifying sexual disorders and has created a new category for women that groups sexual desire and arousal disorders together, **female sexual interest/arousal disorder,** recognizing the continuous nature of sexual desire and response. The following discusses each individual component.

    1. HSDD. Persistently or recurrently deficient (or absent) sexual fantasies and desire for sexual activity. The judgment of deficiency or absence is made by the clinician, taking into account factors that affect sexual functioning, such as age and the context of the person's life.

        a. Prevalence. Multiple studies indicate that this is the most common sexual disorder in women ranging in prevalence from 20% to 40% of the population depending on how the question is asked. The incidence is consistently lower in men but increases with age. The prevalence in men is difficult to determine but estimates range between 1% and 38%. The National Social Life, Health, and Aging Project reports lack of interest in 28% of men between the ages of 57 and 85 years, with 65% of them reporting it as "bothersome." While sexual desire also decreases

TABLE 101–1. COMMON DIAGNOSES

Stage of Cycle	Diagnosis in Women	Diagnosis in Men
Sexual Desire	Female sexual interest/arousal disorder	Hypoactive Sexual Desire Disorder Sexual Aversion Disorder
Sexual Arousal	Sexual Arousal Disorder Genitopelvic pain/penetration disorder (includes dyspareunia and vaginismus)	Erectile Dysfunction
Sexual Orgasm	Female Orgasmic Disorder	Male Orgasmic Disorder Premature Ejaculation

with age in women, the distress about it declines in parallel, keeping the incidence of this disorder relatively stable.

    b. Associated factors

        (1) In women, general well-being and the quality of the emotional relationship with her partner are the two strongest predictors of sexual health. Risk factors for sexual dysfunction include declining health, lower socioeconomic status, emotional distress, and history of a traumatic sexual experience. Women at any age will demonstrate an increased desire in response to new romantic relationships.

        (2) In men, the causes of HSDD are complex and include stress, biologic factors, and relationship stress. Differential diagnoses include depression, generalized anxiety disorder, and erectile dysfunction.

B. Sexual arousal disorders. The definitions of sexual arousal disorders diverge more in both men and women. In men, this category includes erectile dysfunction, which is the dominant sexual complaint in men. In women, the category of sexual arousal disorder is most often secondary to another problem such as trouble lubricating. The sexual pain disorders, dyspareunia and vaginismus, which can lead to trouble with arousal, also fall into this category.

    1. Male erectile disorder (ED) is persistent or recurrent inability to attain or maintain an adequate erection until sexual activity is completed. ED primarily affects men over the age of 40 years. In men aged 40 to 49 years, prevalence ranges from 2% to 9%, increasing to 20% to 40% in men aged 60 to 69 years and to 50% to 100% in men over age 70 years. ED has been linked to diabetes mellitus, hypertension, metabolic syndrome, hyperlipidemia, and depression. A recent meta-analysis found strong evidence that ED is associated with an increased risk of CVD, including coronary heart disease and stroke, and all-cause mortality. Smoking, obesity, and lack of physical activity are thought to be predictors of ED. ED can also be linked to medications and psychogenic factors.

    2. Female sexual arousal disorder (FSAD) is persistent or recurrent inability to attain or maintain until completion of the sexual activity, an adequate lubrication-swelling response of sexual excitement. For women to become aroused involves inclination, sexual stimulation, time, and attention or concentration. It is important to know that the physiologic manifestations of arousal—genital vasocongestion, vaginal lubrication, and perception of genital swelling—are not well correlated with the subjective sensation of arousal, which is strongly associated with emotions and cognition. Estimates of arousal disorders in women range from 14% to 39% depending on how the question is asked. Problems with lubrication increase with age and are common, but other arousal disorders are rarely isolated from problems with other parts of the sexual cycle.

    3. Genito-pelvic pain/penetration disorder is a new classification in the DSM V that merges the categories of dyspareunia and vaginismus, recognizing that these conditions are highly comorbid and difficult to distinguish. These disorders are often considered as part of the arousal stage of the sexual cycle.

        a. Dyspareunia refers to genital pain in either men or women associated with sexual intercourse (before, during, or after). In the National Health and Social Life Survey, 15% of women reported dyspareunia in the past 12 months and the incidence decreased with age ranging from 21% in the youngest group (18–29 years) to 8% in the oldest group (50–59 years) and 5% of men reported dyspareunia in the past 12 months.

            (1) Many medical conditions may cause dyspareunia in women. Sources include the external genitourinary and rectal sites to internal pelvic structures. Common examples include dermatitis, female circumcision, inadequate vaginal lubrication, vaginitis (either atrophic or infectious), pelvic or urinary tract infections, hymenal or vaginal scar tissue, endometriosis, pelvic pathology or masses, and allergic reactions. Localized or generalized vulvodynia may be the most frequent form of chronic dyspareunia in premenopausal women. It is a diagnosis of exclusion that is poorly understood.

            (2) Dyspareunia in men can be caused by structural abnormalities in the penis, Peyronie disease, priapism, urethral stricture, prior genital surgery, or genital infections.

        b. Vaginismus is recurrent or persistent involuntary contraction of the perineal muscles surrounding the outer third of the vagina that interferes with vaginal entry of a penis, a finger, and/or any object, despite the woman's expressed wish to do so. There is often (phobic) avoidance and anticipation/fear/experience of pain, along with variable involuntary pelvic muscle contraction. Structural or other physical abnormalities must be ruled out/addressed. This diagnosis sometimes presents in the office as the inability of the woman to tolerate a speculum examination. Patients with this disorder can have normal sexual desire, arousal, and orgasm.

While descriptions of vaginismus always refer to muscle spasm, this is not well documented and some authors make less of a differentiation from other forms of dyspareunia. Chronic dyspareunia is associated with psychogenic factors including a history of sexual trauma or coercion or negative developmental attitudes toward sexuality.

C. **Orgasmic disorders**
   1. **Female orgasmic disorder** is persistent or recurrent delay, or absence of orgasm following a normal sexual excitement phase. The incidence ranges from a low of 5% to a high in the 40th percentile depending on the specific question.
      a. Only about 25% of women achieve orgasm with stimulation of intercourse alone and 30% achieve it only sometimes or less often in a given sexual encounter. There are many myths about satisfying orgasms, which may contribute to sexual dysfunction including the need for simultaneity with one's partner and that a vaginal orgasm (one obtained with intercourse alone) is somehow different or superior to one that is accomplished with stimulation of the clitoris.
      b. **Etiologies** include a range of psychosocial issues such as negative developmental attitudes toward sex, a history of sexual coercion, spectatoring (consciously watching ones reactions instead of experiencing the sensations), inadequate foreplay, and clumsy partner technique. Chronic diseases including pain and depression can contribute, as can cultural and societal expectations. Difficulty achieving orgasm is a common side effect (up to 45% of patients) of selective serotonin receptor inhibitors (SSRIs) and can also be affected by other medications.
   2. **Male orgasmic disorder** is delayed or absent orgasm following normal sexual excitement. Recent studies indicate a prevalence of 4% to 10%. Many men with this disorder were raised in rigid, puritanical families that considered sex sinful and the genitalia "dirty." These men also experience problems with closeness in relationships. Orgasmic disorders are more common in men with obsessive-compulsive personality disorders and in those with unexpressed hostility toward women. In addition to these psychosocial factors, many of the organic disorders and drugs listed in Table 101–2 interfere with male orgasm and ejaculation.
   3. **Premature ejaculation (PE)** is ejaculation with minimal stimulation before it is wanted (i.e., before, on, or shortly after penetration). An intravaginal ejaculatory latency time (IELT) of 1 to 2 minutes is an accepted definition of premature ejaculation.
      a. It is difficult to determine the true prevalence of PE. Numbers range from 28% to 38% of men reporting concerns with climaxing too early at some point in time; however, lifelong premature ejaculation is thought to be rare at only 2% to 5%. The DSM V divides PE into four categories: lifelong premature ejaculation, acquired premature ejaculation, natural variable premature ejaculation, and premature-like ejaculatory dysfunction. Lifelong premature ejaculation is described as occurring throughout whole life with every partner. Acquired PE begins at some time following normal ejaculation and could be due to biologic reason such as prostatitis or psychosocial reason such as relationship issues. Natural variable PE describes inconsistent or irregular PE which is a normal variant. Premature-like ejaculatory dysfunction describes normal (3–6 minutes) ejaculation time, which the patient perceives as too short.
      b. **The etiology of PE** is thought to be multifactorial and includes organic and psychosocial factors. New evidence shows that PE and IELT are related to low serotonergic transmission, and leptin is being developed as a marker for PE. Other biologic causes include penile hypersensitivity, infection such as prostatitis, a hyper-excitable ejaculatory reflex, and possible endocrinopathy. Psychosocial factors include anxiety about the sex act, societal conditioning about men's sex roles, and stressful relationships.

TABLE 101–2. COMMON ORGANIC AND PSYCHOGENIC FACTORS ASSOCIATED WITH SEXUAL DYSFUNCTION

Chronic Illness
- Congenital illness or malformation
- Endocrine disease (e.g., diabetes mellitus; gonadal dysfunction; pituitary, adrenal, or thyroid disorders)
- Neurologic disorders (e.g., multiple sclerosis, spinal cord injury)
- Vaginal or pelvic pathology (e.g., vaginal atrophy, infections, endometriosis, childbirth injury)
- Genital trauma
- Cardiovascular and peripheral vascular disease
- Postsurgical complications (e.g., after prostatectomy, abdominal vascular surgery, sympathectomy, gynecologic procedures)

Pregnancy (especially in the first and last trimesters)

Psychogenic Factors (can be remote or immediate)[a]
- Personal problems (e.g., depression, anxiety, diminished self-esteem, and intrapsychic conflict)
- Relationship problems (e.g., poor communication, unrealistic marital expectations, unresolved conflict, lost trust, poor relationship models, family system distress, sex role conflicts, and divergent sexual values)
- Psychosexual factors (e.g., prior sexual failure, chronic performance inconsistency, negative learning and attitudes about sex, prior sexual trauma, sexual performance anxiety, gender identity conflict, and paraphilias)

Sexual Enactment Factors (skill and knowledge deficits)
- Examples include inadequate penile stimulation, inadequate clitoral stimulation for orgasm, clumsy or deficient foreplay for vaginal lubrication, unfavorable pelvic position for intercourse.

| | Primarily Affects | | | |
Drugs	Desire	Arousal	Orgasm	Hormones
Pharmacologic Agents				
• Anticholinergics		+		
• Antidepressants	+	+	+	
• Antihistamines	+	+		
• Antihypertensives	+	+	+	+
• Antipsychotics	+	+	+	+
• Anxiolytics	+		+	
• Narcotics	+	+	+	+
• Sedative–hypnotics	+	+	+	
Other Drugs				
• Cimetidine	+	+		+
• Clofibrate	+	+		
• Digitalis	+	+		
• Ethinyl estradiol	+	+		+
• Levodopa			+	
• Lithium	+	+		
• Ketoconazole	+	+		
• Niacin		+		
• Norethindrone	+	+		+
• Phenytoin		+	+	
• Primidone	+			
Drugs of Abuse				
• Alcohol	+	+	+	+
• Amphetamines	+	+	+	
• Cocaine		+	+	
• Heroin	+	+	+	
• Marijuana	+			
• MDMA	+	+	+	
• Methadone	+	+	+	
• Phencyclidine (PCP)	+		+	
• Tobacco		+		

[a]Remote factors have historical origins (e.g., negative sexual learning in childhood, dysthymic depression, prior relationship failures) and immediate factors occur during sexual activity (e.g., sexual anxiety, denial of erotic feelings, ineffective sexual behaviors, failure to communicate desires and feelings).
MDMA, S-methoxy-3,4-methylenedioxy amphetamine.

IV. Signs and Symptoms
A. Sexual desire disorders
1. **Hypoactive sexual desire disorder** can be difficult to define for women as women will frequently engage in sexual encounters without interest or desire for initiation. Other reasons that women will engage in sex include as an expression of love, partner's desire, and to relieve tension. The diagnosis depends on the presence of distress or interpersonal difficulties. As current understanding of normal sexual function includes that desire can follow arousal or emotional intimacy and does not need to occur spontaneously, clarifying all aspects of the sexual response cycle and finding out about the relationship and the patient's general well-being will be important. The diagnosis is based on the history as outlined earlier.
   a. **History.** In both men and women, symptoms should be sought for **evidence of problems with other stages of the sexual cycle** such as pain or an endocrine disorder. A complete history as described earlier including alcohol or substance abuse, medications, depression, the quality of the relationship, and untoward events in their sexual past. Many **medications** for psychiatric illness have sexual side effects. This diagnosis is based primarily on history. About 40% to 70% of patients taking SSRIs report problems with sexual function. Use of validated tools for diagnosing depression and anxiety such as the patient health questionnaire 2 (PHQ-2) and generalized anxiety disorders-2 (GAD-2) can be helpful.
   b. **Physical examination and laboratory testing** should be targeted on diagnosis of concern uncovered in the history. In women, there may be little need for physical examination or laboratory testing. In men, the possibility of hypogonadism should be considered. Laboratory testing may include general blood tests such as complete blood count, fasting glucose, kidney function, and thyroid level. In men, a free and total testosterone level measured first in the morning when levels are highest is also helpful in determining etiology. Not all men who have low testosterone levels will have low desire, and not all men with low desire will have low testosterone levels.
B. Arousal disorders
1. **ED.** A thorough sexual history is important to the diagnosis and should include a psychosocial history from the patient as well as his knowledge about sex, his sexual performance, and his partner's concerns (Table 101–3). Sometimes, patients who complain of problems with erections can be suffering from premature ejaculation. It is important to try to determine whether there is a psychogenic component. A history of rigid morning or night erections or normal sexual function in other settings such as masturbation is suggestive of a psychogenic cause. Other questions include onset and duration, drug and alcohol history, as well as past medical and surgical disorders. ED is a strong predictor of coronary artery disease (CAD), and new recommendations include considering all patients with ED, even if free of cardiac symptoms, to have a cardiac concern. Medical assessment for cardiovascular risk and silent CAD are important (Figure 101–1).
2. **FSAD** rarely occurs as an isolated disorder, but frequently accompanies a concurrent condition that preceded the arousal problem. If genital pain, anorgasmia, or a chronic organic illness exists, those problems should be addressed and treated before attending specifically to arousal as a separate entity. Treating comorbid conditions and underlying disease is the first step for managing FSAD.
3. **Sexual pain disorders.** Adequate evaluation of sexual pain disorders, both dyspareunia and vaginismus, includes a careful pelvic or genitourinary examination in addition to a detailed history. Ascertaining the precise location of the pain and the timing of pain within the sexual encounter, in addition to the questions outlined earlier, are necessary.
C. Orgasmic disorders
1. The diagnosis of **orgasmic disorders** in both men and women should be based on a careful history. As with other sexual diagnoses, overlap with other sexual dysfunctions, for example dyspareunia in women leading to anorgasmia, should be sought.
   Physical examination and laboratory testing should be targeted on diagnosis of concern uncovered in the history. For women, there may be little need for physical examination or laboratory testing.
2. The diagnosis of **premature ejaculation** depends on history. Specific questions regarding the timing of orgasm are essential. The diagnosis of PE is based on the IELT

TABLE 101–3. TAKING A SEXUAL HISTORY

It is often necessary to ask very specific questions when taking a sexual history, initiating the use of words that may be uncomfortable for the clinician as well as the patient. A respectful tone that frames the questions without assumptions will always be important. To adequately diagnose the problem here are the areas that should be covered:

Specific description of the sexual concern including:
- Duration—when did it start or has it always been present? Was the onset gradual or sudden and is it persistent or intermittent?
- Context—is the problem only specific to one partner, during masturbation or in all sexual settings?
- Effect on the patient's life or the level of distress caused by the symptom.
- Attempts at treatment and the outcome.
- Patient's expectations for this encounter.

Aspects of the patient's sexual response cycle. Specific questions that explore include:
- Desire—the experience of fantasy, initiation of sexual contact, self-pleasuring practices.
- Arousal—what physical manifestations does the patient experience such as lubrication for women and erection for men. Quality of the subjective experience.
- Orgasm—frequency, timing, satisfaction, arousal level during intercourse.
- Pain associated with any parts of the cycle and information about where, when.

Sexual practices—what and with whom?
- What sexual habits including: touching and other stimulation that precedes intercourse, oral or anal sex, use of sex toys or objects.
- Who are their sexual partners: specifically asking are they the same or opposite sex, are there multiple partners, even if a patient is married. What about past partners?

Quality of relationship with partner(s) and partner's response.
- Difficulties with communication or trust? Unresolved conflicts or anger? Time and space for intimacy? Is there communication about sexual desires and preferences? Has the patient discussed this issue with the partner and what was the outcome?

Psychosexual History
- General well-being. Current life demands or stressors. Symptoms of depression or other mental illness.
- Developmental beliefs, knowledge, and experiences. What were the messages that patient heard about sex when growing up? Where did they learn about sexuality? Is there a history of disappointing experiences? What were their early sexual encounters like?
- History of abuse, incest, or sexual assault?

General Medical History with attention to:
- Medications
- Recreational drugs and alcohol
- History of surgery or childbirth
- Medical problems, in particular neuromuscular, vascular, or endocrine disorders

being 1 to 2 minutes and the number of thrusts before orgasm being less than 15. The etiology of PE can vary depending on how long it has been occurring, if it is present with every partner, or what else is associated with the concerns. The main differential includes social anxiety disorder/panic attacks, depression, or prostatitis. As the diagnosis of PE is based on history, no laboratory evaluation is necessary unless there is concern of acquired PE and then a urinalysis is obtained to rule out prostatitis and a thyroid-stimulating hormone (TSH) to rule out thyroid problems (see below).

V. Diagnostic Evaluation
A. Questionnaires
    a. The International Index of Erectile Function (IIEF) is a 15-item inventory designed to assess erectile function, orgasmic function, sexual desire, intercourse satisfaction, and overall sexual satisfaction. It demonstrates test reliability, construct validity, and treatment responsiveness. A shortened 5-item version, the **IIEF-5,** is a useful screening instrument for ED, with a sensitivity of 98% and specificity of 88%. (http://www.hiv.va.gov/provider/manual-primary-care/urology-tool2.asp)

    b. While there are several questionnaires assessing sexual dysfunction for women, they are primarily used in research and have not had extensive validation.

B. A directed physical examination may help identify any concurrent acute or chronic illness and any associated physical conditions that could affect sexual functioning or treatment.

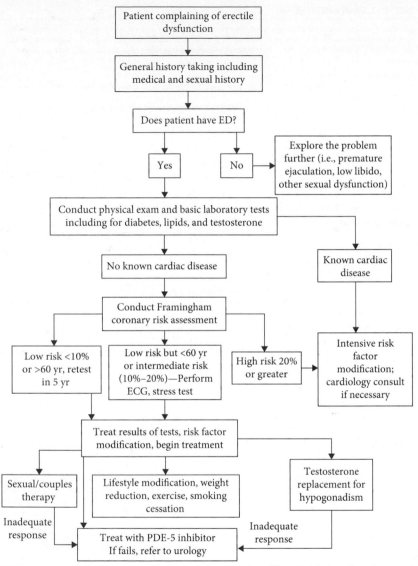

FIGURE 101–1. Approach to the patient with erectile dysfunction. Adapted from Shamloul R, Ghanem H. Erectile dysfunction. *Lancet.* 2013;381(9861):153–165.

1. **General.** Observe for obesity, cachexia, abnormal vital signs, secondary sex characteristics, gynecomastia in men, and galactorrhea in women.
2. **Cardiovascular examination.** Assess for bruits (especially femoral), absent peripheral pulses, evidence of venous stasis or arterial insufficiency (especially in the lower extremities), and a pulsatile epigastric mass.
3. Evaluate the **abdomen** for pain, tenderness, mass, guarding, tympany, and bowel activity.

4. Neurologic examination. Assess gait, coordination, deep tendon reflexes, pathologic reflexes, sensation, motor strength, integrity of the sacral reflex arc (S_2–S_4) with perineal sensation, anal sphincter tone, and bulbocavernosus reflex (clinically present in 70% of normal men).

5. Female pelvic examination

a. External genitalia and introitus. Inspect and palpate the external genitalia looking for dermatitis, inflammation, scars from episiotomy, circumcision or other trauma, clitoral inflammation, and adhesions, and tissue inelasticity or tenderness.

b. Touching the vestibule, vulva, hymen, and minor vestibular glands with a **moistened cotton swab** can help reproduce and localize pain associated with vulvodynia.

c. Vagina. Evaluate for spasm of the vaginal sphincter and adduction of the thighs with attempted vaginal examination, vaginal atrophy, discharge, inflammation, stenosis, relaxation of supporting ligaments, strength of pelvic muscles, and tenderness along the vaginal urethra or posterior bladder wall.

d. Bimanual examination. Assess the cul-de-sac for masses or tenderness; adnexa for masses or tenderness; and uterine position, size, mobility, and tenderness.

e. Rectal examinatiom is performed to identify hemorrhoids, fissures, and tenderness, and a stool specimen can be obtained for occult blood.

6. Male genitourinary examination. Observe the male genitalia for testicular size and consistency, penile size, malformations, and structural lesions. A normal flaccid adult penis is >6 cm in length and >3 cm in width.

C. Laboratory tests, imaging, and procedures

1. Women

a. Laboratory evaluation in women can include urine culture and cultures for sexually transmitted infection (see Chapter 102). Vaginal samples for vaginitis, including saline and potassium hydroxide wet mounts, and a urinalysis can be performed in the office as guided by the clinical evaluation. **Blood tests,** guided by the history and physical examination, can include a TSH, follicle-stimulating hormone, or others.

b. Pelvic ultrasonography can help diagnose adnexal, uterine, or cul-de-sac problems.

c. Laparoscopy can help diagnose, and in some cases treat, adnexal or intraperitoneal disease.

2. Men

a. Basic testing recommended in some diagnoses includes screening for diabetes, hypercholesterolemia, hypothyroidism and hypogonadism; for the latter, a morning **serum bioavailable testosterone** level is obtained. If the level is low, an evaluation for hypogonadism should occur.

b. Nocturnal penile tumescence (NPT) evaluation can be used to differentiate psychogenic from organic ED, although this test is rarely performed. Normally three or four erections occur each night during rapid eye movement sleep with a total night erection time of >90 minutes. Organic interference persists during sleep, disturbing erections. Psychogenic interference should not persist and erections will occur. Several techniques are used to evaluate and quantify NPT, including the snap gauge and the Rigiscan.

VI. Treatment and Management Strategies

A. Psycho-educational treatments are the mainstay of treatment.

1. PLISSIT. This is a psycho-educational framework that grows immediately out of a complete history and can be applied as the initial approach to any sexual dysfunction. The education can begin even as the full picture is being obtained (Table 101–4).

2. Systematic desensitization is an approach that focuses on teaching a woman greater conscious control over her pelvic floor muscles by using relaxation techniques and the gradual introduction of an object (lubricated finger, the patient's or the examiner's, dilators) into the vagina. While systematic desensitization is often recommended as the first step to treatment, there is little evidence that it is effective. (SOR ❸)

a. Perhaps key to this process is the assurance that the woman is in complete control of the process. This very gradual approach can take weeks of practice and/or multiple sessions to demonstrate painless vaginal insertion. Using a mirror throughout the examination so that the physician can teach vulvar and vaginal anatomy and the patient can visualize her own muscle contractions can support the experience

TABLE 101–4. THE PLISSIT MODEL AND EXAMPLES IN CLINICAL PRACTICE

PLISSIT (Permission, LImited information, Specific Suggestions, Intensive Therapy)

Example 1. In the diagnosis of **Hypo Sexual Desire Disorder,** given the huge range of normal and the significant role psychosocial factors play, an initial discussion might include the following:

Listening to the concerns; giving **permission** by encouraging the patient to discuss his/her concerns with his/her partner (sometimes just breaking the ice will engage a new level of emotional intimacy); providing **limited information** by educating the patient about normal expectations and placing the concern in the context of the patient's life, stage of relationship, and other factors. Teaching the patient about the importance of relationship to the level of sexual desire is important as the concept of responsive sexual desire in women as part of sexual function will be new for most people but is helpful in redefining normal sexual behavior; **specific suggestions** can include encouraging a couple to make time for their relationship (e.g., date nights) and finding time for themselves as a couple.

Example 2. In women with anorgasmia, once other disorders (e.g., chronic pain, depression, medication side effects) have been ruled out or addressed, the initial treatment is focused on areas of the history that seem most likely:

Listening to the concerns and asking about the patient's relationship to his/her sexuality, self-stimulation, current sexual activities and the other phases of the sexual cycle, and about the interpersonal relationship (e.g., knowledge and beliefs about sex and any history of coercive or abusive experiences); giving **permission** to be sexual and feel aroused and encouraging the patient to discuss his/her concerns with his/her partner, communicating any specific sexual likes, dislikes or desires; providing **limited information** about sexuality, specifically the role of clitoral stimulation and fantasy and reminding the patient that to experience orgasm requires a degree of release from worry and that they need to feel safe. Also explaining that a minority of women have orgasm with intercourse only and that clitoral stimulation is normal; **specific suggestions** such as encouraging the woman to explore her own body in a comfortable context (see self-directed stimulation in text).

of learning to relax her muscles. This process is the opposite of the Kegel exercises, when the contraction is held, and focuses on the relaxation phase.

   b. The approach to desensitization can focus only on the pelvic examination or incorporate other aspects of sexual responsiveness depending on the needs of the patient. A referral to a physical therapist who specializes in women's health and specifically the pelvic floor may be useful.

3. **Directed self-stimulation.** This is the most effective treatment program to date for **primary orgasmic dysfunction in women.** (SOR **B**) Beginning with basic education in sexual anatomy and physiology, women progress through the stages of tactile and visual self-exploration, manual stimulation to areas of pleasurable sensation, sexual fantasy and image development, sensate focus exercises alone and then with a partner, and finally sharing effective stimulation techniques with a partner. Self-help manuals such as "Becoming Orgasmic: A Sexual and Personal Growth Program for Women" by Heiman and LoPiccolo or "For Yourself" by Lonnie Barbach can be very helpful. There is some literature that supports teaching adolescent women about orgasm and encouraging masturbation as preventive treatment for primary female orgasmic disorder.

4. **Sensate focus.** The original behavioral tasks developed by Masters and Johnson are termed "sensate focus" exercises, since they heighten sensory awareness to touch, sight, sound, and smell. As patients focus on their own sensations, they often relax and overcome barriers that impede natural physiologic responses. Partners first learn to enjoy touching, stroking, exploring, massaging, and fondling all the contours of each other's bodies except for their genitals. When both partners are adept and comfortable exchanging nongenital caresses, they add genital stroking exercises. Specific direction to refrain from intercourse until both partners feel fully ready, which may take many experiences, should be included. Couples learn to use fantasies to distract them from obsessive performance concerns and to communicate mutual needs verbally and nonverbally. (SOR **C**)

5. **The stop–start, or squeeze technique,** was the standard therapy for **PE** before pharmacologic agents became available. It is now used most frequently in combination with pharmacologic agents for men who do not respond optimally to the drugs alone.

   a. Technique. The stop–start technique of Semans and the squeeze technique modification of Masters and Johnson are used to treat **PE**. (SOR **B**) The technique begins as the couple embraces and caresses one another until the man's penis is erect. He then lies on his back, his partner begins stimulating his penis, and he concentrates on his arousal sensations. Just before he reaches the point of imminent ejaculation, he tells his partner to stop stimulation. At this point, Masters and Johnson direct the partner to squeeze the penis firmly between thumb and forefinger, under the corona of the glans. Most current therapists now suggest that the man apply the squeeze himself. When the partner applies the squeeze, it paradoxically suggests that control over erections is the partner's rather than the man's. With or without the squeeze, the couple waits for several minutes until arousal sensations dissipate. This process of stimulation and stopping repeats several times before the man ejaculates.

After four or five successful stimulation–stopping sessions, the couple tries the stop–start process with the penis in the vagina. The woman assumes the woman-superior position and the man glides her slowly up and down the shaft of his penis. As he again almost reaches the point of ejaculation, he ceases moving his partner until the need subsides. This process is also repeated several times before he ejaculates.

When the man can control ejaculation with this level of stimulation, his partner begins to stimulate his penis with vaginal thrusting until the man begins to feel the need to ejaculate. At this point, he tells her to stop stimulation until arousal wanes. This sequence is also repeated several times before he ejaculates.

The couple completes a start–stop sequence at least weekly until they learn to use it automatically during intercourse. Eventually, they use the method with other sexual positions. Most men, however, experience the greatest difficulty controlling ejaculation in the man-superior position.

  b. Although Masters and Johnson report 95% success rates with the start–stop–squeeze technique, others report success rates around 60%. Long-term success, however, is disappointing and recent studies have failed to replicate the success rates that Masters and Johnson report.

6. **Referral for treatment with an experienced sex therapist.** Patients or couples not responding to initial treatment, those who request additional help, or patients with primary arousal disorder should be referred to a sexual therapist or specialist.

  a. Cognitive-behavioral therapy that incorporates behavioral therapy into other treatments is the psychosexual treatment of choice for managing most sexual dysfunctions. Behavior therapists assume that sexual dysfunction is learned maladaptive behavior that causes patients to fear sexual interaction. During treatment, the therapist establishes a hierarchy of anxiety-provoking situations for the patient and then helps him or her master the anxiety through systematic desensitization. This process inhibits the learned anxious response by encouraging antianxiety behaviors.

  b. Traditional couples therapy can also be important, since relationship problems that generate stress, fatigue, and dysphoria commonly underlie sexual dysfunctions. Therapy helps the couple develop communication skills, establish realistic relationship expectations, resolve conflict, and build trust.

B. **Medications for women**
 1. **Testosterone.** For women who have surgically induced menopause and are on estrogen replacement therapy, transdermal testosterone 300 mcg per day can be prescribed. (SOR **B**) It is not FDA approved because of lack of demonstrated long-term safety.

  a. The use of testosterone to treat HSDD in women was initially studied in women who were surgically postmenopausal and already on hormone therapy. For these women, there is a significant postsurgical drop in testosterone. For women undergoing natural menopause, however, there is no clear testosterone decrease although testosterone levels do progressively decline in many women as they age due to a decrease in the adrenal contribution. The epidemiologic literature demonstrates a lack of a correlation between women's testosterone levels and sexual desire.

  b. Studies of testosterone use in premenopausal and naturally postmenopausal women not on estrogen suggest small but statistically significant improvements in measures of sexual function (frequency of satisfying sexual episodes and instruments that measure sexual satisfaction). These studies are limited by short duration and the known benefit that testosterone has on general well-being. The potential benefit of testosterone treatment for women must be weighed against the androgenic side effects (e.g., hair growth, acne) and the potential but still poorly defined risk for more serious consequences (e.g., breast cancer and cardiovascular risks). This is an evolving literature and should also be understood in the context of a pharmaceutical industry that is eager for a female equivalent to the success of the phosphodiesterase-5 inhibitors.

C. Medications for men

  1. Hypogonadism. Testosterone is used in hypogonadal men, as described for HSDD (see later). In men older than 65 years who have low testosterone and have not responded to one of the phosphodiesterase (PDE)-5 inhibitors listed below, testosterone can be taken as an adjunct.

  2. PDE-5 inhibitors

    a. Sildenafil is an orally active inhibitor of the type-V cyclic guanosine monophosphate-specific PDE-5, the predominant isoenzyme in the human corpus cavernosum. It increases levels of nitrous oxide, which relaxes the endothelial muscles, increasing blood flow into the corpora cavernosa. It effectively treats **ED** of organic, psychogenic, and mixed etiology. (SOR **A**) Sildenafil enhances the erectile mechanism with sexual stimulation and does not work without stimulation. Efficacy is greater than 65%.

      (1) Dosing. A man takes a single oral dose starting at 50 mg approximately 1 hour before intercourse. Sildenafil's activity begins in 30 minutes and lasts up to 8 hours.

      (2) The most common **adverse effects** are headache (16%), flushing (10%), and dyspepsia (7%). Drug levels are increased by other drugs that are metabolized by or that inhibit the cytochrome P450 system. Sildenafil also potentiates the hypotensive effects of nitrates and is **absolutely contraindicated** in patients using organic nitrates in any form. Be careful in patients who are on alpha-blockers for blood pressure control.

    b. Vardenafil and **tadalafil** are newer PDE-5 inhibitors that are similar to sildenafil in pharmacologic action and effectiveness (about 65%), but have some unique properties.

      (1) Vardenafil is well tolerated, with pharmacologic and adverse event profiles similar to sildenafil. It is **not recommended for patients taking type 1 or 3 antiarrhythmic drugs** or those who have congenital prolonged QT syndrome. It is administered in a dose of 10 to 20 mg taken 1 hour before intercourse.

      (2) In comparison with the other PDE-5 inhibitors, **tadalafil** has a slower onset of action, but its half-life is prolonged, resulting in a medication effect that lasts as long as 36 hours after administration. Its major unique adverse event is a 6% to 9% incidence of back pain that is usually mild and self-limited. Dosage is 10 to 20 mg taken 1 to 24 hours prior to intercourse.

  3. Intracavernosal injections. Patients can inject **papaverine, PGE$_1$,** or various mixtures into a corpus cavernosum with a 27-gauge needle to induce an erection. This technique is quite successful in men with neurogenic disorders, mild vascular problems, or combined neurogenic and vascular disorders and in selected men with psychogenic causes for whom psycho-sexual treatment has failed. (SOR **A**)

    a. Therapy begins with a low dose of either papaverine or PGE$_1$, gradually titrating the dose to provide an adequate erection that lasts 1 to 2 hours. This usually requires 10 to 80 mg of papaverine or 10 to 40 μg of PGE$_1$. Injections are limited to three times per week and 10 times per month.

    b. Complications include priapism (0.33%), cavernous tissue fibrosis (2.8%), hematoma, cavernositis, pain, and changes in blood pressure (usually orthostatic hypotension). Erections that last more than 4 hours should be reversed by irrigating the corpora cavernosum with diluted phenylephrine.

  4. Intraurethral PGE$_1$ therapy requires a man to insert a PGE$_1$-medicated pellet into his urethra with an applicator following urination. When absorbed through the mucosa, the PGE$_1$ relaxes smooth muscles and dilates arteries. Following insertion, the man must manually stimulate the penis for 10 seconds and then walk around for another 10 minutes to promote erection. The maximal response occurs in 20 to 25 minutes. (SOR **A**) Pellets are available in 125, 250, 500, and 1000 μg dosage strengths. Adverse effects include penile pain (32%), urethral burning (12%), minor urethral bleeding (5%), testicular pain (5%), hypotension (3%), and dizziness (2%).

D. Treatment for specific disorders

1. HSDD. As noted earlier, the mainstay of treatment for HSDD includes treatment of associated or contributing diagnoses, the PLISSIT model, and if needed, cognitive behavioral therapy from a sex therapist. Medication changes may be necessary if a patient is on a drug that typically causes sexual dysfunction such as SSRIs. Testosterone supplementation is rarely used and hypogonadism is infrequent. There have been no trials that support the use of testosterone supplementation in a man with low desire and normal testosterone.

a. There is no specific definition for low testosterone, but general consensus is if total testosterone is <300 ng/dL or free testosterone is <65 pg/mL, supplementation may be of benefit. (SOR **C**) Ways to supplement testosterone include intramuscular testosterone enanthate or cypionate (100–200 mg every 2–4 weeks). (SOR **C**) Transdermal systems are also effective methods for replacing testosterone (Androderm, 2.5–7.5 mg per day or Androgel, 50–100 mg per day). (SOR **A**) Oral agents are less effective and may cause hepatic disorders (e.g., cholestatic jaundice). Potential hazards of testosterone therapy include increased prostate-specific antigen levels and increased prostatic volume. These may increase the risk for prostatic cancer, and men should be screened for cancer at regular intervals of 3 to 6 months for 12 months and then annually. Testosterone is contraindicated in individuals with prostate/breast cancer, untreated sleep apnea, and untreated heart failure. (SOR **C**)

2. ED. After conducting a comprehensive history, physical examination, and evaluation of cardiac risk, considering the most probable etiology of the problem (organic, psychogenic, or a mixture) can help determine treatment. PDE-5 inhibitors and psychoeducation through the PLISSIT model, however, can be useful in all types of ED. Drugs that can be used for patients with ED are listed in Table 101–5.

a. For organic or mixed diagnosis, lifestyle changes should be encouraged including reduced alcohol intake, weight loss if indicated, improved diet, increased exercise, and smoking cessation. After encouraging lifestyle changes, a trial with one of the PDE-5 inhibitors should be attempted. Encourage the patient to try the medication at least four times before calling it a treatment failure. Men respond differently to medication, so a trial of several PDE-5 inhibitors is reasonable.

b. For psychogenic ED, sex therapy with sensate focus is important, but medication can also be tried.

c. If oral therapies fail, referral to an urologist for a range of more advanced treatments is suggested including surgical implants. Penile injections and intraurethral prostaglandins described earlier may best be prescribed by a specialist.

3. PE. The mainstay of medical management for PE are the selective SSRIs (Table 101–6). While they are not FDA approved for this indication, clomipramine, sertraline, fluoxetine, paroxetine, and citalopram are all used. They can be taken on demand or daily, and at a variety of doses. A short-acting SSRI, dapoxetine, showed promising results in studies, but also is not FDA approved for this indication. Topical treatments are also available, and a new aerosol-delivery spray of lidocaine-prilocaine has been shown to improve ejaculatory time.

a. Clomipramine at doses of 25 to 50 mg, taken 12 to 24 hours prior to intercourse, effectively prolonged intravaginal intercourse to at least 2 minutes in 70% of men with **PE** in one study. In another study, clomipramine prolonged ejaculatory latency from 2 to 8 minutes. The minimum time between drug ingestion and the maximum ejaculatory control is not yet known. The shortest studied interval was 4 to 6 hours. (SOR **B**)

b. Paroxetine increased ejaculatory latency when administered following several different protocols: as 20 mg 3 to 4 hours prior to intercourse as needed, as 10 mg once-daily chronic administration, and as 10 mg once daily with an additional 20 mg taken as needed 3 to 4 hours prior to intercourse. All methods increased ejaculatory latency, with the 10 mg per day plus 20 mg as needed protocol showing the greatest improvement. (SOR **B**) **Adding 50 mg of sildenafil to paroxetine** further prolonged ejaculatory latency and the quality of overall sexual activity increased to 87.5% in one study. (SOR **B**)

TABLE 101–5. DRUG TREATMENT OPTIONS FOR PATIENTS WITH ERECTILE DYSFUNCTION

Drug	Dose	Major Side Effects	Contraindications	Drug Interactions
Sildenafil (Viagra) 25, 50, and 100 mg tabs	Start with 50 mg Onset 30 min to 1 h Lasts 4–8 h	Headache, flushing, dyspepsia, insomnia, visual disturbances, priapism, decreased hearing (sudden onset)	Use of nitrate medications,[a] recent serious cardiovascular events (stroke, MI, arrhythmia), CAD with unstable angina	Nitrates,[a] alpha-blockers (hypotension) azole antifungals, HIV protease inhibitors (increased sildenafil adverse effects)
Vardenafil (Levitra) 2.5, 5, 10, and 20 mg	Start with 10 mg Onset 30 min Lasts 4–8 h	Headache, flushing, rhinitis, chest pain/MI prolonged QT, priapism, decreased hearing (sudden onset)	See sildenafil	Nitrates,[a] alpha-blockers (hypotension) quinolone antibiotics, thioridazine, trazodone, fluconazole, cisapride, salmeterol (QT prolongation)
Tadalafil (Cialis) 2.5, 5, 10, and 20 mg	Start with 10 mg Onset 45 min to 2 h Lasts up to 36 h	Flushing, backache, myalgias, headache, dyspepsia, Chest pain/MI priapism, decreased hearing (sudden onset)	See sildenafil	Nitrates,[a] alpha-blockers (hypotension); azole antifungals, macrolide antibiotics, HIV protease inhibitors (increased sildenafil adverse effects); simvastatin (myopathy)
Testosterone	Only use for men with concurrent hypogonadism or used with PDE-5 inhibitors in men older than 65 yr with low testosterone	Increased prostate volume, increased PSA, risk for prostate cancer increased, edema, acne, cholestatic jaundice	Prostate cancer, breast cancer	Warfarin (bleeding); bupropion (seizures)

[a]Whenever prescribing PGE_5 inhibitors, a specific conversation warning about the concomitant use with nitrate medications is mandatory. This should include the hypothetical emergency department evaluation for chest pain and the need to report the medication use.

CAD, coronary artery disease; HIV, human immunodeficiency virus; MI, myocardial infarction; PSA, prostate-specific antigen.

    c. Sertraline delays ejaculation through its serotonergic effects. The usual dose is 50 to 100 mg taken 3 to 5 hours prior to sexual activity.

    d. Fluoxetine is also used to treat PE at doses of 20 to 60 mg.

    e. Dapoxetine is a short-acting SSRI that had promising results in initial trials. In published trials, 30 to 60 mg was taken 1 to 3 hours prior to intercourse and men reported a threefold to fourfold increase in ejaculatory latency time. Although the initial application was not approved by the FDA, the manufacturer intends to continue to working toward approval.

    f. Citalopram can also be used to treat PE. Dosing is 20 to 40 mg daily.

    g. Tramadol is a centrally acting synthetic opioid agonist that has been shown to improve PE through an unknown mechanism. It does have addictive potential.

    h. Nonselective alpha-1 receptor blockers such as **terazosin, phenoxybenzamine,** and **alfuzosin** and the **PDE-5 inhibitors** such as **sildenafil, vardenafil,** and **tadalafil** have all been shown to be helpful in treating PE.

    i. TEMPE, a lidocaine–prilocaine aerosol spray, is a new addition for on-demand topical treatments. It has excellent tissue penetration and the mucosa of the penis is anesthetized rather than the skin. No condom is needed. It is used on demand and in studies improved IELT to 3.8 minutes.

    j. lidocaine–prilocaine cream (EMLA®) can be used in PE; however it is messy, the penis needs to be covered in a condom after the cream is applied, and the entire penis is anesthetized.

TABLE 101–6. DRUG TREATMENT OPTIONS FOR PREMATURE EJACULATION

Drug	Dosing Daily/On-Demand Dose Before Sex	Major Side Effects	Contraindications	Drug Interactions
Clomipramine	25–50 mg daily/25 mg 4–24 h prior to intercourse	Constipation, dyspepsia, weight gain, dizziness, headache, myalgia, fatigue, somnolence, sweating, dry mouth, orthostatic hypotension	Teens, comorbid bipolar disorder, coadministration or within 14 d of use of a MAOI, recent MI	**Multiple Interactions** Quinolone antibiotics, thioridazine, trifluoperazine, chloroquine (QT prolongation); metoclopramide (extrapyramidal reactions); sertraline (serotonin S)
Paroxetine	10–40 mg/20 mg 3–4 h prior to intercourse	Somnolence, dizziness, headache insomnia, tremor, sweating, nausea, diarrhea, constipation	Teens, comorbid bipolar disorder, coadministration or within 14 d of use of a MAOI	**Multiple Interactions** Thioridazine (QT prolongation); metoclopramide (extrapyramidal reactions); tamoxifen (reduced tamoxifen benefit); triptans, dextromethorphan, trazodone (serotonin S); warfarin, ASA, NSAIDs, apixaban (bleeding); tramadol (seizures)
Fluoxetine	5–40 mg/none	Somnolence, dizziness, anxiety, insomnia, nausea, diarrhea, rhinitis	See paroxetine	**Multiple Interactions** Thioridazine, TCAs, Class 1A antiarrhythmics, cyclobenzaprine (QT prolongation); metoclopramide (extrapyramidal reactions); clarithromycin (delirium, psychosis); tramadol (seizures); triptans, trazodone, dextromethorphan (serotonin S); warfarin, ASA, NSAIDs, apixaban (bleeding)
Sertraline	25–200 mg/50 mg 4–8 h prior to intercourse	Nausea, diarrhea, constipation, headache, dizziness, insomnia, tremor, fatigue, somnolence,	See paroxetine; coadministration with disulfiram	**Multiple Interactions** Triptans, TCAs, erythromycin, trazodone, oxycodone, dextromethorphan (serotonin S); tramadol (seizures); warfarin, ASA, NSAIDs, apixaban (bleeding)
Citalopram	20–40 mg daily none	See paroxetine, agitation	See paroxetine	**Multiple Interactions** Amiodarone, azole antifungals, cimetidine, chlorpromazine, clarithromycin, dextromethorphan fluoroquinolones, omeprazole, trazodone, salmeterol (QT prolongation); metoclopramide (extrapyramidal reactions); triptans (serotonin S); warfarin, ASA, NSAIDs, apixaban (bleeding)

(continued)

TABLE 101–6. DRUG TREATMENT OPTIONS FOR PREMATURE EJACULATION (*Continued*)

Drug	Dosing Daily/ On-Demand Dose Before Sex	Major Side Effects	Contraindications	Drug Interactions
Tramadol	/25–50 mg 1–8 h before intercourse	Somnolence, dizziness, headache, insomnia, flushing, pruritus, nausea, vomiting constipation	Severe bronchial asthma, hyper-capnia	**Multiple Interactions** Carbamazepine, TCAs, SSRIs, thioridazine, metoclopramide (seizures, serotonin S); trazodone (serotonin S); warfarin (bleeding); digoxin (digoxin toxicity)
PDE-5 inhibitors (i.e, sildenafil)	/50 mg 1 h prior to intercourse	Headache, flushing, dyspepsia, insomnia, visual disturbances, priapism, decreased hearing (sudden onset)	Use of nitrate medications,[a] recent serious cardiovascular events (stroke, MI, arrhythmia), CAD with unstable angina)	Nitrates,[a] alpha-blockers (hypotension), azole antifungals, HIV protease inhibitors (increased sildenafil adverse effects)
TEMPE-prilocaine/ lidocaine aerosol spray	On demand	Skin irritation	None	Unlikely

[a]Whenever prescribing PGE$_5$ inhibitors, a specific conversation warning about the concomitant use with nitrate medications is mandatory. This should include the hypothetical emergency department evaluation for chest pain and the need to report the medication use.

ASA, acetylsalicylic acid; CAD, coronary artery disease; MAOI, monoamine oxidase inhibitor; MI, myocardial infarction; NSAID, nonsteroidal anti-inflammatory drug; S, syndrome; SSRI, selective serotonin reuptake inhibitor; TCA, tricyclic antidepressant.

E. Treatment of antidepressant-associated sexual dysfunction. Antidepressants commonly cause sexual dysfunction, with 40% to 70% of patients taking SSRIs reporting problems with sexual functioning. One must effectively manage these treatment-emergent dysfunctions so that patients will maintain therapeutic antidepressant treatment. Taking a wait-and-see approach is not recommended, given the risks and the options for alternatives. Asking about sexual side effects specifically when monitoring treatment with SSRIs and seratonin norepinephrine reuptake inhibitor (SNRIs) is the first step. This should be followed by assessing how troublesome the side effect is compared to the benefits of the medication and whether a change in medication or an additional medication is warranted.

   1. Strategies to consider include decreasing the dose of the offending agent, decreasing the dose of the offending agent and adding another agent such as bupropion, or switching medication class altogether such as using a tricyclic or bupropion. Some providers recommend a drug holiday for several days surrounding expected sexual activity with some evidence supporting this practice. However, the risks of withdrawal symptoms and worsening depressive symptoms are present.

   2. Bupropion can be added at a dose of 75 to 150 mg as needed 1 to 2 hours prior to sexual activity, given daily in conjunction with an SSRI or as an initial daily full-dose add-on to relieve sexual dysfunction, followed by a taper and discontinuation of the initial SSRI. (SOR **Ⓑ**)

   3. Evidence shows that sildenafil statistically improves ejaculation and orgasm in men with **ED** who are also taking SSRIs. (SOR **Ⓑ**) Furthermore, depressed men with ED respond to sildenafil as well as any other subgroup of men. (SOR **Ⓑ**) Study doses ranged from 25 to 200 mg taken 1 hour prior to anticipated sexual activity. Using sildenafil allows men to continue therapeutic doses of an effective antidepressant.

VII. Prognosis

A. SDDs. The few published studies indicate that **SDDs** for both men and women resist sustained behavioral change. (SOR **Ⓑ**) Following therapy, authors of one study noted initial improvement that was sustained at 3 months, but that had regressed to below pretherapy levels by 3 years. Prognosis is better if the problem is secondary, the partners are younger, the symptoms are present <1 year, the relationship is stable, the partners are emotionally calm and motivated toward intervention, both partners view each other as loving and attractive, both partners find pleasure in sexual behavior, neither partner has a conflict regarding sexual orientation or major psychopathology, and the couple complies with homework assignments during therapy.

B. ED. The natural history and prognosis of ED depend on many variables, most particularly the underlying problem. Most data on **psychosexual treatment** success were obtained before recent diagnostic advances permitted better differentiation between organic and psychogenic causes. Reported success rates range from 50% to 90%. (SOR **Ⓒ**) Oral agents vary in success. From 70% to 85% of men using **sildenafil** and the other PDE-5 inhibitors achieve erections firm enough for intercourse. (SOR **Ⓐ**) Men with diabetes, and some of those with neurologic dysfunction, spinal cord injuries, prostatic surgery, and pelvic irradiation, report lower response rates, between 35% and 67%. (SOR **Ⓐ**) Success with **intracavernosal injections** varies from 60% to 92%, but only 50% to 80% of men who start on self-injections continue to use them long term. (SOR **Ⓐ**) Reported success rates with **intraurethral PGE₁** are approximately 40%. (SOR **Ⓐ**) Treatment success for **surgical implants** is 85% to 95% in achieving effective erections, with long-term patient satisfaction rates approaching 80% and partner satisfaction rates between 60% and 80%. (SOR **Ⓐ**)

C. Female orgasmic disorder. The natural history of untreated female orgasmic disorder is unknown. Women with primary orgasmic disorder respond rapidly to treatment with a high success rate when therapy focuses specifically on sexual matters. Women with secondary orgasmic disorders do better when traditional couples therapy is combined with sexual therapy. Masters and Johnson report success rates of 83% for primary disorders and 77% for secondary disorders using **dual-gender therapy.** (SOR **Ⓒ**) **Directed self-stimulation** training to treat primary disorders is successful in helping women reach orgasm 90% of the time during self-stimulation and 75% of the time with a partner. (SOR **Ⓒ**)

D. Dyspareunia. Prognosis depends on the nature of any associated organic problems and the success with which they are treated. Women with a pure psychogenic basis for their problem report treatment success rates of around 95%. (SOR **Ⓒ**)

E. Vaginismus is very amenable to treatment. In one group of women who were followed up for 4 years, 95% achieved and maintained sexual functioning. (SOR **Ⓒ**) A desire for childbearing, a husband-initiated consultation, and a couple's perception that the problem was psychogenic predicted successful outcomes. Unsuccessful outcomes were associated with a firm belief that the problem was organic, experience with a previous anatomic problem, abundant sexual misinformation, a negative attitude toward genitalia, fear of sexually transmitted infection, and negative parental attitudes toward sex.

F. Male orgasmic disorder. Outcome studies on treatment for this condition are limited by its relative rarity. Reported success rates range from 46% to 82%. (SOR **C**)

G. Premature ejaculation. While Masters and Johnson reported more than 95% success rate with **start–stop–squeeze technique,** most current studies show about 60% success rate with therapy. With pharmacologic management with SSRIs, men report improved sexual satisfaction (42%–87%) along with a statistically significant increase in ejaculation latency time. (SOR **B**) Other topical treatments such as **TEMPE** have also shown improvement in IELT and are well tolerated. For men with true lifelong PE, the prognosis is poor if it is never treated.

SELECTED REFERENCES

Lamont J. Female sexual health consensus guidelines. *J Obstet Gynaecol Can.* 2012;34(8):769–775.

Melnik T, Althof S, Atallah AN, et al. Psychosocial interventions for premature ejaculation. *Cochrane Database Syst Rev.* 2011;(8):CD008195.

Rosen RC, Riley A, Wagner G, et al. The International Index of Erectile Function (IIEF): a multidimensional scale for assessment of erectile dysfunction. *Urology.* 1997;49:822–830.

Shamloul R, Ghanem H. Erectile dysfunction. *Lancet.* 2013;381:153–165.

Woodis CB, McLendon AN, Muzyk AJ. Testosterone supplementation for hypoactive sexual desire disorder in women. *Pharmacotherapy.* 2012;32(1):38–53.

---

102 Sexually Transmitted Infections

Jessica Dalby, MD, & Jaime Marks, MD

KEY POINTS

- Sexually active women, aged 24 years and younger, should be screened yearly for chlamydia. (SOR **A**)
- Optimal testing for chlamydia and gonorrhea involves nucleic acid amplification tests of vaginal swabs in women and first-catch (start of stream) urine specimens in men. (SOR **C**)
- All adults born between 1945 and 1965 should be offered hepatitis C screening at least once, regardless of identifiable risk factors. (SOR **A**)
- Wet mount has a low sensitivity for trichomonas. If suspicion is high and wet mount is negative, a culture or more sensitive molecular diagnostic test should be obtained when available. (SOR **C**)
- First outbreaks of genital herpes are now more commonly due to HSV-1 than HSV-2. For HSV-1 genital outbreaks, prognosis is better than HSV-2, as recurrent genital outbreaks are less common and daily suppressive therapy is not needed. (SOR **C**)

I. Definition. The term sexually transmitted infections (STIs) encompasses a broad category of diseases transmitted by close interpersonal contact and caused by numerous types of pathogens: viruses, bacteria, protozoa, and parasites. There are nearly 20 million new cases of STIs in the United States each year, half of which occur in young people (aged 15–24 years). The Centers for Disease Control and Prevention (CDC) estimates that there are 110 million STIs nationwide, including both new and chronic infections.

Obtaining a thorough sexual history in a respectful, nonjudgmental way is important for identifying risk factors and providing appropriate screening and education. Guidance on sexual history taking is available through curriculum provided by the CDC STD/HIV Prevention Training Centers (http://www.cdc.gov/std/treatment/SexualHistory.pdf).

II. Common Diagnoses

A. *Chlamydia trachomatis* is the most common STI in the United States with over 1.3 million cases reported in 2010. Chlamydia rates appear to be increasing, but this may be partially due to increased screening in men with urine-based testing. Most cases of chlamydia are reported in sexually active women aged 15 to 24 years, with a prevalence rate of about 7%.

   1. Women are 2.5 times more likely to be diagnosed with chlamydia than men, but this may be due to the higher incidence of screening among women. The difference in rates would indicate that partners are not given the diagnosis of chlamydia.

   2. Rates vary somewhat by location. The highest incidence is found in Washington, DC, and Alaska, with about 9% of the total population being affected.

   3. There is also a difference in rates by ethnic group. African-Americans are roughly eight times and Hispanics and Native Americans are four times more likely to be diagnosed with chlamydia than are Asians and Caucasians.

B. Gonorrhea caused by *Neisseria gonorrhoeae* is the second most commonly reported STI in the United States with over 300,000 cases reported in 2010. The rates of gonorrhea dramatically decreased after implementation of the National Gonorrhea Control Program in the 1970s. However, there is emerging antibiotic resistance that may be contributing to the recent slight increase in cases.

   1. Most cases of gonorrhea are reported in sexually active women aged 15 to 19 years and men aged 20 to 24 years. Rates in women are slightly higher than those in men. African-Americans are six times more likely to be diagnosed with gonorrhea than all other ethnic groups.

C. Genital herpes is a chronic, life-long disease caused by infection with either herpes simplex virus (HSV)-1 or HSV-2. HSV-2 causes the majority of recurrent genital lesions (>90%). However, HSV-1, responsible primarily for recurrent orolabial lesions, now accounts for the majority of first genital outbreaks (50%–60%), but is much less likely to recur than HSV-2. An estimated 24 million people in the United States are infected with HSV-2, making genital herpes second only to human papilloma virus (HPV) in prevalence of infection. There were an estimated 776,000 new cases reported in 2008. Most transmission occurs during viral shedding by asymptomatic partners or those with mild, unrecognized symptoms.

D. HPV is a double-stranded DNA virus that infects human epithelial cells. Low-risk HPV types (including 6, 11, 42, 43, and 44) usually present as verrucous lesions or external genital warts. High-risk types (including 16, 18, 31, 35, 51, and 52) have oncogenic potential in cervical, vulvar, urethral, penile, anal, and oropharyngeal epithelial cells by deactivating tumor suppressors.

   1. Worldwide, HPV subtypes 16 and 18 cause about 70% of all cervical cancers. However, not all women infected with HPV will develop cervical cancer or other cervical lesions. Many infections resolve spontaneously. Cigarette smokers, immunosuppressed patients, and uncircumcised men are at a higher risk for HPV-related cancers.

   2. Most new infections occur in both men and women between the ages of 15 and 24 years, after the onset of sexual activity. An estimated 79 million people are infected with a strain of HPV in the United States. About 80% of sexually active women have had HPV by age 50 years. Despite these high rates, the incidence of strains 6, 11, 16, and 18 is actually on the decline due to use of the HPV vaccine.

E. Syphilis is an STI caused by *Treponema pallidum*. Syphilis is further defined by progression through a series of overlapping stages: primary infection with painless genital ulceration or chancre, secondary infection with skin rash and lymphadenopathy, and tertiary infection involving the cardiovascular system or gummas. Neurologic involvement can occur at any stage. Latent syphilis can also occur where a patient has a positive serologic test without clinical symptoms of disease. There were an estimated 55,000 new cases of syphilis diagnosed in 2008 (see Chapter 30).

F. Hepatitis. Both hepatitis B and C can be transmitted sexually, although this is less common with hepatitis C (see Chapter 72).

G. Human immunodeficiency virus (HIV) is a single-stranded RNA retrovirus that infects the human immune system. There are approximately 50,000 new cases of HIV in the United States every year, with 40,000 cases in men and 10,000 cases in women. Of these cases, 63% occur in men who have sex with men (MSM), 25% in heterosexuals, and 8% injectable drug users.

1. African-Americans are disproportionately affected, comprising 44% of new infections in 2010, despite accounting for only 12% of the population. HIV infection, if untreated, progresses to a severe immunodeficiency state known as AIDS over a variable time course, with median time for progression of 11 years. AIDS, if untreated, is almost universally fatal due to opportunistic infections. There are an estimated 1,100,000 people living with HIV in the United States and approximately 15,500 AIDS-related deaths occur per year, as of 2010. About 636,000 people have died of AIDS in the United States since the epidemic began.

H. **Trichomoniasis** is caused by the protozoan *Trichomonas vaginalis* (see Chapter 63). Trichomoniasis may cause malodorous vaginal discharge and vulvar irritation in women and urethritis in men or be detected in asymptomatic patients during screening. It has been shown to increase the risk of obstetrical complications, including premature rupture of membranes, preterm labor, and low birth weight. Trichomoniasis also increases the risk of acquiring HIV when exposed to the virus.

1. Treatment in women coinfected with *Trichomonas* and HIV reduces HIV shedding, potentially decreasing the risk of transmission. There were an estimated 1,090,000 new infections in 2008, placing trichomoniasis third after HPV and chlamydia for the highest incidence of STI.

I. **Pediculosis pubis.** Pubic lice or "crabs" is an ectoparasitic infection caused by *Pthirus pubis* that is spread through sexual contact, although any close personal contact can result in transmission. This includes shared clothing, linens, and towels used by an infected person.

J. *Mycoplasma genitalium* **and** *Ureaplasma.* These bacteria, generally thought to be less aggressive pathogens or potentially part of normal flora, have emerged as potential pathogens in cases of urethritis and vaginitis or cervicitis, where testing proves negative for gonorrhea and chlamydia. *Mycoplasma genitalium* can also cause upper genital tract disease in females. There are no currently standardized commercial tests available for these infections; thus, data on incidence are limited at this time. Some institutions may have access to nucleic acid amplification tests.

K. **Chancroid** (see Chapter 30). A clinical picture of painful genital ulceration and tender suppurative inguinal adenopathy can be caused by *Haemophilus ducreyi*. Prevalence in the United States as well as worldwide is declining, with most infections occurring in parts of Africa and the Caribbean. Definitive diagnosis can be difficult due to low sensitivity of testing. However, a clinical diagnosis can be made in the presence of typical painful genital ulceration(s) with negative herpes and syphilis testing of ulcer exudate. If dark-field examination is not possible, syphilis serology testing should be done at least 7 days after the appearance of ulcers to exclude syphilis as an alternative diagnosis.

III. **Screening and Prevention**

A. **Screening. United States Preventive Services Task Force (USPSTF) recommendations** are shown in Table 102–1. Optimal screening intervals are unknown. The CDC recommends that patients at increased risk be screened at least annually.

1. **Assessing increased risk** should include consideration of sexual behaviors (i.e., multiple partners, new partners, inconsistent condom use, sex under the influence of alcohol or drugs, transactional sex) and community demographics, such as prevalence of syphilis and gonorrhea in the local population.

a. As per CDC recommendations, MSM are a higher-risk group and should be screened at least yearly for chlamydia, gonorrhea, syphilis, and HIV. Patients with multiple or anonymous partners should be screened more frequently (every 3–6 months).

b. Also per the CDC, HIV-positive women should be screened annually for *Trichomonas* due to increased viral shedding and risk of transmission with coinfection.

c. **Hepatitis B virus screening** should be considered prior to vaccination for patients at increased risk, including close contacts with HBsAg-positive patients, injectable drug users, and MSM.

d. **Hepatitis C virus (HCV) screening** is recommended in high-risk patients by the CDC, including pregnant women at risk. The main risk factor in HCV acquisition is injectable drug use. Additionally, HCV screening is indicated for any HIV-positive patient. The USPSTF recently recommended that all adults born between 1945 and 1965 should be offered HCV screening at least once, regardless of identifiable risk factors. (SOR **Ⓐ**)

TABLE 102–1. USPSTF SCREENING RECOMMENDATIONS FOR ASYMPTOMATIC PATIENTS[a]

Disease	<25-yr Olds	Low Risk	High Risk	Pregnancy
Chlamydia	A (women)	C	A (women)	B (high risk or <25)[b]
	I (men)		I (men)	C (low risk)
Gonorrhea	B (women)	D	B (women)	B (high risk)
	I (men)		I (men)	I (low risk)
HPV	D (<30 yo)	A (30–65 yo)[c]	A (30–65 yo)[c]	A (30–65 yo)[c]
Syphilis	Based on non–age-related risk or pregnancy	D	A	A
HIV	A	A	A	A
Herpes	D	D	D	D
Hepatitis B	D	D	D	A
Hepatitis C	Based on non–age-related risk	B[d]	B	[e]

[a]The USPSTF grades the strength of the evidence as "A" (strongly recommends), "B" (recommends), "C" (no recommendation for or against), "D" (recommends against), or "I" (insufficient evidence to recommend for or against).
[b]Screen high-risk pregnant patients at the first prenatal visit and repeat screening in the third trimester.
[c]HPV testing is indicated as an adjunct to cervical cancer screening cytology in order to lengthen screening interval to every 5 years in women aged 30 to 65 years, regardless of sexual risk or pregnancy status.
[d]Screen all adults born from 1945 to 1965 at least once.
[e]No USPSTF recommendation available.

B. Prevention

1. **Education and counseling.** High-intensity behavioral counseling has been shown to be effective for reducing STI in sexually active adolescents and high-risk adults. (SOR **A**) Successful high-intensity interventions in supporting studies were delivered through multiple sessions, most often in groups, with total durations from 3 to 9 hours. Clinicians should partner with or be aware of community programs that provide high-intensity counseling. Little evidence suggests that single-session interventions or interventions lasting less than 30 minutes are effective in reducing STIs.

   a. Abstinence, mutual monogamy with an uninfected partner, and reduction in the number of sex partners may be an appropriate part of a personalized discussion on patient risk reduction or prevention.

2. **Condoms.** Consistent and correct use of condoms has been shown to reduce the risk of many STIs (see Chapter 97). (SOR **A**) Counseling on correct use should reinforce: using a new condom with each sex act, placing a condom on the erect penis prior to any contact with a partner, using only water-based lubrication if using latex condoms, and holding the condom firmly against the base of the still-erect penis during withdrawal to avoid slipping off.

3. **Vaccination**

   a. **HPV.** Vaccination is recommended routinely for boys and girls starting at age 11 or 12 years (see Chapter 105). The vaccine is most effective in preventing HPV infection that can lead to genital warts or cancer when given prior to the onset of sexual activity. The CDC recommends that previously unvaccinated women through age 26 years and men through age 21 years (age 26 years for MSM) receive the HPV vaccine.

   b. **Hepatitis.** The CDC recommends that any patient presenting for STI screening or treatment should be vaccinated against hepatitis B if not previously done. Additionally, hepatitis A vaccine should be offered to injectable drug users, MSM, and those with chronic liver disease. As a national goal to eliminate hepatitis B transmission, the CDC strategy includes: (1) routine screening of all pregnant women and immunoprophylaxis for infants born to HBsAg-positive mothers, (2) routine infant vaccination, (3) routine childhood vaccination through age 18 years, and (4) vaccination of adults at increased risk.

4. **Male circumcision** has been shown to reduce the risk of HIV infection, along with high-risk HPV and herpes infection, in heterosexual men. These studies were done in sub-Saharan Africa where the HIV epidemic predominantly involves heterosexual transmission. There is little evidence that male circumcision prevents HIV for the female partner or in MSM.

5. Postexposure prophylaxis (PEP). For survivors of sexual assault, compliance with follow-up visits may be suboptimal. The CDC recommends the following PEP measures: (1) Hepatitis B vaccination if not previously vaccinated, (2) empiric treatment for chlamydia, gonorrhea, and trichomonas, and (3) emergency contraception if the assault could result in pregnancy. The benefits of antiretrovirals for HIV prevention in sexual assault victims have been extrapolated from the benefits of healthcare workers with percutaneous exposure to HIV-infected blood. Though the benefits are unproven in assault victims, consideration of risk factors may prompt initiation of antiretrovirals as soon as possible or within 72 hours of the assault.

6. Pre-exposure prophylaxis (PrEP) for high-risk groups. Several studies have shown the safety and efficacy of daily prophylactic use of the antiretroviral combination tenofovir disoproxil fumarate (TDF) and emtricitabine (FTC) for preventing HIV infection in noninfected, high-risk individuals when combined with comprehensive prevention and screening programs. Potential candidates for PrEP include high-risk MSM, heterosexuals with an HIV-infected partner, and injectable drug users. Further guidance on use is available through the CDC.

IV. Symptoms and Signs

A. Asymptomatic. Many STIs can be asymptomatic, which makes prevention and screening essential.

B. Ulcerations (see Chapter 30) can be painful or painless. Depending on the location, dysuria may be the presenting symptom. Ulcerations can also be pruritic instead of painful and misdiagnosed as candidiasis. STIs that can present as ulcerations include the following:

1. HSV is the most common cause of infectious genital ulcers. Patients typically have multiple, painful vesicles that easily rupture and ulcerate. There may be surrounding erythema. The presentation of primary herpes infections vary from asymptomatic to localized lymphadenopathy and fever.

2. Chandroid presents as a single, painful ulcer along with localized, suppurative lymphadenopathy. It is important in these cases to rule out syphilis and HSV.

3. Primary syphilis will present with a single, painless ulcer known as a chancre. Primary syphilis may be missed as the chancre can go unnoticed by the patient. The chancre appears within 3 weeks of infection and lasts for several weeks. Locations include the genitals or mucosal surfaces such as the vagina, mouth, and rectum.

4. Chlamydia trachomatis serovars L1-3 (*lymphogranuloma venereum* [LGV]) cause a single, painless ulcer 3 to 12 days after infection which often goes unnoticed. This progresses to painful inguinal lymphadenopathy.

5. Granuloma inguinale is caused by *Klebsiella granulomatis* and initially presents as small, painless nodules that quickly ulcerate and progress to destroy genital tissue. Lymphadenopathy is usually absent. This condition is rare in the United States.

6. Neoplasms, trauma, Behcet disease, drug reactions, and primary HIV or cytomegalovirus (CMV) infection should also be considered in persons presenting with genital ulcerations.

C. Papules. HPV can cause verrucous papules (genital warts) on the genitals and rectal area. Molluscum, pearly penile papules, infectious causes of ulcerations, and neoplasms should also be considered.

D. Vaginal discharge (see Chapter 63). Normal vaginal discharge is usually clear to white, thick or thin, and odorless. Distinguishing normal from pathologic discharge can be challenging. In general, a change in the volume, color, or odor, or discharge associated with bleeding, burning, dyspareunia, dysuria, irritation or pruritus warrants further evaluation.

1. Pelvic examination is usually part of the evaluation of abnormal vaginal discharge to check for cervical motion tenderness suggestive of pelvic inflammatory disease (PID).

2. STIs that can present as vaginal discharge are chlamydia, gonorrhea, and trichomonas (see Chapter 63).

3. Women with dysuria should also be questioned about vaginal discharge as STIs can mimic urinary tract infections (UTIs). If UTI symptoms persist after adequate treatment, testing for chlamydia and gonorrhea should be considered.

4. Non-STI causes of vaginal discharge such as bacterial vaginosis, candidiasis, foreign body, and physiologic discharge should also be considered in women.

E. Cervicitis and PID. Chlamydia and gonorrhea are STIs that can cause inflammation of the cervix and uterus. These organisms can ascend and cause endometritis or PID. Symptoms include vaginal discharge, intermenstrual or postcoital bleeding, dysuria, dyspareunia, and vulvovaginal irritation.

1. **On examination,** purulent or mucopurulent discharge from the cervix is diagnostic of cervicitis. Cervical motion tenderness in the presence of pelvic or abdominal pain, and/or fever >101°F is consistent with a diagnosis of PID.
    2. **Long-term sequelae of PID** include chronic pelvic pain, infertility, and an increased risk of ectopic pregnancy.
F. **Urethritis in men.** Inflammation of the urethra can cause discharge, dysuria, and penile irritation. Men with STI-induced urethritis have mucopurulent discharge. A positive leukocyte esterase or 10 WBCs per high-powered field are present on microscopy of a first-void urine. If these signs are present, treatment should be initiated. Infectious causes of urethritis include chlamydia, gonorrhea, trichomonas, and *Mycoplasma genitalium*. An organism may not be identified.
G. **Epididymitis** presents as gradual onset of testicular pain and swelling (usually unilateral), urinary urgency and frequency (see Chapter 55). The patient may or may not present with symptoms or urethritis as well. Any male accessory gland may be infected including the epididymis, seminal vesicles, ductus deferens, and prostate. The presentation and treatment are similar for all.
H. **Proctitis** (see Chapter 51). Receptive anal intercourse can cause inflammation of the lining of the rectum that presents as rectal bleeding or blood in the stool, anorectal pain, tenesmus, or discharge. STIs that cause proctitis include chlamydia, gonorrhea, trichomonas, syphilis, *Mycoplasma genitalium*, and LGV. Often an organism cannot be identified. Other diagnoses to consider include autoimmune disorders, HSV ulcerations, genital warts, anal fissures, trauma, radiation treatment, and chemical irritation.
V. **Laboratory Tests.** Recommended tests are displayed in **Table 102–2**.
A. **Repeat testing** should be offered at 3 months following STI treatment due to the high rate of reinfection. A "test of cure" is typically not recommended for asymptomatic patients, except in the case of pregnant women who have a higher risk of neonatal complications with ongoing STI and in penicillin allergic patients being treated for gonorrhea with azithromycin instead of a preferred cephalosporin regimen.
B. **Self-collected vaginal swabs.** Evidence supports allowing women to collect their own vaginal swabs for nucleic acid amplification testing (NAAT) of trichomonas, chlamydia, and gonorrhea as an alternative, less-invasive strategy for screening or diagnosis.
VI. **Treatment** recommendations from the CDC are shown in Table 102–3 (http://www.cdc.gov/std/treatment/2010/). Most treatment can be given in an outpatient setting.
A. **Dual therapy.** For cases of chlamydia, consider treatment for gonorrhea if local prevalence is >5%. For cases of gonorrhea, dual therapy (treatment to cover chlamydia) is required. For recurrent urethritis, consider treatment for trichomonas, especially in areas of high prevalence.
B. **For recurrent genital herpes and recommended regimens for those with HIV,** refer to the CDC treatment guidelines available at http://www.cdc.gov/std/treatment/2010/STD-Treatment-2010-RR5912.pdf.
C. **Indications for treatment of PID as an inpatient** include pregnancy, severe illness (high fever, nausea, vomiting, severe abdominal pain), nonadherence to therapy or inability to take oral medications due to nausea and vomiting, complicated PID with pelvic or tubo-ovarian abscess, possible need for surgical intervention, or diagnostic exploration for alternative etiology such as appendicitis, lack of response or tolerance to oral medications, and no response after 72 hours of oral treatment.
D. **Public health reporting.** State and local requirements for STI reporting vary. All states currently require reporting of syphilis, gonorrhea, chlamydia, chancroid, HIV infection, and AIDS. Because the requirements for reporting other STIs differ by state, clinicians should contact their local public health department and become familiar with local requirements.
E. **Expedited partner therapy (EPT).** Data support patient-delivered partner therapy for heterosexual couples with chlamydia, gonorrhea, and possibly trichomoniasis. In this setting, the partner, who is deemed unlikely to seek testing or treatment themselves, is offered treatment without medical evaluation or counseling. Prescriptions should be accompanied by an informational hand-out reviewing treatment instructions, medication warnings, and advice to seek medical evaluation. EPT may be prohibited in some states, so providers should be aware of laws in their areas, which can be found at http://www.cdc.gov/std/ept/

TABLE 102–2. LABORATORY TESTING FOR SEXUALLY TRANSMITTED INFECTIONS

Disease	Test	Sensitivity (%)	Specificity (%)	Additional Comments
Chlamydia	NAAT	80–91	94–100	Considered first-line
	Nucleic acid hybridization, EIA, DFA	62–75	97–99	No longer recommended due to lower sensitivity than NAAT
	Culture	75	100	Sensitivity is lower on urine compared to endocervical and vaginal swabs
Gonorrhea	NAAT	78–100	94–100	
	Gram stain with GNID	>95	>99	Urethral swab with Gram stain is preferred in men to confirm urethritis (>5 WBCs per high-powered field) and look for gonococcal infection. Not recommended in women or other anatomic sites
	Culture	75	100	Should be performed in cases of treatment failure for antimicrobial sensitivity testing
Trichomonas	Wet mount	44–68	100	Allows for antimicrobial susceptibility testing in resistant cases, unlike NAAT and POC tests
	Culture	44–75	100	
	POC testing: OSOM, Affirm VP III	64–98	99–100	Limited to vaginal specimens in symptomatic women
	NAAT (APTIMA TV only FDA approved test)	76–100	96–100	Vaginal swab with increased sensitivity compared to end ocervical or urine testing. Superior option for testing in men, supported by the CDC though not FDA approved, as wet prep not sensitive and rapid tests not available in men
Herpes	Cell culture	80–90	99	Virologic test for active lesion if NAAT not available, yield is best with first outbreak and early in progression of ulceration
	NAAT	98–100	80–97	Preferred virologic test for active lesion, typically PCR
Serologic tests:	Point-of-care	>91	>94	Differentiating between HSV-1 and HSV-2 is important for patient counseling. More costly than ELISA
	ELISA	94–100	94–98	Some cross-reactivity between types may lead to incorrect typing
	Western blot	99	100	Primarily a research tool. Use for confirmation in select cases
HIV	EIA	>99	>99	Initial screening test for HIV antibodies. Rapid testing available (30 min). Newer generation tests may also detect Ag or IgM in early infection
	Western blot	97–100	96–100	Used to confirm positive EIA. Not useful prior to 5 wk following infection
	RNA assay (direct virus detection)	100	97	Should be used if suspicion for acute infection before Ab formed

Disease	Test	Sensitivity (%)	Specificity (%)	Comments
Syphilis	Non-treponemal: VDRL, RPR	71–100	98	Titers are used to guide patient management decisions in syphilis treatment. Sensitivity varies by syphilis stage, with lower percentages for primary and late latent stages
	Treponemal: FTA-ABS, TP-PA, EIA	76–100	97–99	Should be used to confirm non-treponemal tests. Can remain positive for prolonged period after successful treatment
	Dark-field examination	80	100	Identifies spirochetes in primary lesions
Chancroid	Culture	75	100	
HPV	Cervical cytology	69	92	Sensitivity and specificity relate to detection of CIN2 or greater. Recommended starting at age 21 yr
	Serotype testing	92–97	86–92	Do not use for screening before age 30 yr. Both DNA and RNA based typing exist
Hepatitis C	Anti-HCV IgG (Antibody detection)	86–99	>99	Cannot detect whether infection is active. Used for initial screening, rapid tests have been developed and FDA approved
	HCV RNA (NAT)	>96	>99	Detects active infection. Also used for confirmation of HCV infection when antibody tests are positive (has largely replaced RIBA)
Hepatitis B	Antigen test: HBsAg	79	>99	Present in both acute and chronic infection, may be negative in occult infection
	Antibody testing: Anti-HBs			Present after resolved infection or after vaccination
	Anti-HBc (IgM and total)	>98	>99	Can help differentiate between acute and chronic infection, often positive in occult infection but may be negative early in infection (during "window" period). Used to screen blood donations
	NAAT	>99	>99	Increasingly being used for screening blood donations. Can detect infection during "window" period

NAAT, nucleic acid amplification testing; NAT, nucleic acid test; EIA, enzyme immunoassay; DFA, direct fluorescent antibody test; GNID, gram-negative intracellular diplococcus; POC, point-of-care; PCR, polymerase chain reaction; TMA, transcription-mediated amplification; RIBA, recombinant immunoblot antibody assay.

TABLE 102–3. TREATMENT OF SEXUALLY TRANSMITTED INFECTIONS

Disease	First-Line Treatment	Pregnancy	Alternatives
Chlamydia[a] (Cervicitis, urehritis)	Azithromycin 1 g orally in a single dose OR Doxycycline 100 mg orally twice daily for 7 d	Azithromycin 1 g orally in a single dose OR Amoxicillin 500 mg orally three times daily for 7 d AND test of cure in 4–6 wk	Erythromycin base 500 mg orally four times daily for 7 d OR Erythromycin ethylsuccinate 800 mg orally four times daily for 7 d
Gonorrhea[b] Cervicitis, urehritis, rectal	Ceftriaxone 250 mg IM in a single dose	See first-line and alternative treatments AND test of cure in 4–6 wk	Cefixime 400 mg orally in a single dose AND Azithromycin 1 g orally in a single dose OR Doxycycline 100 mg twice daily for 7 d AND test of cure
Pharyngeal	Ceftriaxone 250 mg IM single dose PLUS Azithromycin 1 g orally in a single dose OR Doxycycline 100 mg orally twice daily for 7 d	See first-line treatments	Alternative regiments not recommended.
Conjunctival	Ceftriaxone 1 g IM single dose		
Children ≤45 kg	Ceftriaxone 25–50 mg/kg IV or IM in a single dose, not to exceed 125 mg		
Trichomonas[c]	Metronidazole 2 g orally in a single dose OR Tinidazole 2 g orally in a single dose	Metronidazole 2 g orally in a single dose	Metronidazole 500 mg orally twice daily for 7 d
Epididymitis	Ceftriaxone 250 mg IM in a single dose AND Doxycycline 100 mg orally twice daily for 10 d	NA	If negative GC culture or NAAT or acute epididymitis most likely due to enteric organisms: Levofloxacin 500 mg once daily for 10 days OR Ofloxacin 300 mg orally twice daily for 10 d
Pelvic Inflammatory Disease (outpatient)	Ceftriaxone 250 mg IM in a single dose AND Doxycycline 100 mg orally twice daily for 14 d AND CONSIDER Metronidazole 500 mg twice daily for 14 d	Hospitalize for parenteral therapy	Cefoxitin 2 mg IM single dose AND Probenecid 1 g orally once AND Doxycycline 100 mg orally twice daily for 14 d AND CONSIDER Metronidazole 500 mg twice daily for 14 d
Pelvic Inflammatory Disease (inpatient) Continue IV therapy for 24 h after the patient begins to improve clinically. Can discharge with oral regiment to complete 14-d course	Doxycycline 100 mg orally or IV twice daily AND Cefoxitin 2 g IV four times daily OR Cefotetan 2 g IV twice daily OR Clindamycin 900 mg IV three times daily AND Gentamicin 2 mg/kg loading does then 1.5 mg/kg IV three times daily	Doxycycline should not be used in pregnancy	Ampicillin-sulbactam 3 g IV four times daily AND Doxycycline 100 mg orally or IV twice daily
lymphogranuloma venerum	Doxycycline 100 mg orally twice daily for 21 d	See alternative therapies	Erythromycin base 500 mg orally four times daily for 21 d

Genital Herpes	For first clinical episode, one of the following for 7–10 d:[d] Acyclovir 400 mg orally three times daily OR Acyclovir 200 mg orally five times daily OR Famcyclovir 250 mg orally three times daily OR Valacyclovir 1 g orally twice daily	Consider prophylaxis after 36 wk until delivery. At delivery, close inspection of genitalia and birth canal for active lesions. If present, C-section indicated	Prophylactic options for recurrent genital herpes and pregnancy: Acyclovir 400 mg orally twice daily OR Famcyclovir 250 mg orally twice daily OR Valacyclovir 500 mg to 1 g orally once daily
Genital Warts — Patient Applied	Podofilox 0.5% solution or gel twice daily for 3 days then rest 4 days, for 4 cycles max OR Imiquimod 5% cream wash off after 6–10 h, every other day, up to 16 wk OR Sinecatechin 15% ointment applied three times daily, up to 16 wk	Cryotherapy, laser removal, acetic acid For small/asymptomatic lesions, consider delay of treatment until postpartum	Intralesional interferon OR Laser/surgical removal
Clinician Applied	Cryotherapy OR Podophyllin resin 10%–25%, wash off after 1–4 h, repeat weekly OR Trichloroacetic acid 80%–90%, wash off after 1–4 h, repeat weekly		
Syphilis — Primary, Secondary, Early Latent	Penicillin G 2.4 million units IM in a single dose	See first-line treatments. If diagnosed after 20 wk, US to evaluate for fetal infection	Doxycycline 100 mg orally twice daily for 14 d OR Tetracycline 500 mg orally four times daily for 14 days
Latent >1 year or duration unknown	Penicillin G 2.4 million units IM weekly × 3 weeks	Follow-up testing for child at 6, 12, and 24 mo	Doxycycline 100 mg orally twice daily for 28 d OR Tetracycline 500 mg orally four times daily for 28 d
Neurosyphilis	Penicillin G 4 million units IV every 4 h × 10–14 d		Procaine penicillin G 2.4 million units IM once daily AND Probenecid 500 mg orally four times daily, BOTH for 10–14 d
Pediculosis Pubis	Permethrin 1% cream rinse OR Pyrethrins with piperonyl butoxide apply to affected area and rinse off after 10 minutes	See first-line treatment	Malathion 0.5% lotion applied 8–12 h then washed off OR Ivermectin 250 µg/kg orally then repeated in 2 wk
Scabies	Permethrin 5% apply to neck down and wash off after 8–14 h OR Ivermectin 200 µg/kg orally then repeated in 2 wk	Permethrin 5% apply to neck down and wash off after 8–14 h	Lindane 1%, 1 oz of lotion or 30 g of cream applied thinly to neck down and wash off after 8 h

[a] Consider treatment for gonorrhea if local prevalence is >5%.

[b] Dual therapy (treatment to cover chlamydia) required.

[c] For recurrent urethritis consider treatment for trichomonas, especially in areas of high prevalence.

[d] For recurrent genital herpes and recommended regimens for those with HIV, please refer to the CDC treatment guidelines available at http://www.cdc.gov/std/treatment/2010/STD-Treatment-2010-RR5912.pdf.

Source: Adapted from the 2010 CDC Treatment Guidelines, http://www.cdc.gov/std/treatment/2010/STD-Treatment-2010-RR5912.pdf. Accessed September 2013.

VII. Patient Education. Counseling should include information about the nature of the disease including symptoms, expected course with and without treatment, transmission, and risk reduction. For treatable infections, patients should be advised to avoid sexual intercourse until "cured." As a "test-of-cure" is not routinely indicated, this is defined as resolved or lacking symptoms following completion of treatment for both the patient and their partner, typically 7 days.

SELECTED REFERENCES

Brill JR. Sexually transmitted infections in men. *Prim Care.* 2010;37(3):509–525.

Centers for Disease Control and Prevention. Sexually Transmitted Diseases Treatment Guidelines, 2010. *MMWR Recomm Rep.* 2010;59(RR-12):1–109. www.cdc.gov. Accessed September 2013.

Satterwhite CL, Torrone E, Meites E, et al. Sexually transmitted infections among U.S. women and men: prevalence and incidence estimates, 2008. *Sex Transm Dis.* 2013;40(3):187–193.

U.S. Preventive Services Task Force. Behavioral Counseling to Prevent Sexually Transmitted Infections: U.S. Preventive Services Task Force Recommendation Statement. AHRQ Publication 08-05123-EF-2, October 2008. http://www.uspreventiveservicestaskforce.org/uspstf08/sti/stirs.htm. Accessed August 2013.

Van Wagoner NJ, Hook EW III. Herpes diagnostic tests and their use. *Curr Infect Dis Rep.* 2012; 14(2):175–184.

Additional references are available online at http://langetextbooks.com/fm6e

SECTION V. Preventive Medicine and Health Promotion

103   Chemoprophylaxis

A. Ildiko Martonffy, MD, & Paul E. Lewis III, MD, MPH

KEY POINTS

- Age of household contacts and extent of exposure are the factors that determine need for meningitis prophylaxis.
- Aspirin has proven efficacy for secondary prevention of myocardial infarction and ischemic stroke and should be considered for primary prevention of MI in men aged 45 to 79 years and stroke in women aged 55 to 79 years when benefits outweigh risks.
- Prophylaxis for endocarditis prior to dental procedures is indicated in only a small subset of patients.
- All women of childbearing age capable of becoming pregnant should consume folic acid daily in order to reduce their risk of having a child with a neural tube defect.
- Patients who have had rheumatic fever need long-term prophylaxis against group A streptococcus.
- All pregnant women should be screened for Group B streptococcal disease and those with a positive test need intrapartum prophylaxis.

I. **Definition.** Prophylaxis is derived from the Greek word *pro phulax*, which means "to put up a guard before it is necessary." Chemoprophylaxis is the use of a chemical or medication to prevent a disease. Chemoprophylaxis is widely utilized in modern medicine from preventing infectious diseases to treating chronic disease states.

II. **Bacterial Meningitis**

   A. **Pathogens**

      1. *Haemophilus influenzae*

         a. The mortality rate of meningitis due to *H. influenzae* is approximately 5%; 20% to 30% of survivors have neurologic sequelae.

         b. The risk of infection in a 1996 national study was 6% in children younger than 1 year, 2.1% in those younger than 4 years, and 0% in those older than 5 years.

         c. In the United States, the incidence is greatest in Native Americans, blacks, those in lower socioeconomic groups, and those with complement or immunoglobulin deficiencies.

         d. The near universal administration of the *H. influenzae* type b vaccine has significantly reduced the incidence of this disease since 1987 and made the need for prophylaxis relatively rare.

      2. *Neisseria meningitidis*

         a. The mortality rate of meningitis due to *N. meningitidis* is approximately 10%; the incidence is highest in children younger than 1 year of age.

         b. Vaccines against serotypes a and c have been developed, but slightly more than 50% of meningococcal infections in the United States are caused by type b, for which there is no vaccine.

         c. Meningococci are carried by 15% of contacts in their throats, but only 3% to 4% will carry a pathogenic strain. Eradication of this pharyngeal carriage and subsequent transmission is the goal of chemoprophylaxis.

   B. **Prophylaxis**

      1. *Haemophilus influenzae* **type b meningitis**

         a. Criteria for prophylaxis

            (1) There is no need for prophylaxis in families with a child with *H. influenzae* meningitis if no one else in the environment is younger than 4 years. (SOR **◯**)

            (2) If there is another child in the household younger than 4 years, the entire family (including the infected child) should receive prophylaxis. (SOR **◯**)

    (3) Personnel of day-care centers **should receive prophylaxis** when **two or more cases** occur within 60 days. (SOR **C**)

    (4) Prophylaxis is not needed when all children in a day-care center are older than 4 years.

    (5) Prophylaxis for day-care contacts >20 hours per week should be considered in a setting where children are younger than 4 years.

  b. Regimen. Rifampin, administered orally at 20 mg/kg/day in one dose for 4 days (maximum dose, 600 mg per day).

2. *Neisseria meningitidis* meningitis

  a. Criteria for prophylaxis

    (1) Household, day-care, and nursery school contacts. (SOR **B**)

    (2) Personnel who have had contact with oral secretions of the index case. (SOR **C**)

    (3) Prophylaxis is not indicated if exposure to the index case is brief. This includes most health-care workers unless they have been directly exposed to respiratory secretions via intubation, suctioning, or oral care. (SOR **C**)

    (4) Travelers on an airplane seated next to the index patient for more than 8 hours. (SOR **C**)

    (5) Protection is only temporary, as colonization rates rise quickly back to baseline by 6 to 12 months post prophylaxis.

  b. Regimen

    (1) Rifampin, administered orally every 12 hours at 5 mg/kg per dose in children younger than 1 year, 10 mg/kg per dose in children aged 1 to 12 years, and 600 mg in adults and children older than 12 years for a total of four doses (maximum 600 mg per day).

    (2) Ciprofloxacin, administered as a single oral 500-mg dose in adults, is equally as effective if rifampin is not tolerated.

    (3) Ceftriaxone, administered as a single intramuscular dose of 125 mg for children younger than 12 years and a dose of 250 mg for adults.

    (4) All three regimens have 90% to 95% efficacy in eradicating nasopharyngeal carriage of *N. meningitidis* and reduce transmission rate to zero. (SOR **B**)

    (5) Prophylaxis is most effective when used within 24 hours and may have some benefit up to 14 days later.

III. Cardiovascular Disease

  A. Primary prevention

    1. The U.S. Preventive Services Task Force (USPSTF) recommends against the use of aspirin for the primary prevention of myocardial infarction (MI) in men younger than 45 years or stroke in women younger than 55 years (Table 103–1). (SOR **B**)

    2. The USPSTF recommends aspirin for men aged 45 to 79 years to reduce risk of MI when the potential benefit of a reduction in MI outweighs the potential harm due to an increase in gastrointestinal (GI) hemorrhage. (SOR **A**)

    3. The USPSTF recommends aspirin for women aged 55 to 79 years to reduce the risk of ischemic stroke when the potential benefit of a reduction in ischemic strokes outweighs the potential harm of an increase in GI hemorrhage. (SOR **A**)

    4. The USPSTF concludes that the current evidence is insufficient to assess the balance of benefits and harms of aspirin for cardiovascular disease prevention in men and women aged 80 years or older.

    5. Net benefit versus risk of daily aspirin use for primary prevention should be assessed at least every 5 years.

    6. Dosage recommendations in primary prevention. Doses of 75 mg to 162 mg per day are as effective as higher doses with a lower risk of GI side effects. (SOR **B**)

TABLE 103–1. FAVORABLE BENEFIT FROM ASPIRIN USE FOR PRIMARY PREVENTION

Age (yr)	10-yr MI Risk in Men (%)	Age (yr)	10-yr Stroke Risk in Women (%)
45–59	≥4	55–59	≥3
60–69	≥9	60–69	≥8
70–79	≥12	70–79	≥11

Source: Adapted from USPSTF at http://www.ahrq.gov/professionals/clinicians-providers/resources/aspprovider.html.

B. Acute MI

  1. The second International Study of Infarct Trial (ISIS-2) randomized patients on aspirin, intravenous streptokinase, both agents, or neither drug during an acute MI. Aspirin was demonstrated to provide a significant mortality reduction (23%) at 5 weeks, which was equivalent to intravenous streptokinase. The absolute mortality reduction was 24 vascular deaths prevented per 1000 patients treated. Aspirin was also demonstrated to significantly reduce the number of nonfatal MIs and strokes. There was no increase in risk of major bleeding/hemorrhage. Aspirin was by far the most cost-effective agent.

  2. Dosage recommendations for acute MI.

  3. A loading dose of preferably 325 mg of uncoated aspirin should be administered within 24 hours of an acute MI. (SOR **Ⓐ**)

  4. If the only preparation available is enteric-coated, then the tablet should be chewed or crushed.

  5. Therapy should be continued at a dose of 75 mg to 162 mg (enteric-coated) indefinitely. (SOR **Ⓐ**)

  6. Several clinical trials have established the efficacy of aspirin therapy in non-ST segment elevation coronary syndromes, in non-Q-wave MIs, and in unstable angina. Aspirin significantly reduced the risk of an acute MI or death at 5, 30, and 90 days and at 1 year of treatment when used in these settings.

  7. Recommendations for aspirin in non-MI coronary syndromes.

   a. Aspirin should be considered for all patients with new-onset angina, angina at rest, or crescendo angina. (SOR **Ⓐ**)

   b. Patients with GI distress may tolerate a lower dose of aspirin or can take clopidogrel or ticlopidine.

C. Secondary prevention

  1. Taking aspirin for secondary prevention after MI or stroke results in fewer MIs, strokes, and deaths and only a small number of bleeding events.

  2. Benefits are seen as early as just over 2 years of aspirin therapy.

  3. Recommended doses are the same as for primary prevention.

D. Acute stroke

  1. The International Stroke Trial (IST) demonstrated that aspirin-treated patients had significant reductions in the 14-day recurrence of ischemic stroke (2.8% versus 3.9%) and in the combined outcome of nonfatal stroke or death (11.3% versus 12.4%) when administered within 48 hours of symptom onset compared to subcutaneous heparin or no treatment.

  2. The Chinese Acute Stroke Trial (CAST) demonstrated a 14% reduction in total mortality at 4 weeks in the aspirin group compared to placebo.

  3. These two trials demonstrate that aspirin therapy is crucial in the acute stroke setting, with an overall reduction of 13 deaths or significant residual impairment per 1000 patients treated at a 6-month follow-up.

  4. Recommendations in acute stroke

   a. Aspirin should be administered to all patients with acute ischemic stroke if no contraindication exists. (SOR **Ⓐ**)

   b. Dosing should be between 162.5 and 325 mg, based on current literature. Enteric-coated preparations should be chewed or crushed initially. (SOR **Ⓐ**)

   c. Therapy should continue indefinitely and the risk–benefit ratio must be examined individually.

   d. Other antiplatelet drugs including clopidogrel, ticlopidine, or the combination of aspirin and dipyridamole may be equally effective after the acute event for those who cannot tolerate aspirin, but aspirin should be used initially. (SOR **Ⓑ**) (See Chapter 88 for dosages.)

E. Atrial fibrillation (AF)

 1. Aspirin

   a. Several trials have attempted to demonstrate the efficacy of aspirin in the prevention of thromboembolic events in patients with AF, with conflicting results.

   b. A meta-analysis of the trials (including the AFASAK trial and the SPAF-I trial) revealed that although there is modest benefit of aspirin, this benefit varies widely with age and risk.

   c. Aspirin should be considered for primary prevention only in patients with no additional risk factors for thromboembolism. Risk factors include a prior embolic event, left ventricular dysfunction, valvular heart disease (especially mitral stenosis), hypertension, age >60 years, and diabetes. (SOR **Ⓐ**)

2. Warfarin

   a. A meta-analysis of five primary stroke prevention trials demonstrates that anticoagulation with warfarin reduces the risk of stroke in patients with AF when compared to aspirin or placebo. Overall, treating 100 patients with warfarin will prevent nearly three strokes per year.

   b. Trials evaluating the additive effect of warfarin plus aspirin therapy demonstrate that the combination is not beneficial. (SOR **Ⓐ**)

   c. Indications for warfarin therapy in AF.

   (1) Warfarin should be administered to patients with AF who are at a higher risk of thromboembolism (see Chapter 48). The International Normalized Ratio (INR) should be maintained at 2.0 to 3.0. (SOR **Ⓐ**)

   (2) For patients with mechanical heart valves, the target INR should be at least 2.5. (SOR **Ⓑ**)

F. Diabetes mellitus

   1. The Antithrombotic Trialist's Collaboration analyzed nine trials evaluating aspirin as a preventive agent in patients with diabetes. Based on these data, aspirin is recommended for all patients with type 2 diabetes mellitus at increased cardiovascular risk. This includes age greater than 40 years, a family history of CVD, hypertension, smoking, dyslipidemia, or albuminuria.

   2. Although no data demonstrate benefit of pharmacotherapy on preventing diabetes, for patients at high risk, pharmacotherapy (i.e., metformin, pioglitazone) appears to be helpful in delaying the diagnosis of diabetes.

IV. Bacterial Endocarditis

A. Pathophysiology

   1. Infective endocarditis (IE) is a localized infection consisting of fibrin, platelets, and microorganisms that adhere to the cardiac valves. The pathogenesis of IE initiates with a bacteremia.

   2. Procedures that result in transient bacteremia include invasive oral and dental surgery where the mucosa is penetrated or traumatized. Invasive genitourinary or GI procedures are less likely to cause significant bacteremia.

   3. Without appropriate treatment, the mortality rate approaches 100%.

   4. Clinical manifestations include fever, cardiac murmurs, anemia, splenomegaly, petechiae, pyuria, and peripheral emboli.

   5. The causative organisms for native valves are *Streptococcus viridans* and other streptococci (60%), *Staphylococcus aureus* (25%), enterococci (10%), and other gram-negative organisms (5%). For prosthetic valves beyond 2 months of placement, *Streptococcus viridans* and other streptococci account for 30% of cases; coagulase-negative staphylococci, 20%; *Staphylococcus aureus*, 15%; and enterococci and gram-negative organisms, 10%.

B. Prophylaxis

   1. In April 2007, the American Heart Association released new guidelines for the prevention of endocarditis. Prophylaxis is now recommended prior to dental procedures only in patients with the following cardiac conditions: (SOR **Ⓒ**)

   a. Patients with prosthetic cardiac valve(s)

   b. Patients with a history of previous infectious endocarditis

   c. Patients with congenital heart disease (CHD)

   (1) Unrepaired cyanotic CHD, including palliative shunts and conduits

   (2) Completely repaired CHD for 6 months after the procedure

   (3) Repaired CHD with residual defects

   d. Cardiac transplantation recipients who develop cardiac valvulopathy.

   2. Administration of antibiotics solely to prevent endocarditis is not recommended for patients who undergo a genitourinary or GI tract procedure. (SOR **Ⓑ**)

   3. The importance of excellent oral hygiene for patients at risk for IE cannot be underestimated. This includes brushing and flossing regularly, using oral antiseptics, providing atraumatic care for acneiform pustules, avoiding nail biting, and careful gum care. (SOR **Ⓒ**)

   4. Amoxicillin is the antibiotic of choice for endocarditis prophylaxis, with other options for patients who are penicillin-allergic or cannot tolerate oral medications (Table 103–2).

TABLE 103–2. PROPHYLACTIC REGIMENS FOR DENTAL, ORAL, RESPIRATORY TRACT, OR ESOPHAGEAL PROCEDURES

Indication	Drug	Dose: Single Dose 30–60 min Before Procedure[a]	Major Side Effects	Contraindications	Drug Interactions
Standard general prophylaxis	Amoxicillin	Adults: 2 g oral Children: 50 mg/kg oral	Nausea, diarrhea, allergic reaction, CNS excitability (rare), agranulocytosis	Serious allergy to beta-lactams; live intravesical BCG	Oral typhoid vaccine, methotrexate (↑ risk of methotrexate toxicity), warfarin (may ↑ risk of bleeding)
Unable to take oral medications	Ampicillin	Adults: 2 g IM or IV Children: 50 mg/kg IM or IV	Nausea, diarrhea (more likely with oral form), allergic reaction	Allergy to penicillins; live intravesical BCG	Oral typhoid vaccine, methotrexate (↑ risk of methotrexate toxicity), warfarin (may ↑ risk of bleeding)
Allergic to penicillin	Clindamycin or	Adults: 600 mg oral Children: 20 mg/kg oral	Diarrhea (Clostridium difficile), pseudomembranous colitis, nausea, thrombocytopenia, granulocytopenia	Allergy to clindamycin, live intravesical BCG	Oral typhoid vaccine, cyclosporine (↑ cyclosporine)
	Cephalexin[b] or	Adults: 2 g oral Children: 50 mg/kg oral	Diarrhea, allergic reaction, pseudomembranous colitis, interstitial nephritis, aplastic anemia, seizures	Allergy to cephalosporins, caution if penicillin allergy; live intravesical BCG	Oral typhoid vaccine, warfarin (↑ risk of bleeding)
	Azithromycin or clarithromycin	Adults: 500 mg oral Children: 15 mg/kg oral	Diarrhea, nausea, dysgeusia (clarithromycin), allergic reaction, pancreatitis, diarrhea (C. difficile), QT prolongation	Allergy to macrolides, long QT syndrome, live intravesical BCG; use of cisapride, dronedarone, phenothiazines, or colchicine (clarithromycin); concomitant use of statin metabolized by CYP3A4[c] (clarithromycin)	Simvastatin (↑ risk of rhabdomyolysis) See contraindications, also many antiarrhythmics antivirals, antifungals, fluoroquinolones, (increase QT prolongation)
Allergic to penicillin and unable to take oral medications	Cefazolin[b] or	Adults: 1 g oral Children: 50 mg/kg IM or IV	Allergic reaction, diarrhea, eosinophilia, aplastic anemia, encephalopathy, renal failure	Allergy to cephalosporins, caution if penicillin allergy, live intravesical BCG	Oral typhoid vaccine
	Clindamycin	Adults: 600 mg oral Children: 20 mg/kg IV	As above for oral dose form	As above for oral dose form	As above oral dose form

[a]Total pediatric dose should not exceed adult dose.
[b]Cephalosporins should not be used in individuals with Type I hypersensitivity reaction (urticaria, angioedema, or anaphylaxis) to penicillins due to risk of cross-reactivity between beta-lactams.
[c]Cytochrome P450 isoenzyme 3A4. Some statins metabolized by this enzyme include simvastatin, pravastatin, and atorvastatin.
BCG, tuberculosis vaccine; IM, intramuscular; IV, intravenous.

V. Neural Tube Defects (NTDs)

A. Studies reveal that 20% of women whose pregnancies ended in miscarriages and up to 30% of women with recurrent miscarriages had an inadequate folate level. Several studies suggest that consumption of folic acid decreases the incidence of NTDs in the fetuses of pregnant women when taken during the first 6 weeks after conception. These studies include trials of folate supplementation, dietary consumption of folate, and folate concentrations in serum and red blood cells.

B. Recommendations for folate supplementation
   1. The US Public Health Service and The Food and Nutrition Board of the Institute of Medicine recommend that all women of childbearing age capable of becoming pregnant consume 0.4 mg of folic acid per day in order to reduce their risk of having a child with an NTD, since nearly half of all pregnancies are unplanned. (SOR **B**)
   2. The USPSTF recommends that all women capable of becoming pregnant or who are planning a pregnancy take a daily supplement containing 0.4 to 0.8 mg (400–800 μg) of folic acid. (SOR **A**)
   3. Women who have delivered a child with an NTD or who are taking certain anti-seizure medications should consume 4 mg per day of folate 1 month prior to conception and for the first 3 months of pregnancy. The minimal effective folate dose is unknown. (SOR **B**)

C. The US Food and Drug Administration decided in 1993 to fortify staple foods by adding 1.4 mg folic acid/kg of cereal grain. Folic acid consumption may mask the hematologic manifestations of pernicious anemia in the elderly. Folate doses should be kept under 1 mg per day in those with low vitamin B_{12} levels, particularly those with achlorhydria and gastric atrophy lacking intrinsic factor.

VI. Rheumatic Fever

A. Rheumatic fever is a **complication of group A β-hemolytic streptococcal infection** of the upper respiratory tract that is most frequently observed in children aged 5 to 13 years.

B. Diagnosis is based on meeting the **Jones criteria:** two major criteria or one major and two minor criteria plus evidence of a preceding streptococcal infection (http://www.medicalcriteria.com/criteria/car_jones.htm).

C. Prophylaxis
   1. The goal of prophylaxis against group A strep is to prevent a recurrence of acute rheumatic fever. Recurrence rates decrease with increasing age, but recurrences have been documented as late as the fifth or sixth decade of life.
   2. **Recommendations for treatment duration**
      a. Patients who have had rheumatic fever with carditis and residual heart disease need prophylaxis for at least 10 years beyond the last episode and until age 40 years or perhaps for life. (SOR **C**)
      b. Patients who have had rheumatic fever with carditis, but without residual heart disease need prophylaxis for at least 10 years since the last episode or well into adulthood, whichever is longer. (SOR **C**)
      c. Patients who have had rheumatic fever without carditis need prophylaxis for at least 5 years since the last episode or until age 21 years, whichever is longer. (SOR **C**)
   3. **Recommended regimen**
      a. Benzathine penicillin G (1,200,000 U intramuscularly every 3–4 weeks).
      b. Penicillin V (250 mg by mouth twice daily).
      c. Sulfadiazine (500 mg per day orally if <60 lbs; 1 g per day orally if >60 lbs).
      d. Erythromycin (250 mg by mouth twice daily).
   4. A possible alternative to long-term prophylaxis in the future may be a streptococcal vaccine that would eliminate primary rheumatic fever by eliminating the causative organism.

VII. Group B Streptococcal (GBS) Disease.
GBS is a Gram-positive bacterium that colonizes the human GI tract and genitourinary tract. It is the most frequently encountered bacterial pathogen in neonates, and prevention of GBS transmission during vaginal delivery is crucial.

A. History of intrapartum prophylaxis (IAP)
   1. Two approaches to IAP existed prior to 2002. The first was risk factor based and the second was screening based.
   2. A 1999 study raised questions about the inconsistency of these two strategies. Infants born to women whose physicians used the risk factor–based approach were 50% more likely to have early-onset GBS disease.

B. Revised 2002 IAP Screening Guidelines (reinforced in 2010 update)
   1. All pregnant women should be screened for GBS colonization with swabs of both the lower vagina and the rectum at 35 to 37 weeks' gestation. (SOR **A**)
   2. Patients with GBS bacteriuria in the current pregnancy or who delivered a previous infant with GBS disease should receive IAP regardless of current carrier status. (SOR **B**)
C. Patients recommended for IAP
   1. Pregnant women with a positive GBS screen unless a planned cesarean section is performed in the absence of labor or rupture of membranes. (SOR **A**)
   2. Pregnant women who had a prior infant with GBS disease. (SOR **B**)
   3. Women with GBS bacteriuria during the current pregnancy. (SOR **B**)
   4. Pregnant women whose culture status is unknown and who also have delivery at <37 weeks, rupture >18 hours, or temperature spike to >100.4°F. (SOR **A**)
D. Regimen
   1. Penicillin G (5 million U intravenously initial dose, then 2.5 million units every 4 hours). (SOR **A**)
   2. Ampicillin (2 g intravenously initial dose, then 1 g every 4 hours). Penicillin has a narrower spectrum and is preferred. (SOR **A**)
   3. Cefazolin (2 g initial dose, then 1 g every 8 hours). (SOR **C**)
   4. If a patient has an anaphylaxis risk to penicillins, the physician can give clindamycin (900 mg intravenously every 8 hours) or erythromycin (500 mg intravenously every 6 hours). (SOR **C**)

SELECTED REFERENCES

Aguilar MI, Hart R, Pearce LA. Oral anticoagulants versus antiplatelet therapy for preventing stroke in patients with non-valvular atrial fibrillation and no history of stroke or transient ischemic attacks. *Cochrane Database Syst Rev.* 2007;(3):CD006186.

Antithrombotic Trialists Collaboration. Aspirin in the primary and secondary prevention of vascular disease: collaborative meta-analysis of individual participant data from randomised trials. *Lancet.* 2009;373(9678);1849–1860.

Antithrombotic Trialists Collaboration. Collaborative meta-analysis of randomised trials of antiplatelet therapy for prevention of death, myocardial infarction, and stroke in high risk patients. *BMJ.* 2002; 324(7329):71–86.

Aspirin for the primary prevention of cardiovascular disease: clinician fact sheet. http://www.ahrq.gov/professionals/clinicians-providers/resources/aspprovider.pdf. Accessed 3/22/13.

Bilukha OO, Rosenstein N. Prevention and control of meningococcal disease. Recommendations of the Advisory Committee on Immunization Practices. *MMWR.* 2005;54(RR-7):1–21.

Braunwald E, Antman EM, Beasley JW, et al. ACC/AHA 2002 Guideline update for the management of patients with unstable angina and non-ST segment elevation myocardial infarction summary article. A report of the American College of Cardiology/American Heart Association task force on practice guidelines. *J Am Coll Cardiol.* 2002;40:1366–1374.

Fuster V, Ryden LE, Cannom DS, et al. ACC/AHA/ESC 2006 Guidelines for the management of patients with atrial fibrillation. *J Am Coll Cardiol.* 2006;48:e149–e246.

Handelsman Y, Mechanick JI, Blonde L, et al. American Association of Clinical Endocrinologists medical guidelines for clinical practice for developing a diabetes mellitus comprehensive care plan. *Endocr Pract.* 2011;17(Suppl 2):1–53.

Prevention of Early-Onset Group B Streptococcal Disease in Newborns. ACOG Practice guideline. http://www.acog.org/Resources%20And%20Publications/Committee%20Opinions/Committee%20on%20Obstetric%20Practice/Prevention%20of%20Early-Onset%20Group%20B%20Streptococcal%20Disease%20in%20Newborns.aspx. Accessed 21 March, 2013.

Sandercock P, Gubitz G, Foley P, Counsell C. Antiplatelet therapy for acute ischaemic stroke. *Cochrane Database Syst Rev.* 2003;(2):CD000029.

Smith SC Jr, Allen J, Blair SN, et al. AHA/ACC guidelines for secondary prevention for patients with coronary and other atherosclerotic vascular disease: 2006 update endorsed by the National Heart, Lung, and Blood Institute. *J Am Coll Cardiol.* 2006;47:2130–2139.

Wilson W, Taubert KA, Gewitz M, et al. Prevention of infective endocarditis. guidelines from the American Heart Association: a guideline from the American Heart Association Rheumatic Fever, Endocarditis, and Kawasaki Disease Committee, Council on Cardiovascular Disease in the young, and the Council on Clinical Cardiology, Council on Cardiovascular Surgery and Anesthesia, and the Quality of Care and Outcomes Research Interdisciplinary Working Group. *Circulation.* 2007;116:1736–1754.

104　　Counseling for Behavioral Change

Mark R. Marnocha, PhD, David C. Pole, MPH, Ryan M. Niemiec, PsyD,
Laura Frankenstein, MD, & Shawn E. Boogaard, MSE

KEY POINTS

- To share advice successfully, providers should understand (1) the patient's goals, (2) what has worked and what has not worked for the patient in the past, and (3) what challenges the patient faces. (SOR ●)
- Providers can develop skills to successfully share information in a way that helps patients understand how to incorporate medical management recommendations, successfully practice self-management, and incorporate prevention behaviors. (SOR ●)
- Creating "Action Plans" with patients and cultivating their self-management skills enhances self-efficacy and positive outcomes. (SOR ●)
- Providers need to use different approaches and communication based upon the patient's readiness for change. (SOR ●)

I. **Introduction.** To achieve optimal counseling for behavior change, providers and patients should negotiate specific goals for illness prevention, risk reduction, and health enhancement. Accomplishing improved health outcomes is dependent upon a collaboration of caregiver and patient that enhances patients' information, activation, and self-efficacy for health behavior change. The following techniques and guidelines are intended to provide a "tool kit" for successfully counseling patients on a variety of health behaviors. Success depends upon a provider–patient relationship in which information is shared clearly, motivation for change is nurtured, and crucial achievements are acknowledged and praised to build self-efficacy.

II. **Characteristics of an Effective Brief Intervention about Lifestyle Change.** The following present features of effective interventions supported by strong evidence (SOR ●):

　A. **Patient-focused.** Whenever possible, frame the intervention to fit well with the patient's needs and interests. Take time to understand and restate accurately those needs and interests in the patient's terms. Use empathy and restatement to better align with the patient's perceptions of obstacles to change as well as hopes for a successful change.

　B. **Health-connected.** Review the rationale and projected power of the intervention on the patient's physical and/or mental health. Encourage a mutual curiosity in what health benefits can be observed even with initial change efforts.

　C. **Behavior-oriented.** Focus on what the patient can "do" differently. Framing the intervention in terms of creating an "action plan" is helpful. Keep behavioral plans closely aligned with the patients' motivations and everyday realities.

　D. **Realistic.** Consider what is within the patient's current capabilities of achieving. Make your interventions "bite-sized" and focus on "being successful at small steps." A commitment to adhere to even a small behavioral change is crucial, and perhaps the most important step toward ultimate success.

　E. **Controllable.** Frame the intervention in terms of what the patient can readily achieve on a short-term basis with daily efforts (e.g., walking 1 mile per day rather than losing 2 lbs per week). Focus on intermediate behavior changes and maintenance of success in such changes.

　F. **Measurable.** Track the progress the patient makes with the intervention, and encourage patient self-monitoring that is efficient and easy to document.

　G. **Practical.** Keep the focus on changes in the patient's daily life and encourage them to begin making changes immediately. Practicality must take into account positive motivations for change along with any obstacles.

III. **The Mindset of the Clinician**

　A. **Consider the life stage and context.** There are numerous factors that can affect a person's present experience such as age, culture, environment, emotions, beliefs, genetics, biology, spirituality, and level of health literacy. These should be considered in designing effective interventions.

B. Stay in the present moment. Let us go of personal concerns, your previous patient, or plans for your next patient, and focus on the patient with whom you are meeting. Do not begin such counseling with a preset behavioral prescription—use the present moment to explore what is feasible.

C. Judge the behaviors and choices, not the person. It is not the patient who is flawed or "wrong," rather it is the choices and behaviors patients engage in that are flawed or problematic. Unhealthy behaviors may have roots in healthy efforts at adaptation and coping in patients' lives. Keep this perspective in the forefront of your efforts. Normalize, but not catastrophize, the strength of unhealthy habits, while eliciting a mutual commitment to work for practical and lasting change.

D. Remember the positive. Despite any current suffering and challenges that patients may have in managing their health, it is likely that there is more going right with each patient than wrong. Part of successful change involves mobilizing and building upon what is positive and what has been proven helpful in patients' lives.

E. Consider strengths. Each patient has strengths that can be tapped into to help them (e.g., creativity, hopefulness, teamwork, compassion, gratitude). Counseling for health behavior change is not the usual problem-focused approach to care—identifying and solving a specific problem. Rather, the focus of care should be upon greater health and salutogenesis, the pursuit of health instead of the fight against illness.

IV. Stages of Change. The Stages of Change model can be applied to virtually any change in lifestyle or behavior (e.g., smoking cessation, weight loss, healthy eating). Diverse meta-analyses cover a range of health-behavior changes and problem areas. Table 104–1 summarizes the stages of change, what they represent for the patient, and the provider's tasks for each stage: precontemplation, contemplation, action, and maintenance.

A. Determining stage or readiness for change. Assess the patient's perceived importance of the behavior and their confidence to engage in behavior change efforts. The patient's rating of importance and confidence allows you to determine the level of intrinsic motivation and readiness for change. Ask the patient the following questions about a specific behavior:

1. On a scale of 0 (not at all) to 10 (extremely), rate how important is it for you to ___ (quit smoking, exercise, disease management, etc.)? What made you choose your rating?

2. On a scale of 0 (not at all) to 10 (extremely), rate how confident are you that if you decided to ___ (i.e., lose weight), you could succeed. What made you choose your rating?

3. What would it take to get your motivation to a 9 or 10?

4. What would it take to get your confidence to a 9 or 10?

5. Utilize the patient answers to guide you in determining an appropriate intervention, Table 104–1.

TABLE 104–1. THE STAGES OF CHANGE

Stage of Change	Description of Patient Intent	Provider Task
Precontemplation	No intention to change, may be unaware of the problem	Education about the health area
Contemplation	Aware of problem, but unwilling to make a change, may feel stuck or says will do in future	Cost–benefit analysis; develop discrepancy between patient goals and behavior
Preparation	Planning to make change, usually within 1 mo	Brainstorm options; assist in developing concrete action plan
Action	Involved in implementing/making a change	Encourage tracking/monitoring actions; validate/provide feedback; discuss/elicit social support
Maintenance	Has sustained change for a while, usually approximately 6 mo	Check progress; trouble shoot slips/concerns of patient; reinforce successes/build patient confidence
Addressing relapse or relapse prevention	Patient behavior starts to slip, falls back to old behaviors	Judge choices, not the patient; focus on past success, progress not perfection; identify new skills or supports that reinforce health behavior

TABLE 104–2. EXAMPLE OF A DECISIONAL BALANCE FOR SMOKING CESSATION

Continue to Smoke		Quit Smoking	
Cost	**Benefit**	**Cost**	**Benefit**
Worry about health	Helps with stress	More stress	Less hacking and cough in
Tired of smell	Been a "best friend"	Weight gain	the morning
Cannot smoke anywhere	Enjoy smoking with friends	Lose my only pleasure	More energy
Social stigma		Withdrawal symptoms	Have more money
Get winded, cannot do			Better role model to kids
some activities			Get people off my back

B. Addressing precontemplation stage
   1. Educate the patient about their condition and potential negative health outcomes.
   2. Revisit and explore patient perceptions of potential benefits of change.
   3. Provide literacy level appropriate education materials regarding the health condition (see **Bibliotherapy and Accessible Handouts** section).
   4. Continue to ask about the behavior at each subsequent visit with the patient.
   5. Explore obstacles to change and perceived efficacy for overcoming them.

C. Moving from contemplation to action
   1. Use a Decisional Balance Sheet/Cost–Benefit of Change to help identify and high-light any conflict or ambivalence that the patient may have about the change. See Table 104–2 for an example.
   2. Summarize patient statements and highlight mixed feelings (e.g., "I hear that quit-ting smoking feels like losing a friend, but that you are also very worried about your health").
   3. Acknowledge "cost" of change and determine patient's motivation/confidence to move toward "benefits" of change. Accept both obstacles and motivations.

D. Creating an action plan that includes:
   1. Target behavior (exercise, medications, quit smoking, change diet, etc.).
   2. Specific goal within that behavior (I will begin walking for exercise).
   3. Quantity and frequency of the behavior (walk for 20 minutes, 3 days per week on Mondays, Wednesdays, and Fridays).
   4. Detailed specifics of the behavior (I will walk in the morning before work Mondays, Wednesdays and Fridays, outdoors in good weather, on treadmill in bad).
   5. Confidence in their action plan on a scale of 1 to 10.
   6. For additional information and suggestions on creating an Action Plan, go to www.improvingchroniccare.org (select Practice Change; select Self-Management Support; select Clinician Toolkit-see bibliography).

E. Maintenance and relapse prevention
   1. Ask about patient Action Plan and progress, and review any tracking tools or log the patient has been keeping.
   2. Make positive comments about any/all improvements in behavior. Clarify patient's positive and negative perceptions of efforts.
   3. Acknowledge and help patient see any links between behavior changes and health outcomes or clinical measures.
   4. Slips and relapses occur naturally as part of behavior change. Explore triggers for going off-track, barriers to change, and supports for maintaining the desired changes. Note and underscore patients' previous successful efforts. When needed, refresh/revise action plans.
   5. Encourage patient reflection upon choices and values, and exploration of what has worked and what has not. Avoid problem-solving for the patient. Open-ended questions can elicit patient problem-solving and self-affirmation as well as identifi-cation of resources and positive steps. Encourage monitoring progress to stay on track. Open-ended questions that may help with reflection and motivation include the following:
      a. What happened?
      b. What worked and what did not?
      c. What was helpful?

      d. What's missing?

      e. What's next?

V. Understanding and Addressing Low Health Literacy

  A. Health Literacy refers to the capacities of individuals to obtain, process, understand, and apply health-related information to make informed health decisions. According to the most recent National Assessment of Adult Literacy (2003), more than one-third of patients may have difficulty understanding and acting on the health information provided–regardless of the "grade level" they completed. To address such difficulties (SOR **Ⓒ**):

    1. Speak clearly and at a moderate pace.

    2. Use plain nonmedical language. Take note of and use words the patient uses to describe their condition.

    3. Limit content, repeat key points, and encourage questions.

    4. Use Teach-Back Techniques (have patient explain key points to you).

    5. Draw pictures, use diagrams, or demonstrate with models.

VI. Health Behavior-Specific Recommendations

  A. Tobacco use. The effectiveness of clinician counseling in the prevention and cessation of tobacco use is well documented for adults. The Public Health Service Guideline "Treating Tobacco Use and Dependence 2008 Update" recommends the "5 A's" approach to screening and intervention: At every visit, **Ask** about tobacco use, **Advise** to quit, and **Assess** willingness to make an attempt to quit. For patients ready to attempt quitting, **Assist** in the quit attempt, and **Arrange** follow-up. All nonpregnant adults should be asked about tobacco use and provide intervention as needed (SOR **Ⓐ**), and physician intervention for prevention of smoking in children and adolescents is recommended (SOR **Ⓑ**). The AAFP strongly recommends that clinicians screen all pregnant women for tobacco use and provide 5 to 15 minutes of smoking cessation counseling using messages and self-help materials tailored for pregnant smokers. (SOR **Ⓐ**) Continue to ask the patient if they have considered quitting at each visit and provide information/education on smoking as it relates to their specific health condition. When the patient is ready to make a change, use the Brief Intervention principles already discussed as well as the following strategies:

    1. Examine the patient's prior successes or failures with quitting. Use past successes in developing action plans and in deciding whether to taper or "cold turkey" quit from current level of use. If tapering, consider reduction to six to seven cigarettes per day prior to cessation. Set dates and plans for taper and quitting for which the patient finds fewest obstacles and most benefit and self-efficacy.

    2. Instruct/encourage the patient to eliminate all smoking-related paraphernalia in the house and car.

    3. Encourage the patient to set up "No Smoking" signs in areas where previously smoking. Suggest other response-cost techniques such as outdoor smoking only; keeping cigarettes on hand only in limited numbers; storing cigarettes where it requires effort to obtain them, for example in a plastic bag with multiple rubber bands stored on a high shelf; or other patterns that interrupt automatic smoking behaviors.

    4. Encourage the patient to tell others they have quit and to ask for specific support. It can be helpful for patients to invite significant others to commit to quitting also. However, this needs to be a comfortable mode of change, and others' declining to make such a commitment could become an obstacle to or a diversion from personal change.

    5. Suggest the patient make a list of the costs and impact of continued smoking and post it where it can be seen daily. Update list as adverse effects are more evident.

    6. Suggest the patient make a list of the health and personal benefits of stopping smoking and keep it posted. Update it as additional benefits are observed in the tapering/quitting processes.

    7. Encourage the patient to practice a daily stress management activity (e.g., relaxation, self-hypnosis, journaling, or mindfulness meditation). Maintain work breaks and stress management routines that normally would have included a cigarette, but establish different behaviors and habits during those breaks.

    8. Encourage the patient to start or increase daily exercise, keeping intensity and expectations moderate.

    9. Consider nicotine replacement therapy (e.g., nicotine patch, gum, inhaler; E-cigarettes have no evidence-based recommendations at present for use as a form of replacement therapy) (see Chapter 71).

    10. Consider medication (e.g., varenicline, bupropion) (see Chapter 71).

11. For patients who are ready to quit or initiate some behavior change around tobacco use, there are self-help websites:

    a. American Academy of Family Practice link = http://familydoctor.org/familydoctor/en/diseases-conditions/tobacco-addiction.html

    b. American Lung Association—www.lungusa.org; scroll down to *Freedom From Smoking* program. Current site: http://www.lung.org/stop-smoking/ Tips for adults, parents, and kids ("Not On Tobacco" program): http://www.lung.org/stop-smoking/how-to-quit/getting-help/ Quitline resources are provided at a state level throughout the United States and provide information and coaching for patients initiating change.

B. Nutrition. Nutrition and dietary patterns affect many chronic conditions as well as obesity. Take a complete dietary history including a food diary. The *Choose My Plate.gov* USDA website has assessment tools and guidelines.

    1. Adolescents and adult women may need additional calcium, though the USPSTF has found insufficient evidence to recommend vitamin D and calcium supplementation for fracture prevention in men and women.

    2. Pregnant women, infants, and young children have unique dietary requirements. See AAP and AAFP recommendations.

    3. There is insufficient data to recommend routine vitamin supplementation to prevent cancer or cardiovascular disease and use of beta-carotene is not advised.

    4. See general dietary recommendations in the next section.

C. Weight management

    1. All adults and children older than 6 years of age should be screened for obesity. (SOR **B**) For those with a BMI equal to or greater than 30, offer or refer to registered dietitians, nutritionists, or other trained staff (e.g., Diabetic Educator) for comprehensive intervention when available. (SOR **B**) Intensive behavioral dietary counseling is recommended for adults with hyperlipidemia and other risk factors. (SOR **B**) Behavioral counseling for diet and exercise has some evidence for reducing risk of cardiovascular disease in adults (SOR **C**) and should be tailored to the needs and risks of the individual patient.

    2. Recommend a balanced diet based on the *Choose My Plate.gov* template. Dietary patterns should take into account personal preferences and lifestyles. The DASH diet and several Mediterranean style diets have shown health benefits. (SOR **B**)

    3. Encourage an increase in physical activity level to at least 150 minutes per week of moderate intensity exercise for "modest weight loss" and to over 225 minutes per week for greater weight loss. (SOR **B**)

    4. Help the patient identify easy ways to reduce added sugars and fat calorie intake, while increasing plant-based foods. Reduce sodium and refined grain intakes, especially when combined with less sugar, solid fat, and sodium.

    5. Advise the patient to eat smaller meals more frequently.

    6. Suggest the patient practice a daily stress management activity (e.g. relaxation, self-hypnosis, focused breathing). Practice mindful eating and self-monitoring. (SOR **C**)

    7. Assist the patient in setting a behavior-specific Action Plan and track patient efforts. (SOR **B**)

D. Exercise. Evidence remains somewhat equivocal for benefits of primary care interventions. AAFP observes that "although the correlation among healthful diet, physical activity, and the incidence of cardiovascular disease is strong, existing evidence indicates that the health benefit of initiating behavioral counseling in the primary care setting to promote a healthful diet and physical activity is small. Clinicians may choose to selectively counsel patients rather than incorporate counseling into the care of all adults in the general population." (SOR **C**) However, sports medicine provides a strong evidence base for exercise prescriptions.

    1. Advise all patients on the benefits of regular moderate aerobic exercise. (SOR **A**) In older adults regular physical activity increases average life expectancy, reduces the risk of developing a large number of chronic diseases and conditions, and reduces risk of clinical depression or anxiety. (SOR **A/B**) Recommendations for regular physical activity should be tailored to the health status and lifestyle of each patient. (SOR **C**)

    2. Adults should perform 30 to 60 minutes daily of moderate-intensity physical activity 5 or more days of the week including walking, gardening, dancing. (SOR **A**)

    3. Provide instructions on the safe performance of exercise and educate about warning signs or symptoms of cardiovascular difficulty. (SOR **C**) Those at increased risk of injury or medical complications should be advised about appropriate physical activity. If medically indicated, refer to disease-specific exercise guidelines, and/or refer the patient to an exercise specialist, and/or seek consultation for diagnostic exercise testing for CHD to reduce risks. (SOR **Ⓒ**) Supervision by an experienced health and fitness professional may enhance adherence. (SOR **Ⓒ**) The AAFP has exercise prescription guidelines for older adults: http://www.aafp.org/afp/2006/0801/p437.html.

4. Discuss the three components of F.I.T.—frequency, intensity, and time—for any form of exercise: cardiorespiratory, resistance, flexibility, or neuromotor (e.g., yoga, Tai Chi).

5. Warm-up, cool down, flexibility exercise, and gradual progression of exercise volume may reduce risk of musculoskeletal injury or cardiovascular events during exercise. (SOR **Ⓒ**) Standard cardiovascular warm-up and cool-down periods may be helpful, with longer time periods for patients with additional risks.

6. Recommend daily strengthening activities. Flexibility exercises can maintain or improve joint range of motion. (SOR **Ⓐ**)

E. Intentional injuries

1. **Suicide** (see Chapter 94).

   a. Routine suicide screening in the general population has insufficient evidence of actual reductions in suicide rates to recommend for or against (AAFP; USPSTF). However, screening and community awareness programs may increase detection of and interventions provided to those with conditions that increase risk for suicide. There is some evidence for suicide prevention via primary care education, improved access to care for those at risk, and restricting access to means of suicide.

   b. Suicide risk may increase as a result of recent divorce, separation, unemployment, depression, alcohol and other drug abuse, major medical illnesses, living alone, recent bereavement, and with initiation of antidepressants (especially among young adults). Young adults have an increased risk of suicide; risk factors include declines in school performance or attendance, isolation or changes in peer relations, excessive anger or fighting behavior, and bullying or being bullied. Online bullying or harassment is an emerging risk factor, and well-child visits should include consideration of screen time, the degree and quality of youth involvement in social media, and the degree of parental monitoring of online socialization. Older adults are also at excess suicide risk.

   c. Patients with suicidal ideation should be questioned about the extent of their plans (e.g., distribution of possessions, obtaining a weapon, writing a suicide note) and their prior history of suicide plans and attempts. If suicidal intent is considered serious, clinicians should make immediate referrals to mental health professionals and consider emergent hospitalization. Means of emergency detention due to danger to self or others vary by state and community, and practitioners should be familiar with applicable practice patterns and medico-legal standards. Persons with suicidal thoughts should also be informed about community resources such as local mental health agencies and crisis intervention centers. Clinical interventions may reduce risk factors for suicide, but there is little evidence that prevention programs will reduce rates of suicide attempts or completions.

   d. There is little evidence that risk factors can predict whether a specific patient will attempt or reattempt suicide. Contracts for safety in and of themselves show no clinical effectiveness, though arranging a follow-up plan, soliciting patient commitment for adherence, and documenting compliance or lack thereof may set the stage for further intervention and risk monitoring. A Safety Plan Template is available through the Suicide Prevention Resource Center (http://www.sprc.org/for-providers/primary-care).

   e. Routinely screen for depression in adolescents and adults when systems for referral and treatment are in place. (SOR **Ⓑ**)

2. **Violence**

   a. The AAFP and USPSTF recommend screening all women of childbearing age for intimate partner violence, even those without signs or symptoms of such abuse, and providing or referring to intervention services. (SOR **Ⓑ**)

   b. Both the history (discussion of previous violent experiences and current risk factors, such as weapons in the home and discord in the peer group and community) and the physical examination (detection of burns, bruises, and other traumatic injuries) can be used to identify victims of abuse or neglect. Clinicians who suspect violence among patients should refer both the victim and the perpetrator to mental health professionals and other community resources to prevent future episodes.

   c. Certain physical, behavioral, and medical signs indicate child neglect and abuse (see Chapter 93). Physicians must report probable cases of such abuse to local child protective service agencies. In addition, clinicians should be alert to risk signs for adolescent violence such as fighting, bullying, chronic victimization, weapon-carrying, history of domestic violence, and changes in peer relationships.

   d. Clinicians should screen for undetected previous exposure to sexual or physical violence or assault, and provide or refer to intervention services. Trauma-informed care is supported by SAMHSA (www.samhsa.gov/nctic) as a way to engage people with histories of trauma in a comprehensive approach to healthcare, and can form a useful component of patient-centered medical homes.

F. Unintentional injuries

   1. Motor vehicle-related injuries. Urge all patients to use federally approved occupant restraints (e.g., safety belts and child safety seats), to wear safety helmets when riding motorcycles and bicycles, horses, roller skates, and ice skates or snowboarding (high risk of head injury with falls).

   2. Advise patients to avoid driving or riding with a driver under the influence of alcohol or other psychoactive drugs. Help patients develop, with family/friends, a plan for safe alternative transportation with no adverse consequences as an alternative to riding with intoxicated driver.

   3. Counsel individuals at increased risk of motor vehicle injury, such as adolescents and young adults, alcohol and other drug users, and patients with any medical conditions that affect driving skills, to find transportation alternatives. For those with altered perception, cognition, coordination, or movement, referral for functional assessment, typically through rehabilitation services, may be useful for guiding medical recommendations or limitations for driving.

   4. Advise patients to always use car seats for children in an appropriate fashion. (SOR ❸) Anticipatory guidance includes the following:

     a. Always ask if the patient is using a car seat for their child.

     b. Never use a rear-facing car seat in the front seat of a vehicle with an air bag.

     c. All children younger than 13 years should be restrained in the rear seat for optimal protection.

     d. All infants should be in a rear-facing seat until they have reached 2 years of age or until they reach the highest weight or height allowed by their car seat's manufacturer.

     e. A forward-facing car seat or a belt-positioning booster seat should be used until the child reaches 4'9" in height AND is between 8 and 12 years old.

     f. When old enough and large enough to use vehicle seat belts, children should always use lap and shoulder seat belts.

G. Environmental and household injuries. Although passive interventions (e.g., child-resistant containers to prevent poisoning) are the most effective measures to control injuries, clinician counseling may help patients reduce their risks of household and environmental injuries (e.g., falls, drowning, fire, poisoning, suffocation, and firearm mishaps). (SOR ❻) Encourage patients to do the following:

   1. Install smoke detectors and check them monthly, change batteries annually, or with time change if applicable.

   2. Lower the temperature setting on hot-water heaters to 48.4°C (120°F).

   3. Encourage patients with **children in the home** to store all medications, toxic substances, matches, and firearms out of the reach of children and display emergency numbers prominently near telephones (e.g., the police department, the fire department, 911, the local Poison Control Center).

   4. Patients with pools should install four-sided fencing with self-latching and self-closing gates around swimming pools and spas.

   5. Recommend the installation of window guards on all windows not designated as emergency fire exits.

   6. Bicyclists and parents of children who ride bicycles/scooters should be made aware of the importance of wearing **safety helmets and protective gear**.

   7. To prevent falls among **older patients,** consider clinical factors suggesting an elevated risk of falls. These include a history of falls, a history of mobility problems, and poor performance on behavioral measures such as the timed Get-Up-and-Go test (http://www.youtube.com/watch?v=sOnqzvt9JSs).

   a. The USPSTF does not recommend routinely performing an in-depth multifactorial risk assessment for falls, but patients and clinicians should consider benefits versus harms based on history of prior falls, comorbid medical conditions, and patient values. (SOR **❸**)

   b. When indicated for specific patients, home visits could be used to assess the possible utility of home modifications such as tacking down carpets and arranging furniture so that pathways are not cluttered; lowering kitchen items to prevent over-reaching; testing visual acuity periodically; and closely monitoring use of drugs, such as those with sedative, amnestic or anticholinergic effects, that can increase the risk of falls.

   c. Older patients may benefit from **appropriate physical exercises** to maintain and improve strength, flexibility, and mobility; and community-dwelling adults aged 65 years or older who are at increased risk for fall should receive exercise or physical therapy and vitamin D supplementation. (SOR **❸**) Recommended daily allowance, set in 2010 by the institute of medicine, are based on age as follows: for those 1 to 70 years of age, 600 IU daily; for those 71 years and older, 800 IU daily.

H. Sexual behavior

  1. Sexually transmitted infections (STIs) (see Chapter 102).

    a. Take a complete sexual history from all adolescent, adult, and older adult patients and offer STI screening according to recommended guidelines. Clinicians should discuss sexual behavior with respect, compassion, and confidentiality. Remember that seniors are also at high risk of infection and may not be aware of protective measures for safe sex.

    b. The AAFP recommends high-intensity behavioral counseling to prevent STIs for all sexually active adolescents and for adults at increased risk for STIs. (SOR **❸**) Sexually active patients should be counseled that the most effective strategy to prevent infection with human immunodeficiency virus (HIV) or other STIs is to abstain from sex or maintain a mutually monogamous sexual relationship with a partner known to be uninfected and use contraception. Patients should be counseled to engage in routine screening since many STIs are asymptomatic. Encourage patients to decrease the number of sexual partners and counsel on how to discuss infection status with their partners. Counsel women of childbearing age on the dangers of HIV and STI infection during pregnancy. (SOR **❸**)

    c. The AAFP recommends that clinicians screen adolescents and adults aged 18 to 65 years for HIV infection. Younger adolescents and older adults who are at increased risk should also be screened. Clinicians should screen all pregnant women for HIV, including those who present in labor whose HIV status is unknown. (SOR **❹**) Patients should be alerted that a nonreactive HIV test does not rule out infection if the sexual partner has engaged in sexual intercourse during the 6 months before testing. Safe (or "safer") sexual practices (e.g., massage, hugging, or dry kissing) should be encouraged.

    d. Counsel patients on the consistent and proper use of condoms (see Chapter 97).

  2. Unintended pregnancy. Discuss the efficacy, limitations, and proper use of available contraceptive techniques (see Chapter 97).

I. Dental disease

  1. Counsel patients to visit a dentist regularly, to brush their teeth daily with fluoride-containing toothpaste, and to use dental floss daily to clean between teeth.

  2. Young children should have their first dental visit no later than their first birthday. Children 2 years and older should be taught to spit out rather than swallow toothpaste containing fluoride, to prevent dental fluorosis. Not rinsing after brushing leaves a small amount of fluoride to help prevent decay. Parental assistance with tooth brushing is helpful until fine motor skills progress sufficiently, typically by age 7 or 8 years. Children and other with dental abnormalities found through visual examination (e.g., nursing bottle tooth decay, crowding or misalignment of teeth, dental caries, or periodontal infections) should be referred to their dentist for further evaluation. Dental visits should be scheduled twice a year.

  3. Patients should be advised to limit their intake of foods containing refined sugar, particularly between-meal snacks and/or keep a tooth brush and tooth paste available at work.

4. To reduce the risk of early childhood caries, infants should not be put to bed with a bottle. If a bedtime bottle is necessary, encourage use of water only.

5. Children living in areas with inadequate fluoride in their drinking water should be prescribed daily fluoride drops or tablets according to recommended guidelines. Clinicians prescribing fluoride supplements for children must know the concentration of fluoride in the child's drinking water. Dental sealants reduce frequency of decay on some tooth surfaces, and some schools may have sealant programs available in lower income communities. Dental consultation may be helpful.

6. Urge patients to reduce their risk of oral cancer by eliminating tobacco use and limiting alcoholic beverage consumption.

7. Oral health problems have been shown to adversely affect school performance and adjustment, with increased risk for anxiety, depression, and absences. http://www.mchoralhealth.org/PDFs/learningfactsheet.pdf

J. Alcohol and other drugs (see Chapter 90).

1. The routine history for adults aged 18 years and older should include screening for quantity, frequency, and other patterns of use of wine, beer, and liquor, and provide persons engaged in risky or hazardous drinking with brief behavioral counseling interventions to reduce alcohol misuse. (SOR **B**) Questionnaires are available for more systematic detection of problem drinking. The AAFP concludes that the current evidence is insufficient to assess the balance of benefits and harms of screening adolescents, adults, and pregnant women for illicit drug use. (USPSTF update is in progress as of 2013.)

2. The AAFP recognizes that avoidance of alcohol products by adolescents aged 12 to 17 years is desirable. The effectiveness of the physician's advice and counseling in this area is uncertain.

3. Negotiate safe drinking amounts—Recommendations for healthy, nonpregnant women in standard drinks are no more than 7 drinks per week or 3 per occasion; recommendations for healthy men are no more than 14 drinks per week or 4 per occasion. For patients older than 65 years, recommend no more than 1 drink per day. For patients who drink over those amounts, an Action Plan to reduce or stop drinking should be developed. (SOR **B**) Those patients with a history of substance abuse should consume less than these amounts.

4. There are **no documented safe levels** of alcohol intake during pregnancy. To reduce the risk of Alcohol Exposed Pregnancy (AEP) and Fetal Alcohol Spectrum Disorders (FASD), pregnant women or those wish to become pregnant should be counseled not to drink. (SOR **B**) Women at risk of becoming pregnant who choose to drink, should be counseled on consistent and proper use of contraceptives. (SOR **B**)

   a. For additional information on AEP and FASD, visit the website for the Midwest Region Fetal Alcohol Syndrome Training Center at http://ssw.missouri.edu/MRFASTC/. To order a FASD Prevention Tool Kit, go to the American College of Obstetricians and Gynecologists website at www.acog.org and search for "FASD Prevention Tool Kit." Or enter the following: http://www.acog.org/~/media/Department%20Publications/FASDToolKit.pdf?dmc=1&ts=20130831T1528156377

5. Provide substance-abusing patients with information about chemical dependence, the effects of the drug, and its effect on health. Intravenous drug users should be referred for treatment and counseled against the use of contaminated or shared needles, which can transmit HIV, hepatitis B virus, and other organisms. Harm reduction programs are available in some regions, including needle exchange programs and distribution of naloxone to patients for field administration. Treatment plans should be tailored to the drug of abuse and the individual needs of the patient and his or her family (see Chapter 90).

K. Cancer screening and self-examination (see Chapters 69 and 106). Although widely practiced, self-examinations have not been proven to be an effective maneuver for reducing cancer mortality. The USPSTF recommends against teaching of breast self-examination (BSE) as a means of reducing cancer risk.

1. Skin cancer. Although the ACS recommends screening for skin cancer, the AAFP and USPSTF conclude that the current evidence is insufficient concerning use of a whole-body skin examination by a primary care clinician or patient skin self-examination for the early detection of cutaneous melanoma, basal cell cancer, or squamous cell skin cancer in the adult general population.

   a. To prevent skin cancer, counsel youth and young adults, aged 10 to 24 years, who have fair skin about minimizing their exposure to ultraviolet radiation to reduce risk for skin cancer. (SOR **B**) Such counseling for adults older than 24 years has insufficient supporting evidence according to AAFP.

   b. Patients with increased occupational or recreational exposure to sunlight as well as those who live in tropical climates should be counseled to regularly apply broad-spectrum sunscreen with UVA/UVB protection and use sunglasses with 99% UV blockage. They should also be advised to wear protective clothing, such as wide-brimmed hats and long-sleeved shirts and slacks, and to try to reduce outdoor activity between 10 AM and 4 PM.

   c. Parents should limit their children's exposure to ultraviolet light through similar measures, especially children with fair skin. (SOR **B**)

   d. Use of tanning beds should be discouraged due to association with increased risk of skin damage and cancer.

SELECTED REFERENCES

ACSM and American Diabetes Association Joint Position Statement: Exercise and Type 2 Diabetes. Web reference made August 2013. http://www.ncbi.nlm.nih.gov/pmc/articles/PMC2992225/pdf/zdce147.pdf

AHRQ Health Literacy Toolkit. Web reference made August 2013. http://www.ahrq.gov/professionals/quality-patient-safety/quality-resources/tools/literacy-toolkit/index.html

American Cancer Society Chronological History of Recommendations for Prevention. Web reference made August 2013. http://www.cancer.org/healthy/findcancerearly/cancerscreeningguidelines/chronological-history-of-acs-recommendations

American College of Sports Medicine (ACSM) Public position stands. Web reference made August 2013. http://www.acsm.org/access-public-information/position-stands

Holt K, Barzel R. *Oral Health and Learning: When Children's Health Suffers, So Does their Ability to Learn.* 3rd ed. Washington DC: National Maternal and Oral Health Resource Center; 2013.

Lorig K, Laurent DD, Plant K, Krishnan E, Ritter PL. The components of action planning and their associations with behavior and health outcomes. *Chronic Illn.* 2014;10(1):50–59.

Miller W, Rollnick S. *Motivational Interviewing: Preparing People for Change.* New York, NY: Guilford Press; 2002.

Ozer E, Urquhart B, Brindis C, Park J, Irwin C. Young Adult Preventive Health Care Guidelines: There But Can't Be Found. *Arch Pediatr Adolesc Med.* 2012;166(3):240–247.

Schaefer J, Miller D, Goldstein M, Simmons L. *Partnering in Self-Management Support: A Toolkit for Clinicians.* Cambridge, MA: Institute for Healthcare Improvement; 2009. Web reference made August 2013. Available at http://www.ihi.org/knowledge/Pages/Tools/SelfManagementToolkitforClinicians.aspx

US Public Health Service Clinical Practice Guideline Treating Tobacco Use and Dependence: 2008 Update. Web reference made August 2013. http://www.ctri.wisc.edu/Researchers/Guideline_update/cpg_full2008.pdf

USPSTF: *Guide to Clinical Preventive Services, 2012.* Web reference made August 2013. Agency for Healthcare Research and Quality (AHRQ), Rockville, MD. http://www.ahrq.gov/professionals/clinicians-providers/guidelines-recommendations/guide/index.html

BIBLIOTHERAPY AND ACCESSIBLE HANDOUTS

American Academy of Family Physicians: www.aafp.org Treatment recommendations: http://www.aafp.org/patient-care/clinical-recommendations/a-z.html Patient Education resources: http://familydoctor.org/familydoctor/en.html Smoking Cessation info: http://familydoctor.org/familydoctor/en/diseases-conditions/tobacco-addiction.html Guideline for Tobacco Cessation: http://www.aafp.org/dam/AAFP/documents/patient_care/clinical_recommendations/TreatingTobaccoUseandDependence-2008Update.pdf

WebMD for diverse health topics: www.webmd.com

Women's Health resources: www.womenshealth.gov

Kids Health resources for parents, children, teens: www.kidshealth.org .

Oral Health Guide http://www.mchoralhealth.org/pocket.html

Education Resources: Medline Plus: www.nlm.nih.gov/medlineplus/tutorial.html

Health Information for diverse audiences: http://www.fda.gov/ForConsumers/default.htm Click on "consumer information by audience": Health Resources in diverse formats to accommodate health literacy levels: http://www.healthliteracy.worlded.org/healthinfo.htm

AMA Health Literacy resources: http://www.ama-assn.org/ama/pub/about-ama/ama-foundation/our-programs/public-health/health-literacy-program.page?

Consumer Updates, FDA: http://www.fda.gov/ForConsumers/ConsumerUpdates/default.htm Tanning
   bed cautions, FDA, May, 2013 http://www.fda.gov/downloads/ForConsumers/ConsumerUpdates/
   UCM351054.pdf
USDA Dietary Guidelines, 2010 (revision due in 2015): http://www.cnpp.usda.gov/dietaryguidelines.
   htm *Choose My Plate* 2-page handout: http://www.choosemyplate.gov/downloads/mini_poster_
   English_final.pdf
Overview of Health Promotion GOALS: Healthy People 2020: http://healthypeople.gov/2020/default.
   aspx
American Cancer Society skin CA prevention: http://www.cancer.org/acs/groups/cid/documents/
   webcontent/003184-pdf.pdf
Car Seat Information http://www.healthychildren.org/English/safety-prevention/on-the-go/Pages/
   Car-Safety-Seats-Information-for-Families.aspx (2013)

---

105   Immunizations

William E. Cayley, Jr., MD, MDiv

KEY POINTS

- Immunizations are among the most cost-effective preventive health measures, significantly reducing rates of infectious disease. (SOR **A**)
- Every health visit is an opportunity to update immunization status. Immunizations should be given according to the current schedules on CDC's National Immunization Program's website. http://www.cdc.gov/vaccines/. (SOR **A**)
- Contraindications to vaccine usage should be checked in every patient. A full discussion of risks and benefits, including benefits to society, should be done with every patient or guardian to ensure informed consent. (SOR **C**)

I. Introduction
   A. Overview. Immunizations have significantly reduced rates of infectious disease and are among the most cost-effective preventive health measures. (SOR **A**) Nevertheless, vaccine coverage of the general population is less than optimal because of missed opportunities and misconceptions by parents and clinicians.
   B. Timing. Every healthcare visit is an opportunity to update a patient's immunization status. Routine immunizations should be given according to the current schedules posted on the website of the Centers for Disease Control and Prevention (CDC) (http://www.cdc.gov/vaccines/schedules/index.html). Separate schedules for birth to18 years and for adults are reviewed and revised annually. Administering multiple vaccines at the same visit is both safe and effective. (SOR **A**) Inactivated vaccines can be given any time before or after other live or inactivated vaccines. Live vaccines not administered at the same time should be separated by at least 4 weeks. Interruptions or delays in a vaccination series do not require restarting that series since delays in dosing do not reduce final antibody response. If past records cannot be located, the patient should be considered nonimmune and started on the appropriate schedule of doses.
   C. Administration. Routes of administration are recommended by the manufacturer of each vaccine. Descriptions and illustrations of appropriate immunization sites and techniques are provided in the General Recommendations on Immunization (http://www.cdc.gov/mmwr/preview/mmwrhtml/rr6002a1.htm). If two or more vaccinations are given, each should be given at a different anatomic site.
   D. Safety. Patients with a history of severe allergic response to a vaccine or one of its components should not receive further doses of that vaccine. Since no vaccine is completely safe or completely effective, administration of vaccines requires an understanding of the risks and benefits involved; the benefits to the individual and to society at large weighed against the risks to the individual.

1. Anaphylactic reactions after vaccination are rare, but potentially life-threatening and all personnel and facilities providing vaccinations need proper training, equipment, and office procedures for cardiopulmonary resuscitation and management of anaphylaxis.

2. Illness. Mild illnesses are not contraindications to vaccination and research has generally demonstrated adequate antibody response to vaccinations given at the time of mild illness. Patients with more severe illness should be immunized once the acute phase of the illness is over, to avoid confusing effects of the illness with vaccine side effects.

3. Immunocompromise. Inactivated vaccines (e.g., pneumococcal, meningococcal, and inactivated influenza vaccines) generally are safe and live vaccines generally are avoided in persons with immunocompromising conditions. Live vaccines may pose some risk for immunosuppressed family members, and in this context an inactivated vaccine may also be preferred.

4. Reporting. Any adverse events following vaccination should be reported to the Vaccine Adverse Event Reporting System (http://vaers.hhs.gov/).

II. Recommended Immunization Schedules for Persons Aged 0 to 18 Years

A. Hepatitis B (HBV). Approximately 600,000 people globally die each year of HBV-related liver disease, including cirrhosis and hepatocellular carcinoma. Universal immunization of infants against HBV is recommended (1) to protect children younger than 5 years, who are at higher risk of chronic disease if they become infected, and (2) to increase immunity among the general population.

1. Infants born to hepatitis B surface antigen (HBsAg) negative mothers should receive a dose of single-antigen HBV vaccine prior to hospital discharge. Infants born to HbsAg positive mothers should receive a first dose of HBV vaccine in the first 12 hours of life, along with 0.5 cc of hepatitis B immune globulin (HBIG) injected IM at another site. If the mother's HbsAg status is unknown, HBV vaccine should be given in the first 12 hours of life, and if the infant weighs less than 2000 g, also administer HBIG in the first 12 hours of life. The mother's HbsAg status should be tested, and HBIG should be given within 1 week of birth if the mother tests HbsAg positive. The three-dose series is completed with a minimum interval between dose 1 and dose 2 of 4 weeks and between dose 2 and 3 of 8 weeks.

2. Adolescents not previously vaccinated against HBV should receive a complete series of three doses with a single-antigen HBV vaccine. There should be at least 1 month between doses 1 and 2, and 4 months between doses 2 and 3.

3. Adverse events/effects. Local pain and a mildly elevated temperature are the most common reactions. There appears to be no association between HBV immunization and Guillain–Barré syndrome.

B. Rotavirus. Rotavirus is responsible for one-third of the cases of childhood death from diarrheal disease worldwide and over 550,000 hospitalizations annually in the United States. The virus is common, hardy, and highly contagious, thus even proper attention to hygiene and contact precautions may not prevent transmission. An earlier quadrivalent human-rhesus vaccine (RRV-TV) was removed from the market in 1999 after reports of increased rates of intussusception. The newer oral Rotavirus vaccine is a live-virus vaccine that appears to be effective in reducing rates of disease with no increased rates of intussusception.

1. There are currently two Rotavirus vaccines, RV-1 given as a two-dose series at 2 and 4 months of age, and RV-5 given as a three-dose series at 2, 4, and 6 months of age. The vaccine series should not be started after 15 weeks of age.

2. Adverse events/effects. Approximately 2% to 3% of infants will experience mild vomiting or diarrhea after Rotavirus vaccination. The vaccine does not appear to increase the rate of intussusception. Because the vaccine is a live virus, it should not be given to children of mothers with human immunodeficiency virus (HIV) until it has been determined that the infant does not have HIV. The safety of using this vaccine for infants with other immunosuppressive conditions is currently unknown.

C. Diphtheria–tetanus–acellular pertussis (DTaP), Tetanus–diphtheria–acellular pertussis (Tdap), and Tetanus-diphtheria (Td). Childhood vaccination against diphtheria, tetanus, and pertussis has been routine in the United States since the 1940s. The older DTP vaccine with inactivated whole-cell pertussis has been replaced by the newer DTaP using an acellular pertussis toxin. Immunity to pertussis wanes, with little protection after 5 to 10 years, but childhood DTaP vaccines should not be used for immunizing adults.

1. DTaP is administered by IM injection at ages 2, 4, 6, 15, to 18 months, and 4 to 6 years. Patients who do not receive their fourth dose until after the age of 4 years do not need a fifth dose.

2. **Adverse events/effects.** Mild reactions (fever, drowsiness) or more severe reactions (high temperatures >105°F, or febrile seizures) are much less common after DTaP administration than with the older DTP vaccine. If encephalopathy, such as unresponsiveness or seizures, occurs within 7 days of DTaP administration and cannot be attributed to another cause, DT (diphtheria and tetanus toxoids alone) should be used for all subsequent immunizations. Stable neurologic conditions, or a family history of seizures, are not contraindications to pertussis immunization.

3. **Immunity to pertussis from childhood DTaP vaccination wanes with age** and reimmunization of adolescents against pertussis is important. The Tdap vaccine contains the same dose of Tetanus toxoid as the pediatric DTaP, the acellular pertussis component, but a lower dose of Diphtheria toxoid. A single dose of Tdap is recommended at age 10 or 11 years (depending on the manufacturer) for individuals who completed the primary pediatric series of immunizations. Children aged 7 to 10 years who did not receive a full childhood series of DTaP, should be given one dose of Tdap, then complete any remaining catch-up doses with the tetanus-diphtheria (Td) vaccine. Adolescents aged 11 to 18 years who have not received Tdap, should be given one dose of Tdap, followed by Td boosters every 10 years.

   a. **Adverse events/effects.** Headache, injection site pain, myalgias, and fatigue are the most commonly reported adverse effects. Patients experiencing an Arthus hypersensitivity reaction or a temperature over 103°F after any dose of Tetanus toxoid should not receive further doses of Tetanus toxoid more frequently than every 10 years.

D. *Haemophilus influenzae* **Type B (Hib).** Before development of effective vaccinations, 1 in 200 children developed invasive Haemophilus disease before age 5 years, often leading to meningitis, hearing loss or mental retardation. Vaccines against *H. influenzae* type B have been 95% to 100% effective in preventing invasive Hib disease.

1. Two Hib vaccines are available: *Haemophilus* B Meningococcal Protein Conjugate (PRP-OMP), and Haemophilus B Tetanus Toxoid Conjugate (PRP-T). Hib vaccines should not be given to infants younger than 6 weeks. The recommended schedule is a dose of Hib at 2, 4, and 6 months and a booster at 12 to 15 months. Children who have received PRP-OMP at 2 and 4 months do not require a dose at 6 months but should receive the booster at 12 to 15 months.

2. **Adverse events/effects** from Hib vaccination are rare, usually occur after the third dose if at all, and are usually limited to mild fever or local redness, swelling, or warmth.

E. **Pneumococcal conjugate vaccine (PCV13).** *Streptococcus pneumoniae* is a major cause of pediatric otitis media, pneumonia, meningitis, and bacteremia. Rates of disease are higher among children younger than 5 years and are highest in infants. PCV13 contains antigens from 13 serotypes of pneumococcus conjugated to a carrier protein and is effective in reducing invasive disease and pneumonia.

1. PCV13 should be given at 2, 4, 6, and 12 to 15 months of age. Since the highest risk of invasive disease is in children younger than age 2 years, catch-up vaccination with PCV13 between the ages of 2 and 5 years is recommended only for children with increased risk of disease because of HIV, sickle-cell disease, asplenia, or chronic illness. Local redness and tenderness at the injection site are the only reported adverse effects of PCV13.

2. **The 23-valent pneumococcal polysaccharide vaccine** (PPSV23) should be given at least 8 weeks after the last dose of PCV13 to children 2 years or older with chronic heart disease, chronic lung disease (including asthma if treated using oral corticosteroids), diabetes, cerebrospinal fluid leaks, or a cochlear implant, and a single booster dose of PPSV23 should subsequently be given to children with anatomic or functional asplenia, or any immunocompromising condition. Details of catch-up vaccination scheduling for incompletely immunized individuals are given in the annually updated immunization schedules.

F. **Inactivated poliovirus vaccine (IPV).** Routine vaccination has led to control of polio in the Western Hemisphere. Since the live oral polio vaccine (OPV) carries a small but real risk of vaccine-associated paralytic polio, it has been replaced in the United States by the inactivated polio vaccine (IPV). Recommended doses of IPV are at ages 2 months,

4 months, between 6 and 18 months, and between 4 and 6 years. Any adolescent who has not already received a complete primary series of polio vaccine should be immunized. No serious adverse events have been associated with the use of IPV.

G. Influenza. Influenza virus is second only to respiratory syncytial virus (RSV) in causing hospitalizations among children with chronic illness. Even among healthy children younger than 2 years, influenza hospitalization rates are as high as 187 per 100,000 children.

1. All children older than 6 months should be vaccinated annually against influenza, and anyone 8 years or younger receiving influenza immunization for the first time should receive two doses at least 4 weeks apart. The vaccine is not recommended for children younger than 6 months, though they may be protected from influenza by vaccination of household contacts. Only the trivalent inactivated influenza vaccine (IIV) should be used for children between the ages of 6 months and 2 years, but either the (IIV) or the intranasal live attenuated influenza vaccine (LAIV) may be used for healthy, nonpregnant individuals of age 2 years or older.

2. Patients who are concerned about the influenza vaccine causing disease should be educated that the vaccine contains noninfectious killed virus. It cannot cause disease, but will not protect against coincident infection with other viruses.

3. **Adverse events/effects.** Local reactions of redness and tenderness are the most common adverse reactions, though anaphylactic reactions to residual egg protein from the virus culture process have rarely been reported.

H. Measles–mumps–rubella (MMR) vaccination has reduced rates of measles, mumps, rubella (german measles) and congenital rubella syndrome by 99% over the last century, although occasional outbreaks continue to occur among unimmunized persons. The MMR vaccine combines attenuated strains of all three viruses.

1. The first dose of MMR vaccine is given at 12 to 15 months of age, and the second dose at 4 to 6 years. One dose of MMR should be given to infants aged 6 to 11 months before departure from the United States for international travel, followed by the routine doses at 12 to 15 months and 4 to 6 years. Any school-aged child not previously immunized should receive two doses of MMR vaccine at least 4 weeks apart.

2. **Adverse events/effects.** Pain, redness, and local irritation can occur with all three vaccines. Rubella vaccine rarely causes generalized lymphadenopathy in children or a transient arthralgia in young women, and mumps vaccine rarely causes transient orchitis in young men. Egg allergy is not a contraindication to MMR vaccine, but the vaccine should not be given to persons with severe allergy to gelatin or neomycin. Patients with HIV can be given MMR unless they have low age-specific CD4 counts.

I. Varicella vaccine (VAR). The live attenuated VAR vaccine is 97% effective against moderate or severe varicella and at least 44% protective against any varicella for at least 7 years; antibody response has been documented for up to 20 years. Approximately 1% of vaccinees per year develop mild, breakthrough infection that does not appear to be contagious.

1. The first dose of VAR should be given between 12 and 15 months of age and a second dose between 4 and 6 years of age, although the second dose may be given before age 4 years if at least 3 months have passed since the first dose. Varicella immunization is recommended for all persons aged 7 to 18 years without a reliable history of immunity (such as documentation of prior age-appropriate vaccination, laboratory confirmation of immunity or varicella disease, or healthcare provider diagnosis of chickenpox or zoster). Two doses of vaccine are given, spaced 3 months apart for those younger than 13 years of age and spaced 4 weeks apart for those 13 years or older.

2. The vaccine is contraindicated in immunosuppressed individuals. Transient zoster in recipients and transmission to susceptible contacts of vaccinees has been reported.

J. Hepatitis A (HAV) is usually transmitted by the fecal-oral route. While acute disease is more common in adults, children generally have asymptomatic infection and so can be an important reservoir and source of infection for older individuals. Hepatitis A immune globulin has been available for several years for inducing passive immunity, and since 1995, inactivated-virus vaccination conferring active immunity against HAV has been available.

1. Immunization against HAV is recommended for all children between 12 and 23 months of age, as well as older children for whom immunity is desired. Two doses

are given, separated by at least 6 months. Onset of immunity is in 15 to 30 days and protection lasts for at least 10 years. No booster doses are recommended. The only reported adverse effects from HAV vaccination are local warmth, soreness, and occasional headache.

K. Human papilloma virus (HPV2 and HPV 4). Most HPV infections are asymptomatic and 90% clear within 2 years. However, persistent HPV infection can cause cervical cancer in women, throat cancer in men, and genital warts in both men and women. The quadrivalent vaccine (HPV4, Gardasil) against HPV types 6, 11, 16, and 18 (which cause 90% of genital warts) is licensed for use in males and females aged 9 to 26 years. Quadrivalent vaccine has also been shown to protect against cancers of the anus, vagina, and vulva. The bivalent vaccine (HPV2, Cervarix) against HPV types 16 and 18 (which cause 70% of cervical cancers) is licensed for females aged 9 to 25 years. Ideally, the series should be given before the onset of sexual activity. However, if a patient has become infected with HPV, the vaccine may provide some protection against further infection with other HPV serotypes.

1. Routine HPV vaccination is recommended for **all adolescents at age 11 or 12 years,** with catch-up doses recommended for previously unimmunized individuals between the ages of 13 and 26 years. The vaccine series can be started at age 9 years. HPV vaccine is also recommended for gay and bisexual men (or any man who has sex with men) and persons with compromised immune systems (including HIV) through age 26 years, if they did not get fully vaccinated when they were younger. There should be 1 to 2 months between doses 1 and 2, and 4 months between doses 2 and 3.

2. **Adverse events/effects.** Local pain, swelling, and redness are not unusual, and approximately 4% of patients experience a mild fever. Severe adverse events have not been reported.

3. Although there has been a dramatic decrease (56%) in the rate of HPV infection since the vaccination program began, is important to realize that HPV vaccination will not eliminate the risk of cervical cancer or the need for screening since the vaccine does not include all HPV types causing cancer. The long-term duration of immunity has not been established.

L. Meningococcal conjugate vaccine (MCV4). The newer meningococcal conjugate vaccine (MCV4) provides longer-lasting immunity than the older meningococcal polysaccharide vaccine (MPSV4), but is only approved for individuals aged 11 to 55 years. MCV4 is recommended at age 11 or 12 years, with a booster dose at age 16 years. Adolescents aged 13 to 18 years not previously immunized should receive MCV4 at age 13 to 15 years, with a booster dose (at least 8 weeks after the prior dose) at ages 16 to 18 years.

1. Since crowded living conditions are a risk factor for meningococcal disease, MCV4 vaccination is recommended for college freshmen who will be living in dormitories and for military recruits. No booster is needed if the first dose is given at age 16 years or older. Adolescents aged 11 to 18 years with HIV infection should receive two doses of MCV4, separated by 8 weeks.

2. The CDC immunization schedules give specific additional details for immunizations for children at higher risk of meningococcal disease due to anatomic or functional asplenia, complement deficiency, or travel to or residence in an area of high risk.

3. **Adverse events/effects.** Mild fever and local pain, redness, or swelling may occur after MCV4 vaccination, but there is minimal risk of severe side effects.

III. Recommended Immunization Schedules for Adults Older Than 19 Years of Age

While immunizations are ideally given at routine health maintenance visits, many adults seek medical care only for acute injury or illness and may not have had all recommended immunizations. Thus, episodes of acute care also are important times for assessing and updating immunization status. The adult immunization schedule is published on the CDC website and is updated annually.

A. Influenza. Annual influenza vaccination is now recommended for all adults. In addition, healthcare workers should be vaccinated annually to reduce the risk of transmitting influenza to susceptible individuals. Persons who contract influenza following immunization usually have a milder course and are less likely to have complications. Healthy nonpregnant adults younger than 50 years who are not close contacts of immunocompromised individuals in special care units can receive LAIV or IIV. All other individuals should only be given IIV, and for adults aged 65 years or older there is an option to use an alternative high-dose IIV.

B. Tetanus, diphtheria, and acellular pertussis (Tdap/Td). Adults who have completed a primary series of pediatric tetanus and diphtheria vaccinations should continue to receive a tetanus booster every 10 years. Adult immunization against pertussis has recently been added to standard recommendations to help reduce transmission from nonimmune and mildly infected adults to children and adolescents who are more vulnerable to pertussis. All adults who have not previously received Tdap or for whom vaccine status is unknown should receive Tdap regardless of interval since the most recent tetanus or diphtheria-toxoid containing vaccine, then continue with Tetanus–Diphtheria Td booster immunizations every 10 years. Tdap should also be given to all pregnant women during each pregnancy (ideally between 27 and 36 weeks' gestation), regardless of number of years since prior Td or Tdap vaccination. Those who have not completed a primary series should receive three doses of Tetanus toxoid (two doses Td and one dose Tdap), with the second dose 4 weeks after the first, and the third dose 6 months after the second.

   1. Wounds. During routine wound management, tetanus toxoid administration is not required unless more than 10 years has elapsed since the last dose for clean, minor wounds. For contaminated or deep wounds, a booster is recommended if it has been longer than 5 years since the last dose or the immunization history is unclear. Tetanus immune globulin (250 IU intramuscularly) is also indicated for contaminated wounds in those with uncertain histories or with less than three primary Td doses.

C. Varicella. All adults without a reliable history of varicella immunity should be assumed susceptible and offered immunization with two doses at least 4 weeks apart to decrease the risk of severe varicella, pneumonia, hepatitis, or encephalitis. Pregnant women without evidence of immunity should receive a first dose of varicella vaccine upon completion of pregnancy and before discharge from the healthcare facility, with a second dose 4 to 8 weeks later. A reliable history of varicella immunity includes documentation of prior age-appropriate vaccination, laboratory confirmation of immunity or of varicella disease, birth in the United States before 1980 (except for healthcare personnel and pregnant women), or healthcare professional diagnosis of chickenpox or zoster.

D. Human papilloma virus (HPV2 and HPV4). HPV2 (for females) or HPV4 (for males or females) should be offered to all individuals aged 26 years or younger who have not previously been vaccinated against HPV, at the same intervals as recommended for adolescents.

E. Zoster vaccine is a live attenuated varicella zoster virus (VZV) used to boost active immunity to VZV to reduce the risk of developing Zoster (shingles) and postherpetic neuralgia in older adults. It is not recommended for individuals who have received prior immunization with the varicella vaccine. A single dose of zoster vaccine should be given to all adults aged 60 years or over, whether or not they have had a prior episode of zoster (shingles). Chronic medical conditions are not a contraindication to zoster vaccination, unless there is a specific contraindication such as severe immunodeficiency or pregnancy. The vaccine may be given to patients as young as age 50 years, but the CDC recommends administration at age 60 years or older.

F. Measles–mumps–rubella (MMR). All persons born in 1957 or later who lack evidence of immunity to measles, mumps, or rubella or do not have documentation of having received MMR on or after their first birthday should receive one dose of MMR vaccine. Persons born in 1956 or before are generally assumed to be immune. MMR or other live-virus vaccines should not be given during pregnancy. Any woman who is not pregnant and who has no history of MMR vaccination or evidence of immunity to rubella should be immunized with MMR or rubella vaccine and agree to avoid pregnancy for 3 months. Susceptible pregnant women should be immunized in the immediate postpartum period, with the same instructions.

G. Pneumococcal polysaccharide vaccination (PPSV23). The 23-valent PPSV23 should be given to all adults aged 65 years or older because of their high risk of complications from pneumococcal disease. Adults younger than 65 years who smoke, have chronic cardiovascular disease, chronic pulmonary disease (chronic obstructive pulmonary disease or asthma), diabetes mellitus, alcoholism, chronic liver disease, cerebrospinal fluid leaks, cochlear implants, depression, absent spleen function (e.g., caused by sickle cell disease or splenectomy), immunosuppression, or anyone living in a chronic-care facility are also at risk of pneumococcal disease and should be vaccinated. Immunocompromised adults should be given both PCV13 and PPSV23 vaccines, the latter given at least 8 weeks after the PCV13 (see below).

1. One-time **revaccination** after an interval of 5 years is recommended for: (1) those younger than 65 years who received the vaccine because of chronic renal failure or nephrotic syndrome, functional or anatomic asplenia, or any immunocompromising condition, and (2) those aged 65 years or older whose first dose was before age 65 years.

H. Pneumococcal conjugate vaccine (PCV13). The PCV13 vaccine should be given to anyone aged 19 years or older with chronic renal failure or nephrotic syndrome, functional or anatomic asplenia, CSF leaks or cochlear implants, and who have not previously been vaccinated with PCV13 or PPSV23. Vaccination is followed by a one-time dose of PPSV23 at least 8 weeks later.

I. Meningococcal conjugate vaccine (MCV4). MCV4 is recommended for first-year college students up through age 21 years living in dormitories and for military recruits, if not previously vaccinated on or after their 16th birthday. Individuals should also be vaccinated if they are at increased risk of disease because of depressed or absent spleen function (e.g., caused by sickle cell disease or splenectomy), terminal complement component deficiencies, occupational exposure in a research or clinical setting, or travel to an endemic area (especially the "meningitis belt" of sub-Saharan Africa from Senegal to Ethiopia). MCV4 is recommended for anyone younger than 55 years, although MPSV4 is an acceptable alternative. MPSV4 should be used for all adults older than 55 years, and revaccination after 5 years can be considered for adults previously vaccinated with MPSV4 who remain at high risk for infection.

J. HAV. Immunization against HAV should be given as two doses separated by at least 6 months to adults who live in endemic areas or travel internationally to countries with endemic HAV. Other groups at risk who should be immunized are men who have sex with men, users of illegal drugs, patients with clotting factor disorders, patients with chronic liver disease, and those with occupational exposure to HAV.

1. **Immediate postexposure protection** against HAV can be achieved with immune serum globulin (ISG) given within 2 weeks of exposure to close household and sexual contacts of persons with HAV and to healthcare workers and patients in centers with active cases of HAV. ISG affords protection against HAV for 3 to 6 months, depending on the dose given.

2. The protective effect of HAV immunization takes 4 weeks to develop, but protection lasts for at least 10 years. For international travelers, it may be necessary to administer ISG at a different site, in addition to the vaccine, if travel is anticipated before 4 weeks has elapsed.

K. HBV vaccination should be offered to persons with occupational risk (healthcare workers and public service workers), persons with lifestyle risk (sexually active persons who are not in a long-term mutually monogamous relationship, men who have sex with men, persons seeking treatment for sexually transmitted infection, and injectable drug users), persons with hepatitis C or hemophilia, hemodialysis patients, and those with environmental risk factors (including household or sexual contacts of HBV carriers, prison inmates, and immigrants from HBV-endemic areas). All pregnant women should be screened prenatally for active HBV infection (HBsAg positive).

1. HBV vaccine is administered in three doses, with a second dose given 1 month later and the third dose given at 6 months. Though not routinely recommended, booster doses of HBV vaccine and pre- and postimmunization serologic testing may be considered, based on the patient's risk factors.

2. Postexposure prophylaxis using HBIG, in addition to the HBV vaccine series, should be offered to persons with percutaneous or mucous-membrane exposure to blood or secretions known to be HBsAg positive, as soon as possible after exposure (within 72 hours).

IV. Combination Vaccines

Combination vaccines allow adequate administration of recommended vaccines with fewer total injections, but only US Food and Drug Administration-licensed combination vaccines should be used. Combination vaccines are appropriate when any component vaccine is indicated and none of the component vaccines are contraindicated. Whenever possible, a vaccine series should be completed with all doses coming from the same manufacturer.

SELECTED REFERENCES

Centers for Disease Control and Prevention: Adult Immunization Schedules. http://www.cdc.gov/vaccines/schedules/hcp/adult.html. Accessed June 2013.

Centers for Disease Control and Prevention: Birth-18 Years & "Catch-up" Immunization Schedules. http://www.cdc.gov/vaccines/schedules/hcp/child-adolescent.html. Accessed June 2013.

Centers for Disease Control and Prevention: Vaccines and Immunizations. http://www.cdc.gov/vaccines./ Accessed June 2013.

General Recommendations on Immunization. Recommendations of the Advisory Committee on Immunization Practices (ACIP). *MMWR Recomm Rep.* 2011;60(RR2):1–64. Available at http://www.cdc.gov/mmwr/preview/mmwrhtml/rr6002a1.htm. Accessed June 2013

Shots Online (sponsored by the Group on Immunization Education of the Society of Teachers of Family Medicine and the Centers for Disease Control and Prevention). http://www.immunizationed.org./ Accessed June 2013.

---

106   Screening Tests

Larry L. Dickey, MD, MPH

KEY POINTS

- The following screening tests and examinations should be considered for children and adults.
  - **A.** Children
    - **1.** Body measurement
      - **a.** Head circumference (until age 2 years) (SOR **C***)
      - **b.** Height and weight (SOR **B**)
      - **c.** Blood pressure (beginning at age 3 years) (SOR **C**)
    - **2.** Blood tests
      - **a.** Hypothyroidism, phenylketonuria, hemoglobinopathies (newborns) (SOR **A**)
      - **b.** Anemia (at 6–12 months, adolescent girls at risk) (SOR **C**)
      - **c.** Glucose (high risk) (SOR **C**)
      - **d.** Lead (universal or high risk at 12 and 24 months) (SOR **C**)
      - **e.** Cholesterol (between ages 9–11 years and 17–21 years) (SOR **C**)
    - **3.** Sensory screening
      - **a.** Hearing (newborns, children, and adolescents) (SOR **B**, SOR **C**, SOR **C**)
      - **b.** Vision (amblyopia/strabismus until age 3–4 years, acuity beginning at age 3–4 years) (SOR **B**)
    - **4.** Mental health screening
      - **a.** Depression (adolescents) (SOR **C**)
    - **5.** Infectious diseases tests
      - **a.** Hepatitis C (high risk) (SOR **B**)
      - **b.** Human immunodeficiency virus (HIV) (age 15–17 years and high risk at other ages) (SOR **A**)
      - **c.** Chlamydia (all sexually active adolescents) (SOR **A**)
      - **d.** Gonorrhea/syphilis (high-risk adolescents) (SOR **B**/SOR **A**)
      - **e.** Tuberculosis (high risk) (SOR **A**)
  - **B.** Adults
    - **1.** Body measurement
      - **a.** Height and weight (SOR **B**)
      - **b.** Blood pressure (SOR **A**)
      - **c.** Bone density (women, beginning at age 65 years) (SOR **B**)
      - **d.** Abdominal aortic ultrasound once (men, smokers, age 65–75 years) (SOR **B**)
    - **2.** Blood tests
      - **a.** Anemia (pregnant women) (SOR **B**)
      - **b.** Cholesterol (men ≥35 years of age, women over age 44 years at high risk) (SOR **A**)

    c. Cholesterol (men aged 20–34 years at high risk, women over age 20–44 years at high risk) (SOR **B**)

    d. Glucose (adults with sustained high blood pressure) (SOR **B**)

    e. Glucose (adults over age 44 years and younger adults at high risk) (SOR **C**)

    f. Thyroid (high risk) (SOR **C**)

3. Sensory screenings

    a. Hearing (beginning at age 65 years) (SOR **C**)

    b. Vision (age 65 years and older) (SOR **B**)

    c. Glaucoma (high risk) (SOR **C**)

4. Mental health screening

    a. Depression (adults if management systems in place) (SOR **B**)

5. Infectious diseases tests

    a. Hepatitis C (high risk and once if born between 1945 and 1965) (SOR **B**)

    b. HIV (age 18–65 years and high risk at other ages) (SOR **A**)

    c. Chlamydia (sexually active females <25 years and high risk) (SOR **A**)

    d. Gonorrhea/syphilis (high risk, pregnant women) (SOR **B**/SOR **A**)

    e. Tuberculosis (high risk) (SOR **A**)

6. Cancer tests

    a. Clinical breast examination (women ≥50 years) (SOR **C**)

    b. Mammogram every 2 years (women aged 50–74 years) (SOR **B**)

    c. Cervical—Pap smear (women aged 21–65 years with a uterus) (SOR **A**)

    d. Colorectal screening (stool guaiac cards, flexible sigmoidoscopy, barium enema, or colonoscopy age 50–75 years) (SOR **A**)

    e. Prostate examination and prostate-specific antigen (discuss with black men aged 45–70 years and other men aged 50-70 years) (SOR **C**)

    f. Skin examination (high risk) (SOR **C**)

    g. Thyroid examination (high risk) (SOR **C**)

*Expert opinion by at least one national advisory body other than the USPSTF (I rating for these).

I. Definitions

The strength of recommendations for this chapter is given using the rating system of the US Preventive Services Task Force (USPSTF). The meaning of the A, B, C, D, and I ratings are explained in Table 106–1. For screening tests that have not been rated by the USPSTF, strength of recommendations ratings is not given. The strength of recommendation ratings of other organizations for screening tests, if available, is not provided since the USPSTF is widely recognized as the leading authority in accessing the strength of scientific evidence for preventive services.

Characteristics of a good screening test include the following:

- The test is acceptable to the patient (i.e., not particularly painful, easy to do).
- Confers minimal risk at a reasonable cost.
- Is accurate (i.e., has a high sensitivity and specificity).
- Can detect the disease when it is asymptomatic.
- The condition is such that early diagnosis affects outcome (e.g., treating early improves outcome).

II. Body Measurement Screening

A. Head circumference. The American Academy of Pediatrics (AAP) has recommended measurement of head circumference at every visit until a child is 2 years old. Other authorities have not made recommendations for or against this. Measuring head circumference can help identify microcephaly (<2 SDs below the mean or <10th percentile) and macrocephaly (<2 SDs above the mean or >90th percentile) which are associated with a number of conditions that require additional investigation.

B. Height and weight. Most major authorities recommend regular measurement of height and weight at all ages (USPSTF B for children and adults). For children and adolescents, these can be plotted using age-specific growth curve charts. For adults, standard height and weight or body mass index (BMI) charts can be used for assessing norms. Several authorities recommend periodic calculation and charting of body mass index (BMI = weight [kg]/height^2 [m]), since BMI is believed to be more reflective of total body fat than weight for height norms. According to the US Department of Agriculture, BMI of 25 or more constitutes overweight for adults, the point at which negative health consequences begin.

TABLE 106–1. U.S. PREVENTIVE SERVICES TASK FORCE (USPSTF) RATINGS: WHAT THE GRADES MEAN AND SUGGESTIONS FOR PRACTICE

Grade	Definition	Suggestions for Practice
A	The USPSTF recommends the service. There is high certainty that the net benefit is substantial.	Offer or provide this service.
B	The USPSTF recommends the service. There is high certainty that the net benefit is moderate or there is moderate certainty that the net benefit is moderate to substantial.	Offer or provide this service.
C	The USPSTF recommends selectively offering or providing this service to individual patients based on professional judgment and patient preferences. There is at least moderate certainty that the net benefit is small.	Offer or provide this service for selected patients depending on individual circumstances.
D	The USPSTF recommends against the service. There is moderate or high certainty that the service has no net benefit or that the harms outweigh the benefits.	Discourage the use of this service.
I Statement	The USPSTF concludes that the current evidence is insufficient to assess the balance of benefits and harms of the service. Evidence is lacking, of poor quality, or conflicting, and the balance of benefits and harms cannot be determined.	Read the clinical considerations section of USPSTF Recommendation Statement. If the service is offered, patients should understand the uncertainty about the balance of benefits and harms.

Source: Adapted with permission from USPSTF at http://www.ahrq.gov/professionals/clinicians-providers/resources/aspprovider.html.

Underweight is BMI <18.5 and very severely underweight is BMI <15. The AAP classifies children with BMIs >95th percentile as obese and children with BMIs between the 85th and 95th percentiles to be at risk of being overweight. Growth charts and BMI calculators can be found on the Centers for Disease Control and Prevention websites http://www.cdc.gov/growthcharts/ and http://www.cdc.gov/healthyweight/assessing/bmi/index.html.

C. Waist/hip measurement. Some authorities, such as the US Department of Health and Human Services, recommend measurement of waist and hip circumferences and calculation of waist/hip ratio (WHR) for adults. By some reports, this may be a more accurate predictor of negative health consequences than height/weight or BMI values. Upper limits of healthy WHR values are usually cited as 0.8 for women and 1.0 for men. According to the National Heart, Lung, and Blood Institute, an abdominal circumference of >40 inches for men and >35 inches for women constitutes abdominal obesity and should be considered a cardiovascular disease risk factor.

D. Blood pressure

1. Children and adolescents. The AAP and National Heart Lung and Blood Institute (NHLBI) recommend yearly blood pressure screening of all children beginning at age 3 years. For children, values above the 95th percentile are considered elevated (Table 106–2). The USPSTF found insufficient evidence to recommend for or against

TABLE 106–2. 95TH PERCENTILE OF BLOOD PRESSURE BY SELECTED AGES IN GIRLS AND BOYS, BY THE 50TH AND 75TH HEIGHT PERCENTILES

Age (years)	Girls' SBP/DPB		Boys' SBP/DBP	
	50th Percentile for Height	75th Percentile for Height	50th Percentile for Height	75th Percentile for Height
1	104/58	105/59	102/57	104/58
6	111/73	112/73	114/74	115/75
12	123/80	124/81	123/81	125/82
17	129/84	130/85	136/87	138/88

DBP, diastolic blood pressure; SBP, systolic blood pressure.
Source: Reprinted from National Institutes of Health. *The Sixth Report of the Joint National Committee on Prevention, Detection, Evaluation, and Treatment of High Blood Pressure.* US Department of Health and Human Services; 1997. NIH publication 98-4080.

routine screening of children and adolescents, stating that evidence is poor that routine blood pressure measurement accurately identifies children and adolescents at increased risk for cardiovascular disease or that treatment of elevated blood pressure in children or adolescents decreases the incidence of cardiovascular disease (USPSTF I).

2. Adults. All authorities recommend regular routine screening of adults for elevated blood pressure (USPSTF A). The NHLBI recommends screening every 2 years for persons with systolic blood pressure <130 mm Hg and diastolic blood pressure <85 mm Hg, with more frequent screening for adults with higher pressures. The USPSTF has found insufficient evidence to recommend an optimal screening interval.

    a. For adults, systolic pressures ≥140 mm Hg and diastolic pressures ≥90 mm Hg are considered elevated. Target (or goal) blood pressure, however, may be lower than <140/90 for individuals with certain health conditions such as diabetes (<140/80; American Diabetes Association [ADA]) or chronic kidney disease (<130/80; Joint National Commission [JNC]).

    b. Elevated values should be confirmed on at least one or two additional visits before hypertension is diagnosed.

    c. The NHLBI classifies adult systolic pressures >120 mm Hg or diastolic pressures >80 mm Hg as "prehypertension," for which lifestyle modifications should be considered.

E. Bone density. The USPSTF recommends routine screening for normal-risk women aged 65 years or older (USPSTF B). The USPSTF has found insufficient evidence to recommend screening for men (USPSTF I). The National Osteoporosis Foundation recommends bone density testing for all women aged 65 years or older and all men aged 70 years or older. It also recommends bone density testing for postmenopausal women younger than 65 years and men aged 50 to 69 years if there is a concern about osteoporosis based on their risk factor profile. Although the optimal interval screening is not determined, intervals of at least 2 years may be necessary to detect changes.

F. Abdominal aortic ultrasound. The USPSTF recommends one-time screening for abdominal aortic aneurysm (AAA) by ultrasonography in men aged 65 to 75 years who have ever smoked (USPSTF B). For this group, the moderate magnitude of net benefit from surgery outweighs the potential harms. The USPSTF has made no recommendation for or against screening for AAA in men aged 65 to 75 years who have never smoked (USPSTF C) and recommends against screening for women (USPSTF D).

III. Blood Test Screening

  A. Cholesterol

    1. Children and adolescents. An expert panel convened by the NHLBI issued recommendations in 2011 for routine screening between the ages of 9 and 11 years and again between 17 and 21 years with a non-fasting, non-HDL-C level. The rationale for this new guideline is that early atherosclerosis is present in some young patients with elevated cholesterol and early treatment of cardiovascular risk factors in youth can be effective. In addition, with increasing numbers of obese children, lipid disorders are becoming more common in children and are often missed using the traditional selective screening methods. The USPSTF has not issued recommendations for cholesterol screening of children and adolescents.

    2. Adults. Recommendations vary regarding screening of adults. The most aggressive recommendations are those of the National Cholesterol Education Program (NCEP), which recommends screening all adults at least once every 5 years for total cholesterol and at the same time, if accurate results are available, for high-density lipoprotein (HDL) cholesterol. The USPSTF recommends screening for all men aged 35 years and older (USPSTF A) and for men aged 20 to 35 years who are at an increased risk for coronary heart disease (USPSTF B). Screening women ages 20–45 years (USPSTF B) and over 45 years (USPSTF A) if they are at increased risk of coronary heart disease. The USPSTF does not make recommendations about screening men aged 20 to 35 years or women who are not at an increased risk (USPSTF C).

      a. The USPSTF states that the optimal interval for screening is uncertain. On the basis of other guidelines and expert opinion, reasonable options include every 5 years, with shorter intervals for people who have lipid levels close to those warranting therapy and longer intervals for those not at an increased risk who have had repeatedly normal lipid levels.

b. The NCEP has classified cholesterol level in adults without coronary artery disease as follows: desirable (total <200 mg/dL, LDL <130 mg/dL); borderline (total 200–239 mg/dL, LDL 130–159 mg/dL); and high (total ≥240 mg/dL, LDL ≥160 mg/dL). The NCEP considers HDL levels <35 and ≥60 mg/dL to be positive and negative risk factors, respectively, for coronary artery disease.

B. Glucose

1. Children and adolescents. Because of the growing prevalence of type II diabetes in children and adolescents, the ADA recommends plasma glucose screening at 2-year intervals for overweight children and adolescents (BMI >85th percentile) beginning at age 10 years with any two of the following risk factors: a family history of type II diabetes in first- or second-degree relatives; belonging to a high-risk race/ethnic group (Native American, African American, Hispanic American, and Asian/South Pacific Islander); or having signs of insulin resistance or conditions associated with insulin resistance (acanthosis nigricans, hypertension, dyslipidemia, and polycystic ovary syndrome). The USPSTF has not evaluated diabetes screening in children.

2. Adults. The USPSTF recommends screening for type 2 diabetes in asymptomatic adults with sustained blood pressure (either treated or untreated) greater than 135/80 mm Hg (USPSTF B). The USPSTF found that the current evidence is insufficient to assess the balance of benefits and harms of screening for type 2 diabetes in asymptomatic adults with blood pressure of 135/80 mm Hg or lower (USPSTF I).

a. The ADA recommends screening at 3-year intervals for adults aged 45 years or older. Younger adults should be screened if they have a BMI of >25 kg/m² and have at least one of the following risk factors for diabetes: physical inactivity, first-degree relative with diabetes, high-risk race/ethnicity (e.g., African-American, Latino, Native American, Asian-American, Pacific Islander), women who delivered a baby weighing ≥9 lbs or who were diagnosed with gestational diabetes mellitus, hypertension, HDL cholesterol level <35 mg/dL and/or a triglyceride level >250 mg/dL, women with polycystic ovary syndrome, A1C ≥5.7%, other clinical conditions associated with insulin resistance such as severe obesity or acanthosis nigricans, or a history of coronary vascular disease.

b. The ADA recommends the following thresholds for diagnosing diabetes mellitus: A1C ≥6.5%, fasting blood glucose ≥126 mg/dL, 2-hour plasma glucose ≥200 mg/dL, or in a patient with classic symptoms of hyperglycemia or hyperglycemic crisis, a random plasma glucose level of ≥200 mg/dL. In the absence of hyperglycemic symptoms, abnormal test results should be confirmed by repeat testing on a second occasion.

C. Hemoglobin/hematocrit

1. Children and adolescents. The AAP recommends screening all children for anemia once between 9 and 12 months of age and then annually for children and adolescents at high risk for anemia. According to the Centers for Disease Control and Prevention (CDC), the cutoff points for defining anemia in children aged 6 months to 2 years are hemoglobin ≤11.0 g/dL and hematocrit ≤33.0%. The USPSTF has found insufficient evidence to recommend for or against screening for anemia in children (USPSTF I). The American Congress of Obstetricians and Gynecologists (ACOG) recommends screening adolescents beginning at age 13 years belonging to a high-risk race/ethnic group (Caribbean, Latin American, Asian, Mediterranean, or African ancestry) or with a history of excessive menstrual flow.

2. Adults. No major authority recommends routine screening of asymptomatic, non-pregnant adults for anemia. The USPSTF recommends screening pregnant women (USPSTF B). ACOG recommends periodic screening of women with a history of excessive menstrual flow and women of Caribbean, Latin American, Asian, Mediterranean, or African ancestry. In nonpregnant women and adolescent girls older than 15 years, the cutpoints for anemia are hemoglobin ≤12 g/dL and hematocrit ≤36%.

D. Lead. In 1997, the **CDC** recommended that state health officials develop plans for targeted blood lead level (BLL) screening of children based on assessments of the lead exposure and screening capacity in specific regions of the state. For targeted screening, the CDC recommends screening of children who reside in a zip code in which >27% of housing was built before 1950; receive services from public assistance programs for the poor, such as Medicaid or the Supplemental Food Program for Women, Infants, and Children; or whose parents answer "yes" or "don't know" to any of the three questions of a personal-risk questionnaire (Table 106–3). In areas where exposure to lead

TABLE 106–3. BASIC LEAD PERSONAL RISK PROFILE

1   Does your child live in or regularly visit a house that was built before 1950? This question could apply to a
    facility such as a home day-care center or the home of a babysitter or relative
2   Does your child live in or regularly visit a house built before 1978 with recent or ongoing renovations or
    remodeling (within the last 6 months)?
3   Does your child have a sibling or playmate who has or did have lead poisoning?

Source: Reprinted from Centers for Disease Control and Prevention. *Screening Young Children for Lead Poisoning:
Guidance for State and Local Public Health Officials.* US Department of Health and Human Services; 1997.

from older housing is unlikely, the CDC states that the personal-risk questionnaire could
contain questions about other risk factors, such as parental occupation or use of lead-
containing ceramic ware or traditional remedies. In the absence of a targeted screening
plan or other formal guidance from state health officials, the CDC recommends universal
screening of all children aged 12 and 24 months and of children aged 36 to 72 months
not previously screened. In 2010, the CDC deleted the recommendation for universal
screening of Medicaid-eligible children.

1. **Diagnostic testing** of venous blood should be performed for children with elevated BLLs >5 μg/dL at a follow-up interval based on degree of elevation of BLL (see
   Table 106–4).

2. **The USPSTF found insufficient evidence** to recommend routine screening for
   high-risk children 1 to 5 years of age (USPSTF I) and recommends against screening
   of normal-risk children and asymptomatic pregnant women (USPSTF D).

E. **Newborn screening.** The AAP and other authorities recommend that newborn screening be performed according to each state's regulations. Using new tandem mass spec-
   troscopy technology, several states have recently expanded required screening to 30
   or more conditions. National authorities have made recommendations for the following
   important conditions:

   1. **Hypothyroidism.** The AAP, American Thyroid Association (ATA), and USPSTF
      (USPSTF A) recommend that all neonates be screened for congenital hypothyroidism
      between 2 and 6 days of life. Care should be taken to ensure that infants born at
      home, ill at birth, or transferred between hospitals in the first week of life are screened
      before 7 days of life.

   2. **Phenylketonuria (PKU).** The American Academy of Family Physicians (AAFP) and
      USPSTF (USPSTF A) recommend that all infants be screened for PKU prior to discharge
      from the nursery. Premature infants and those with illnesses should be tested at or
      near 7 days of age. Infants tested before 24 hours of age should receive a repeat
      screening. According to the USPSTF, this should occur by the time the infant is 2 weeks
      of age.

**TABLE 106–4. SCHEDULE FOR DIAGNOSTIC TESTING OF A CHILD WITH AN ELEVATED BLOOD LEAD
LEVEL ON A SCREENING TEST[a]**

If Result of Screening Test (μ/dL) Is:	Perform Diagnostic Test on Venous Blood Within:
10[b]–19	3 months
20–44	1 month–1 week[a]
45–59	48 h
60–69	24 h
≥70	Immediately as an emergency laboratory test

[a]The higher the screening blood lead level, the more urgent the need for a diagnostic test.
[b]In 2012, the CDC issued guidance that children with BLLs greater than 5 μg/dL undergo ongoing monitoring of
BLLs. These children should also be assessed for iron deficiency and general nutrition (e.g., calcium and vitamin C
levels), consistent with American Academy of Pediatrics (AAP) guidelines. Iron-deficient children should be provided
with iron supplements.
Source: Reprinted from Centers for Disease Control and Prevention. *Screening Young Children for Lead Poisoning:
Guidance for State and Local Public Health Officials.* Washington, DC: US Department of Health and Human
Services; 1997.

3. Hemoglobinopathies. The Sickle Cell Disease Guideline Panel of the Agency for Health Care Policy and Research, US Public Health Service, has recommended universal screening of newborns for sickle cell disease. This recommendation has been endorsed by the AAP, American Nurses Association, and AMA. The USPSTF has also recommended neonatal screening for sickle hemoglobinopathies (USPSTF A), but it has stated that whether screening should be universal or targeted to high-risk groups should depend on the proportion of high-risk persons in the screening area. All screening must be accompanied by comprehensive counseling and treatment services.

F. Thyroid function. No authorities recommend screening of asymptomatic adults for thyroid dysfunctions. ACOG recommends measurement of thyroid-stimulating hormone (TSH) levels in adult women with a strong family history of thyroid disease or autoimmune disease. The USPSTF has found insufficient evidence for screening of asymptomatic persons, stating that although the yield of screening is greater in certain high-risk groups (e.g., postpartum women, people with Down syndrome, and the elderly), there is poor evidence that screening these groups leads to clinically important benefits (USPSTF I).

IV. Sensory Screening
A. Hearing
1. Children. The Joint Committee on Infant Hearing (composed of the AAP, American Speech-Language-Hearing Association, American Academy of Otolaryngology—Head and Neck Surgery, and American Academy of Audiology) has endorsed universal screening of all neonates. These authorities recommend screening neonates for hearing impairment prior to hospital discharge, but before 3 months of age. The USPSTF recommends screening all newborns for hearing loss (USPSTF B). The AAFP is in the process of updating its recommendation. The AAP recommends routine screening of asymptomatic children with pure-tone audiometry at ages 3, 4, 5, 10, 12, 15, and 18 years. The Joint Committee on Infant Hearing has identified recurrent or persistent otitis media with effusion for at least 3 months to be a risk factor requiring screening.

2. Adults. The USPSTF in 2012 found insufficient evidence to recommend screening adults aged 50 years or older for hearing impairment (USPSTF I). The American Speech-Language-Hearing Association recommends that adults be screened once per decade and every 3 years after age 50 years.

B. Vision
1. Children. Recommendations regarding vision screening for children vary among authorities. The AAP recommends questioning parents regarding a child's vision at well-child visits, with the first objective test of visual acuity at age 3 years. If the child is uncooperative, this should be rescheduled 6 months later. Subsequent objective testing is recommended at 4, 5, 10, 12, 15, and 18 years of age. The USPSTF recommends screening to detect amblyopia, strabismus, and defects in visual acuity in children younger than 5 years (USPSTF B) and states that the choice of tests should be influenced by the child's age.

   a. During the first year of life, **strabismus** can be assessed by the cover test and the Hirschberg light reflex test. Screening children younger than 3 years for visual acuity typically requires testing by specially trained personnel. Newer automated techniques can be used to test these children. In children older than 3 years, **stereopsis** (the ability of both eyes to function together) can be assessed with the Random Dot E test or Titmus Fly Stereotest; **visual acuity** can be assessed by tests such as the HOTV chart, Lea symbols, or the tumbling E.

   b. The USPSTF has found insufficient evidence to recommend for or against routine visual acuity testing of schoolchildren (USPSTF I), because refractive errors of consequence present symptomatically and respond to corrective lenses without lasting effects.

2. Adults. Recommendations for vision screening of adults vary considerably among authorities.

   a. Visual acuity. All major authorities recommend routine visual acuity screening for normal-risk adults beginning at age 65 years (USPSTF B).

   b. Eye examination. The American Academy of Ophthalmology recommends a comprehensive eye examination for normal-risk adults every 5 to 10 years until age 39 years, every 3 to 4 years 40 to 54 years of age, and every 1 to 2 years 65 years of age and older. The National Eye Institute recommends comprehensive eye examinations every 2 years starting at age 60 years, with examinations beginning at age 40 years for African Americans. All authorities recommend frequent, yearly, comprehensive eye examinations by eye care specialists for patients with diabetes mellitus. The USPSTF has not assessed comprehensive eye examinations but has found insufficient evidence to recommend routine screening for glaucoma (USPSTF I), stating that it is unclear whether earlier detection and treatment of people with increased intraocular pressure or early primary open-angle glaucoma reduces impairment in vision-related function or quality of life.

V. Mental Health and Cognition

A. Depression. The USPSTF recommends screening adults for depression in clinical practices that have systems in place to assure accurate diagnosis, effective treatment, and follow-up (USPSTF B). The USPSTF found limited evidence on the accuracy and reliability of screening tests and on the effectiveness of therapy in children and adolescents identified in primary care settings (USPSTF I).

    1. Although formal **screening tools** (such as the Beck Depression Inventory or the Zung Self-Assessment Depression Scale) are available, the USPSTF states that **asking two simple questions** ("Over the past 2 weeks, have you felt down, depressed, or hopeless?" and "Over the past 2 weeks, have you felt little interest or pleasure in doing things?") may be as effective as using long instruments.

    2. The AAP recommends that clinicians ask questions about depression in history-taking with **adolescents,** and the AMA recommends screening for depression and treating adolescents who may be at risk because of family problems, drug or alcohol use, or other risk factors.

B. Dementia. Although instruments such as the Mini-Mental State Examination are often used for screening older adults, the USPSTF has found insufficient evidence to recommend for or against routine screening of asymptomatic older adults for dementia (USPSTF I). The USPSTF recommends that clinicians assess cognitive function whenever cognitive impairment or deterioration is suspected.

VI. Infectious Disease

A. Hepatitis C. In recognition of the heavy burden of disease caused by hepatitis C (1.8% of the US population infected, >US $600 million in medical and work-loss expenses annually), the CDC has recommended screening of high-risk populations. The USPSTF recommends screening for hepatitis C virus (HCV) infection in persons at a high risk for infection. The USPSTF also recommends offering one-time screening for HCV infection to adults born between 1945 and 1965 (USPSTF B).

B. Human immunodeficiency virus. The USPSTF recommends that clinicians screen for HIV infection in adolescents and adults aged 15 to 65 years. Younger adolescents and older adults who are at increased risk should also be screened (USPSTF A). Because of the high efficiency of anti-viral treatment for preventing maternal-fetal transmission, the USPSTF and other major authorities recommend that clinicians screen all pregnant women for HIV, including those who present in labor who are untested and whose HIV status is unknown (USPSTF A). All major authorities recommend that HIV screening be offered to patients at risk: those with another sexually transmitted infections (STIs), homosexual and bisexual men; past or present injectable drug users; persons with a history of prostitution or multiple sexual partners; persons whose past (or present) sexual partners are HIV-infected or injectable drug users, or both; patients with a history of blood transfusion between 1978 and 1985; and persons born in, or with long-term residence in, a community in which HIV is prevalent.

C. Other STIs (see Chapter 102).

    1. Chlamydia. The AAP and AMA advocate screening all sexually active adolescents for STIs. The USPSTF recommends screening all sexually active females younger than 25 years and other high-risk adult women for chlamydia (USPSTF A). Chlamydia risk factors include a history of prior STIs, a new partner or multiple sex partners, inconsistent barrier contraceptive use, cervical ectopy, and being unmarried. The USPSTF has made no recommendation for screening women aged 25 years or older who are not at high risk (USPSTF C) and has found insufficient evidence to recommend screening men (USPSTF I).

    2. Gonorrhea. All major authorities recommend screening women at high risk for gonorrhea (USPSTF B). Women at risk include commercial sex workers, those with repeated episodes of gonorrhea, and women younger than 25 years with two or more sex partners in the last year. The USPSTF has found insufficient evidence to recommend for or against screening asymptomatic males at high risk for gonorrhea (USPSTF I) and has recommended against screening individuals not at high risk for gonorrhea (USPSTF D). Although dipstick leukocyte testing is convenient and inexpensive, its positive predictive value has been found to be as low as 11% for chlamydia and 30% for gonorrhea. Thus, confirmation with more specific tests is required for all positive results.

3. Syphilis. All major authorities recommend that screening be performed for persons at high risk for infection (USPSTF A). These persons include sexual partners of known syphilis cases, those with multiple sexual partners—especially in high-prevalence areas, prostitutes or those who trade sex for drugs, and males who engage in sex with other males. The USPSTF has recommended against the routine screening of normal-risk populations (USPSTF D). In 2009, the USPSTF recommended screening for all pregnant women (USPSTF A).

  a. Because the causative agent of syphilis cannot be cultured, screening relies on serology. A nontreponemal test, either the Venereal Disease Research Laboratory (VDRL) or rapid plasma reagin (RPR), is recommended for initial screening. Because the specificity of these tests is limited, follow-up testing with a treponemal test, such as the FTA (fluorescent treponemal antibody), is required for positive results.

  b. Because the sensitivity of nontreponemal tests may be as low as 75% in primary syphilis, **patients who have had recent sexual contact with a person with a documented case of syphilis should be treated,** even if serologic tests are negative.

D. Tuberculosis (TB). All major authorities recommend screening persons at high risk for TB (USPSTF A). In general, authorities have not specified how often high-risk persons should be screened, although the AAP has recommended annual screening for children at risk. Populations at risk include (1) medically underserved, low-income populations, including those of African American, Hispanic, Asian, Native American, and Alaskan Native heritage; (2) foreign-born persons from high-prevalence countries (e.g., Asia, Africa, and Latin America); (3) persons in close contact with infectious TB cases (sharing accommodations as well as playing or working in the same enclosed area); (4) alcoholics and injectable drug users; (5) residents of high-risk environments including long-term care facilities, correctional institutions, and mental institutions; and (6) persons with medical conditions known to substantially increase the risk of TB, such as HIV infection, diabetes mellitus, and chronic renal failure.

1. The appropriate **criterion for defining a positive skin-test reaction** depends on the likelihood of TB exposure and the risk of TB if exposure has occurred. For persons with HIV infection, close contacts of infectious cases, and those with fibrotic lesions on chest radiograph, a reaction of ≥5 mm is considered positive. For other at-risk persons, including all infants and children younger than 4 years, a reaction of ≥10 mm is considered positive. Persons who are not likely to be infected with *Mycobacterium tuberculosis* should generally not be skin tested because the predictive value of a positive skin test in low-risk populations is poor. If a skin test is performed on a person who is not in a high-risk category or who is not exposed in a high-risk environment, a cutoff point of ≥15 mm is considered positive, although prophylaxis with isoniazid is not necessarily recommended for these persons.

VII. Cancer Screening

A. Breast cancer

1. Clinical breast examination (CBE). Most major authorities recommend regular CBEs for women aged 50 years and older. The American Cancer Society (ACS) recommends CBE every 3 years for women aged 20 to 39 years and annually thereafter. The USPSTF has found insufficient evidence to recommend for or against CBE for screening at any age (USPSTF I). In performing a CBE, the examiner should be systematic, palpating every portion of the breast with the patient in both upright and supine positions. One of the best indicators of examiner accuracy is thought to be the amount of time spent.

2. Mammography and MRI. The USPSTF recommends mammography every 2 years for all women aged 50 to 74 years (USPSTF B) and states that "The decision to start regular, biennial screening mammography before the age of 50 years should be an individual one and take patient context into account, including the patient's values regarding specific benefits and harms." According to the USPSTF, the evidence is insufficient (USPSTF I) for recommending routine screening of women over 75 years of age. Other major authorities recommend routine mammography for women aged 40 years and older and this is now covered by Medicare under the Affordable Care Act. The ACS recommends annual screening beginning at age 40 years. In 2007, the American College of Physicians recommended that clinicians base screening mammography decisions for women aged 40 to 49 years on benefits and harms of screening, as well as on a woman's preferences and breast cancer risk profile.

   a. The clinician should keep in mind that the sensitivity of a mammogram is limited—approximately 90%—and is worse in women with dense breasts. Thus, symptoms and positive physical findings should not be dismissed strictly on the basis of a negative mammogram result. The specificity is similarly limited; thus, women should be counseled against alarm based strictly on a positive mammogram result.

   b. The ACS recommends that women with a 20% to 25% lifetime risk of breast cancer should receive MRI screening as an adjunct to mammography. Women at such high risk include those with BRCA genetic mutations, a strong family history of breast or ovarian cancer, and women who have been treated for Hodgkin disease with radiation to their chest. Evidence regarding when to start such dual screening is unclear, although ACS stated that most women at such high risk should begin annual screening by 30 years of age. The USPSTF has found insufficient evidence to assess the additional benefits and harms of MRI or digital mammography compared to film mammography screening.

   3. Genetic testing. In 2005, the USPSTF recommended that women whose family history is associated with an increased risk for deleterious mutations in BRCA1 or BRCA2 genes be referred for genetic counseling and evaluation for BRCA testing (USPSTF B). Women with a BRCA1 or BRCA2 mutation have a high risk (35%–84%) of developing breast cancer by 70 years of age. See Table 106–5 for risk factors indicating the need for BRCA testing. The USPSTF has recommended against genetic testing for women not at increased risk (USPSTF D).

B. Cervical cancer. The USPSTF recommends screening for cervical cancer in women aged 21 to 65 years with cytology (Pap smear) every 3 years or, for women aged 30 to 65 years who want to lengthen the screening interval, screening with a combination of cytology and human papillomavirus (HPV) testing every 5 years (USPSTF A). The USPSTF recommends against screening for cervical cancer in women younger than age 21 years; women older than age 65 years who have had adequate prior screening and are not otherwise at high risk for cervical cancer; and women who have had a hysterectomy with removal of the cervix and who do not have a history of a high-grade precancerous lesion (i.e., cervical intraepithelial neoplasia [CIN] grade 2 or 3) or cervical cancer (USPSTF D). The USPSTF also recommends against screening women younger than 30 years for HPV (with or without Pap smear). These same basic screening recommendations are also supported by the ACS, but the ACS states that combination HPV and PAP testing every 5 years is the preferred screening method for women 30 to 65 years of age.

C. Colorectal cancer (CRC). The USPSTF recommends screening for CRC using fecal occult blood testing, sigmoidoscopy, or colonoscopy, in adults, beginning at age 50 years and continuing until age 75 years (USPSTF A). According to the USPSTF, the following three regimens provide similar benefits: (1) annual high-sensitivity fecal occult blood testing, (2) sigmoidoscopy every 5 years combined with high-sensitivity

---

TABLE 106–5. RISK FACTORS FOR BRCA MUTATION TESTING

Ashkenazi Jewish
- First-degree relative with breast or cervical cancer
- Two second-degree relatives on the same side of the family with breast or ovarian cancer

Others:
- Two first-degree relatives with breast cancer, one of whom received the diagnosis at age 50 years or younger
- A combination of ≥3 first- or second-degree relatives with breast cancer regardless of age at diagnosis
- Both breast and ovarian cancers among first- or second-degree relatives
- A first-degree relative with bilateral breast cancer
- ≥2 first- or second-degree relatives with ovarian cancer
- A first- or second-degree relative with both breast and ovarian cancers
- A male relative with breast cancer

fecal occult blood testing every 3 years, and (3) screening colonoscopy at intervals of 10 years. The USPSTF recommends against routine screening for CRC in adults aged 76 to 85 years, although there may be considerations that support CRC screening in an individual patient (USPSTF C). The USPSTF recommends against screening for CRC in adults older than 85 years (USPSTF D). The USPSTF found insufficient evidence to assess the benefits and harms of computed tomographic colonography and fecal DNA testing as screening modalities for CRC (USPSTF I).

    a. The ACS recommends screening for CRC with annual fecal occult blood/immunochemical testing, flexible sigmoidoscopy every 5 years, computed tomographic colonography every 5 years, double contrast barium enema every 5 years, OR colonoscopy every 10 years.

    b. A US multi-society task force recently published consensus guidelines for colonoscopy surveillance after screening and polypectomy, based on type, number, and size of polyps (http://www.gastrojournal.org/article/S0016-5085(12)00812-8/fulltext).

D. Oral cancer. The ACS recommends periodic oral cavity examinations beginning at 20 years of age as part of a cancer-related check-up. The USPSTF states that there is insufficient evidence to recommend for or against screening examinations (USPSTF I), but states that clinicians should be alert to the possibility of oral cancer when treating patients who use tobacco or alcohol.

E. Ovarian cancer

    1. Bimanual pelvic examination. The USPSTF does not recommend screening for ovarian cancer with bimanual pelvic examination (USPSTF D). The ACS and ACOG continue to recommend that bimanual examination be performed as a part of the routine gynecologic examination. The main limitation of pelvic examination for screening is its limited sensitivity, with many tumors becoming large in size before becoming detectable by examination.

    2. Tumor markers. No major authorities recommend screening normal-risk women using tumor markers such as CA-125 (USPSTF D). A National Institutes of Health consensus conference has recommended using annual CA-125 measurements and transvaginal ultrasonography to screen women at particularly high risk because of hereditary cancer syndrome. Because of limited specificity and low prevalence of the disease, the use of tumor makers for screening in normal-risk populations results in large numbers of false-positive results.

    3. Ultrasonography. No major authority currently recommends the use of ultrasonography to screen normal-risk women, largely because of its poor positive predictive value (USPSTF D). As previously described, some authorities recommend its use in combination with tumor marker measurement to screen high-risk women.

    4. Genetic testing. The USPSTF has recommended that women at high risk for *BRCA1* or *BRAC2* (see Table 106–5) genetic mutations be counseled regarding genetic testing (USPSTF B). Women with *BRCA1* or *BRCA2* mutations are at a 10% to 50% risk of ovarian cancer by 70 years of age and may benefit from intensive screening or prophylactic surgery.

F. Prostate cancer. The USPSTF recommends against prostate specific antigen (PSA)-based screening for prostate cancer (USPSTF D). Other authorities such as the ACS, recommends that men be informed of the uncertain benefits and possible harms of prostate cancer screening. The DRE has limited sensitivity (33%–69%) and positive predictive value (6%–33%) for detecting prostate cancer in asymptomatic men. The positive predictive value of PSA testing is estimated to be 10% to 35%, thus leading to many unnecessary biopsies. Efforts to refine PSA testing using age, prostate size based on ultrasound findings, and rates of change in PSA over time may lead to improvements in sensitivity and specificity. No major authority currently recommends using transrectal ultrasonography (TRUS) to screen for prostate cancer. Because TRUS cannot distinguish between benign and malignant nodules, its positive predictive value is lower than that of PSA testing. The ACS recommends that discussions about PSA testing begin at 45 years of age for men who are African-American, or have a brother or father with prostate cancer diagnosed before 65 years of age. The American Urological Association recommends against screening before 55 years of age and after 70 years of age in average-risk men.

G. Skin cancer. The ACS recommends skin examinations periodically beginning at 20 years of age as part of cancer-related check-ups. The USPSTF has found insufficient evidence to recommend for or against routine skin examinations by primary care clinicians, while recommending that they remain alert for skin lesions with malignant features, particularly in patients at risk (USPSTF I). Risk groups include fair-skinned men and women older than 65 years, patients with atypical moles, and those with >50 moles. Major characteristics that make a lesion suspicious for malignant melanoma may be remembered by the ABCDs: A, asymmetry; B, irregular borders; C, variation in color; and D, diameter greater than 6 mm.

H. Testicular cancer. The ACS recommends testes examinations periodically beginning at 20 years of age as part of cancer-related check-ups. The USPSTF recommends against routine screening (USPSTF D), stating that better evaluation of testicular problems may be more effective than widespread screening as a means of promoting early detection. A major factor against screening is the excellent prognosis of testicular cancer, regardless of how it is detected.

I. Thyroid cancer. The ACS recommends thyroid palpation periodically beginning at 20 years of age as part of cancer-related check-ups. The USPSTF has found inadequate evidence to recommend for or against routine screening by thyroid palpation (USPSTF I), while stating that screening of persons at high risk because of a history of external upper body radiation in infancy and childhood may be justified on other grounds, such as patient preference or anxiety.

J. Lung cancer. The USPSTF has found insufficient evidence to recommend routine screening of smokers or nonsmokers for lung cancer. The ACS has recommended that persons with the following risk factors be considered for screening with low-dose CT scan: 55 to 74 years of age, in fairly good health, have at least a 30 pack-year smoking history, and are currently smoking or have quit within the last 15 years.

SELECTED REFERENCES

Advisory Committee on Childhood Lead Poisoning Prevention of the Centers for Disease Control and Prevention. *Low Level Lead Exposure Harms Children: A Renewed Call for Primary Prevention.* January, 2012. http://www.cdc.gov/nceh/lead/acclpp/final_document_030712.pdf. Accessed September 3, 2013

American Academy of Family Physicians, Commission on Science. *Summary of Recommendations for Clinical Preventive Services.* October, 2012. http://www.aafp.org/online/etc/medialib/aafp_org/documents/clinical/CPS/rcps08-2005.Par.0001.File.tmp/October2012SCPS.pdf. Accessed July 22, 2013.

American Academy of Pediatrics, Committee on Practice and Ambulatory Medicine. Recommendations for preventive pediatric health care. *Pediatrics.* 2007;120:1376. http://pediatrics.aappublications.org/content/120/6/1376.full.h. Accessed June 20, 2013.

American Academy of Ophthalmology. *Preferred Practice Pattern Guidelines: Comprehensive Adult Medical Eye Evaluation.* San Francisco, CA: American Academy of Ophthalmology; 2010. http://one.aao.org/CE/PracticeGuidelines/PPP_Content.aspx?cid=64e9df91-dd10-4317-8142-6a87eee7f517. Accessed July 30, 2013.

American Cancer Society. *Guidelines for Early Detection of Cancer.* American Cancer Society. http://www.cancer.org/healthy/findcancerearly/cancerscreeningguidelines/american-cancer-society-guidelines-for-the-early-detection-of-cancer. Accessed April, 2014.

American College of Obstetricians and Gynecologists. Committee Opinion No. 477. The role of the generalist obstetrician–gynecologist in the early detection of ovarian cancer. *Gynecol Oncol.* 2011; 117:742–746.

American College of Obstetricians and Gynecologists: Routine Cancer Screening. ACOG Committee Opinion 356. *Obstet Gynecol.* 2006;108:1611–1613.

American College of Obstetricians and Gynecologists. Primary and Preventive Care: Periodic Assessments. Committee Opinion 483. *Obstet Gynecol.* 2011;117:1008–1015.

American College of Physicians. Screening mammography for women 40 to 49 years of age: a clinical practice guideline from the American College of Physicians. *Ann Intern Med.* 2007;146:511–515.

American Diabetes Association. Standards of Medical Care in Diabetes—2012. http://care.diabetesjournals.org/content/35/Supplement_1/S11.full.pdf+html?sid=a6c7945d-96ec-468f-a53d-59e2b73eedcb. Accessed July 18, 2013.

American Urological Association. AUA Issues New Guidelines on Prostate Cancer Screening. http://www.auanet.org/advnews/press_releases/article.cfm?articleNo=290. Accessed July 18, 2013.

Centers for Disease Control and Prevention. Screening tests to detect *Chlamydia trachomatis* and *Neisseria gonorrhoeae* infections—2002. *MMWR.* 2002;51(RR-15):1–27. http://www.cdc.gov/STD/LabGuidelines. Accessed July 22, 2013.

Centers for Disease Control and Prevention. *Screening Young Children for Lead Poisoning: Guidance for State and Local Public Health Officials.* http://www.cdc.gov/nceh/lead/publications/screening. htm Accessed September 3, 2013.

Lieberman DA, Rex DK, Winawer SJ, et al. Guidelines for colonoscopy surveillance after screening and polypectomy: a consensus update by the US Multi-Society Task Force on Colorectal Cancer. *Gastroenterology.* 2012;143(3):844–857.

National Eye Institute. NEI Statement on the Difference Between Screening and Comprehensive Dilated Eye Exams in Detecting Glaucoma. http://www.nei.nih.gov/news/briefs/detecting_glaucoma.asp. Accessed July 22, 2013.

National Osteoporosis Foundation. *Having a Bone Density Test.* http://www.nof.org/articles/743. Accessed July 22, 2013.

USDA Center for Nutrition Policy and Promotion. Body Mass Index and Health. *Nutrition Insights* March 2000. http://www.cnpp.usda.gov/publications/nutritioninsights/insight16.pdf. Accessed July 22, 2013.

US Department of Health and Human Services. *The Seventh Report of the Joint National Committee on Prevention, Detection, Evaluation, and Treatment of High Blood Pressure (JNC 7).* http://www.nhlbi. nih.gov/guidelines/hypertension/index.htm. Accessed July 7, 2013.

US Department of Health and Human Services. *Third Report of the Expert Panel on Detection, Evaluation, and Treatment of High Blood Cholesterol in Adults (Adult Treatment Panel III).* http://www.nhlbi. nih.gov/guidelines/cholesterol/. Accessed July 7, 2013.

US Department of Health and Human Services. *Full Report of the Expert Panel on Integrated Guidelines for Pediatric Cardiovascular Health and Risk Reduction.* http://www.nhlbi.nih.gov/guidelines/ cvd_ped/. *Accessed July 22, 2013.*

US Preventive Services Task Force. *US Preventive Services Task Force Recommendations.* http://www. uspreventiveservicestaskforce.org/recommendations.htm. Accessed July 6, 2013.

---

107 Travel Medicine

Mark K. Huntington, MD, PhD, FAAFP

KEY POINTS

A. Know your traveler!
  1. Age, gender, chronic illnesses, or pregnancy.
  2. Destination, duration, modes of travel.
  3. High-risk activities or behaviors.
B. Nonpharmacologic interventions.
  1. Arthropod bite prevention. The following measures can afford nearly 100% protection from ticks and mosquitoes:
  • Limiting the amount of exposed skin.
  • Proper coverage of exposed areas of skin with 30% to 35% N,N-diethyl-3-methylbenzamide.
  • Use of permethrin-impregnated clothing and bednets.
  2. Food and water precautions.
  • "Boil it, peel it, cook it, or forget it."
  • Avoid unpasteurized milk.
  • Avoid reheated foods (especially from street vendors). Food should be served and eaten piping hot.
  • Consume seafood with caution.
  • Drink bottled, boiled, carbonated, or treated water only and use a straw to drink from a beverage container.
  3. Sunscreen. Use Sun Protection Factor (SPF) of 15 or greater. Use of clothing (long sleeves, hats, etc.) to protect from the sun is even more effective.
C. Pharmacologic interventions.
  1. Malarial chemoprophylaxis. See Table 107–2.
  2. Travelers' diarrhea. See Table 107–3.
  3. Motion sickness and jet lag. See Tables 107–4 and 107–5.

> **D.** Vaccinations. CDC's National Immunization Program (www.cdc.gov/vaccines) and Table 104–1.
> **E.** Geopolitical issues. Keep abreast of current events. The State Department webpage (www.travel.state.gov) aids in keeping up-to-date on destination-specific events, customs, and other hazards.

I. Introduction. Over 1 billion international journeys occur annually. Despite economic downturns, terrorism, regional conflicts, and emerging diseases, international travel is increasing. Travel medicine, also known as emporiatrics, addresses the travel-specific health concerns of travelers. The majority of travelers can be appropriately cared for by their family physician.

    A. The pretravel visit (Figure 107–1). The clinic visit should be as far in advance of travel as possible to ensure adequate time for vaccinations. A clinic visit just days prior to travel, while not ideal, can still be beneficial. The visit involves both traveler- and itinerary-dependent risk identification and stratification. This is followed by counseling to

---

Patient schedules appointment

The staff member scheduling the appointment obtains:
- Dates of travel
- Destination country (including region within country, rural or urban, etc.)
- Reason for travel or anticipated activities (business, mission work, extreme sports)
- Current medications
- Current vaccinations
- History of prior international travel

and communicates this information to the physician *prior to the day of the appointment*.

↓

Physician researches destination

Identifies medical, geopolitical, logistical, and activity-related risks prior to appointment.

Potential resources for identifying destination-specific risks:[2]
- Public information: www.cdc.gov/travel, www.travel.state.gov
- Subscription-based information: www.exodus.ie, www.travax.com, www.tropimed.com, etc.

↓

Patient arrives at appointment

Physician focuses history and physical on identifying:
- Current medical conditions, medications, or past history that could alter risk of travel
- Patient activities (and attitudes) that could alter risk
- Patient's level of risk tolerance

Physician provides education on:
- Destination-, patient-, and activity-specific risks
- Available risk-reduction interventions

Via shared decision-making, physician and patient decide on appropriate interventions:
- Administration of vaccinations
- Prescribing of malaria prophylaxis medications
- Prescribing of other special medications (altitude sickness, traveler's diarrhea, etc.)

FIGURE 107–1. Travel Clinic Flowsheet.

make the patient aware of and comfortable with travel risks, recognizing that individual traveler's "risk tolerance" can vary as widely as risks inherent at different destinations.
   B. **Vaccinations for travel** (Table 107–1).
      1. **Routine vaccinations.** All routine vaccinations should be current according to established guidelines. An accelerated vaccination schedule can be used to catch-up children who are not up-to-date prior to travel (see Chapter 105 and www.cdc.gov/vaccines/schedules/index.html).
      2. **Travel-specific vaccinations** are summarized in Table 107–1. Careful review of travel plans is required to ensure adequate protection without administering unnecessary vaccinations, some of which are quite expensive and have potential for adverse effects. The CDC website, www.cdc.gov/travel, is a valuable source for this information.
   C. **Medications for travel**
      1. **Malaria.** Malarial prophylaxis can be critical. (SOR **Ⓐ**) Local resistance patterns should be considered prior to prescribing prophylaxis (Table 107–2A). Table 107–2B provides dosage instructions. For travel to areas endemic with Plasmodium vivax or ovale, terminal prophylaxis with primaquine may be needed.
      2. **Travelers' diarrhea (TD)**
         a. **Prophylaxis.** The CDC does not recommend prophylactic antibiotics for TD for most travelers. Nevertheless, some may elect to take prophylactic antibiotics, particularly if even a portion of a lost day to illness would be catastrophic (e.g., diplomats, athletes, business people). Ciprofloxacin (500 mg per day), norfloxacin (400 mg/d), ofloxacin (400 mg/d), levofloxacin (500 mg/d), and Pepto-Bismol (two tablets or two ounces four times daily) are all reasonable choices. (SOR **Ⓒ**) Rifaximin (200 mg taken once a day) is also a useful agent, with studies demonstrating prevention of up to 80% of TD. (SOR **Ⓑ**)
         b. **Treatment.** Most TD is self-limited. Antibiotics can hasten recovery in most cases. (SOR **Ⓑ**). Dosages can be found in Table 107–3. Maintaining adequate hydration is critical, particularly for children. (SOR **Ⓑ**)
      3. **Symptomatic medications.** Travelers should be instructed to bring any nonprescription medications that they might use with them. Examples include acetaminophen, ibuprofen, topical antibiotics and antifungals, and antihistamines. Not all medicines readily available in the United States are available abroad, and those that are available may have unfamiliar trademarks and generic names.
 II. **Illness and Injury Prevention**
   A. **Arthropod bite prevention**
      1. **N,N-Diethyl-3-methylbenzamide (DEET)** is the most effective and best studied insect repellent; used as directed, its safety profile is unmatched. (SOR **Ⓐ**). While some newer agents such as picaridin are of similar efficacy, most plant-based repellents (Bite Blocker™, Skin-so-Soft™, citronella) and electronic "repellants" are much less effective. For the vast majority of travelers, including pregnant women and children, a concentration of 30% to 35% provides adequate protection. Reapply every 4 hours, more often when perspiring heavily or after swimming. When using sunscreen and insect repellent together, the sunscreen should be applied first. Round-the-clock protection is necessary; while the *Anopheles* and *Culex* species of mosquitoes are nighttime feeders, *Aedes,* responsible for yellow and dengue fevers, are daytime feeders.
      2. **Permethrin** is a contact insecticide that is applied to clothing. Insecticidal effects linger through several launderings. Combined with DEET, permethrin affords nearly 100% protection from ticks and mosquitoes. (SOR **Ⓐ**)
      3. **Other measures.** Using permethrin-impregnated mosquito netting for sleeping, having air-conditioned sleeping quarters, spraying sleeping quarters with an insecticide for flying insects (e.g., Raid™), wearing light-colored clothing, and avoiding colognes and perfumes can reduce the risk of arthropod bites. (SOR **Ⓑ**)
      4. **Special note of caution.** A variety of insect vectors of disease such as the tsetse fly, sandfly, and black fly are not well repelled by DEET. Barrier protection against their bite is essential.
   B. **Food and drinking water safety.** TD and other food-borne illnesses are the most common causes of morbidity among travelers to developing countries.
      1. **Water.** Avoid consuming tap water in developing countries. Water that has been brought to boil or properly treated with water filtration systems or halogen additives (chlorine or iodine) may be safe. Using ice in beverages and using tap water to brush teeth are common lapses. (SOR **Ⓒ**)

TABLE 107–1. TRAVEL-SPECIFIC IMMUNIZATIONS[a,b]

Vaccinations (Earliest Effective Date)	Indication	Administration	Booster Requirements	Contraindications[c]	Miscellaneous Comments
Hepatitis A immune globulin (Immediately effective)	Travelers to areas of high endemicity with contraindications to vaccine, or did not receive the vaccine >1 month pretravel	Short-term (1–2 mo) coverage: 0.02 mg/kg IM Long-term (3–6 mo) coverage: 0.06 mg/kg IM	Booster dependent on length of continued stay; *not needed if vaccine given just prior to travel.*		For children <12 mo of age, can be administered IM in the anterolateral thigh.
Japanese encephalitis (after two doses)	Adult travelers for >1 mo to endemic rural areas of eastern Asia including the Indian subcontinent	0.5 mL IM, two injections, 4 wk apart	Once if primary series >1 yr prior to potential exposure.	Hypersensitivity reactions occur up to 10 d postvaccination: delay travel if going to area with poor medical access	Endemic to rural Southeast Asia, *most travelers are at low risk for this disease,* consider if traveling in rural areas for more than 1 mo. No pediatric dosing available
Meningococcal (10 d)	Travelers to Saudi Arabia Travelers to sub-Saharan Africa, especially those with asplenia.	Single injection for adults; IM or SC, depending on the specific vaccine (see package insert) 1- or 2-dose series for children, IM or SC, depending on the specific vaccine (see package insert)	Every 3–5 yr		Entry into Saudi Arabia for the Hajj, Umbra, or work requires proof of quadrivalent (A, C, W-135, Y) vaccination >10 d but <3 yr prior to arrival. The quadrivalent vaccine is poorly immunogenic in young children, but is still recommended for children traveling to high-risk areas. A monovalent vaccine to serogroup C is available in Canada, Australia, and Europe, but not against the predominant serotype in sub-Saharan Africa (serogroup A). There is no effective vaccine for serogroup B.
Rabies (1 wk after final dose) Human Diploid Cell Vaccine (HDCV) 1cc IM dose or 0.1cc intradermal dose. Purified Chick Embryo Cell (PCEC). 1 cc IM only Rabies Vaccine Absorbed (RVA) 1 cc IM only	Preexposure prophylaxis is recommended for high-risk travelers including animal handlers, trekkers, cyclists, veterinarians, spelunkers, field biologists, children, and missionaries	Series of three injections at 0, 7, and 21–28 d for preexposure prophylaxis	2–3 y depending on risk of exposure. *Preexposure vaccination does not eliminate need for postexposure management*		Preexposure vaccines should never be given in the gluteal muscle because of decreased efficacy with this route Concomitant dosing of HDCV with chloroquine or mefloquine can dampen the immune response; should not be given within 1 wk of them Preexposure rabies vaccination simplifies the post-bite regimen but does *not* eliminate the need for prompt medical care.

Disease (interval)	Indication	Schedule	Booster	Contraindications	Comments
Typhoid fever (1 wk)	Recommended for high-risk areas if duration of stay is over 1 mo. Parenteral age >2 yr. Oral age >6 yr	Parenteral, one dose IM. Oral, four doses on d 1, 3, 5, and 7.	Parenteral—2 yr. Oral—6 yr	Parenteral vaccine more likely to cause a systemic reaction	Breastfeeding may confer passive immunity. Stop antimalarials and antibiotics 1 wk before and after administration of oral vaccine.
Yellow fever (10 d)	Sub-Saharan Africa and tropical South America	Single injection	10 years	Egg allergy. Immunocompromise. Infants younger than 6 mo; only use in children from 6 to 9 mo of age if traveling to an area with an active yellow fever outbreak. Pregnancy	Closely regulated: available only through an approved yellow fever vaccination center. Must be properly recorded on the International Certificate of Vaccination (Form PHS-731) for entry into some countries.

[a] Additional travel-specific vaccines—such as tick-borne encephalitis, BCG, and cholera—exist but are not available in the United States.

[b] All routine vaccinations should be up to date for all travelers (cf. Chapter 105). This includes hepatitis A and hepatitis B, a single polio booster as an adult (in addition to childhood series), and influenza (indicated for travel at any time to tropical areas, though due to seasonal variations between hemispheres, may need to receive vaccination at destination).

[c] Hypersensitivity can occur with any vaccine. Previous hypersensitivity is a contraindication to further vaccination.

TABLE 107–2. MALARIA CHEMOPROPHYLAXIS DRUGS

A. Selection of Appropriate Agent

Geographic Resistance/Susceptibility	Drug Choices in Order of Preference (SOR ⑥)
Chloroquine-*susceptible* areas	Chloroquine, doxycycline, mefloquine, atovaquone-proguanil
Chloroquine-resistant areas	Mefloquine, doxycycline, atovaquone-proguanil
Mefloquine-resistant areas	Doxycycline, atovaquone-proguanil

B. Dosages of Prophylactic Agents

Drug	Adult Dosing	Pediatric Dosing/Concerns	Pregnancy/Lactation Concerns	Side Effects, Precautions, and Miscellaneous Concerns
Chloroquine (Aralen)	500 mg weekly beginning 1–2 wk before travel and continuing 4 wk after return	5 mg/kg up to adult dose. Liquid formulation available in some countries. May require pharmacy compounding. Fatal overdoses of young children have been reported at doses as little as 300 mg. Accurate dosing in young children is critical	Safe in pregnancy and lactation. Concentrations in breast milk are not protective for infant	Usually minor: itching, skin eruptions, headache. Contraindicated in patients with severe hepatic insufficiency. The therapeutic window is fairly narrow
Mefloquine (Lariam)	250 mg weekly beginning 1–2 wk before travel and continuing 4 wk after return	<15 kg: 5 mg/kg weekly (will require pharmacy compounding into liquid form for accurate dosing) 15–19 kg: ¼ tablet weekly 20–30 kg: ½ tablet weekly 31–45 kg: ¾ tablet weekly >45 kg: adult dose	Safe in second and third trimesters	25%–40% will experience mild side effects (nausea, headaches). Neuropsychiatric side effects uncommon in prophylactic dosages. Contraindicated in patients with epilepsy, serious psychiatric illness, or cardiac conduction disturbance. Concomitant use with beta-blockers increases risk of cardiac arrest
Atovaquone-proguanil (Malarone)	250 mg/100 mg daily beginning 1–2 d before travel and stopping 1 wk after return	<11 kg: not recommended at this time 11–20 kg: 1 pediatric tablet (62.5/25) orally daily 21–30 kg: 2 pediatric tablets po daily 31–40 kg: 3 pediatric tablets po daily >40 kg: 1 adult tablet po daily	First trimester usage unstudied. Concentrations in breast milk are not protective for nursing infant	Contraindicated in patients with severe renal insufficiency (creatinine clearance <30 mL/min)

Doxycycline (Vibramycin and others)[a]	100 mg po *daily* beginning 1–2 d before travel and continuing for 4 wk after return	**>8 y:** 2 mg/kg/d up to adult dose. Contraindicated in children 8 y old and younger	Contraindicated in pregnancy and lactation	A photo sensitizer. Increases risk for sunburn. Recommend sunscreen. Those anticipating considerable sun exposure and women prone to vaginal yeast infections when taking antibiotics may prefer a different medicine
Primaquine (Palum)	26.3 mg po *daily* for 14 d after departure *from an endemic area* for those with prolonged exposure to *P. vivax* and *P. ovale* Start drug 1–2 d prior to travel until 7 d after	0.5 mg/kg up to adult dose	Contraindicated in pregnancy.	Contraindicated in G6PD deficiency The most effective medicine for preventing *P. vivax* so a good choice for travel to places with >90% *P. vivax*

[a]Doxycycline also can prevent other infections (e.g., Rickettsiae and leptospirosis) and may be preferred by people planning to do lots of hiking, camping, or wading and swimming in fresh water.

TABLE 107–3. TREATMENT OF TRAVELERS' DIARRHEA (TD)

Drug	Adult Dosing	Pediatric Dosing/ Concerns	Pregnancy/Lactation Concerns	Precautions, and Miscellaneous Concerns
Azithromycin (Zithromax™)	200–500 mg/d for 3 d or 1000 mg once	10 mg/kg/d × 3 d after onset of diarrhea	May use in pregnancy	
Bismuth subsalicylate (e.g., Pepto-Bismol™)	524 mg (two tablets or 30 cc) four times daily	**9–12 yr:** 1 tablet or 15 cc four times daily **6–8 yr:** ²/₃ tablet or 10 cc four times daily **3–6 yr:** ¹/₃ tablet or 5 cc q four times daily Not recommended for children <3 y	Should avoid during last half of pregnancy	Not recommended for travel longer than 3 wk Contraindicated in aspirin allergy, renal insufficiency, or gout
Ciprofloxacin (Cipro™)	500 mg orally twice daily for 3 d	Some experts recommend for severe TD/ dysentery: 15–20 mg/kg/dose twice daily up to adult dose	Relative contraindication in preg-nancy: Some experts recommend for severe TD/dysentery	Relative contraindication in childhood and in pregnancy due to studies showing arthropathy in immature animals
Levofloxacin (Levaquin™)	500 mg orally daily for 1–3 d	Not recommended	Relative contraindication in pregnancy	Avoid use with serious illness such as fever or bloody diarrhea, as this may worsen/ prolong illness
Loperamide (Imodium™)	4 mg followed by 2 mg for each unformed stool Maximum of 8 mg/d	**30–45 kg:** ¹/₂ adult dose Maximum 6 mg/d **22–29 kg:** ¹/₄ adult dose, Maximum 4 mg/d **<22 kg or <6 y old:** not recommended	May use in pregnancy	
Rifaximin (Xifaxan™)	200 mg orally three times daily for 3 d	Not recommended	Not absorbed systemically, may be used in pregnancy/lactation	Not for use in bloody diarrhea, severe or systemic symptoms
Trimethoprim/ sulfamethoxazole (Bactrim™)	One double-strength 160/800 mg tablet orally every 12 h for 5 d	**>2 mo:** 10 mg/kg/d divided twice daily up to adult dose	Safe in pregnancy	Resistance is increasingly a problem

2. **Vegetables and fruits.** Raw, unpeeled vegetables and salads should be avoided. (SOR **Ⓑ**). Melons and other fruits should be closely inspected for puncture marks, as unscrupulous vendors may inject fruit with water to increase the weight.
3. **Dairy products.** Unpasteurized dairy products should be avoided. (SOR **Ⓒ**)
4. **Seafood.** Fish and shellfish can harbor both pathogens and toxins. Proper cooking eliminates most pathogens, but not toxins.

C. **Unintentional injuries during travel.** Nearly one quarter of overseas fatalities are because of accidents; the most common causes are motor vehicle accidents and drowning. Falls and water recreation-related injuries are the most common nonfatal injuries.
   1. Alcohol consumption correlates with an increased risk of injury and death while traveling.
   2. Travelers should **bring personal protective gear** such as helmets if they intend to ride bicycles or motorbikes, and become familiar with road conditions and laws and customs of the road. If travelers are going to be participating in water-based recreation during their travel, encourage them to know the area well before engaging in these activities, particularly higher-risk activities like scuba diving.

D. **Deep vein thromboses** (see Chapter 64). Deep vein thromboses and pulmonary emboli associated with long airline flights are rare, but there appears to be a transient increased risk (OR 2.2 for flights >4 hours, OR 2.76 for flights >12 hours). Travelers should stretch and walk frequently about the plane, taking into consideration flying conditions and air turbulence. Compression stockings may offer some protective benefit in these patients. Aspirin has not been shown to reduce the risk of thromboembolic events in travelers, but has demonstrated efficacy for thromboembolic prevention in other settings. Low-molecular-weight heparin is unstudied for this indication.

E. **Motion sickness.** Several medications, including the herb ginger, have been shown to be effective in preventing or reducing the symptoms of motion sickness (see Table 107–4). Scopolamine appears most effective (SOR **Ⓐ**), with the older sedating antihistamines also showing benefit. (SOR **Ⓑ**) The herb ginger has shown efficacy in well-designed trials (SOR **Ⓑ**).

TABLE 107–4. MOTION SICKNESS PROPHYLAXIS

Drug	SOR	Dosages	Side Effects	Additional Comments
Scopolamine hydrobromide (Transderm Scop™, Scopace™)	A	1.5 mg transdermal patch behind ear every 3 d 0.4 mg tablet, 1–2 tabs orally every 8 h	Dry mouth (66%), drowsiness (33%)	Tablets better suited for shorter outings Patch costs 10× more than tablets Patch is effective 6–8 h after it is placed Oral forms are effective within 1–2 h Efficacy may be enhanced and drowsiness reduced by concurrent use of sympathomimetics such as ephedrine, D-amphetamine, and methylphenidate
Dimenhydrinate (Dramamine™)	B	50–100 mg orally every 4–6 h (12 yr and older; max 400 mg/d); 25–50 mg orally every 6–8 h (6–12 yr old); 12.5–25 mg orally every 6–8 h (2–6 yr old)		Most effective nonprescription medication Chewable tablet formulations available
Meclizine (Antivert™, Bonine™) 12.5–, 25–, 50-mg tablets	B	25–50 mg orally daily (12 y and older) or 12.5–25 mg every 12–24 hr up to 50 mg in 24 hours		Pregnancy category B Chewable tablet formulations available
Ginger	B	940 mg powdered root every 8 h Ginger powder/capsule: 0.5 to 1 g every 4 h		

TABLE 107–5. STRATEGIES FOR LESSENING JET-LAG SYMPTOM

Direction of Travel	Pre-travel Bedtime Adjustments	Wakefulness During Flight	Bright Light Exposure at Destination	Vigorous Exercise at Destination
Eastward	Go to bed 1 h earlier each night for three nights prior to departure	Try to sleep on plane Avoid caffeinated beverages	Bright light in early morning—avoid sunglasses for first few days	Mid-morning exercise
Westward	Go to bed 1 h later each night for three nights prior to departure	Try to stay awake during flight. Drink caffeinated beverages	Bright light in late afternoon—avoid sunglasses for first few days	Late afternoon exercise

Nonsedating antihistamines, antiemetics, and nonpharmacologic methods (e.g. acupressure bracelets) have not been shown to be effective in clinical trials and should be avoided. (SOR **B**) Motion sickness can be reduced by sitting in the front seat of the car or over the wings in an aircraft. (SOR **C**)

F. **Jet lag.** Rapidly crossing multiple time zones disrupts a traveler's normal sleep–wake cycle. This effect increases as more time zones are crossed and is particularly troublesome for travelers traveling in an easterly direction. Adjustment to a new time zone usually requires 1 day for every time zone crossed. Strategies to reduce jet lag are summarized in Table 107–5.

   1. Several trials have demonstrated the effectiveness of **melatonin** in reducing the symptoms of jet lag. (SOR **B**) The benefit is greater the more time zones are crossed and for eastward flights. Many pretravel, en route, and posttravel melatonin-dosing regimens have been described—some can be quite complicated. Melatonin is an unregulated substance, and formulations vary considerably. A simplified dosing regimen is 5 mg en route taken at the destination bedtime and 5 mg orally nightly for 3 to 5 nights posttravel. Short-acting agents such as zolpidem (Ambien™) and benzodiazepines can be used in a similar manner.

G. **Sun protection.** Sun exposure has short- and long-term consequences, including sunburn, photoaging, and skin cancer. Wearing protective clothing and hats, avoiding exposure during the daytime when the sun's rays are most intense (10:00 AM to 3:00 PM), and applying sufficient sunscreen reduce the untoward consequences of sun exposure. (SOR **B**) While a sunscreen with a sun protection factor (SPF) of 15 can afford more than 90% protection when applied as directed, most people apply sunscreen more sparingly and less frequently than recommended; recommending a higher SPF can partially compensate for this deficiency. (SOR **C**)

H. **Sexually transmitted disease (STD) prevention.** Nearly 20% of international travelers report at least one new sexual encounter during their travels. Human immunodeficiency virus (HIV) and hepatitis B infection rates are very high in some countries, particularly among prostitutes.

   1. Abstinence should be strongly encouraged. Latex condoms, consistently and correctly used, may afford some protection to those unwilling to abstain. (SOR **A**)
   2. Pretravel hepatitis B vaccination and a posttravel examination to screen for STDs of travelers engaging in sexual encounters with locals are recommended. (SOR **C**)

III. **Special Populations**

A. **Pregnant travelers**

   1. **Air travel.** Commercial air travel generally does not pose a significant risk to the pregnant patient or her fetus. (SOR **B**) Pregnancy increases risk of thromboembolism, so it is recommended that the pregnant traveler walk about frequently while traveling, flying conditions, and turbulence permitting. (SOR **C**) Each airline has defined policies regarding the pregnant traveler. US domestic and intra-European travel is usually allowed until the 36 weeks' gestation in uncomplicated pregnancies. Many airlines require medical authorization before permitting travel by pregnant women beyond 36 weeks' gestation. Pregnant travelers should carry a copy or summary of the prenatal record. Blood type and due date are particularly important data to carry. (SOR **C**)
   2. **Vaccines in pregnancy.** Most vaccines are safe during pregnancy. Measles–mumps–rubella, varicella, and yellow fever are the notable exceptions and should be

avoided until the postpartum period. Other live viral/bacterial vaccines (oral typhoid, oral polio, and Japanese encephalitis virus vaccine) have relative contraindications but can be given if travel to areas with active outbreaks or high levels of endemicity cannot be avoided and the vaccine's benefit outweighs any perceived risks. (SOR **C**)

3. TD and food-borne illnesses during pregnancy. While quinolones are a pregnancy category C, many experts believe that these medications should not be withheld from the pregnant women for cases of severe TD (dehydration or dysentery). Azithromycin, cefixime, and furazolidone are also reasonable choices. Hepatitis E, which is not vaccine-preventable, is usually contracted from contaminated food or water. This infection carries a 17% to 33% case fatality rate among pregnant women. Strict food and water discipline is critical for the pregnant traveler. (SOR **C**)

4. Malaria and the pregnant traveler. Malaria can be catastrophic to the pregnant woman and her fetus. Maternal mortality can approach 10%. Recreational travel to malarious areas during pregnancy should be avoided. (SOR **C**) In the event that travel to malarious areas is unavoidable, malarial prophylaxis and vector avoidance are paramount.

- Chloroquine and mefloquine, though pregnancy category C, **are generally considered safe throughout pregnancy**. (SOR **C**) Travel to mefloquine-resistant areas should be avoided during pregnancy because no proven safe prophylaxis exists at this time. Doxycycline has a relative contraindication during pregnancy; there is little evidence of a class effect in this regard. Data on the safety of atovaquone-proguanil (Malarone™) are incomplete at this time and cannot be formally recommended for use in the pregnant traveler.
- **Primaquine is contraindicated during pregnancy** because the glucose-6-phospate dehydrogenase (G6PD) status of the fetus is unknown. In cases where primaquine terminal prophylaxis is necessary, chloroquine should be continued until delivery (even if it requires months of treatment after return). (SOR **C**) Primaquine can begin in the postpartum period.
- DEET and permethrin, used as directed, are safe in pregnancy.

5. Miscellaneous travel hazards in pregnancy. Scuba diving and water skiing are contraindicated during pregnancy. (SOR **C**) Acetazolamide for high-altitude illness prophylaxis is not recommended during the first trimester. Nifedipine and dexamethasone are safe throughout pregnancy but are also pregnancy category C.

B. The pediatric traveler

1. Air travel. The WHO recommends that children younger than 48 hours old, and preferably those younger than 7 day old, should avoid air travel. (SOR **C**) Although most US carriers have no age restrictions for air travel, contacting the airline well in advance is wise. Ear pain during ascent and descent affects over half of children. Bottle-feeding, nursing, and decongestants have been advocated to ameliorate these symptoms, but multiple small studies have shown minimal benefit.

2. Vaccinations in childhood. All routine immunizations should be up-to-date. An accelerated vaccination schedule can be used to catch-up children who are not up-to-date prior to travel. See Section I.B and Table 107–2 for discussion of travel-specific immunizations.

3. Malarial chemoprophylaxis in childhood. Children are at an increased risk for mortality from *P. falciparum* malaria. Chloroquine, mefloquine, and atovaquone-proguanil, in appropriate doses, are safe for all ages. (SOR **C**) Overdoses of these medications can be fatal; proper compounding of suspensions and accurate dosing are *critical*. Doxycycline is contraindicated in children. When a mosquito-free microenvironment can be assured (e.g., permethrin-impregnated netting over a bassinet, stroller, playpen, or car seat, combined with DEET), one may forgo chemoprophylaxis. Refer to Table 107–3.

4. TD in childhood. Prophylaxis is not recommended. (SOR **C**) Nonantibiotic treatments are preferred. (SOR **C**) Quinolones are the most effective treatment for severe TD in all age groups, including children (See Table 107–3 for dosage). Azithromycin, cefixime, and furazolidone can also be used.

Vigorous rehydration is essential. The WHO recommends rehydration with reconstituted prepackaged WHO Oral Rehydration Salts in the following amounts:

a. Children younger than 2 years: 1/4 to 1/2 cup (50–100 mL) after each loose stool.

b. Children 2 to 10 years: 1/2 to 1 cup (100–200 mL) after each loose stool.

    c. Older children and adults: unlimited amount. (As a substitute to the prepackaged WHO Oral Rehydration Salts: 6 level tsp of sugar plus 1 level tsp of salt and 1 level tsp of baking soda in 1 L/quart of safe drinking water can be used.)

C. The elderly traveler. While there are no age-specific travel issues, per se, mobility and physical fitness level, mental acuity, and the presence of chronic diseases (see section below) vary between individuals. These issues may complicate travel logistics and warrant thorough evaluation during the pretravel consultation.

D. Travelers with chronic diseases

    1. General considerations. Prescribed medications should be hand-carried in sufficient quantity to last the duration of the trip. A reserve supply of medications should be packed in a separate, checked bag. Medications should be in their original containers and labeled with generic names. A letter on official letterhead from the physician explaining dosages and indications of medications, particularly scheduled medications and diabetic needles and syringes, may avert legal problems at some international borders and assist with replacement, if needed. (SOR **C**)

    2. Immunosuppressed travelers. The risk of infectious disease is increased in the immunocompromised traveler, including those with diabetes, transplant patients, chemotherapy patients, those with rheumatologic disorders, and those who are infected with HIV.

        a. TD in the immunocompromised traveler. Prophylaxis for TD is essentially the same as for the immunocompetent. Acute treatment plans as outlined in Table 107–3 are also effective in this group, but may need to be extended for 7 days. (SOR **C**)

        b. Immunizations in the immunocompromised traveler

            (1) HIV-positive travelers. Vaccine immunogenicity may be decreased in HIV-positive patients with CD4$^+$ peripheral cell count <300 cells/μL. Generally, live vaccines should be avoided in the severely immunocompromised traveler, defined as the presence of opportunistic infections or a CD4$^+$ peripheral cell count <200 cells/μL. Inactivated vaccines should be used in place of live vaccines wherever possible (e.g., poliomyelitis, typhoid). Measles and yellow fever vaccines should only be given to those with CD4$^+$ peripheral cell count >200 cells/μL. Killed vaccines are generally considered safe. (SOR **C**)

            (2) Other immunocompromised travelers. Travelers who have recently received high-dose steroids for >14 days should delay vaccination for 2 weeks after the completion of high-dose steroid therapy. (SOR **C**) Similarly, cancer patients undergoing radiation or chemotherapy may be immunosuppressed and should avoid vaccinations during this time. Cancer patients who are not actively being treated may be vaccinated. Travelers with leukemia who have been in remission for 3 months or transplant patients no longer needing immunosuppression can be vaccinated. (SOR **C**)

        c. Travel restrictions for the HIV-positive patient. In most countries, travelers staying <1 month are not required to show proof of being HIV-negative, but some countries will deny entry to travelers carrying antiretroviral medications. For HIV-positive travelers, consult the US State Department web site (www.travel.state.gov/travel/cis_pa_tw/cis/cis_4965.html) for further country-specific information. Since regulations change frequently, contacting the consulate of the country in question prior to travel planning is also recommended.

    3. Travelers with diabetes. It is critical that the travelers with diabetes carry adequate medications and monitoring supplies on the trip. This equipment and medication should be hand-carried during travel. Insulin vials can be stored at room temperature for up to 30 days without losing effectiveness, but exposure to sunlight and temperature extremes should be avoided.

        a. Travel across time zones can shorten or lengthen the "24-hour day," changing insulin and meal requirements. Travel in an easterly direction shortens the day and may decrease insulin and meal requirements; westward travel lengthens the day and can increase requirements. Frequent blood glucose monitoring is essential. Having ready access to a glucose source (e.g., glucose tablets, hard candies) is recommended. Coordinating premeal insulin dosing with unpredictable meal times during air-travel can be simplified by using short-acting insulins. (SOR **C**)

        b. Insulin concentrations may vary from the standard U100 concentration prescribed in North America: U80 and U40 concentrations with corresponding syringes can be found in other countries. Mixing syringes with different concentrations of insulin increases the chances of overdosing or underdosing. Bringing adequate diabetic supplies can minimize this risk.

TABLE 107–6. CARDIOVASCULAR CONTRAINDICATIONS TO AIR TRAVEL

Myocardial infarction
• Uncomplicated (within 2–3 wk)
• Complicated (within 6 wk)

Unstable angina
• Stable angina CCS class III–IV acceptable with in-flight oxygen

Decompensated congestive heart failure
• Stable NYHA class III–IV with PaO_2 <70 mm Hg acceptable with in-flight oxygen

Uncontrolled severe hypertension

Coronary artery bypass grafting (within 10–14 d)
• PCI acceptable, unless PCI was complicated, then wait 7–14 d

Stroke (within 2 wk)

Uncontrolled ventricular or supraventricular tachycardia
• Pacemakers and ICDs are low risk once patient is medically stable

Eisenmenger syndrome

Severe symptomatic valvular disease

Source: Reproduced with permission from Aerospace Medical Association MGTF: *Medical Guidelines for Airline Travel,* 2nd ed. Aviat Space Environ Med 2003;74(5, Section II):A1.

   c. Severe TD can predispose the diabetic traveler to wildly fluctuating blood glucoses and adverse sequelae such as diabetic ketoacidosis; it should be aggressively treated. (SOR ☉)
4. Travelers with cardiovascular disease. Cardiac conditions are the most common reasons for in-flight medical emergencies and aircraft diversions on international flights. Hypobaric hypoxemia due to altitude can increase the risk of cardiac events. Cardiovascular contraindications to air travel are summarized in Table 107–6. Special considerations for air travelers with cardiac disease include the following:
   a. Those with compensated congestive heart failure, stable angina, or a sea-level PaO_2 <70 mm Hg should arrange for in-flight oxygen. (SOR ☉)
   b. Carrying a recent copy of electrocardiogram (ECG) results is recommended (with and without magnet ECG for pacemakers).
   c. A wallet card documenting pacemaker/AICD placement can speed transit through airport security.
5. Travelers with pulmonary disease. As with travelers with cardiac disease, those with pulmonary disease are also susceptible to the hypobaric hypoxemia of air travel. The British Thoracic Society (BTS) lists as contraindications to commercial airline travel the following: infectious tuberculosis, ongoing pneumothorax with persistent air leak, major hemoptysis, and baseline oxygen requirements >4L/min. (SOR ☉)
   a. For those in whom airline travel is not contraindicated, BTS recommends **doubling the usual flow rate** for those on long-term oxygen therapy (LTOT). Those not on LTOT with baseline saturations <95% should consider a hypoxic challenge test (see below): those with saturations <85% at the test should use in-flight oxygen at 2 L/min, those above that level do not require in-flight oxygen. (SOR ☉)
      (1) Hypoxic challenge test. The patient breathes 15% FiO_2 for 20 minutes and pulse oximetry (or arterial blood gas) is checked. Levels of PaO_2 <6.6 kP_a, or saturations <85% indicate the need for in-flight oxygen.
      (2) Functional capacity test. A traveler who can walk up a flight of stairs or walk 50 m at a brisk pace without becoming severely dyspneic will usually tolerate flight without supplemental oxygen. An exercise challenge test, with some additional calculations, can be closely correlated with performance on the hypoxic challenge test.
   b. If in-flight supplemental oxygen is required, special arrangements must be made. Although airline policies vary considerably, several generalizations can be made:
      (1) Filled personal oxygen bottles are not permitted on commercial aircraft. Personal O_2 bottles must be purged and transported as checked luggage.
      (2) In-flight oxygen can be arranged through each airline. It is recommended that the traveler contact the airline well in advance of travel. Most airlines will require a letter or prescription from a physician.

(3) If supplemental oxygen is needed during layovers, arrangements for oxygen must be made with venders in that particular locale. The airline usually does not provide this service.

6. Travelers with mental illness. As a general rule, individuals with pre-existing significant mental illness should be encouraged to refrain from international travel. (SOR ❸) The definition of "significant" is murky, given the proportion of the population been treated with antidepressants, anxiolytics, or stimulants. Unfamiliar cultures and accommodation, strange languages, and the effects of jet lag all increase the risk of psychological decompensation, and certain antimalarial medications are contraindicated in those with pre-existing psychiatric diagnoses. (SOR ❸) There is also a risk of mental illness developing while abroad, whether it is young adults of the age at which schizophrenia has its onset or older adults with early dementia that could present as delirium. Extremely limited literature is available on the topic of mentally ill travelers; it is an area warranting much more study.

IV. Health Care Abroad

A. Obtaining care. Consular officers at embassies can assist in locating appropriate medical services, but the costs of care and, if necessary, air evacuation, are usually the traveler's responsibilities. Travelers should carry the name, phone number, and e-mail address of their personal physician for consultation if needed. Lists of English-speaking health-care providers by country can be obtained from the following sources:

1. Office of Overseas Citizens Services, 2201 C Street NW, SA-29, 4th Floor, Washington, DC, 20520. (888)407-4747, (202)501-4444. Indicate country or region of interest when you write.

2. International Association for Medical Assistance to Travelers (IAMAT), www.iamat. org, 1623 Military Rd. #279, Niagara Falls, NY 14304-1745. (716)754-4883

3. International Society of Travel Medicine, www.istm.org. 315 W. Ponce de Leon Ave., Suite 245, Decatur, GA 30030. 404.373.8282

B. Affording care

1. Medical insurance. If the traveler's insurance plan provides for international coverage, it is important to bring an insurance card as proof of coverage and a claim form. Many insurance plans do not provide coverage at the point of service, and the traveler may be responsible for payment even before services are rendered. Some plans will offer partial or complete reimbursement upon return, so it is critical to save all receipts. **Medicare does not cover health expenses incurred outside of the United States.** Seniors may want to contact their insurance agent about a Medicare supplement that provides international coverage.

2. Evacuation insurance. Since medical care in most of the developing world is below Western standards, the most prudent thing in the event of severe illness or injury may be air evacuation. This can be prohibitively expensive; evacuation insurance should be strongly recommended. While some domestic health insurance policies include evacuation insurance, travelers should confirm their coverage with their agent rather than assuming it is included.

3. Sources. Medical and evacuation insurance can be purchased at a reasonable cost through a travel agent or online. See the US State Department web site at http://travel. state.gov/travel/tips/brochures/brochures_1215.html for a list of private insurance and air evacuation companies. Most policies include both medical and evacuation coverage.

V. Special Activities

A. High-altitude destinations. Altitude illnesses can occur in travelers who travel to high-altitude destinations. The risk of occurrence is dependent on rate of ascent, sleeping altitude, the traveler's home altitude, and other aspects of individual physiology. Acute mountain sickness (AMS), the most common and least severe type of high-altitude illness, occurs in roughly one quarter of travelers to elevations of 7000 to 9000 feet (1850–2750 m) and >40% of travelers to elevations of 10,000 feet (3000 m). The incidence of more severe conditions is 0.1% to 4.0%. High-altitude renal syndrome (HARS), a recently described clinical entity, affects long-term inhabitants of high altitude; it does not appear to be a significant condition for travelers.

1. The most important advice in avoidance of altitude sickness is slow ascent. (SOR ❸)

2. Historically, acetazolamide has been the main pharmacologic intervention, but recent studies suggest that ibuprofen is just as effective (SOR ❸). Table 107–7 summarizes the symptoms, signs, prevention, and treatment of high-altitude illnesses.

TABLE 107–7. SUMMARY OF SYMPTOMS/SIGNS, PROPHYLAXIS, AND TREATMENT FOR HIGH-ALTITUDE ILLNESSES

	Symptoms/Signs	Prophylaxis	Treatment
Acute mountain sickness (AMS)	Headache (most common) Nausea	Gradual ascent (<300 m/daily) at elevations >3000 m with rest day every 2–3 days	Rest Avoid further ascent until symptoms resolve
	Difficulty sleeping	Sleeping altitudes most critical Climb high but sleep low	Descent for severe AMS
	Fatigue	Acetazolamide 250 mg orally twice daily starting 1 day prior to ascent Ibuprofen 600 mg orally 3 times daily starting 6 hours prior to ascent	Antiemetics Oxygen
	Anorexia	Dexamethasone 4 mg orally twice daily starting 1 day prior to ascent Gingko biloba 120 mg orally twice daily starting 5 days prior to ascent	Acetazolamide 250 mg orally 2–3 times daily Dexamethasone 4 mg oral/ IM every 6 hours
High altitude cerebral edema (HACE)	Ataxia—inability to walk heel-to-toe (tandem walk test) Altered level of consciousness ± Symptoms of AMS	Avoid hypothermia Keep well hydrated Avoid sedatives/narcotics that result in hypoventilation during sleep	Immediate descent to lower altitude Oxygen Acetazolamide or dexamethasone in doses noted above Portable hyperbaric chamber
High altitude pulmonary edema (HAPE)	Dyspnea on exertion Cough	Gradual ascent, avoidance of hypothermia, hydration, and avoidance of sedatives and narcotics	Immediate descent Reduce exertion
	Blood-tinged sputum	Nifedipine SR 20 mg orally 3 times daily	Oxygen
	Often coexists with AMS/HACE	Salmeterol MDI 1–2 puffs twice daily	Continuous positive airway pressure
	Crackles, especially right middle lobe early on	Persons with prior history of HAPE are at extremely high risk of recurrence. Avoidance of rapid altitude increases in these individuals should be strongly encouraged Risk is increased in patients with patent foramen ovale.	Portable hyperbaric chamber Nifedipine 10 mg orally followed by 20–30 mg SR daily to twice daily Inhaled β-adrenergic agonists may be helpful
High-altitude retinal hemorrhage (HARH)	Usually asymptomatic May have visual disturbances	Similar to HACE	Patients with symptomatic HARH should not continue to ascent. Upon return from altitude, most HARH spontaneously resolve in 2–8 wk

(continued)

TABLE 107–7. SUMMARY OF SYMPTOMS/SIGNS, PROPHYLAXIS, AND TREATMENT FOR HIGH-ALTITUDE ILLNESSES (*Continued*)

	Symptoms/Signs	Prophylaxis	Treatment
High-altitude seizure (HAS)	• New-onset seizure at altitude	• Travelers with history of central apnea or obstructive sleep apnea should consider avoiding high altitude. • Gradual ascent (<300 m/d) at elevations >3000 m with rest day every 2–3 d. • Sleeping altitudes most critical. Climb high but sleep low. • CPAP may help	• Anti-seizure medication (treat as any other seizure). • Oxygen • Descent
High-altitude renal syndrome (HARS)	• Systemic hypertension and microalbuminuria with preserved GFR, polycythemia, and hyperuricemia	• Affects only long-term inhabitants of high-altitude locales.	• ACE inhibitors at normal therapeutic doses appear to reverse proteinuria and polycytemia

B. Water sports

1. Fresh water. As a general rule, swimming in nonchlorinated freshwater should be discouraged for travelers to the tropics. (SOR **Ⓒ**) A variety of bacterial and parasitic infections, ranging from Vibrio and coliforms to schistosomiasis and leptospirosis, present in tropical waters present a hazard.

Doxycycline prophylaxis (200 mg orally weekly beginning 1 to 2 days prior to activity and continuing for the duration of the activity) can be protective against leptospirosis for at-risk adventure travelers (kayaking, canoeing, whitewater rafting). (SOR **Ⓒ**)

2. Ocean activities. Salt water activities are generally safer than those in fresh water, but attention must be paid to risks such as marine life and rip currents.

3. Scuba diving. Popular dive sites in underdeveloped countries may not be well regulated, and instruction/supervision of novice divers may be rudimentary at best. Obtaining certification prior to travel, and diving with experienced divers, should be strongly recommended. (SOR **Ⓒ**)

a. Air travel after diving increases the risk of decompression sickness. A minimum surface interval of 12 hours prior to air travel after a single dive is recommended. For repetitive dives in a single day, a longer surface interval (at least 17 hours) prior to flying is recommended. (SOR **Ⓒ**)

b. The Divers Alert Network (www.diversalertnetwork.org) is a reputable resource for other medical concerns associated with diving.

VI. Geopolitical Concerns. Since the 9/11 attacks, no one is unaware of the hazard posed by terrorist elements. An attentiveness to one's surroundings, including checking with one's embassy/consulate or www.state.gov for official "alert levels," can decrease one's risk of becoming a victim of terrorism-induced ill-health.

A. At any given time, regions of our planet are war zones. In some places, de facto governments have been established by rebel forces who may not recognize visas issued by the official government (and vice versa). In other places, criminal elements may present a grave risk to travelers. Areas of instability may deteriorate into civil war in relatively short order. Wars, declared or undeclared, can rapidly render a traveler unhealthy. Checking the Travel Advisories and Consular Information Sheets at www.state.gov can aids the traveler in monitoring the pulse of their intended destination.

B. Politics may inhibit travel. For example, holders of passports bearing entry stamps for Israel are denied entry to most Arab nations. Similar situations exist between a significant number of states; Consular Information Sheets can provide valuable direction in this regard. Travelers with dual citizenship should be aware that they may be subject to *both* governments' laws and requirements, including military conscription. The one nation may not be able to intervene on behalf of its citizen who is detained in another nation of which that individual is also a citizen.

VII. Travel After-Care. Between 22% and 64% of travelers to developing countries will have an illness or injury associated with their travel, nearly 10% of whom will seek medical care during travel or shortly after return. It is critical that the primary care clinician recognize the potential link between the current illness and the recent travels. This holds true whether ultimate care will be rendered in the medical home or by consultation with specialists. Unfortunately, this connection is often missed. Travelers, particularly those to developing nations, are advised to seek medical attention upon return in the following situations:

A. Fever in a returning traveler is malaria until proven otherwise. (SOR ❸) This is the most commonly missed diagnosis; the average time of presentation-to-diagnosis for malaria is nearly a week in North America.

   1. Fever with severe retrobulbar pain is strongly suggestive of dengue fever; if accompanied by petechiae, ecchymoses, and shock, dengue hemorrhagic syndrome or other hemorrhagic fevers should be considered.

   2. Other febrile illnesses that can rapidly lead to death and must be considered include meningococcemia, leptospirosis, African trypanosomiasis, arboviral encephalitides, rickettsial disease, and typhoid. Many other causes of fever that are not immediately life threatening may be acquired abroad. A full discourse on each of these is beyond the scope of this chapter and the reader is referred to the "general references" listed in the bibliography. Additionally, a useful web tool for determining the etiology of a fever in an otherwise healthy, nonpregnant adult traveler can be found at www.fevertravel.ch.

B. Persistent diarrhea or vomiting. Nearly half of travelers develop diarrhea; though usually self-limiting, in 10% it persists for more than 2 weeks, and for some it lasts a month or more.

   1. In evaluating persistent diarrhea, it is important to be aware of associated signs and symptoms. Arthralgias may be associated with *Campylobacter, Shigella, Salmonella,* and *Yersinia* infections. Fevers, bleeding, and severe pain are suggestive of invasive causes of diarrhea such as *Campylobacter, Clostridium, Entamoeba, Escherichia coli* O157:H7, *Listeria, Aeromonas, Vibrio,* and *Yersinia.* Explosive, malabsorptive diarrhea is suggestive of *Giardia* or tropical sprue; eosinophilia is seen with the parasitic worms.

   2. Laboratory evaluation of those with diarrhea lasting more than a week is warranted. (SOR ❸) Fecal leukocytes and occult stool hemoglobin are indicative of invasive diarrhea. Routine stool culture typically includes only *Salmonella, Shigella,* and *Campylobacter,* so it is important to alert the laboratory if clinical suspicions suggest other organisms.

   a. Microscopic examination for ova and parasite may be helpful; three samples collected at 24- to 48-hour intervals are necessary to have adequate sensitivity, and cryptosporidia must be specified if suspected, as special staining techniques are employed.

   b. Both stool and serum enzyme-linked immunosorbent assay testing is available for many pathogens. Rarely, endoscopic visualization of the colon may be useful.

   c. There also exists prolonged yet self-limiting postinfectious irritable bowel and postinfectious malabsorptive syndromes, which affect a quarter of patients following acute infectious gastroenteritis. Failure to recognize this results in fear of "occult" infectious processes and excessive (and expensive) testing that is of no benefit to the patient.

C. Jaundice, with or without other symptoms, following a trip to the tropics requires evaluation. (SOR ❸) The most common cause of jaundice is **infectious hepatitis**. Hepatitis A is food borne and is not rare among unvaccinated travelers. Travelers who have had sexual encounters or other body fluid exposures while abroad are at significant risk for the development of hepatitis B. Serology for acute viral hepatitis is indicated in the workup of jaundice in returning travelers.

   1. Parasitic infections may also cause jaundice or other hepatobiliary symptoms. The liver and biliary flukes are naturally found in the relevant anatomical sites, and *Ascaris* or other roundworms may occasionally be found there. Stool ova or serological testing may be employed in the diagnosis of these organisms.

   2. Excessive hemolysis, such as that encountered in malaria or its treatment, can present with jaundice. Mefloquine and atovaquone/proguanil are known to elevate transaminase levels, and primaquine causes severe hemolysis in patients with G6PD deficiency. The underlying cause must be identified and addressed.

3. Other infectious causes may range from leptospirosis to yellow fever. An assortment of noninfectious causes of liver toxicity, including things such as aflatoxin, hepatotoxic herbal remedies, or industrial toxins, may be encountered while traveling in developing nations and should also be included in the differential diagnosis.

D. **Newly acquired skin disorders.** The three most common skin disorder presented by returning travelers in a 2011 study were bacterial skin infections, leishmaniasis, and myiasis. The characteristics of a rash can direct the diagnostic directions undertaken.

1. **Ulcers** may be due to leishmaniasis, anthrax, or leprosy, as well as other more common things such as venous stasis.

2. Onchocerciasis, leprosy, myiasis, scabies, pinta, insect bites, and phytodermatitis are among the causes of **maculopapular rashes**.

3. **Diffuse rashes** are suggestive of rickettsial infections (e.g., the spotted fevers), typhoid, multiple insect bites, drug reactions, or viral conditions ranging from measles to the hemorrhagic fevers. Appropriately obtained biopsies, cultures, and serologies are of great value in reaching the diagnosis. (SOR ⊙)

SELECTED REFERENCES

Centers for Disease Control and Prevention. *Yellow Book 2013.* Atlanta: CDC; 2013. http://wwwnc.cdc.gov/travel/yellowbook/2012/table-of-contents.htm . Accessed 4 February, 2013.

Keystone JS, Freedman DO, Kozarsky P, Northdurft HD, Connor BA. *Travel Medicine: Expert Consult.* 3rd ed. Philadelphia, PA: Saunders; 2013

Magill AJ, Ryan ET, Solomon T, Hill DR. *Hunter's Tropical Medicine and Emerging Infectious Diseases.* 9th ed. Philadelphia: Saunders; 2012.

U.S. State Date Department. www.travel.state.gov/travel/cis_pa_tw/cis/cis_4965.html. Accessed 20 February 2013.

World Health Organization. *International Travel and Health.* Geneva: WHO; 2012.

Additional references are available online at http://langetextbooks.com/fm6e

---

108   Preoperative Evaluation

Jaime D. Marks, MD

KEY POINTS

- The purpose of the preoperative evaluation is to identify and manage risk, not to guarantee a problem-free surgery. (SOR ⊙)
- The most common complications of surgery are infectious, cardiac, and pulmonary problems. (SOR ⊕)
- Preoperative testing should be customized to the findings of the history and physical examination. No test is recommended for every patient. (SOR ⊕)
- The preoperative evaluation begins with assessing surgical urgency and risk followed by optimizing control of chronic medical problems and testing for suspected undiagnosed disease (Figure 108–1). (SOR ⊙)
- The final important step in a preoperative evaluation is communication of your findings to both the patient and the consulting surgeon. The operative plan should include measures to decrease the patient's operative risk as much as possible. (SOR ⊙)

I. Introduction

A. **Role of the Primary Care Physician.** Primary care physicians (PCPs) are frequently asked to perform preoperative evaluations on surgical patients. When this consultation is made, the task is to identify and quantify the patient's risk for adverse outcomes.

1. Preoperative evaluations should include medical history, comprehensive medication review, and physical examination (Table 108–1). Further evaluation, if appropriate,

TABLE 108-1. COMPONENTS OF THE PREOPERTIVE EVALUATION

Patient Medical History
Type of surgery and indication to assess surgical risk level
Known medical problems and current status
Current medications including nonprescription drugs and herbal supplements
Allergies and intolerances with the type of reaction
Surgical history including bleeding risk and reactions to anesthesia
Family history including bleeding risk and reactions to anesthesia
Social history including smoking, alcohol, and illicit drug use
ROS to assess for cardiac and pulmonary function, hemostasis, anemia, DM, pregnancy

Cardiac Evaluation
Prior revascularization or recent MI
Current symptoms
Functional capacity

Physical Exam
Physical Examination
Height, weight, BMI
Vital signs
Cardiopulmonary exam
Other pertinent exam

Results
Identify areas that place this patient at higher risk and discuss with the patient
Preoperative testing if indicated
Communicate results to the surgeon with suggestions for minimizing risks

ROS, review of systems; DM, diabetes mellitus; MI, myocardial infarction; BMI, body mass index.

may include ECG, chest radiograph, hemoglobin, potassium, and coagulation studies (Table 108-2).

2. The consultation allows the surgeon and the PCP to work together to minimize the known risks before, during, and after the procedure.

3. The preoperative evaluation cannot, "clear," the patient for surgery, as all surgeries involve some level of risk. Rather, this evaluation allows the patient to balance the need for surgery against the risk of adverse outcome in order to make an informed decision.

4. While the PCP should be familiar with the indications for surgery and the procedure itself, these are not part of the preoperative evaluation. A member of the surgical team should conduct informed consent for surgery with the patient after discussing the risks, benefits, and indications of the specific surgery.

5. The effectiveness of preoperative evaluation has not been well demonstrated in the literature. Nonetheless, preoperative evaluation is recommended by most organizations. Operative risks that are identified and controlled in the outpatient setting may result in shorter hospital stays and fewer surgeries that are cancelled or postponed. (SOR **G**)

B. Timing

1. The ideal timing for the preoperative assessment is several weeks before the procedure. This allows the provider time to evaluate problems and initiate therapy without having to postpone a scheduled surgery.

2. The Joint Commission on Accreditation of Healthcare Organizations requires all surgical patients to have a medical history and physical examination within 30 days of surgery. (SOR **G**)

C. Outcomes

1. Surgical morbidity and mortality rates vary depending on the type of surgery, the anatomical location of the procedure, and the condition of the patient.

2. Between 15% and 20% of surgeries have at least one complication. The most common complications are summarized in Table 108-3.

3. The most common adverse outcomes of surgery are infection and cardiac and pulmonary events.

   a. Cardiovascular complications are uncommon in children. In adults, they are the events most likely to be fatal.

TABLE 108–2. SUMMARY OF PREOPERATIVE TESTING

Test	Indications[a]
ECG	Signs or symptoms of cardiovascular disease High-risk surgery Intermediate risk surgery with one or more RCRI risk factor Some experts recommend for all patients 65 years or older
Chest radiograph	Signs or symptoms of pulmonary disease Not recommended in asymptomatic individuals
Pulmonary function tests	Suspected asthma or COPD
CBC	Surgery with anticipated significant blood loss History or symptoms of anemia History of chronic kidney disease or inflammatory disease
Coagulation tests	History or symptoms of coagulation disorders History of liver disease Family history of inheritable coagulation disorder Patients on anticoagulants
Creatinine and potassium	History of uncontrolled hypertension, heart failure, chronic kidney disease, complicated DM, or liver disease Currently taking diuretics, angiotensin-converting enzyme inhibitors, angiotensin receptor blockers, digoxin, or regular use of nonsteroidal anti-inflammatory drugs
Glucose	Signs or symptoms of DM High risk of DM
HbA1c	History of DM
Urinalysis	Surgery with implantation of foreign material (heart valve, joint replacement) Major urologic surgery New urinary symptoms
Pregnancy Test	All sexually active women of child-bearing age

[a]Most recommendations are based on low-level evidence and consensus opinion.
RCRI, revised cardiac risk index; COPD, chronic obstructive pulmonary disease; DM, diabetes mellitus.

> **b.** Pulmonary complications are most frequently seen after abdominal or thoracic surgery and among obese patients. They are the most common adverse events for children.
>
> **c.** Diagnosis of postoperative venous thromboembolism can be difficult as they are often asymptomatic.

4. Guidelines are available to aid in preoperative evaluations. However, most of them are based on expert opinion and consensus statements. Nevertheless, preoperative evaluation can help the physician predict and manage complications even if the evaluation cannot prevent complications.

> **a.** A 2012 Cochrane review of randomized control trials for cataract surgery shows no difference in morbidity and mortality by performing preoperative testing, but

TABLE 108–3. POTENTIAL SURGICAL COMPLICATIONS

Category	Examples
Infectious	Surgical site infections, pneumonia, urinary tract infections, bacterial endocarditis, and sepsis
Cardiac	Myocardial infarction, cardiac arrest, pulmonary edema, and congestive heart failure
Pulmonary	Pneumonia, atelectasis, bronchitis, respiratory failure with unplanned intubation, inability to wean from the respirator, and pulmonary embolus
Thrombosis	Peripheral venous thromboembolism, cardiac or pulmonary thromboses, and renal or mesenteric arterial thrombosis
Adverse reaction to anesthesia	Malignant hyperthermia and drug or materials (e.g., latex) allergy including anaphylaxis. More commonly nausea, sore throat, and sleepiness
Gastrointestinal	Gastritis, peptic ulcer disease, postoperative constipation, ileus, and hyperemesis
Psychological	Postoperative delirium, confusion, and exacerbation of latent psychiatric disease
Musculoskeletal	Muscle atrophy, deconditioning, and fatigue
Social	Financial or professional ramifications of missed work and possibly altered functional level. Increased burden on caregivers

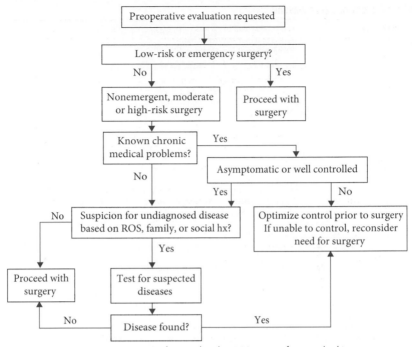

FIGURE 108–1. Preoperative Evaluation Algorithm. ROS, review of systems; hx, history.

increased costs. Therefore, routine preoperative testing for cataract surgery is not advised. (SOR **Ⓐ**)

    b. More studies are needed to determine if preoperative evaluation reduces the rate of complications for other surgeries.

II. Preoperative Assessment Algorithm (Figure 108–1). (SOR **Ⓒ**)

    A. Consider urgency of surgery. If the risk of delaying surgery outweighs the benefits of preoperative evaluation then the patient should proceed to surgery. Such situations are innately high risk for the patient regardless of underlying medical conditions. Surgery for acute trauma often falls into this category, as do surgeries for ruptured intraperitoneal organs such as the spleen, bowel, or bladder. In general, preoperative evaluations are requested for procedures that are elective or nonemergent.

    B. Evaluate risks of surgery (Table 108–4). As a general rule, the preoperative workup should be more thorough for patients undergoing high-risk surgeries.

        1. A high-risk surgery is defined as one in which the risk of cardiopulmonary complications is >5% (See Revised Cardiac Risk Index [RCRI], Table 108–5).

        2. The literature about surgical risk is difficult to assess because of constant improvements in surgical and anesthesiology techniques. Thus, results may be inaccurate for all but the most recent publications.

        3. Intrathoracic surgeries, major spinal surgeries, and vascular surgeries are usually considered high risk.

        4. Potentially prolonged surgery (more than 4 hours) or surgery involving large blood loss or fluid shift should also be considered high risk.

        5. Lower-risk surgeries include superficial dermatologic and ophthalmologic surgeries.

    C. Check status of known chronic conditions

        1. Perform testing and examination as appropriate to establish whether chronic conditions are as well controlled as possible.

        2. When practical, optimize control before proceeding to surgery.

TABLE 108–4. RISK OF CERTAIN SURGERIES

High-risk surgeries	High anticipated blood loss Aortic or major vascular surgery Peripheral vascular surgery
Moderate-risk surgeries	Intraperitoneal or intrathoracic surgery Head and neck surgery Carotid endarterectomy Orthopedic surgery Prostate surgery
Low-risk surgeries	Breast surgery Cataract surgery Superficial dermatologic surgery Endoscopy

    D. Scrutinize review of systems, family and social history, and physical examination findings for evidence of undiagnosed disease. As with known chronic conditions, new conditions identified at the preoperative evaluation should be worked up and stabilized prior to surgery whenever possible.

III. Evaluate Risks for the Patient

    A. Previous surgical experience. Patients who have had bleeding complications, anesthesia reactions (such as malignant hyperthermia), or other adverse responses to surgery should have their previous history investigated carefully. This history should strongly influence the perioperative care plan. For example, work-up of a patient with prior bleeding complications may show a clotting disorder, which can be treated with preoperative supplementation of clotting factor or fresh frozen plasma immediately before surgery.

    B. Cardiac evaluation. Because of the high morbidity and mortality associated with perioperative cardiac problems, every patient should have a careful cardiac evaluation.

        1. Well-known **preoperative algorithms** can be used to evaluate cardiac risk. These include Goldman's Risk Index, Detsky's Modified Cardiac Risk Index, the American Society of Anesthesiology's preoperative guideline, the Lee Risk Index, the American College of Physicians guideline, and the American College of Cardiology/American Heart Association (ACC/AHA) guideline. Comparative studies have not established the superiority of any one of these guidelines, and incorporating them into clinical practice can be challenging.

        2. Factors that have been shown to predispose a patient to coronary artery disease are summarized in Table 108–5; the presence of two or more risk factors indicates a need for additional cardiac evaluation.

        3. Functional Capacity. Cardiac risk can also be predicted by the intensity of physical effort that the patient is capable of performing regularly. (SOR **Ⓐ**)

            a. Typically functional capacity is measured in METs (metabolic equivalents of oxygen consumption) according to the Duke Activity Status Index (Table 108–6).

            b. A patient who is able to perform moderate intensity activity (>4 MET equivalent) is unlikely to have significant coronary artery disease and can likely proceed to surgery.

            c. Poor functional capacity correlates highly with coronary artery disease and may require further preoperative workup. Intermediate functional capacity should be

TABLE 108–5. REVISED CARDIAC RISK INDEX (RCRI)

Cerebrovascular disease
Congestive heart failure
Insulin dependent diabetes
Ischemic heart disease
Serum creatinine >2 mg/dL
Intraperitoneal or intrathoracic surgery

Number of Risk Factors	Risk of Major Cardiac Event
0	0.4%
1	0.8%
2	6.6%
≥3	≥11%

TABLE 108–6. DUKE ACTIVITY STATUS INDEX

Functional Class	METs	Activity
I	7.5–8	Heavy housework Strenuous sports Can run a short distance
II	4.5–5.5	Climb one flight of stairs Sexual relations Light yard work
III	2.5–3.5	Light housework Walk two level blocks Self-care (dressing, bathing)
IV	1.75	Walk short distances indoors

METs, metabolic equivalents of oxygen consumption.
Source: Data from Hlatky MA, Boineau RE, Higginbotham MB, et al. A brief self-administered questionnaire to determine functional capacity (the Duke Activity Status Index). *Am J Cardiol.* 1989;64:651–654.

considered for evaluation, particularly if one or more risk factors are also present.

    d. Functional capacity cannot be evaluated in a number of patients because of non-cardiac factors that limit exercise. For example, a patient with mobility impairment because of osteoarthritis cannot run, but may have intact coronary vasculature. When functional capacity is unknown, it is advisable to err on the side of caution.

4. Surgical complications. Certain surgical procedures are associated with a higher risk of perioperative myocardial infarction (MI) (Table 108–4). The physician's threshold for cardiac testing should be lower for the patient preparing to undergo a high-risk surgery.

5. A summary of **guidelines for cardiac evaluation is shown in Figure 108–2**. According to the AHA algorithm, the initial evaluation should divide the patients into the following groups (SOR **C**):

    a. High-risk patients are those with clearly established, uncontrolled coronary disease. This includes MI within the past 6 weeks, decompensated congestive heart failure, significant arrhythmia, or severe valvular disease. Surgery should be deferred until better control is achieved.

        (1) Patients with recent MI are at high risk for another attack during or after surgery. The risk for recurrent MI decreases after 6 weeks and the patient should be re-evaluated at that time. (SOR **B**)

        (2) Patients who have undergone cardiac revascularization in the past 6 months should defer surgery or have repeat evaluation of their coronary arteries prior to surgery. (SOR **B**)

        (3) Even under optimal medical management patients with congestive heart failure, previous MI, or coronary artery obstruction that is not amenable to repair are at higher risk of perioperative cardiac events. This risk has to be balanced against the benefits of surgery on a case-by-case basis. (SOR **C**)

        (4) Assessment of left ventricular function (such as echocardiogram) does not change the management patients with congestive heart failure and is not recommended. (SOR **A**)

    b. Patients at **intermediate risk** include those with stable or mild coronary artery disease or cardiac disease equivalents such as compensated heart failure, renal insufficiency, or diabetes mellitus. Patients with signs and symptoms consistent with previously undiagnosed heart disease such as exertional chest pain, dyspnea, and poor functional capacity are also at intermediate risk.

        (1) Insufficient data exist to determine whether preoperative EKG is predictive of intraoperative cardiac risk. (SOR **B**)

        (2) If the review of systems reveals symptoms consistent with angina or anginal equivalent, the patient should undergo noninvasive (stress) testing to clarify the likelihood of coronary artery disease. (SOR **C**)

        (3) Patients with ongoing or recurrent symptoms that have been previously established to be angina should have evaluation of their coronary arteries (catheterization or angiography) prior to surgery, to determine whether revascularization should be performed before elective surgery is scheduled. (SOR **C**)

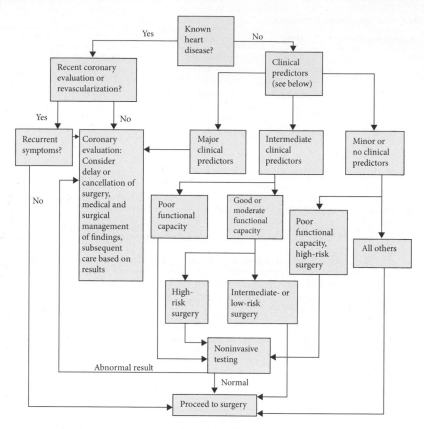

FIGURE 108–2. American College of Cardiology/American Heart Association Guidelines for Perioperative Cardiac Evaluation (Summarized). CHF, congestive heart failure.

Major Clinical Predictors	Intermediate Clinical Predictors	Minor Clinical Predictors
Unstable coronary syndromes Decompensated CHF Significant arrhythmias Severe valvular disease	Mild angina pectoris Prior myocardial infarction Compensated CHF Diabetes mellitus Renal insufficiency	Advanced age Abnormal electrocardiogram Rhythm other than sinus Low functional capacity History of stroke Uncontrolled hypertension

    c. Patients who have no concerning history or symptoms are considered **low risk;** if they have fewer than two risk factors they can proceed to surgery.
        (1) Some experts suggest screening EKG in asymptomatic patients older than 65 years. (SOR **C**)
        (2) Asymptomatic patients who have had a normal stress test in the past 2 years, bypass surgery in the past 5 years, or angioplasty in the past 5 years are unlikely to have developed significant new disease. These patients may proceed to surgery without further cardiac workup. (SOR **B**)

C. Pulmonary evaluation
    1. Pulmonary complications of surgery are most common in surgeries that are anatomically close to the diaphragm.

2. Preexisting respiratory disease increases the chance of bad outcomes. This includes asthma, chronic obstructive pulmonary disease (COPD), sarcoidosis, pneumonia, and tuberculosis.

3. Smoking, obesity, and a history of dyspnea or cough are risk factors for pulmonary problems after surgery.

4. Patients with obstructive sleep apnea are at an increased risk for difficult intubations and postoperative complications.

5. Evaluation.
   a. Chest X-ray is indicated for evaluation of physical examination abnormalities or reported symptoms of dyspnea or cough. **Routine baseline chest x-rays for all patients undergoing surgery has been shown to be unhelpful.** (SOR **A**)
   b. **Pulmonary function testing** is useful for evaluation of patients with suspected asthma or COPD. This testing may also be useful for demonstrating the status of these problems prior to surgery. (SOR **B**)
   c. **Arterial blood gases** are rarely useful in the preoperative patient. (SOR **B**) Patients whose pulmonary function is diminished enough to affect blood oxygenation are at inherently high surgical risk; these patients should be easily identifiable from the history and physical alone.

6. Pulmonary medication, including steroids, should be continued perioperatively. Patients with severe COPD or asthma may benefit from a course of prophylactic steroid therapy prior to surgery. (SOR **C**)

7. Nasogastric decompression may reduce the risk of pulmonary complications after abdominal surgery. (SOR **A**)

8. High-risk patients can be taught to perform **incentive spirometry** before, during, and after the procedure to minimize the chances of pulmonary complications. (SOR **B**)

D. **Diabetes mellitus** can increase the risk of cardiac events as well as perioperative infection.

1. Perioperatively, blood sugar should be maintained as close to euglycemia as possible, avoiding both hyper- and hypoglycemia. (SOR **B**) The best regimen for accomplishing this has not been established. **Intense perioperative control has not been demonstrated to improve outcomes** and is associated with increased rates of hypoglycemia. (SOR **A**)

2. Patients with previously diagnosed diabetes should be evaluated for current diabetic control and presence of secondary organ damage. If not recently done hemoglobin A_{1C} and renal function testing should be performed. Patients with diabetes should be **considered high risk for cardiac disease and evaluated as such**. (SOR **A**)

3. All patients undergoing surgery should be screened for the signs and symptoms of diabetes mellitus including polyuria, thirst, weight loss, blurring vision, acanthosis nigricans, and truncal obesity. All patients older than 50 years, patients with a family history of diabetes, or patients whose history or physical examination suggests the possibility of diabetes mellitus should have a fasting blood glucose test performed. (SOR **C**)

4. New or uncontrolled diabetes mellitus should be brought into good glycemic control prior to surgery. (SOR **C**)

E. **Additional conditions that affect perioperative risk**

1. **Immunocompromise.** Certain patients are at a high risk for infectious complications, including patients with genetic immune deficiencies, rheumatologic disease requiring immunosuppressive therapy, HIV, and diabetes mellitus, as well as chemotherapy recipients. In addition, patients with asplenia and valvular heart disease are at an increased risk for catastrophic bacterial infection. These patients should be considered for prophylactic antibiotic therapy during the procedure and should be closely monitored throughout the operative period. (SOR **C**)

2. **Anemia** can result from a number of causes and can be particularly dangerous when the proposed surgery is likely to result in significant blood loss. Review of systems may reveal fatigue, syncope, or cold intolerance, and examination may reveal pallor, pale mucus membranes, rapid pulse, or a functional heart murmur. A hemoglobin level should be checked in any patient with a history of anemia or a suggestive history or physical examination; hemoglobin may also be a useful test prior to surgeries that often cause significant bleeding. (SOR **C**) Any finding of anemia warrants work-up to determine the cause prior to surgery. Transfusion may be necessary prior to any surgery that cannot be deferred. The optimal hemoglobin level is unclear and probably varies by patient and by procedure.

3. **Malnutrition.** Individuals with protein-calorie malnutrition or specific vitamin or mineral deficiencies have a much higher rate of postoperative complications. Weight loss, edema, fatigue, syncope, pallor, dental disease, financial or social deprivation, anemia, or frequent illness can be warning signs of malnutrition. Laboratory tests used to evaluate malnutrition include a blood count, prealbumin level, and specific vitamin assays. Supplements prior to and immediately after the procedure are helpful. For surgeries that require a fasting patient, parenteral nutrition can be considered to sustain a malnourished patient. (SOR **C**)

4. **Peripheral vascular disease.** In general, the risk of peripheral vascular disease closely parallels that of ischemic cardiac disease. Thus, the presence of one should promote evaluation for both, and all patients with claudication symptoms or abnormal peripheral pulses should receive both peripheral vascular and cardiac evaluation. Noninvasive peripheral arterial evaluation may include Doppler or Duplex scanning, high-resolution computed tomography, or magnetic resonance angiography (MRA). If the testing shows evidence of peripheral vascular disease, the **postoperative plan should include prevention of pressure ulcers**. (SOR **C**)

5. **Hypercoagulable or hypocoagulable state.** The patient should be questioned about a personal or family history of hypercoagulable conditions as well as rheumatologic disease. At-risk patients should receive **perioperative prophylaxis against venous thromboembolism** including subcutaneous heparin (5000 U subcutaneously every 8 hours) or low-molecular-weight heparin (such as enoxaparin, 40 mg subcutaneously once daily), and intermittent limb compression. There is no indication for routine checking of coagulation studies. (SOR **B**)

6. **Peptic ulcer disease.** Most postoperative gastrointestinal complications are new-onset, so all patients should be monitored closely. However, patients who have a prior history of peptic ulcer, or who are experiencing symptoms of dyspepsia or reflux, should receive prophylactic therapy in the preoperative and perioperative periods. (SOR **B**)

7. **Renal or hepatic failure.** Patients with end-stage liver or kidney disease face unique surgical challenges. Maintenance of blood pressure and fluid balance is more difficult in such patients, and many medications are metabolized at different rates in these patients. In addition, patients with renal failure often have disrupted hematopoiesis and concurrent anemia. Liver failure leads to decreased synthesis of important proteins including clotting factors. Prior to end-stage disease, the physiologic stress of surgery may worsen the organ's function either temporarily or permanently. Patients with significant renal disease should consider preparation for dialysis prior to surgery, including placement of long-term or permanent venous access. Patients with significant liver failure should not undergo surgery except in life-threatening situations.

8. **Psychiatric disease.** Symptomatic control should be evaluated in all patients with known psychiatric disease. In addition, all patients should be monitored for signs of active psychiatric disease, and their social support system assessed. Patients with evidence of or predisposition for psychiatric disturbance should delay surgery until acute problems are controlled and should be monitored during and after surgery for exacerbation. (SOR **C**)

9. **Drug or alcohol use/abuse.** Patients who abuse alcohol or drugs must be evaluated for use-associated organ damage such as alcoholic hepatitis. In addition, the perioperative period presents **risks for withdrawal symptoms**. Ideally, the addicted patient should undergo medically monitored detoxification prior to surgery (see Chapter 90). If a history of intravenous drug use is elicited, testing for HIV and hepatitis C is warranted.

10. **Cigarette smoking.** Smokers have a higher risk of cardiovascular and pulmonary disease and should be evaluated carefully for those problems. In addition, smokers should be advised that **smoking cessation at least 8 weeks before surgery** can improve their mucociliary capacity considerably and thus decrease their chances of postoperative pneumonia. Fewer than 8 weeks of smoking cessation has not been associated with an improvement in operative morbidity or mortality. Smokers also have a higher risk of surgical site infection.

11. **Sexual behavior.** Brief questioning about sexual behavior can uncover female patients at risk for pregnancy and will help identify patients at risk for HIV. A urine pregnancy test should be performed in all sexually active, premenopausal women (SOR **C**)

IV. Medications. In general, continue medications for chronic medical conditions. Special considerations are discussed below.

A. Beta-Blockers

1. Continue beta-blockers in patients already on beta blockers. Adjust dose to target heart rate of 60 to 65 beats per minute. In known coronary artery disease, perioperative beta-blocker therapy reduces risk. (SOR **A**)

2. The initiation of beta-blockers in the perioperative period is controversial. Some experts recommend initiating selective beta-blockers at least 2 weeks before surgery for patients with cardiac risk factors or undergoing high-risk surgery. A recent cohort analysis found that perioperative β-blocker exposure was associated with lower rates of 30-day all-cause mortality in patients with 2 or more RCRI factors. If initiated, continue postoperatively for at least 1 month. (SOR **C**)

3. Perioperative beta-blockers have not been found to be advantageous in lower-risk patients. (SOR **B**)

4. A high-dose intravenous beta-blocker before a surgical procedure is no longer recommended. While this has been shown to decrease cardiac mortality, all-cause mortality is increased, most often due to the increase risk of stroke. (SOR **A**)

B. Alpha2-Agonists

1. Consider as an alternative to beta-blockers in patients who cannot take them.

2. For patients with known cardiovascular disease and at least one risk factor, alpha-blockers may reduce mortality for noncardiac surgery. (SOR **B**)

C. Angiotensin-converting enzyme (ACE) inhibitors and **angiotensin receptor blockers (ARBs)**

1. There is controversy over stopping these medications for patients who are already on them. More randomized controlled studies are needed to show if there is benefit or harm. If the medication is stabilizing a chronic medical condition, such as heart failure, it should probably be continued.

2. The addition of ACE to beta-blocker and aspirin therapy in patients undergoing high-risk surgeries has not been shown to be beneficial. (SOR **B**)

D. Calcium channel blockers and **nitrates** have not been shown to influence perioperative cardiac risk. (SOR **A**)

E. Statins

1. Continue statins in patients already on statins. (SOR **A**)

2. Adding statin therapy in patients with vascular disease at least 2 weeks before surgery is reasonable as it has been shown to decrease cardiac risk in patients having noncardiac vascular surgery. (SOR **A**)

3. Consider adding statins in patients with one or more risk factors undergoing moderate- or high-risk surgeries.

F. Antiplatelets

1. Continue aspirin if the patient is at moderate to high risk for cardiac events. (SOR **B**)

2. Stop aspirin 7 to 10 days before surgery if patient is at low risk for cardiac events. (SOR **B**)

3. For patients with drug-eluting stents, delay elective procedures for at least 6 months post-stent placement.

4. If unable to delay surgery and must discontinue thienopyridine, then continue aspirin and restart thienopyridine as soon as possible. (SOR **C**)

G. Anticoagulants

1. Should be stopped at least 1 week before surgery.

2. For some patients, the risk of short-term discontinuation exceeds the risk of surgery. These patients can be changed to low-molecular weight heparin at 1 mg/kg twice daily one week before surgery. This is typically stopped the day before surgery or the morning of surgery and the patient can be started on intravenous unfractionated heparin. IV heparin can be discontinued several hours before the procedure.

H. Insulin should be continued, but the morning of the surgery only half the usual dose is given.

I. Oral hypoglycemic agents should be held the morning of surgery and restarted as soon possible.

J. Nonprescription anti-inflammatory drugs and some herbal remedies (e.g., fish oil, garlic, ginkgo, ginseng, melatonin) also cause a predisposition for excess bleeding. Many can be held 1 to 2 weeks before surgery.

V. Special Cases

A. Children are far less likely to have coronary artery disease but are at higher risk of having undiagnosed pulmonary, immunologic, anatomic, or genetic abnormalities. The preoperative history should include the prenatal and birth history and a history of recent infections. Upper respiratory infections or pneumonia should be allowed to completely resolve prior to surgery. (SOR ❸)

B. Patients who are unable to give a history. Evaluation of functional capacity and current symptoms is impossible if a patient is unconscious or incapable of communicating with the physician. In this case, a careful physical examination becomes the only tool the primary care physician has to identify risks. In this situation, a lower threshold for ordering preoperative tests should be employed. (SOR ❸)

C. Pregnancy. Except in life-threatening situations, surgery should be avoided in pregnant women. (SOR ❸) By consensus opinion, the American Congress of Obstetrics and Gynecology recommends that elective surgery be postponed until after delivery and that, if possible, nonurgent surgery is performed in the second trimester.

D. Elderly patients. The likelihood of serious medical problems increases with age, and thus the perception arises that older patients are at higher risk during surgery. In fact, healthy geriatric patients do not have a higher surgical morbidity. These patients should be carefully evaluated for medical problems or social support issues, but can expect to undergo surgery quite successfully. Because of the high prevalence of dementia, the primary care examiner should perform a mental status examination on geriatric patients. (SOR ❸)

VI. The Perioperative Plan

A. Communication of results to the surgeon. The primary care consultation to the surgeon should include the following:
1. A listing of the patient's known risk factors and medical conditions.
2. Appraisal of how these factors will affect the patient's overall surgical risk.
3. Suggestions for controlling, minimizing, or eliminating risks discovered in the preoperative evaluation.

B. Patient counseling. The primary care physician should discuss the risks and benefits of surgery clearly with the patient. The patient should understand:
1. That all surgeries may include unanticipated complications.
2. Any factors that create particularly high risk for this patient.
3. Your suggestions to the patient for minimizing risk.
4. Your suggestion for long-term follow-up of any medical problems found in the examination.

SELECTED REFERENCES

American College of Obstetricians and Gynecologists. Nonobstetric surgery during pregnancy. Committee Opinion No. 474. . *Obstet Gynecol.* 2011;117:420–421.

Buchleitner AM, Martínez-Alonso M, Hernández M, et al. Perioperative glycaemic control for diabetic patients undergoing surgery. *Cochrane Database Syst Rev.* 2012;(9):CD007315.

Danielson D, Bjork J, Card R, et al. Guideline Summary: Preoperative Evaluation. Bloomington, MN. *Institute for Clinical Systems Improvement (ICSI).* 2012, July. 61p. http://www.guideline.gov/content.aspx?id=38289&search=preoperative+evaluation. Accessed May 2013.

Fleisher LA, Beckman JA, Brown KA, et al. American College of Cardiology; American Heart Association Task Force on Practice Guidelines; American Society of Echocardiography. ACC/AHA 2007 guidelines on perioperative cardiovascular evaluation and care for noncardiac surgery. *J Am Coll Cardiol.* 2007;50(17):e159–e241.

Keay L, Lindsley K, Tielsch J, et al. Routine preoperative medical testing for cataract surgery. *Cochrane Database Syst Rev.* 2012;(3):CD007293.

London MJ, Hur K, Schwartz GG, et al. Association of perioperative β-blockade with mortality and cardiovascular morbidity following major noncardiac surgery. *JAMA.* 2013;309(16):1704–1713.

Rivera RA, Martinez-Osoria JI, Mansi IA. Preoperative medical consultation: maximizing its benefits. *Am J Surg.* 2012;204:787–797.

Thomsen T, Villebro N, Møller AM. Interventions for preoperative smoking cessation. *Cochrane Database Syst Rev.* 2010;(7):CD002294.

Index

A

abdominal films, 9, 285
abdominal pain
  acute, causes of, 2
  in children, 7–8
  chronic, 6–7
  defined, 1
  diagnoses of, 1–3
  eating disorders and, 871
  in elderly, 8
  laboratory tests and imaging, 6
    barium enema/colonoscopy, 10
    endoscopic retrograde cholangiopancrea-
      togram, 10
    initial, 8–9
    magnetic resonance angiography, 9
    radiologic tests, 9
    radionuclide scanning, 9
  physical examination in, 5
  signs, 5–6
  symptoms, 3–5
  treatment, 10–12
abdominal wall pain, 6
abnormal Pap smears
  evaluation, 14–16
  laboratory tests, 14
  postcolposcopy treatment, 16
  treatment, 14–16
acamprosate, for substance abuse, 815–816
ACD. See anemia of chronic disease (ACD)
acetaminophen, 178, 182
  for chronic persistent pain, 598
  for myalgia, 369
  for osteoarthritis, 731
acetic acid application, 14
achilles tendon rupture, 209
acne rosacea
  common diagnoses
    ocular rosacea, 533
    papulopustular rosacea, 532
    phymatous/rhinophymatous rosacea, 533
  definition, 532
  pathophysiology, 532
  risk factors, 532
  signs, 533
  symptoms, 533
  treatment, 533–534
acne vulgaris
  acne conglobata, 526
  acne fulminans, 526
  common diagnoses
    mild acne, 528
    moderate acne, 528
    severe acne, 528
  definitions, 525–526

  epidemiology, 526
  inflammatory lesions, 526
  iPledge Program, 531
  laboratory tests, 531
  management, 528
  management strategies, 531
  noninflammatory (obstructive) lesions, 525
  pathophysiology, 526–527
  treatment
    oral contraceptives, 530
    systemic agents, 530–531
    topical agents, 528–529
acoustic damage, 275–276
acoustic neuroma, 145, 274. See also hearing loss
  audiometric findings, 274
  treatment for, 274
acrochordon, 125, 129
acromioclavicular (AC) injuries, 37
  treatment, 43
actinic keratoses, 124, 129
action tremors, 461
active TB, 102
acupressure, 152
acupuncture
  for asthma, 558
  for dysmenorrhea, 152
  for nausea and vomiting, 376
  for osteoarthritis, 734
acute abdominal pain
  causes of, 2
  laboratory tests in, 8–9
  x-rays in, 9
acute anal fissure, 413
acute angle-closure glaucoma, 424
  laboratory tests/diagnostics, 430
  symptoms, 429
  treatment, 431
acute appendicitis, Alvarado scoring system
    for, 10
acute brachial plexus neuritis, 40–41
acute cholecystitis, HIDA scan in, 9
acute coronary syndrome (ACS)
  definition, 697
  diagnosis, 699–702
  epidemiology, 697
  pathogenesis, 697, 699
  prevention, 699
acute fracture, 34
acute hemorrhage, 26
  treatment, 30
acute interstitial nephritis, 283, 773. See also
    renal failure
  hematuria and, 283
acute labyrinthitis, 146
acute lymphadenitis, 364

acute torticollis, and neck pain, 383
acute tubular necrosis, 773. *See also* renal failure
acyclovir treatment, pediatric fever, 399
ADA. *See* American Diabetes Association (ADA)
adapalene, 529
adenomyosis
    dysmenorrhea and, 149
    signs, 150
    symptoms, 150
adhesions
    chronic pelvic pain (CPP), 402
    treatment, 408
adhesive capsulitis, 40, 41
    treatment, 43
adjuvant therapy, for breast cancer, 571
adnexal mass, 404
adolescents. *See also* children
    HPV infections in, 16
adult-onset congenital adrenal hyperplasia, 240
AGCs. *See* atypical glandular cells (AGCs)
AIDS
    definition, 535–536
    epidemiology
        prevalence, 536
        risk factors, 536
        transmission, 536
    laboratory tests, 540
    management strategies, 547
    opportunistic infections and other
            manifestations
        CMV retinitis, 545
        cryptococcal meningitis, 545
        diarrhea, 545–546
        esophageal candidiasis, 546
        Kaposi's sarcoma (KS), 546
        mycobacterium avium complex (MAC), 546
        oropharyngeal candidiasis, 546
        PCP, 546–547
        prophylaxis, 545
    prevention
        biomedical, 537
        primary, 536
    prognosis, 547–548
    screening
        risk-based, 536
        routine, 536
    signs and symptoms
        eye diseases, 537
        gastrointestinal conditions, 539
        genitourinary disease, 539
        lymph nodes, 537
        neurologic problems, 539–540
        oral cavity, 537
        pulmonary involvement, 537–539
        skin conditions, 537
    treatment, 540–547
air-contrast barium enema, nausea and vomiting,
        375
alanine aminotransferase (ALT), 606
albuterol, for asthma, 558
albuterol sustained-release, 556
alcohol
    behavioral change counseling, 958
    peptic ulcer disease and, 754
    sleep disorder and, 293

alcohol abuse, 3
    Alcoholics Anonymous (AA)
        effectiveness, 817
        12-step recovery program, 816–817
    breast cancer and, 564
    CAGE questionnaire, 809
    clinical clues, 810
    colon cancer, 565
    defined, 808–809
    detoxification, 814
    differential diagnosis, 809
    epidemiology, 808
    heart failure and, 620
    laboratory tests, 810–812
    management strategies, 816–817
    prenatal care, 899
    preoperative evaluation, 1004
    prevalence, 808
    prognosis, 817–818
    screening, 809
    SOAPE glossary, 813
    symptoms and signs, 810
    treatment, 813–816
    withdrawal symptoms, 810
alcoholic cirrhosis, 606, 608, 611
Alcoholics Anonymous (AA), 816–817
    effectiveness, 817
    12-step recovery program, 816–817
Allen test, 260, 261
allergic reaction, insect bite, 45
    treatment, 51
allergic vaginitis, 507, 511
allergy tests, for nasal disorders, 435, 436
alopecia, 237
    androgenetic, 238
    areata, 238
        nail disorders and, 238
        signs, 243, 244
        treatment, 247–248
    cicatricial, 237
    diagnoses and etiologic classifications of,
            238
    infectious, 238
    laboratory tests, 244–246
    noncicatricial, 237
    nonscarring, 237
    physiologic, 238
    signs, 242–244
    symptoms, 242
    totalis, 243
    traumatic, 238
    treatment, 246–250
    universalis, 243
alosetron, 10
alpha-adrenergic blockers, 484, 487
alpha-1-antitrypsin (AAT) deficiency, 608
alpha-glucosidase inhibitors, for diabetes
        mellitus, 653
Alzheimer disease (AD). *See also* dementia
    costs, 629
    diagnosing and assessing, 631–632
    incidence, 629
    screening tools for, 634
amantadine, 465, 466
ambulatory monitoring, 389

amenorrhea
  defined, 17, 23
  diagnoses, 17–19
  diagnostic tests, 20–21
  hypergonadotropic, 19
  hypogonadotropic, 17
  hypothalamic, 17
  normogonadotropic, 18
  patient education, 23
  primary, 17–18, 21–22, 23
  secondary, 17, 18–19, 22–23
  symptoms/signs, 19–20
  treatment, 21–23
  vaginal bleeding symptoms, 503
American Diabetes Association (ADA), 644
amitriptyline, 369
amnesia, 297
amoxicillin, 49
  for Lyme disease treatment, 53
amoxicillin-clavulanate, 68, 69
ampicillin-sulbactam, 69
amylase, 8
amylin mimetics, diabetes mellitus, 654
anal fissure, 411
  acute, 413
  chronic, 413
  LGI bleeding and, 223
  signs, 413
  symptoms, 412
  treatment, 415
anal fistulas, 413
analgesics
  for fractures treatment, 36
  for migraine, 270
  for myalgia, 369
  for osteoarthritis, 731–732
  for tenosynovitis treatment, 36
anaphylaxis, 519, 524
androgen testing, 21
anemia, 8. See also red blood cell (RBC)
  aplastic, 26
  defined, 24
  diagnoses, 25–27
  diagnostic tests
    invasive testing, 29
    laboratory tests, 27–28
  pernicious, 25
  preoperative evaluation and, 1003
  screening and prevention, 24–25
  symptoms/signs, 27
  treatment, 29–30
anemia of chronic disease (ACD), 26
  treatment, 30
angina, chest pain treatment and, 76–77
angiography
  cerebral, 790
  for GI bleeding, 226
  for headaches, 268
  for IHD, 702
  mesenteric, 9
angiotensin-converting enzyme inhibitor (ACE-I)
  and cough, 92, 96, 102
angiotensin II receptor blockers (ARBs), 622
animal bites, 44. See also mammalian bites
  treatment, 49, 50

ankle fractures
  treatment, 220
ankle injuries
  anatomy, 31
  defined, 31
  diagnoses, 32–33
  imaging, 34–35
  patient education, 36
  prevention of sprains, 31
  symptoms/signs, 33–34
  treatment, 35–36
anorexia nervosa. See also eating disorders
  definition, 865
  epidemiology, 866
anoscopy, 413
anterograde amnesia, 297
antianginal drug therapy, for IHD, 702–707
antibacterial drugs for asthma, 557
antibiotics treatment
  acne vulgaris, 529
  acute bacterial cystitis, 169
  AOM, 175, 177
  bacterial skin infections, 68–70
  for COPD, 585, 586–588
  cough, 98–102
  diarrhea, 139
  dysuria without pyuria, 169
  foot complaints, 215
  genital lesions, 233
  for inflammatory bowel disease, 691
  pertussis, 101
  for proteinuria, 422
  sinusitis, 441–442
  sore throat, 452
  testicular scrotal complaints, 447–448
  urinary symptoms in men, 484
antibiotic therapy, for mammalian bites
  treatment, 49
anticholinergic treatment, 187
  nausea and vomiting, 381
anticoagulation therapy, 393–394
  hematuria, 283
anticonvulsants, for chronic persistent pain,
  603–604
antidepressants therapy
  for chronic persistent pain, 603
  for eating disorders, 871
  generalized anxiety disorder (GAD),
    822, 826
  myalgia, 369
antiemetics therapy
  migraine, 270
  peripheral vestibular disorders, 148
antiepileptic drug (AED)
  for migraine, 271
antihistamines therapy
  allergic rhinitis, 438
  for asthma, 557
  earache, 178
  nasal disorders, 439
  for nausea and vomiting, 381
  peripheral vestibular disorders, 148
  pruritus, 115–117
  sinusitis, 441
  urticaria, 492

antihypertensive therapy, proteinuria, 422–423
anti-inflammatory medications, for osteoarthritis, 732–734
antioxidants, for IHD, 707
antiplatelet therapy, for IHD, 702
antipsychotics, for nausea and vomiting, 376, 381
antipyretics, 398
antispasmodics, for chronic persistent pain, 604
antithrombotic therapy, 394
antiviral agents for asthma, 557
anxiety, 819–828
    generalized anxiety disorder (GAD), 819–820
        diagnoses, 820–821
        management strategies, 827
        prognosis, 827
        treatment, 822–826
    intimate partner violence and, 852
    overview, 819
    panic disorder, 820
        diagnoses, 821
        management strategies, 827
        prognosis, 828
        treatment, 826–827
    phobia, 820
        diagnoses, 821
        management strategies, 827
        prognosis, 828
        treatment, 827
    posttraumatic stress disorder (PTSD), 820
        diagnoses, 821
        management strategies, 827
        prognosis, 828
        treatment, 827
    prognosis, 827–828
anxiolytics, 166
aortic dissection, thoracic, 71. See also chest pain
aplastic anemia, 26
appendectomy, 10
appendicitis, 8
    and abdominal pain, 1, 4
    acute, Alvarado scoring system for, 10
    and leukocytosis, 8
    signs, 6
    treatment, 10
arachnid bites, 44
    diagnosis, 45
    wounds, 46–47
arm/shoulder complaints, 37
    diagnoses, 37–40
    evaluation, maneuvers used in, 42
    laboratory tests, 38–39, 41
    signs, 38–39, 41
    symptoms, 38–39, 41
    treatment, 42–43
aromatase inhibitors/inactivators (AIs)
    for breast cancer, 565
arrhythmia, 455
arterial blood gases (ABG), 164
    asthma, 552
    COPD, 580
arterial insufficiency, 367

arteriovenous malformations, 283
arthritis. See also joint pain
    hand and wrist complaints and, 256
arthropod bite prevention, for travelers
    DEET, 981
    permethrin, 981
    special note, 981
arthroscopy, for osteoarthritis, 729
5-ASA compounds
    for inflammatory bowel disease, 691
ascites, 610
ASCs. See atypical squamous cells (ASCs)
Asherman syndrome, 19
aspiration
    acute cough and, 92, 101
    suspected breast cyst, 56
    wheezing and, 519, 523–524
aspirin (ASA)
    for colon cancer, 566
    for hypertension, 686
    for myalgia, 369
    for stroke, 794
asthma, 548–562
    cough and, 96
    definition, 549
    diagnosis, 549–553
    diagnostic tests, 552
    differential diagnosis, 552–553
    epidemiology, 549
    exacerbation, 92, 95
    management strategies, 559–561
    pathophysiology, 549
    prognosis, 561–562
    pulmonary function tests, 552
    signs, 549
        chronic changes, 551
        pulsus paradoxus, 550
        severe asthma, 550
    symptoms, 549
        atelectasis, 549
        coughing, 549
    treatment, 553–559
    wheezing and, 518
asymmetric FTT, 192
asymptomatic bacteriuria (ASB), 171
asymptomatic inflammatory prostatitis, 480
ataxia, 470
atelectasis, 549
atherosclerotic disease
    gastrointestinal bleeding and, 225
atrial fibrillation (AF)
    antithrombotic therapy in, 394
    palpitations treatment and, 390–394
atrophic vaginitis, 507, 511
attention deficit hyperactivity disorder (ADHD), 829–845
    diagnosis, 831–836
    differential diagnosis
        adult conditions, 835–836
        behavioral rating forms, 836–837
        continuous performance tasks, 837
        laboratory tests, 836
        medical conditions, 834
        mental status examination, 837
        pediatric conditions, 835

primary care, 836–837
psychiatric conditions, 835–836
DSM-5, 832–834
DSM-IV, 833–834
epidemiology, 830
etiology, 830
overview, 829–830
prognosis, 845
risk factors, 830
treatment, 837–845
  atomoxetine, 841
  behavioral parent training, 843
  child interventions, 844
  clonidine, 841
  complementary and alternative medicines,
    844–845
  dexmethylphenidate, 839
  dextroamphetamine, 839
  guanfacine, 841, 842
  lisdexamfetamine, 839
  mixed amphetamine salts, 839
  MPH, 839
  nonpharmacologic treatment for children
    and adolescents, 843–844
  nonstimulant medications, 840–842
  pharmacotherapy, 837–842
  psychoeducation, 843
  psychotherapy, 844
  special education services, 844
  special issues in pharmacotherapy, 843
  stimulants, 838–840
atypical glandular cells (AGCs), 13
  symptoms, 14
  treatment, 16
atypical mole syndrome, 121
atypical squamous cell cannot exclude HSIL
    (ASC-H), 13
  treatment, 15
atypical squamous cell of uncertain significance
    (ASC-US), 13
  treatment, 15
atypical squamous cells (ASCs)
  causes of, 13
  symptoms, 13
audiometry, 278
auditory brainstem response (ABR), 279
auscultation, 74
autoimmune hemolytic anemia, 26
autoimmune hepatitis, 608–609, 613
azapirones
  for generalized anxiety disorder (GAD), 822
azathioprine
  for inflammatory bowel disease, 695
azithromycin, 68, 69, 101, 453, 485
azo compounds
  for inflammatory bowel disease, 691

B
back pain. *See* low back pain (LBP)
bacteremia, 395
bacteria, 13
bacterial skin infections
  deep
    carbuncle, 61
    cellulitis, 59–61

ecthyma, 61
erysipelas, 61
furuncle (boil), 61
signs, 63–66
treatment, 68–69
definition, 58
diagnostic tests, 66–68
  bone scans, 68
  cultures, 66–68
  sonograms, 68
  special procedures, 68
  wood lamp illumination, 68
pathogenesis, 58–59
patient education, 69–70
signs
  carbuncle, 66
  cellulitis, 63–66
  erysipelas, 66
  erythrasma, 63
  folliculitis, 66
  furuncle (boil), 66
  hidradenitis suppurativa, 66
  impetigo, 63
  sebaceous cyst abscess, 66
specialized skin structure
  folliculitis, 62
  hidradenitis suppurativa, 62
  sebaceous gland abscess, 62
  signs, 66
  treatment, 69
superficial
  erythrasma, 59
  impetigo, 59
  signs, 63
  treatment, 68
symptoms, 62–66
treatment
  antibiotics, 68–70
  carbuncles, 69
  cellulitis, 68–69
  ecthyma, 69
  erysipelas, 69
  erythrasma, 68
  folliculitis, 69
  hidradenitis suppurativa, 69
  impetigo, 68
  necrotizing fasciitis, 69
  sebaceous cyst abscess, 69
bacterial vaginosis (BV), 507, 509–510
β_2-agonists for asthma
  long-acting, 556
  short-acting, 558–559
balanitis
  laboratory tests for, 234
  pruritic lesions and, 228
  signs, 232
  symptoms, 229
  treatment, 236
balanitis xerotica obliterans (BXO), 229
  laboratory tests for, 234
  signs, 232
  symptoms, 229
  treatment, 236
banding, wrist, 376
bariatric surgery, 724–725

barium enema/colonoscopy, 10
barotrauma
   earache and, 172
   symptoms, 173
   treatment, 182
barrier methods, contraception, 888–889
   cervical cap, 888
   diaphragms, 888
   female condoms, 888
   male condoms, 888
   sponge, 888–889
Bartholin's gland cysts
   cystic lesions and, 229
   laboratory tests for, 234
   signs, 233
   symptoms, 229
   treatment, 236
basal cell cancer (BCC), 124, 129–130
bedbugs bites, 45
   prevention from, 44
bee sting, 45
behavioral change counseling, 950–959
   brief intervention about lifestyle change, 950
   health behavior-specific recommendations,
         953–959
      cancer self-examination, 958–959
      dental disease, 957–958
      drugs, 958
      environmental and household injuries,
            956–957
      exercise, 954–955
      intentional injuries, 955–956
      motor vehicle-related injuries, 956
      nutrition, 954
      sexually transmitted infections (STIs), 957
      skin cancer, 958–959
      suicide, 955
      tobacco use, 953–954
      unintentional injuries, 956
      violence, 955–956
      weight management, 954
   overview, 950
   practitioner mindset, 950–951
   stages of change
      action plan creation, 952
      contemplation to action, moving from, 952
      maintenance and relapse prevention,
            952–953
      precontemplation stage, addressing of, 952
      stage/readiness for change, determining, 951
   understanding and addressing low health
         literacy, 953
behavioral therapy
   fatigue, 196
   incontinence, 473–474
   for obesity, 721
   for osteoarthritis, 731
benign neoplasms, 127–129
benign positional vertigo, 146
benign prostatic hypertrophy (BPH), 247, 281
   laboratory tests, 482
   signs, 481
   symptoms, 481
   treatment, 487
   urinary symptoms in men, 480

benign supraventricular or ventricular
      ectopy, 389
Bennett fractures, 255
benzodiazepines
   for delirium, 82
   for generalized anxiety disorder (GAD), 822
beta-blockers
   generalized anxiety disorder (GAD), 822
   for IHD, 703
   phobia, 827
   for systolic dysfunction HF, 624
Bethesda system, 12
bibasilar crackles, 81
bile acid sequestrants, 672
biliary colic, 4
   treatment, 11
biliary peritonitis, 5
binge eating disorders. See also eating
      disorders
   definition, 866
   epidemiology, 866
biofeedback therapy, 87
biologics, for inflammatory bowel disease, 695
biopsy, 14
   arterial, 268
   bone, 68
   bone marrow, 29
   breast condition
      excisional/incisional, 56
      fine needle aspiration, 56
   endometrial (EB), 503
   excisional, 128
   excisional or incisional, 334
   hair disorder, 236, 245
   liver, 307, 350
   lymph node, 362–363
   myalgia, 368
   nail disorder, 246
   proteinuria, 422
   pruritic dermatoses, 114
   pruritic lesions and, 234
   punch, 128, 334
   renal, 286
   shave, 334
   skin, 66
   urinary symptoms in men, 483
   verrucous/papillomatous lesions and, 234
bipolar disorder, 857. See also depression
bisphosphonates, for osteoporosis, 743–744
bites/stings
   arachnid, 44
      diagnosis, 45
      spider. See spider bites
      wounds, 46–47
   diagnoses, 44–45
   insect, 44
      diagnosis, 45
      treatment, 49, 51–54
      wounds, 45–46
   laboratory tests, 48
   mammalian
      defined, 44
      diagnosis, 44
      treatment, 48–49, 50, 51
      wounds, 45

spider, 44, 45
    treatment, 53–54
    wounds, 47
    symptoms and signs, 45–47
    treatment, 48–54
black widow spider bite, 45
    treatment, 54
    wounds, 47
bladder cancer, 480. *See also* urinary symptoms
        in men
    hematuria and, 281
    treatment, 488
blepharitis, 424
    laboratory tests/diagnostics, 429
    symptoms, 427
    treatment, 431
blood cultures, 66, 397
blood tests
    cholesterol, 970–971
    glucose, 971
    hemoglobin/hematocrit, 971
    hemoglobinopathies, 973
    hypothyroidism, 972
    lead, 971–972
    newborn, 972
    phenylketonuria (PKU), 972
    and proteinuria, 421–422
    thyroid function, 973
blunt trauma, 369
BMD (bone mineral density), for osteoporosis,
        739–740
BNP (brain or b-type natriuretic peptide) test, 165
body lice, 46
body lice *(pediculosis humanus)*, 105
body measurement screening
    abdominal aortic ultrasound, 970
    blood pressure, 969–970
    BMD, 970
    head circumference, 968
    height and weight, 968, 969
    waist/hip measurement, 969
Bonacini Cirrhosis Discriminant Score, 610
bone densitometry, 21
bone marrow biopsy, 29
bone scans, 35, 385
Borrelia burgdorferi, 46–47
bowel obstruction, 2
    included nausea and vomiting, 381
    signs, 6
    symptoms, 5
    treatment, 11
boxer's fracture, 218, 255
bradyarrhythmia, 455
bradykinesia, 462
breast cancer, 54
    diagnosis, 569
    differential diagnosis, 568–569
    epidemiology, 563
    genetic testing for, 56–57
    male, 575
    prevention, 565–566
    prognosis, 574
    risk factors, 563–564
        aging, 563
        alcohol consumption, 564

endogenous estrogen, 564
        genetic history, 564
        obesity, 564
        personal history, 563
    screening, 566–567
    screening tests, 975–976
    signs and symptoms, 567–568
    staging, 570
    treatment, 571
breast condition
    breast lumps, 54–58
    breast surface
        retraction, 55
        skin edema, 55
        venous pattern, 55
    cancer. *See* breast cancer
    fibroadenomas, 55
    fibrocystic changes, 55
    gynecomastia, 55
    laboratory tests, 56–57
    mastalgia, 55
    mastitis, 55
    patient education, 58
    screening and prevention, 54–55
    signs, 55
    symptoms, 55
    treatment
        breast cancer, 57
        fibroadenoma, 57
        fibrocystic changes, 57
        gynecomastia, 58
        mastitis, 58
breast-conserving therapy (BCT), 571
breastfeeding
    breast cancer, 564
    postpartum care, 914
breastfeeding jaundice, 303
Breast Imaging Reporting and Data System
        (BI-RADS), 56
breast inflammation, 55
bromocriptine, 22, 466
bronchial thermoplasty, for asthma, 559
bronchiolitis
    treatment, 523
    wheezing and, 518
bronchitis. *See also* chronic obstructive
        pulmonary disease (COPD)
    acute, 92, 95
        treatment, 100
    wheezing and, 518
bronchodilators
    for COPD, 580–585
    for dyspnea, 165
bronchoprovocative testing, 97
bronchoscopy, 98
brown recluse spider bite, 45
    laboratory tests for, 48
    treatment, 53–54
    wounds, 47
buckle fracture, 216, 218
bulimia nervosa. *See also* eating disorders
    definition, 865–866
    epidemiology, 866
bulk-forming agents, 90
buprenorphine, for substance abuse, 816

bupropion
  for eating disorders, 871
  for obesity, 722
burners/stingers, 40

C
caffeine, 57
calcitonin, for osteoporosis, 745
calcium channel blockers
  dysmenorrhea, 152
  for IHD, 703
  migraine, 271
  for systolic dysfunction HF, 623
calcium citrate, for osteoporosis, 743
calcium supplements, for osteoporosis, 740, 743
calculi, hematuria, 281
Canadian cervical spine rules, for neck
        pain, 386
canalith repositioning maneuver, 148
cancer. *See also* specific cancer
  referred otalgia and, 172
Candida, 13, 63
  perianal complaints and, 417
cannabinoids, 376
carbamazepine, for chronic persistent pain, 604
carbidopa, 464–466
carbuncle, 61
  signs, 66
  treatment, 69
cardiac auscultation, 74
cardiac biomarkers, 74
cardiac syncope
  laboratory tests, 457
  signs, 457
  symptoms, 457
cardiomegaly, 74, 618
cardiovascular complications, eating disorders
      and, 872
carotid Doppler ultrasonography, 790
carotid endarterectomy (CEA), 793
carotid sinus hypersensitivity, 457
carotidynia, 451
carpal tunnel syndrome, 256
  testing, 260
  treatment, 262–263
cast or splint immobilization, 221
cataplexy, 290
catechol-O-methyltransferase (COMT) inhibitors,
    466
cat-scratch disease, 364
cefaclor, 69
cefadroxil, 69
cefixime, 69
ceftriaxone, 484
cefuroxime, 69
cellulitis, 59–61
  foot/leg, 65
  gas gangrene, 66
  hand, 65
  necrotizing fasciitis, 66
  postseptal orbital, 65
  preseptal orbital, 65
  signs, 63–66
  treatment, 68–69
central nervous system diseases, 145, 148

central sleep apnea (CSA), 290
cephalexin, 68, 69
cephalosporins, 68
cerebral angiography, for stroke, 790
cerebral edema, 793
cerebrovascular syncope, 455
  symptoms, 457
cervical cancer, 13
  screening, 976
  symptoms, 14
  treatment, 16
cervical cap, 888
cervical nerve root irritation/radiculopathy, 386
cervical spine, 729. *See also* osteoarthritis
cervicitis
  treatment, 511
  vaginal discharge and, 507
cetirizine, 117, 492
chancre, 228, 230–231
  multiple, 231
  of syphilis, 229
chancroid, 228, 231, 235. *See also* genital
    lesions
charcot triad, 5
chemoprophylaxis, 943–949
  bacterial endocarditis, 946
  bacterial meningitis, 943–944
  cardiovascular disease, 944–945
  definition, 943
  group B streptococcal (GBS) infection,
    948–949
  neural tube defects (NTDs), 948
  rheumatic fever, 948
chemotherapy
  for breast cancer, 571
  for colon cancer, 573
  induced nausea and vomiting (CINV), 382
  for lung cancer, 573
cherry angiomas, 121–122, 128
chest pain
  aortic dissection, 71
  common diagnoses
    cardiovascular (CV) conditions, 71
    chest wall pain, 71
    GI sources, 71
  definition, 70
  laboratory testing, 74–76
  pericarditis, 71–72
  pulmonary embolism (PE), 72
  signs, 74
  symptoms, 72–74
  treatment
    angina, 76–77
    miral valve prolapse, 77
    oral NSAIDs, 76
    psychiatric disease, 77
    pulmonary sources, 77
chest radiographs (CXR), 9, 618
  for dyspnea laboratory testing, 164
  for wheezing, 518, 522
chest radiography, 74–75
  and pediatric fever, 398
chest wall pain, 71, 73
chiggers bites, 45. *See also* arachnid bites
  wounds, 46

child abuse. *See also* family violence
  definition, 847
  diagnosis, 848–850
  emotional, 847, 849
  epidemiology, 847–848
  as intergenerational cycle, 850
  neglect, 847
  physical, 847, 848–849
  prognosis, 850
  sexual abuse, 847, 849–850
  specialized child abuse assessment programs, 850
  treatment strategies and intervention, 850
children. *See also* adolescents
  abdominal pain in, 7–8
  screening and prevention for anemia in, 24–25
chlamydia, 13
  conjunctivitis, 424, 427, 431
  screening tests, 975
chloramphenicol, for Rocky Mountain spotted fever treatment, 53
chlorpheniramine, 492–493
cholecystitis, 4–5
  acute, 9
  and leukocytosis, 8
  signs, 6
  treatment, 11
cholelithiasis, 4–5
  dyspepsia and, 155
  vomiting and, 372
cholesteatoma, 173
cholinergic urticaria, 489
chorea, 469
chronic abdominal pain, 6–7
  treatment of, 7
chronic anal fissure, 413
chronic diseases, travelers with, 990–992.
        See also travel medicine
  cardiovascular disease, 991
  diabetes, 990
  HIV-positive patient, 990
  mental illness, 992
  pulmonary disease, 991–992
  TD, 990
chronic endometritis, 402, 404
chronic fatigue syndrome (CFS), 194
chronic narcotic therapy, 735–736
chronic obstructive pulmonary disease (COPD)
  clinical assessment, 578–580
  death rate, 595
  definition, 576
  diagnosis, 577–580
  differential diagnosis, 577
  epidemiology, 576
  exacerbation, 92, 96
  management of stable, 589–590
    exercise, 590
    nutrition, 589–590
    pharmacotherapy, 589
  management strategies, 592–595
    environmental control, 593
    home oxygen therapy, 593–594
    pulmonary rehabilitation, 594–595
    smoking cessation, 592–593
    surgery, 593

pathology and pathophysiology, 577
  risk factors, 576–577
  screening and prevention, 577
  symptoms and signs, 577–578
  treatment, 101, 580–592
  wheezing and, 519
chronic pancreatitis
  treatment, 11
chronic pelvic pain (CPP)
  adhesions, 402
  clinical findings with common causes of, 401
  diagnostic testing in, 405
  dysmenorrhea, 402
  dyspareunia, 402
  endometriosis, 402
  Mittelschmerz, 402
  psychogenic pain, 402
  symptoms, 403
  syndrome (CPPS)
    inflammatory, 480
    non-inflammatory, 480
  treatment, 408–409
  uterine leiomyomas, 402
chronic pelvic pain syndromes (CPPS)
  laboratory tests, 482
  symptoms, 481
  treatment, 484, 487
  urinary symptoms in men and, 480
chronic persistent pain, 596–604
  diagnosis
    assessment, 597
    measure, 597
    pain rating scales, 597
  management strategies, 604
  treatment, 597–604
    acupuncture, 598
    cognitive therapy, 598
    occupational therapy, 598
    pharmacologic therapy, 598–604
    physical therapy, 597–598
Chvostek sign, 200
cigarette smoking. *See also* smoking cessation
  preoperative evaluation and, 1004
ciprofloxacin, 11
circumcision, 236. *See also* genital lesions
cirrhosis, 605–614
  alcoholic, 606, 608, 611
  alpha-1-antitrypsin (AAT) deficiency, 608, 613
  autoimmune hepatitis and, 608–609, 613
  diagnosis, 606–610
  diagnostic tests, 609–610
  hemochromatosis and, 608, 612
  management strategies, 613
  managing complications, 610–611
  nonalcoholic steatohepatitis (NASH) and, 608, 613
  primary biliary, 608, 612
  prognosis, 613–614
  symptoms and signs, 606
    hepatocellular dysfunction, 606
    portal hypertension, 606
  treatment, 609–613
  Wilson disease and, 608, 612–613
clarithromycin, 68

clindamycin, 68, 69, 529
clitoromegaly, 19
clomiphene, for ovulatory dysfunction, 895
clonazepam, for chronic persistent pain, 604
clopidogrel, for stroke, 794
Clostridia perfringens, 66
Clostridium difficile proctitis, 416
cluster headache, 264, 267
　signs, 267
　symptoms, 267
　treatment, 273
coagulopathy, 611
cocaine, 3, 814, 818
codeine
　for cough, 437
　for myalgia, 369
cognitive behavioral therapy (CBT)
　for GAD, 822
　for myalgia, 369
　for panic disorder, 826
　for PTSD, 827
coitus interruptus, 890
colchicine, 493
cold urticaria, 489
colitis, 223. *See also* inflammatory bowel disease
collagen vascular disease, 366, 370.
　　　　See also myalgia
colon cancer
　diagnosis, 569–570
　differential diagnosis, 569
　epidemiology, 563
　prevention, 566
　prognosis, 575
　risk factors
　　alcohol consumption, 565
　　genetic syndromes, 565
　　inflammatory bowel disease, 565
　　obesity, 565
　　tobacco use, 565
　screening, 567
　screening tests, 976
　signs and symptoms, 568
　staging, 570–571
　treatment, 573–574
colonic imaging, 86
colon ischemia, 133
colonoscopy. *See also* barium enema/colonoscopy
　for perianal complaints, 414
colposcopy, 14, 15, 16
combination therapy, 187
comedo extraction, 532
common bile duct, stone in, 5
common cold, 433
　signs, 434
　treatment, 436–437
complementary alternative medicine (CAM)
　for ADHD, 844–845
　for asthma, 558
　for chronic persistent pain, 604
　for dementia, 637, 638
　fatigue, 198
　inflammatory bowel disease, 691
　for menopause, 714
　nausea and vomiting, 376
　peptic ulcer disease and, 754

for premenstrual syndrome, 759, 762
complete blood count, 8, 27
computed tomography (CT), 9, 35, 68, 82, 97,
　　175, 255, 268, 305–306, 375, 414,
　　422, 436, 459
　cirrhosis, 609
　dementia, 634
　inflammatory bowel disease, 690
　for osteoarthritis, 729–730
　for stroke, 788
condoms
　female, 888
　male, 888
condyloma acuminata, 417
　genital lesion and, 228
　laboratory tests for, 234
　signs, 231
　symptoms, 229
　treatment, 235
condyloma lata
　laboratory tests for, 234
　signs, 229
　symptoms, 229
confusion. *See also* delirium
　definition, 78
Confusion Assessment Method (CAM), 81
congenital nevi, 121
　signs, 127
　treatment, 130
congenital sensorineural hearing loss, 276
congestive heart failure (CHF), cough and, 75,
　　92, 96
conjugated hyperbilirubinemia, 302
conjunctival cultures, 66
conjunctivitis
　infectious
　　bacterial, 424, 427, 430–431
　　chlamydia, 424, 427, 431
　　viral, 424, 427, 430
　laboratory tests/diagnostics
　　bacterial, 429
　　chlamydial, 429
　　viral, 429
　noninfectious, 424
　symptoms
　　allergic, 427
　　bacterial, 427
　　chlamydial, 427
　　viral, 427
　treatment
　　allergic, 431
　　bacterial, 430–431
　　chlamydial, 431
　　herpes, 430
　　viral, 430
　viral, 427, 429
　　adenovirus, 424
　　herpes, 426
constipation
　common diagnosis
　　fecal impaction, 85
　　normal-transit constipation (NTC), 83–84
　　pelvic floor dysfunction, 84
　　secondary causes, 84–85
　　slow-transit constipation (STC), 84

definition, 83
laboratory tests, 86
signs, 85–86
symptoms, 85–86
treatment
  biofeedback therapy, 87
  bowel training, 86
  bulk-forming agents, 90
  enemas, 90–91
  fluid intake, 87
  laxatives, 90
  lifestyle modifications, 86–87
  lubiprostone, 90
  methylnaltrexone, 91
  pharmacologic therapy, 87–91
  surfactants, 90
contact dermatitis, 104, 117
contraception, 881–891
barrier methods, 888–889
  cervical cap, 888
  diaphragms, 888
  female condoms, 888
  male condoms, 888
  sponge, 888–889
birth control method, selection, 881–883
hormonal, 883–888
  injectable, 885–886
  oral contraception, 883–885
  postcoital contraceptives, 887–888
  subdermal implant, 887
  transdermal patch, 886
  vaginal ring, 886–887
intrauterine devices (IUD), 889–890
natural family planning
  coitus interruptus, 890
  lactation amenorrhea method (LAM), 890
  periodic abstinence, 890
spermicide, 889
sterilization, 891
  implants, 891
  transabdominal surgical, 891
  vasectomy, 891
contraceptives
for PMS, 759
for vaginal bleeding, 503
contusions, 31. See also ankle injuries
diagnosis, 32
fracture and, 216
core temperature, 395
corneal abrasion, 424
laboratory tests/diagnostics, 429
sysmptoms, 427
treatment, 431
coronary angiography, 76
coronary artery bypass graft (CABG)
  surgery, 708
coronary CT angiography (CCTA), 702
corticosteroid injection, for osteoarthritis, 734
corticosteroid therapy
for asthma, 553
for COPD, 581–584, 585
GI bleeding and, 225
for inflammatory bowel disease, 691, 696
low back pain, 358
nausea and vomiting treatment, 382

proteinuria, 423
pruritus, 115, 117
sinusitis, 441
systemic, 559
for tenosynovitis, 36
for urticaria, 493
Corynebacterium minutissimum, 63
costovertebral angle tenderness, 284
cough
ACE inhibitors, 102
acute, 91
  pneumonia and, 92
  sinusitis, 92
  symptoms and signs, 95–96
  treatment, 100–101
  viral URIs, 91
chronic, 91, 92–95
  symptoms, 96–97
  treatment, 101–102
definition, 91
laboratory tests
  barium swallow, 97
  CT and MRI, 97
  endoscopy, 98
  esophageal pH monitoring, 98
  hematologic tests, 97
  nasal smear, 98
  polymerase chain reaction, 98
  pulse oximetry, 98
  purified protein derivative (PPD), 98
  radiography, 97–98
  skin testing, 98
  spirometry, 97
  sputum cytology, 98
  sweat chloride testing, 98
subacute, 91, 92–95
  symptoms, 96–97
  treatment, 101–102
treatment, 98–102, 437
  antibiotics, 98–102
  COPD, 101
  eosinophilic bronchitis (nonasthmatic), 101
  gastroesophageal reflux disease (GERD),
    101
  hospitalization, 100
  irritant-related cough, 100
  postnasal drainage (PND), 101
  psychogenic cough, 102
  supportive treatment, 100
  tuberculosis, 102
  vaccine, 101
coughing, 549. See also asthma
cow's milk hypersensitivity, 134
COX-2 inhibitors
for dysmenorrhea, 152
c-reactive protein, 9
Crohn's disease
chronic diarrhea and, 133–134
symptoms, 136
cromolyn sodium
for asthma, 556
cryosurgery, for lung cancer, 573
cryotherapy, 235, 236
cryptorchidism, 445
cryptosporidium, 135

CT. *See* computed tomography (CT)
culture test
  for bacterial skin infections, 66–68
    blood culture, 66
    conjunctival culture, 66
curcumin, for inflammatory bowel disease, 691
cyclophosphamide, 422
cyclosporine, for inflammatory bowel disease, 695
cyproterone, 249
cystic fibrosis (CF), 519
cystitis, 167, 281
  signs, 167
  treatment, 169
cystoscopy, 286
cytology, 15
cytomegalovirus, 133

D
dairy products safety, 987. *See also* travel
    medicine
danazol, 152
dapsone, 493
David Letterman sign, 260
D-dimer, 512, 514
deafness, sudden, 275. *See also* hearing loss
decongestants
  for earache, 178
deep venous thrombosis (DVT), 512–513
  laboratory tests, 512–513
  model for clinical prediction of, 513
  signs, 512
  symptoms, 512
dehydration, severe, 139
delayed hypersensitivity reaction, 46
  treatment, 51
delayed pressure urticaria, 489
delirium, 635. *See also* dementia
  common diagnoses
    change in environmental setting, 79
    depression, 79
    drug intoxication, 78
    general medical conditions, 78
    prescription medications, 78
    structural brain disease, 79
    substance-induced delirium, 78
    substance-withdrawal delirium, 78
  laboratory tests, 81–82
  risk factors for, 79
  signs
    agitated confusional state without focal
      signs, 81
    Confusion Assessment Method (CAM), 81
    diastolic blood pressure, 81
    eye examination, 81
    fever, 81
    mini-mental state examination (MMSE),
      80–81
    systolic blood pressure, 81
    tachycardia, 81
    tachypnea, 81
    vital signs, 81
  symptoms, 79–80
  treatment
    benzodiazepines, 82
    drugs with anticholinergic properties, 82

drug therapy, 82
haloperidol, 82
open communication, 82
prevention, 82
supportive care, 82
delusions, 638. *See also* dementia
  of parasitosis, 109
dementia, 627–643
  abnormal neurologic signs and importance,
    633
  behavioral and psychological symptoms, 635
  brain imaging, 634
  causes, 628, 629
  cognitive assessment, 634, 635
  CSF analysis, 633
  definition, 627–628
  delirium, 635
  diagnosis and evaluation, 629–635
  diagnostic tests, 632–634
  driving and, 643
  genetic testing, 633
  laboratory tests, 632
  pathophysiology, 629
  patient care, 640
  physical assessment, 632
  risk factors, 628
  safety, 640–643
  screening and prevention, 629
  staging and typing, 635
  syndromes, 629
  treatment, 635–640
Dennie's pleats, 522
denosumab, for osteoporosis, 745
dental complications, eating disorders and, 872
dental diseases, 172
depo-medroxyprogesterone acetate, 152
depression
  definitions, 856–857
  delirium and, 79
  diagnosis, 858–859
  epidemiology, 857
  etiology, 857
  intimate partner violence and, 852
  laboratory tests, 859
  management strategies, 863–864
  osteoarthritis and, 735
  screening, 858
  symptoms and signs, 858–859
  treatment, 859–863
de Quervain tenosynovitis, 251–252
dermatitis
  contact, 104, 117
  definition, 103
  facial seborrheic, 119
  infantile seborrheic, 119
  patient education, 119
dermatofibromas, 125, 129
dermatologic neoplasm
  common diagnoses
    macular lesions, 121
    nodular lesions, 125–126
    papular lesions, 121–122
  definition, 120
  laboratory tests, 127
  nevi macular lesions, 121

signs, 126–127
  epidermoid cysts, 127
  melanomas, 126
  warts, 126
symptoms, 126
treatment
  benign neoplasms, 127–129
  malignant lesions, 129–130
  premalignant lesions, 129
dermatomyositis, 365, 367
dermatophyte infection, 108, 118–119
dermatosis
  atopic, 117
  definition, 103
dermographism, 489
desmopressin (DDAVP), 185
detoxification, 814
dexamethasone, 270
dextromethorphan, 437
diabetes mellitus, 643–659
  control, 644–645
  early detection of complications, 657–658
  health literacy, 657
  heart failure treatment and, 620
  office management, 658–659
  patient-centered care, 656
  preoperative evaluation and, 1003
  prevention, 657–658
  prognosis, 659
  with proteinuria, 423
  psychosocial factors, 657
  self-management skills, 656
  self monitoring of blood glucose, 656
  symptoms and signs, 648
  treatment, 648–656
    insulin therapy, 655–656
diaphoresis, 374
diaphragms, 888. See also contraception
diarrhea
  acute, 131, 136
  bacterial infections, 131, 135
  chemical contamination of water, 131
  chronic, 131–132
    in children, 134
    diagnostic tests, 136–137
    fatty, 132
    inflammatory, 132
    nonspecific, 134
    symptoms, 135
    treatment, 139
    watery, 131
  colon ischemia, 133
  definition, 131
  food poisoning and, 135
  noninfectious causes, 131
  parasitic infections, 131, 135
  patient education, 144
  persistent, 131–132
  prevention of, 132
  sexually transmitted proctitis, 133
  signs, 136
  symptoms, 134–136
  treatment
    antibiotic treatment, 139
    in children and elderly, 138–139

diet, 139
hydration and rehydration maintenance, 138
probiotics, 144
symptomatic treatment, 139
viral infections, 131, 135
diarrhea (TD). See also travel medicine
  childhood, 989–990
  immunocompromised traveler, 990
  prophylaxis, 981
  treatment, 981, 986
diastolic blood pressure, 81
diastolic dysfunction HF, 624, 625–626
dicloxacillin, 69
dietary supplements for obesity management, 723
diets, for obesity management, 720–721
  low-calorie, 721
  low-carbohydrate, 721
  lower-fat, 721
  South Beach diet, 721
  very low-calorie, 721
  zone, 721
diet therapy, 197
digital rectal examination, 284
digoxin, for systolic dysfunction HF, 624
dilated cardiomyopathy, 389
dipeptidyl peptidase 4 (DPP-4) inhibitors
  for diabetes mellitus, 652–653
diphenhydramine, 115, 492, 493
diphenoxylate hydrochloride with atropine, 10
dipstick test, 419
direct trauma, 173, 182
direct trauma, arm/shoulder complaints, 37
disability assessments, osteoarthritis, 735
discolored nails, 240, 242
disequilibrium, 146
dislocations
  fracture and, 216
  phalangeal, 262
  treatment, 217–218
dislocations, shoulder, 37
  treatment, 42–43
distal fractures, 219
disulfiram
  for substance abuse, 815
diverticular disease, 2
  peritonitis in, 6
  symptoms, 5
  treatment, 11
diverticulosis, 222
Dix-Hallpike (Nylen-Barany) maneuver, 147
dizziness
  common diagnoses
    acoustic neuroma, 145
    central nervous system diseases, 145
    peripheral vestibular disorders, 145
    systemic diseases, 145
  definition, 145
  laboratory tests, 147
  patient education, 148
  symptoms, 145–147
  treatment
    central nervous system diseases, 148
    peripheral vestibular disorders, 148
    systemic diseases, 148
  types, 146

donepezil, for dementia, 536–537
doxazosin, 485
doxepin, 115, 117, 493
doxycycline, 69, 484
    for acne vulgaris, 530
    for Lyme disease treatment, 53
    for mammalian bites, 49
    for urinary symptoms in men, 484
driving, and dementia, 643
droperidol, 382
drug use disorders. *See* substance abuse
duloxetine, 477
duplex ultrasonography, 9
dutasteride, 484, 486, 487
dynamic shoulder stability, 37
dysfunctional uterine bleeding (DUB)
    anovulatory bleeding, 503
    ovulatory bleeding, 503
dyshidrosis
    pruritic dermatoses and, 106
    signs, 113
    treatment, 118
dyshidrotic eczema, 107
dyslipidemias, 660–675
    acute pancreatitis, 674
    diagnosis, 662–664
    hyperbetalipoproteinemia, 662
    hypercholesterolemia, 660–661
    hyperlipidemia, 660
    hypertriglyceridemia, 661
    hypoalphalipoproteinemia, 661
    laboratory tests, 663–664
    management strategies
        children and adolescents, 673–674
        elderly patients, 673
        long-term adherence, 673
        patient education, 673
        secondary prevention, 674
        systematic follow-up, 674
    metabolic syndrome, 661–662
    primary, 660
    prognosis, 674
    screening and prevention, 662
    secondary, 660
    treatment, 664–673
dysmenorrhea
    chronic pelvic pain (CPP), 402
    common diagnoses, 149–150
    definition, 149
    primary, 149
    secondary, 149–150
        adenomyosis, 149
        endometriosis, 149
        leiomyomas, 149–150
    treatment, 408
        COX II inhibitors, 152
        exercise, 152
        nonpharmacologic approaches,
            151–152
        NSAIDs, 152
        oral contraceptives for, 152
        physical treatments, 152
        surgical therapies, 154
dyspareunia, chronic pelvic pain (CPP),
    402

dyspepsia
    common diagnoses
        cholecystitis, 155
        gastroesophageal reflux disease (GERD), 155
        medications, 155
        nonulcer dyspepsia (NUD), 155
        peptic ulcer disease (PUD), 155
    definition, 154
    laboratory tests, 157
    signs, 155
    symptoms, 155
    treatment, 157–160
dysphagia, 5
dyspnea, 92, 96
    causes, 162
    common diagnoses
        cardiac dyspnea, 161
        mixed cardiopulmonary dyspnea, 161
        noncardiopulmonary causes, 161–162
        pulmonary disorders, 161
    definition, 161
    laboratory tests, 163–165
    signs, 162
    symptoms, 162
    treatment, 165–166
dystonia, 469–470
dysuria
    asymptomatic bacteriuria (ASB), 171
    causes, 166–167
    common diagnoses, 167
        acute bacterial cystitis, 167
        dysuria without pyuria, 167
        urethritis, 167
        vulvovaginitis, 167
    definition, 166
    psychogenic, 167
    signs, 167–168
    symptoms, 167
    treatment, 169–171
    without pyuria, 168, 169

E
earache
    common diagnoses
        acute otitis media (AOM), 172
        barotrauma, 172
        direct trauma, 172
        otitis externa (OE), 172
        referred otalgia, 172
    treatment
        AOM, 175–181
        barotrauma, 182
        direct trauma, 182
        OE, 181–182
    definition, 172
    laboratory tests, 175
    signs, 173
    symptoms, 173
eating disorders
    anorexia nervosa
        definition, 865
        epidemiology, 866
    binge
        definition, 866
        epidemiology, 866

bulimia nervosa
  definition, 865–866
  epidemiology, 866
  differential diagnosis, 868
  female athlete triad, 866
  laboratory findings, 868
  management strategies, 871–872
  pathophysiology, 867
  prognosis, 872–873
  risk factors, 866–867
    cultural, 866
    familial, 867
    psychiatric illness, 867
  symptoms and signs, 867–868
  treatment, 869–871
    antidepressants, 871
    inpatient hospitalization, 869
    nutritional rehabilitation, 869
    outpatient treatment, 869
    psychosocial interventions, 869, 871
    psychotropic medications, 871
echocardiography (ECG)
  for chest pain, 74
  exercise stress, 76
  for stroke, 790
econazole, 236
ecthyma, 61
  treatment, 69
ectopic pregnancy, 406–407
  acute pelvic pain (APP) and, 402
  methotrexate protocols for, 407
eczema
  atopic, 103, 117
  dyshidrotic, 107
  nummular, 108, 119
educational notes and suggestions, Pap smears
    report, 14
eflornithine HCl, 249
elder abuse. See also family violence
  definition, 853
  diagnosis, 854
  epidemiology, 854
  ethical and legal obligations, 855
  management, 854–855
  material or financial abuse, 853
  physical, 853
  physical neglect, 853
  psychological abuse, 853
  psychological neglect, 853
  self-neglect, 853–854
  sexual abuse, 853
  violation of personal rights, 853
elderly
  abdominal pain in, 8
  acute abdominal pain in, causes of, 2
  bowel obstruction in, 2
  with chronic mesenteric ischemia, 5
elderly women with asymptomatic bacteriuria,
    171
electrocardiogram (ECG), 457–458
  for dyspnea, 165
  IHD, 701, 702
  in joint pain, 314
  for palpitations, 389
  for syncope, 457–458

electrocautery, for lung cancer, 573
electroencephalography (EEG)
  for delirium testing, 82
  for stroke, 790
  for syncope, 459
electromyography
  for foot complaints, 212
  for perianal complaints, 414
electronystagmography, 147
elliptocytosis, hereditary, 26. See also anemia
emotional abuse, of child, 847, 849
emotional stress, peptic ulcer disease and,
    754
endocrine complications, eating disorders
    and, 872
endometrial ablation, 154
endometrial biopsy, 715
  for vaginal bleeding, 503
endometrial cells
  treatment, 16
endometriosis
  chronic pelvic pain (CPP), 402
  dysmenorrhea and, 149
  signs, 150
  symptoms, 150
  treatment, 408
endometritis
  chronic, 402, 404
endoscopic retrograde cholangiopancreatogram,
    10
endoscopy
  for cough
    bronchoscopy, 98

    esophagogastroduodenoscopy (EGD),
        98
    nasopharyngoscopy, 98
  gastrointestinal, 29
  for GI bleeding, 225–226
  for inflammatory bowel disease, 690
  for nausea and vomiting, 375
  for perianal complaints, 414
  video capsule, 226
  for wheezing, 523
enemas, 90–91
entacapone, 464–466
entrapment neuropathies, 256, 262
enuresis
  definition, 183
  important history in children with, 184
  interventions for, 186
  laboratory tests, 184–185
  non-monosymptomatic, 183
  primary monosymptomatic, 183
  secondary monosymptomatic, 183
  signs, 183–184
  symptoms, 183
  treatment, 185–187
eosinophilia-myalgia syndrome (EMS), 366.
    See also myalgia
eosinophilic bronchitis (nonasthmatic), 101
ephedrine, 493
ephedrine, for obesity, 723
ephelides, 121
epidermal cysts, 126, 127

epididymitis
  scrotal complaints and, 444
  signs, 445
  traumatic, 448
  treatment, 447
epiglottitis, 450
epinephrine
  for immediate hypersensitivity reaction
    treatment, 51
  for urticaria, 493
episcleritis, 424
  laboratory tests/diagnostics, 430
  simple, 429
  symptoms, 429
  treatment, 431
episodic migraine, 264–265, 266, 268
epithelial cell abnormalities, Pap smears report, 14
eplerenone, for heart failure, 621
ergot alkaloids, 270
eructation, 371
erysipelas, 61
  signs, 66
  treatment, 69
erythema chronicum migrans, 48
erythrasma, 59
  pruritic lesions and, 228, 234
  signs, 63, 232
  symptoms, 229
  treatment, 68, 236
erythromycin
  for acne vulgaris, 529
  for mammalian bites, 49
  for pertussis, 101
  for sore throat, 453
Escherichia coli, 395
esophageal varices, 225
esophagitis
  UGI bleeding and, 222
esophagogastroduodenoscopy (EGD), 98
essential tremor, 461, 467, 468
estrogen
  for incontinence treatment, 477
  replacement therapy
    for vaginal bleeding, 505
estrogen-progestin challenge test, 21
estrogen–progestin pills, 883–885
ethmoid sinusitis, 435
evaluation for cervical nerve root lesions, neck
    pain, 385
excisional biopsy, 56
  for perianal complaints, 416
excision or electrodesiccation and curettage
    (ED&C), 129
exenatide, for obesity, 723
exercise
  for asthma, 553
  for breast cancer, 564
  for COPD, 590
  for diabetes mellitus, 650
  for dyslipidemias, 666
  for dysmenorrhea, 152
  induced hematuria, 283
  low back pain and, 358
  for menopause, 714
  for myalgia, 369

  for obesity, 719, 721
  for osteoarthritis, 730
  supervised, 316
  for systolic dysfunction HF, 624
  weight-bearing, 346
exercise-induced hematuria, 283
exercise stress echocardiography, 76
exercise stress electrocardiography, 75–76
exercise treadmill test (ETT)
  IHD, 701
exfoliating agents, 529
expectorants for asthma, 557
expedited partner therapy (EPT), 937
external auditory canal, 173
extrahepatic obstruction
  jaundice and, 302, 309
extratesticular scrotal complaints
  signs, 446–447
  symptoms, 446–447
  treatment, 448
ezetimibe, for dyslipidemias, 673

F
facial seborrheic dermatitis, 119
failure to thrive (FTT)
  asymmetric, 192
  calorie requirements for catch-up growth,
    192
  definition, 187–188
  differential diagnoses, 188–191
    constitutional growth delay, 188
    familial short stature, 188
    intrauterine growth restriction, 188
    midparental height, 188
  epidemiology, 188
  laboratory tests, 189–191, 192
  presentation, 189–191
  prognosis, 192
  signs, 191–192
  symmetric, 192
  symptoms, 191
  treatment, 192
familial atypical mole and melanoma syndrome
    (FAMMS), 121
  signs, 126
family violence
  child abuse
    definition, 847
    diagnosis, 848–850
    epidemiology, 847–848
    as intergenerational cycle, 850
    prognosis, 850
    treatment strategies and intervention, 850
  elder abuse
    definition, 853
    diagnosis, 854
    epidemiology, 854
    ethical and legal obligations, 855
    management, 854–855
    material or financial abuse, 853
    physical, 853
    physical neglect, 853
    psychological abuse, 853
    psychological neglect, 853
    self-neglect, 853–854

sexual abuse, 853
violation of personal rights, 853
intimate partner violence
anxiety disorders, 852
chronic pain, 852
definition, 850
depression, 852
diagnosis, 851
epidemiology, 850
management strategies, 851–852
prevention, 852–853
prognosis, 852
PTSD, 852
violent relationships, 851
overview, 847
fatigue
common diagnoses
chronic fatigue syndrome (CFS), 194
mixed fatigue, 193
physical fatigue, 193
physiologic fatigue, 193
psychological illness, 193
definition, 193
diet therapy, 197
drug therapy, 196
laboratory tests, 195
natural history of fatigue complaint, 198
patient education, 198
signs, 194
symptoms, 194
treatment, 195–198
fatty chronic diarrhea, 132
febrile exanthems, 395
febrile seizures, 399
fecal occult blood testing, 86
female condoms, 888. See also contraception
fenofibrate, for dyslipidemias, 673
fever. See also pediatric fever
definition, 395
of unknown origin (FUO), 395
fexofenadine, 115, 492, 493
fiberoptic rhinoscopy, 435
fibric acid derivatives, 673
fibroadenoma, 55, 57
fibrocystic changes
breast condition, 55
breast pain and, 55
treatment
dietary changes, 57
pharmacologic therapy, 57
supportive measures, 57
surgery, 57
fibromyalgia
syndrome (FMS), 365
treatment, 369
fibular fractures at/above/below tibial dome,
220
finasteride, 484, 486, 487
for hair disorder treatment, 247, 249
fine needle aspiration (FNA) biopsy, 56
finger fractures
distal phalangeal fractures, 218
metacarpal fractures, 218
middle and proximal phalangeal, 218
PIP joint dislocations, 218

Finkelstein test, 260, 261
fire ants bites, 45, 46
fistula-in-ano, 411
fistulas
hematuria and, 283
perianal complaints sign, 413
Flagyl. See metronidazole
flat warts
signs, 126
treatment, 128
fleas bites, 45
fleeting pain, 74
fluconazole, 236, 247, 250
fluid, electrolyte, and acid-base disturbances
definition, 199
diagnostic tests, 200
hypercalcemia, 200
hyperkalemia, 199
hypernatremia, 199
hypocalcemia, 200
hypokalemia, 199
hyponatremia, 199
patient education, 205–206
signs, 200
symptoms, 200
treatment, 200–205
fluoride, for osteoporosis, 745
fluoroquinolones, 69
flush, 711
flutamide, 249
folate deficiency, 25, 28
treatment, 30
follicle-stimulating hormone (FSH)
level, in amenorrhea, 21
folliculitis, 62
signs, 66
treatment, 69
food poisoning, bacterial diarrhea and, 135
food safety, 981, 987. See also travel medicine
foot care, 730
foot complaints
common diagnoses
achilles tendon rupture, 209
forefoot, 206–207, 209–210
hindfoot, 208
lisfranc injury, 208
midfoot, 207–208
tarsal navicular bone fractures, 208
definition, 206
evaluation and management, 209–212
foot and toe fractures, 220–221
forefoot, 206–207
laboratory tests, 209–212
signs, 209–211
symptoms, 209–211
treatment, 212–215
appropriate footwear, 212–213
orthotics, 214
of pain and inflammation, 213
stretching exercises, 213–214
systemic antibiotics, 215
systemic antifungal drugs, 215
foot/leg cellulitis, 65
forefoot complaints, 206–207, 209–210
formoterol for asthma, 556

fractures, 31. *See also* ankle injuries
  acute, 34
  in adult, 216
  in childhood, 216
  clavicle, 219
  common diagnoses
    contusion, 216
    dislocations, 216
    sprain, 216
    strain, 216
    subluxations, 216
  definition, 216
  diagnosis, 32
  in elderly, 216
  growth plate injuries, 221
  hand and wrist
    Bennett fracture, 255
    Boxer's, 218, 255
    scaphoid fractures, 255
  imaging, 217
  immobilization time and, 218
  intra-articular, 221
  laboratory tests, 217
  neurovascular compromise situation in, 221
  occult, 34
  open, 221
  signs, 216–217
  simple torso, 219
  stress, 35
  symptoms, 216–217
  symptoms/signs, 34
  treatment, 36
    ankle fractures, 220
    clavicle fractures, 219
    finger fractures, 218
    foot and toe fractures, 220–221
    fractures requiring referral, 221
    leg fractures, 219–220
    metacarpal fractures, 218
    pediatric, 221
    torso fractures, 219
    wrist and arm fractures, 218–219
  unstable, 221
  wrist and arm, 218–219
Francisella tularensis, 47
frontal sinusitis, 435
FSH. *See* follicle-stimulating hormone (FSH)
fumigation, 51
functional incontinence, 471
fungi, 13
furosemide, 422
furuncle (boil), 61
  signs, 66

G
gabapentin, for chronic persistent pain, 603
galactorrhea, 19
galantamine, for dementia, 537
gallbladder pain, 73
gallstone ileus, 5
gallstones, 1, 4–5
  chemical dissolution of, 11
gas gangrene, 66
gastric banding, 724
gastric cancer, 160
gastric varices, 222

gastritis, 222
gastroenteritis, acute, 372
gastroesophageal reflux disease (GERD)
  pediatric, 160
  testing for wheezing, 523
  treatment, 155, 160
  vomiting and, 372
gastrointestinal bleeding
  common diagnoses
    LGI bleeding, 222–223
    LGI bleeding in children, 223
    obscure GI bleeding, 223
    UGI bleeding, 222
    UGI bleeding in children, 223
  definition, 222
  initial predictors of poor clinical outcome in, 227
  rare but serious conditions, 223
  signs
    abdominal examination, 225
    bleeding history, 223–224
    general history, 224–225
    mentation, 225
    nasogastric (NG) tube, 225
    rectal examination, 225
    sequelae of chronic liver disease, 225
    vital signs, 225
  symptoms, 223–225
  tests, 225–226
    angiography, 226
    barium studies, 226
    double-balloon enteroscopy, 226
    electrocardiogram, 226
    endoscopy, 225–226
    hematologic studies, 226
    technetium red cell scan, 226
    video capsule endoscopy, 226
  treatment, 226–227
    hospitalization, 226–227
    risk stratification, 226
gastrointestinal complications, eating disorders
    and, 872
gastrointestinal (GI) endoscopy, 29
gastrointestinal obstruction, vomiting and, 372, 374
gastrointestinal pain (GI), 73, 76
gemfibrozil, for dyslipidemias, 673
gender differences, in sexual function, 916
generalized anxiety disorder (GAD), 819–820
  diagnoses, 820–821
  management strategies, 827
  prognosis, 827
  treatment, 822–826
    antidepressants, 822, 826
    azapirones, 822
    benzodiazepines, 822
    beta-blockers, 822
    cognitive behavioral therapy (CBT), 822
    hydroxyzine, 822
genital lesions, 228
  chancroid, 228, 231, 235
  common diagnoses
    cystic lesions, 229
    other causes, 229
    pruritic lesions, 228–229
    ulcerative lesions, 228
    verrucous/papillomatous lesions, 228
  cystic

laboratory tests, 234
    signs, 233
    symptoms, 229
    treatment, 236
  definition, 228
  pruritic
    laboratory tests, 234
    signs, 232–233
    symptoms, 229
    treatment, 236
  ulcerative
    laboratory tests, 233–234
    signs, 229–231
    symptoms, 229
    treatment, 234–235
  verrucoid/papillomatous, 228–236
    laboratory tests, 234
    signs, 231–232
    symptoms, 229
    treatment, 235–236
gestational diabetes, 646
  screening for, 647
giant cell arteritis, 370
ginger extract, 376
glabella tap reflex, 463
glenohumeral instability, 37, 41
  treatment, 43
glomerular disease. See also renal failure
  hematuria treatment, 285
  prognosis, 773
  symptoms and signs, 765
  tests, 766
  treatment, 768
GLP-1 mimetics
  for diabetes mellitus, 654
glucose-6-phosphate dehydrogenase (G6PD)
    deficiency, 26
glyceryl trinitrate, 152
golfer's elbow. See medial epicondylitis
gonadotropin levels, postpartum, 910
gonadotropin-releasing hormone analogs, for
    PMS, 759
gonococcal infection, 480. See also urinary
    symptoms in men
gonococcal urethritis, 480
gonorrhea, 933
  screening tests, 974–975
Goodsall rule, 413
G6PD deficiency. See glucose-6-phosphate
    dehydrogenase (G6PD) deficiency
gram stain, 66
Group A beta-hemolytic streptococcal infection
    (GABHS), 449
group A streptococcal (GAS) vaginitis, 507
growth plate injuries, 216, 221
guttate psoriasis, 106
gynecomastia, 55, 57

H
HA. See hypothalamic amenorrhea (HA)
Haemophilus ducreyi, 228, 231
Haemophilus influenzae, 395
Haemophilus influenzae type b (Hib), 65
hair diorders
  alopecias, 237–238
    alopecia areata, 238

androgenetic, 238
    diagnoses and etiologic classifications of, 238
    infectious, 238
    physiologic, 238
    systemic processes, 238
    traumatic, 238
  baldness, 238, 243
  definition, 237
  hair definition
    terminal hair, 237
    vellus hair, 237
  hirsutism, 238–240
    adult-onset congenital adrenal hyperplasia,
        240
    causes of, 240
    cushing syndrome, 240
    idiopathic hirsutism, 240
    medications, 240
    ovarian or adrenal tumors, 240
    polycystic ovarian syndrome (PCOS), 238
    laboratory tests, 244–246
    signs, 242–244
    symptoms, 242
    treatment, 246–250
hallucinations, 638. See also dementia
haloperidol, 82
hand and wrist complaints
  common diagnoses
    arthritis, 256
    Bennett fracture, 255, 258
    boxer's fractures, 218, 255
    dislocations, 256
    entrapment neuropathies, 256
    ganglia injuries, 256
    metacarpal fractures, 255
    phalangeal fractures, 256
    scaphoid fractures, 255
    scapholunate dissociation, 255
    sprains and contusions, 252–255
    tendon injuries, 251–252
  definition, 251
  differential diagnosis and management, 257–260
  laboratory tests, 260
  signs, 256–260
  special tests
    Allen test, 260, 261
    Finkelstein test, 260, 261
    froment sign, 260, 262
    gamekeeper test, 260, 261
    grind test, 260, 261
    Phalen test, 260, 261
    Spurling test, 260, 261
    TFCC compression test, 260, 262
    Tinel test, 260, 261
    two-point discrimination, 260, 262
    Watson, 260, 261
  symptoms, 256–260
  treatment, 262–263
    entrapment neuropathies, 262
    injections for, 262–263
    mallet deformity, 262
    nonpharmacologic, 262–262
    patient follow-up, 263
    phalangeal dislocations, 262
    phalangeal fractures, 262
    pharmacologic, 262

hand cellulitis, 65
handcuff neuropathy, 256
hands, 728–729. *See also* osteoarthritis
headaches
    common diagnoses
        analgesic rebound, 265
        cluster, 264, 267
        episodic migraine, 264–266, 268
        secondary, 264–265, 267, 273
        tension-type (TTH), 264, 266
    definition, 264
    laboratory tests, 268
        angiography, 268
        arterial biopsy, 268
        blood analysis, 268
        computed tomography (CT), 268
        electroencephalography, 268
        magnetic resonance imaging (MRI), 268
        radiologic evaluation, 268
        radionucleotide imaging, 268
    neck pain and, 384
    primary headache disorders, 264
        cluster, 264
        episodic migraine, 264
        tension-type headache (TTH), 264
        unusual primary headache disorders, 264
    rebound or withdrawal, 265
    secondary, 265
    signs, 267–268
    snoop, 267
    symptoms, 265–267
    treatment
        analgesic rebound headaches, 265
        cluster, 273
        episodic migraine (with or without aura), 268–271
        migraine, 268–271
        secondary headaches, 273
        TTH, 271, 273
head lice *(pediculosis capitis)*, 45, 46, 105
    bites, treatment of, 52
hearing loss
    acoustic neuroma and, 274
    central, 274
    common diagnoses
        central hearing loss, 277
        conductive loss, 276–277
        sensorineural loss, 275–276
    common etiologies of, 276
    conductive, 274
        laboratory testing, 279
        obstruction, 277
        otitis media, 277, 280
        otosclerosis, 277
        symptoms, 277
        treatment, 280
    definition, 274
    earache symptoms and, 173
    laboratory tests, 278–279
        audiometry, 278–279
        OAE and ABR, 279
        tympanometry, 279
    mixed, 274
    prevention, 275
    screening, 275

    sensorineural, 274
        acoustic damage, 275–276
        congenital, 276
        laboratory tests, 278
        Meniere's disease, 276
        ototoxicity, 276, 280
        presbycusis, 276, 277
        treatment, 279–280
    signs, 277–278
        developmental milestones, 278
        otoscopic examination, 277
        tuning fork tests, 278
    sudden deafness, 275
    symptoms, 277
        associated, 277
        reduced hearing acuity, 277
        timing/onset of, 277
    treatment, 279–280
    tuning fork tests, 278
heart failure (HF), 614–627
    classification, 615
    definition, 615
    diagnosis, 617–619
    epidemiology, 615–616
        cardiomyopathy, 616
        coronary artery disease, 616
        etiology, 616
        hypertension, 616
        prevalence, 615
        valvular disease, 616
    management strategies, 626
    palpitations and, 389
    pathophysiology, 616–617
    prevention, 617
    prognosis, 626–627
    treatment, 619–626
        diastolic dysfunction, 624, 625–626
        systolic dysfunction, 620–624
heat urticaria, 489
Helicobacter pylori, 74, 750, 751, 754
    pathophysiology, 747
hematemesis, 223
hematochezia, 223
hematologic complications, eating disorders and, 872
hematologic studies, 226
hematologic tests
    for chest pain, 74
    for cough, 97
    for GI bleeding, 226
    for hair disorders, 245
    jaundice, 306–307
    joint pain, 313
hematomas, 182
    perianal, 411
        symptoms, 412
        treatment, 415
hematuria
    common diagnoses
        calculi, 281
        glomerular causes, 283
        infections, 283
        neoplasms, 281–283
        nonglomerular causes, 281–283
    definition, 281

diagnostic tests, 284–286
  blood work, 285
  cystoscopy, 286
  imaging studies, 285–286
  renal biopsy, 286
  screening, 284
  urinalysis, 284–285
  urine collection, 285
  urine culture, 285
  urine cytology, 286
  urine dipstick, 284
exercise-induced, 283
signs, 284
symptoms, 283–284
treatment, 286
  calculi, 286
  glomerular disease, 286
  infections, 286
hemochromatosis, 608
hemoglobin (Hb) electrophoresis, 28
hemorrhagic pancreatitis, 6
hemorrhoids
  LGI bleeding and, 223
  perianal complains and, 411
    hemorrhoidectomy, 415
    sign, 413
    symptom, 412
    treatment, 414
heparin therapy, VTE, 517
hepatic encephalopathy, 611
hepatic iminodiacetic acid (HIDA) scan
    in acute cholecystitis, 9
hepatitis, 606
hepatitis B, 606, 612
  prevention, 44
hepatitis C, 606, 612
hepatitis D, 606
hepatojugular reflux, 618
hepatomegaly, 618
herbal remedies, for asthma, 558
herb ma huang (ephedra), for asthma, 558
hereditary elliptocytosis, 26
hereditary nephritis, 283
hereditary spherocytosis, 26
hernias
  extratesticular scrotal complaints and, 445
  treatment, 448
herpes conjunctivitis, 426, 430
herpes simplex virus (HSV)
  pediatric fever and, 395
HIDA scan. See hepatic iminodiacetic acid
    (HIDA) scan
hidradenitis suppurativa, 62
  signs, 66
  treatment, 69
high-grade squamous intraepithelial lesion (HSIL), 13
  symptoms, 14
  treatment, 16
hindfoot complaints, 208, 212
hip complaints, 338
  in adults, 343
  in children and adolescents, 341
  definition, 338
  evaluation, 340–341
  hip impingement, 345
  imaging, 345

Perthes disease, 345
SCFE, 343, 345
septic arthritis, 311
signs, 344–345
symptoms, 344–345
transient synovitis, 345
treatment, 345–347
hips, 728. See also osteoarthritis
hirsutism, 19
  adult-onset congenital adrenal hyperplasia, 240
  from androgen excess, 242
  causes, 240
  cushing syndrome, 240
  defined, 237
  hair disorder and, 249–250
  hair growth and, 249–250
  idiopathic, 240, 242
  laboratory tests, 245
  medications causing, 240
  moderate or severe, 245
  ovarian or adrenal tumors, 240
  polycystic ovarian syndrome (PCOS), 238–239
  signs, 242–243
  symptoms, 242
  treatment, 249–250
hollow viscus perforation, 3
  signs, 6
  symptoms, 5
  treatment, 11–12
home monitoring, for hypertension, 686
homocysteine, 28
hormonal contraception, 883–888
  injectable, 885–886
  oral contraception, 883–885
  postcoital contraceptives, 887–888
  subdermal implant, 887
  transdermal patch, 886
  vaginal ring, 886–887
hot flash, 711
HPV. See human papilloma virus (HPV)
HSIL. See High-grade squamous intraepithelial
    lesion (HSIL)
HSV-1 or 2
  genital lesions
    signs, 229–230
    symptoms, 229
  ulcerative lesions and, 228
human bites
  injuries from, 44. See also mammalian bites
  treatment, 48
human immunodeficiency virus (HIV), 16. See
    also AIDS
  antiretroviral agents, 540–545
  definition, 535–536
  screening, 974
  testing
    vaginal discharge complaints and, 509
  travelers with, 990
human papilloma virus (HPV), 12–13
  and low-grade squamous intraepithelial
    lesions, 13
  prevention of, 13
  testing, 14
humeral head fractures, 218–219
humidification, 441
hydration and rehydration, 138. See also diarrhea

hydroceles
extratesticular scrotal complaints and, 445
treatment, 448
hydrochlorothiazide, for osteoporosis, 745
hydrocodone
for chronic persistent pain, 602
for myalgia, 369
hydrotherapy, for asthma, 558
hydroxyzine, 115, 492
for generalized anxiety disorder (GAD), 822
hymenoptera, 44
treatment, 51
hymenoptera venom allergy, 45
hyperandrogenism, 19
hyperbetalipoproteinemia, 662. See also
dyslipidemias
hypercalcemia, 200
laboratory test for, 200
signs, 200
symptoms, 200
treatment, 205
hypercholesterolemia, 660–661. See also
dyslipidemias
hypercoagulable
preoperative evaluation and, 1004
hypergonadotropic amenorrhea, 19
vitamin D supplementation for, 23
hyperkalemia, 199
laboratory test for, 200
symptoms, 200
treatment, 204
hyperkeratinization, 526
hyperkinesias, 461
hyperlipidemia, 660. See also dyslipidemias
hypernatremia, 199
signs, 200
symptoms, 200
treatment, 203–204
hyperosmolar agents, 90
hyperprolactinemia, 18–19
brain MRI for, 20–21
medication causes of, 18
treatment, 22
hypersensitivity, wheezing and, 519
hypersensitivity reaction
delayed, 46
immediate, 45–46
hypertension
causes, 677
definition, 676
diagnosis, 677
epidemiology, 676
heart failure and, 616
laboratory tests, 679
physical examination, 678–679
signs, 677
symptoms, 677
systemic venous, 618
treatment, 679–686
hyperthyroidism, 801–805
diagnosis, 801
management strategies, 805
signs and symptoms, 798
treatment
antithyroid drugs (ATD), 801–803

β-adrenergic antagonists, 804–805
calcium channel blockers, 805
methimazole (MMI), 802
propylthiouracil (PTU), 802
radioactive iodine (RAI), 803–804
surgery, 804
thyroiditis, 805
types, 801
hypertrichosis, 237
causes of, 240
medications causing, 240
symptoms of, 242
hypertriglyceridemia, 661. See also
dyslipidemias
hypertrophic obstructive cardiomyopathy, 389
hypertrophic pyloric stenosis
children with, 374
vomiting and, 371
hyperventilation, 73
hyperventilation therapy, 793
hypoalphalipoproteinemia, 661. See also
dyslipidemias
hypocalcemia, 199
symptoms, 200
treatment, 204–205
hypoestrogenic states
in amenorrhea, 19
vaginal discharge and, 507
hypogonadism, 503
hypogonadotropic amenorrhea, 17
treatment, 21–22, 23
hypokalemia, 199
laboratory test for, 200
symptoms, 200
treatment, 204
hypokinesias, 461
hyponatremia
hyperosmolar, 199
hypo-osmolar euvolemic, 199
hypo-osmolar hypervolemic, 199
hypo-osmolar hypovolemic, 199
iso-osmolar, 199
symptoms, 200
treatment, 200, 203
hypothalamic amenorrhea (HA), 17
treatment, 21–22, 23
hypothenar eminence, 251
hypothermia, 81
hypothyroidism
diagnosis, 799
management strategies, 800–801
signs and symptoms, 798
treatment, 799–800
types, 799
hysterectomy, 154, 505–506
treatment, 409
hysterosalpingogram, 150
hysteroscopy, 21

I

ibandronate, for osteoporosis, 744
IBS. See irritable bowel syndrome (IBS)
ibuprofen, 484
for common cold, 436–437
for myalgia, 369

idiopathic fatigue, 194
idiopathic hirsutism, 240, 242
idiopathic inflammatory bowel disease,
  133–134
idiopathic syncope, 455
IgA nephropathy
  hematuria and, 283–284
imidazole, 236
imipenem-cilastatin, 69
imipramine, 187
imiquimod, 235
immediate hypersensitivity reaction, 45–46
  treatment, 51
immobilization, myalgia, 369
immunizations, 960–966
  administration, 960
  diphtheria–tetanus–acellular pertussis,
    961–962
  haemophilus influenzae Type B (Hib),
    962
  hepatitis A (HAV), 963–964, 966
  hepatitis B (HBV), 961, 966
  human papilloma virus (HPV2 and HPV 4),
    964, 965, 966
  illness, 961
  immunocompromise, 961
  inactivated poliovirus vaccine (IPV),
    962–963
  influenza, 963, 964–965
  measles–mumps–rubella (MMR),
    963, 965
  meningococcal conjugate vaccine (MCV4),
    964, 966
  overview, 960
  pneumococcal conjugate vaccine (PCV13),
    962, 966
  pneumococcal polysaccharide vaccination
    (PPSV23), 965–966
  reporting, 961
  Rotavirus, 961
  safety, 960–961
  tetanus–diphtheria–acellular pertussis (Tdap),
    961–962, 966
  tetanus-diphtheria (Td), 961–962
  timing, 960
  varicella vaccine (VAR), 963, 965
  zoster virus, 965
immunocompromise patients, 507
immunohemolysis, 28
immunomodulators, for inflammatory bowel
  disease, 695
immunosuppressive drugs for asthma,
  557
immunotherapy for asthma, 558
impetigo, 59
  signs, 63
  treatment, 68
implants, sterilization, 891
incarcerated hernia, 374
incisional biopsy, for breast condition, 56
inclusion conjunctivitis, 427
infantile seborrheic dermatitis, 119
infectious mononucleosis (IM), 453–454
infectious urticaria, 489
inferior vena cava (IVC) filters, 517

infertility
  common diagnoses, 892
  definition, 892
  diagnosis, 893–894
    laboratory tests, 893
      male factors, 893
      ovulatory dysfunction, 893–894
      tubal factors, 894
  management strategies, 895–896
  pathophysiology
    male factors, 892
    ovulatory dysfunction, 892
    tubal and pelvic pathology, 892
    unusual problems, 892–893
  prognosis, 896
  signs and symptoms, 893
  treatment, 894–895
    assisted reproductive technology (ART),
      895
    male factor, 894
    ovulatory dysfunction, 894
    tubal and pelvic pathology, 895
    unusual problems, 895
inflamed pingueculum, 424
  laboratory tests/diagnostics, 429
  symptoms, 427
  treatment, 431
inflammation, symptoms, 13
inflammatory bowel disease, 687–696
  definition, 687–688
  epidemiology, 688
  imaging/diagnostics, 689–690
  laboratory assessment, 689
  management strategies, 695–696
  prognosis, 696
  risk factors, 688
    appendectomy, 688
    diet, 688
    genetics, 688
    geography, 688
    smoking, 688
  signs and symptoms, 688
  treatment, 690–695
inflammatory chronic diarrhea, 132
inflammatory CPPS, 480
  laboratory tests, 482
  treatment, 484
inflammatory markers
  and rapid viral testing, 398
inflammatory prostatitis, 480
infrared coagulation, 414
ingrown nails, 240
  signs, 244
  toenail removal, 210
  treatment, 250
inhaled corticosteroids (ICS)
  for asthma, 553
injectable hormones, contraception,
  885–886
insect bites, 44
  diagnosis, 45
  outdoor, prevention, 44
  treatment, 49, 51–54
  wounds, 45–46
insecticides, to treat pets with fleas, 51

insomnia. *See also* sleep disorder
  additional tests and studies, 291
    laboratory testing, 291–292
    patient reporting tools, 291
  chronic, 288
  cognitive-behavioral interventions for, 294
  definition, 287–288
  follow-up, 299
  obstrucive sleep apnea, 292
  pathophysiology, 288
  prevalence, risk factors, and impact, 288
  signs, 291
  sleep maintenance, 287
  summary of pharmacologic agents for, 297–298
  symptoms and sleep history
    additional history, 290–291
    associated nocturnal symptoms, 290
    daytime activities and function, 290
    primary complaint, 288–290
  treatment
    complementary medicine, 295
    goals of, 293
    nonpharmacologic management of chronic
      insomnia, 293–294
    pharmacologic agents, 295–299
    relaxation therapy, 294
insulin therapy
  diabetes mellitus, 655–656
  long-acting insulins, 655
  rapid-acting insulins, 655
  in type 1 DM, 655–656
  in type 2 DM, 656
International Prostate Symptom Score (IPSS), 481
interstitial cystitis (IC), 167
  treatment, 171, 408
intestinal angina, 5
intimate partner violence. *See also* family
      violence
  anxiety disorders, 852
  chronic pain, 852
  definition, 850
  depression, 852
  diagnosis, 851
  epidemiology, 850
  management strategies, 851–852
  prevention, 852–853
  prognosis, 852
  PTSD, 852
  violent relationships, 851
intra-articular diseases
  fractures, 315
  joint pain
    crystal-induced, 310
    gouty arthritis, 310, 313–315
    immune-complex, 310–311
    pseudogout, 310, 311, 313–314, 316
    rheumatoid arthritis (RA), 310
    signs, 312–313
    synovitis, 310–311
    joint pain and, 315
intractable diarrhea of infancy, 134
intractable incontinence, 478
intrauterine devices (IUD), 889–890. *See also*
      contraception
intravaginal administration, 152

intravenous magnesium sulfate, for asthma, 559
intravenous pyelogram (IVP), 285
intussusception
  children with, 374
  LGI bleeding and, 223
  vomiting and, 371
iPledge Program, 531
ipratropium bromide, for asthma, 559
ipriflavone, for osteoporosis, 745
iritis, 425
iron deficiency, 25
  treatment, 29–30
irritable bowel syndrome (IBS)
  chronic diarrhea and, 133, 135–136
  symptoms, 4
  treatment, 10
irritants, cough, 92, 96, 100
ischemic bowel disease, 5
  treatment, 11
ischemic colitis, 2
ischemic heart disease (IHD)
  annual influenza vaccination, 699
  chest pain symptom, 72
  definition, 697
  diagnosis, 699–702
  diagnostic tests, 701–702
    angiography, 702
    electrocardiogram (ECG), 701, 702
    exercise treadmill test (ETT), 701
    laboratory studies, 702
    x-ray, 702
  epidemiology, 697
  pathogenesis, 697, 699
  prevention, 699
  prognosis, 708–709
  treatment, 702–708
ischemic pain, 73
isotretinoin (Retin A), 68, 531
itching, as symptom of insect bite, 45
itraconazole, 215, 236, 250

J
jaundice
  bilirubin overproduction and, 301
  common diagnoses
    adult conjugated hyperbilirubinemia,
      302
    adult unconjugated hyperbilirubinemia, 302
    breastfeeding jaundice, 303
    childhood conjugated hyperbilirubinemia,
      302
    childhood jaundice, 301–302
    childhood unconjugated hyperbilirubinemia,
      301–302
    conjugated hyperbilirubinemia, 302
  definition, 301
  intrahepatic excretion in, 302
  laboratory tests, 303–307
    basic tests, 303–305
    hematologic testing, 306–307
    imaging studies, 305–306
    liver biopsy, 307
  signs, 303
    cutaneous xanthomas, 303
    in infants, 303

Kayser-Fleischer rings, 303
large, palpable, nodular liver, 303
in newborns, 303
palpable gallbladder, 303
spider angiomata, 303
splenomegaly, 303
urticaria, 303
symptoms
abdominal pain as, 302
fever with chills as, 302–303
in neonates, 303
obstructive jaundice, 303
onset, 302
pruritus, 302
treatment
of breastfeeding jaundice, 307
of breast milk jaundice, 307
of cholestatic jaundice, 309
exchange transfusion, 308
extrahepatic obstruction, 309
of neonates with hemolytic jaundice,
308
of other hepatocellular disease, 309
phototherapy, 308
of physiologic jaundice, 307
unconjugated hyperbilirubinemia, 309
of underlying diseases contributing to,
309
of viral hepatitis, 308
Jersey finger
hand and wrist complaints and, 251
treatment, 257
jet lag
sleep disorder and, 295, 298
travel medicine, 988
joint pain, 310. See also arthritis
common diagnoses
degenerative disease, 311
intra-articular joint pain, 310–311
periarticular processes, 311
definition, 310
diagnostic tests, 313–315
electrocardiography (ECG), 314–315
hematologic tests, 313–314
joint fluid examination, 314
radiology, 314
growing pains, 317
psychogenic pain, 311, 312
signs, 312–313
intra-articular processes, 313
periarticular processes, 313
vital signs/general appearance, 312
symptoms, 311–312
associated symptoms, 312
chronology, 311–312
exacerbating/alleviating factors, 312
location/number of joints involved, 311
treatment
chronic management, 315–316
gouty arthritis, 315
growing pains, 317
intra-articular diseases, 315–317
NSAIDs for, 315
oral colchicine for, 316
patient education, 315

periarticular diseases, 317
preventive medication, 315–316
pseudogout, 316
rheumatoid arthritis (RA), 316
rheumatic fever (RF), 316–317
septic arthritis, 315
supportive therapy, 316
transient synovitis, 315
urate-lowering therapy, 316
joints, shoulder, 37
juvenile polyps, 223

K
Kallmann syndrome, 17
karyotyping, 21
Kegel exercises, 474
keratitis, 426
laboratory tests/diagnostics, 430
symptoms, 429
treatment, 431
keratoacanthoma, 123, 129
kinetic tremor, 461
knee braces, 730
knee complaints
acute, 318
chronic, 318
common diagnoses
arthritis, 321
Baker cyst, 321
bursitis, 320
fractures, 321
iliotibial band (ITB) syndrome, 321
ligament injuries, 319
meniscal injuries, 319
Osgood-Schlatter disease, 320–321
osteochondritis dissecans (OCD), 320
pain referred from hip, 321
patellar dislocation, 320
patellar tendinopathy, 320
patellofemoral dysfunction, 1
patellofemoral pain syndrome (PFS),
319–320
plica syndrome, 321
Sinding-Larsen-Johansson disease, 321
definition, 318
diagnostic testing, 324–326
patient education, 331
prevention, 321
ACL injuries, 321
MCL, 321
signs, 321–324
Baker cyst, 324
bursitis, 322–324
ITB, 324
ligament injuries, 321–322
meniscal injuries, 322
osteochondritis dissecans, 324
Osgood-Schlatter disease, 324
patellar dislocation/subluxation, 322
patellar tendinopathy, 322
patellofemoral pain syndrome, 322
plica syndrome, 324
Sinding-Larsen-Johansson disease, 324
special maneuvers in, 321, 323
symptoms, 321–324

knee complaints (*continued*)
  treatment
    Baker cyst, 328
    bursitis, 328
    iliotibial band syndrome, 328
    indications for orthopedic referral, 326
    mild soft-tissue injuries, 326
    nonpharmacologic treatment, 327
    NSAIDs for, 328
    Osgood-Schlatter disease, 328
    Sinding-Larsen-Johansson syndrome, 328
knees, 728. *See also* osteoarthritis

L
lacerations
  common diagnoses
    clean lacerations, 333
    puncture wounds, 333
    superficial wounds, 333
    wounds with extensive tissue loss or injury, 333
  definition, 332
  laboratory tests, 333
    deep wound culture, 333
    x-rays, 333
  signs
    compound lacerations, 333
    dirty lacerations, 333
    tissue damage, 333
  symptoms, 333
  treatment
    anesthesia, 334
    infection prevention, 337
    patient education, 337–338
    patient follow-up, 338
    skin biopsy for, 334
    staples, 337
    tissue adhesive for closure, 336–337
    wound repair, 334–336
lactase deficiency, primary, 134
lactation, and hyperprolactinemia, 18
lactation amenorrhea method (LAM), 890
lactose intolerance, 133, 136
laparoscopic cholecystectomy, 11
laparoscopic uterosacral nerve ablation
      (LUNA), 154
laparoscopy
  for pelvic pain (PP), 406
  for secondary dysmenorrhea, 150
large bowel obstruction, treatment, 11
latent autoimmune diabetes in adults (LADA),
      645–646, 647
latent TB, 102
lateral epicondylitis, 40, 41
  treatment, 43
laxatives, 90
leg complaints
  in adolescents, 343
  in adults, 343
  in athletic adolescents and adults, 343
  bilateral leg edema, 344
  in children, 343
  definition, 338–339
  evaluation, 340–341
  in infants and toddlers, 343
  osteomyelitis, 343

peripheral arterial disease (PAD), 344
peripheral neuropathies, 343–344
  signs, 344–345
  spinal stenosis, 353, 359
  symptoms, 344–345
  treatment, 345–347
leiomyomas
  dysmenorrhea and, 149–150
  signs, 150
  symptoms, 150
lentigines, 128
leukocytosis, 8
leukotriene modifiers for asthma, 557
leuprolide, 152, 249
levalbuterol, for asthma, 559
levator ani syndrome, 412
  laboratory tests for, 414
  signs, 413
  symptoms, 412
  treatment, 416
levodopa, 464–466
levofloxacin, 484
levonorgestrel intrauterine devices, 152
lice bites
  body, 46
  head, 45
  public, 45
  treatment options for patients with, 52–53
lichen planus, 106, 118
lichen sclerosus et atrophicus (LSA), 228
  laboratory tests for, 234
  signs, 232
  symptoms, 229
  treatment, 236
lichen simplex chronicus, 105, 118
ligaments, ankle, 31, 32
lightheadedness, 146
linaclotide, 10
  for constipation, 90
linezolid, 69
lipase, 8
lipomas, 125, 129
liquid nitrogen method, 210
liraglutide, for obesity, 723
lisfranc injury, 208
liver biopsy, 609
liver function tests (LFT) abnormalities
  common diagnoses
    elevated alkaline phosphatase, 349
    elevated aminotransferases, 348–349
    hyperbilirubinemia, 350
  definition, 347–348
  diagnostic tests, 350–351
    alcoholic liver disease, 350
    bilirubin fractions, 350
    cytotoxic reactions, 351
    GGT test, 350
    Gilbert syndrome, 351
    hemolysis, 351
    infiltrative diseases, 351
    intrahepatic or extrahepatic obstruction,
      351
    liver biopsy, 350
    medications, 351
    prothrombin time (PT), 350

serum albumin, 350
stepwise approach to evaluating, 350
ultrasound, 350
viral hepatitis, 350
screening, 348
signs, 350
sore throat and, 284
symptoms, 350
treatment, 351–352
liver transplantation, for cirrhosis, 613
loop diuretics
for proteinuria, 422
loperamide hydrochloride, 10
loratadine, 115, 492–493
lorazepam, 82
lorcaserin, for obesity, 722
low back pain (LBP), 352
common diagnoses
acute, 353
subacute, 353–354
definition, 352–353
diagnostic testing, 355–356
nonspecific, 353
prevention and screening, 353
signs, 354–355
specific, 353
symptoms, 354
treatment, 356–359
activity, 356
exercise, 358
major evidence-based recommendations,
357–358
nonrecommended therapies, 359
NSAIDs for, 356
osteopathic manipulation treatment (OMT),
358
patient education, 358–359
physical modalities, 358
surgery, 359
lower GI (LGI) bleeding, 222–223
in children, 223
lower urinary tract symptoms (LUTS),
481–482
low-grade squamous intraepithelial lesion (LSIL),
13
symptoms, 14
treatment, 15–16
lubiprostone for constipation, 90
lumbar disk herniation, 353
lumbar puncture
delirium testing and, 82
and pediatric fever, 398
for stroke, 790
lumbar spine, 729. See also osteoarthritis
lung cancer
diagnosis, 569
differential diagnosis, 569
epidemiology, 563
prevention, 566
prognosis, 574–575
risk factors, 564–565
asbestos exposure, 565
cigarette smoking, 564
family history, 565
radon exposure, 564

screening, 567, 978
signs and symptoms, 568
staging, 570
treatment, 571–573
lung function tests for wheezing, 522
lung volume reduction surgery, for COPD,
593
Lyme disease, 46–47
treatment, 53
lymphadenopathy, 136
causes, 360
common diagnoses, 360
definition, 360
differential diagnosis, 362
laboratory tests, 361
location, 361
peripheral, 363
signs, 361
size, 361
symptoms, 360–361
texture, 361
treatment
acute lymphadenitis, 364
cat-scratch disease, 364
mycobacterial disease, 364
neoplasm, 364
viral infections, 363
lymph node evaluation, 571
lymph nodes
biopsy, 362–363

M

macrolide antibiotics, 101
Macroprolactin, 20
macular lesions in dermatologic neoplasm
congenital nevi, 121
ephelides, 121
FAMMS, 121
lentigines, 121
malignant melanomas, 121
magnetic resonance angiography (MRA), 9,
268, 459
magnetic resonance imaging (MRI), 68, 97,
147, 208, 212, 217, 268, 326, 356,
362, 406, 414, 436, 447, 459
and abdominal pain evaluation, 9
in ankle injuries, 35
inflammatory bowel disease, 690
for osteoarthritis, 729–730
for stroke, 788
major depressive disorder (MDD), 856. See also
depression
malabsorption syndrome, 134
malaise, 63
male breast cancer, 575
male condoms, 888. See also contraception
malignant melanoma
nails disoders and, 243
treatment, 130
mallet deformity, 251, 262
hand and wrist complaints and, 251, 257
treatment, 262
Mallory-Weiss tear, 222
malnutrition, preoperative evaluation and,
1004

mammalian bites
 defined, 44
 diagnosis, 44
 laboratory tests, 48
 treatment, 48–49, 50
  antibiotic therapy, 49
  closure, 48–49
  hospitalization, 49
  rabies postexposure prophylaxis, 49, 51
  tetanus prophylaxis, 49
  thorough cleansing, 48
 wounds, 45
mammography, 56
manipulation under anesthesia, 43
mastalgia, 55
mastectomy, 571
mastitis
 breast condition, 55
 breast inflammation, 55
 nipple discharge and, 55
 signs, 55
 treatment, 58
maxillary sinusitis, 435
MDS. See myelodysplastic syndrome (MDS)
Meckel diverticulum, 223
medial epicondylitis, 40
 treatment, 43
medication, and hyperprolactinemia, 18
medroxyprogesterone acetate, 22
medullary cystic kidney disease, 283
melanomas, 126, 130
melatonin, 295
melena, 223
memantine, for dementia, 537
memory-assist device, for hypertension, 685
Meniere disease, 276
 dizziness and, 146
 hearing loss and, 275, 276
menopause
 definition, 709–710
 epidemiology, 710
 laboratory tests, 711–712
 management strategies, 714–715
 pathophysiology, 710
 perimenopause, 710
 postmenopausal, 710
 premature, 710
 signs, 711
 symptoms, 710–711
 treatment, 712–714
menstrual cycle. See also vaginal bleeding
 abnormal bleeding and, 500
 bleeding symptoms, 503
 early secretory phase, 500
 late secretory phase, 500
 proliferative phase, 500
6-mercaptopurine
 for inflammatory bowel disease, 695
meropenem, 69
mesalamine, for inflammatory bowel disease, 691
mesenteric angiography, 9
mesenteric ischemia, 6
mesenteric vascular occlusion, 2
mesenteric vein thrombosis, 2
metabolic acidosis, 9
 treatment, 205

metabolic alkalosis, 205
metabolic complications, eating disorders and, 872
metacarpal fractures
 first, second, and third metacarpals, 218
 fractures of neck of fifth metacarpal, 218
 of shaft of fourth and fifth metacarpal, 218
 treatment, 259
metatarsal fractures
 fifth, 221
 second, third, and fourth, 220–221
metformin
 for diabetes mellitus, 648
 for hirsutism, 351
 for ovulatory dysfunction, 895
methotrexate, 407
 for inflammatory bowel disease, 695
methylnaltrexone for constipation, 91
metolazone, for heart failure, 621
metronidazole, 11
microalbuminuria, 418. See also proteinuria
MIDAS questionnaire, 265. See also headaches
middle third (midclavicular) fractures, 219
midfoot complaints, 207–208
migraine
 episodic, 264, 266
 medications for acute migraine headaches, 269
 prophylaxis for recurrent migraine headaches, 272
 strength of recommendation for prophylactic
  treatment options in migraine, 270
 treatment, 268–271
  ergot alkaloids, 269, 270
  prophylactic therapy, 270–271, 272
  triptans for, 269, 270
mini-mental state examination (MMSE), 80–81
minoxidil
 for alopecia, 246–247
 for hair disorders, 246–247
mitral valve prolapse (MVP), 389
 chest pain symptom, 72
 chest pain treatment and, 77
Mittelschmerz
 chronic pelvic pain (CPP), 402
 treatment, 409
mixed cardiopulmonary dyspnea, 161, 165
mixed fatigue, 193
mixed headache, 264
mixed hearing loss, 274, 279
mixed incontinence, 471
mobility assessments, osteoarthritis and, 735
moist crackles, 618
molluscum contagiosum, 228
 laboratory tests for, 234
 signs, 232
 symptoms, 229
 treatment, 236
monoamine oxidase inhibitor (MAOI)
 for Parkinson disease, 464
monosymptomatic enuresis, 183
Morton's neuroma injection, 210
mosquitoes bites, 45
motility disorders, vomiting and, 372
motion sickness, 987
movement disorders. See also tremors
 ataxia, 470
 chorea, 469
 definition, 461

dystonia, 469–470
hyperkinesias, 461
hypokinesias, 461
myoclonus, 469
sleep-related, 287
tic disorders, 468–469
treatment, 290
Wilson disease, 470
MRI. See magnetic resonance imaging (MRI)
mucolytics for asthma, 557
mupirocin, 68
Murphy sign, 6
muscle relaxants, 273, 356
musculoskeletal complications, eating disorders and, 872
musculoskeletal pain, 73
musculoskeletal ultrasound (MSUS), 730
myalgia
    collagen vascular disease, 366
    common diagnoses
        collagen vascular diseases, 365
        eosinophilia-myalgia syndrome (EMS), 366
        fibromyalgia and myofascial pain, 365
        ischemia, 365
        major or minor trauma/exertional, 365
        primary muscle malignancy, 366
        statin-induced myalgia (SIM), 366
        substance-induced, 366
        vascular insufficiency, 365
        viral syndromes, 365
    definition, 365
    EMS, 366
    fibromyalgia syndrome (FMS), 366
    laboratory tests, 368
    myalgia from trauma, 366
    myalgia from viral syndromes, 366
    myofascial pain syndrome, 366
    statin-induced myalgia (SIM), 368
    thoracic outlet syndrome, 368
    treatment
        collagen vascular diseases, 370
        EMS, 370
        fibromyalgia, 369
        SIM, 370
        trauma, 369
        viral syndromes, 369
    vascular insufficiency, 368
myalgias, 671
mycobacterial disease, 364
myelodysplastic syndrome (MDS), 26
myocardial infarction (MI)
    epidemiology, 697
myoclonus, 469
    focal, 469
    generalized, 469
myofascial pain syndrome, 365
myopathy, 671

N
nafcillin, 69
nail disorders
    common diagnoses
        discolored nails, 240, 242
        ingrown nails, 240
        onychomycosis, 240
        paronychia, 240

hypertrichosis, 237, 240
laboratory tests, 244–246
normal nail anatomy, 237
signs, 242–244
treatment, 246–250
naltrexone, for substance abuse, 815
naproxen sodium
    for myalgia, 369
narcolepsy, 290, 292
narcotics, for osteoarthritis, 732
nasal disorders. See also rhinitis; sinusitis
    antihistamines therapy, 439
    common cold or viral upper respiratory infection, 433
    laboratory tests, 435, 436
    signs, 433–435
    symptoms, 433–435
    treatment, 436–443
nasogastric tube aspiration, nausea and vomiting, 375
nasopharyngeal wash (NP wash), 522
nasopharyngoscopy, 98
National Diabetes Education Program website, 659
natriuretic peptides, 616–617. See also heart failure (HF)
natural family planning. See also contraception
    coitus interruptus, 890
    lactation amenorrhea method (LAM), 890
    periodic abstinence, 890
nausea. See also vomiting
    acupuncture for, 376
    definition, 371
    diagnosis using symptoms of, 374
    diagnostic testing, 375–376
    differential diagnosis, 372
    medications associated with, 373
    relative costs, benefits, and risks of diagnostic tests, 375
    symptoms, 373–374
    treatment, 376–382
        CINV, 382
        clinical situation, 381–382
        pharmacologic, 376–381
        PONV, 382
        RINV, 382
neck pain
    acute torticollis and, 383
    Canadian cervical spine rules, 386
    common diagnoses, 383–384
    definition, 383
    differential diagnosis of common causes, 384
    evaluation for cervical nerve root lesions, 385
    and headaches, 384
    laboratory tests, 385–386
    mechanical, 383
    nonmechanical, 383
    OA, 386
    signs, 385
    Spurling test and, 385
    symptoms, 383–384
    treatment, 386
    whiplash injury and, 384
necrotizing fasciitis, 66
    treatment, 69
necrotizing otitis externa, 182

needle aspiration
  for bacterial skin infections, 66
  for breast lumps, 56
neglect
  child abuse, 847
  elder
    physical, 853
    psychological, 853
    self-neglect, 853–854
Neisseria meningitidis, 395
neoplasms. *See also* dermatologic neoplasm
  benign, 127–129
  definition, 120
  hair and nail disorders, 243
  hematuria and, 281, 286
  LGI bleeding and, 223
  lymphadenopathy, 364
  malignant, 353
  osteoporosis or bony, 353
  testicular, 445, 448
nephrolithiasis, 281
nephrotic syndrome
  proteinuria and, 418
neurally mediated syncope
  signs, 457
  symptoms, 457
  treatment, 459–460
neuromuscular diseases, 161
neuropathic pain, 597. *See also* chronic
      persistent pain
neuropathies
  dysproteinemic, 344
  entrapment, 256, 262
  peripheral, 343–344
nevi
  macular lesions in dermatologic neoplasm, 121
  signs, 127
  treatment, 127
New York Heart Association (NYHA) Functional
      Classification, 619
niacin, for dyslipidemias, 666
nifedipine, 493
nightmares, 290
night terrors, 290
nimodipine, for stroke, 793
nipple discharge, 55
nitrates, for IHD, 703
nitric oxide test system, 552
nociceptive pain, 597. *See also* chronic
      persistent pain
nocturnal leg cramps, 343, 347
nodular episcleritis, 429
nodular lesions in dermatologic neoplasm
  dermatofibromas, 125
  epidermal cysts, 126
  lipomas, 125
  sebaceous hyperplasia, 126
noise-induced hearing loss
  screening and prevention, 275
  symptoms, 277
nonalcoholic steatohepatitis (NASH), 608
noncardiopulmonary dyspnea
  causes, 161–162
  examination, 165
  testing for, 165

nondisplaced pelvic fractures, 219
nonexcisional therapy, 416
nongonococcal urethritis (NGU). *See also*
      urinary symptoms in men
  symptoms, 480
noninflammatory CPPS, 480
  laboratory tests, 482
non-monosymptomatic enuresis, 183
nonspecific abdominal pain (NSAP), 1
  signs, 5
  symptoms, 4
  treatment, 10
nonsteroidal anti-inflammatory drugs (NSAIDs)
  for ankle sprains treatment, 35
  for APP, 408
  for chest pain treatment, 76
  for chronic persistent pain, 598
  for CPP, 409
  for dysmenorrhea, 152
  for fractures treatment, 36
  for GI bleeding, 222, 225
  for glenohumeral instability treatment, 43
  for hand and wrist complaints, 262
  for hematuria, 283
  for joint pain, 315
  for knee complaints, 316, 328, 331
  for leg and hip complaints, 345–346
  for low back pain, 356–357
  for myalgia, 369
  peptic ulcer disease and, 748, 751, 754
  for rotator cuff injuries treatment, 42
  for tenosynovitis treatment, 36
  topical, 328
  for urinary symptoms in men, 484
  for vaginal bleeding, 505
non-sulfonylureas secretagogues
  for diabetes mellitus, 653
nonsustained ventricular tachycardia (NSVT),
      389
nonulcer dyspepsia (NUD), 155
  symptoms, 155
  treatment, 157, 160
normal sinus rhythm (NSR), 390–391. *See also*
      palpitations
  maintenance of, 391
normal-transit constipation (NTC), 83–84
normogonadotropic amenorrhea
  PCOS and, 18
  treatment, 22
NSAIDs. *See* nonsteroidal anti-inflammatory
      drugs (NSAIDs)
NSAP. *See* nonspecific abdominal pain (NSAP)
nummular eczema, 108, 119
nutrition
  for COPD, 589–590
  for dementia, 637
  for inflammatory bowel disease, 690
nystatin, 236

O

obesity, 716–725
  comorbidities, 719
  definition, 717
  diagnosis, 718–719
  dietary history and, 719

endocrine disorders and, 719
epidemiology
    health effects, 717
    prevalence, 717
    risk factors, 717
etiology, 717–718
    environmental factors, 717–718
    gene–environment interaction, 718
    genetic factors, 718
exercise and, 719
and hypogonadotropic/hypothalamic amenor-
    rhea, 17
laboratory evaluation, 719
treatment, 720–725
obstructive disease, dyspnea, 161, 165
occult fractures, 34
ocular rosacea, 533
office cystometrography, 473
ofloxacin, 484
olecranon bursitis, 40, 41
    treatment, 43
oligomenorrhea, 19. See also amenorrhea
omalizumab for asthma, 557
onychomycosis. See also nail disorders
    antifungal therapy for, 248
    distal, 243
    nails disorders and, 240, 243, 250
    proximal, 243
    symptoms, 242
    treatment, 250
    white superficial, 243
open fractures, 221
opioid analgesics, for chronic persistent pain, 602
opioids, for dyspnea, 166
opioid withdrawal, 814
    treatment for, 815
oral antihistamines
    for atopic dermatitis, 117
    for pruritus, 115–117
    for urticaria, 492
oral cancer, screening tests, 977
oral contraceptives (OCPS)
    for acne vulgaris, 530
    for alopecia, 238
    for dysmenorrhea, 152
    estrogen–progestin pills, 883–885
    for hair disorder, 247
    for headaches, 272
    hormonal, 883–885
    for nail disorder, 249
    progestin-only pills, 885
oral corticosteroids
    for pruritus, 117
    for sinusitis, 441
oral decongestants, 440, 441
oral medications for pruitus, 115–117
oral rehydration solutions (ORS), 138
orchiectomy, 448, 487
orchitis, 444
orlistat, for obesity, 722
orthostatic hypotension, 457, 460
orthostatic proteinuria, 418
    treatment, 422
orthostatic syncope, 455, 457
orthotics for foot complaints, 214–215

osmotherapy, 793
osmotic laxatives, 90
osteoarthritis (OA)
    definition, 726–727
    diagnosis, 728
    epidemiology, 727
    laboratory tests, 729
    management strategies, 734–736
    neck pain, 386
    pathophysiology, 727
    prognosis, 736
    radiographic findings, 729–730
    risk factors, 727
    signs, 728–729
    symptoms, 728
    treatment, 730–734
osteopenia, 739
osteoporosis, 737–746
    diagnosis, 738–739
    eating disorders and, 871
    imaging studies, 739–740
    involutional, 737
    laboratory tests, 739
    management strategies, 746
    postmenopausal, 737
    prognosis, 746
    risk factors, 737–738
    screening and prevention, 738
    secondary, 737
    treatment, 740–746
osteoporosis, vitamin D supplementation for, 23
osteoporosis management, 715
otitis externa (OE)
    earache and, 172
    necrotizing, 182
    signs, 173
    symptoms, 173
    treatment, 181–182
otitis media (OM), 277
    acute (AOM)
        in infants, 178–181
        symptoms, 173
        treatment, 175–177
    signs, 277
    treatment, 280
otoacoustic emission (OAE), 279
otorrhea, 173
otosclerosis, 277, 280
ototoxicity, 276, 280
    sensorineural loss CD and, 276
    treatment, 280
Ottawa Ankle and Foot Rules, 34–35
outdoor insect bites, prevention of, 44
outpatient therapy, for PID, 407
ovarian cancer, screening, 977
ovarian remnant syndrome, 405
overflow incontinence, 471, 477–478
overload proteinuria, 418
overuse, and arm/shoulder complaints, 37
ovulatory bleeding, 503
ovulatory dysfunction, 894–895
    clomiphene for, 895
    laboratory tests, 893–894
    metformin for, 895
    pathophysiology, 892

oxybutynin, 474, 475
oxycodone, for chronic persistent pain, 602
oxygen
    for COPD, 591–592, 593–594
    for dyspnea, 165

P

PA. *See* pernicious anemia (PA)
palpitations
    common diagnoses
        cardiac, 387
        psychiatric, 387
    decision tree for evaluation of, 390
    definition, 387
    electrocardiographic clues, 391
    etiologies, 388
    laboratory tests, 389
    neck pain and, 385
    perianal complaints sign, 413
    signs, 389
    symptoms, 388–389
        description, 388
        onset and offset, 388
        positional, 388–389
        syncope or presyncope, 389
    treatment, 389–394
        atrial fibrillation (AF), 390–394
        NSVT patients, 389
        SVT patients, 389
pancreatic cancer, 160
pancreatitis, 1, 2, 8
    chronic, treatment of, 11
    hemorrhagic, 6
    signs, 6
    symptoms, 5
    treatment, 11
    vomiting and, 372
panic disorder, 820
    diagnoses, 821
    management strategies, 827
    prognosis, 828
    treatment, 826–827
        benzodiazepines, 826
        CBT, 826
        SSRIs, 826
        tricyclic antidepressants, 826
Pap smears. *See also* abnormal Pap smears
    defined, 12
    diagnoses by, 13
    reports, content of, 14
    results, systems for reporting, 12
    screening, 13
papular lesions in dermatologic neoplasm
    acrochordon, 125
    actinic keratoses, 124
    basal cell carcinoma, 124
    cherry angiomas, 121–122
    keratoacanthoma, 123
    nevi, 121
    pyogenic granulomas, 123
    seborrheic keratoses, 123
    squamous cell carcinoma, 125
    warts, 123
papulopustular rosacea, 532
paracentesis, 611

parasitic infections
    causing diarrhea, 131
    diarrhea and, 133, 135
parasitosis
    delusion of, 109
parasomnias, 292, 294
paring of calluses, 210
Parkinson disease (PD)
    MAOI for, 464
    signs, 461–462
    treatment, 464–467
        neuroprotective therapy, 464
        supportive care, 467
        surgical treatment of, 466–467
        symptomatic therapy, 464–466
        tremors and, 461–462
paronychia, 66, 240
    acute, 243
    chronic, 243, 250
    signs, 243
    treatment, 250
partial ileal bypass surgery, 673
Pasteurella multocida, 65
patch testing, 114
pathophysiology, 532
peak expiratory flow rate (PEFR), 97,
        163, 552
peak flow–zone system, 552
pearly penile papules, 228
    laboratory tests for, 234
    signs, 232
    symptoms, 229
    treatment, 236
pediatric fever, 395
    blood cultures, 397
    cell count, 397
    chest radiography, 398
    common diagnoses, 395
    definition, 395
    and febrile seizures, 399
    laboratory tests, 397–398
    lumbar puncture test, 398
    and rapid viral testing, 398
    signs, 396–397
    symptoms, 396–397
    treatment, 398–399
        acyclovir, 399
        antipyretics, 398
        empiric antibiotic, 398–399
        and UA, 398
pediatric fractures, 221
pediatric GERD, 160
pediatric traveler. *See also* travel medicine
    air travel, 989
    malaria, 989
    vaccinations, 989
pediculosis capitis. *See* head lice (pediculosis
        capitis)
pediculosis corporis, treatment of, 52
pediculosis humanus, 105
pediculosis pubis, 105
pediculosis pubis, treatment of, 52–53
pelvic congestion syndrome, 404
pelvic floor dysfunction constipation, 84
pelvic fractures, 219

pelvic inflammatory diseases (PID)
  acute pelvic pain (APP) and, 400–401, 402
  outpatient therapy for, 407
  treatment, 406
pelvic pain (PP)
  acute (APP), 400–401, 402
    ectopic pregnancy and, 402
    findings with common causes, 401
    PID, 400, 402
    treatment, 406–408
    uterine leiomyomas, 402
  adnexal mass and, 404
  chronic (CPP), 402–403, 408–409
  chronic endometritis and, 404
  common diagnoses
    APP, 400–401, 402
    CPP, 402–403
  definition, 400
  diagnostic criteria for pelvic inflammatory
      disease, 403
  laboratory tests for, 405–406
  laparoscopy for, 406
  ovarian remnant syndrome, 405–406
  pelvic congestion syndrome, 404
  signs, 404–405
  symptoms
    APP, 403
    associated symptoms, 403
    CPP, 403
    location and quality, 403
    onset/chronology, 403
  treatment
    APP, 406–408
    CPP, 408–409
pelvic ultrasound, 21
  for secondary dysmenorrhea, 150
penicillin
  for sore throat treatment, 452–453
penicillin V, for animal bites treatment, 49
pentosan, 484
peptic ulcer disease, 747–754
  definition, 747
  diagnosis, 749–750
  epidemiology, 748
  pathophysiology, 747–748
  preoperative evaluation and, 1004
  prevention, 748–749
  prognosis, 754
  treatment, 750–752
peptic ulcer disease (PUD), 155. See also gastro-
      esophageal reflux disease (GERD)
  symptoms, 155
  UGI bleeding and, 222, 227
  vomiting and, 372
percutaneous coronary interventions (PCIs),
      708
perforations, 3, 5
perianal complaints
  anal fissure, 411
  anorectal abscesses, 411
  anorectal infections, 411
  anoscopy and, 413
  definition, 410
  fistula-in-ano, 411
  hematoma, 411

hemorrhoids, 411
  laboratory tests, 413–414
  levator ani syndrome, 411
  pilonidal cysts, 411
  pilonidal disease, 411
  proctalgia fugax, 411
  proctitis, 411
  pruritus ani, 411
  signs, 413
  symptoms, 412
    bleeding, 412
    discharge, 412
    perianal mass, 412
    prolapse, 412
  treatment
    anal fissures, 415
    anorectal abscess, 415–416
    hemorrhoids, 414
    levator ani syndrome, 416
    perianal fistulas, 416
    pilonidal sinus disease, 416
    proctalgia fugax, 416
    proctitis, 416–417
    pruritus ani, 417
perianal fistulas, 416
pericarditis, 71–72. See also chest pain
periodic abstinence, 890
peripheral edema, 618
peripheral lymphadenopathy, 363
peripheral vestibular disorders, 145, 148
peritonitis, in diverticular disease, 6
peritonsillar abscess, 451
periungual warts
  signs, 126
  treatment, 128
permethrin, 44
  for genital lesions, 236
  for scabies bite treatment, 53
pernicious anemia (PA), 25
persistent depressive disorder, 856. See also
      depression
persistent diarrhea, 131–132, 139
persistent proteinuria, 418
  treatment, 422
pertussis
  antibiotics for, 101
  and cough, 95, 96
Phalen test, 260, 261
pharmacologic stress testing, 76
phenylephrine, 182
phimosis, 232–233
phobia, 820
  diagnoses, 821
  management strategies, 827
  prognosis, 828
  treatment, 827
    behavioral treatment techniques, 827
    beta-blockers, 827
    SSRIs, 827
photodynamic therapy, for lung cancer, 573
Phthirus pubis
  genital lesions and, 228
  laboratory tests for, 234
  pruritic lesions and, 229
  signs, 232

phymatous/rhinophymatous rosacea, 533
physical abuse
  child, 847, 848–849
  elder, 853
physical fatigue, 193
physical urticaria
  cholinergic, 489
  cold, 489
  delayed pressure, 489
  dermographism, 489
  heat, 489
  solar, 489
physiologic
  fatigue, 193
  tremor, 462
physiologic jaundice, 307
physiologic stress, 244
pilonidal
  abscess, 412
  cysts, 411
  disease, 411
  sinus, 416
pimecrolimus, 117
pinworms, 417
pituitary macroadenoma, treatment of, 22
pityriasis rosea, 113–114
  pruritic dermatoses and, 106
  signs, 113–114
  treatment, 118
plain radiographs, 68
plantar fasciitis, 213, 214
plantar warts
  signs, 126
  treatment, 128
pleurisy, 77
pleuritic pain, 73, 74
PMR treatment, 370
pneumonia
  acute cough and, 96
  and dyspnea, 161
  wheezing and, 518
pneumonitis, 77
pneumothorax, 75
podofilox, 235
podophyllin, 235
polycystic kidney disease, 283
polycystic ovarian syndrome (PCOS), 238–239.
  See also amenorrhea
  and normogonadotropic amenorrhea, 18
polymyositis, 367
polyps
  hematuria and, 281
  juvenile, 223
  LGI bleeding and, 223
  neoplasms and, 223
polyvalent pneumococcal vaccine, 181
postcoital contraceptives, 887–888. See also
  contraception
postinfectious cough, 92, 95, 96
postinfectious diarrhea, 134
postnasal drainage (PND), 95, 96,
  101
postoperative induced nausea and vomiting
  (PONV), 382
postpartum care
  definition, 909

diagnosis and treatment
  antepartum, 910
  baby blues, 913
  depression, 913
  emotional disorders, 913
  endometritis, 910, 912
  Group B streptococcal sepsis, 912
  hematomas, 913
  intrapartum, 910
  lacerations, 913
  mastitis, 912
  parametritis, 912
  perineal infection, 912
  postpartum hemorrhage, 913
  puerperal infection, 910
  thromboembolic disease, 913
  thrombophlebitis, 912–913
  urinary tract infections, 912
  uterine atony, 913
management strategies
  breastfeeding, 914
  discharge instructions, 914
  immunizations, 914
  postpartum examination, 915
  sexual intercourse, 914
  sitz baths, 914
  suppression of lactation, 914
pathophysiology and epidemiologic data
  abdominal wall, 909
  breasts, 910
  cardiovascular changes, 910
  cervix, 909
  hypothalamic–pituitary–ovarian function, 910
  lochia, 909
  reproductive hormones, 910
  urinary tract, 909
  uterus, 909
  vagina, 909
  weight change, 910
postpartum hemorrhage (PPH)
  defined, 913
  hematomas, 913
  lacerations, 913
  uterine atony, 913
postseptal orbital cellulitis, 65
posttraumatic stress disorder (PTSD), 820
  diagnoses, 821
  intimate partner violence and, 852
  management strategies, 827
  prognosis, 828
  treatment, 827
    CBT, 827
    SSRIs, 827
postural tremors, 461
postvoid residual urine (PVR), 473, 483
pramipexole, 465, 466
pramlintide, for obesity, 723
PRE. See progressive resistive exercise (PRE)
pre- and postbronchodilator testing, 97
preconception care
  definition, 897
  health promotion, 898
  immunization history, 898
  laboratory tests, 898
  medical history, 897–898
  physical examination, 898

pregnancy planning, 898
psychosocial history, 898
prediabetes, 645, 647
treatment for, 648–649
prednisone
for delayed hypersensitivity reaction
treatment, 51
for proteinuria, 422
for urticaria, 493
pregabalin, for chronic persistent pain, 603
pregnancy, 16
asymptomatic bacteriuria (ASB) during, 171
ectopic
treatment, 406–407
HIV and, 547
and hyperprolactinemia, 18
induced nausea and vomiting, 381–382
screening and prevention for anemia during, 24
symptoms, 19
test
for pelvic pain (PP), 405
trichomonas vaginitis in pregnant patients, 511
vaginal bleeding and, 502
Prehn's sign, 445
premenstrual symptoms, vaginal bleeding and,
504
premenstrual syndrome (PMS), 755–762
definition, 755
diagnosis, 756–758
epidemiology, 755
management strategies, 762
pathophysiology, 755–756
prognosis, 762
screening and prevention, 756
treatment, 758–762
prenatal care
alcohol use and, 899
between 14 and 28 weeks' gestation (second
trimester), 901–902
beyond 28 weeks of gestation (third trimester),
902
blood pressure, 902
fetal position, 902
caffeine and, 899
cocaine use and, 899
common symptoms, 902–904
headache, 903
nausea and vomiting, 902–903
definition, 897
D (Rh)-negative women, 902
first prenatal visit, 899
initial diagnosis of pregnancy, 898–899
nutrition and weight gain, 899–900
opiates use and, 899
patient education, 899
patient history, 899
physical examination, 899
prior to 14 weeks, 900–901
sexual intercourse and, 900
smoking and, 899
preoperative evaluation, 996–1006
algorithm, 999–1000
components, 997
medications
ACE inhibitors, 1005
alpha2-agonists, 1005

anticoagulants, 1005
antiplatelets, 1005
ARBs, 1005
beta-blockers, 1005
calcium channel blockers, 1005
insulin, 1005
oral hypoglycemic agents, 1005
statins, 1005
perioperative plan, 1006
primary care physicians and, 996, 997
risks, 1000–1004
alcohol use/abuse, 1004
anemia, 1003
cardiac evaluation, 1000–1002
cigarette smoking, 1004
diabetes mellitus, 1003
hypercoagulable, 1004
immunocompromise, 1003
malnutrition, 1004
peptic ulcer disease, 1004
peripheral vascular disease, 1004
psychiatric disease, 1004
pulmonary evaluation, 1002–1003
renal or hepatic failure, 1004
sexual behavior, 1004
special cases
children, 1006
elderly patients, 1006
patient unable to give a history, 1006
pregnancy, 1006
presbycusis, 275, 276, 277
hearing loss
laboratory tests, 278
symptoms, 277
treatment, 279–280
preseptal orbital cellulitis, 65
presyncope, 146
PRICEM. See protection, rest, ice, compression,
elevation, and medications (PRICEM)
primary
complaint, 288–289
headache disorders, 264–265, 267
insomnia, 288
lactase deficiency, 134
monosymptomatic enuresis, 183
muscle malignancy
myalgia and, 368
treatment, 370
psychiatric disorders, 114
renal disease, 418, 422
syphilis
laboratory tests for, 233–234
signs, 230
symptoms, 229
treatment, 234–235
ulcerative lesions and, 228
ulcerative lesion, 228
primary amenorrhea
defined, 17, 23
diagnoses, 17–18
treatment, 21–22
primidone, 467, 468
probiotics, 132
for diarrhea, 144
for inflammatory bowel disease,
691

proctalgia fugax
  perianal complaints, 411
  treatment, 416
proctitis
  laboratory test, 413–414
  perianal bleeding symptom, 412
  perianal complaints, 411
  perianal complaints sign, 413
  symptoms, 412
  treatment, 416–417
progestin challenge test, 21
progestin-only pills, 885
progestins, 713–714
  for vaginal bleeding, 505
progressive resistive exercise (PRE), 35
prokinetic agents for nausea and vomiting, 381
prolapse, 412
propanolol, 467
prostate cancer. *See also* urinary symptoms in men
  advanced, 487
  hematuria and, 281
  laboratory tests for, 483
  screening, 977
  treatment, 487
  urinary symptoms in men, 480
prostate-specific antigen (PSA) testing, 483
prostatitis, 281
  acute, 482, 484
  asymptomatic inflammatory, 480
  chronic bacterial, 480, 482, 484
  extratesticular scrotal complaints and, 445
  laboratory tests, 482–484
  signs, 447, 482
  symptoms, 447, 481
  treatment, 448, 484
  urinary symptoms in men, 480
prostatodynia, 480
protection, rest, ice, compression, elevation, and
      medications (PRICEM), 35
  for fractures treatment, 36
  for tenosynovitis treatment, 36
proteinuria. *See also* microalbuminuria
  and blood tests, 421–422
  definition, 418
  diabetic patients with, 423
  drugs and toxins causing, 418, 419
  evaluation, 422
  laboratory tests, 419–422
  orthostatic, 418
  overload, 418
  persistent, 418
  signs, 419
  symptoms, 419
  systemic illnesses causing, 418, 419
  transient, 418, 422
  treatment, 422–423
  and UA, 421
prothrombin time (PT)
  liver function tests (LFT) abnormalities and, 347
proton-pump inhibitors, 133
protozoa, 13
proximal
  fractures, 219
  onychomycosis, 243
  phalangeal fractures, 218
  radial head fractures, 218

pruritic dermatoses
  atopic eczema, 103
  body lice *(pediculosis humanus)*, 105
  contact dermatitis, 104
  diagnostic tests
    biopsy, 114
    microscopic examination, 114
    patch testing, 114
    Wood's light examination, 114
  dyshidrosis, 106
  head lice *(pediculosis capitis)*, 105
  lichen planus, 106
  lichen simplex chronicus, 105
  nummular eczema, 108
  pityriasis rosea, 106
  pruritus symptoms in, 109–114
  psoriasis, 106
  scabies, 104–105
  seborrhea, 108
  signs, 109–114
    delusions of parasitosis, 114
    dyshidrosis, 113
    pityriasis rosea, 113–114
    PUPP, 114
  treatment
    atopic dermatitis, 117
    contact dermatitis, 117–118
    dermatophyte infection, 118–119
    dyshidrosis, 118
    facial seborrheic dermatitis, 119
    lichen planus, 118
    lichen simplex chronicus, 118
    nummular eczema, 119
    pityriasis rosea, 118
    psoriasis, 118
    seborrhea, 119
    tinea corporis, 118–119
    tinea pedis, 118
    xerosis, 118
  xerosis (dry skin), 106
pruritus. *See also* dermatitis
  ani, 411
    laboratory tests, 413
    treatment, 417
  definition, 103
  oral corticosteroids for, 117
  with prominent psychogenic component,
    109
    delusions of parasitosis, 109
    localized psychogenic pruritus, 109
    puritic urticarial papules and plaques of
      pregnancy, 109
  symptoms in pruritic dermatoses, 109–114
  in systemic disease, 108–109
  treatment
    nonmedication measures, 114–115
    oral medications, 115–117
    topical antihistamines, 115
    topical steroids, 115
pseudoephedrine, 182, 437
psoriasis
  guttate, 106
  nail disorders and, 242, 244
  pruritic dermatoses and, 106
  treatment, 118
psychiatric assessment, 376

psychiatric disorders
  sleep disorder and, 291
psychogenic
  chest pain, 73
  cough, 97, 102
  dyspnea, 161
  dysuria, 167
  pain
    chronic pelvic pain (CPP) and, 402
  pruritus
    delusions of parasitosis, 109
    localized, 109
  vomiting, 373
psychogenic pain, 311, 312
psychogenic pain, CPP, 402
psychological illness, 193
psychotherapy, and irritable bowel syndrome
    treatment, 10
psyllium hydrophilic mucilloid
  for dyslipidemias, 666
pterygium, 424
  laboratory tests/diagnostics, 429
  symptoms, 429
  treatment, 431
public lice, 45
pulmonary diseases
  chest pain and, 74, 77
  dyspnea and, 161
  embolism (PE). See also chest pain
    prediction rules for suspected, 72
  pulmonary auscultation, 74
pulmonary edema, 618
pulmonary embolism (PE), 512
  laboratory tests, 513–514
  signs, 512
  symptoms, 512
pulmonary function tests (PFTs)
  for chest pain, 76
  for wheezing, 522
pulmonary rehabilitation, for COPD, 594–595
pulse oximetry
  for cough, 98
  dyspnea laboratory testing and, 164
pulsus paradoxus, 550
punch biopsy, 66
PUPP signs, 114
purified protein derivative (PPD), 98
pyelonephritis, 281
  acute/subclinical, 167
  signs, 168
  treatment, 169
pyogenic granuloma, 123, 129
pyruvate kinase deficiency, 26

R
rabies
  postexposure prophylaxis, 49
  prevention, 44
radiation therapy
  induced nausea and vomiting (CINV), 382
radiation therapy, for breast cancer, 571
radioallergosorbent (RAST) testing, 436
radiography
  for chest pain, 74–75
  for cough, 97–98
  for earache, 175

for foot complaints, 211–212
  for mammalian bites, 48
  for proteinuria, 422
radiologic tests, abdominal pain, 9. See also
    specific tests
radionuclide scanning, 9
radionuclide testing
  for nausea and vomiting, 376
raloxifene, for osteoporosis, 744
range of motion (ROM), 35, 385. See also neck
    pain
  for rotator cuff injuries treatment, 42
ranolazine, for IHD, 703
Ranson criteria, 11
rapid eye movement (REM) sleep, 288, 296,
    298–299
rapid viral testing
  and inflammatory markers, 398
  and pediatric fever, 398
rasaligine, 464
RBC. See red blood cell (RBC)
rectal examination, 225
recurrent
  AOM, 181
  UTIs, 168, 169
recurrent abdominal pain syndrome, 8
recurrent sinusitis, 433
red blood cell (RBC). See also anemia
  destruction, disorders of, 26
  loss, disorders of, 26–27
  production, disorders of, 25–26
  transfusion, 30
red eye
  clinical feature in diagnosis of, 428
  common diagnoses
    acute angle-closure glaucoma, 424
    blepharitis, 424
    conjunctivitis, 424
    corneal abrasion, 424
    episcleritis, 424
    inflamed pingueculum, 424
    keratitis, 426
    pterygium, 424
    scleritis, 425
    subconjunctival hemorrhage, 424
    uveitis, 425–426
  definition, 424
  laboratory tests/diagnostics, 429–430
  symptoms
    acute angle-closure glaucoma, 429
    allergic conjunctivitis, 427
    anterior uveitis, 429
    bacterial conjunctivitis, 427
    blepharitis, 427
    chlamydial conjunctivitis, 427
    corneal abrasion, 427
    episcleritis, 429
    inflamed pingueculum, 427
    keratitis, 429
    pterygium, 429
    scleritis, 429
    subconjunctival hemorrhage, 427
    viral conjunctivitis, 427
  treatment, 430–431
referral criteria, osteoarthritis, 736
referred otalgia, 173

referred pain, 73
regurgitation
children with, 374
definition, 371
vomiting and, 371
rehabilitation, ankle sprains treatment, 35–36
Reiter syndrome, 135
renal
biopsy, 286, 422
cell carcinoma, 281
colic, 445, 446
cysts, 283
dialysis, 422
function, 285
and gastrointestinal toxicity, 262
infarction, 283
transplantation, 422
tumors, 281
ultrasonography, 285
ultrasound (US), 285
renal complications, eating disorders and,
872
renal failure
definition, 763–764
diagnosis, 764–767
entity-specific tests
glomerular disease, 766
postrenal disease, 767
prerenal disease, 766
tubulointerstitial disease, 766–767
vascular disease, 766
etiology, 764
laboratory tests, 765–766
management strategies, 768, 771–773
acute renal failure, 771
anemia, 772–773
calcium metabolism, 772
chronic kidney disease, 771
dialysis, 773
metabolic acidosis, 772
nutritional imbalance, 773
phosphorus metabolism, 772
potassium metabolism, 772
volume overload, 772
prognosis
glomerular disease, 773
postrenal disease, 773
prerenal disease, 773
tubulointerstitial disease, 773
vascular disease, 773
symptoms and signs
glomerular disease, 765
postrenal disease, 765
prerenal disease, 764
tubulointerstitial disease, 765
vascular disease, 764–765
treatment, 767–768
cirrhosis, 768
glomerular disease, 768
heart failure, 767, 768
hypotension, 767
hypovolemia, 767
postrenal disease, 768
tubulointerstitial disease, 768
vascular disease, 768

renin–angiotensin–aldosterone blocker therapy,
for IHD, 707
renin–angiotensin–aldosterone system (RAAS),
616. See also heart failure (HF)
repetitive overuse injuries
myalgia, 369
reproductive complications, eating disorders
and, 872
respiratory acidosis, 205
respiratory alkalosis
laboratory test for, 200
signs, 200
symptoms, 200
treatment, 205
respiratory distress, 518. See also wheezing
restless legs syndrome, 290
restrictive diseases, 161, 165
rest tremors, 461
retapamulin, 68
retching, 371
retinoids, 528–529
retropharyngeal abscess, 450
rhinitis
allergic, 433
acute cough and, 92, 96
signs, 434
symptoms, 434
treatment, 437–440
atrophic
signs, 434
symptoms, 434
treatment, 440
definition, 432
medicamentosum, 434
signs, 434
treatment, 440
vasomotor
signs, 434
symptoms, 434
treatment, 440
rhinorrhea, 437
rib fractures, 219
Rickettsia rickettsii, 47
rifampin, 68
Rinne test, 278
Risk Evaluation and Mitigation Strategy (REMS),
602
rivaroxaban, 517
rivastigmine, for dementia, 637
Rocky Mountain spotted fever, 47
laboratory tests for, 48
treatment, 53
ROM. See range of motion (ROM)
ropirinole, 466
Rotarix, 132
RotaTeq, 132
rotator cuff, 37
impingement, 41
injuries, treatment of, 42
Roux-en-Y gastric bypass, 724
rubber band ligation, 414

S
salicylates, for chronic persistent pain, 598
salicylic acid paste method, 235

saline laxatives, 90
salmeterol for asthma, 556
Salter-Harris classification of pediatric fractures, 220, 221
scabies
  patient education, 119
  pruritic dermatoses and, 104–105
scabies bite, 45. *See also* arachnid bites
  treatment options for patients with, 52, 53
  wounds, 46
scaphoid fractures, 255
  hand and wrist, 255
  treatment, 258
scapholunate dissociation, 255
scleritis, 425
  laboratory tests/diagnostics, 430
  symptoms, 429
  treatment, 431
sclerotherapy, 414–415
screening tests, 966–978
  blood test
    cholesterol, 970–971
    glucose, 971
    hemoglobin/hematocrit, 971
    hemoglobinopathies, 973
    hypothyroidism, 972
    lead, 971–972
    newborn, 972
    phenylketonuria (PKU), 972
    thyroid function, 973
  body measurement screening
    abdominal aortic ultrasound, 970
    blood pressure, 969–970
    bone density, 970
    head circumference, 968
    height and weight, 968, 969
    waist/hip measurement, 969
  cancer screening
    breast, 975–976
    cervical, 976
    colorectal, 976–977
    lung, 978
    oral, 977
    ovarian, 977
    prostate, 977
    skin, 977–978
    testicular, 978
    thyroid, 978
  infectious disease
    chlamydia, 975
    gonorrhea, 974–975
    syphilis, 975
    tuberculosis (TB), 975
  mental health and cognition
    dementia, 974
    depression, 974
  for pediatric fever, 397–398
  sensory
    hearing, 973
    vision, 973–974
scrotal complaints
  definition, 444
  differential diagnosis, 446
  extratesticular causes
    signs, 446–447

symptoms, 446–447
    treatment, 448
  laboratory tests, 447
  testicular causes, 444–445
    signs, 445
    symptoms, 445
    treatment, 447–448
seafood
  ingestion syndromes, acute diarrhea and, 133
  safety, 987
sebaceous cyst
  abscess, 62
    signs, 66
    treatment, 69
  treatment, 129
sebaceous hyperplasia, 126, 129
seborrhea
  pruritic dermatoses and, 108
  treatment, 119
seborrheic
  dermatitis, 119
  keratoses, 123, 128
sebum production, excessive, 526
secondary
  headaches, 264, 265
    signs, 267–268
    symptoms, 267
    treatment, 273
  insomnia, 288
  monosymptomatic enuresis, 183
  syphilis
    genital lesion and, 228
    treatment, 236
secondary amenorrhea
  defined, 17, 23
  diagnoses, 18–19
  treatment, 22–23
seizure disorders, 774–785
  brain imaging, 777–778
  causes, 776–777
  definition, 774
  diagnosis, 776–779
  electroencephalogram (EEG), 778–779
  epidemiology, 775–776
  febrile, 775
  focal, 774–775
  generalized, 774
  laboratory tests, 777
  lumbar puncture (LP), 777
  management strategies, 784
  nonepileptiform seizure (NES), 775
  prognosis, 784–785
  signs, 777
  status epilepticus, 775
  symptoms, 776
  treatment, 779–784
selective estrogen receptor modulators (SERMs)
  for breast cancer, 565
selective serotonin reuptake inhibitors (SSRIs)
  for chronic persistent pain, 603
  for depression, 859
  for eating disorders, 871
  panic disorder, 826
  phobia, 827
  for posttraumatic stress disorder (PTSD), 827

selegiline, 464
self-monitoring of blood glucose (SMBG), 656
self-neglect of elder, 853–854
serotonin-norepinephrine reuptake inhibitors
        (SNRIs)
    for chronic persistent pain, 603
serotonin receptor antagonists for nausea and
        vomiting, 381
serum
    test
        for pelvic pain (PP), 405
        for proteinuria, 421
serum chemistry, 8–9
serum sickness. See delayed hypersensitivity
        reaction
sexual abuse
    child, 847, 849–850
    elder, 853
sexual behavior, and preoperative evaluation,
        1004
sexual dysfunction, 915–932
    biopsychosocial condition, 916
    definition, 915
    diagnostic evaluation, 921–923
    gender differences, 916
    orgasmic disorders, 918–919
        signs and symptoms, 920, 921
    prevention and screening, 915
    prognosis, 931–932
    sexual arousal disorders, 917–918
        signs and symptoms, 920
    sexual desire disorders (SDDS), 916–917
        signs and symptoms, 920
    treatment and management, 923–931
sexually transmitted diseases (STDs)
    proctitis, 133
    vaginal bleeding and, 502
    vaginal discharge and, 507
sexually transmitted infections, 932–942
    definition, 932
    diagnoses, 933–934
        chancroid, 934
        chlamydia trachomatis, 933
        genital herpes, 933
        gonorrhea, 933
        hepatitis, 933
        HIV, 933–934
        HPV, 933
        mycoplasma genitalium, 934
        pediculosis pubis, 934
        syphilis, 933
        trichomoniasis, 934
        ureaplasma, 934
    laboratory tests, 937, 938–939
    patient education, 942
    prevention
        condoms, 935
        education and counseling, 935
        male circumcision, 935
        postexposure prophylaxis (PEP), 936
        pre-exposure prophylaxis (PrEP), 936
        vaccination, 935
    screening, 934–935
        HBV, 934
        HCV, 934

symptoms and signs
    asymptomatic, 936
    cervicitis, 936–937
    epididymitis, 937
    papules, 936
    PID, 936–937
    proctitis, 937
    ulcerations, 936
    urethritis in men, 937
    vaginal discharge, 936
    treatment, 937, 940–941
sexual response cycle, 915
short stature, 192. See also failure to thrive (FTT)
shoulder
    anatomy, 37
    complaints. See arm/shoulder complaints
    function, 37
sialorrhea, 374
sickle cell disease, 26
    hematuria and, 283, 285
    treatment, 30
sinuses
    signs, 435
    transillumination, 435
sinusitis, 92, 95
    acute, 432
    antibiotics treatment, 441–442
    chronic, 433
    complications, 442–443
        intracranial, 443
        local, 442
        orbital, 442–443
    conditions mimicking sinus pain, 433
    definition, 432
    ethmoid, 435
    frontal, 435
    laboratory tests, 435, 436
    maxillary, 435
    recurrent, 433
    signs, 435–436
    sphenoid, 435
    subacute, 432–433
    symptoms, 435–436
    treatment, 440–441
        antibiotics for, 441–442
        oral corticosteroids, 441
situational syncope
    signs, 457
    symptoms, 457
    treatment, 459–460
skin
    biopsy, 414
skin cancer
    screening, 977–978
skin complications, eating disorders and, 872
sleep
    history, 289
    hygiene, 289
    hygiene education, 293
    initiation, 287
    maintenance, 287
    nonprescription sleep aids, 296
    polysomnogram, 291
    prescription sleep aids, 296
    REM, 296, 299

sleep disorder. *See also* insomnia
  alcohol and, 293
  central sleep apnea (CSA), 290
  jet lag and, 295, 298
  psychiatric disorders and, 291
sleep phases
  advanced, 289
  delayed, 290
sleepwalking, 294
SLGT2 inhibitors
  for diabetes mellitus, 653–654
slow-transit constipation (STC), 84
small-bowel obstruction, 374
  risk factors for, 2
  treatment, 11
SMBG. *See* self-monitoring of blood glucose
      (SMBG)
smoking
  and cough, 101
smoking cessation
  for COPD, 592–593
  for diabetes mellitus, 657
  hypertension, 686
  for osteoarthritis, 731
sodium restriction, in heart failure, 621
solar urticaria, 489
somatization
  definition, 873
  diagnosis, 874–877
  epidemiology, 873–874
  management strategies, 879–880
  pathophysiology, 874
  prognosis, 880
  risk factors, 874
  treatment, 877–879
somnambulism, 290
sonograms, 68
sore throat
  common diagnoses
    irritants, 449
    viral infections, 449
  definition, 449
  GABHS and, 449
  laboratory tests, 451–452
  signs
    carotidynia, 451
    epiglottitis, 450
    GABHS pharyngitis, 449–450
    peritonsillar abscess, 451
    retropharyngeal abscess, 450
  symptoms, 449
  treatment, 452–454
South Beach diet, 721
soy protein hypersensitivity, 134
specialized child abuse assessment programs, 850
specimen adequacy, Pap smears report, 14
spermatoceles
  extratesticular scrotal complaints and, 445
  treatment, 448
spermicide, 889
sphenoid sinusitis, 435
spherocytosis, hereditary, 26. *See also* anemia
spider bites, 44, 45
  treatment, 53–54
  wounds, 47

spinal stenosis, 353, 359
spirometry, 97
spironolactone, 247, 249
  for acne vulgaris, 531
spironolactone, for heart failure, 621
splint, 217
spondylosis, 386
sponge, 888–889. *See also* contraception
spontaneous bacterial peritonitis (SBP), 611
sprains, 31, 252. *See also* ankle injuries
  diagnosis, 32
  hand and wrist complaints and, 252
  prevention of, 31
  symptoms/signs, 34
  treatment
    acute management, 35
    rehabilitation, 35–36
Spurling test, 260, 261
Spurling test and neck pain, 385
sputum cytology, 98
squamous cell carcinomas, 125, 130
Staphylococcus aureus, 55, 59, 61. *See also*
      bacterial skin infections
stapled gastroplasty, 724
static shoulder stability, 37
statin-induced myalgia (SIM), 366
  laboratory tests for, 368
  symptoms and signs, 368
  treatment, 370
statins
  for dyslipidemias, 671
  for hypertension, 686
sterilization, 891
  implants, 891
  transabdominal surgical, 891
  vasectomy, 891
steroids
  for asthma, 556
  for atopic dermatitis, 117
  for dyspnea, 166
  for genital lesions, 236
  intra-articular, 315
  nasal sprays, 438
  for pruritic dermatoses, 115
stimulants
  laxatives, 90
stingers. *See* burners/stingers
stings. *See* bites/stings
stool, 224
  currant jelly, 224
  examination of retrieved, 225
  false-positive, 225
  formed, 224
strains, 31. *See also* ankle injuries
  diagnosis, 32
  symptoms/signs, 34
  treatment, 36
streptococcal infection, 449, 451, 452. *See also*
      sore throat
Streptococcus pneumoniae, 395
Streptococcus pyogenes, 59, 60–61. *See also*
      bacterial skin infections
streptomycin, for tularemia treatment, 53
stress fractures, 35
stress incontinence, 471, 474, 477

stress test for urinary incontinence, 472
stress testing. *See also* chest pain
  exercise stress echocardiography, 76
  exercise stress electrocardiography, 75–76
  pharmacologic stress testing, 76
stretching program
  for myalgia, 369
strictures, 283
stroke, 786–796
  diagnosis, 786–790
  differential diagnosis, 786
  laboratory tests, 788
  management strategies, 795–796
    acute stage, 795
    chronic stage, 796
    subacute stage, 795–796
  prognosis, 796
  treatment, 790–795
    anticoagulation therapy, 794
    antiplatelet therapy, 794–795
    BP control, 790–791
    carotid endarterectomy (CEA), 793
    cerebral edema, 793
    glucose control, 791
    immediate management, 790
    intravenous fluids, 791
    nimodipine, 793
    reperfusion, 790, 792
  types, 786
structural heart disease
  cardiac syncope and, 455
  syncope
    signs, 457
subacromial bursitis, 37, 41
  treatment, 43
subacute sinusitis, 432–433
subclavian steal syndrome, 455
subclinical pyelonephritis, 167
subconjunctival hemorrhage, 424
  laboratory tests/diagnostics, 429
  symptoms, 427
  treatment, 431
subdermal implant, 887
subluxation, shoulder, 37
  treatment, 43
subluxations, 216
substance
  induced-delirium, 78
  withdrawal-delirium, 78
substance abuse
  CAGE questionnaire, 809
  clinical clues, 810
  defined, 808–809
  and delirium symptoms, 80
  detoxification, 814
  differential diagnosis, 809
  epidemiology, 808
  heart failure and, 620
  laboratory tests
    AST/ALT, 810
    CDT, 811
    EtG, 812
    GGT, 810
  prevalence, 808
  screening, 809

SOAPE glossary, 813
  symptoms and signs, 810
  treatment, 813–816
  withdrawal symptoms, 810
subungual hematomas, 250
sudden deafness, 275. *See also* hearing loss
  barotrauma, 275
  head trauma, 275
  localized lesions, 275
  systemic diseases, 275
suicide, 863
  eating disorders and, 872
sulfamethoxazole/trimethoprim, 69
sulfonylureas
  for diabetes mellitus, 651–652
sun protection
  dermatologic neoplasm treatment and, 129
  travel medicine, 988
surfactants, 90
surgery
  for breast condition treatment, 57
  for colon cancer, 573
  for COPD, 593
  for incontinence, 474
  for inflammatory bowel disease, 695
  for lung cancer, 573
  for obesity, 723–725
  for Parkinson disease (PD), 466–467
  preoperative assessment, 999
  for sinusitis, 442
sustained supraventricular tachycardia (SVT), 389
swan-neck deformity, 252, 254
sycosis barbae, 69
symmetric failure to thrive (FTT), 192
sympathetic nervous system, 616
syncope
  common diagnoses, 455
    cardiac syncope, 455
    cerebrovascular, 455
    classic vasovagal, 455
    idiopathic, 455
    neurally mediated, 455
    orthostatic, 455
    signs, 457
    situational syncope, 455
    symptoms, 455, 457
  definition, 454–455
  differential diagnosis, 456
  laboratory tests, 457–459
  treatment, 459–460
syndrome of inappropriate antidiuretic hormone
    release (SIADH) treatment, 202
syphilis
  chancres of, 229
  primary
    laboratory tests for, 233
    ulcerative lesions and, 228
  screening tests, 975
  secondary, 228
  vaginal discharge complaints and, 509
systemic
  antibiotics
    for acne vulgaris, 530
    for foot complaints, 215
  antifungal drugs, 215

corticosteroids, 559
steroids, 556
systemic diseases, 108–109
dizziness and, 145, 148
dyspnea and, 162
hair loss and, 243
nail disoders and, 240, 244
proteinuria, 418, 422–423
sudden deafness and, 275
systolic blood pressure, 81
systolic dysfunction HF, 620–624
ACEIs for, 622
ARBs for, 622
beta-blockers for, 624
calcium channel blockers for, 623
digoxin for, 624
exercise training for, 624
HYD-ISDN for, 622

T
tachyarrhythmia, 455
tachycardia, 81, 618
tachypnea, 81
tacrolimus, 117
tamsulosin, 484, 487
tapentadol, for chronic persistent pain, 602
tarsal navicular bone fractures, 208
tazarotene, 529
technetium red cell scan, 226
tegaserod, 10
telogen effluvium, 238, 247, 910
temporomandibular joint dysfunction, 172
tenderness, 216, 385. See also fractures; neck pain
costovertebral angle, 284
joint, 284
local, 354
point, 354
tendon injuries, 251, 260
tennis elbow. See lateral epicondylitis
tenosynovitis, 31. See also ankle injuries
de Quervain, 251–252
diagnosis, 32
symptoms/signs, 34
treatment, 36
tension night splint for plantar fasciitis, 214
tension-type headache (TTH), 264
episodic, 266
signs, 267
symptoms, 267
treatment, 271, 273
terazosin, 487
terbinafine, 215, 236, 247–248, 250
terbutaline, 493
terbutaline, for asthma, 558
teriparatide, for osteoporosis, 744–745
terminal hair, 237
Terry Thomas sign, 256, 260
testicular scrotal complaints, 444–445
signs, 445
symptoms, 445
treatment, 447–448
tetanus
for mammalian bites treatment, 49
tetracycline
for acne vulgaris, 530

for mammalian bites, 49
for tick-borne relapsing fever treatment, 53
thalassemia, 26
thenar eminence, 251
theophylline for asthma, 557
thiazolidinediones (TZDs)
for diabetes mellitus, 653
thin basement membrane nephropathy, 283
thoracic aortic dissection, 71
thoracic outlet syndrome, 40
myalgia and, 368
thrombocytopenia, 8
thrombophlebitis
pelvic, 912–913
postpartum care, 912–913
superficial, 912
thyroid cancer
screening, 978
thyroid disease, 797–807
diagnostic evaluation, 797–798
hyperthyroidism, 798, 801–805
hypothyroidism. See hypothyroidism
physiology, 797
screening, 797
thyroid dysfunction, 503
thyroid nodules, 805–807
diagnosis, 806
management strategies, 806–807
treatment, 806
thyroid-stimulating hormone (TSH), 504
level, in amenorrhea, 20
tic disorders, 468–469
tick bites, 45. See also arachnid bites
treatment, 53
wounds, 46–47
tick-borne relapsing fever
treatment, 53
tinea
capitis, 108, 118, 238, 243, 247–248
corporis, 108, 118–119
cruris, 108
pedis, 108
perianal complaints and, 417
Tinel test, 260, 261
tinnitus, 173
toe fractures, 220–221
toenail avulsion, 215
tolcapone, 466
tolterodine, 474, 475
topical agents
antibiotics, 529
antihistamines, 115
immunosuppressants, 117
for psoriasis treatment, 118
topical gel and emulsion, for menopause, 713
topiramate, for obesity, 722–723
torsion. See also scrotal complaints
signs, 445
testicular, 444
treatment, 448
torso fractures
nondisplaced pelvic fractures, 219
rib fractures, 219
treatment, 219
vertebral compression fractures, 219

torticollis
  acute, 383
  neck pain treatment, 386
trachoma, 427
traditional Chinese medicine, for asthma, 558
tramadol, for chronic persistent pain, 602
tramadol hydrochloride, for osteoarthritis, 731
trancutaneous electrical nerve stimulation (TENS), 152
transcranial Doppler (TCD) ultrasonography, 790
transdermal patch, 886. *See also* contraception
transdermal patches, for menopause, 713
transient
  incontinence, 471, 473
  insomnia, 293
  proteinuria, 418, 422
  synovitis, 310, 311, 313–315, 341, 345–346
transillumination, sinuses, 435
transitional cell carcinomas, 281
transrectal ultrasound (TRUS), 483
traumatic myalgia
  symptoms and signs, 366
  treatment, 369
travel medicine, 979–996
  after-care
    diarrhea or vomiting, 995
    fever, 995
    jaundice, 995–996
    skin disorders, 996
  arthropod bite prevention
    DEET, 981
    permethrin, 981
    special note, 981
  care abroad, 992
  chronic diseases, travelers with, 990–992
    cardiovascular disease, 991
    diabetes, 990
    HIV-positive patient, 990
    mental illness, 992
    pulmonary disease, 991–992
    travelers' diarrhea (TD), 990
  deep vein thromboses, 987
  diarrhea (TD)
    childhood, 989–990
    immunocompromised traveler, 990
    prophylaxis, 981
    treatment, 981, 986
  elderly traveler, 990
  geopolitical concerns, 994–995
  jet lag, 988
  malaria, 981, 984
  motion sickness, 987
  pediatric traveler
    air travel, 989
    malaria, 989
    vaccinations, 989
  pregnant travelers
    air travel, 988
    malaria, 989
    vaccines, 988–989
  pretravel visit, 980, 981

  special activities
    high-altitude illness, 992–994
    water sports, 994
  STD prevention, 988
  sun protection, 988
  symptomatic, 981
  unintentional injuries during travel, 987
  vaccinations for travel, 981
    hepatitis A, 982
    Japanese encephalitis, 982
    meningococcal, 982
    pediatric traveler, 989
    pregnant travelers, 988–989
    rabies, 982
    routine, 981
    travel-specific, 981
    typhoid fever, 982
    yellow fever, 982
tremors. *See also* movement disorders; Parkinson disease (PD)
  action, 461
  common diagnoses
    essential tremor, 461
    PD, 461–462
    physiologic tremor, 462
  definition, 461
  differential diagnosis of, 462
  evaluation, 463
  kinetic, 461
  physiologic, 462
  postural, 461
  rest, 461
  signs, 462–463
  symptoms, 462–463
  treatment
    essential tremor, 467
    PD, 464–467
tretinoin, 529
triamcinolone, 247, 346
  for myalgia, 370
triamcinolone acetonide, 438
triangular fibrocartilage complex (TFCC) tears, 255
trichomonas, 13
  vaginitis, 507, 511
tricyclic antidepressants (TCAs)
  for chronic persistent pain, 603
  for depression, 859
  for eating disorders, 871
  for low back pain, 358
  for migraine, 271, 272
  for pruritus, 117
trigger finger, 251, 254
trigger point injection, 370
triptans, 269, 270
TSH. *See* thyroid-stimulating hormone (TSH)
tuberculosis (TB)
  cough treatment and
    active TB, 102
    latent TB, 102
  screening tests, 975
tubulointerstitial disease, 773. *See also* renal failure
tularemia, 47
  laboratory tests for, 48
  treatment, 53

tuning fork tests
  Rinne test, 278
  Weber test, 278
Turner syndrome, 17
two-point discrimination test, 260,
  262
tympanic membrane, 173
tympanometry, 175, 279
tympanostomy tube, 181
type 1 DM. *See also* diabetes mellitus
  insulin therapy, 655–656
  overview, 645
  pharmacologic treatment, 650
  symptoms and signs, 648
type 2 DM. *See also* diabetes mellitus
  insulin therapy, 656
  overview, 645
  pharmacologic treatment, 650–651
  risk factors, 645
  screening criteria
    in adults, 646
    in children, 647
    in pregnancy, 647
  symptoms and signs, 648
Tzanck test, 233

U
ulcerative
  colitis, 133, 136
  lesions, 228–235
ulnar collateral ligament (UCL) injuries
  hand and wrist complaints and, 252
  testing of, 260
  of thumb MCP joint, 258
ulnar neuropathy of hand, 256
ultrasonography
  of biliary tree and liver, 609
  for breast cancer, 56
  for proteinuria, 422
ultrasound, 9
  and ankle sprains, 35
  nausea and vomiting, 375
  pelvic, 21
  for perianal complaints, 414
  for scrotal complaints, 447
  for urinary incontinence, 473
  for urinary symptoms in men, 482
unstable angina (UA), 707
upper airway causes of dyspnea,
  162
upper extremity DVT, 513
upper gastrointestinal series, 375
upper GI (UGI)
  bleeding, 222, 223
urethral smear, 447
urethritis, 167, 281
  causes, 167
  dysuria laboratory testing and, 168
  gonococcal, 480
  nongonococcal, 480
  signs, 168
  symptoms, 480
  treatment, 171, 484
  urinary symptoms in men, 480
urge incontinence, 471, 473–474

urinalysis (UA), 284, 304, 356
  for dysuria, 168
  for enuresis, 184
  for low back pain, 356
  and pediatric fever, 398
  and proteinuria, 421
  for scrotal complaints, 447
  for secondary dysmenorrhea, 150
  for urinary incontinence, 473
  for urinary symptoms in men, 482
urinary incontinence
  common diagnoses
    mixed incontinence, 471
    overflow incontinence, 471
    stress incontinence, 471
    transient incontinence, 471
    urge, 471
  definition, 471
  laboratory tests, 473
  signs, 472
  symptoms, 472
  treatment, 473–478
    intractable, 478
    overflow, 477–478
    stress, 474, 477
    transient, 473
    urge, 473–474
urinary symptoms in men
  common diagnoses
    bladder cancer, 480
    BPH, 480
    CPPS, 480
    prostate cancer, 480
    prostatitis, 480
    urethritis, 480
  definition, 479–480
  laboratory tests, 482–484
  signs, 480–482
  symptoms, 480–482
    irritative, 481
    obstructive, 481
    urethral discharge, 480
  treatment, 484–488
    acute prostatitis, 484
    bladder cancer, 488
    BPH, 487
    chronic bacterial prostatitis, 484
    CPPS, 484, 487
    prostate cancer, 487
    urethritis, 484
urinary tract infections (UTI)
  dysuria and, 166
  elderly women with symptomatic, 171
  hematuria and, 283, 284
  pediatric fever and, 395
  recurrent, 168
  treatment, 169
urine
  collection, 285
  culture, 285
  cytology, 286
  dipstick, 284
  microscopic examination of the sediment of,
    284
  output, 284

urolithiasis, 281
urticaria
    acute, 490–491
    common diagnoses
        emotional and psychogenic factors,
            490
        foods and food additives, 490
        infections, 489
        medications, 490
        physical factors, 489
    definition, 489
    laboratory tests, 490–491
    signs, 490
    symptoms, 490
    treatment, 491–499
US. See ultrasound (US)
uterine leiomyomas
    acute pelvic pain (APP) and, 402, 408
    chronic pelvic pain (CPP) and,
        402, 408
uveitis, 425–426
    symptoms, 429
    treatment, 431

V
vaccinations for travel, 981
    hepatitis A, 982
    Japanese encephalitis, 982
    meningococcal, 982
    pediatric traveler, 989
    pregnant travelers, 988–989
    rabies, 982
    routine, 981
    travel-specific, 981
    typhoid fever, 982
    yellow fever, 982
vaccines
    for cough, 101
    for diarrhea, 132
vaginal bleeding. See also abnormal pap
        smears
    abnormal, 500
    common diagnoses
        chronic or acute conditions, 502
        dysfunctional uterine bleeding (DUB),
            503
        pregnancy and its complications,
            502
        STDs, 502
        trauma and foreign bodies, 502
    definition, 500
    laboratory tests, 504–505
    signs, 503–504
    symptoms
        menstrual pattern, 503
        premenstrual symptoms, 504
    treatment, 505–506
vaginal creams, 713
vaginal discharge
    common diagnoses
        allergic vaginitis, 507
        atrophic vaginitis, 507
        BV, 507
        cervicitis, 507

GAS vaginitis, 507
        physiologic discharge, 507
        trichomonas vaginitis, 507
        VVC, 507
    definition, 506–507
    in dysuria, 167
    laboratory tests, 508–509
    symptoms and signs of, 508
    treatment
        allergic vaginitis, 511
        atrophic vaginitis, 511
        BV, 509–510
        cervicitis, 511
        general measures, 509
        trichomonas vaginitis, 511
        VVC, 510–511
vaginal infections, treatment, 16
vaginal rings, 886–887. See also
        contraception
    for menopause, 713
vaginitis. See also cervicitis
    allergic, 507, 511
    atrophic, 507, 511
    GAS, 507
    treatment, 511
    trichomonas, 507, 511
valproic acid, for chronic persistent
        pain, 604
vancomycin, 69
varicoceles
    extratesticular scrotal complaints
        and, 445
    treatment, 448
vascular diseases
    hematuria and, 283
    LGI bleeding and, 225
vascular insufficiency, 365
    symptoms and signs, 367–368
    treatment, 370
vasectomy, 891
vasovagal syncope
    signs, 457
    treatment, 459–460
vellus hair, 237
venous insufficiency
    myalgia and, 368
venous thromboembolism (VTE)
    complications, 517
    deep venous thrombosis (DVT), 512
    definition, 512
    laboratory tests, 512–514
    pulmonary embolism (PE), 512
    risk factors for, 512
    signs, 512
    symptoms, 512
    treatment, 514–517
        acute management, 514
        complications, 517
        subsequent management, 514–517
vertebroplasty, 746
vestibular dysfunction
    nausea and vomiting, 372
    for nausea and vomiting, 381
    neuronitis, 146

viral diarrhea, 135
viral hepatitis
    liver function tests (LFT) abnormalities and,
        302, 309
viral infections
    acute diarrhea and, 132
    causing diarrhea, 131, 135
    lymphadenopathy, 363
    sore throat and, 449, 452
viral syndromes, myalgia from, 365
    symptoms and signs, 366
    treatment, 369
viral upper respiratory illnesses (URIs), 91, 95,
        100. See also cough
vitamin B$_{12}$ deficiency, 25, 28
    treatment, 30
vitamin D supplementation
    for hypergonadotropic amenorrhea, 23
    for hypocalcemia, 205
    for osteoporosis, 23, 743
Vitex agnus castus, 762
vomiting
    acupuncture for, 376
    in adolescents and adults, 372–373,
        374
    in children, 371, 374
    definition, 371
    diagnosis using symptoms of, 374
    diagnostic testing, 375–376
    differential diagnosis, 372
    in infants, 371, 374
    medications associated with, 373
    psychogenic, 373
    reaction to drugs, 372
    relative costs, benefits, and risks of diagnostic
        tests, 375
    signs, 374–375
    symptoms, 373–374
    treatment, 376–382
        CINV, 382
        clinical situation, 381–382
        pharmacologic, 376–381
        PONV, 382
        RINV, 382
    in women, 371–372
vulvar dystrophy
    pruritic lesions and, 228–229
    signs, 232–233
    symptoms, 229
    treatment, 236
vulvovaginal candidiasis (VVC), 507
    complicated infection, 510
    recurrent, 510–511
    uncomplicated infection, 510
vulvovaginal pruritus, 713
vulvovaginitis, 167

W
waist circumference, 718–719
warfarin therapy, VTE, 517
warts, 123
    signs, 126
    treatment, 128
wasp sting, 45

water safety, 981. See also travel medicine
water-soluble contrast medium, 10
water sports, 994. See also travel medicine
watery chronic diarrhea, 131
Watson "click" test, 260, 261
Weber test, 278
weight loss
    complications of, 725
    osteoarthritis and, 731
weight management, for diabetes mellitus,
        650
wheezing
    common diagnoses
        acute bronchitis and pneumonia,
            518
        acute viral RTIs, 518
        adults (young age to middle age), 519
        anaphylaxis or hypersensitivity, 519
        aspiration, 519
        asthma, 518
        bronchiolitis, 519
        children age 2 years to teenage, 519
        congestive heart failure (CHF), 519
        COPD, 519
        cystic fibrosis (CF), 519
        elderly (older than 50 years), 519
        hypersensitivity, 519
        infants younger than 2 years,
            518–519
    definition, 518
    laboratory tests, 522–523
    signs
        auscultation, 520
        Dennie's pleats, 522
        percussion, 520
        respiratory rate, 520
    symptoms, 520–522
    treatment
        anaphylaxis, 524
        aspiration, 523–524
        bronchiolitis, 523
        pulmonary embolus, 524
whiplash injury
    acute, 386
    chronic, 386
    and neck pain, 384
    neck pain treatment, 386
white blood cells (WBC), 285, 397
Wilms tumor (nephroblastoma), 281
Wilson disease, 470
    and cirrhosis, 608
withdrawal symptoms. See also substance
        abuse
    alcohol abuse, 810
    substance abuse, 810
wounds
    arachnid bites, 46–47
    insect bites, 45–46
    mammalian bites, 45
        treatment, 48–49
    spider bites, 47
wrist. See also hand and wrist complaints
    and arm fractures, 218–219
    banding, 376

X
xerosis, 106, 118
X-ray
  in acute abdominal pain, 9
  in ankle injuries, 35
  asthma, 552
  COPD, 580
  for cough, 97
  fractures, 217
  hand and wrist complaints, 260
  for IHD, 702

for lacerations, 333
for leg and hip complaints, 345
nausea and vomiting, 375
for osteoarthritis, 729
for osteoporosis, 739

Z
Zelnorm. *See* tegaserod
zoledronic acid, for osteoporosis, 744
zone diet, 721
zonisamide, for obesity, 723